Exercise Therapy

Principles and Practice

THIRD EDITION

Request for Your Suggestions, Criticism and Ideas

This book is an attempt to bring basic, applied and related knowledge for exercise therapy.

We have done the best we can, given or limitations. We know the book is not perfect and that it has weaknesses and perhaps some mistakes.

We would appreciate any **S**uggestions, **C**riticism and **I**deas you may have for ways that this book might be improved to serve the patients.

⇓

Mail at:

roshan7leo@yahoo.com

Exercise Therapy

Principles and Practice

THIRD EDITION

Roshan Lal Meena
BPT, MPT (Ortho)
Lecturer in Physiotherapy
Pandit Deendayal Upadhyaya
National Institute for Persons with Physical Disabilities (Affiliated to the University of Delhi)
Department of Empowerment of Persons with Physical Disability
Ministry of Social Justice and Empowerment
Government of India
4, Vishnu Digambar Marg
New Delhi - 110002, India

PEEPEE PUBLISHERS AND DISTRIBUTORS (P) LTD.®

Exercise Therapy
Principles and Practice

Published by
Pawaninder P. Vij and Anupam Vij

Peepee Publishers and Distributors (P) Ltd.
***Head Office:* 160, Shakti Vihar, Pitam Pura, Delhi-110 034 (India)**

Correspondence Address:
7/31, First Floor, Ansari Road, Daryaganj
New Delhi-110 002 (India)
Ph: 41512412, 23246245, 9811156083
e-mail: peepee160@yahoo.co.in
e-mail: peepee160@gmail.com
www.peepeepub.com
join us on facebook.com/pp.publishers

First Edition: 2006

Second Edition: 2014

Third Edition: 2020

ISBN: 978-81-8445-269-3

Dedicated to

My parents, my wife,
my son Hardik and daughter Mayara for
their appreciation and encouragement

FOREWORD

The twin disciplines of physical therapy and occupational therapy are two of the most upcoming health related professions in our country. Exercise therapy is an integral part of treatment in majority of the disabling conditions that physiotherapists and occupational therapists are dealing with in their day-to-day practice.

The present textbook titled **"Exercise Therapy: Principles and Practice"** covers the entire subject of exercise therapy in a very lucid manner. The contents of book succinctly describe the systematic meaning of exercise therapy and its importance in the rehabilitation of person with impairments. Its illustration provides visual image and help in understanding of various methods and concepts of exercise therapy.

This will definitely prove to be one of the most comprehensive presentation of a subject which has so far failed to receive the attention of practising physical therapists and occupational therapists in India.

I have no hesitation in stating that this book will act as a guide book for physical therapists and occupational therapists. They can easily look up to the contents of this book which will help them in selecting the appropriate regimen when faced with different problems requiring exercise therapy.

Dharmendra Kumar
MS (Orthopaedic)
DNB (Physical Medicine and Rehabilitation)
Director, Pt. DUIPH, New Delhi-2
Former Dy. Director (Technical) and Officiating Director
NIRTAR, Cuttack, Orissa

PREFACE TO THE THIRD EDITION

The **Exercise Therapy: Principles and Practice** is divided into two parts. The first part of the book explains principles of the exercises and the advance therapeutic approaches advocated to improve functional limitations and symptoms of various ailments. This part comprises twenty-one chapters. The second part of the book describes the various conditions and diseases practiced by the physical therapists across the globe. The conditions are described with the pathophysiology, clinical feature, assessment, physical tests and advance therapeutic exercises administered to the conditions.

I am particularly excited by this third edition because it brings the book to another level in the journey to become the best comprehensive textbook for the learners as well as for the practitioners. Third edition is actually an extension of the first and second editions.

The first biggest change in the third edition is manual muscle strength testing which previously in the first edition was covered briefly with the principles and basic concepts. The third edition of the book explains manual muscle testing with the full color presentation designed to maximize text and images quality, clarity and accuracy. This chapter covers the MMT of upper extremity, lower extremity and spine with emphasis on the position of the patient, position of therapist, substitution of the muscles and placement of the hands of the examiner for testing of the strength of the muscles and to minimize errors. I have tried my best to explain the deformities occur following individual muscle weakness or paralysis along with images and clinical manifestations.

The second biggest change in this new edition is the addition of the goniometry. The chapter of goniometry describes range of motion, planes, axes, end feels, placement of arms of goniometer, position of the patient and examiner to minimize the errors in measuring range of motion. The third change in this edition is the introduction of some common conditions practiced by the physiotherapists worldwide such as lateral epicondylitis, carpal tunnel syndrome and deQuervain tenosynovitis.

The whole arrangement makes reading a pleasure and time effective experience.

Roshan Lal Meena

PREFACE

"**Exercise Therapy: Principles and Practice**" is divided into Two Parts. Part-I consists of two sections. First Section covers the principles and basic concepts of the therapeutic exercises. Second Section covers advanced therapeutic approaches. Part-II covers pathomechanics, assessments, differential diagnosis and therapeutic interventions of different conditions, commonly administered by the therapists in their day-to-day practice.

This book includes all the aspects of exercise therapy which are used by Physical therapists and Occupational therapists in the management of patients with musculoskeletal disorders, neurological disorders, pediatric and geriatric ailments, sports injuries and cardiovascular diseases.

It has been observed that the importance of exercises in the rehabilitation field is decreasing day-by-day and therapists are relying more on electrotherapy. This book empowers professionals and students by giving them knowledge about various exercises as well as all other related aspects without which comprehensive management through exercise therapy is not possible.

This book is useful for Physical therapists, Occupational therapists, Orthopaedic surgeons, Physiatrists and all other health care professionals concerned with the rehabilitation of persons with physical disability. As this book is written in simple and clear form it is also useful for the students of aforesaid professionals.

Roshan Lal Meena

ACKNOWLEDGEMENTS

The first edition of the book titled "**Concise Exercise Therapy: Principles and Practice**" with my Co-Author Dr. Kamal Narayan Arya published in 2006 was appreciated by many of physical therapists and students of physiotherapy and occupational therapy. This appreciation has inspired me to write its second and third edition in 2014 and 2019 respectively.

I would like to thank my wife Manju, my son Hardik and my daughter Mayara, who supported and encouraged me in spite of all the time it took me away from them. I thank my parents who have encouraged me to work hard to accomplish the task and objective to achieve peace of mind.

I express my deep sense of gratitude towards my head of physiotherapy department, Mrs Manda Chauhan, Associate Professor, Mrs Rajni Kalra, Assistant Professor and other seniors and colleagues for their kind support and cooperation in writing this third edition of the book.

My special thank to Mr. Anupam Vij for taking photographs that has helped me in relating and expressing the text with the images. I extend my sincere thanks to Mr. Pawaninder Pal Vij, Director, Peepee Publishers and Distributors (P) Ltd. and his team Mr. Pawan Sharma and Mr. S.K. Sharma for their valuable support in editing the text and getting the book printed and published.

Last but not the least, I beg forgiveness of all those who have been with me over the course of the years and whose name I have failed to mention.

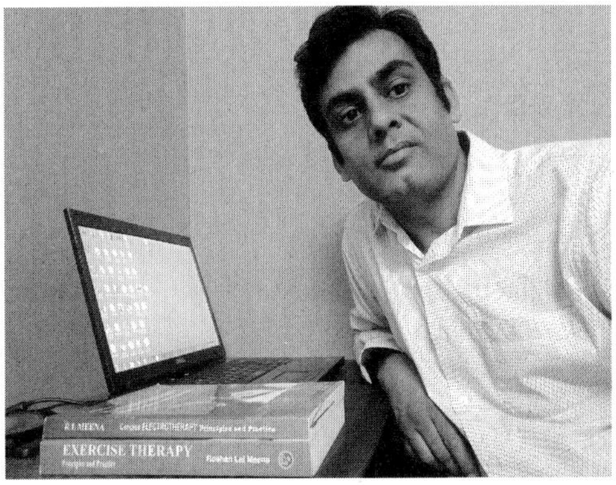

ABOUT THE AUTHOR

Roshan Lal Meena, BPT, MPT (Orthopedics) is a physical therapist, a teacher, researcher and author, and the primary author of this book, **Exercise Therapy: Principles and Practice**. Roshan has also recently authored a new textbook, Concise Electrotherapy: Principles and Practice. He has attended and participated and presented papers in many workshops, national and international conferences.

He has done his Bachelor in Physiotherapy from Calcutta University in 1998, and Master in Physiotherapy (Orthopedics) from Chaudhary Charan Singh University in 2006. He had joined Pandit Deendayal Upadhyaya National Institute for Persons with Physical Disabilities, Government of India affiliated to the University of Delhi in 1998 and has been teaching the students of Physiotherapy since then. Roshan has been awarded ACADEMIC EXCELLENCE AWARD from Neuraxis in 2018.

Roshan has been elected and served the office of Faculty Association of Pandit Deendayal Upadhyaya National Institute for Persons with Physical Disabilities as a President for the consecutive five terms from 2011 to 2016 and 2018 to 2019. He has been given additional responsibilities of Nodal Office, National Scholarship Portal and Incharge Library.

His presentation on minimum standards for clinical establishment before National Accreditation Board for Hospitals and Health Care Providers and Scope of Physiotherapy and Code of Ethics in the meeting of Delhi Council for Physiotherapists and Occupational Therapists are few of the eminent presentations.

CONTENTS

PART I

Section I
Basic Concepts

Section II
Therapeutic Approaches

PART II

PART I

Section I : Basic Concepts

1

INTRODUCTION TO EXERCISE THERAPY

Before discussing the field of exercise therapy, the concept of exercise must first be defined and explained. When we contract skeletal muscles to cause movement, or maintain a given posture, it is generally explained that we are being active. This is in contrast to being inactive, where we are not voluntarily contracting our skeletal muscles.

The Webster's dictionary provides three important definitions of exercise:

i. "Regular or repeated use of a faculty or body organ."

ii. Bodily exertion for the sake of developing and maintaining physical fitness.

iii. Something performed or practised in order to develop, improve, or display a specific power or skill.

The term exercise therefore can be used to denote activity that is performed for the purpose of improving, or expressing a particular type of physical fitness.

The organised and purposeful implication of exercise that separates it from activity is a complication, when going to market to get vegetables, we are being active, simply we are performing this act for a task rather than for physical fitness means that it does not suit the previous definition of exercise. Similarly, when workers lift object or force to exert themselves with repeated periods of muscular contraction (e.g., Labourers, farmers, construction workers, hawkers), they are active yet once again are not exercising. This definitional inadequacy of exercise has caused the term physical activity to be more widely used. Physical activity pertains to the activity performed by the body for purpose other than the specific development of physical fitness. Research has shown that physical fitness is improved from regular physical activity, just as it is from exercise. Thus individuals who are physically active in general lifestyle and vocation can be physically fit without (necessarily completing what we know to be exercised) exercise.

Exercise: Activity that is performed for the purpose of improving maintaining or expressing a particular type of physical fitness.

Physical Activity: The activity performed by the body for purpose other than the specific development of physical fitness.

Physical Fitness: A state of bodily function that is characterized by the ability to tolerate exercise stress. Exercise training is the repeated use of exercise to improve physical fitness.

Exercise Therapy: Is the systematic and planned performance of bodily movement postures or physical activities intended to provide a patient or client with means to:

- Remediate or prevent impairment.
- Improve, restore or enhance physical function.
- Prevent or reduce health-related risk factors.
- Optimise overall health status fitness or sense of well-being.

Therapeutic exercise programs designed by therapist are individualized to the unique needs of each patient or client. A patient is an individual with impairment and functional limitations diagnosed by a therapist, receiving therapeutic care to improve functions and prevent disability.

A client is an individual without diagnosed dysfunction who is engaged in therapeutic services to promote health and wellness to prevent dysfunction.

EFFECTS OF THERAPEUTIC EXERCISES

Every normal muscular contraction affects not only the musculoskeletal system but also neuromuscular and cardiopulmonary system of human body. These systems respond according to the force and stress created by such contractions. An external and constant force, i.e., gravity also affects these systems. These forces and stresses altogether are essential for normalcy of the body and its system. When these forces and stresses decrease or increase than the normal requirement, bodily dysfunction occur in the form of osteoporosis, muscle atrophy, deformity, pain and poor cardiopulmonary fitness etc.

Therapeutic exercises are not only controlled, progressive and planned but are also as per the capability of the patient resulting into the improvement of their functional ability.

Therapeutic exercise affects the development, improvement and maintenance of normalcy.

Goals of Exercise Therapy

To improve or maintain the following:

- Muscular strength.
- Muscular power.
- Muscular endurance.
- Cardiorespiratory endurance.
- Joint mobility.
- Joint flexibility.
- Agility.
- Body and mental relaxation
- Coordination.
- Motor control.
- Balance.

TYPES OF MUSCULAR CONTRACTION/ ACTION

Traditionally the word contraction has been used to describe different muscle actions, i.e., isometric, isotonic, concentric and eccentric contraction.

Recently a suggestion has been made to replace the word contraction with the term action. The proposed change in terminology was made on the base that the term "contraction" (which means drawing together) does not adequately or accurately reflect what happens to the entire muscle during activity and is contradictory when used to describe eccentric muscle activity, that is lengthening contraction.

Isotonic (iso = equal, tonic = muscle tone, the tone of muscle remains same throughout the contraction of muscle)

This is the contraction in which the intramuscular tension or tone remains same/constant as the muscle shortens or lengthens. The intramuscular tension is accompanied by a change in the length of the muscle.

The use of the term isotonic "contraction" is not used by some authors, because it refers to equal or constant tension which is unphysiological. The tension generated in a muscle cannot be controlled or kept constant.

Isometric (iso = equal, metric = length, the length of muscle remains same throughout the contraction of muscle)

When both the distal and proximal attachments of a muscle are fixed and the torque produced by a muscle is equal to the torque of the resistance the visible muscle length will remain unchanged, although shortening occurs at the myofibrils level. When there is no noticeable change in the length of muscle that is developing tension in the muscular action is called an isometric contraction. No mechanical work is performed in an isometric contraction because work is equivalent to the product of $F \times d$ (F = force, d = distance). There is no distance involved in an isometric contraction because both bony components are fixed and do not move during the contraction. However energy is being expended to produce cross-bridge cycling.

Static

The muscle remains in partial or complete contraction without changing its length. These are two different conditions under which this type of contraction is likely to occur:

1. Muscles which are antagonistic to each other contract with equal strength, thus balancing or counteracting each other (co-contraction of the agonist and the antagonist). The part affected is held tensly in place without moving. Tensing the Biceps to show off its bulge is an example of this. The contraction of the triceps prevents the elbow from further flexing.
2. A muscle is held in either partial or maximal contraction against another force such as the pull of gravity or an external mechanical or muscular force. Examples of this are holding a book at stretched hand, a tug of war between two equally matched opponents and attempting to move an object which is too heavy to move.

Concentric–Toward the Centre

The muscles contract isotonically in shortening to produce movement.

The attachments of the muscles are drawn closer together and movement is in the direction of the muscle pull (Fig. 1.1).

Usually during functional activities, one attachment of a bone is stabilized and the other attachment is free to move. If the proximal attachment is fixed and the distal attachment is free (as in an open kinematic chain) the muscle

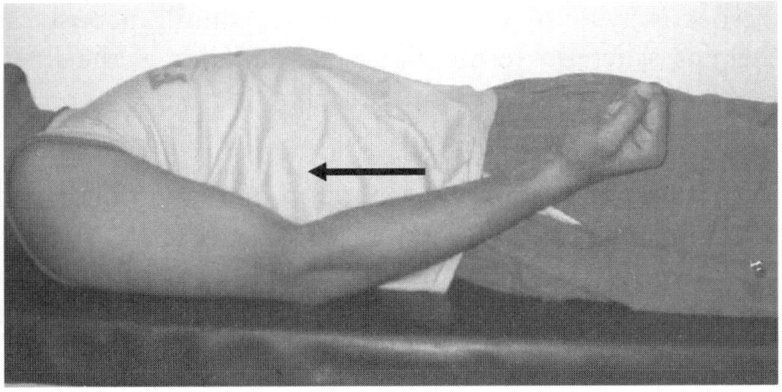

Fig. 1.1: Concentric contraction of elbow flexors

action will pull the distal bony component toward the proximal component. If the distal component is fixed and proximal bony component is free (in a closed kinematic chain), reverse action will occur and the proximal bony component will be pulled toward the distal bony component.

Positive muscular work is done during concentric exercise because when a concentric contraction occurs the muscular moment acts in the same direction as the angular velocity of the joint and by convention both are considered to be positive.

Eccentric–Away from the Centre

When a force that a muscle generates is insufficient to offset an opposing force on a lever, the muscle will undergo a lengthening or eccentric contraction. In this type of contraction the muscle acts as a brake and controls the movement of a bony component (Fig. 1.2).

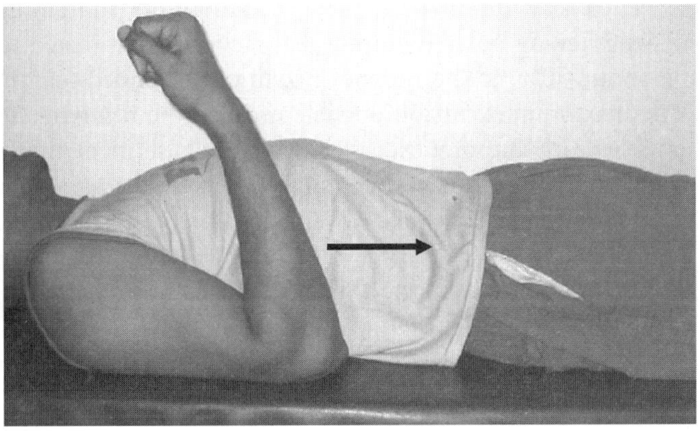

Fig. 1.2: Eccentric contraction of elbow flexors

When the hand holding a glass moves from the face to the table the flexor muscle of the elbow undergo a lengthening or eccentric contraction as they control the gravity-produced descent of the hand. In this activity the two ends of the muscle move apart or away from each other. The muscle acts as the resistance to the gravitational effect and a second class lever is formed. Eccentric muscle action like concentric muscle action can occur as motion of either the distal or proximal bony lever or normal and reverse actions, respectively. The mechanical work that is done by a muscle during an eccentric contraction is called negative work because work is done on the muscle rather than by the muscle. The energy cost of an eccentric contraction is considerably less than that of a concentric contraction when equal loads are used.

THE GROUP MUSCLE ACTION

Under normal circumstances a smooth purposeful desired movement cannot be produced by a single muscle action. To produce such type of efficient movement, and to maintain the stability of the joint during movement, integrated activity of many/several muscles is required. This is known as group muscle action.

Group of muscles are categorized on the basis of either the action they perform or the particular role they serve during specific action. When muscles are categorized on the basis of action, muscles that cause flexion at a joint are categorized as flexors. Similarly muscles that cause either extension/rotation are referred to as extensors or rotators. Individual muscle or group of muscles are described in terms of they demonstrate the specific role during action or movement.

Functionally muscles work together in groups, although each muscle may have some specific part to play in relation to the action of the whole group.

For example, Determining the precise direction of the movement or by maintaining its progress in a particular part of the range.

Movers

Mover is a muscle which is directly responsible for producing a movement. In the majority of movements there are several movers some of them have greater importance than others.

Principal Movers

When a movement is performed by several muscles, some of them have greater importance than other. These are known as prime or principal movers.

For example, Dorsiflexors of ankle joint are: tibialis–anterior, extensor hallucis longus, extensor digitorum longus. But principal mover is tibialis anterior.

Assistant Movers

The muscles which help to perform the movement but which seem to be less important, or which contract only under certain circumstances are assistant movers.

Emergency Muscles

Muscles which help only when an extra amount of force is needed, as when a movement is performed against resistance are sometimes called emergency muscles.

Agonist and Antagonists

Agonist is used to designate a muscle that is responsible for producing a desired motion at a joint. If flexion is the desired action, the flexor muscles are the agonists and extensors that are working directly opposite to the desired motion are called the *antagonists.* The desired motion may not be opposed by antagonists but these muscles have the potential to oppose the action.

Ordinarily when antagonist is called to perform a desired motion, the agonist is inhibited (reciprocal inhibition) if however, the agonist and potential antagonist contract simultaneously, then *co-contraction* occurs. Co-contraction of muscles around a joint can help to provide stability for the joint and represents a joint synergy that may be necessary in certain situations. Co-contraction of muscles with opposing function can be undesirable when a desired motion is prevented by involuntary co-contraction such as occurs in disorders affecting the control of muscle function.

Synergists

Muscles that help the agonist to perform desired action are called *synergists.*

For example, If flexion of the wrist is the desired movement/action, the flexor carpi radialis and flexor carpi ulnaris would be referred to as the "agonists" or "prime movers" because these muscles produce flexion. The wrist extensors would be the potential antagonists. The synergists that might directly help the wrist flexors would be the finger flexors.

Synergists may assist the agonist directly by helping to produce the desired movement such as in the wrist flexion, or indirectly either by stabilizing a part or by preventing an undesired action.

True Synergists

True synergists act, for example, when using the long finger flexors as agonists to grip an object in the hand. The unwanted action of these muscles in flexing the wrist needs to be controlled or opposed. This is done by the simultaneous contraction of the wrist extensors acting as true synergists.

Helping Synergists

Helping synergists act simultaneously. Flexor carpi radialis and extensor carpi radials longus are usually antagonistic to each other in producing wrist flexion and extension, respectively. However, they can act simultaneously as helping synergists to produce radial deviation at the wrist.

Neutralizer

Neutralizer is a muscle which acts to prevent an undesired action of one of the movers. Thus if a muscle both flexes and abducts, but only flexion is desired in the movement, an adductor contracts to neutralize the abductor actions of the mover.

Mutual Neutralizers: Occasionally two of the movers have one action in common but can also perform second action which are antagonistic to each other. For instance one muscle may upward rotate and adduct the scapula while the other may downward rotate and adduct. When they contract together to cause adduction, their rotatory function counter act each other. Muscles which behave this way in a movement are mutual stabilizers as well as movers.

Stabilizers or Fixators

Stabilizers or fixators are muscles which contract to control the position of a bone so that it may act as a steady base from which the agonist can act. They thus provide a fixed attachment for another muscle.

For example, during elbow flexion the shoulder girdle muscles act as fixators to control the position of the arm.

RANGE OF MUSCLE WORK

The range of muscle work is the extent of the muscular contraction which result in joint movement.

The excursion of muscle, i.e., the amount of shortening or lengthening possible during contraction, is estimated to be about 50% of the muscles maximum extended length. The maximum excursion possible is called the full range of muscle work and any excursion which falls short of this is called inner, outer or middle range to specify the particular part of the range in which movement takes place (Fig. 1.3).

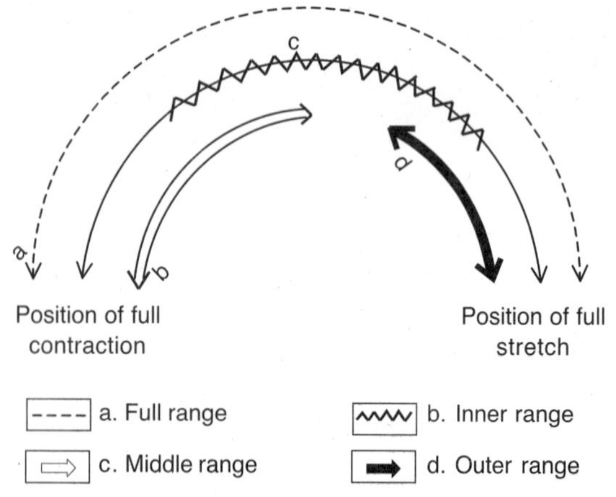

Fig. 1.3: Range of muscle work

Full Range

The joint is moved as the muscles work concentrically from the position in which they are fully stretched to the fully contracted, or concentrically, from the position of the fully contracted to the fully stretched (Fig. 1.4).

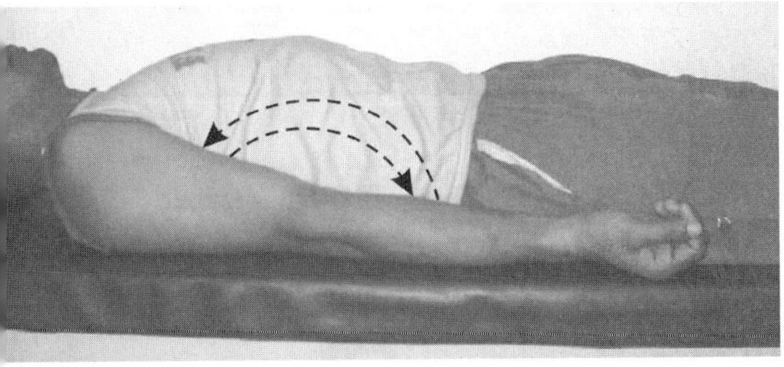

Fig. 1.4: Range of muscle work (full range) of elbow flexors

Under ordinary circumstances muscles are rarely required to work in full range, but in emergencies they may have to do so. Active full range of exercises are used for patients as they maintain its mobility, increase the circulation and ensure that the emergency reserve of powers and mobility is preserved.

Inner Range

The muscle works either concentrically from a position in which it is partially contracted (approximately half-way between the limit of full range) to position of full contraction, or vice versa if it works eccentrically (Fig. 1.5). The inner range for the joint which has 0° to 140° normal range will be 40° to 140°.

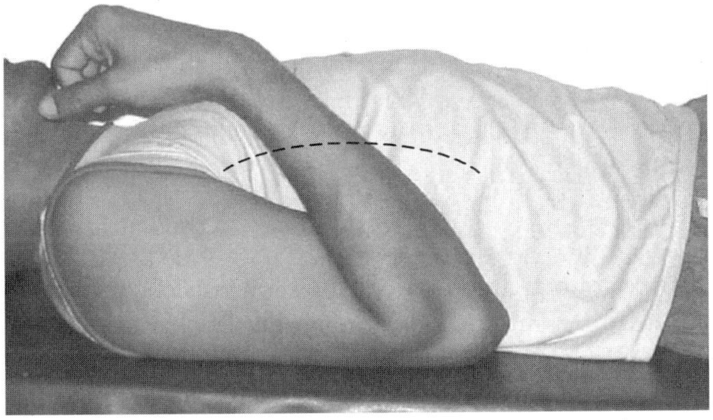

Fig. 1.5: Inner range of elbow flexors

Exercises in inner range is used to gain or maintain movement of a joint in the direction of the muscle pull, and to train some extensor muscles responsible for stabilizing joints.

Middle Range

The muscles are usually neither fully stretched nor fully contracted, this is the range in which muscles are most often used in everyday life. Generally speaking, they are most efficient in this range (Fig. 1.6). The middle range for the joint which has 0° to 140° normal range will be between 40° and 100°.

Exercises in this range maintain muscle tone and muscle power.

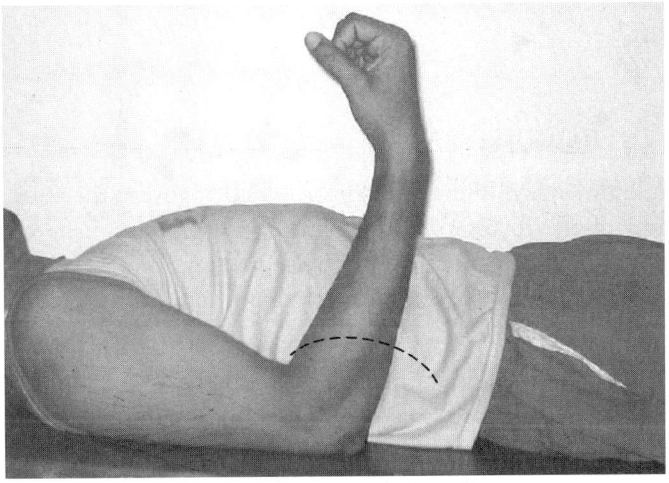

Fig. 1.6: Middle range of elbow flexors

Outer Range

The muscles work concentrically from the position in which they are fully stretched to a position in which they are partially (held) contracted, or vice versa if working eccentrically. The outer range for the joint which has 0° to 140° normal range will be between 0° and 120°.

The outer range work is used extensively in muscle re-adduction as a contraction is initiated more easily from stretched position in most muscles (Fig. 1.7).

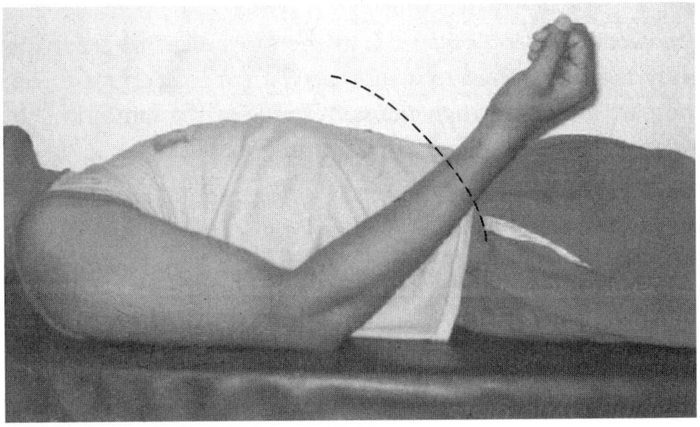

Fig. 1.7: Outer range of elbow flexors

2

SIMPLE AND APPLIED BIOMECHANICS

INTRODUCTION

A knowledge of the physical principles that govern the body and of the forces that affect the body is prerequisite to understand the concept of exercise therapy. Biomechanics the study of mechanics in the human body can give this knowledge.

Biomechanics consists of kinematics and kinetics. Kinematics is the area of biomechanics that include description of motion without regard for the forces producing the motion.

Kinetics is the area of biomechanics concerned with the forces producing motion or maintaining equilibrium.

KINEMATICS

Kinematics consists of:

- Type of motion.
- Location of motion.
- Direction and magnitude of motion.

Type of Motion

Angular or rotatory motion: It is the movement of a part of body around a fixed axis in a curved path. Each point on the part moves through the same angle at the same time at a constant distance from the axis of rotation.

Translation/Linear motion: It is the motion of a part of body in a straight line. Each point on the part moves through the same distance at the same time in parallel paths.

Angular and translatory motion combine to produce the third pathway of motion known as *curvilinear motion.*

Location of Motion (Fig. 2.1)

Consists of various planes and axis.

The movements of the shafts of bones (osteokinematics) takes place in one of the three cardinal planes of the body around their corresponding axes. These planes lie at right angles to one another, whereas the three axes lie at right angles both to one another and to their corresponding planes.

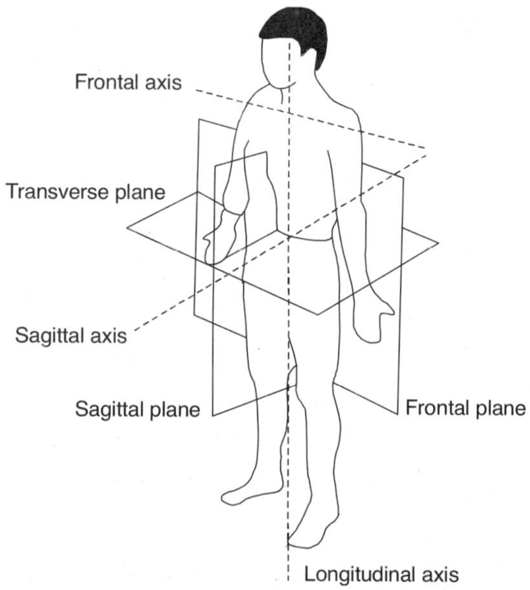

Fig. 2.1:

Sagittal Plane

It proceeds from anterior to the posterior aspect of the body and divides it into two equal right and left halves. Flexion and extension of the joints occurs in the sagittal plane around its frontal axis (medial lateral) which is perpendicular to the sagittal plane. The frontal axis proceeds from one side of the body to the other side.

Frontal Plane

It proceeds from one side of the body to the other side and divides it into two equal halves anterior and posterior. Abduction and adduction movements occur in the frontal plane around its sagittal axis (anterior posterior) which lies perpendicular to the frontal plane. Sagittal axis proceeds from anterior to the posterior aspects of the body and lies in the sagittal plane.

Transverse Plane

It is a horizontal plane and divides the body into two equal upper and lower portions. Rotations such as internal and external occurs in the transverse plane around its vertical axis which lies perpendicular to transverse plane.

Exceptional

The flexion and extension of carpometacarpal and metacarpophalangeal occurs in the frontal plane around its sagittal axis when the subject is in the anatomical position. The abduction and adduction of carpometacarpal joint occurs in the sagittal plane around its frontal axis when the subject is in the anatomical position.

Direction and Magnitude

Direction is basically the movement in terms Flexion/ Extension, Abduction/Adduction and rotations (Internal/ External).

While magnitude is the measure of movement in degrees or radians.

KINETICS

It is the study of forces which can make body or its part to move or at rest.

External forces: Come from outside the body, gravity is one of the important external forces which greatly influence human body position and motion.

Internal forces: Come from within the body. Muscles are the structures which provide such forces.

Center of gravity: While gravity acts at all points or segment of an object, its centre point of application is given as the gravity (COG).

It is a hypothetical point at which all mass would appear to be concentrated and is the point at which the force of gravity would appear to act.

The action line and direction of the force of gravity on an object are always vertical downward toward the center of the earth regardless of the orientation in space of the object.

The gravity vector is commonly referred to as the line of gravity (LOG).

COG of the Human Body

When all the segments of the body are combined and the body is taken as a single solid object in anatomic position, the COG of the body lies approximately anterior to the second sacral vertebrae.

Also each segment in the body is acted on by the force of gravity and has its own COG.

Stability and COG

For an object to be stable the COG must fall within the base of support, when the COG falls outside the base of support, the object will tend to fall.

Other factors which affect stability:

i. The larger the base of support of an object, the greater the stability of that object.
ii. The closer the COG is to the base of support, the more stable is the object.

   For e.g., In cricket wicketkeeper widely opens his legs (larger base of support) and flexes his knees (COG closer to base of support).

Newton's Laws of Motion

These laws are also applicable to human motion and therefore their concept should be reviewed to understand exercise therapy.

First Law: States that an object will remain at rest or in uniform motion unless acted upon by an unbalanced force.

Inertia is the property of an object that makes the object resist both in initiation of motion and a change in motion.

Second Law: States that the acceleration of an object is proportional to the unbalanced forces acting on it and inversely proportional to the mass of that object

$$a = F/m$$

(a–acceleration, F–force, m–mass)

i.e., the greater the force more will be acceleration and on contrary greater the mass lesser will be accleration.

Third Law: States that for every action there is an equal and opposite reaction.

Pulleys

Pulleys are frequently used in exercise and traction equipment to change the direction of a force or to increase or decrease the magnitude of a force.

Anatomic Pulley: Muscles or muscle tendons are found to be wrapped or deflected by bony prominences or sesamoid bone like patella.

When the direction of pull of a muscle is altered the bone or bony prominences causing the deflection from an anatomical pulley. Pulley changes the direction.

Example: The tendon of the quadriceps not only changes its direction of pull as a result of the interposed patella but its leverage also improves.

They are commonly used in two forms:

1. Single fixed pulley.
2. Movable pulley.

Single Fixed Pulley: The line of action of force may be changed by means of a pulley, such pulley does not provide any mechanical advantage to the force, but only changes its direction (Fig. 2.2).

Example: Cervical traction.

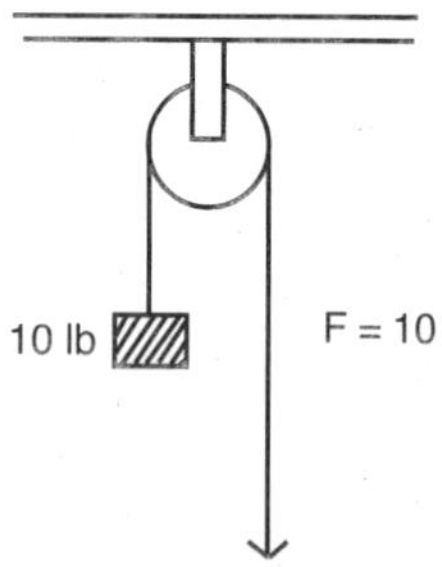

Fig. 2.2: Fixed pulley (*example*–cervical traction)

Movable Pulley: If a weight is attached to a movable pulley, half of the weight is supported by the rope attached to stationary hook and half by the rope on the other side of the pulley. Therefore, there is a mechanical advantage of the force F is 2. The rope, however, must be moved twice the distance that the weight is raised, and what is gained in force is lost in distance (Fig. 2.3).

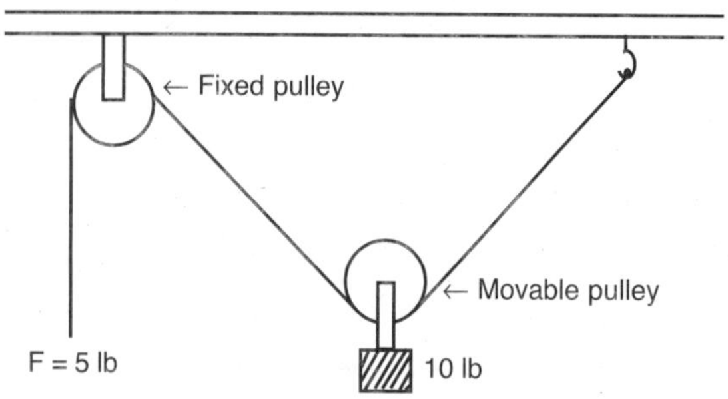

Fig. 2.3: Movable pulley (*example*–Leg traction, russal traction)

LEVERS

A lever is a simple machine that magnifies force and speed of the movement, and commonly defined as rigid bar that rotates about a fixed point, the fulcrum. In biomechanics the principles of the lever are used to visualise the more complex system of forces that produce rotatory motion in the body. In the human body levers are primarily the bones and axis (fulcrum) are the joints where bones meet.

There are three elements of the lever (Fig. 2.4):

a. *The fulcrum (F):* It is represented by the joint or is a point on the axis about which the rigid mass rotates.
b. *The effort arm (EA):* Effort (E) is the point where contracting muscle is attached to the moving bone. EA includes all parts of the rigid mass between the fulcrum and the point at which energy is applied to the rigid bar.

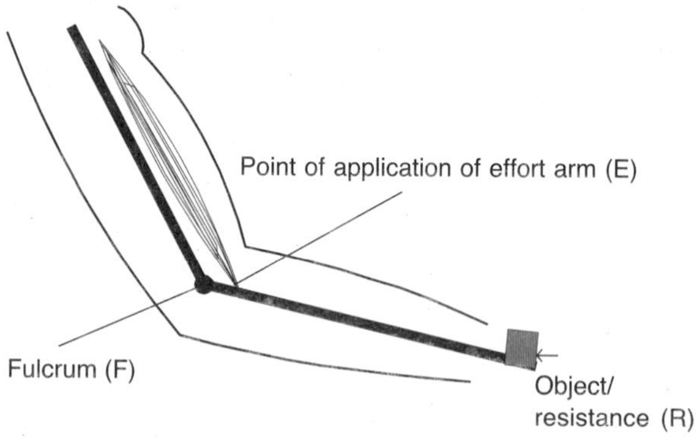

Fig. 2.4: Elements of Lever–Fulcrum (F). Point of application of Effort Arm (E) and Resistance or weight of the body (R)

c. *The resistance arm (RA):* Resistance (R) is the point where object is held. RA includes all parts of the rigid mass between the fulcrum and the point at which energy is applied to the object to be moved by the lever.

These three elements may be found in any arrangement and any one of the three may be between the other two.

Classification of Levers

Basically three types of levers are found in the body and are classified on the basis of arrangement of the three elements, i.e., Fulcrum (F), point of application of effort (E) and point of application of resistance (R).

- If the fulcrum is in between the point of application of effort (E) and point of application of resistance (R) or EFR it is termed as first class lever.
- If the point of application of effort is between fulcrum and point of application of resistance or FER it is termed as third class lever.
- If the point of application of resistance is between fulcrum and point of application of effort or FRE it is termed as second class lever.

First Class Lever

As the Figure 2.4 shows that the fulcrum lies between two resultant forces one applied on either side. In description of body levers the EFR will not be exactly located (Fig. 2.5).

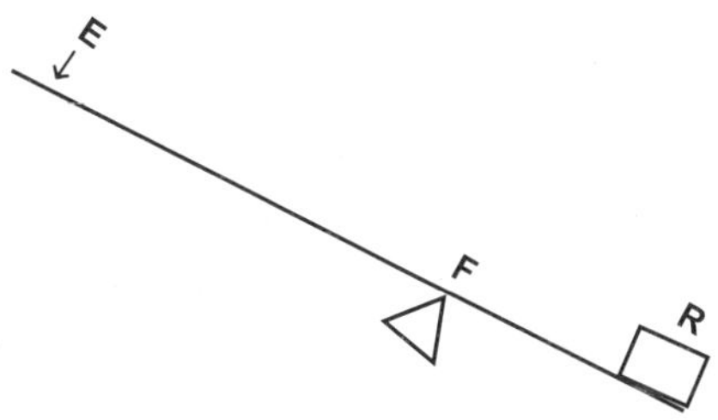

Fig. 2.5: First class lever. A first class lever is commonly exemplified by a seesaw

Examples of 1st class lever: Atlanto occipital joint where the weight of the head is balanced by posterior neck muscle force. Similarly at the intervertebral joints where the weight of the trunk is balanced by the erector spinal muscle forces. The first class lever is also seen during extension of elbow (Fig. 2.6).

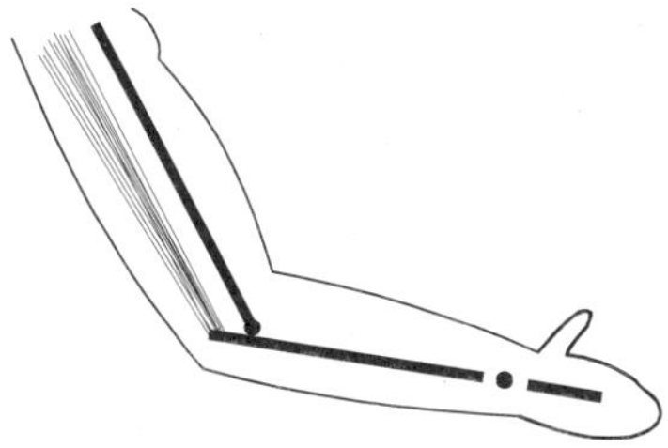

Fig. 2.6: Example of first class lever. The fulcrum (F) lies between the point of application of resistance (R) and effort (Triceps), or EFR

The first class lever are used for maintaining postures and balance.

Second Class Lever

In the second class the resistance arm lies between the fulcrum and effort arm (FRE) or whenever two parallel forces are applied at some distance from the fulcrum or axis (F) with the resistance arm closer to the fulcrum. In a second class lever effort arm is always greater than the resistance arm (Fig. 2.7).

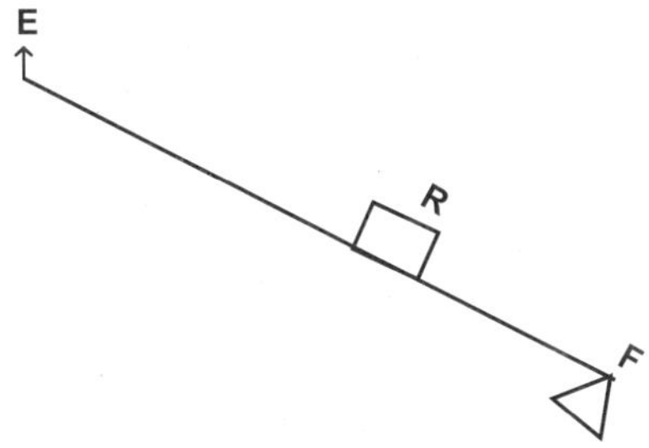

Fig. 2.7: Second class lever. In a second class lever, the Weight (Resistance) is located between the Axis (Fulcrum) and the Force

In the human body there are limited examples of the second class lever. It commonly occurs when gravity is the effort force and muscles are the resistance. The only muscle example is the pull of the brachioradialis and wrist extensors to maintain the position of elbow joint, therefore the resistance arm lies between the fulcrum (elbow joint) and point of application of effort arm. The lever includes the radius and ulna; the effort arm includes the length of the bones which extends from the axis to the point of attachment of the muscle, a length of 10 inches. If a weight were suspended at the mid point of the forearm, the resistance arm would then include that portion of the radius and ulna, which extends from the axis to the weight a distance of 5 inches. However, this system changes to a third class lever if any heavy object is held in the hand. This example of lever is because in case of paralysis of the biceps brachii and brachialis, patient can use the brachioradialis and wrist extensors to hold the elbow in a flexion position. Normally however, brachioradialis and wrist extensors do not act in this isolated manner.

There are no apparent examples of second class lever in the body.

Third Class Lever

It is the most common lever formed in the body. The effort arm lies between the fulcrum and resistance (Fig. 2.8).

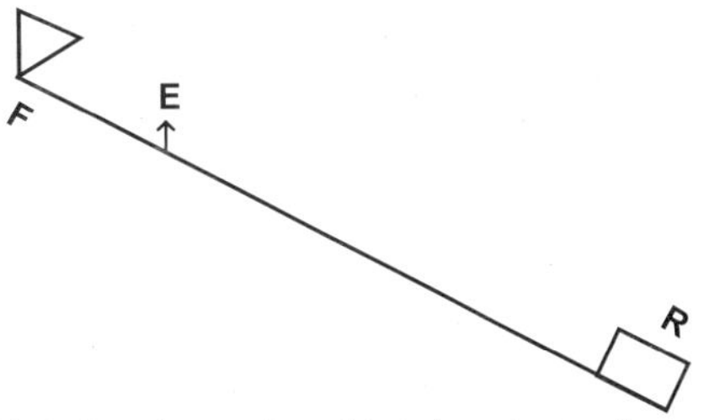

Fig. 2.8: Third class lever. In a third class lever, the most common in the human body, Force is applied between the Resistance (Weight) and the Axis (Fulcrum).

The point of application of effort is always closer to the fulcrum therefore effort arm is smaller and resistance arm is larger and mechanical advantage may be 0.1 or even low. This arrangement is designed for producing speed of the distal segment or for moving a small weight a long distance (Fig. 2.9).

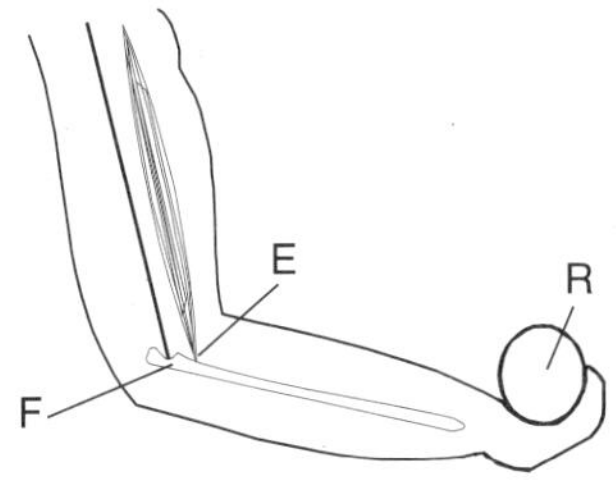

Fig. 2.9: Example of third class lever, the point of application of effort (E) is located between fulcrum (F) and resistance (R), (or FER) therefore it forms the third class lever

Example: Forces on the forearm. The fulcrum will be a point on the axis and in the joint. The point of application of effort is at point where the brachialis attaches to the bone and the effort arm is between the fulcrum and point where the brachialis attaches to the bone which may be approximately 1 inch in length.

The resistance is the object held in the hand and the resistance arm extends from fulcrum (F) to the object or the resistance arm includes the total length of the radius and ulna, the wrist and metacarpal and the portion of the proximal phalanges, approximately 16 inches in length.

Mostly third class lever is common in open chain motions of the activities.

Mechanical Advantage of Lever

Is a measure of the efficiency of the lever. It is the ratio of the effort arm to the resistance arm or

$$MAd = EA/RA$$

MAd	:	Mechanical Advantage
EA	:	Effort Arm
RA	:	Resistance Arm

Whenever mechanical advantage is greater than one, the magnitude of the effort force can be smaller than the magnitude of resistance. That is, a small effort can create more torque and overcome a large resistance.

- In all second class lever, the mechanical advantages of the lever will always be greater than one as effort arm is larger than resistance arm (EA > RA).
- In all third class lever mech. advantage will always be less then one. Hence more effort force is required to overcome resistance force (as RA > EA).
- 1st class lever follows no rules relative to mech advantage. EA can be greater than, less than, or equal to RA.

Use of Levers in Exercise Therapy

By learning the concepts of various types of lever these principles can be applied in almost all aspects of therapy.

To make exercises more resistive long lever arm can be selected. Contrary in the beginning short lever arm is preferred.

These concepts are also be used in gait training with crutches, canes etc.

3

ACTIVE AND PASSIVE MOVEMENTS

ACTIVE MOVEMENTS/EXERCISES

Movement which is performed by the patient on his own efforts with little or without external support.

All the activities of daily living (ADL) done without the help of external support such as combing hair, shaving, fastening bras, sitting on toilet, bringing hand to the mouth for eating or drinking are all the active movements. Activities such as jogging, brisk walk, running, lifting dumbbells, raising one leg alternately in supine or prone, and bringing single knee or both the knees to the chest performed to the purpose of improving, maintaining or expressing particular type of physical fitness known as active exercise. Active movements or exercises are classified into four groups:

- Active free movement/exercise.
- Active assisted movement/exercise.
- Active assisted and resisted movement/exercise.
- Active resisted movement/exercise.

Free Exercises

Free exercises are those exercises which are performed by the patient's voluntary muscular effort in the absence of any assistance or resistance of external force except gravity.

Effects of Free Exercises

- Relaxation.
- Maintenance of muscle tone.
- Improving strength and power (depends upon speed, leverage and duration of the exercise).
- Improving co-ordination maintaining flexibility and mobility.

Advantage:

After learning the concept of the exercise patient can perform and practice it on his own.

Disadvantage:

- Neurologically affected patients who have poor voluntary control cannot perform it.
- Weak muscles can be strengthened upto certain extent only.

Classification of Free Exercises

Free exercise can be classified on the basis of the extent of the area involved into localized and generalized forms.

Localized free exercises are those which are to mobilize a particular joint or to strengthen a particular muscle/muscle group, e.g., Active movements of shoulder joint; pendular movement of shoulder.

Generalized free exercises are those which involve the use of many joints and muscles all over the body and the effect is generalized as in running, jogging, cycling etc.

Free exercise can also be classified on the basis of character of a particular exercise. They may be subjective or objective free exercises.

Subjective free exercises are usually formal and consist of more or less anatomical movements performed in full range, the emphasis is on form and pattern of the exercise.

Objective free exercises are those in which patient's aim is to achieve a particular goal during performance, e.g., to reach a point marked on the wall, here goal is a stimulating factor for the performance. But care should be taken to maintain the accuracy of movement. The movement should not be compromised in an effort to reach for the goal.

Indications and Uses of Free Exercises

The indication and use of any particular free exercise depend on the nature of exercise, its extent, intensity and duration of its performance.

1. *Relaxation:* Rhythmical swinging and pendulum movements are used for relaxation of muscles in the region of the joint moved. The alternating and reciprocal contraction and relaxation of the opposing muscle group cause state of relaxation which is prerequisite for contraction.

   Active free movements or exercises are used for relieving wasteful tension in the muscles which limits joint mobility and reduces the efficiency of neuromuscular coordination.

2. *Joint mobility and flexibility* are maintained and improved by free exercises (Figs. 3.1a to c).
3. *Muscle strength power and endurance* are maintained or increased in response to the tension created in the muscles (Figs. 3.2a to d).

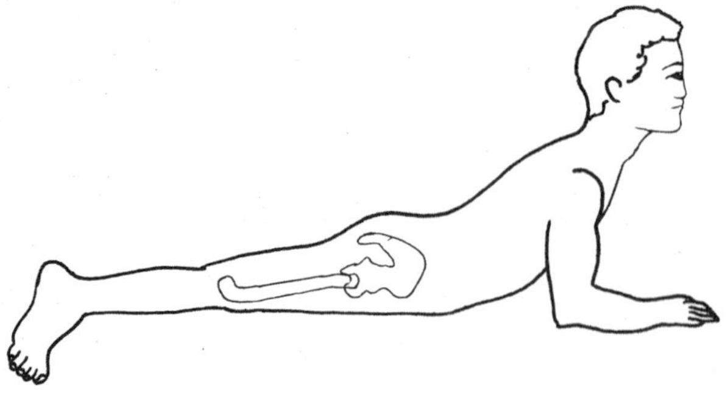

Fig. 3.1c: Prone on elbows

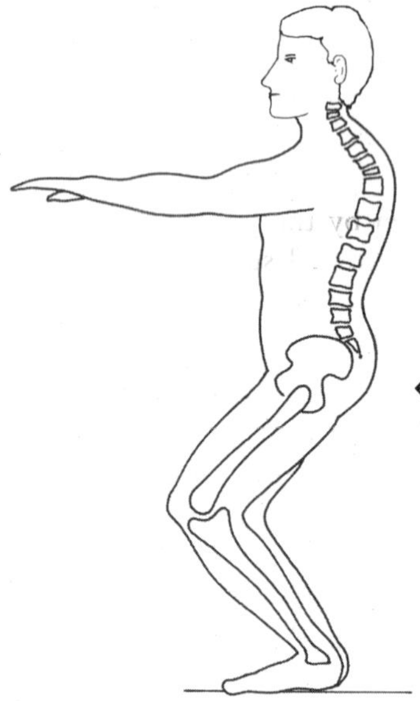

← **Fig. 3.2a:** Squatting

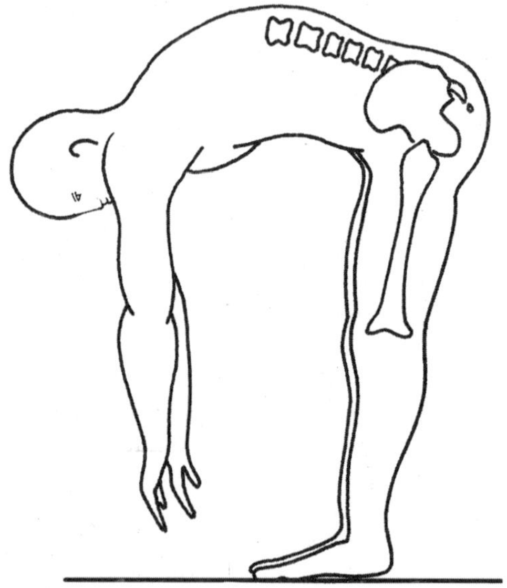

Fig. 3.1a: Forward bending

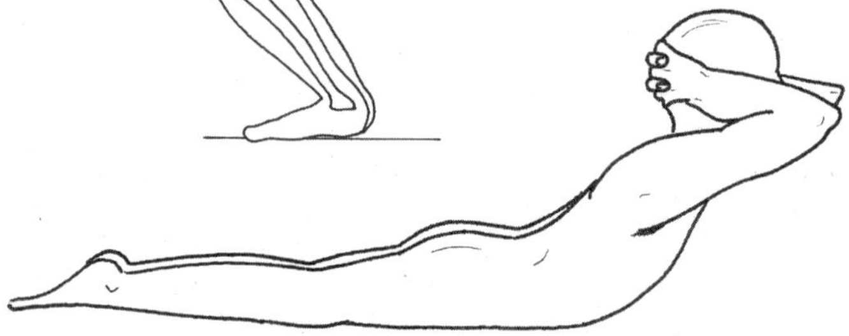

Fig. 3.2b: Spinal extension

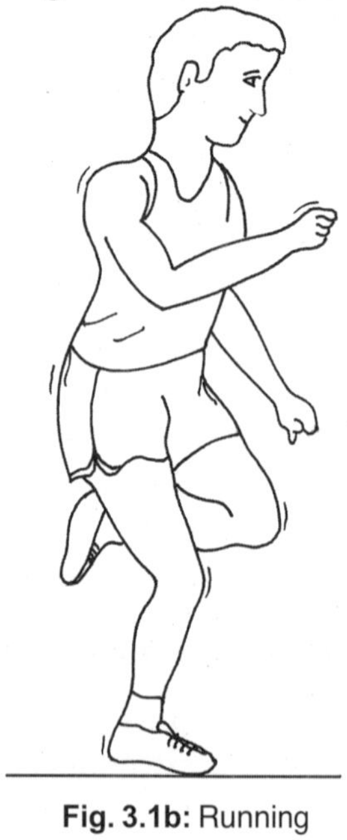

Fig. 3.1b: Running

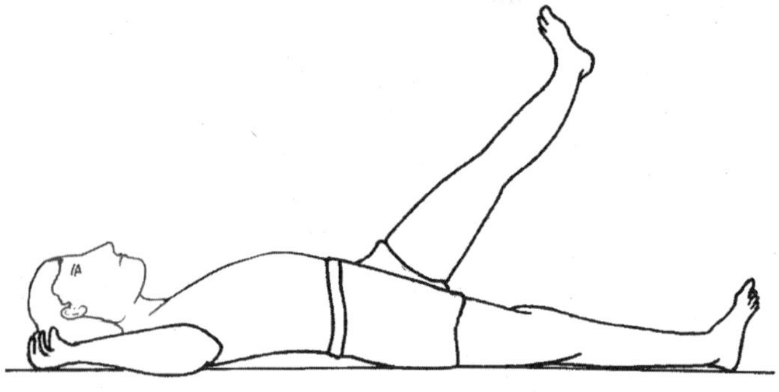

Fig. 3.2c: Straight leg raise (Single leg)

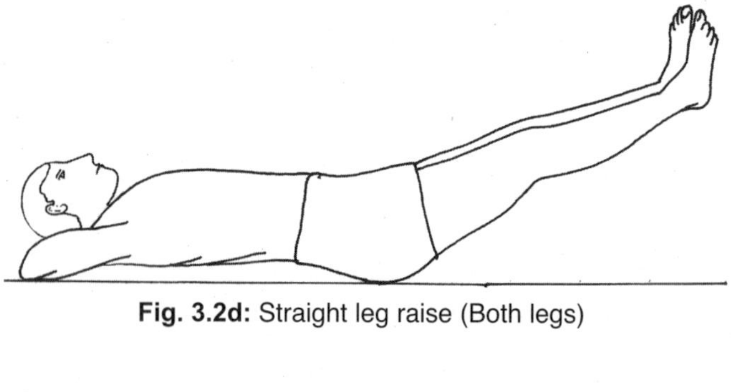

Fig. 3.2d: Straight leg raise (Both legs)

Free exercises which are performed against resistance of body weight or gravity and/or with long leverage, mainly improve strength and power. While those which are performed for longer duration with slow speeds tends to improve endurance.

4. *Tone:* Muscles are toned up; when free exercises performed. On contrary it also reduces the tone in hypertonic muscle groups.
5. *Neuromuscular coordination* is improved by practising free exercises or movement. As the pattern of movement is established it is simplified and it becomes more efficient, and the conduction of the necessary impulses along the neuromuscular pathways is facilitated. With repetition and practice, exercises which at one time required good amount of effort and concentration become easier for the performer (Figs. 3.3a to 3.3c).

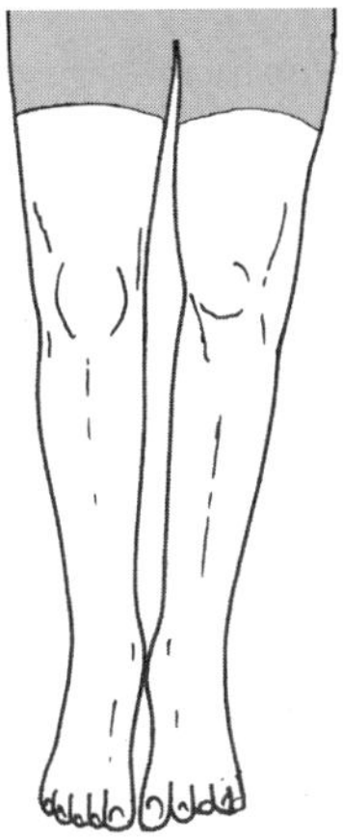

Fig. 3.3a: Close standing

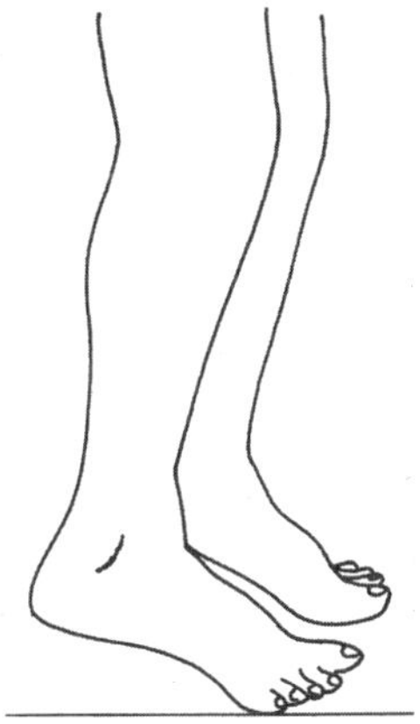

Fig. 3.3b: Raise heels off the ground

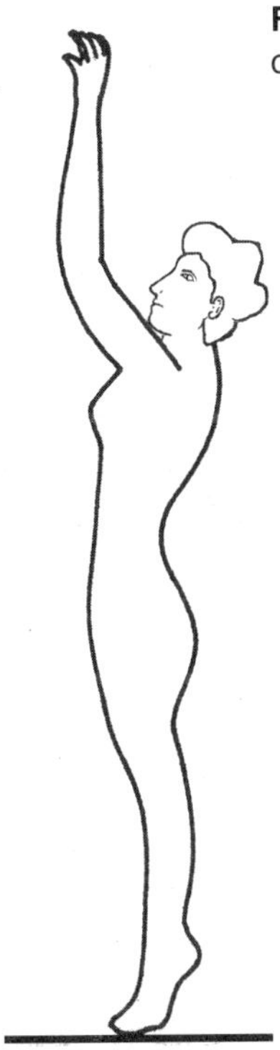

Fig. 3.3c: Raise arms overhead

6. *Confidence:* Coordinated and efficient performance of movement gives confidence to the patient to carry out other and new activities with full voluntary control.
7. *Cardiopulmonary effect:* Free exercise increases cardio-respiratory work, it increases both local and the general circulation providing work for the heart muscles (Fig. 3.4).

   Any type of free exercise causes increase in blood demand during contraction of muscles working which gets fulfilled during relaxation period of that muscle. This leads to fresh oxygenation of blood and removal of metabolic products. Overall all type of free exercises improve the cardiopulmonary endurance of the patient.

Active Assisted Movement/Exercise

Voluntary contraction of a muscle, which is able to produce little movement but not sufficient enough to produce the movement in full range of motion. In order to produce the movement in full range of motion an external assistance is provided by the therapist, along with voluntary contraction of the muscle. The patients with weak or paralized muscles find difficulty in initiating the movement. These patients require an assistance for initiating the movement. Therapist provides assistance to the patient in initiating the movement. Therapist may assist the patient throughout the range of motion, if required (Fig. 3.4).

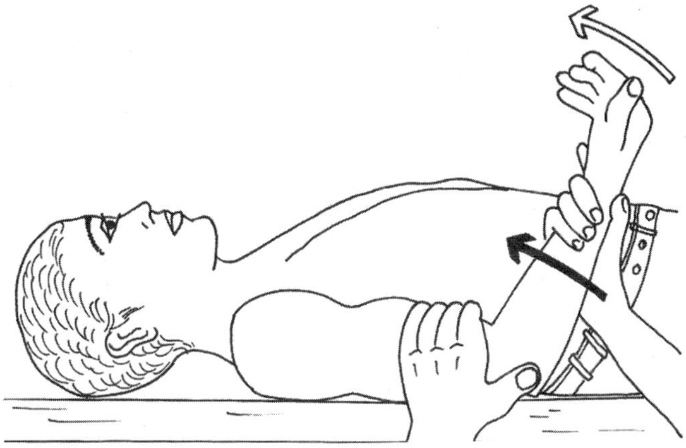

Fig. 3.4: Active assistive elbow flexion (initial ROM) white arrow shows movement and black assistance toward the movement

Techniques of Active Assisted Movements

1. *Position of the Patient:* Patient should be relaxed and comfortable and the joint should be placed in such a position so that the tension of the antagonistic muscles can be eliminated.
2. *Stabilisation of the Proximal Part of the Joint:* To avoid trick movements and achieve accurate movement, the proximal part of the joint should be stabilised adequately.

3. *Stretch stimulus:* Stretching of agonist muscles prior to movement facilitates the contraction of the agonist muscles and more contraction can be achieved. For e.g., a stretch stimulus is given to the agonist (dorsiflexors) before the active assisted dorsiflexion.
4. *Direction of movement:* Patient may have difficulty to perform the movement in desired direction. Therefore, it is important to explain the direction of movement and it can be taught by active movement of the contralateral limb or passive movement of the same joint.
5. *Suspension* (discussed in Chapter 10).
6. *Assisting force:* Therapist's hand(s) provide assistance to the agonist muscles to perform the movement in full range of motion. An assistance force should not be higher than the contraction of the agonist muscles as it is given to augment the contraction of muscle.

   An assistance is given in the direction of movement and patient is given command to contract the muscle as maximum as possible. A muscle is formed by number of muscle fibres and different muscle fibres work in different range of the movement. Generally more assistance is required in initial and end ROM because the middle ROM is completed by more muscle fibres than the initial and end range.
7. *The nature of the movement:* The movement is performed in smooth manner in the anatomical range. When an assistance is given to strengthen the muscles in gravity eliminated position, great support is required to perform the movement.

   Assistance is always given to facilitate the contraction of muscle fibres, therefore, therapist must keep observing the patient whether he/she is contracting the muscle or not. There will not be any use of assisting the movement if patient does not contract the muscle while performing the movement.
8. *Repetitions* of active assisted movement depends on the condition of patient and age. In order to strengthen the muscles, three sets of 30 repetitions may be performed. Each set consists 20 repetitions. A brief rest between the sets required to avoid fatigue of the muscle.

Indications of Active Assisted Exercises/ Movements

1. *Strengthening of the weak muscles:* Prolonged immobilisation of joint can cause disuse atrophy of muscles and patient finds difficulty to perform the movement in available ROM against gravity or in gravity eliminated positions. An external assistance by the hands of therapist or suspension therapy unit is given to complete the ROM. To strengthen the muscles an assistance is given to support the movement and during this period patient is asked to contract the muscle as maximum as possible. After 1-2 weeks an external assistance may be eliminated as patient starts moving the joint without any assistance against the gravity or in gravity eliminated position.

   Example: Post fracture disuse atrophy, post tendon transfer muscle weakness, and peripheral nerve injuries.
2. *Co-ordination of movement:* It has been observed that prolonged immobilisation of joint can cause loss of memory of brain to the movement and patient finds difficulty to initiate the movement. Passive or Active movement of the same joint of contralateral limb is performed to stimulate motor pathway. The patient may re-learn the movement as the conduction of impulses is facilitated in the neuromuscular pathway. As patient re-learns the movement an external assistance is given to perform the movement in available range of movement.

Active Assisted Resisted Movement

Muscle is formed by number of muscle fibres and different muscle fibres work at different ranges (outer range, middle range and inner range). Some muscle fibres initiate the range, while others are engaged to perform the movement in middle and end range.

Trauma or pathology in the muscle can hamper the movement at different ranges. Patient finds difficulty in initiating the movement, but has strong contraction of the muscle in the middle range.

Active assisted resisted is a combination of both assisted and resisted movement in which an assistance is given to initiate the movement and resistance is given in the middle range where patient has strong contraction of muscle (Figs. 3.5 and 3.6).

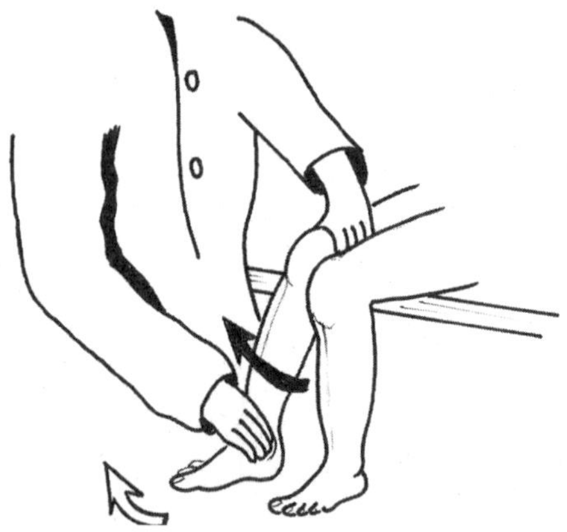

Fig. 3.5: Active assistive movement, white arrow shows movement (extension) and black arrow shows assistance toward the movement (initial) extension of knee joint

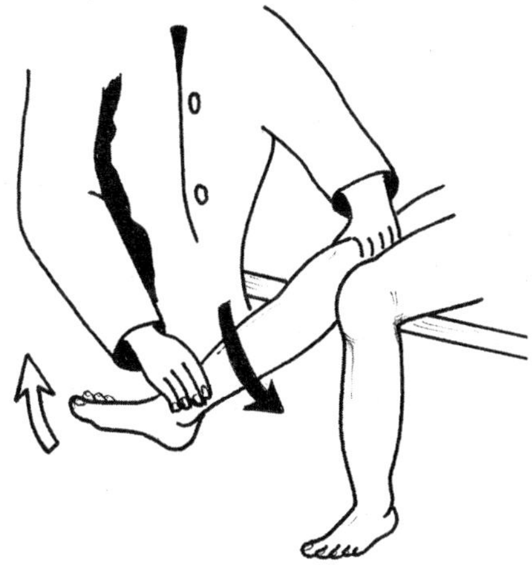

Fig. 3.6: Active assistive movement, white arrow shows movement and black arrow shows resistance against movement at the terminal extension of the knee joint

Resisted Movement or Exercise

A movement or exercise is carried out against the resistance in available range of motion. The intramuscular tension is increased as the resistance is applied against isometric or isotonic contraction of muscle (Fig. 3.7).

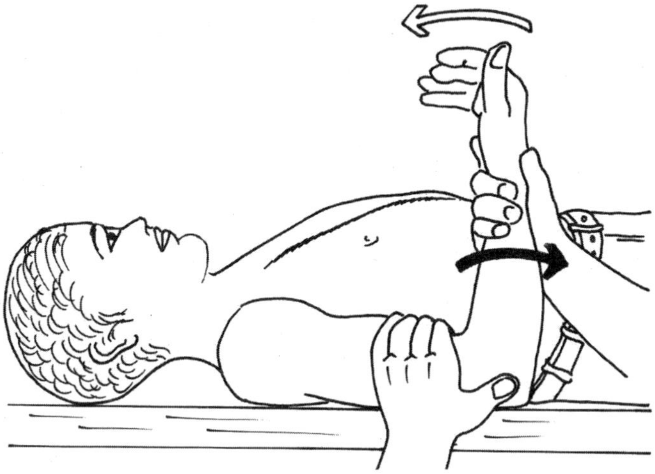

Fig. 3.7: Active resistive elbow flexion white arrow shows movement and black arrow shows resistance against the movement (flexion)

Methods/Apparatus Used to Provide Resistance

1. Multigymnasium apparatus–weights, pulley, dumbells.
2. Highly sophisticated computer driven-isokinetic.
3. Suspension therapy unit.
4. Hydrotherapy.
5. Therabands.
6. Sponge balls and medicinal ball.

Resistance can also be applied by:

- Therapist (Manual resistance).
- Patient (auto resistance).
- Springs.

1. Resistance by the Therapist

a. *Position of the Patient:* Should be comfortable.

b. *Stabilization:* The proximal part of the joint should be stabilised by straps or therapist's hand, or body weight.

c. *Pattern of Movement:* Explain the direction of movement to the patient to perform the smooth and coordinated movement in anatomical range. This can be taught by passive or active movement of same limb.

d. *Resisting Force:* Therapist stabilizes the proximal part of joint by one hand while other hand is used to apply resistance.

2. Resistance by the Patient

The patient can apply resistance by his/her contralateral limb.

3. Resistance by Weight

The apparatus which are used to apply resistance are sandbags, dumbell, metal weights, medicinal ball etc. In U/E while stabilising the proximal part of the joint patient is asked to hold the weight and lift it in full ROM (isotonic resisted exercise). In L/E straps can be used to attach the weight to a shoe or quadriceps table can also be used. This technique is also known as Heavy Resistance Training.

4. Resistance by Springs

The springs and therabands in sports physiotherapy clinic is widely used to provide resistance.

- *Advantage:* Can be arranged easily.
- *Disadvantage:* Resistance which is applied by spring does not remain same, increases gradually and becomes very high in the end range of movement. The resistance which is calculated for the particular muscle cannot be achieved by the springs as the resistance does not remain same throughout the range of motion.

5. Resistance by Therabands

The resistance is also applied by therabands. Therabands are elastic straps which are specially designed to strengthen a particular group of muscles.

Example: Theraband kit for tennis elbow, this type of theraband kit contains therabands which are used to strengthen the extensors of the wrist to prevent tennis elbow. Different sizes of *theraband exercise balls* are inflatable balls used for strengthening and *balance training.* Each ball comes with two plugs and an inflation adapter alongwith poster illustrating 24 exercise. *Five sizes* are available which are *prescribed according* to the *height* of *patient.* Theraband exercise balls also have specific role on cerebral palsy patient to strengthen *spinal extension* and *abdominals against gravity* and to improve balance.

6. Resistance by Medicinal Ball

Medicinal weighted ball is another means of giving resistance during the management of weak muscle groups. These are available in different sizes and weight, prescribed according to the strength of particular group of muscles and mainly given for upper extremity and spinal muscles.

Muscles are strengthened by giving the weighted medicinal ball in various forms of movement and activities.

Example: Hold the weighted medicinal ball in both hands, with extended elbow and raise it over the shoulder (strengthening exercise for shoulder flexors).

Further it can also be used to develop coordination and balance in standing and sitting position by throwing and catching activities.

7. Resistance by Water

Water possesses the property of viscosity–the resistance of fluid flow. It is the friction that occurs between individual molecules as they attempt to move by each other. Because water has greater viscosity than air, there is more resistance when one is moving through water than air.

As a body moves through the water the pressure is increased in front of the body and decreased behind it. Water runs to the area of decreased pressure causing turbulence that tend to drag the body backward. The faster the movement the greater the turbulence and the longer the drag force or resistance to movement. This property of water may be used along with streamlined or blunt object for less or more resistance respectively.

Types of Resisted Exercises

1. Isotonic resistance exercise.
2. Isometric resistance exercise.
3. Isokinetic resistance exercise.

1. Isotonic Resistance Exercise

During isotonic resistance exercise, muscle contracts concentrically or eccentrically it means length of muscle keeps changing but the intramuscular tension remains same. Positive muscular work is done during concentric exercise because when concentric contraction occurs the muscular moment acts in the same direction as the angular velocity of the joint and by convention both are considered to be positive. The mechanical work that is done by a muscle during an eccentric contraction is called negative work because work is done on the muscle rather than by the muscle. The energy cost of an eccentric contraction is considerably less than that of a concentric contraction when equal loads are used.

Uses of isotonic resistance exercise—Isotonic resisted exercise is designed to increase:

- Muscle power.
- Muscle strength.
- Muscle endurance.
- Cardiopulmonary endurance.

2. Isometric Resistance Exercise

Iso means equal and metric means length—it is the types of resistance exercise in which the length of muscle remains same or constant but an intramuscular tension changes.

Types of isometric resistance exercise: An isometric resistance exercise is devised on the basis of its amount of resistance, duration of exercise, degree of movement and contraction. The following isometric exercises are practised by the physical therapists.

- Muscle setting exercises.
- Stabilization exercises.
- Multiple angle isometric exercise.

Muscle Setting Exercises: It is a type of isometric exercise in which little or no resistance is applied. Exercise is generally indicated after an injury at the acute stage (although the application of this exercise depends on the severity of injury), to promote muscle relaxation (by decreasing muscle spasm), blood circulation and decrease pain. The purpose of exercise is to increase or restore the vital functions of the muscle and increase the healing process. It is a low intensity exercise carried out against no or little resistance, thus exercise does not improve the muscle strength although some weak muscles may show improvement in muscle strength but not much markable.

Stabilization Exercise: It is a type of isometric exercise which is carried out against submaximal resistance, generally at the mid range to enhance postural stability. The muscles contract isometrically against the gravitational resistance (force) or resistance applied by the hands of therapist.

Multiple-Angle Isometric Exercise: This exercise is indicated to improve the strength of muscle when the isotonic resistance exercise is not recommended because of pain or instability. Isometric contraction of muscle is carried out against resistance applied by the hands of therapist or mechanical devices at different angles in the available range of motion. This exercise is carried out against maximal resistance for at least 6 seconds or count of 10. An alternate method of multiple-angle isometric exercise is isokinetic machine, where desired angles, resistance, duration of resistance during single angle and duration of whole treatment session are set, and exercise is carried out smoothly. The equipment offers an accurate resistance against the movement at different angles. This helps in strengthening of muscles without provoking pain.

3. Isokinetic Resisted Exercise

It is a type of isotonic resisted exercise in which resistance is applied by mechanical device so that the speed of movement remains same throughout the range of motion. The speed of movement cannot be maintained same through the range of motion against the resistance applied by the hands of therapist, therefore this type of exercise is performed by highly sophisticated equipment, known as isokinetic machine (*Kincom, Biodex* etc.).

Progressive Resisted Exercises (PRE)

PRE was developed by De Lorme in 1946, which is based on *10 RM* (RM = Repetition maximum). He calculated 10 RM and executed on soldiers suffering from muscle weakness following trauma in Second World War. A set of exercise was repeated from 7 to 10 times during treatment session. Exercises prescribed 5 days a week and in the last day of week (Friday) 10 RM was to be calculated and new exercise programme used to introduce for the next week. De Lorme called this method "Heavy Resistance Exercises".

The muscles strengthened by him were not disused but they had lost muscle strength from disuse. Later De Lorme implemented same exercises on poliomyelitis patients.

In 1948 De Lorme revised his original method and adopted the name PRE because he believed the original name bore false implications since even muscles which could not contract against the force of gravity could be strengthen by this method. PRE has been explained in Chapter 20.

Active movements of upper and lower extremities (Figs. 3.8a to z)

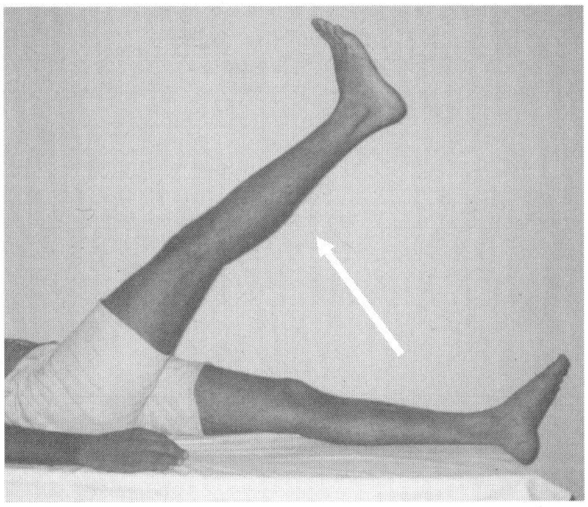

Fig. 3.8a: Hip flexion with knee extended

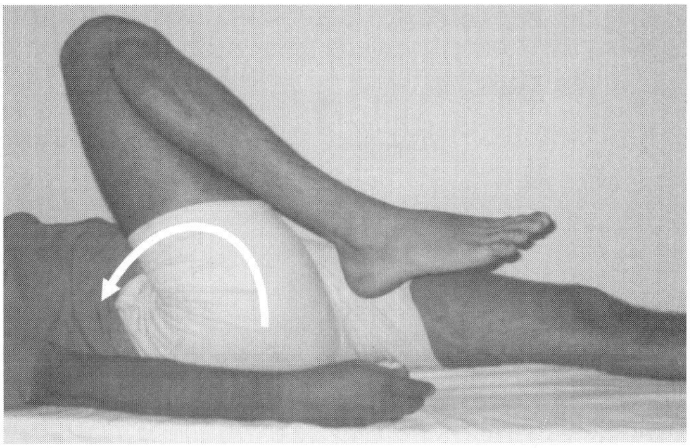

Fig. 3.8b: Hip flexion with knee flexion

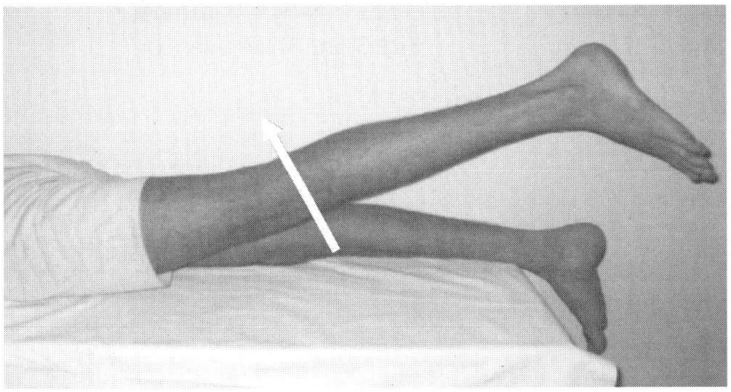

Fig. 3.8c: Hip extension

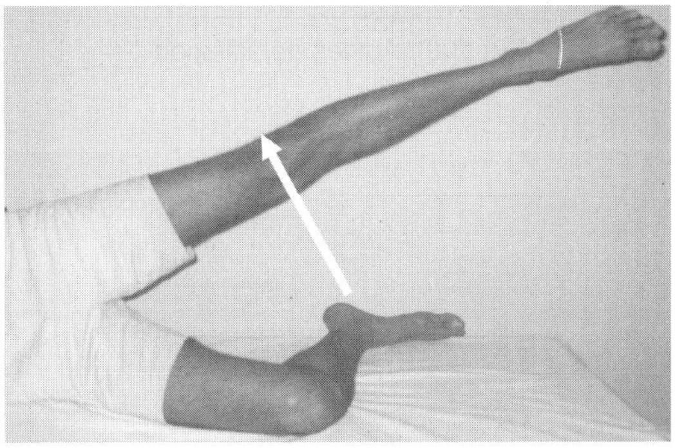

Fig. 3.8d: Hip abduction

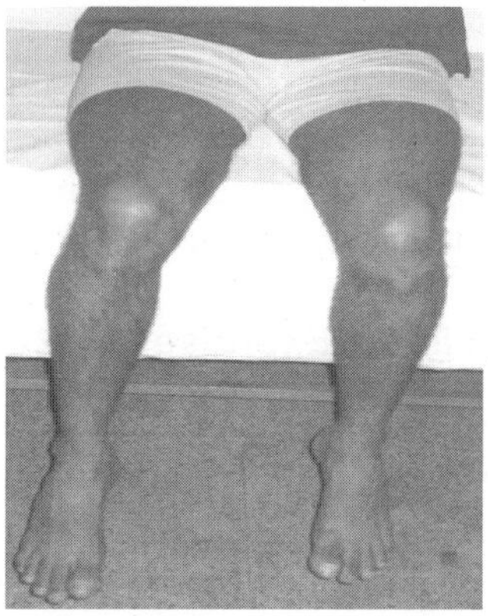
Fig. 3.8e: Hip at neutral position

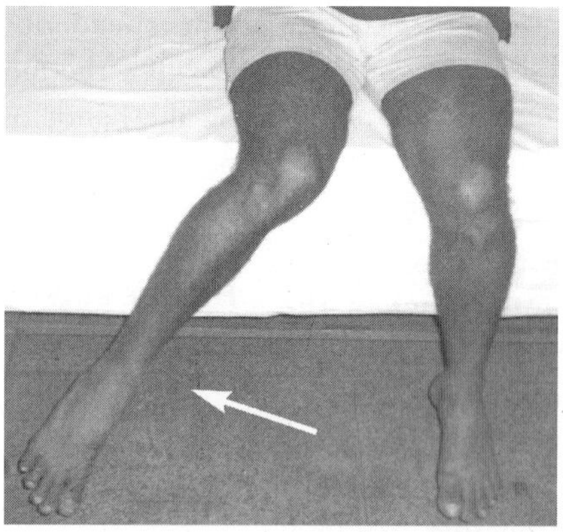
Fig. 3.8f: Hip internal rotation

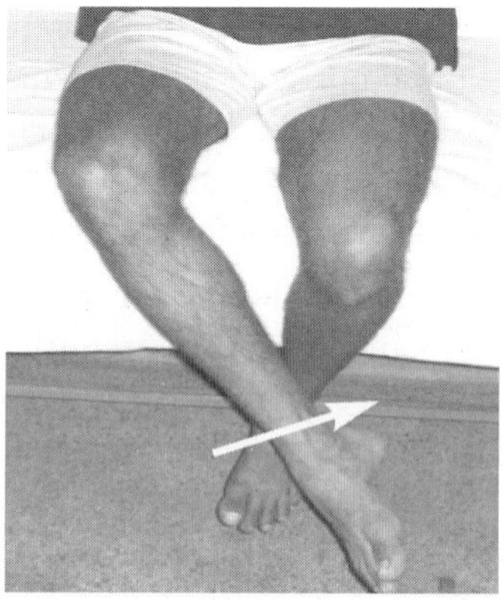
Fig. 3.8g: Hip external rotation

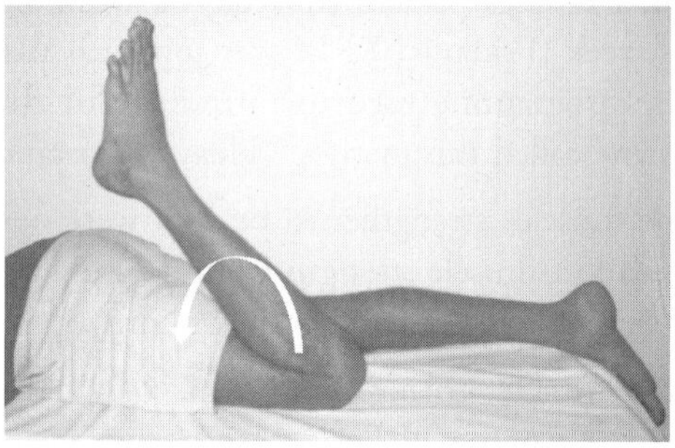
← Fig. 3.8h: Knee flexion

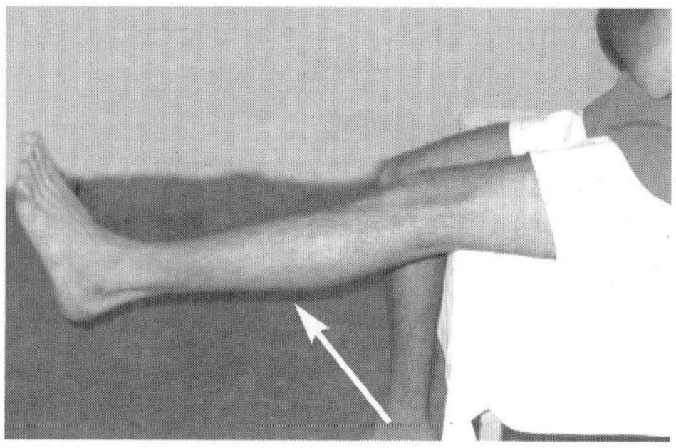
Fig. 3.8i: → Knee extension

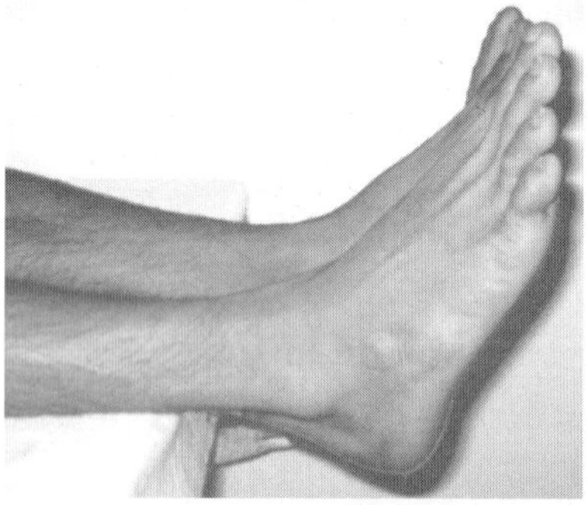
← Fig. 3.8j: Ankles at neutral position

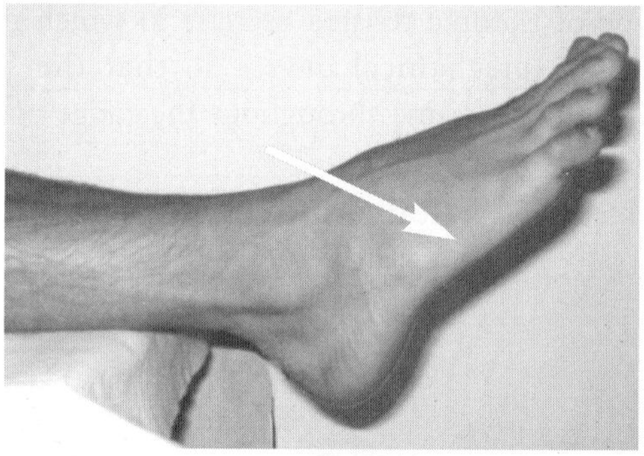
Fig. 3.8k: → Ankles plantar flexion

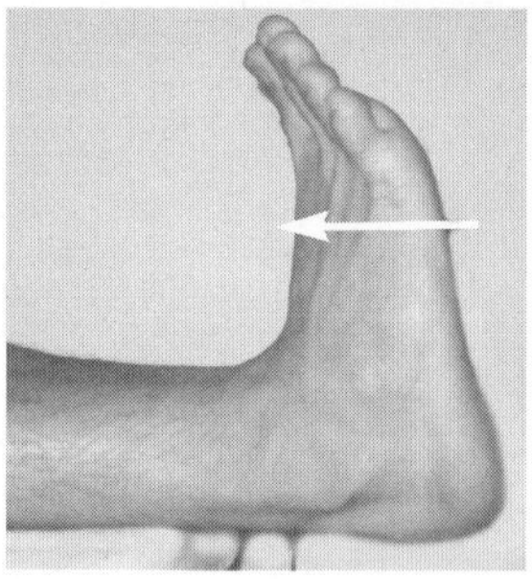
Fig. 3.8l: Ankles dorsiflexion

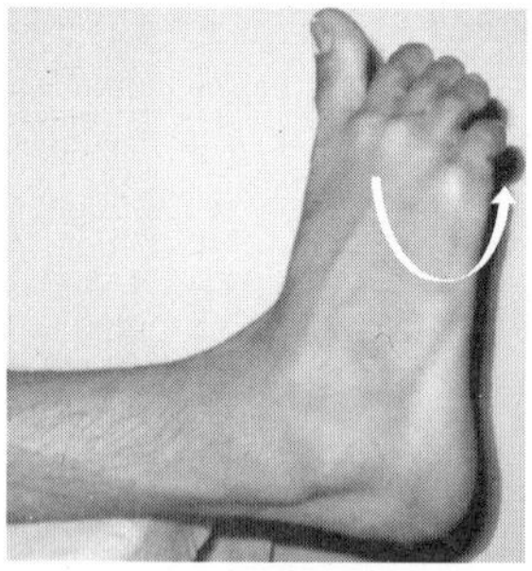
Fig. 3.8m: Ankle inversion

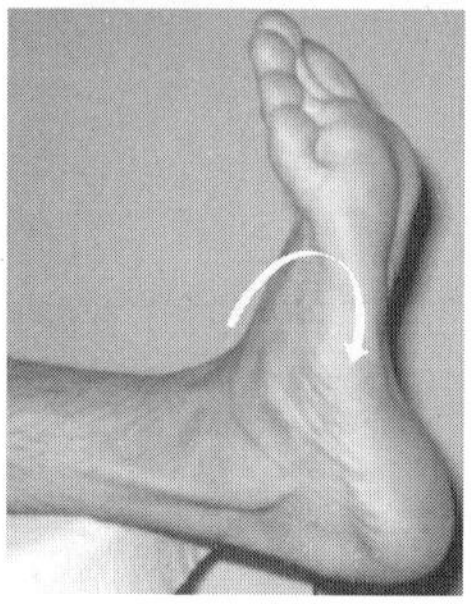
Fig. 3.8n: Ankle eversion

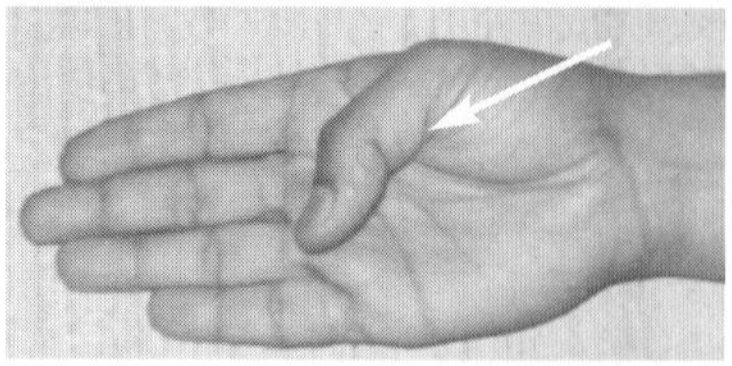
Fig. 3.8o: Thumb flexion

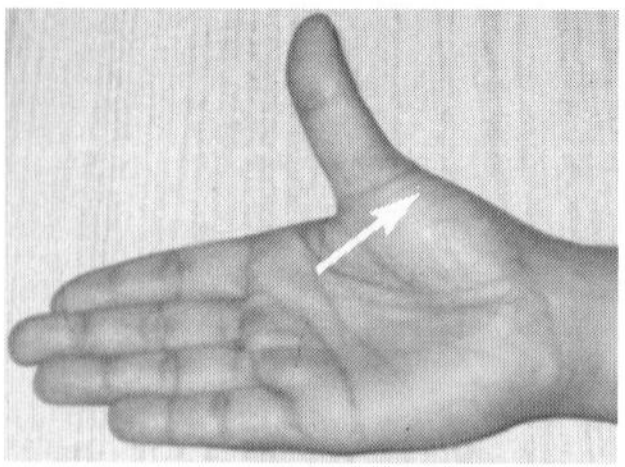
Fig. 3.8p: Thumb extension

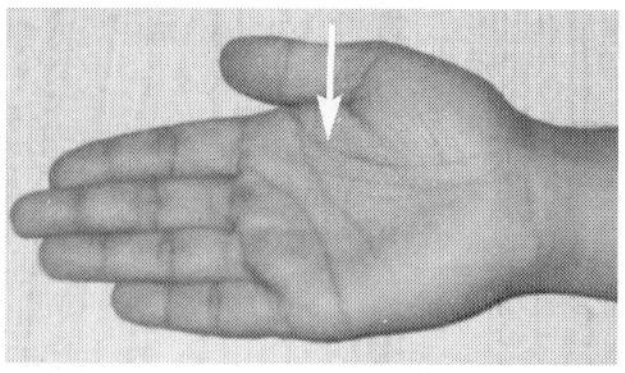
Fig. 3.8q: Thumb adduction

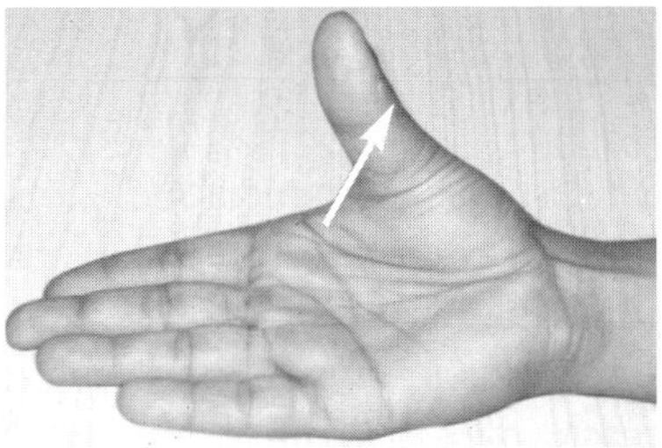

Fig. 3.8r: Thumb abduction (Perpendicular to palmar plane)

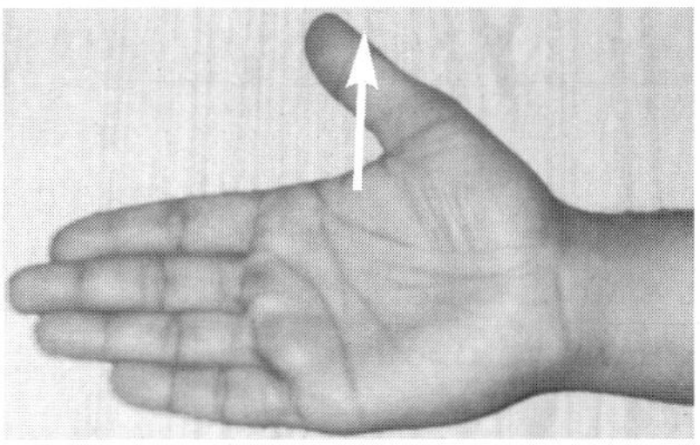

Fig. 3.8s: Thumb abduction (Parallel to palmar plane)

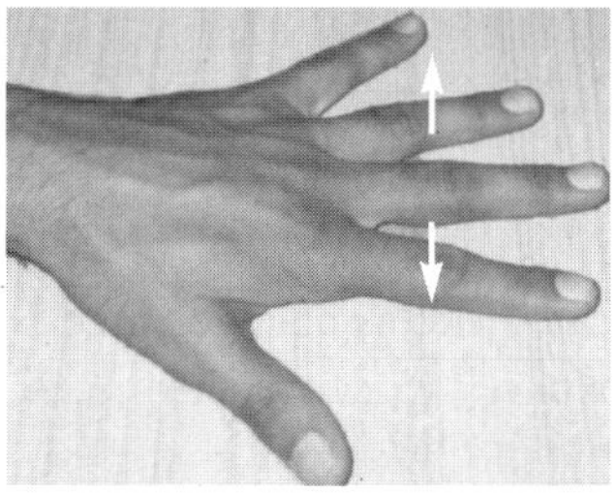

Fig. 3.8t: Finger abduction

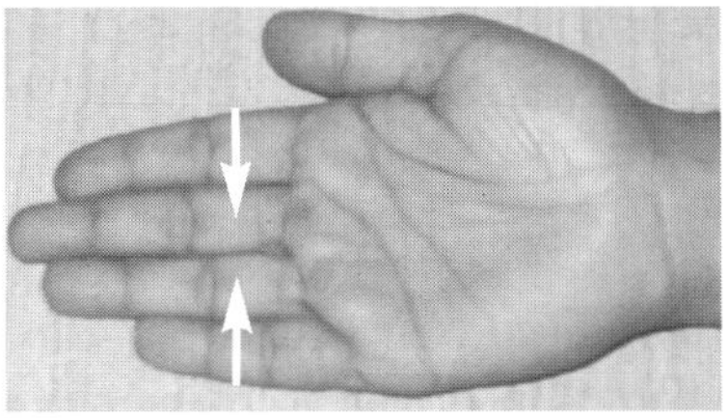

Fig. 3.8u: Finger adduction

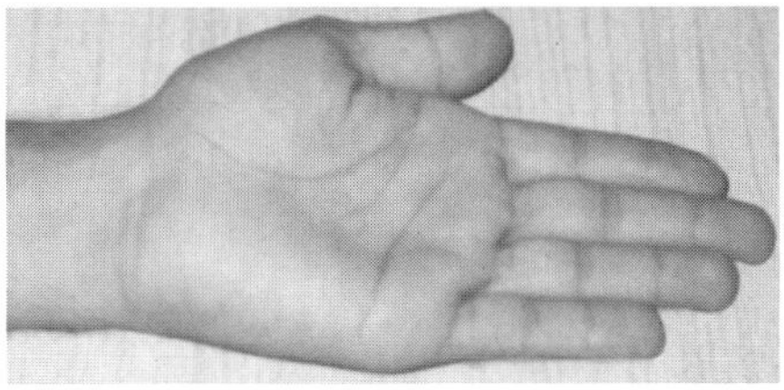

Fig. 3.8v: Wrist (Neutral)

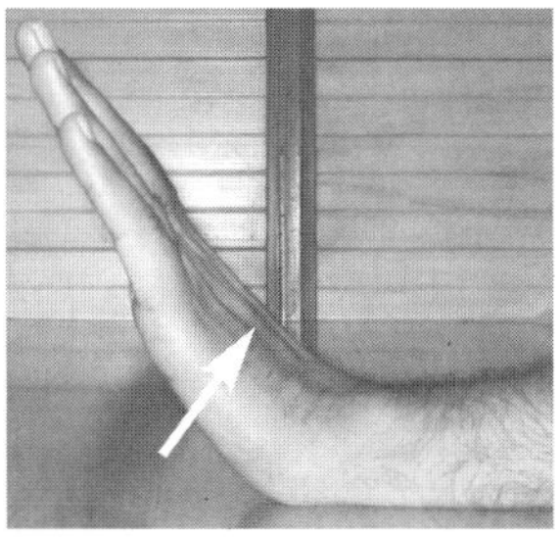

Fig. 3.8w: Wrist extension

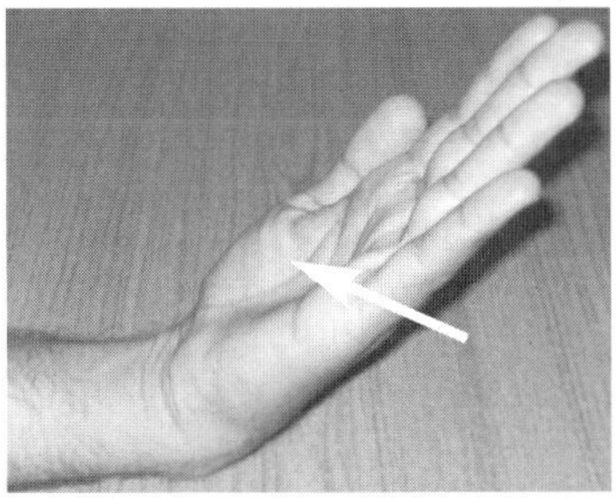

Fig. 3.8x: Wrist flexion

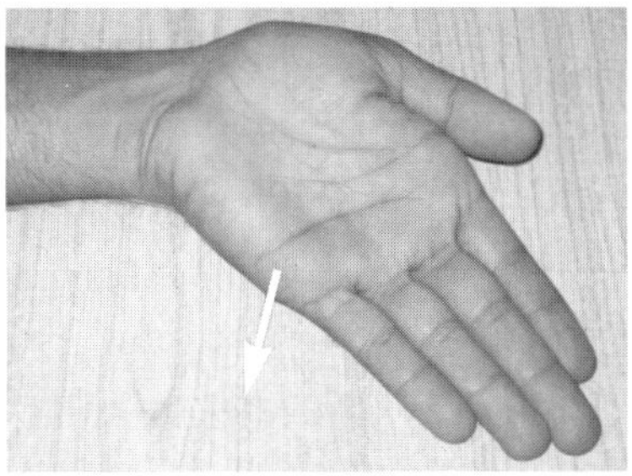

Fig. 3.8y: Wrist ulnar deviation

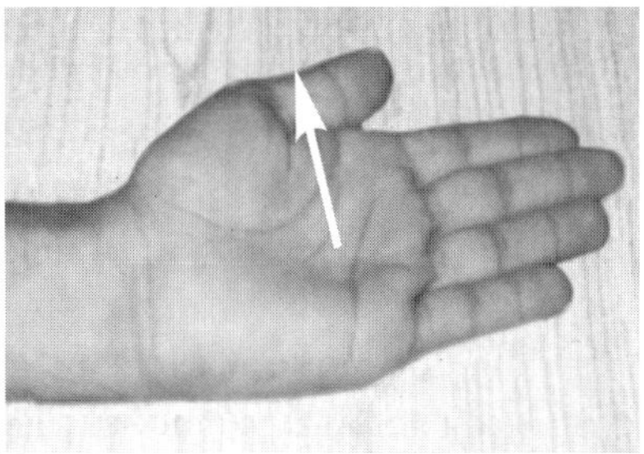

Fig. 3.8z: Wrist radial deviation

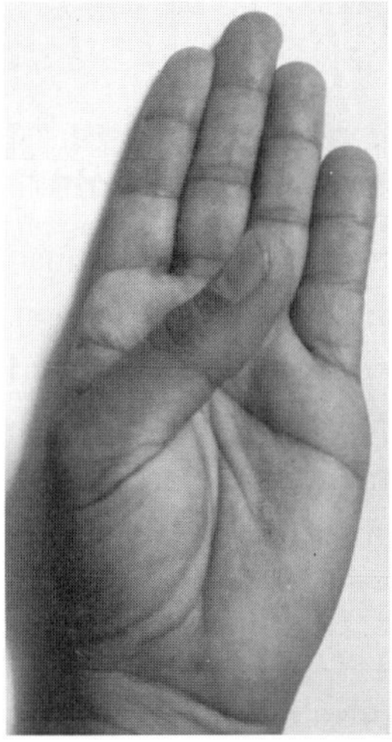

Fig. 3.8za: First Metacarpophalangeal (MCP) flexion

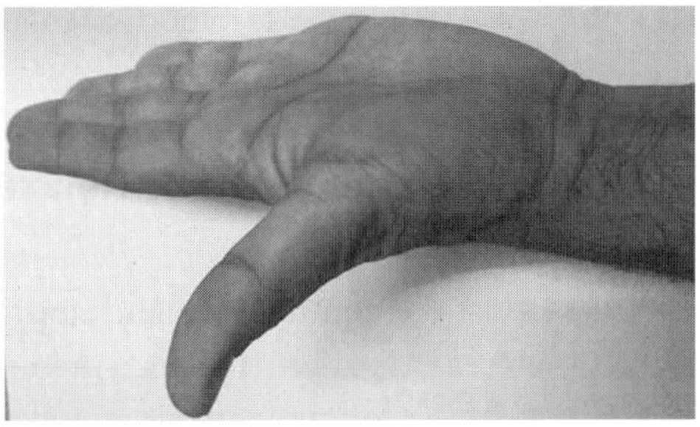

Fig. 3.8zb: First Metacarpophalangeal (MCP) extension

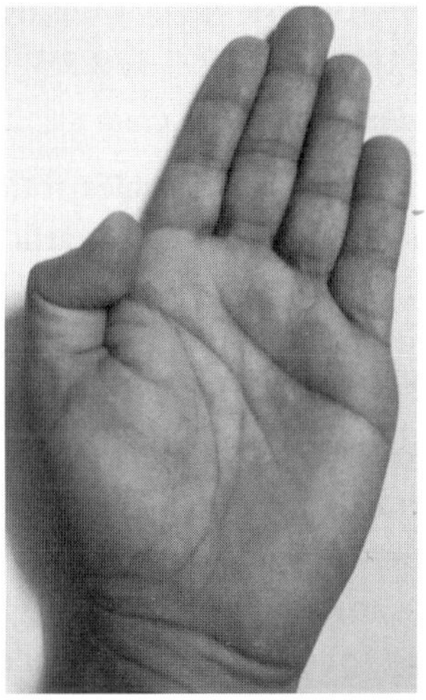

Fig. 3.8zc: PIP flexion (Thumb)

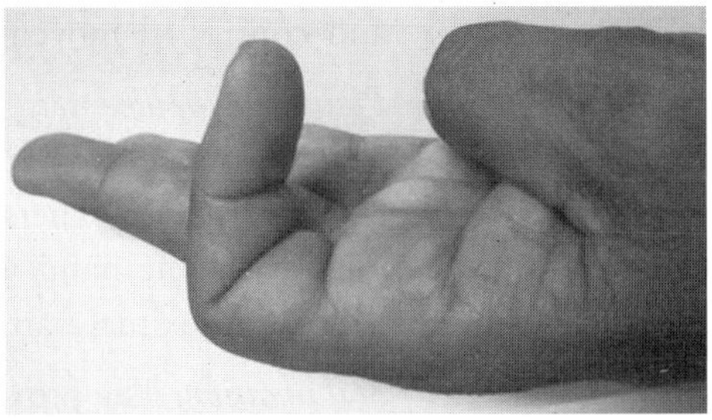

Fig. 3.8zd: PIP flexion (Index)

PASSIVE MOVEMENTS

INTRODUCTION

The movement which is not produced by a voluntary effort, requires an external force to perform. An external force can be applied by the hands of therapist, mechanical device and/or patient itself.

Classification of Passive Movements

- Relaxed passive movements.
- Forced passive movements.
- Passive manipulation.
- Passive accessory movements.

Uses, Goals and Indications of Passive Movements

1. *Maintain range of motion of the joint:* Patients with chronic inflammatory conditions such as rheumatoid arthritic, ankylosing spondylitis and acute injuries find difficulty in performing an active movement due to pain and muscle spasm. Prolong avoidance of active movements may result in disuse atrophy and limitation in the range of motion. Passive range of motion exercises help in improving pain, muscle spasm and in maintaining range of motion. Movements should be performed in available range of motion. Forced passive movements in this stage may increase the inflammation and pain. Ice can be applied for 15-20 minutes prior to relaxed passive movements to avoid pain.
2. *Increase joint range of motion:*
   a. Tightness of the muscles followed by trauma or immobilization restricts the articular surfaces to move in full range of motion actively and prevents functional activities. Forced passive movements, stretches the muscles and increases the plasticity and extensibility of the muscle fibres.
   b. Tightness of joint capsule followed by immobilization of the joint restricts the range of motion. Passive accessory movements (glides) of the articular surfaces stretch the joint capsule thus increase range of motion of the joint.
3. *Decrease pain:* Activates pain inhibiting receptors (mechano receptors).
4. *Relaxation:* Relaxed passive movements decrease the muscle spasm and fatiguability. These movements give soothing effects to the joint if performed with soft tissue manipulation (massage) techniques.
5. *Decrease spasticity:* In upper motor neurone lesion spasticity is the most dominant clinical feature, where patient can not move the joint voluntarily. This causes tightness and contracture of the spastic muscles and lengthening of antagonistic muscles over the time in long standing cases. Relaxed passive movements decrease the spasticity temporarily and helps in the rehabilitation programmes. To decrease the spasticity, movement should be fairly slow, controlled and rhythmical. If the movement is preformed with high speed this can increase further spasticity by stimulating the spastic muscle fibres.

Relaxed Passive Movements

These are slow, rhythmical movements performed in the available range of motion of the joint by the hands of therapist.

Relaxed passive movements are generally given to:

- Maintain joint range of motion and connective tissue mobility.
- Prevent adhesion in the joint space.
- Enhance synovial movements for articular cartilage nutrition.
- Minimize the tightness of myofibrils.
- Decrease the spasticity temporarily.
- Increase blood circulation.
- Decrease pain.

Techniques of Relaxed Passive Movements

- *Position of the Patient:* Position of the patient must be comfortable and appropriate instructions are given to patient to relax the antagonistic muscles. Contraction of antagonistic muscles can change the accuracy, speed, force and rhythm of the movement, therefore patient is asked to relax the antagonistic muscles to allow smooth and controlled movement.
- *Position of the Therapist:* Position of the patient also should be comfortable and as close as possible to the part which is being treated. Therapist grasps the distal end of the joint with one hand while other hand may be placed over the proximal part of the joint to stabilize it.
- *Stabilization:* The proximal part of the joint is stabilized with the straps, weight of the body, or by the hand of the therapist. Straps should not be too tight to allow the contraction of muscles.

- *Traction:* Minimal traction may be given to draw the articular surfaces apart, which is given in the longitudinal axis of the joint. The traction is maintained throughout the range of motion and is not released unless the distal part of the joint comes to the original or starting position.
- *Repetitions:* The number of time the movement is performed depends upon the goal for which it is applied.
- *Speed of movement:* The speed of movement must be slow, uniform, controlled and rhythmical.

Forced Passive Movement

It is a movement which is performed by the therapist with force at the end range of motion, which can be resisted or controlled by the patient. The movement is directed at the joint without any high velocity within the range of motion. These type of movements are commonly used to stretch the joint capsule and periarticular structures to increase range of motion and decrease pain. The forced passive movements are described in Chapter 13.

Passive Accessory Movement

These are the movements which take place between the joint surfaces and cannot be performed voluntarily by the patient. The accessory movements which are performed by the therapist or with the help of an external force is known as passive accessory movements. The metatarsal movements cannot be performed by the patient voluntarily but these movements can be performed passively by the therapist. These movements are commonly used to stretch the joint capsule and subsequently to increase range of motion and decrease pain (Passive accessory movements are described in Chapter 7).

Passive Manipulation

It is a rapid, passive movement performed at the end rang of a joint. It is far more forceful than mobilization and cannot be controlled by the patient.

Relaxed Passive Movements of Upper Extremity

Shoulder Joint

Flexion and Extension: Patient is in supine position and therapist stands close to the shoulder joint. One hand of therapist grasps the arm at the elbow joint while other hand stabilizes the shoulder joint.

- *Movement:* The extremity is raised with the one hand and is moved slowly and rhythmically in the available flexion of the shoulder then returns to the starting position. Several repetitions may be performed as per the condition (Fig. 3.9a).

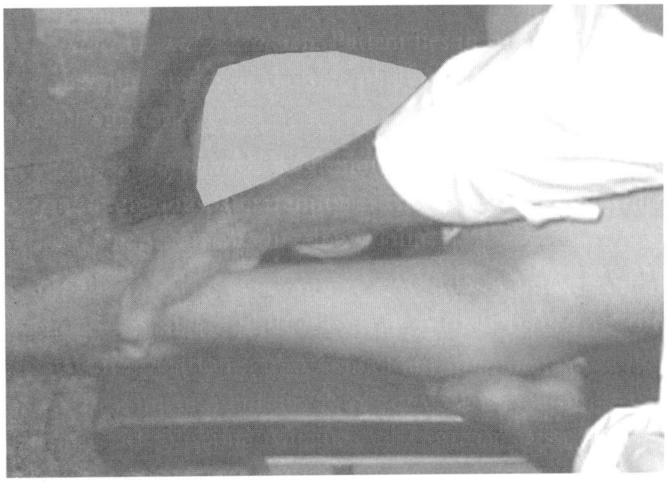

Fig. 3.9a: Flexion

Hyperextension: Patient lies on unaffected side, therapist stands behind the patient, faces the posterior aspect of the joint. The shoulder joint remains at the neutral position, elbow is flexed 45° to 60° for the convenient of therapist.

- *Placement of hands*: The upper hand is placed over the shoulder joint while lower hand grasps elbow and forearm of patient rests on therapist's forearm.
- *Movement*: Joint is moved from neutral position to the hyperextension (toward the therapist's body) in available range (Fig. 3.9b).

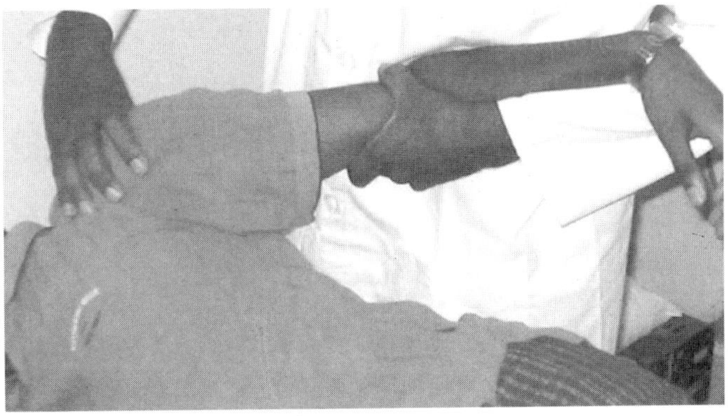

Fig. 3.9b: Shoulder hyperextension

Abduction and Adduction: Patient lies in supine position, and therapist stands at the side of shoulder joint with wide base of support.

- *Placement of hands:* Like flexion and extension movement one hand grasps extremity at the shoulder joint while other hand grasps the elbow joint.
- *Movement:* The extremity is moved with little traction in the available abduction range then return to the starting position.

Note: During abduction the extremity is rotated externally after 90° to avoid impingement between head of humerus and acromion process of scapula. Traction is maintained throughout abduction range till it comes to the starting position (Fig. 3.10).

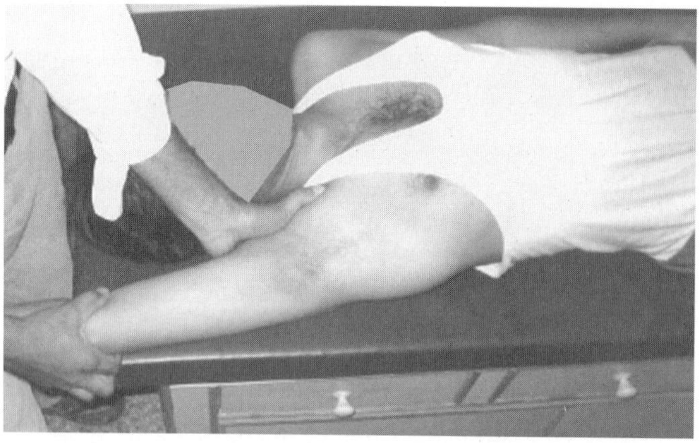

Fig. 3.10: Abduction and adduction

Horizontal Adduction and Abduction: Patient lies in supine position and therapist stands close to the body and faces the patient's face. Starting position of shoulder is 90° of abduction.

- *Placement of hands*: Remains same as shoulder flexion-extension.
- *Movement:* Extremity is moved by one hand horizontally across the body in available range (Fig. 3.11).

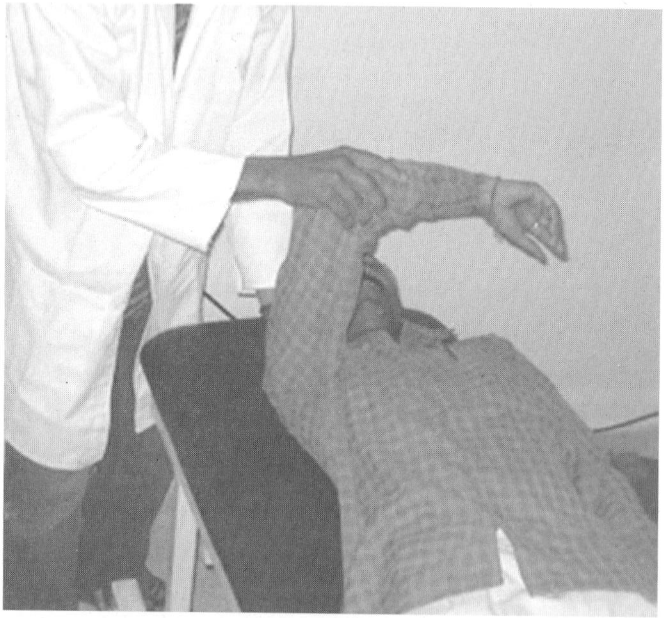

Fig. 3.11: Horizontal abduction and adduction

Internal (Medial) and External (Lateral) Rotation: The patient is placed supine or in sitting position and therapist remains at side of patient, the shoulder joint is abducted at 90° and elbow flexed at 90°.

- *Placement of hands:* One hand grasps the extremity at wrist while other hand holds the flexed elbow joint.
- *Movement:* While maintaining above position, traction is applied by the lower hand and upper hand moves the arm in the available external rotation (taking hand to the head with maintaining elbow flexion) then brings to the neutral position. Now hand is moved towards the hip joints with traction in the available internal rotation, then returns to the neutral position (Figs. 3.12a to c).

(a)

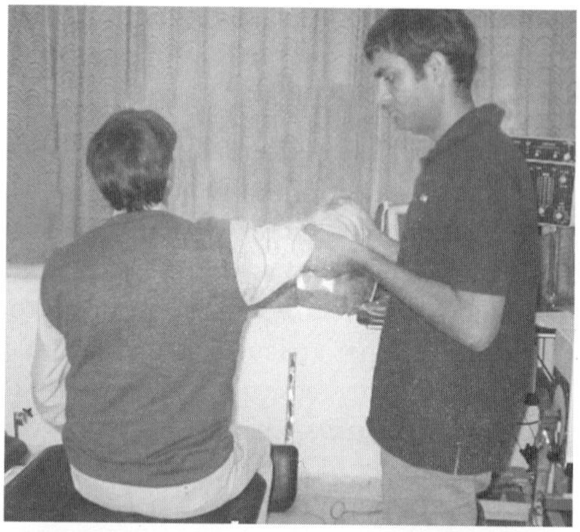

(b)

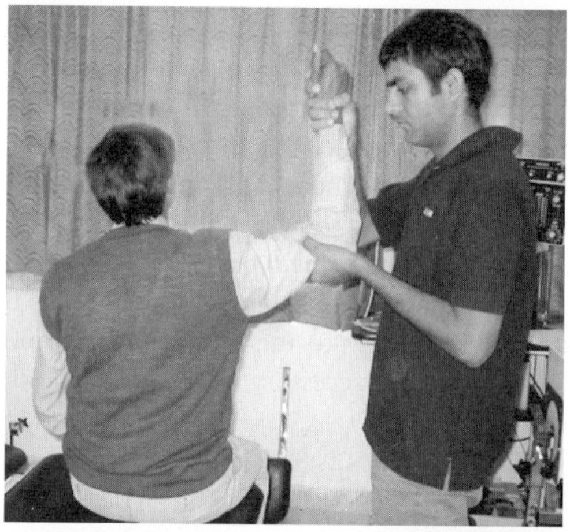

(c)

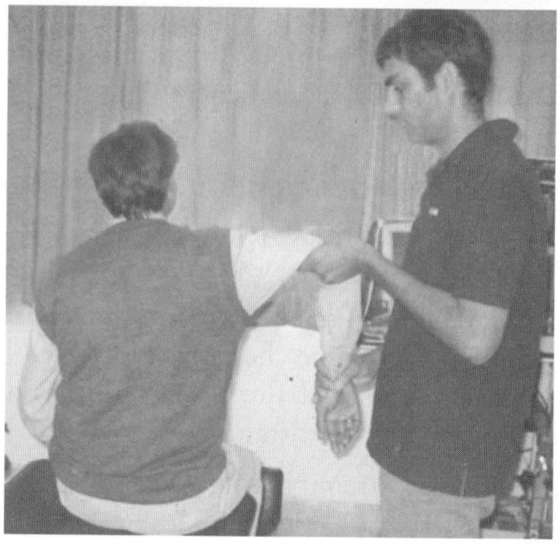

Figs. 3.12a to c: Internal and external rotation

Elbow Joint

Flexion and extension: Patient lies in supine position, and therapist stands at the side of patient. The proximal part of the elbow may be stabilized by the hand of therapist, the other hand grasps the wrist joint and moves the elbow in available range of flexion, i.e., extension (Figs. 3.13a to d).

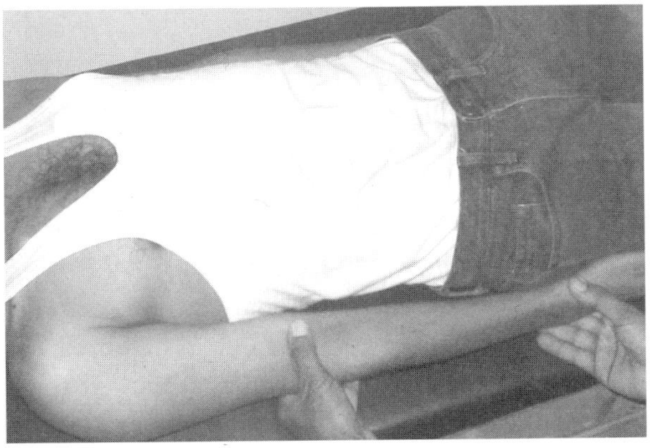

Fig. 3.13a: Elbow (neutral)

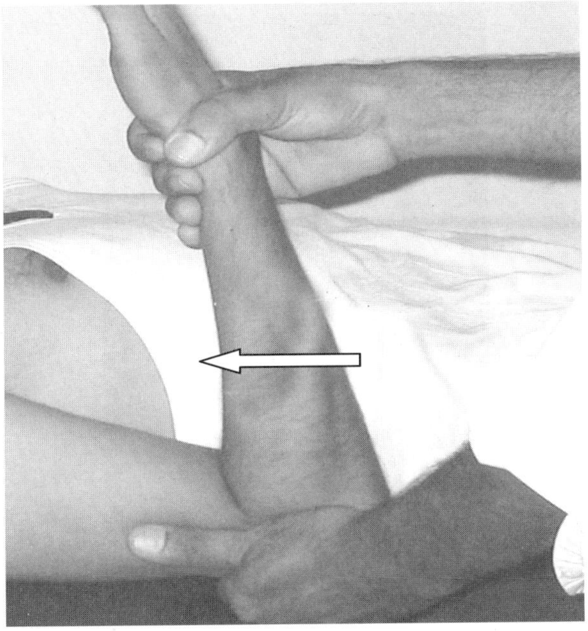

Fig. 3.13b: Elbow flexion (mid range)

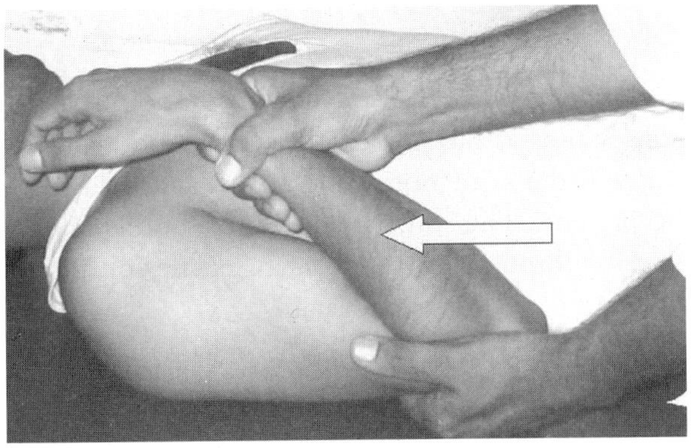

Fig. 3.13c: Elbow flexion (end range)

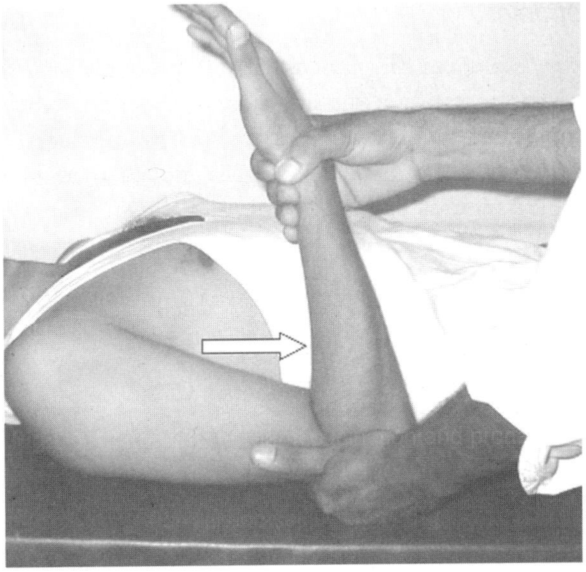

Fig. 3.13d: Elbow extension

Radioulnar Joint

Forearm pronation and supination: The position of patient and therapist remains same as elbow flexion and extension. Therapist holds the distal forearm and rotates it alternately into supination and pronation. The other hand stabilizes the elbow joint (Figs. 3.14a and b).

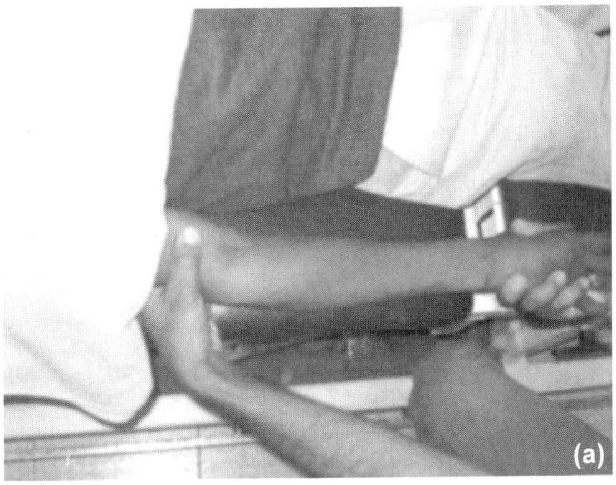

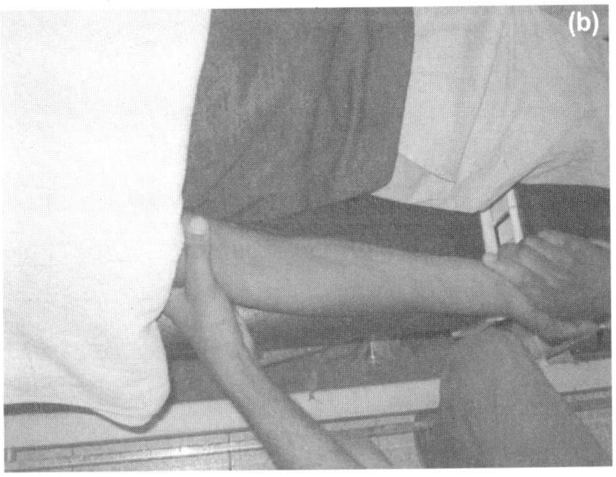

Figs. 3.14a and b: Forearm supination and pronation

Wrist Joint

Palmar flexion and dorsiflexion: Patient lies supine or sitting, and therapist stands at the side close to the wrist joint, the proximal part of the wrist is stabilized by the therapist's upper hand while distal segment is moved through the available range of palmar flexion and dorsiflexion (Figs. 3.15a and b).

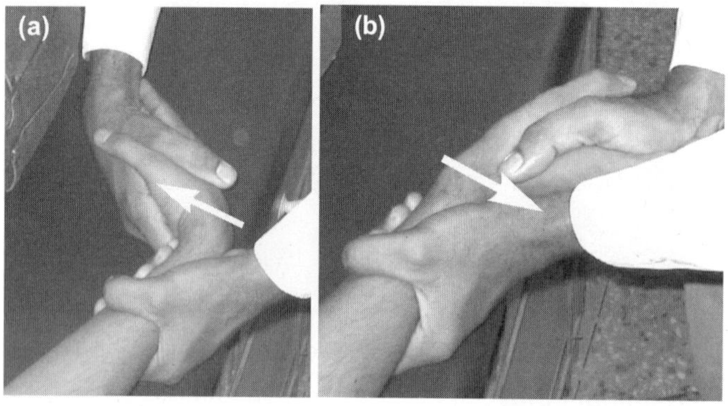

Figs. 3.15a and b: (a) Wrist flexion (palmar flexion) and (b) Wrist extension (dorsiflexion)

Radial and ulnar deviation: Position of therapist and patient remains same as above, therapist stabilizes the proximal segment of wrist by upper hand while lower hand grasps the patient's hand and moves into radial deviation and ulnar deviation (Figs. 3.16a to c).

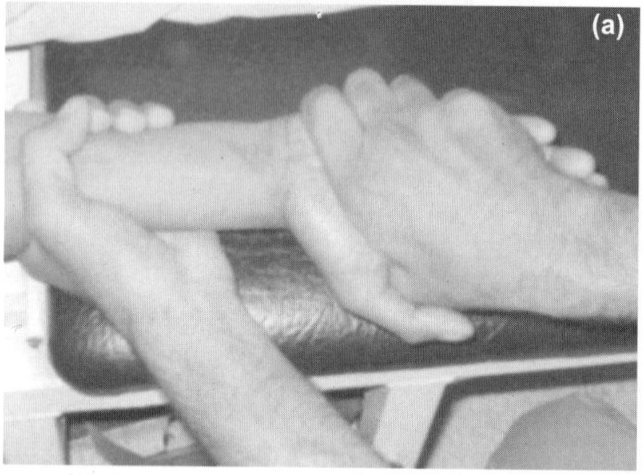

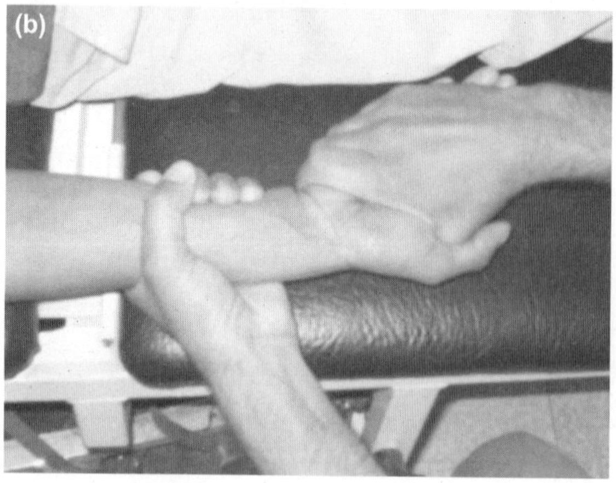

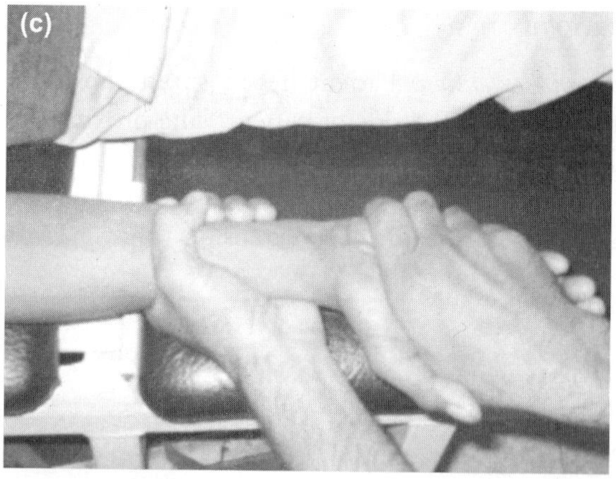

Figs. 3.16a to c: Wrist radial/ulnar deviation

Metacarpophalangeal and interphalangeal joint: The position of patient and therapist remain same as wrist flexion and extension. Proximal part of joint is stabilized by one hand while other hand grasps the distal part of the joint and moves in available range of flexion and extension (Fig. 3.17).

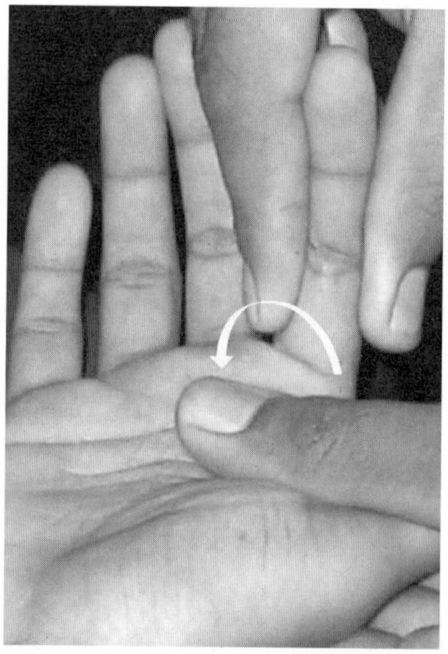

Fig. 3.17: Metacarpal joint flexion-extension

Relaxed Passive Movements of Lower Extremity

Hip Joint

Flexion and extension: Patient lies in supine position, the therapist stands at the side of hip joint, upper hand grasps extremity at the knee joint while other hand holds the heel of the patient. The joint is moved by both hands with knee flexion through the available range of flexion and return to the neutral position (extension).

Note: Full flexion of hip joint cannot be performed with the knee extended, because hamstring muscles get stretched and do not allow the joint to move beyond 80° (Figs. 3.18a and b).

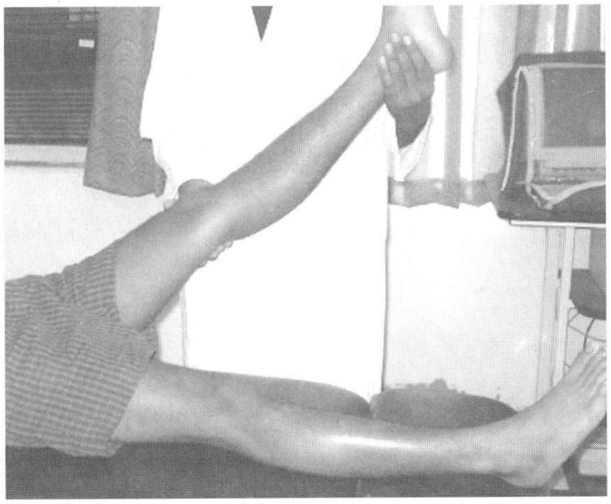

Fig. 3.18a: Hip flexion with knee extension

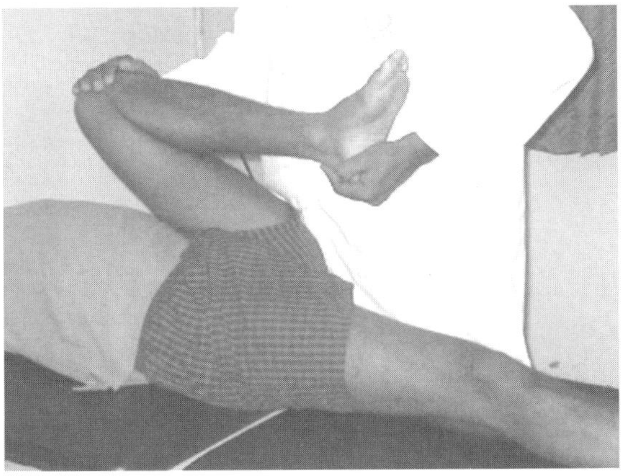

Fig. 3.18b: Hip flexion with knee flexion

Hyperextension: Patient lies on unaffected side therapist stands behind the patient close to the hip joint. The upper hand is placed over the pelvis to stabilize it, while lower hand grasps the knee, the patient's leg rests on the forearm of therapist (knee flexes at 90°). While maintaining above position therapist hyperextends the hip joint by bringing the leg toward his or her body, in the available range of motion (Fig. 3.19).

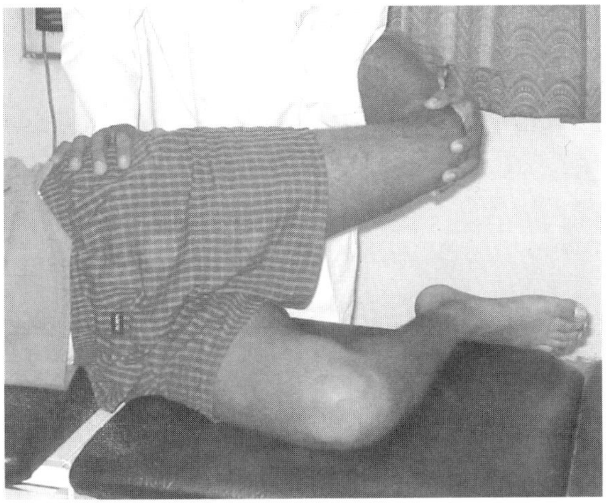

Fig. 3.19: Hip hyperextension

Note: Knee joint should not be flexed beyond 80° as rectus femoris gets stretched and prevents the hyper-extension.

Abduction and adduction: Patient lies in supine position, therapist stands at the side of patient. The upper hand of therapist grasps the extremity at knee joint while other grasps at the ankle joint (Fig. 3.20).

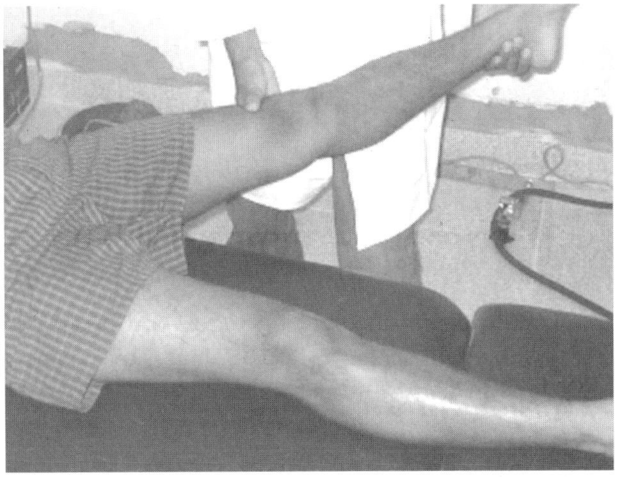

Fig. 3.20: Hip abduction-adduction

- *Movement:* Therapist moves the limb by taking toward his or her body in the available range of abduction then brings back to the neutral position (adduction).

Internal and external rotation: The patient lies in supine position and therapist stands at the side of patient. The knee and hip is flexed at 90°, therapist grasps the knee joint and ankle joint (Figs. 3.21a and b).

- *Movement:* While maintaining above position the leg is rotated inward (external rotation) and outward (internal rotation).

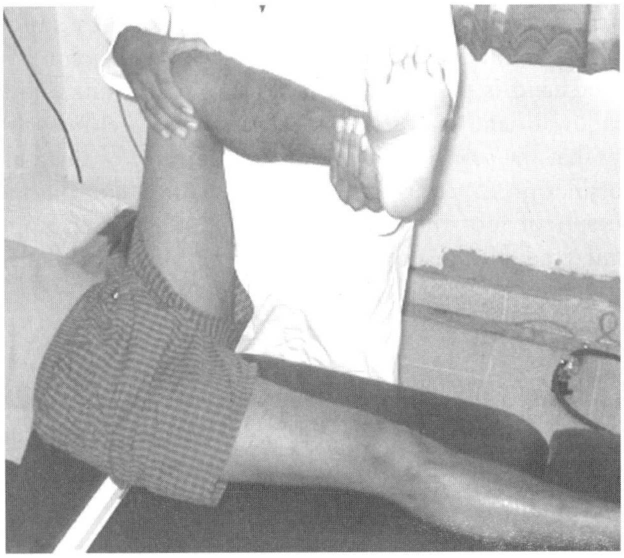

Fig. 3.21a: Hip external rotation

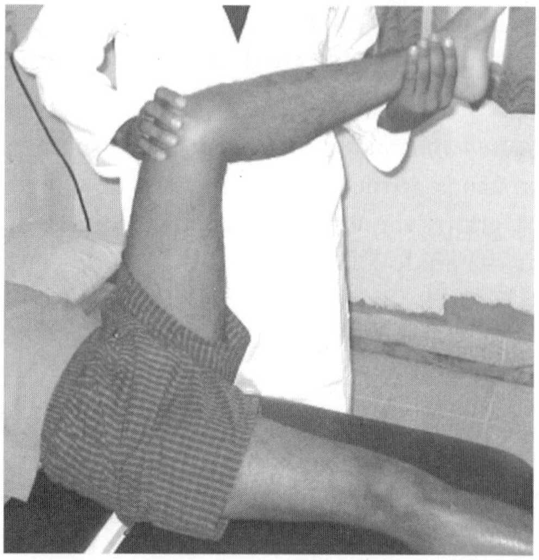

Fig. 3.21b: Hip internal rotation

Note: During inward and outward rotation hip and knee should remain at 90° of flexion. This movement may also be done in high sitting position.

Knee Joint

Flexion and extension: The procedure remains same as flexion and extension of the hip joint.

Patient is placed in the supine position. Therapist stands at the side of patient and grasps the extremity at knee joint and ankle joint. Therapist flexes the knee joint with the hip flexion in the available range of motion. Knee flexion and extension can also be performed in the prone lying position. Examiner stabilizes the leg with one hand and grasps the ankle joint with other hand. The ankle is brought to the thigh (flexion) and then return to the neutral position (extension) in a smooth rhythmical manner.

Ankle Joint

Dorsiflexion and plantar flexion: Patient lies in supine position and therapist stands at the side of ankle joint. The upper hand is placed over the dorsum of the ankle joint and lower hand grasps the plantar aspect of heel in such a way that the sole of foot rests on the forearm of therapist. Dorsiflexion is performed by pulling the heel and pushing the sole of foot through the available range then upper hand gradually pushes the dorsum of foot into plantar flexion (Figs. 3.22a and b).

Subtalar Joint

Varus and valgus: The ankle joint is placed out of the edge of table, therapist holds the heel with both the hands and moves inward (varus) and outward (valgus) (Figs. 3.23a and b).

- *Movement:* Therapist moves the heel inward (varus) and outward (valgus).

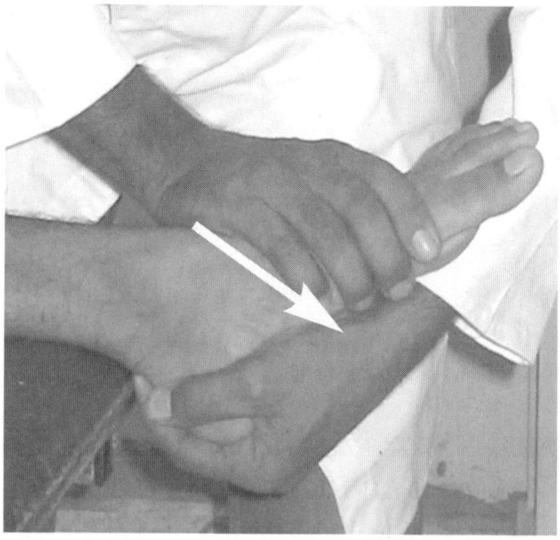

Fig. 3.22a: Ankle plantar flexion

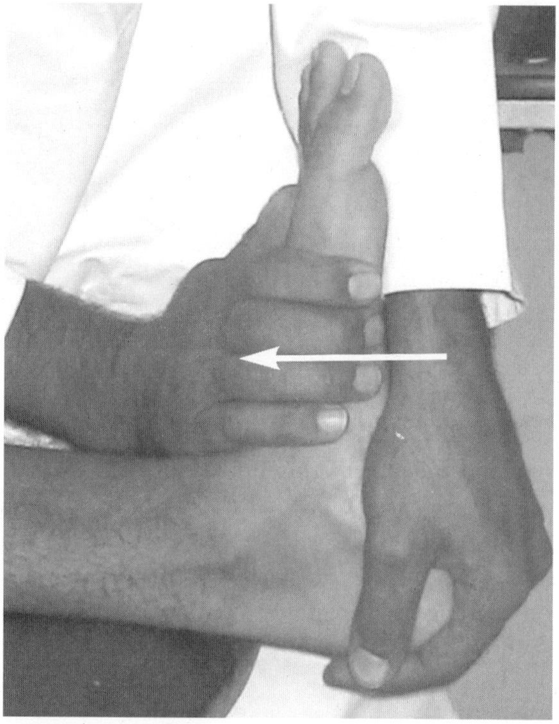

Fig. 3.22b: Ankle dorsiflexion

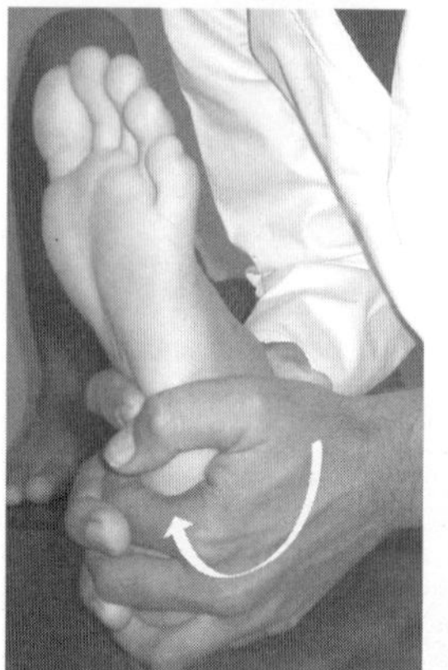

Fig. 3.23a: Varus

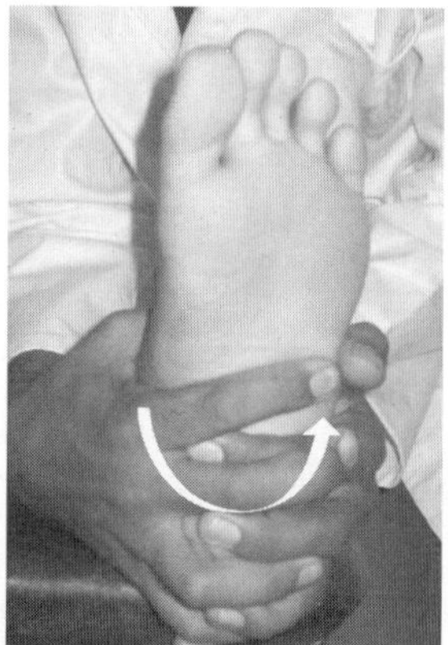

Fig. 3.23b: Valgus

Transverse Tarsal Joints

Supination and pronation: Position of patient and therapist remain same as dorsiflexion and plantar flexion of ankle joint. Therapist places both the hands over the dorsum of foot in such a way that the thenar surface of both the hands rest on dorsum and fingers grasp the plantar surface. The thenar aspect of other hand lies on the dorsum of foot and fingers grasp the plantar surface.

- *Movement:* The forefoot is taken inward by raising the middle arch (supination) and after performing available range of supination it is taken back to the normal then into outward by raising the lateral arch (pronation) of foot and back into the neutral position (Figs. 3.24a and b).

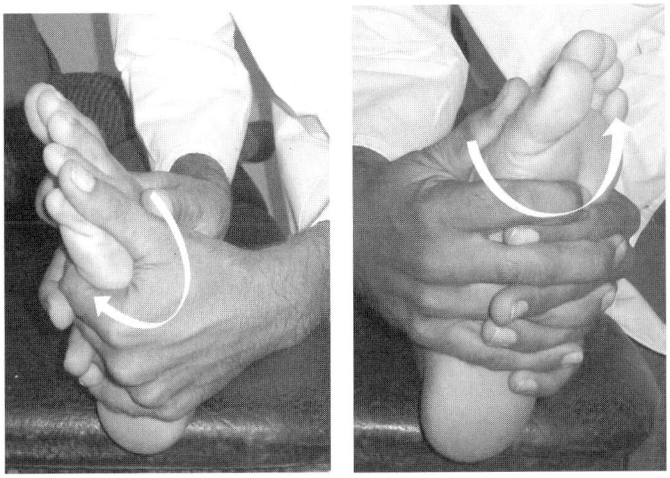

(a) (b)

Figs. 3.24a and b: (a) Ankle supination and (b) Ankle pronation

Metatarsophalangeal and Interphalangeal Joint

Flexion and Extension:

- *Metatarsophalangeal (MTP) joint:* The proximal part of the joint is stabilized by one hand and the distal part moved by the other hand into available range of flexion and extension (Figs. 3.25a and b).

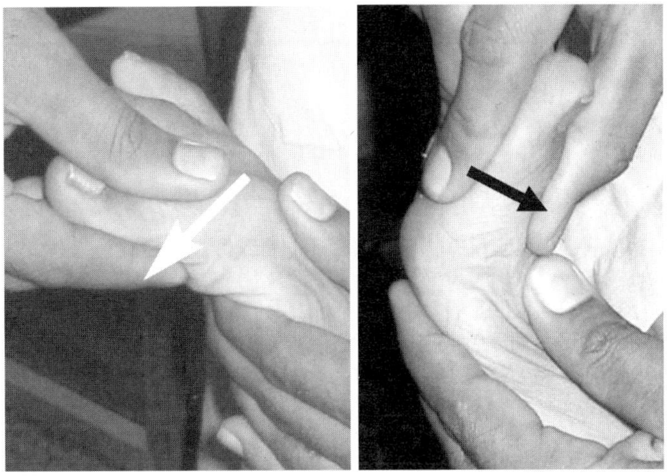

Fig. 3.25a: MTP joint flexion **Fig. 3.25b:** MTP joint extension

- *Interphalangeal (IP) joint:* Procedure remains same as MTP flexion extension (Fig. 3.26).
- *Interphalangeal (IP) joint (flexion and extension):* The patient lies in supine or sitting position, therapist stabilized the proximal phalange with one hand, while other hand grasps the distal phalange. The distal phalange is moved in flexion and extension. Each interphalangeal joint is mobilized separately.

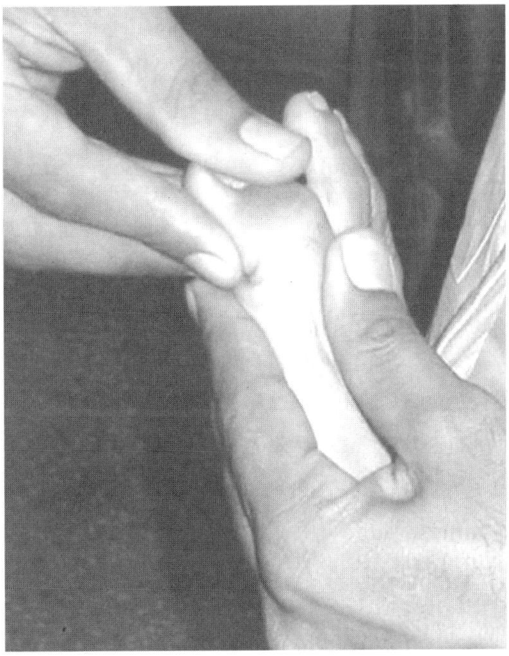

Fig. 3.26: IP flexion

4

BASIC AND DERIVED POSITIONS

INTRODUCTION/BASIC FUNDAMENTAL POSITION

Mobility depends upon stability or success of every movement lies on its posture. Postures are fundamental to movements.

Many authors have given five basic positions (along with their derivatives) in which exercises may be given. These are lying, sitting, kneeling, standing and hanging. Out of these hanging is rarely used in clinical practice, hence first four and its derivative are discussed.

1. Lying (Supine)

The body is supine, with the arms by the sides and legs straight. The body is fully supported with a longer base of support and low centre of gravity. The muscle work is minimal and body is fully relaxed.

The derived positions are:

a. *Side lying:* Clinically this position is used for exercise therapy by bending the under arm with slight hip and knee flexion of under leg. The base of support is smaller as compared to supine lying (Fig. 4.1).

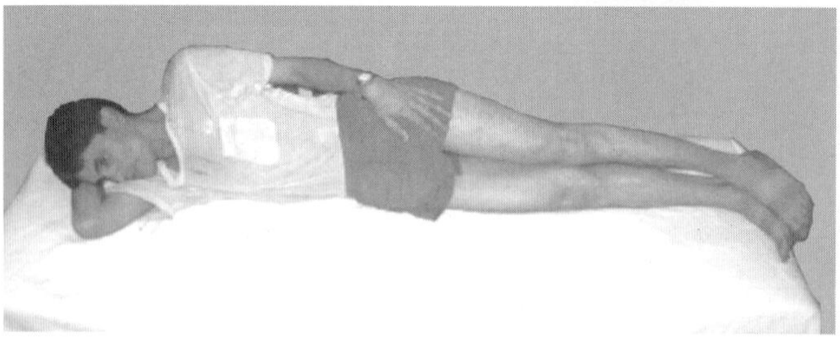

Fig. 4.1: Side lying

b. *Prone lying:* The base of support is almost same as of supine lying. Neck may be rotated to one side or pillows may be used to support forehead. This position is mainly used for spinal extensors, hip extensors and knee flexors exercises (Fig. 4.2).

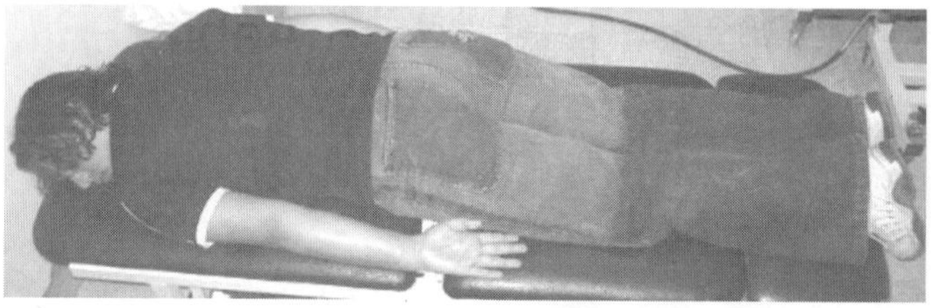

Fig. 4.2: Prone lying

c. *Across-prone lying:* It is further modified form of prone lying position in which the upper body with arms lie outside the supporting surface and the anterior superior iliac spine just off the front edge of the support. This position is usually used in pediatric group for spinal extensor exercise. The hands may be supported on stool bars or by therapist. The therapist may also hold the legs of the patient (paediatric) just above the ankle (Fig. 4.3).

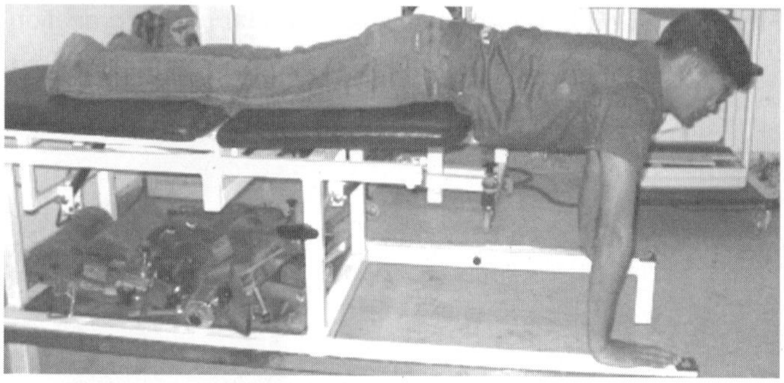

Fig. 4.3: Across prone lying

d. *Crook lying:* Lying with the soles of the feet resting on the floor. The knees are flexed to varying degrees (usually 90°) (Fig. 4.4).

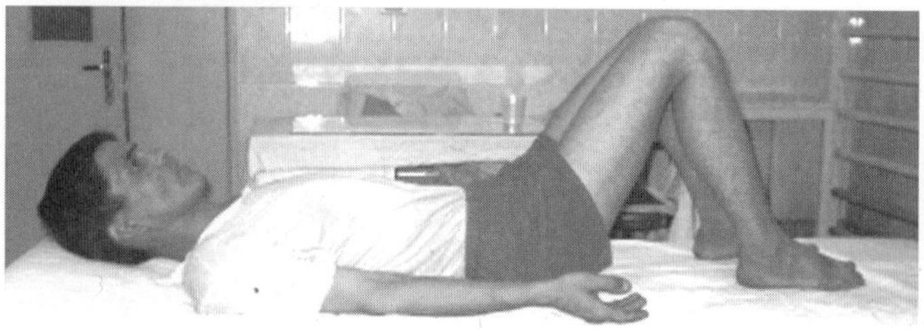

Fig. 4.4: Crook lying

e. *Stride crook lying:* As crook lying, but the legs and feet are placed astride apart, with the heels about 45 cm apart. The feet point obliquely outward in line with the legs (Fig. 4.5).

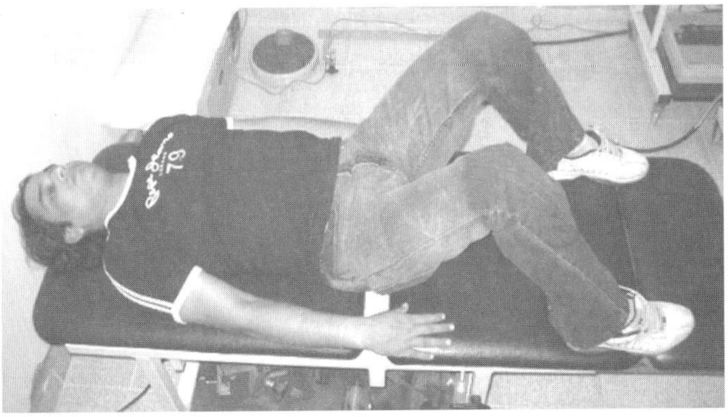

Fig. 4.5: Stride crook lying

f. *Crook lying with pelvis raised:* From crook lying position the pelvis is raised until there is a straight line between the trunk and thighs (Fig. 4.6).

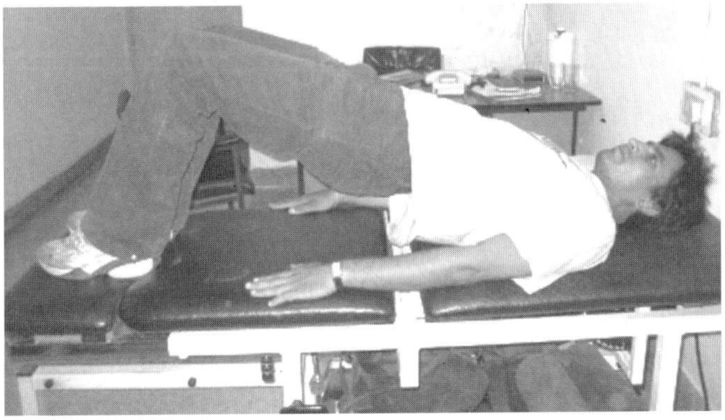

Fig. 4.6: Crook lying with pelvis raised

g. *Leg lift lying:* Lying with the legs raised (the range of movement must be indicated) (Fig. 4.7), also known as straight leg(s) raising.

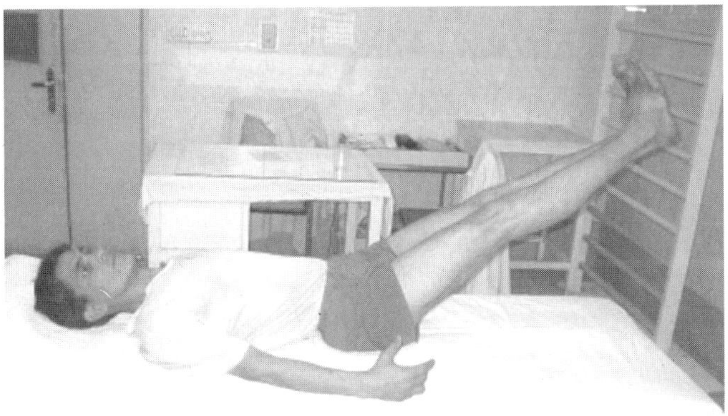

Fig. 4.7: Leg lift lying

h. *Stride lying:* Lying with feet astride apart (Fig. 4.8).

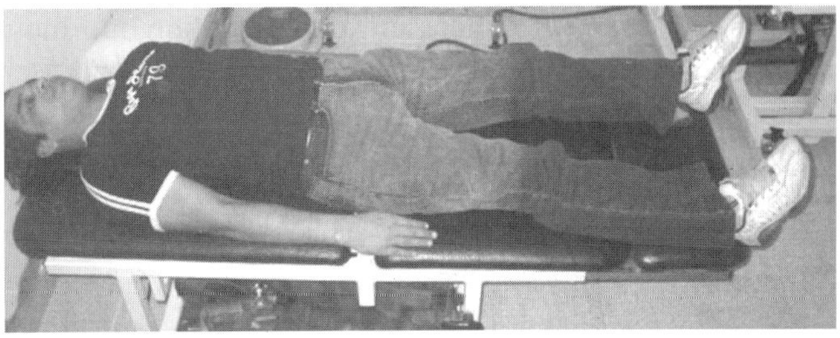

Fig. 4.8: Stride lying

i. *Half lying:* Lying on a plinth or bed with the trunk supported by a back rest or pillows in a position midway between lying and sitting upright. The legs are straight and fully supported (Fig. 4.9).

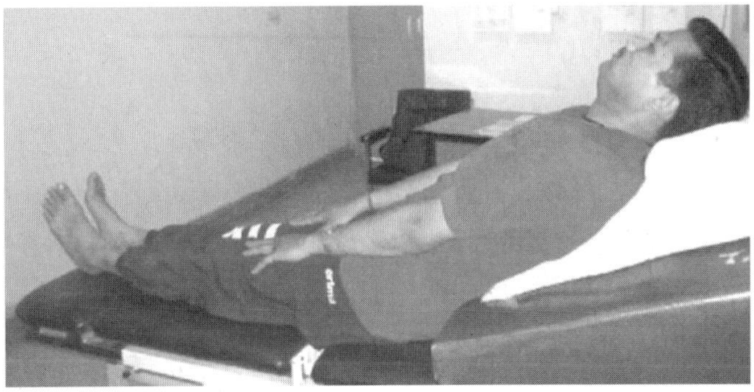

Fig. 4.9: Half lying

j. *Crook half lying:* As half lying, but the knees are flexed and the feet rest on the plinth or bed as in crook lying (Fig. 4.10).

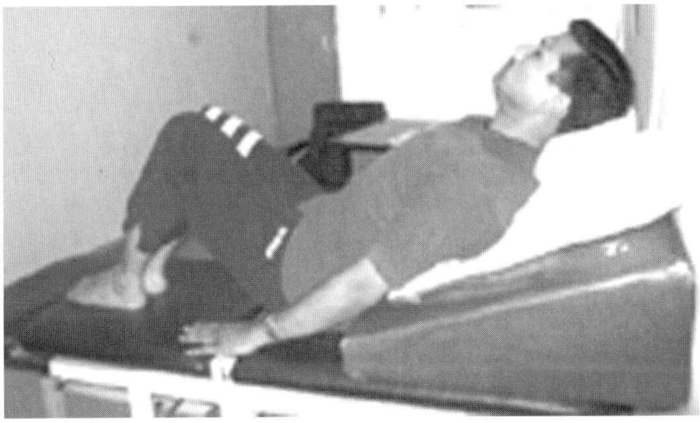

Fig. 4.10: Crook half lying

2. Sitting

Chair or stool should be used for this position. Height of chair or stool should be adjusted to keep the hip and knee 90° flexed and ankle in plantigrade position. Stools are better for movements which occurs posterior such as shoulder hyper extension. In this position muscular work of lower extremity is zero as these are fully supported on the floor. Hip flexors are in stage of static contraction to maintain hip in flexion.

This is also very comfortable and stable position and most commonly used position for therapy.

The practice derived positions are:

a. *Long sitting:* Legs are straight with hips flexed at 90° and knees extended trunk is erect, commonly used for stretching purposes (Fig. 4.11).

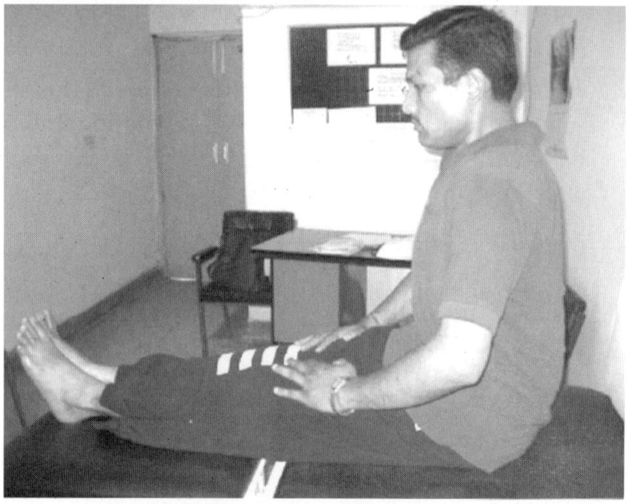

Fig. 4.11: Long sitting

b. *Sitting with legs unsupported:* The position is commonly sitting position only difference is that the legs are not supported on the floor instead they dangle in the air. The position is used mainly for knee and ankle exercises (Fig. 4.12).

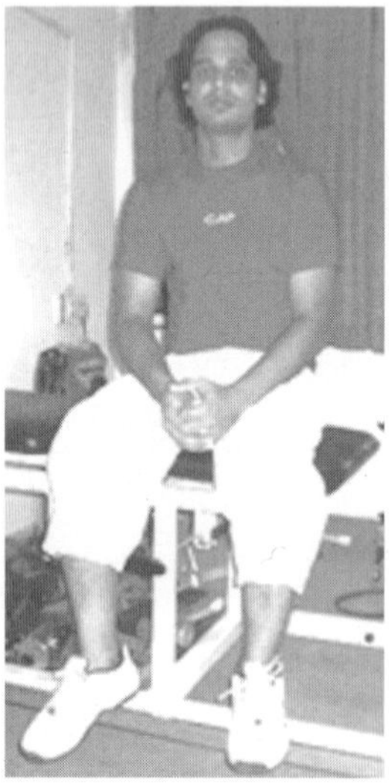

Fig. 4.12: Sitting with leg unsupported

c. *Half sitting:* Subject sits only with one buttock supported on the sitting surface. The knee of unsupported is usually flexed (Fig. 4.13).

d. *Forward lean sitting:* The trunk is bent forward and head supported on table with pillows (Fig. 4.14), while sitting on stool.

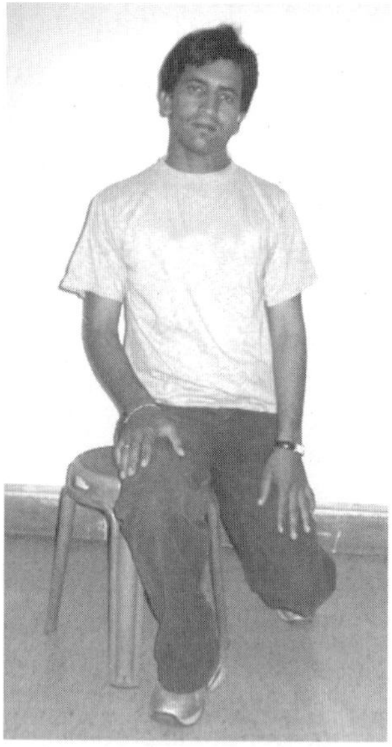

Fig. 4.13: Half sitting

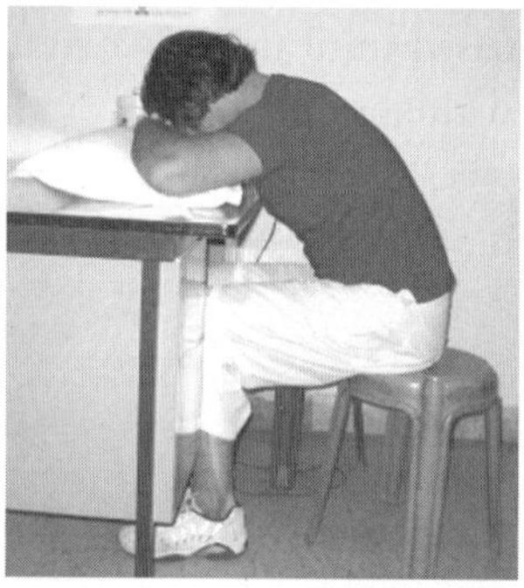

Fig. 4.14: Forward lean sitting

e. *Stride sitting:* The feet and ankles are placed apart (one foot distance between the heels). The knees are flexed to 90° and the feet point obliquely outward in line with the legs (Fig. 4.15).

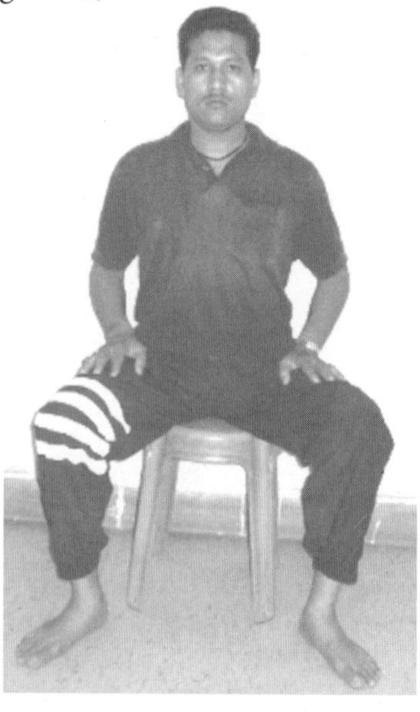

Fig. 4.15: Stride sitting

f. *Long sitting with trunk inclined backwards:* As long sitting, trunk inclined backwards supported with the hands, a widely used position for leg exercises such as quadriceps contraction and single leg raising (Fig. 4.16).

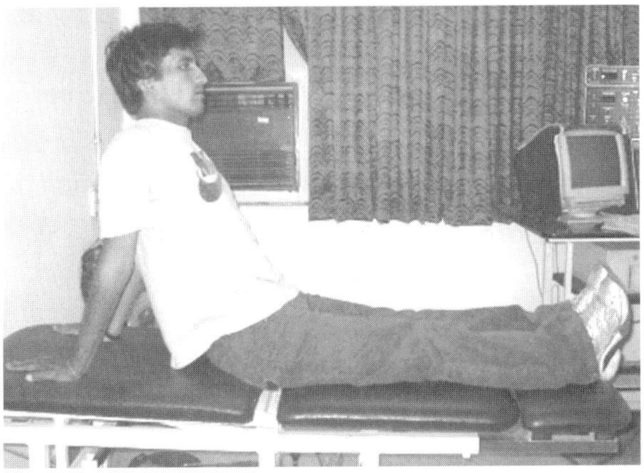

Fig. 4.16: Long sitting with trunk inclined backward

3. Kneeling

The position is like standing the only difference is that the knees are flexed and are in contact with the surface (ground/ plinth). The whole body weight comes on the knees.

The muscles below knee are in rest while others contract to maintain the posture. Extensors of the hip and flexors of the lumbar spine contract strongly to maintain the proper alignment of pelvis. This position is slightly stable than standing but uncomfortable for the subject. This is the preparatory position for the standing and used to strengthen the extensors of the hip and trunk.

The derived positions are:

a. *Kneel sitting:* It is a sitting position adopted from knee standing position with lower legs coming under the thigh (when legs are the part of body which are in contact with ground/sitting surface) (Fig. 4.17).

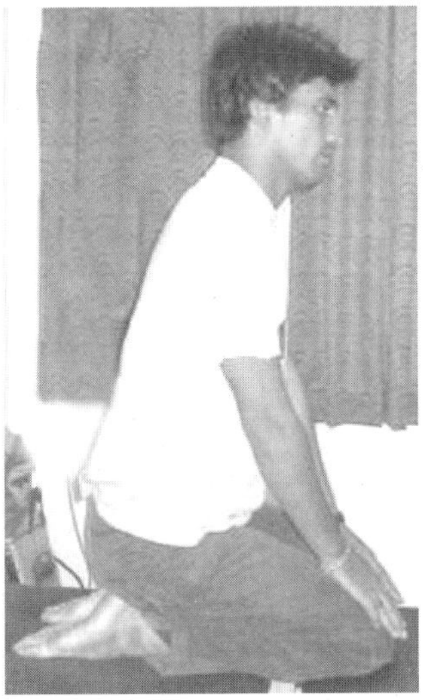

Fig. 4.17: Kneel sitting

b. *Side sitting:* From kneel sitting position the buttocks are moved side ways so that one or both buttocks are moved sideways so that one or both buttocks rest on the ground/sitting surface (Fig. 4.18).

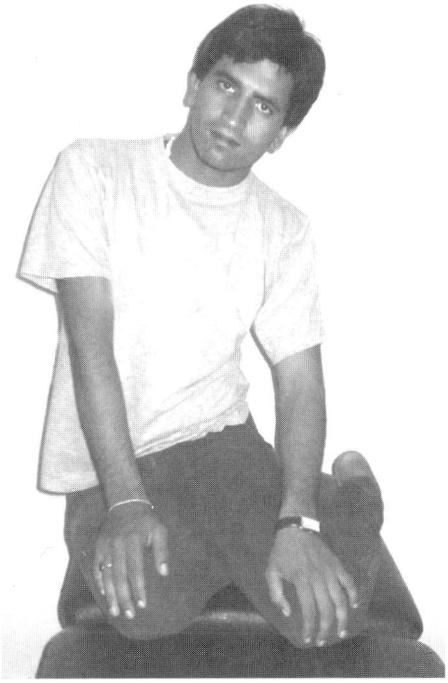

Fig. 4.18: Side sitting

c. *Half kneeling:* From kneeling position one leg is taken forward to be flexed at 90° at the hip, knee and ankle. This is a transfer stage position of standing from kneeling (Fig. 4.19).

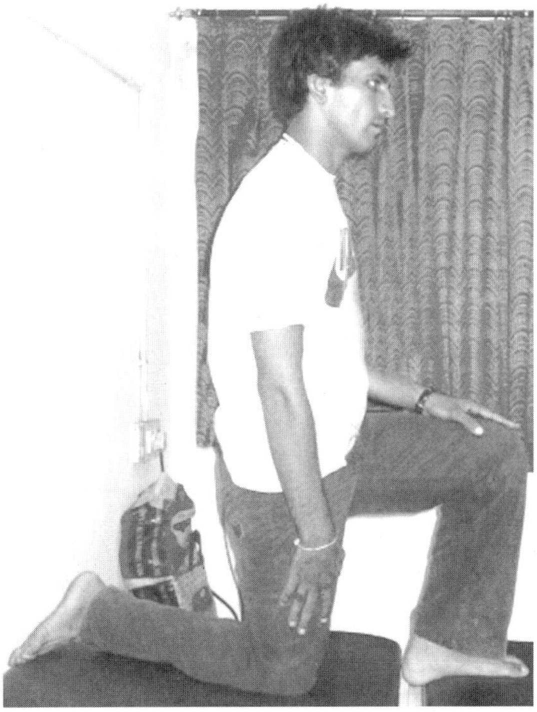

Fig. 4.19: Half kneeling

d. *Prone kneeling:* or quadruped position in which body weight is equally supported on all four limbs. Shoulder should be flexed at 90° elbow fully extended and wrist dorsiflexed with finger extended (Fig. 4.20).

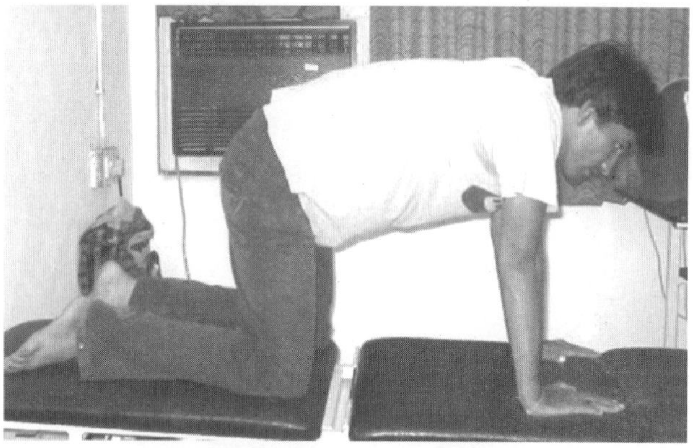

Fig. 4.20: Prone kneeling

The hip and knee should be at 90° flexion and the ankles may be plantarflexed or dorsiflexed.

4. Standing

Ideally normal standing position should have following component (Fig. 4.21):

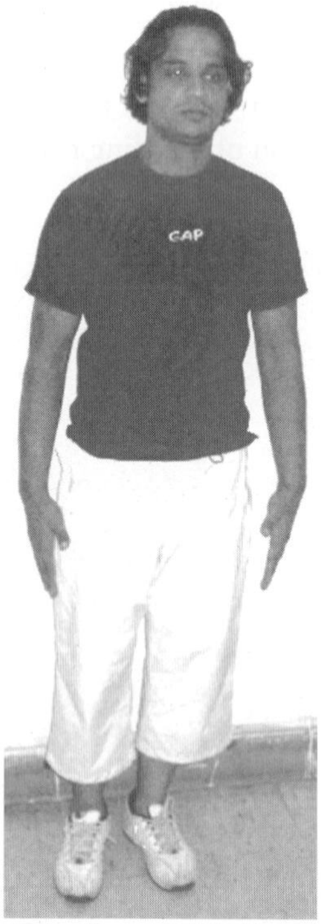

Fig. 4.21: Standing

- The head should be erect.
- The shoulders are down and back.
- The arms hanging by the sides palm facing medially towards the body.
- Spine in normal curvature (i.e., normal thoracic kyphosis and normal lumbar lordosis).
- The pelvis should not tilted anteriorly or posteriorly.
- The hips are extended and slightly in external rotation.
- The knees are fully extended.
- The heels are together with feet apart at angle not more than 45°.

The muscles of the body part contract to maintain the normal standing posture. The main groups participating are:

1. Neck extensors.
2. Spinal flexors and extensors.
3. Hip extensors.
4. Plantar and dorsi flexors of ankle.
5. Intrinsic foot muscles.

(*Note:* Other muscles such as retractors of scapulae, knee extensors etc. also participate but in less amount).

The standing position is most difficult of all basic positions as base of support is small and COG is higher as compared to other positions.

The derived positions are:

a. *Standing with feet apart/together:* With feet apart there is a larger base of support and the subject is more stable to stand up with less muscular effort (Fig. 4.22).

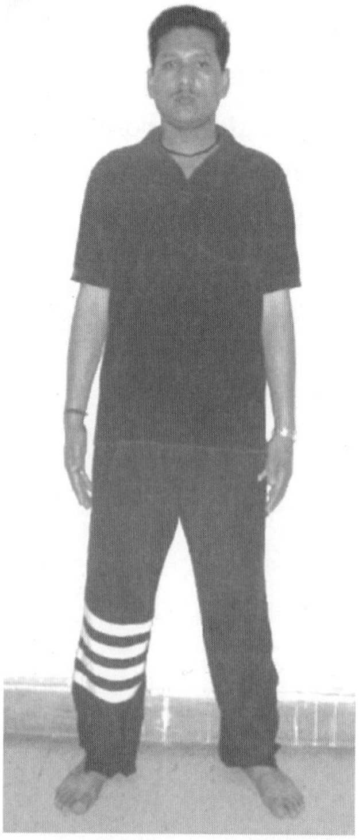

Fig. 4.22: Standing with feet apart

While with feet together base of support is narrower and the subject needs more muscular energy to maintain stability (Fig. 4.23).

b. *One leg standing:* Base of support is more narrower and leg which is in contact with ground has to bear whole body weight. One of the hand can be used to support the body (Fig. 4.24).

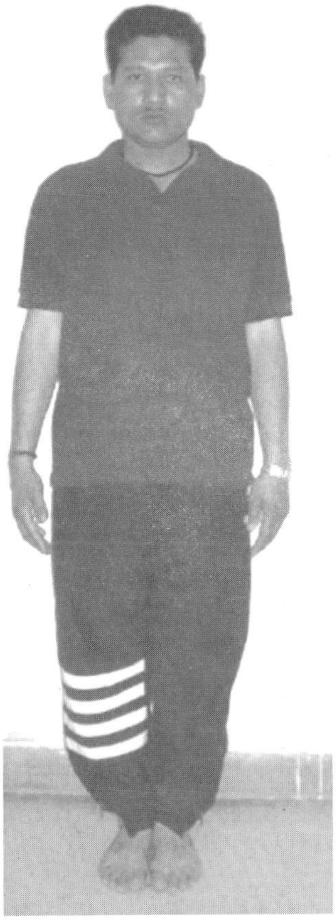

Fig. 4.23: Standing with feet together

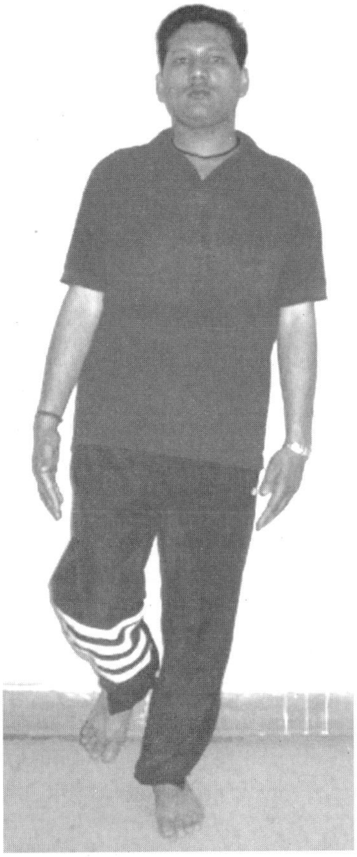

Fig. 4.24: One leg standing

c. *Toe and heel standing:* Smallest base of support is there. Toe standing is mainly used for increasing muscular strength of plantar flexors and also for improving balance (Figs. 4.25a and b).

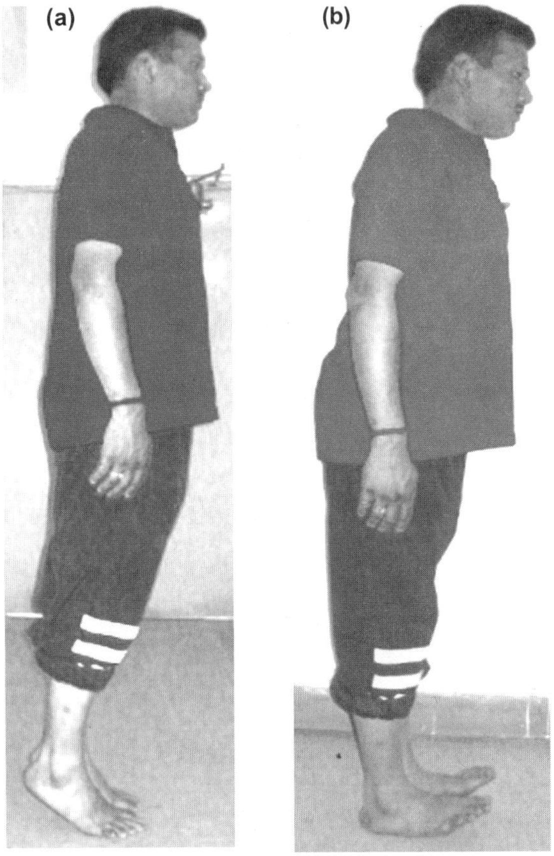

Figs. 4.25a and b: (a) Toe standing and (b) Heel standing

d. *Step standing:* Standing with one foot on a higher level than the other, as in standing on stairs with one leg on one step while other leg on other step. Foot stools or steps can also be used for this position. This position is usually used for teaching weight shift (Fig. 4.26), for stair climbing/descending.

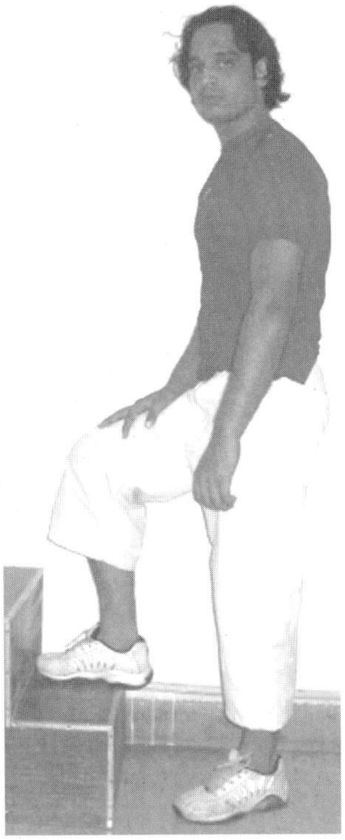

Fig. 4.26: Step standing

e. *Walk forward standing:* One leg is moved/placed directly forward, so that there is a distance of 1.5 to 2 feet length between the heels (Fig. 4.27).

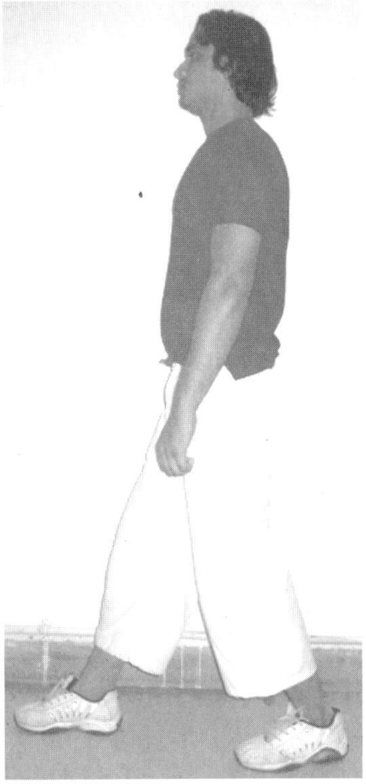

Fig. 4.27: Walk forward standing

f. *Stoop standing:* The trunk is inclined forward from the hip joints with the spine kept straight. The movement is generally taken as far as the length of the hamstring muscles allows. The hips are inclined backwards by plantar flexion at ankle joints (Fig. 4.28).

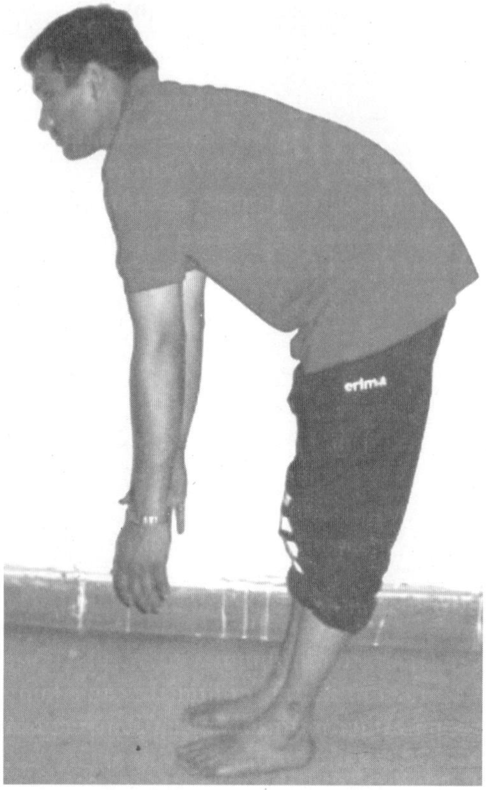

Fig. 4.28: Stoop standing

g. *Lax stoop standing:* The spine and hip joints are flexed in a completely relaxed manner. The arms hang loosely downward, and the hips are inclined backward by plantar flexion at ankle joints (Fig. 4.29).

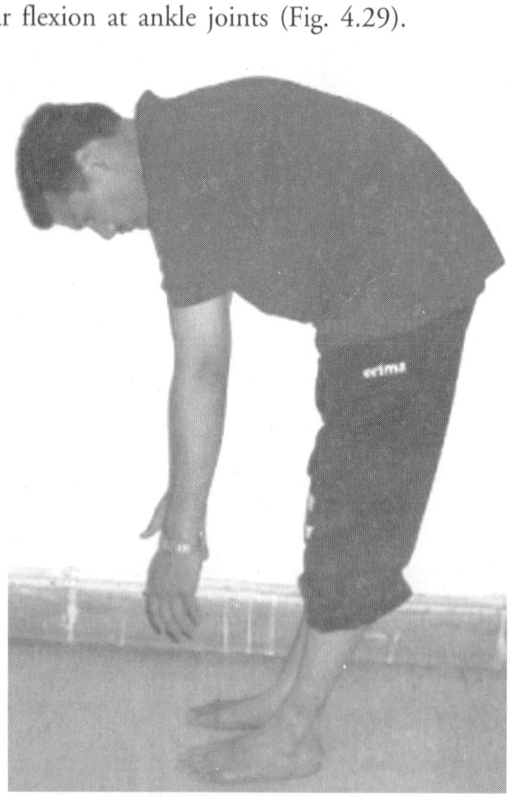

Fig. 4.29: Lax stoop standing

h. *Wing standing:* Hand rests on iliac crest, with fingers pointing forward and thumbs behind. The shoulders are dropped and the elbows kept in line with the trunk (Fig. 4.30).

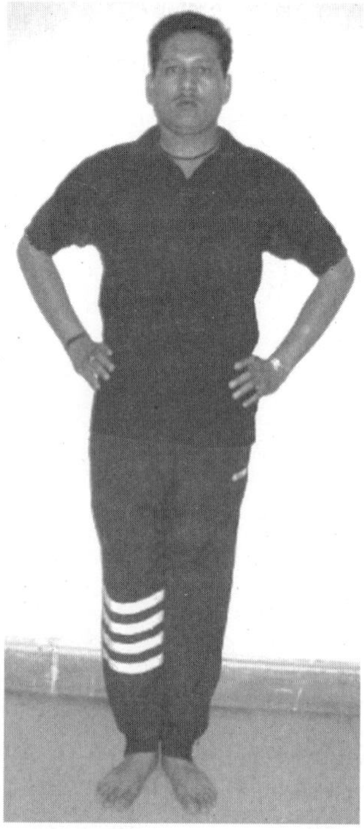

Fig. 4.30: Wing standing

i. *Neck rest standing:* Arms are held sideways in line with trunk, with shoulder joints laterally rotated and elbow joint flexed, so that fingers are placed on occiput. Palms face forward, tips of fingers touch each other, wrist and fingers are straight (Fig. 4.31).

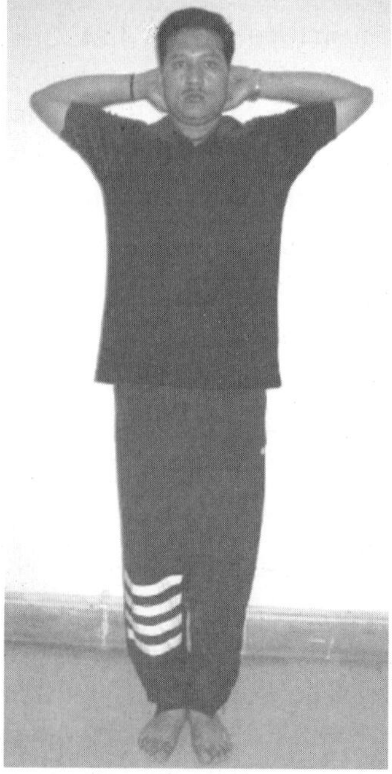

Fig. 4.31: Neck rest standing

j. *Head rest standing:* As neck rest standing but hands are placed on top of the head, with palms facing downward (Fig. 4.32).

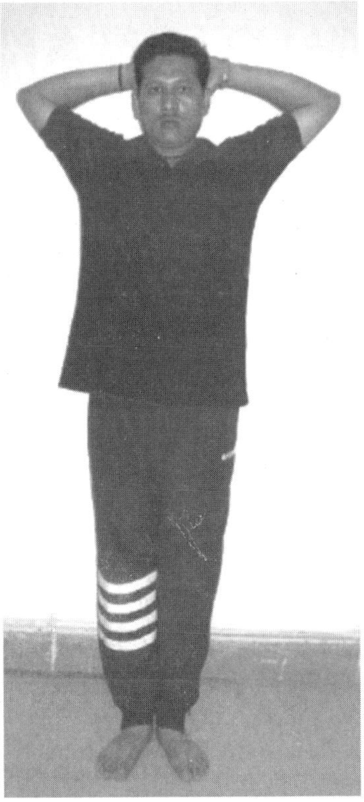

Fig. 4.32: Head rest standing

k. *Lumbar rest standing:* As neck rest standing but shoulder joints are rotated medially and hands are placed behind lumbar spine, palm facing backward (Fig. 4.33).

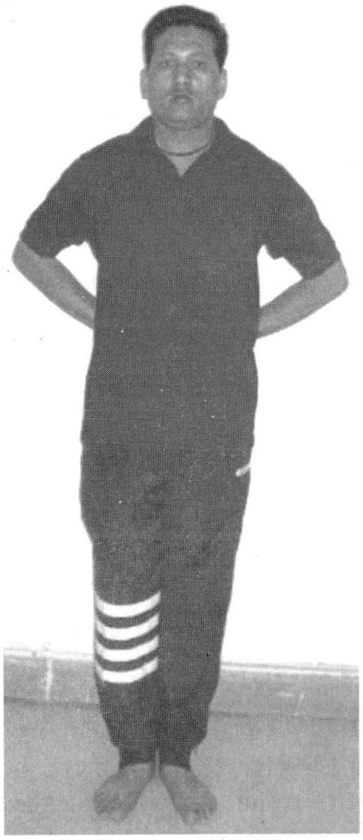

Fig. 4.33: Lumbar rest standing

l. *Reach standing:* The arms are held parallel with each other in front of the body at shoulder level, with palm facing each other. The elbows, wrists and fingers are straight (Fig. 4.34).

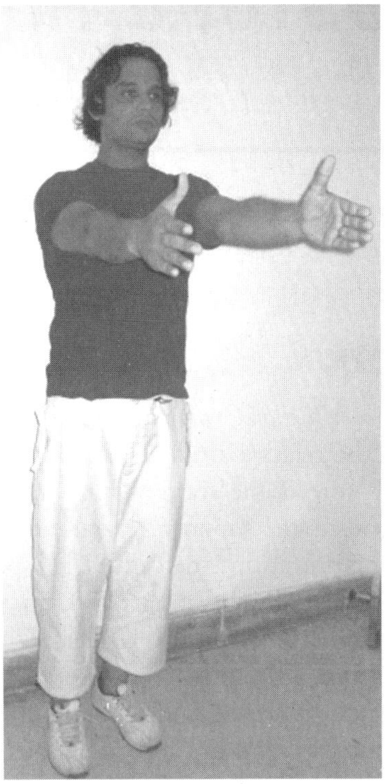

Fig. 4.34: Reach standing

Reach standing can be low or high depending upon the position of arms below or above horizontal respectively.

m. *Yard standing:* The arms are held sideways at shoulder level, with palm facing downwards (Fig. 4.35).

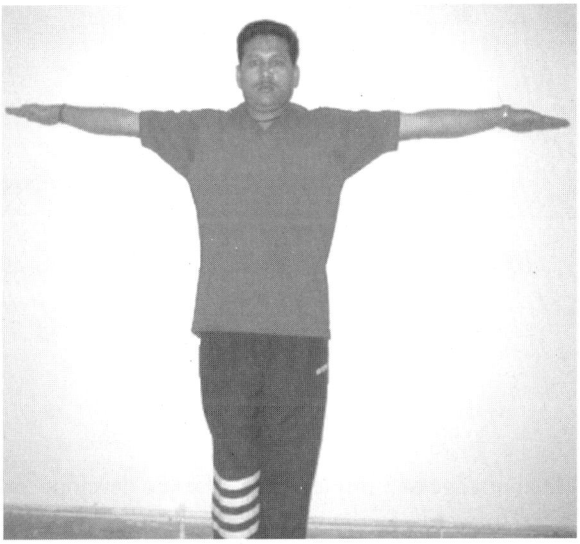

Fig. 4.35: Yard standing

Yard standing can be low or high depending upon the position of arms below or above horizontal respectively.

5

POSTURE, HUMAN LOCOMOTION AND WALKING AIDS

POSTURE

INTRODUCTION

The Posture Committee of Orthopaedic Surgeons has defined the posture as: the relative arrangement of the parts of the body. Good posture is the state of muscular and skeletal balance that protects the supporting structures of the body against injury or progressive deformity irrespective of the attitude (e.g., erect, lying, squatting), in which these structures are working or resting. Under such conditions, the muscles function efficiently, and the optimum positions are afforded for the thoracic and abdominal organs. Poor posture is a faulty relationship of the various parts of the body, which produces increased strain on the supporting structures and in which there is less efficient balance of the body over its base of support.

Development

At birth the spine is flexed or concave forward. **Primary curve** is found at birth, secondary curves appear as the child grows and starts convexing forward or in extension (Fig. 5.1).

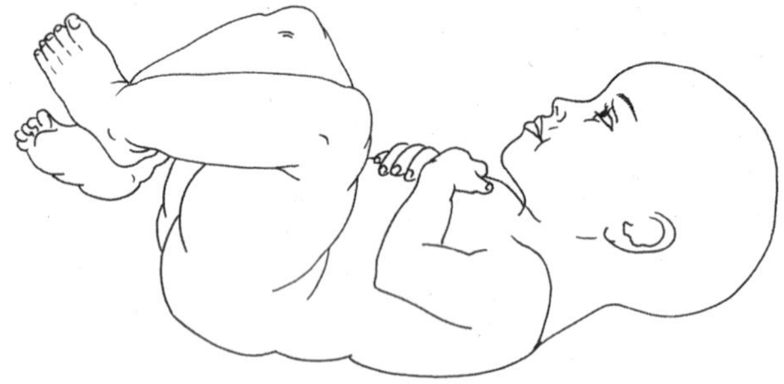

Fig. 5.1: Flexed posture in newborn

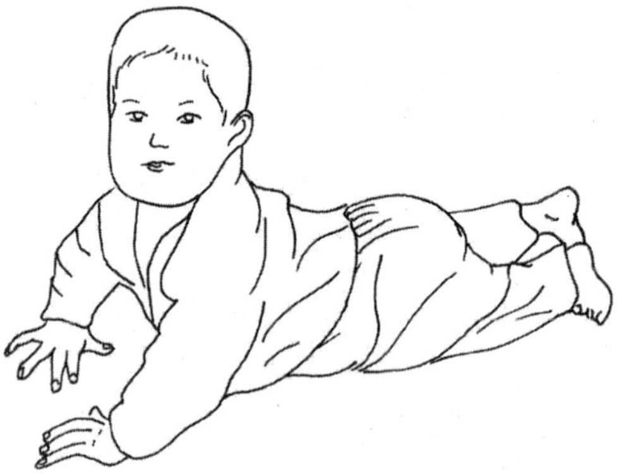

Fig. 5.2: Development of secondary curve of cervical spine

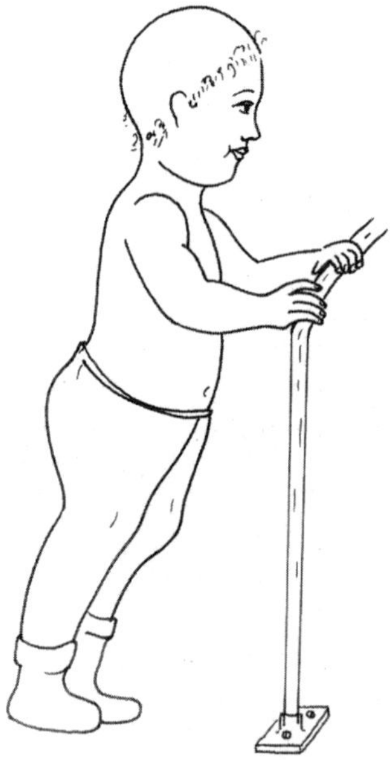

Fig. 5.3: Development of secondary curve of lumbar spine

At about age of 3 months cervical spine develops lordosis (convex forward) as the child starts lifting the head, but the lumbar spine develops secondary curve lumbar lordosis (convex forward) slightly later as the child begins to sit up and walk (Figs. 5.2 and 5.3). The centre of gravity passes through the T_{12} vertebra but as the child grows older, the centre of gravity drops, eventually reaching the level of the S2 vertebra in adult. It remains slightly higher to S2 in males. The lordosis of spine increases as the weakness of muscles of abdominal and presence of large abdominal contents, and the small pelvis characteristic of children at this age (Figs. 5.4a to f).

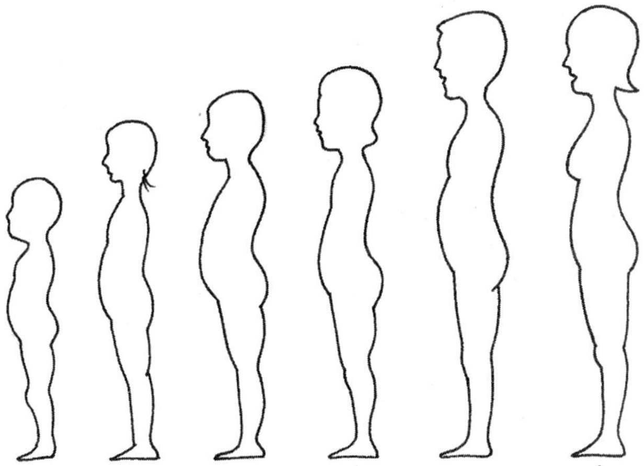

Figs. 5.4a to f: Postural changes at age—(a) 2 years, (b) 4 years, (c) 6 years, (d) 10 years, (e) 14 years and (f) 18 years

Child starts standing at the age of 11 months with knees flexed and wide base to maintain balance. Knees remain bowed (genu varum) until about 18 months of age, then become knocked (genu valgum) until the age of 3 years, and then straighten by the age of 6 years. Feet do not develop any arch and remains flat at the birth but as the child grows medial arch develops by the age of three to five years and gradually fat pad increase in size, and muscles become strong.

Types of Posture

Static and Dynamic Posture

Static: Lying, kneeling, sitting: The body and its segments are aligned and maintained in certain position.

Dynamic Posture: Walking running, jumping, thrusting and lifting—refers to postures in which the body and its segments do not remain static/constant.

Postural Control

Maintenance of Body and Its Segments

Stability either in static or dynamic posture is known as postural control. Postural control requires activity of different systems of body. Mainly postural control depends on the integrity of central nervous system, visual system, vestibular and musculoskeletal system. Proprioceptors which are situated in the joints give information about the joints to central nervous system and intact central nervous system detects, predicts and receives *inputs*, and responds to all of these inputs with appropriate output to maintain the posture (equilibrium) of the body.

According to Horak the ability to maintain stability in the erect standing posture is a skill that the central nervous system learns using information from passive biomechanical elements, sensory system and muscles. The central nervous system interprets and organizes inputs from the various structures and systems and selects responses based on past experience of the goal of the response.

Role of Muscles in Posture Control

Muscles play an important role to maintain the center of gravity of the body in its position. In erect standing the center of gravity passes through the S2 vertebra and requires minimal muscle interaction. The center of gravity passes from lumbar/vertebra through the S2 to between the feet.

Stabilization of the Spinal Column by the Muscles of Trunk

The trunk muscles including: The abdominals, erector spinae, psoas major, quadratus lumborum and the muscles of the neck such as trapezius, scalenes, and levator scapulae all serve as a stabilizing guide wire. These muscles provide dynamic control of the posture against the force of the gravity as the weight of various segments shift away from the base of support.

- When the body moves forward, the center of gravity shifts anteriorly, the extensor muscles such as the erector spinae, and posterior neck muscles such as trapezius contract eccentrically and provide the stability to the spine.
- When the body moves backward, the center of gravity shifts posteriorly, the flexor muscles such as rectus abdominals, and intercostals as well as psoas major, anterior scalenes, the capitis musculature and sterno-cleidomastoid (SCM) contract eccentrically and provide the stability to the spine.
- When the body moves to one side, the center of gravity shifts to the lateral side, the muscles of contralateral side such as psoas major, quadratus lumborum, erector spinae, the internal and external oblique, the sternomastoid, scalenes, and intercostal muscles provide the stability to the spine.

Standard Posture

It refers to an ideal posture rather than an average or normal posture. The standard posture is examined from two views (back and side). In the back view, a line of reference represents a plane that coincides with the midline of the body. This begins from a point in between the heels and extends upward between the lower extremities through the mid point of the pelvis, spine and skull, and divides the body into right and left halves. Both right and left of the skeletal structures are essentially symmetrical. The two halves of the body are assumed in equilibrium.

In the side view, the vertical line of reference begins at the calcaneocuboid joint and extends to a point slightly anterior to the center of the knee joint, slightly posterior to the center of the hip joint, through the sacral promontory, through the bodies of the lumbar vertebrae, through the dens, through the external auditory meatus and slightly posterior to the apex of the coronal sutures. This vertical line of reference divides the body into anterior and posterior parts. Around this line of reference, the body is hypothetically in a position of equilibrium.

Any deviation from the standard posture, changes the equilibrium of the body and is considered as an abnormal posture. Factors such as pain, muscle weakness (hypertrophy and shortening), anatomical impairments and developmental factors predispose the standard posture to an abnormal posture.

FAULTY OR ABNORMAL POSTURES

1. An Excessive Lordosis (Fig. 5.5)

Lordosis is the normal curve (anterior covexity) of the cervical and lumbar spine which can be observed in all normal individuals. In normal lumbar lordosis the angle of pelvis is found approximately 30°. In excessive lumbar lordosis the pelvis tilts anteriorly and the angle of pelvis increases to 40°. In excessive cervical lordosis there is sagging of the shoulders, medial rotation of the arms and poking forward of the head so that it is in front of the center of gravity.

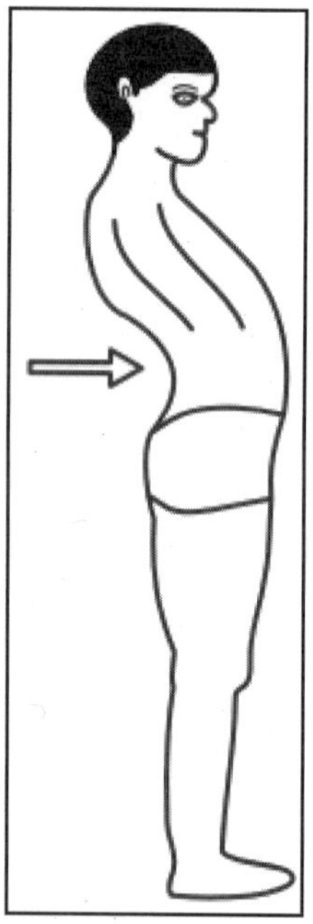

Fig. 5.5: Excessive lumbar lordosis

Common Causes of Excessive Lumbar Lordosis

1. Weakness of muscles (Abdominals).
2. Tightness or contracture of hip flexors (Iliopsoas).
3. Congenital problems, such as bilateral congenital dislocation of the hip.
4. Pregnancy.
5. High heel shoes/footwears.
6. Spondylolisthesis.
7. Postural deformity.
8. Anterior tilt of pelvis as result of weak extensor of hip and abdominals.
9. Tightness or shortening of cervical extensors.

2. Kyphotic Lordotic Posture

It's a faulty posture in which lumbar spine and cervical spine get hyperextended while thoracic spine gets flexed and head becomes slightly forward. The pelvis tilts anteriorly and hip joints get flexed. Slight hyperextension of knees and plantar flexion of ankle joints may also be noted (Fig. 5.6).

Causes

1. Shortening or tightness of extensors of cervical spine and lumbar spine and flexors of hip joint.
2. Weakness of neck flexors, upper back extensors (Erector spinae) and hamstring muscles.
3. Bony anomaly.

Generally, in individuals with anterior tilt of pelvis, abdominals get elongated but excessive flexion of thoracic spine offsets the effect of the anterior pelvic tilt.

3. Sway Back Posture

Sway back is a faulty posture in which head becomes slightly forward, there is extension of the cervical spine, flexion of thoracic and loss of lordosis of lumbar spine. Extension of hip and knee joint can also be observed in individuals with sway back posture. Ankle joints remain in neutral position (Fig. 5.7). Pelvis rotates posteriorly.

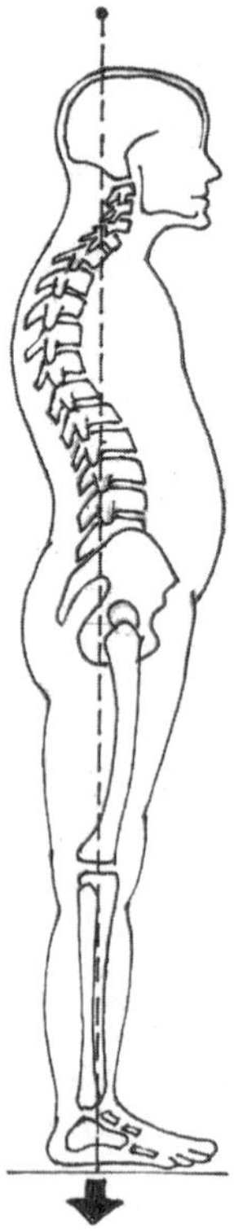

Fig. 5.6: Kyphosis-Lordosis posture

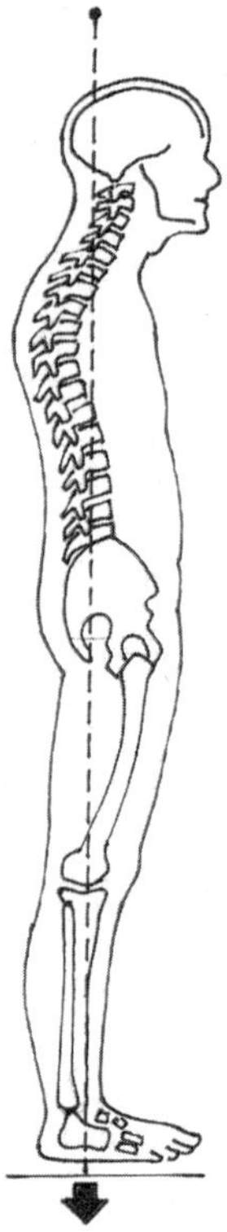

Fig. 5.7: Sway back posture

Causes of Sway Back

1. Tightness of hamstrings, and abdominal muscles.
2. Weakness of one joint iliopsoas.
3. Bony anomaly.

Mechanisms of Sway Back Posture: Shortening of hamstring muscles pull the pelvis posteriorly, that results in hyperextension at the hip and, flexion at the lumbar spine. Flexion or decreased lordosis of lumbar spine causes compensatory curve in the thoracic spine that results in increased lordosis and deviation into backward.

4. Flat Back Posture (Fig. 5.8)

Flat back is a faulty posture in which whole lumbar and thoracic spine gets flattened. Although the causes and symptoms of both flat back and sway back are common but can be differentiated by excessive flexion and backward deviation of the upper thoracic spine in sway back posture, while in flat back posture spine becomes almost straight.

5. Forward Head Posture

It is a faulty posture which is characterized by excessive extension of the cervical spine and flexion of the lower cervical and upper thoracic spine (Fig. 5.9).

Common Causes

This posture is generally caused by occupational activities which require forward head posture such as:

1. Working on computer which is slightly higher than the position of head.

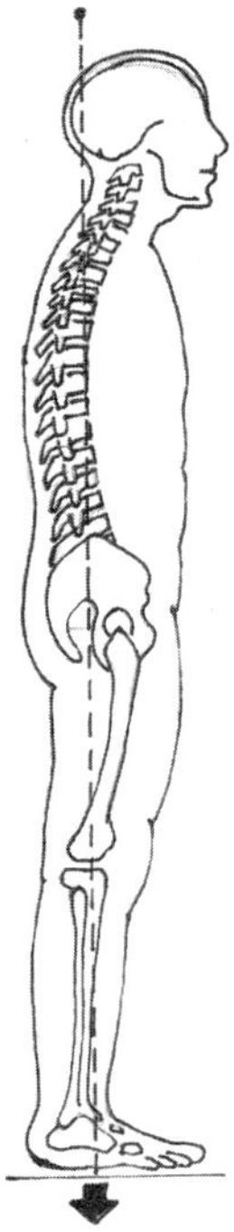

Fig. 5.8: Flat back posture

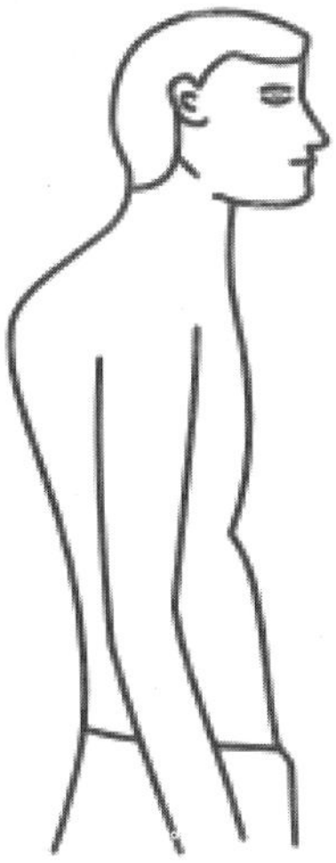

Fig. 5.9: Forward head posture

2. Enthusiastically watching match on television for prolonged time also predisposes to this type of faulty posture.
3. Using of high pillow under the neck.

6. Flat Neck Posture

It is an abnormal posture which is characterized by any increased flexion of the occiput on atlas and decreased lordosis of the cervical spine.

Common Causes

Activity which requires straightening of cervical spine predisposes to this type of posture. Such as soldiers keep their upper back straight (attention position) for prolonged period of time, using high pillow under the head, and spasm of cervical muscles.

7. Scoliosis

Bending of the vertebral column to one side, combined with rotation of the vertebral bodies toward the convexity, and the spinous processes toward the concavity. It may be single structural curve, double structural curve, S-shaped curve and gravity collapsed C curve. Scoliosis can be measured on X-rays by using cobes and rib-vertebral angle methods (Fig. 5.10). Rib prominence usually associated with thoracic scoliotic curves makes the deformity easier to

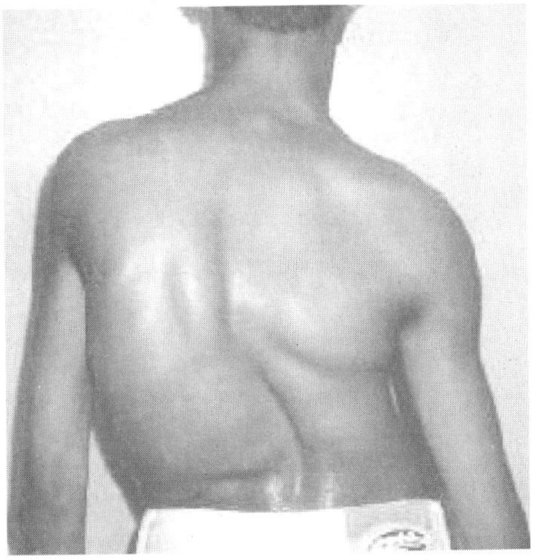

Fig. 5.10: Scoliosis

detect. The rib prominence is a reflection of a rotational component of scoliosis. Ribs articulate with the transverse processes of the corresponding vertebra. The ribs on the convex side are more prominent as the transverese processes of the convex side rotates posteriorly. The rib prominence becomes more prominent on the convex side if the patient is asked to bend the trunk forward as much as possible.

ASSESSMENT OF POSTURE (ADULT)

It is always difficult to assess the posture, as patient *(usually females)* feels uncomfortable while undressing. Ideally male patient should be in shorts and female patients be in a bra and shorts, without wearing shoes. For privacy of female patient sometimes male therapist can be assisted by female therapist. On observation, therapist must observe the bony anomalies, muscle wasting/atrophy, muscle tightness, position of joints, range of motion, swelling and curve of spine (Fig. 5.11).

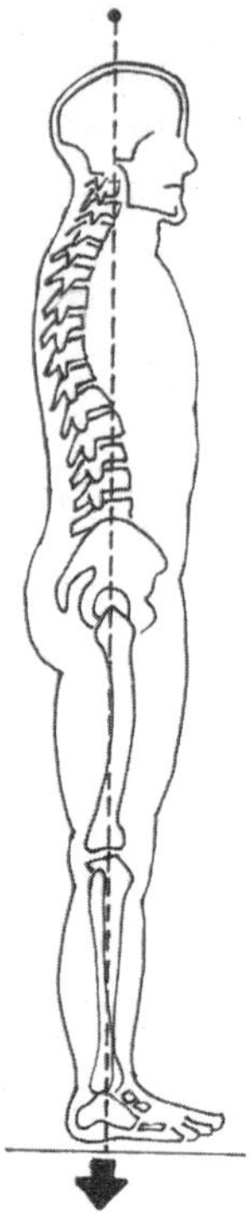

Fig. 5.11: Normal posture

Assessment of Posture in Standing

The whole posture is assessed from head to toes in different views such as lateral view, posterior view and anterior view.

Anterior View

Position of Head: Any deviation of head should be noted. Muscle tightness or contracture (sternocleidomastoid) can cause the head to rotate to one side. This condition is known as torticollis (Fig. 5.12).

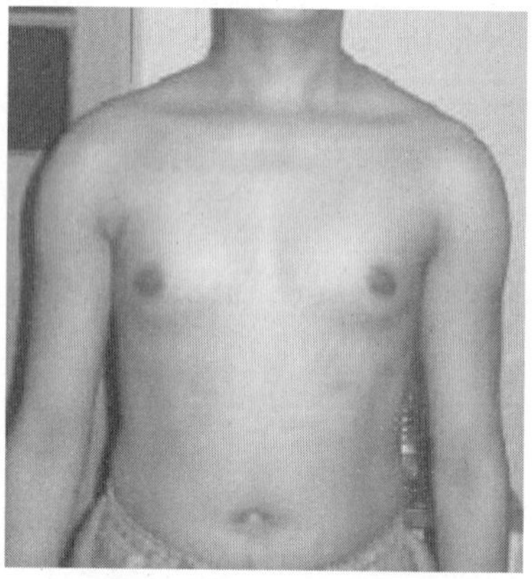

Fig. 5.12: Anterior view

In normal individual when line is drawn from tip of the nose it passes through the manubrium, sternum, xiphisternum, and umbilicus. Any deviation should be noted and considered as abnormal.

The sternoclavicular and acromioclavicular joint should be in symmetry. Any abnormality, swelling, subluxation or dislocation should be noted.

Shoulders: Should be in level, generally dominant shoulder lies slightly lower.

Muscle atrophy of upper trapezius (bilateral) and pectoralis should be observed carefully.

Any protrusion, depression and lateral deviation of the sternum, ribs, or costocartilage should be noted.

Waist angles should be equal and the arms should be equidistance from the waist. In scoliosis waist angle is disturbed and it should be measured carefully.

- The carrying angle at each elbow should be observed carefully, normal carrying angle varies from 5° to 15°.
- The high points of the iliac crest should be at the same height on each side. In scoliosis iliac crest of one side becomes higher than the other.
- In normal person when he or she is standing, both the ASIS should have same distance from umbilicus. The distance changes with scoliosis and limb length discrepancy.
- Both knees should be straight and any deviation such as genu valgum and varus should be noted. In normal person while standing, when both feet are together both knees should not touch each other.

'Q' Angle

In normal person the quadriceps angle is found 14° in males and 18° in females. In valgus the quadriceps angle is increased and is associated with lateral deviation of the tibia. The quadriceps angle is decreased in varus and is associated with internal rotation of the tibia. Examination of quadriceps angle → a line is drawn from anterior superior iliac spine to the tip of patella and another line is drawn from tip of patella to the tibial tuberosity, the goniometer's fulcrum is placed over the tip of patella, the static arm over the line above the patella and movable arm is placed over the line which is drawn from tip of patella to tibial tuberosity. The angle formed on the goniometer is known as 'Q' angle.

Bilateral bow legs can be recorded by measuring the distance between the knees with the legs held in full extension and heels touching. It should be less than 6 cm.

- Bow legs in babies and knock knees in 4-year-old children are so common that they are considered to be normal stage of development.

The feet angle: It is usually measured as 10° (both tibias are normally rotated laterally at 10°) which is considered normal.

Medial arch which is present in the medial border of the foot should be equal on both feet, decreased arch is known as flat foot (Pes planus) and increased arch is known as Pes cavus.

The medial malleolus is placed slightly anterior to the lateral. Any deviation should be noted.

Posterior View

Clinician should observe the following structures carefully (Fig. 5.13):

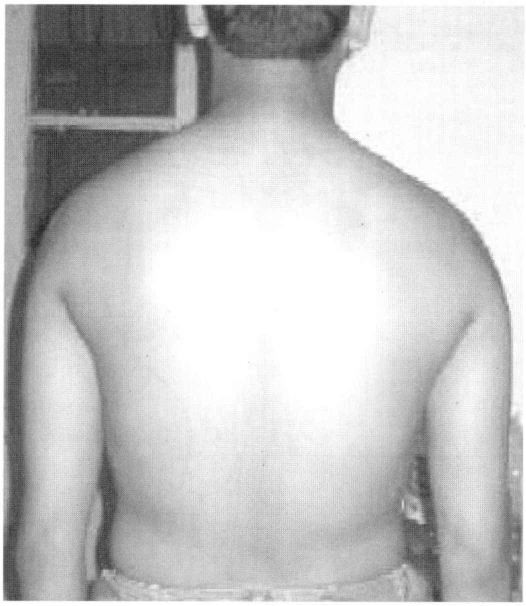

Fig. 5.13: Posterior view

Cervical spine: Lateral deviation and rotation.

Shoulder girdle:

- Subluxation and dislocation.
- Level of tip of acromion process.
- Muscle wasting—trapezius, rhomboides, serratus anterior etc.

Thoracic spine-level of scapula: The inferior angle of both scapula should be at the same level. In scoliosis the convexity side's scapula and the shoulder become higher than the concavity side scapula and shoulder. When the distance is measured from mid thoracic to the arms, the convexity side arm is closer than the concavity side arm.

Pelvis and Lumbar Spine

- Normal curve of the lumbar spine.
- Level of both PSIS.
- Level of iliac crests.
- Drooping of pelvis.

Hip Joints

May be observed in single and both limb loading to see the muscular imbalance. Trendelenburg sign is observed in single limb loading.

Knees

Any deviation such as valgus or varus should be noted.

Feet

Any deviation such as pronation, supination, valgus or varus should be noted.

Lateral View

Head

The ear lies in line with the tip of the acromion process (Fig. 5.14).

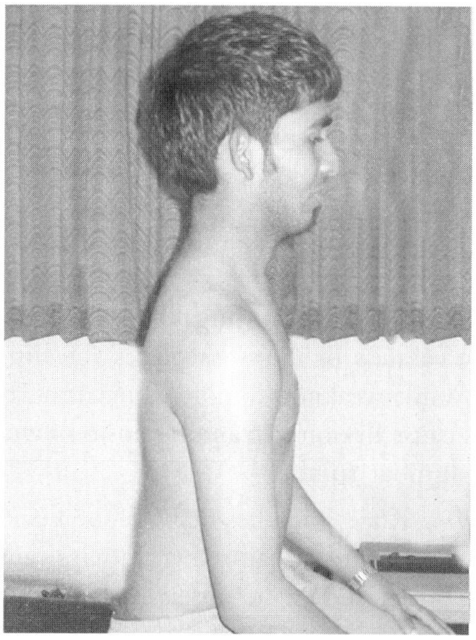

Fig. 5.14: Lateral view of posture

Neck

The curvature of cervical spine—the cervical spine has got lordotic curve at the upper region, which is considered as a normal curve of the cervical spine. Normally when a line is drawn from ear it passes in the line of tip of acromion process. In excessive lordosis of cervical spine, line passes anterior to the tip of acromion process and posteriorly in case of straightening of cervical spine.

Shoulder Girdle

Alignment of glenohumeral joint: Sulcus appearance between the head of humerus and acromion process gives clues about inferior subluxation of the glenohumeral joint. To confirm it, a finger is placed on the sulcus (between head of humerus and acromion process) and is pushed into the joint. The normal joint does not allow the finger to move into the joint. If finger moves slightly into the joint and allows the articular surfaces (head of humerus and glenoid fossa) to get separated, a subluxation is considered. A large sulcus between head of humerus and acromion process gives appearance of dislocation.

Thoracic spine and chest: Thoracic spine has got the normal kyphotic curve. Excessive kyphosis of the thoracic spine places head forward (decreases lumbar lordosis).

Lumbar spine and pelvis: Lumbar spine has got normal lordotic curve. Normal pelvic angle is considered as 30°. Weak abdominals and tight iliopsoas muscle causes excessive lumbar lordosis and anterior tilt of pelvis. While spasm or tightness of lower back extensors and hamstring muscles flatten the lumbar spine (posterior tilt of the pelvis).

Forward Bending
During this movement 70° flexion occurs at hip joint and 40° at lumbar spine and is known as lumbopelvic rhythm. Patients with restriction of lumbar spine movement flexes hip joint excessively and compensates the lumbar movement. Similarly restriction in the hip joint, compensates by excessive flexion of the lumbar spine. Clinician must observe the abnormal movement of lumbopelvic rhythm. Patient is allowed to stand up in erect standing position, or sitting (if not able to stand up).

Hip joint: In erect standing hip joint lies in neutral position. Weakness of iliopsoas places the hip joint into extension. While weakness of gluteus maximus or tightness of iliopsoas cause flexion in standing position with excessive lordosis of lumbar spine.

Knee joint: Knee joint lies at 0°-5° of flexion in erect standing. Contracture of hamstring muscles causes flexion. Genu recurvatum should be observed carefully.

Ankle joint: Remains slightly everted in individuals.

ASSESSMENT OF POSTURE (INFANT)

When a baby's posture is assessed an examiner must keep the normal limits of the developmental milestones in mind. Normally baby starts standing and walking at the age of 12 months soon after the crawling. To assess the posture of baby before the age of 12 months an examiner needs to hold the baby at both the axilla. In abnormal cases where developmental milestones are delayed examiner has to hold the baby even after 12 months.

The head, trunk, upper extremities and lower extremities are observed carefully when the baby stands with or without support (0-12 months). Detection of abnormal developmental milestones helps the therapist to make an appropriate scheme of management.

If child does not poses normal posture, it may have one of three types of abnormal posture:

a. Floppy.
b. Spastic.
c. Athetoid.

Head

Normal Development

0-03 months: Hold the baby at the both axilla your fingers lies at the axilla while the thumb over the anterior aspect of the shoulder joint.

Response: Bobbing of head (Fig. 5.15).

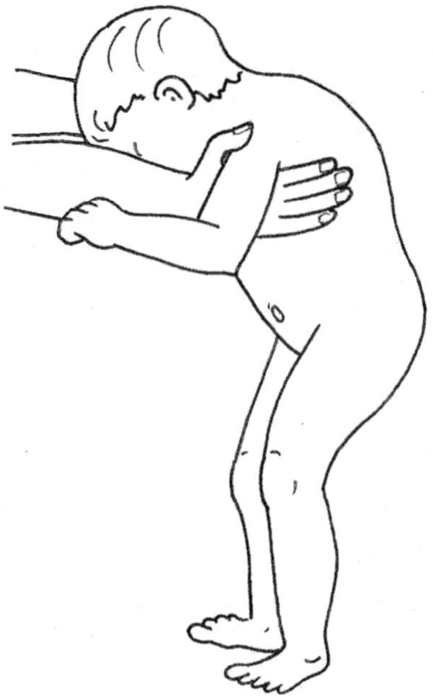

Fig. 5.15

03 months and above: The baby is held in the same position as 03 months.

Response: The baby is able to hold the head upright in mid position (Fig. 5.16).

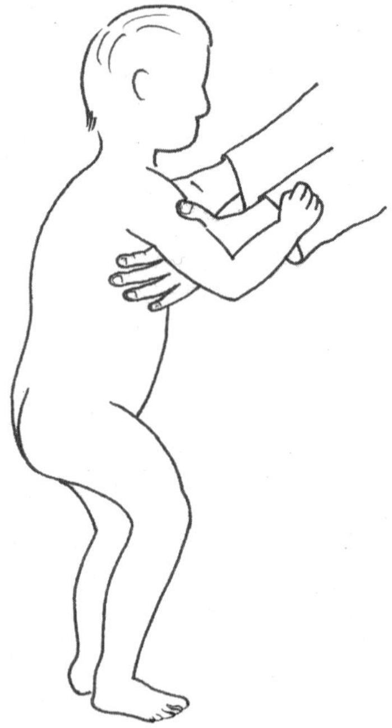

Fig. 5.16

Abnormal Development

Following abnormal responses of head may be observed by an examiner when baby is held at the axilla:

1. Flopping of head backward (Fig. 5.17).
2. Flopping of head forward (Fig. 5.18).

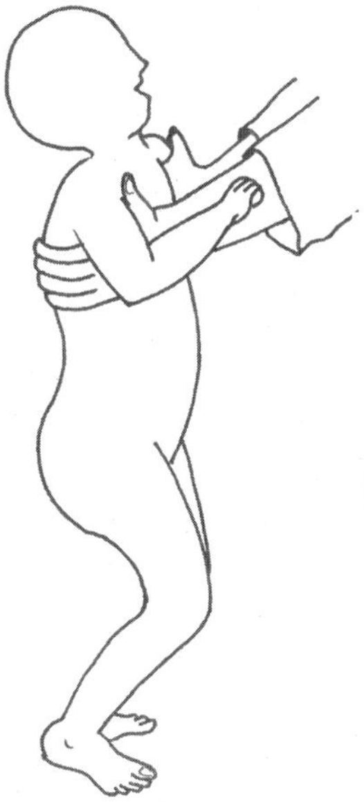

Fig. 5.17

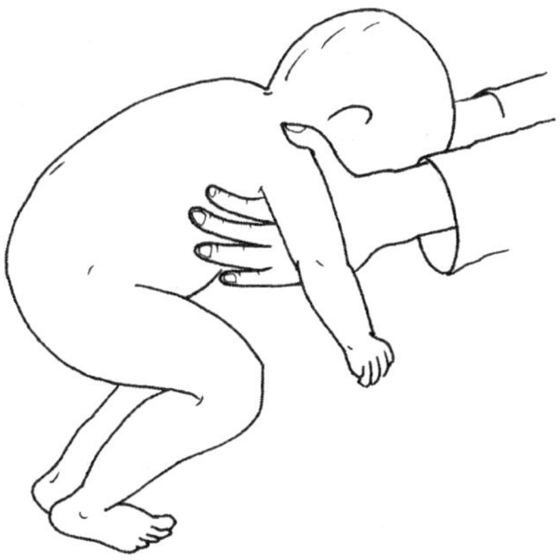

Fig. 5.18

3. Retraction of the head to either the right or the left side (Fig. 5.19).
4. Head stiffly flexed (Fig. 5.20).

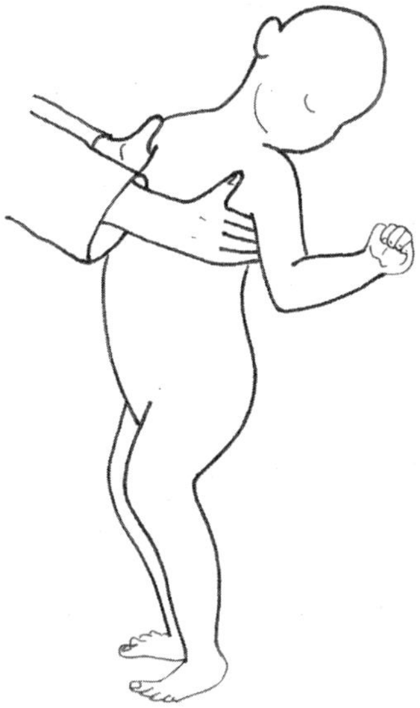

Fig. 5.19

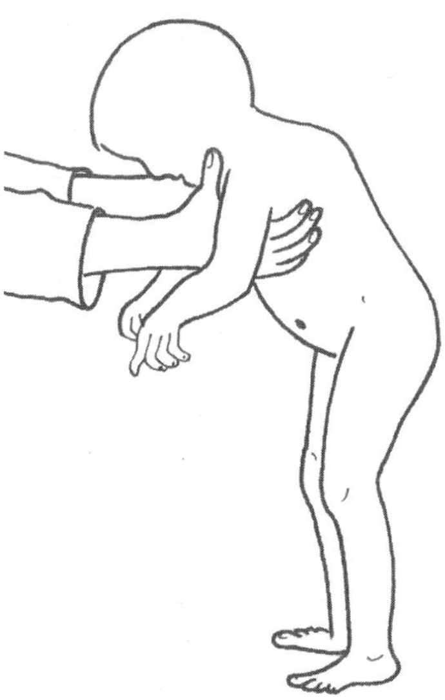

Fig. 5.20

Shoulders

Normal Development

0-03 months baby is held in standing position.

Response: Elevation of both shoulders (Fig. 5.21).

0-03 months and above baby is held in standing position.

Response: Both shoulders are kept in neutral alingment with head upright position (Fig. 5.22).

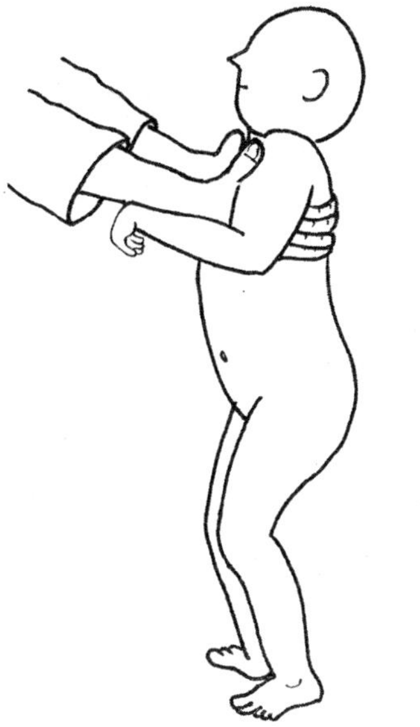

Fig. 5.21

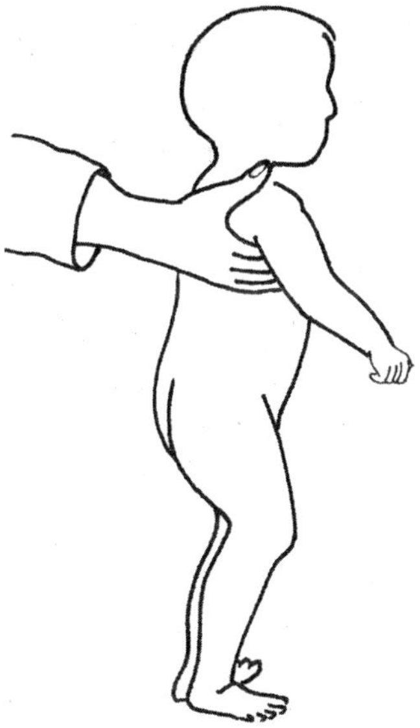

Fig. 5.22

Abnormal Development

Baby is held in standing position by the examiner, the following abnormal response of shoulders may be noted:

1. Retraction of one or both shoulders (Fig. 5.23).
2. Protraction of one or both shoulders (Fig. 5.24).

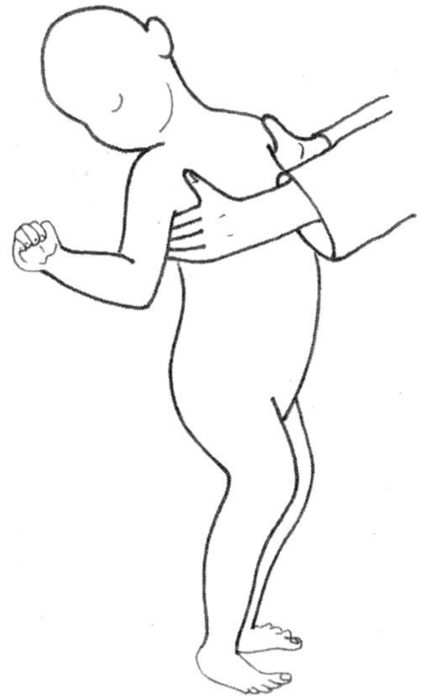

Fig. 5.23

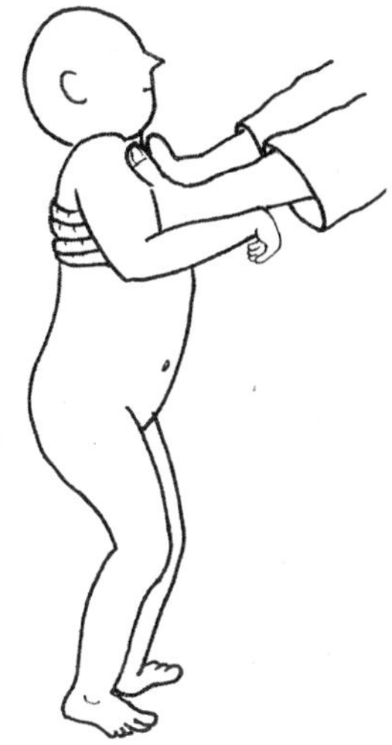

Fig. 5.24

3. Elevation of the shoulders because of hypotonicity of the muscles (Fig. 5.25).

Arms

Normal Development

0-03 months baby is held in standing position.

Response: Arms remain at semiflexed position (at shoulders, elbows and wrist joints).

03 months and above baby is held in standing position.

Response: Arms at the side of body with neutral position at shoulders, elbows and wrist joints (Fig. 5.26).

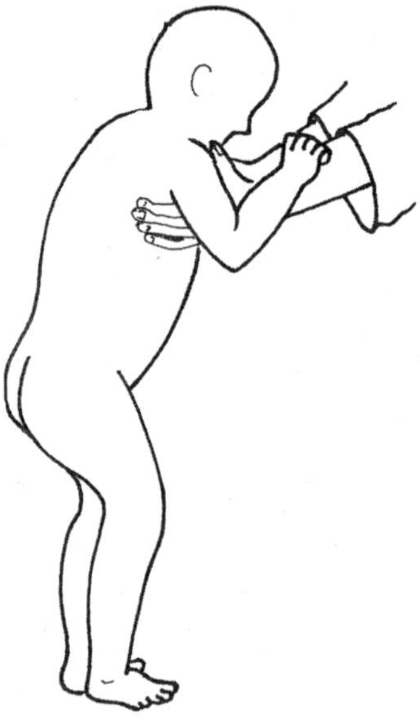

Fig. 5.25

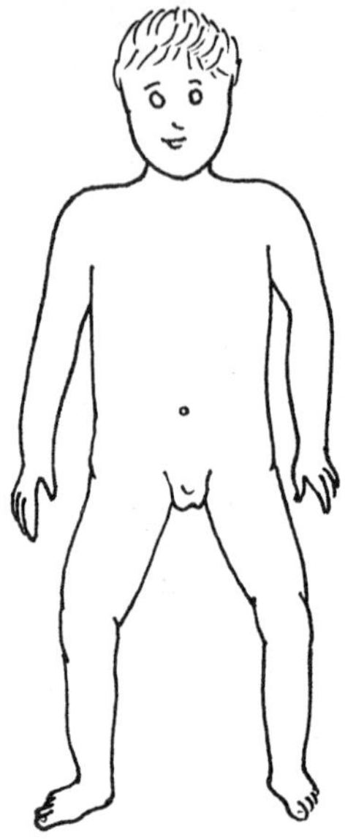

Fig. 5.26

Abnormal Development

The examiner holds the baby in standing position and observes the following abnormal responses of the arms:

1. Baby positions the arms in flexion, adduction and internal rotation of the shoulder joints, keeps elbow extended, forearm pronated and wrist flexed. If the examiner attempts to abduct the shoulder joint, flex the elbow, supinate the forearm and extends the wrist joint, the baby offers resistance to all these movements (Fig. 5.27).

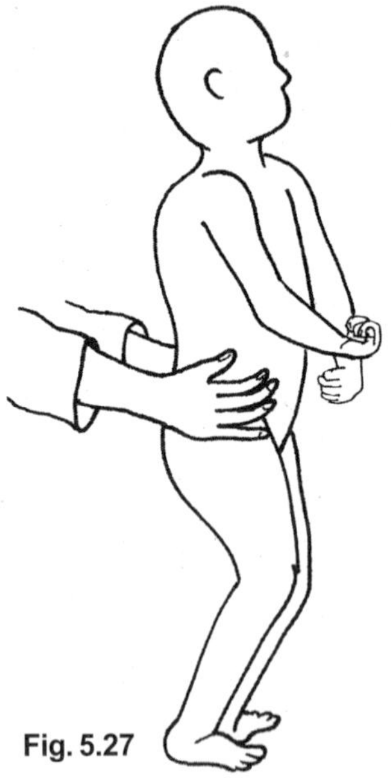

Fig. 5.27

2. Wide abduction of the shoulder with flexion of elbows, pronation of forearm and flexion of wrist. If examiner attempts to extend the elbow joint, supinates the forearm and extends the wrist joint the baby offers resistance to all these movements (Fig. 5.28).

Trunk

Normal Development

0-03 months baby is held at the axilla in standing position.

Response: Generalized flexion of the trunk in symmetrical alignment with the head and the limbs.

0-03 months and above baby is held in standing position.

Response: Upright symmetrical alignment of the trunk in relation to the head and extremities (Fig. 5.29).

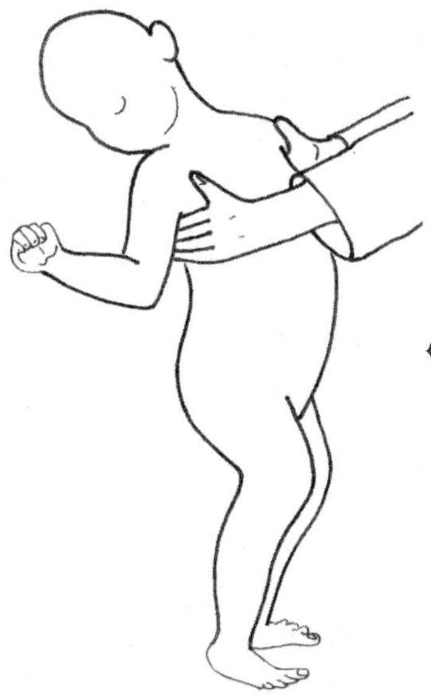

Fig. 5.28

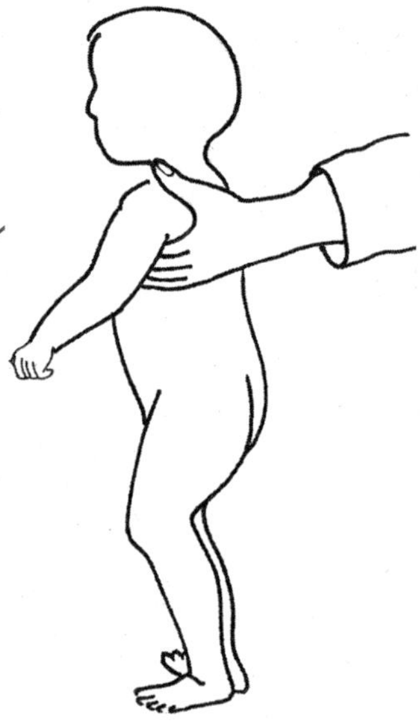

Fig. 5.29

Abnormal Development

The examiner holds the baby at the axilla in standing position and observes the following abnormal responses:

1. The infant tends to fall forward or sideways caused by *flexor* hypertonicity. Hypotonicity of the *extensors* of the trunk are unable to hold the trunk in upright symmetrical alignment (Fig. 5.30). This posture is very uncommon.

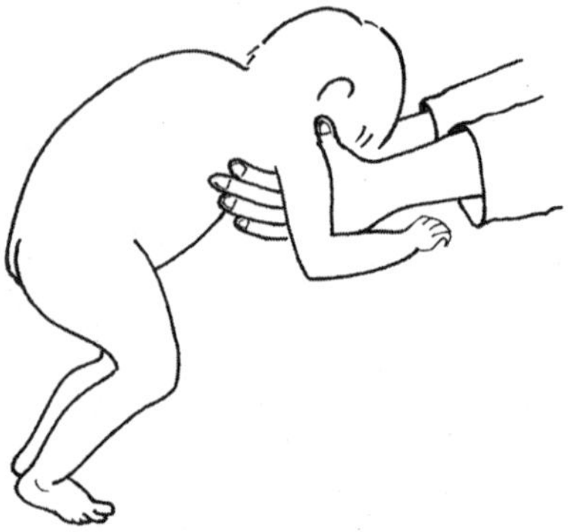

Fig. 5.30

2. The infant attempts to fall backward.

   Cause: Hypertonicity (spasticity) in the extensors of back (extensor synergy-cervical, dorsal and lumbar) causes excessive extension of the trunk (Fig. 5.31).

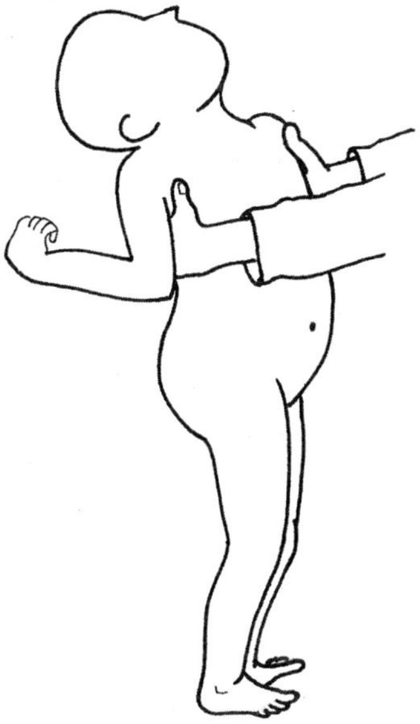

Fig. 5.31

3. The infant shows dystonic pattern by a sudden excessive extension of the trunk which is followed by trunk flexion (Figs. 5.32a and b).

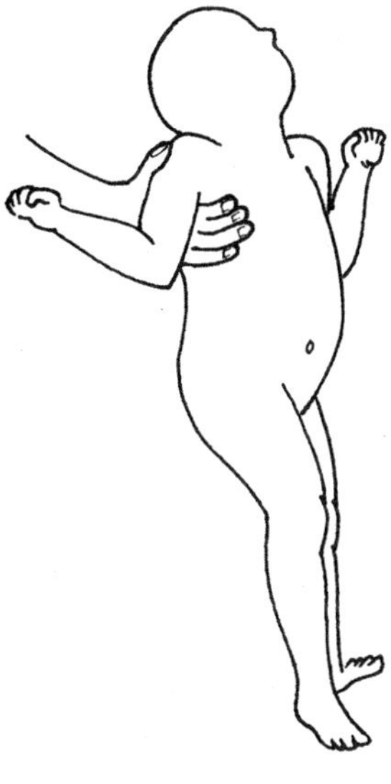

Fig. 5.32a

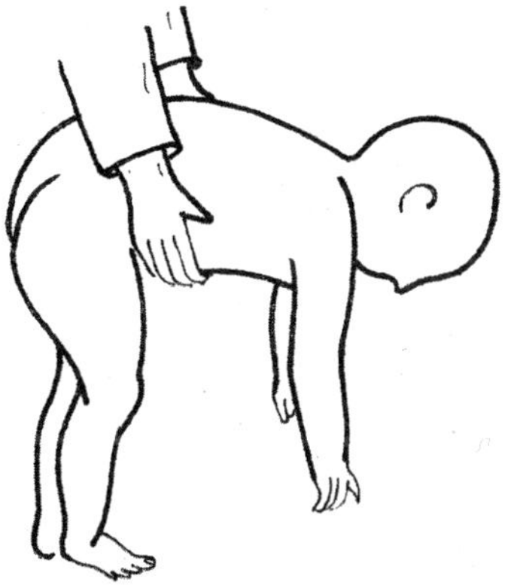

Fig. 5.32b

Pelvis

Normal Development

0-03 months: Anterior tilt of the pelvis (Fig. 5.33).

03 months and above baby is held in standing position.

Response: No anterior or posterior tilt, pelvis remains in neutral symmetrical alignment (Fig. 5.34).

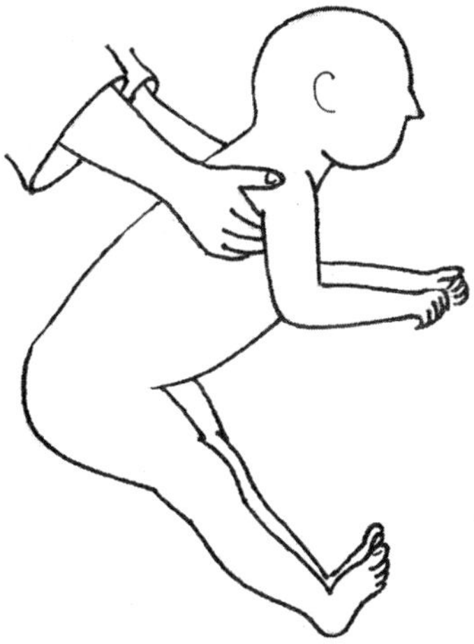

Fig. 5.33

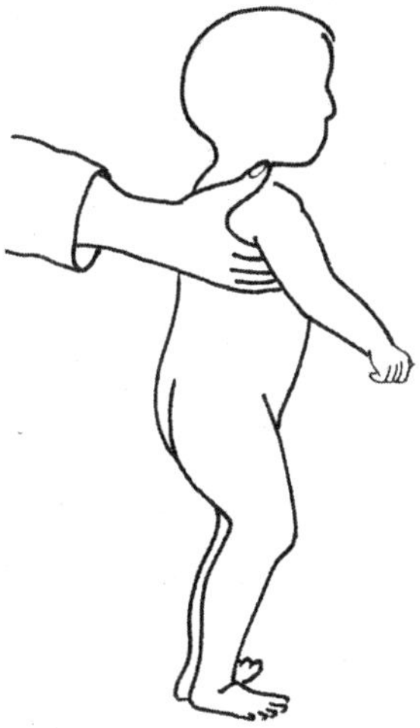

Fig. 5.34

Abnormal Development

1. Anterior pelvic tilt caused by increased flexor spasticity.
2. Posterior pelvic tilt (Fig. 5.35).
3. Retraction of pelvis (Figs. 5.36a and b).

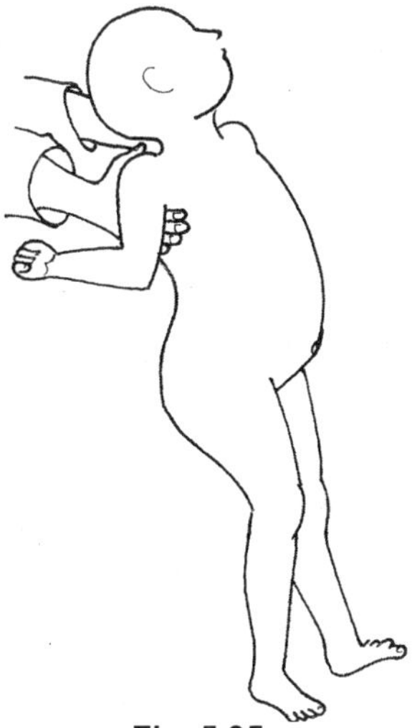

Fig. 5.35

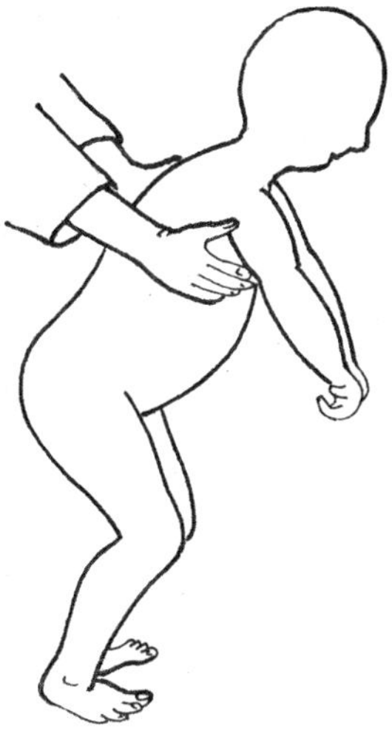

Fig. 5.36a

Hip Joints

Normal Development

0-03 months: The infant is held at axilla in standing posture.

Response: Flexion (45°) abduction and external rotation.

03 months and above: The baby is held in standing position.

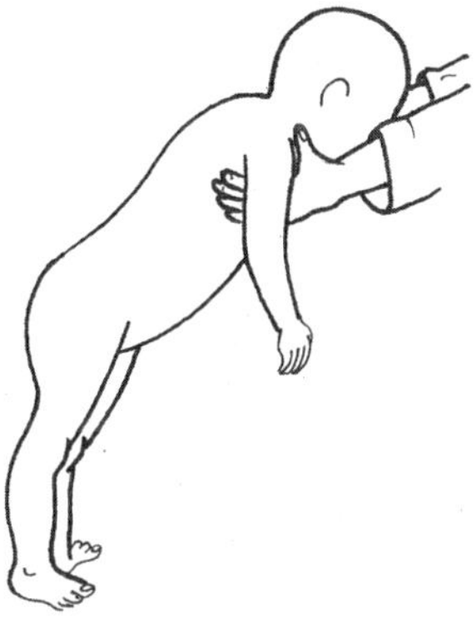

Fig. 5.36b

Response: The baby keeps hip joints at semiflexed position till the age of six months and starts keeping the hip joints in neutral position gradually by contraction of hip extensors. The baby keeps the hip slightly in abduction and external rotation (Fig. 5.37).

Abnormal Development

1. Flexion, abduction and external rotation of the hip joint when examiner attempts to extend the hip joint, baby offers resistance to extension cause-flexor hypertonicity (Fig. 5.38).

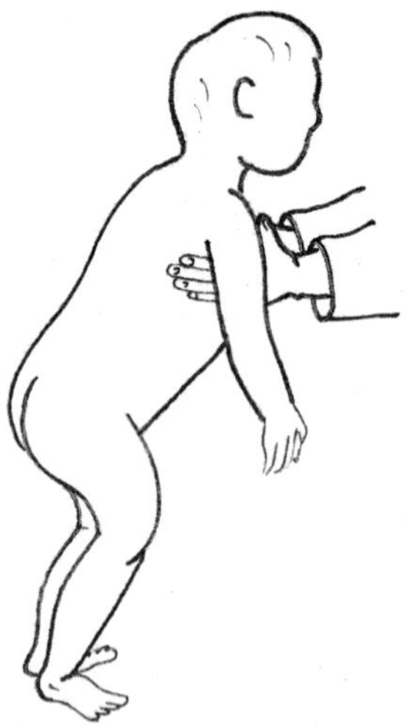

Fig. 5.37

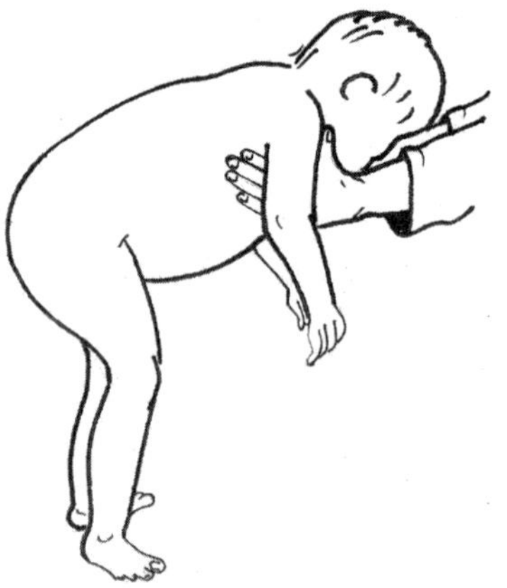

Fig. 5.38

2. Extension adduction and internal rotation of the hip joint. When examiner attempts to flex, abduct and externally rotate the hip joint, baby offers resistance to all these movements cause hypertonicity of the adductors (extensor hypertonicity) (Fig. 5.39).

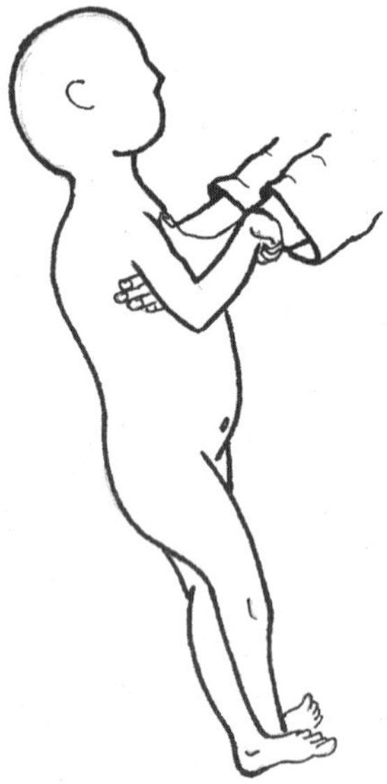

Fig. 5.39

Knees

Normal Development

0-03 months: The infant is held at axilla in standing position.

Response: Baby keeps the knees in extended position.

03 months and above: After three months baby may flex the knees but as the baby starts bearing weight on his feet voluntarily at the age of 5-6 months he shows extension of the knees.

Abnormal Development

1. When baby is held in neutral position, knees go into the flexion. Attempts made to extend the knee joints cause resistance (Fig. 5.40).

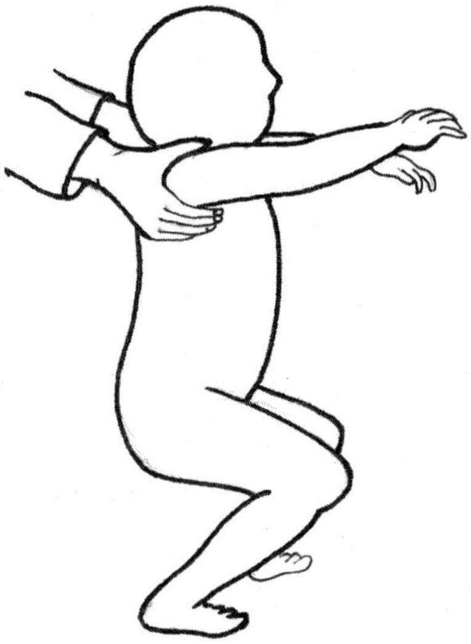

Fig. 5.40

2. When examiner holds the baby in standing position knees go into the flexion. Attempts made to extend the knee joints cause resistance.

Feet

Normal Development

0-03 months: Baby shows plantar flexion when held at axilla in standing position (Fig. 5.41).

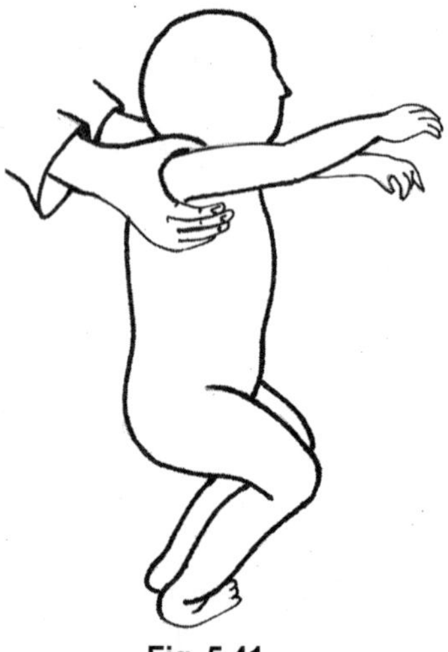

Fig. 5.41

03 months and above: At the age between 3 and 6 months the feet go into dorsiflexion and baby starts bearing weight on heels, keeps the ankle joints dorsiflexed (5-6 months) and after this the ankle joints are kept in neutral position. The infant offers no resistance against plantarflexion/dorsiflexion (Fig. 5.42).

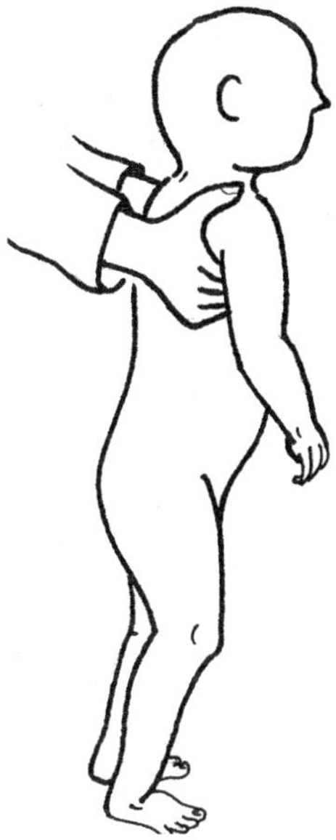

Fig. 5.42

Abnormal Development

The infant bears whole weight of body on toes with eversion or inversion and offers resistance to dorsiflexion (Fig. 5.43).

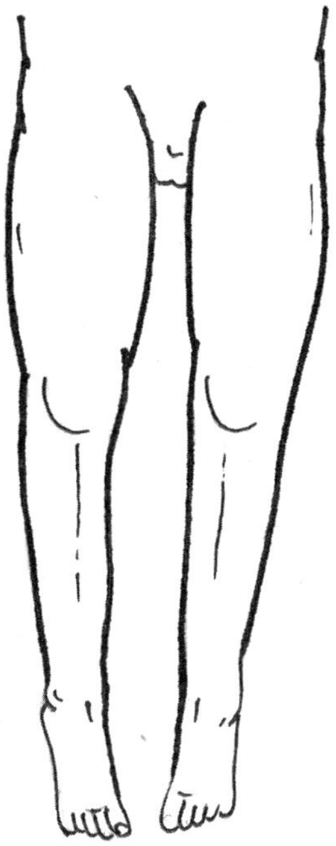

Fig. 5.43

HUMAN LOCOMOTION

GAIT

Human locomotion or gait is defined as a series of smooth, rhythmic, alternating movements of the limbs and trunk which result in the forward progression of the center of gravity. When the gait of one normal person is compared with another normal person there may be slight difference in walking patterns, this difference falls within comparatively narrow range which is considered as a normal gait.

Gait Cycle

The gait cycle is the time interval or sequence of movement that occurs between heel strike of one limb and subsequent heel strike of the same side, or between two consecutive initial contacts of the same foot. For example, time interval between one heel strike (initial contact) of the right foot to the next heel strike of the same foot consists of a gait cycle. Gait cycle is divided into two phases (i) stance and (ii) swing.

A. Stance Phase

Stance phase is the phase of gait cycle which begins with heel strike (touching of heel with the ground) and ends with toe off of the same foot. The stance phase contributes 60% of the gait cycle.

Subdivisions of stance phase: (Table 5.1)

1. Heel strike (initial contact).

Table 5.1: ROM and contraction of muscles during stance phase (right lower limb)

	Heel Strike	*Foot Flat*	*Mid Stance*	*Push Off*
Sub-phase of Stance Phase	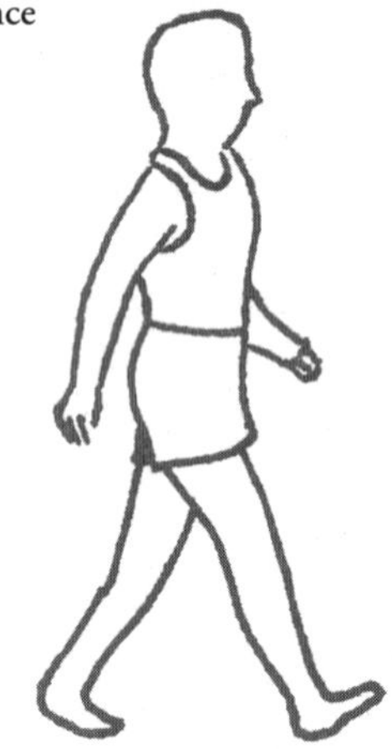	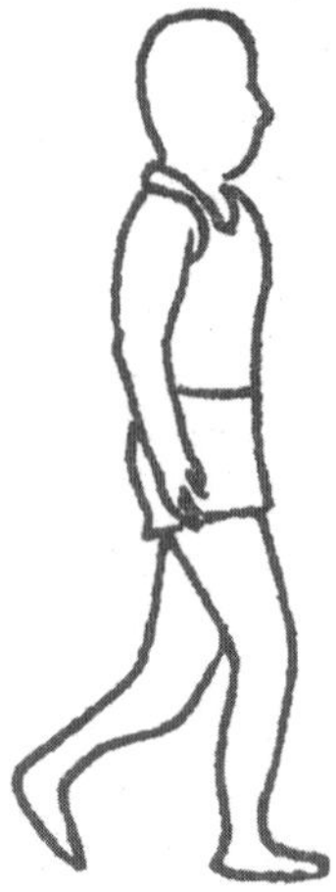	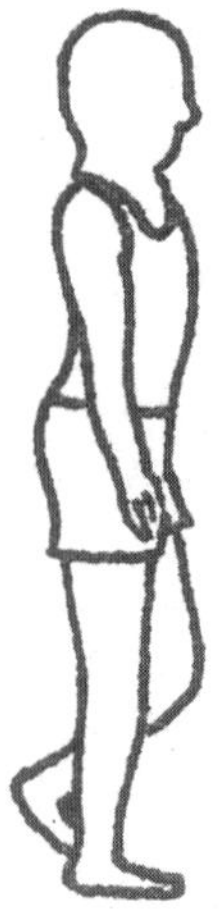	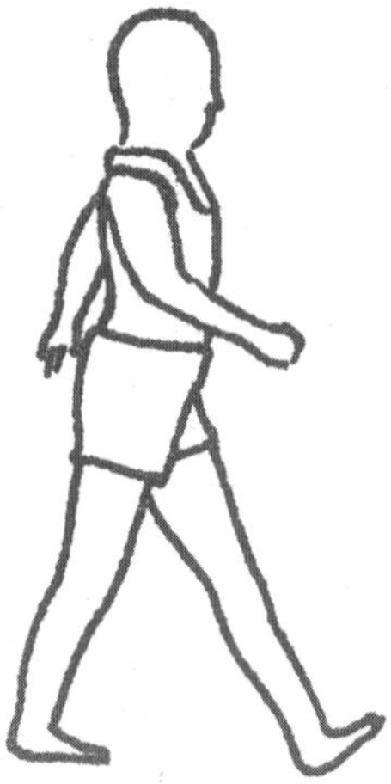
ROM of:				
– Ankle joint	Neutral	15° Plantar flexion	10° Dorsiflexion	Neutral
– Knee joint	Full extension	15° Flexion	Neutral	Full extension
– Hip joint	30° Flexion	30° Flexion	Neutral	10° extension
– Pelvis	5° Foward rotation	Decrease forward rotation	Neutral	5° Backward rotation
– Trunk	Erect neutral	Erect neutral	Erect neutral	Erect neutral
Contraction of muscles required	Dorsiflexors Quadriceps Gluteus maximus Hamstrings Erector spinae	Plantar flexors Quadriceps Gluteus maximus	Plantar flexors Quadriceps Gluteus maximus Iliopsoas Gluteus medius Quadratus magnus Adductor longus Gluteus medius	Plantar flexors Toe flexors Hamstrings Quadriceps Iliopsoas
Weakness of muscles causes	Foot drop	Excessive dorsiflexion	Excessive dorsiflexion	No sequence from heel off to toe off

2. Foot flat (load response).
3. Mid stance (single leg stance).
4. Push off (heel off and toe off).

- *Heel Strike*—The stance phase begins as soon as the heel of the limb touches the floor, or the heel touches the ground and starts accepting the weight of the body, at the same time the other foot prepares to leave the ground so that during the heel strike both feet are in contact with the floor, it is thus a period of double leg support or double leg stance, and contributes 10% of the gait cycle (Fig. 5.44).
- *Foot Flat*—Shortly after heel strike, the whole sole (heel to toes) of the foot touches the floor (Fig. 5.45).

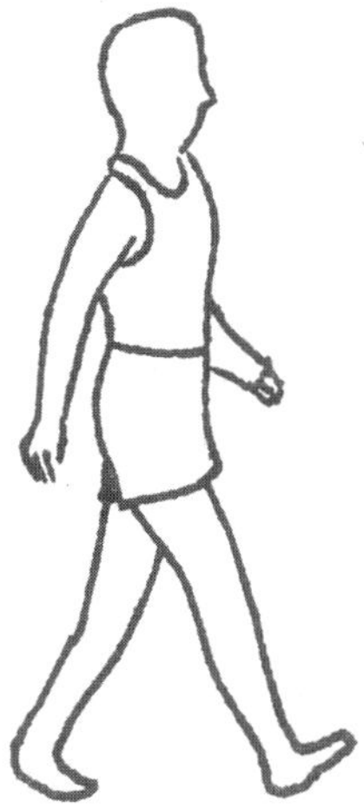

Fig. 5.44: Heel strike

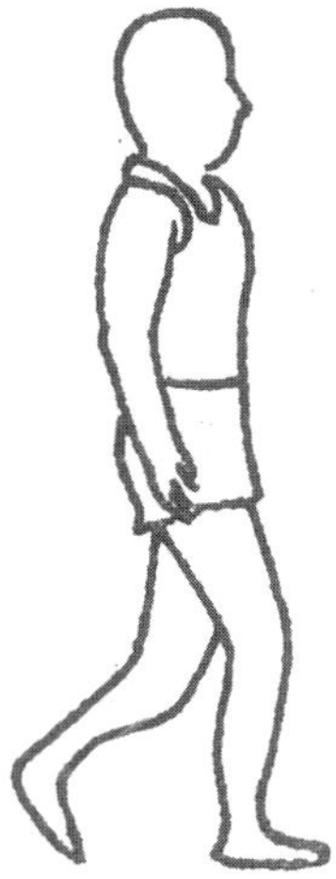

Fig. 5.45: Foot flat

- *Mid Stance*—It begins with foot flat and ends with heel off. During mid stance one leg alone carries the weight of whole body, while the other leg passes beneath the body, and this is known as single leg support or single leg stance (Fig. 5.46).

  The foot flat and mid stance contributes 40% of the gait cycle.
- *Push Off*—Begins with heel off and ends with toe off of the same foot. This subphase of stance is the interval between heel off and toe off position of the same foot. This phase is known as push off because it pushes the weight of body to the another leg and prepares for swing phase (Fig. 5.47).

  Heel off is the end stage of mid stance where heel leaves the ground and prepares for push off, while the weight of body is being transferred to contralateral leg.

  Toe off is the end stage of push off and of course stance phase where body weight is propelled to the contralateral leg. During toe off the contralateral limb's heel strikes the ground and both feet are again in contact with the floor so that double stance occurs for the second time during gait cycle. The push off contributes 10% of the gait cycle.

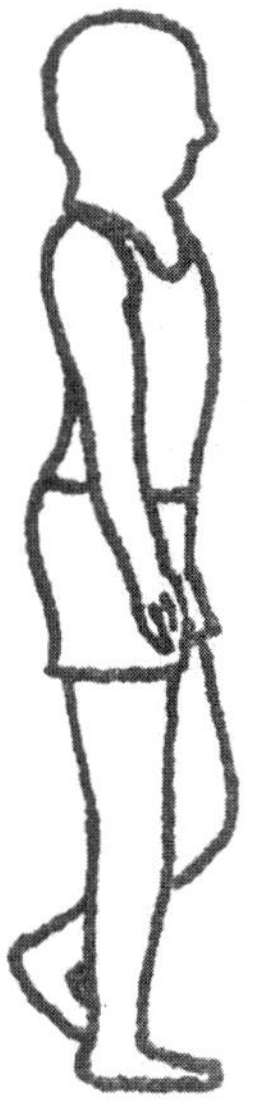

Fig. 5.46: Mid stance

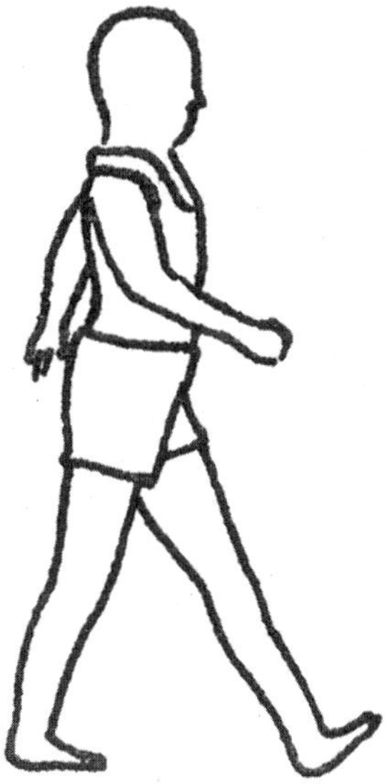

Fig. 5.47: Push off

B. Swing Phase

Swing phase begins with toe off and ends with heel strike of the same foot, during this phase leg swings forward bearing no weight of the body, and contributes 40% of the gait cycle. Swing phase consists of three sub phases:

1. Acceleration (Initial swing).
2. Mid swing.
3. Deceleration (Terminal swing).

- *Acceleration (Initial Swing)*–It begins at the instant the toe leaves the ground. After leaving the ground the leg accelerates forward, with knee flexion and dorsiflexion of the same limb (Fig. 5.48).
- *Mid Swing*–This begins after initial swing. The accelerated leg (swing leg) passes directly beneath the body. During this stage rapid knee flexion and dorsiflexion occur and shorten the limb to clear the ground for mid swing (Fig. 5.49).
- *Deceleration (Terminal Swing)*—Begins after mid swing and the leg slows down in preparation for heel strike with the floor. During this phase the moving leg is controlled by extensors and flexors of the knee joint (Fig. 5.50).

Muscular Activity During Stance Phase

The Ankle Joint

Heel Strike–At the instant of heel strike the dorsiflexors (tibialis anterior, extensor digitorum longus and extensor hallucis longus) of the ankle joint generate great force. The

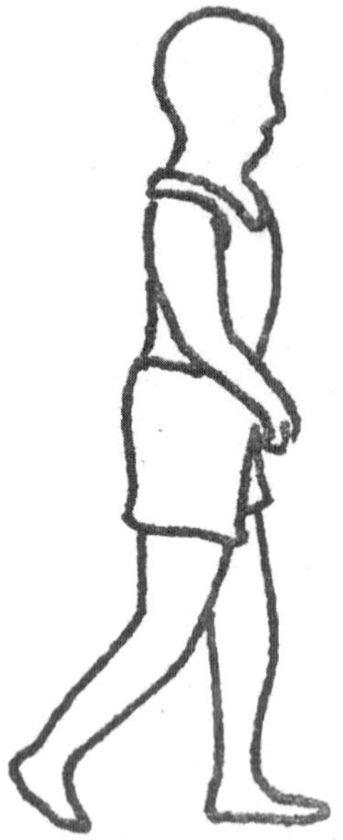

Fig. 5.48: Acceleration (Initial swing)

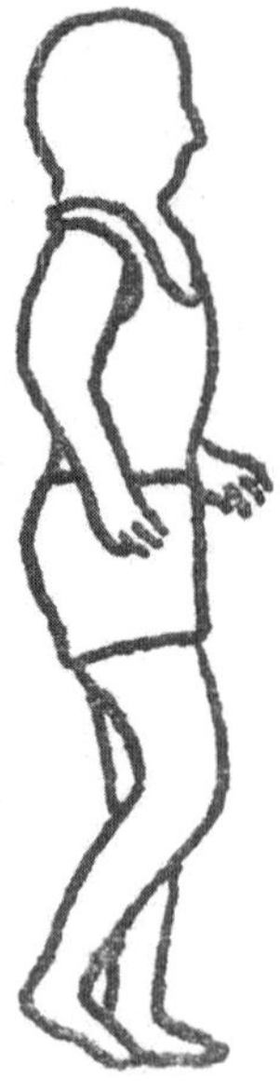

Fig. 5.49: Mid swing

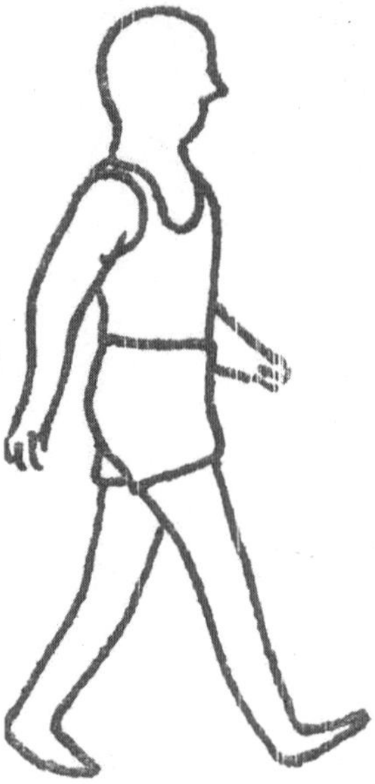

Fig. 5.50: Deceleration

EHL and EDL show the greater activity than the tibialis anterior (according to the electromyography studies).

Following heel strike the above three dorsiflexors of ankle joint relax in a contracted manner or eccentrically and allow the whole sole of foot to make contact with the ground or floor (foot flat) without slapping. During heel strike the ankle joint remains in neutral position and after that it goes into the plantar flexion and by the time the sole makes contacts with the floor 15° of plantar flexion may be measured (Fig. 5.51).

Mid Stance—The dorsiflexors become inactive and the plantar flexors (gastrocnemius, soleus, tibialis posterior, flexor digitorum longus) start contracting and the activity of plantar flexors continues beyond the point of mid stance. During end of mid stance the ankle joint remains approximately two to three degrees in dorsiflexion.

Push Off—In mid stance the plantar flexors contract eccentrically; from mid stance to heel off, plantar flexors of ankle joint contract concentrically while the flexors of toes contract eccentrically.

The Knee Joint

At heel strike the quadriceps (knee extensors) contract eccentrically in order to control the knee joint as it moves from complete extension to position of 15° to 20° of flexion.

At the point of heel strike the knee joint remains straight which is controlled by quadriceps. From heel strike to foot flat, the quadriceps contract eccentrically and allow the knee joint to flex from 0° to 15–20° of flexion. The nature of the contraction as soon as the whole foot approaches to the ground changes and quadriceps muscles contract concentrically which allows the knee joint to extend from 15°–20° to full extension.

The Hip Joint

At the heel strike the contraction of gluteus maximus and hamstrings resist the moment of force that tends to flex the hip joint following heel strike. Concentric contraction of these muscles extend the hip joint at the heel strike. The erector spinae muscle also contracts to resist the tendency of the trunk to go into forward flexion. Abductors of the hip stabilize the hip joint during mid stance and prevent the pelvis to drop to the opposite side.

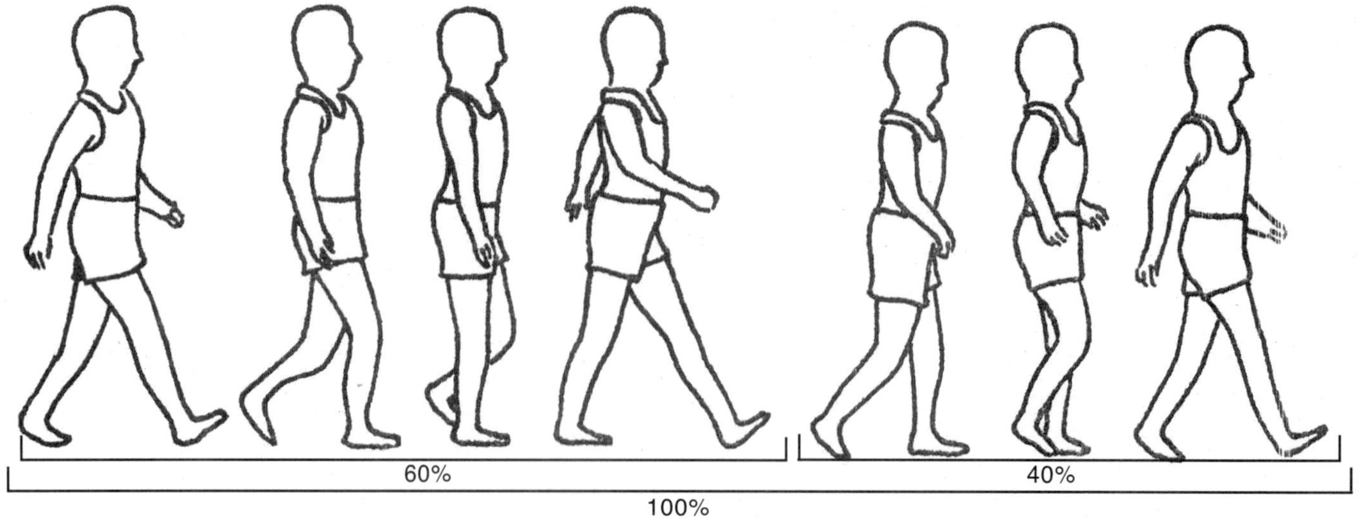

Fig. 5.51: The distribution of time in percentage spends during one gait cycle (Stance = 60%) (Swing = 40%)

Muscular Activity During Swing Phase

The Ankle

As soon as the toes leave the ground the dorsiflexors start contracting to bring the ankle joint from plantar flexion to neutral position and prevent the toes from dragging on the floor. The dorsiflexors keep contracting from acceleration to the end of swing phase (Table 5.2).

The Knee Joint

The hamstring muscles (biceps femoris–short head), gracilis and sartorius contract concentrically from acceleration to mid swing while quadriceps remain inactive and knee is flexed between 40° and 60°. After mid swing the quadriceps contract concentrically and prepare the leg for heel strike.

The Hip Joint

At the beginning of swing phase the joint remain close to the neutral position. As soon as toes leave the ground the iliacus, and psoas major muscles contract concentrically and flexes the hip joint to 25° at the time of mid swing.

General Characteristics of a Normal Gait

1. *Vertical displacement of the centre of gravity (Pelvic tilt)*—During normal walking pattern the vertical pelvic shift (pelvic tilt) keeps the centre of gravity (COG) moving rhythmically upwards and downwards. Total amount of pelvic displacement adult male rarely exceeds 50 mm. The highest vertical displacement (50 mm) occurs during the mid stance (single limb support) and lowest point occurs at the heel strike (double leg support). In patients with knee ankylosis vertical pelvic displacement increases more than 50 mm as the person requires more vertical pelvic displacement to clear the ground (Figs. 5.52a and b).
2. *Lateral pelvic shift or pelvic list (Lateral displacement of the centre of gravity)*–During normal walking the pelvis moves side to side as it is necessary to keep the body weight over the stance leg for balance. The normal lateral pelvic shift is 2.5 to 5 cm (Figs. 5.53a and b).

Table 5.2: ROM and contraction of muscles during swing phase

	Acceleration	*Mid swing*	*Deceleration*
Sub-phase of swing phase	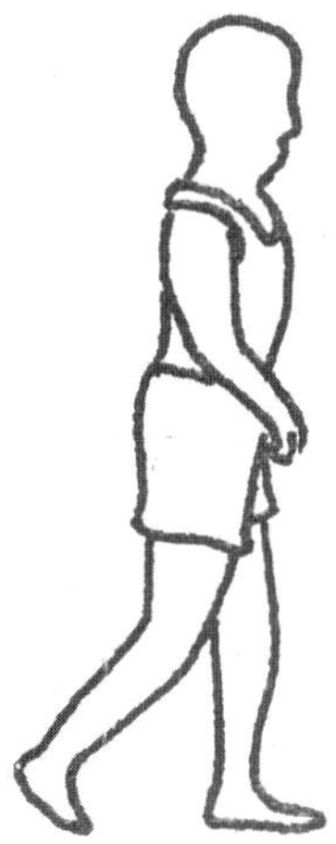	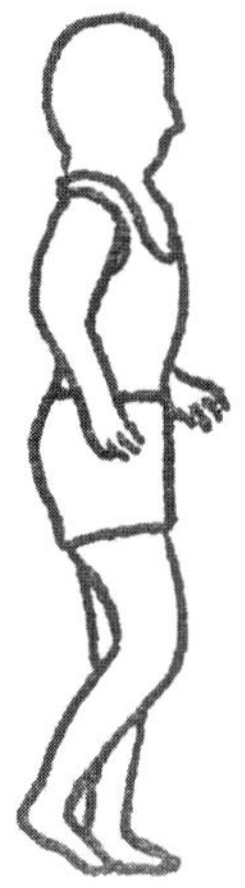	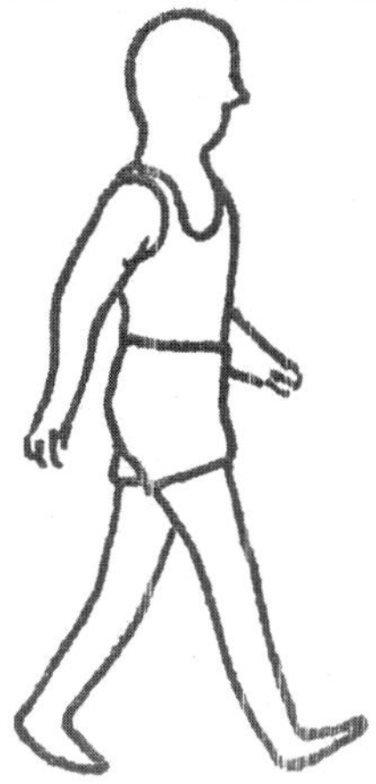
ROM of:			
– Ankle joint	10° Plantar flexion	Neutral	Neutral
– Knee joint	60° Flexion	60°–30° Flexion	Neutral
– Hip joint	20° Flexion	20°–30° Flexion	30° Flexion
– Pelvic joint	5° Backward rotation	Neutral	5° Forward rotation
– Trunk	Erect neutral	Erect neutral	Erect neutral
Contraction of muscles requires	Dorsiflexors Biceps femoris (Short head) Gracilis and sortorius	Dorsiflexors Hamstrings	Dorsiflexors Quadriceps Iliacus and Psoas major
Weakness of muscles causes	Dragging of foot (toes) Unable to flex the knee joint Unable to flex the hip joint	Dragging of foot (toes) No forward progression of leg	Dragging of foot (toes) No forward progression of leg

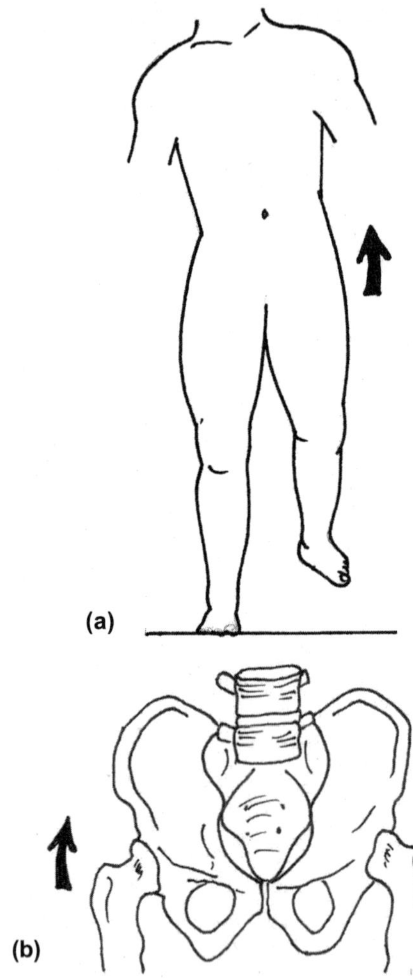

Figs. 5.52a and b: Vertical shift of pelvis

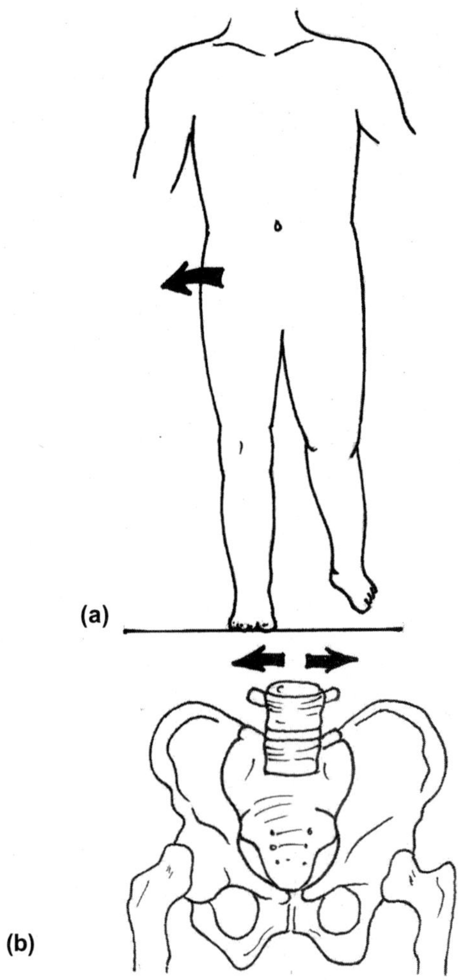

Figs. 5.53a and b: Lateral shift of pelvis

3. *Horizontal dip of the pelvis*—Anterior and posterior rotation of pelvis during gait is necessary to lessen the angle of the femur with the floor, result lengthening of the femur. It decreases the centre of gravity path amplitude of displacement and thus decreases the centre of gravity dip. 5° forward and 5° backward rotation is considered as a normal pelvic rotation during gait. To maintain the balance the thorax rotates in the opposite direction of the pelvis. Thus when the pelvis rotates clockwise, the thorax rotates counter clockwise and vice versa.
4. *Flexion of the knee joint during stance*—Immediately after heel strike knee begins flexing which is continued till it reaches to approximately 15°. This motion is coordinated with the motions at the ankle, and keeps the centre of gravity approximately at the same level for some time as it moves forward. **Knee flexion during stance phase is of special importance in minimising the vertical displacement of the centre of gravity in walking.**
5. *Cadence*—The number of steps taken per minute is known as cadence. It varies from slow walking to fast running (70 to 140 per min respectively). An average cadence for a normal adult male is considered as 90 steps per minute and he can cover four kilometer in an hour.
6. *Double support*—When both feet are simultaneously in contact with the ground it is known as double support. For example, when a stance phase commences the heel contacts (heel strike) with the ground, at the same time the toes of the contralateral limb make contact with the ground. Each gait cycle consists two double supports. Double support is a characteristic feature of normal gait when person walks. The double support decreases as the walking speed increases, and it disappears when person runs (Fig. 5.54).
7. *Single support*—It is a part of stance phase where one limb bears whole weight of the body while another

limb swings forward for preparation of stance phase without carrying weight of the body. During a gait cycle only one single support occurs (Fig. 5.55).

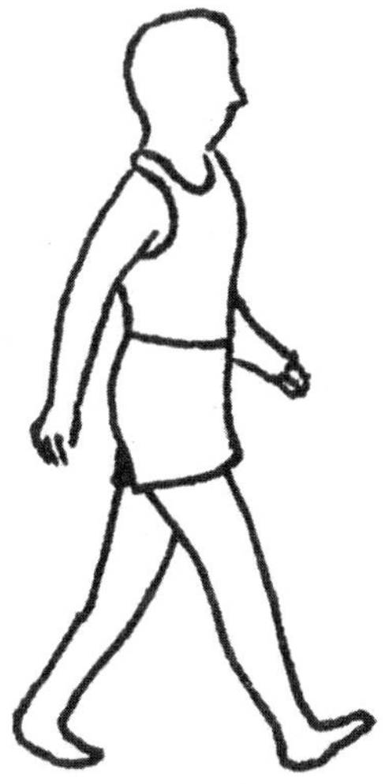

Fig. 5.54: Double support

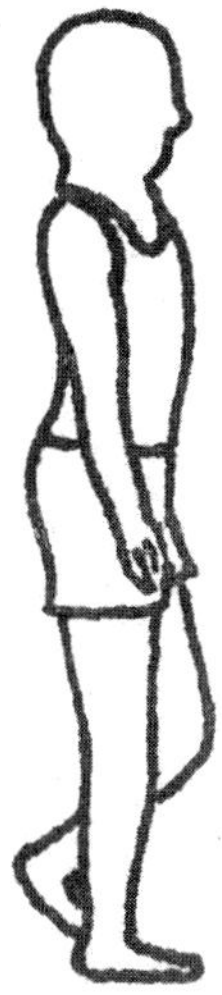

Fig. 5.55: Single support

8. *Base width*—It is the distance between the two feet when person is in erect standing posture. 5 to 10 cm distance between the feet is considered normal range of base width, more than 10 cm and below 5 cm width is considered as abnormal base width (Fig. 5.56).
9. *Step length or gait length*—It is the distance between two successive contact points. For example—the distance between right heel strike to the left heel strike is known as step length. 35 to 41 cm between two successive contact points is considered as a normal step length and should be equal for both legs. The step length varies with age and sex. Children take smaller steps than the adult, and females take smaller steps than males (Fig. 5.57).
10. *Stride length*—It is the linear distance in the plane of progression between two successive points of the same foot. (For example—the distance between two successive right heel strikes is known as stride length). Between 70 and 82 cm length between two successive points of the same foot is considered as a normal stride length. 70-82 cm covers one gait cycle. (Stride length = one gait cycle) (Fig. 5.58).

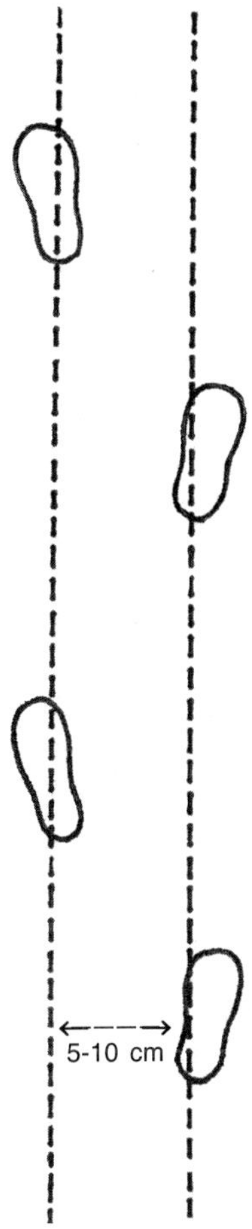

Fig. 5.56: Base width

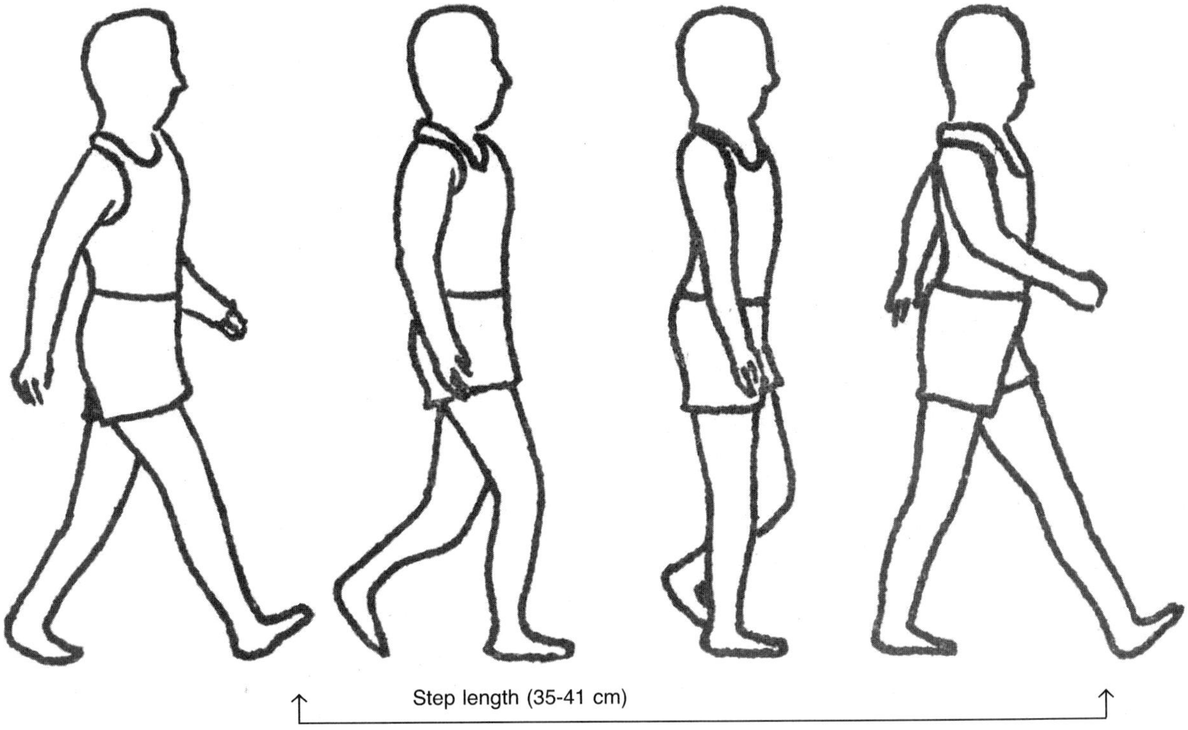

Fig. 5.57: Step length or gait length—distance between two successive points (right heel strike to the left heel strike)

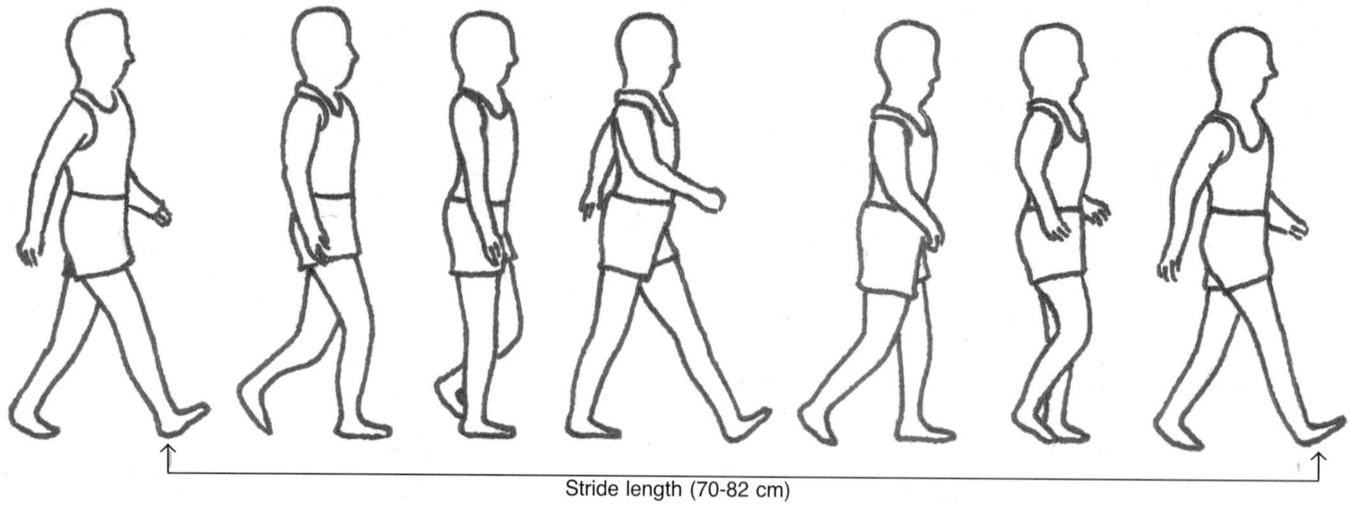

Fig. 5.58: Stride length (Gait cycle)—distance between right heel strike to the next right heel strike

Pathological Gait or Abnormal Human Locomotion

1. *Trendelenburg gait or Lateral trunk bending*—During mid stance the gluteus medius and minimus of the weight bearing side contract eccentrically to prevent the displacement of pelvis (drop of the contralateral pelvis. Weakness or inadequate contraction of the gluteus medius and minimus causes inability to stabilise the pelvis on femur, as a result contralateral pelvis drops, this does not allow the swing leg to clear the ground. Therefore person leans or bends the trunk toward the side of weakness which minimizes the external torque (hip abduction force) demand due to body weight on the abductor muscles of the stance leg.

When an individual has one side hip abductors weakness then he or she bends the trunk only toward the involved side during stance phase. Weakness of one side hip abductors is known as Trendelenburg sign.

If both sides of hip abductors are weak then an individual leans the trunk on both sides alternately which is called as waddling gait (Figs. 5.59a and b).

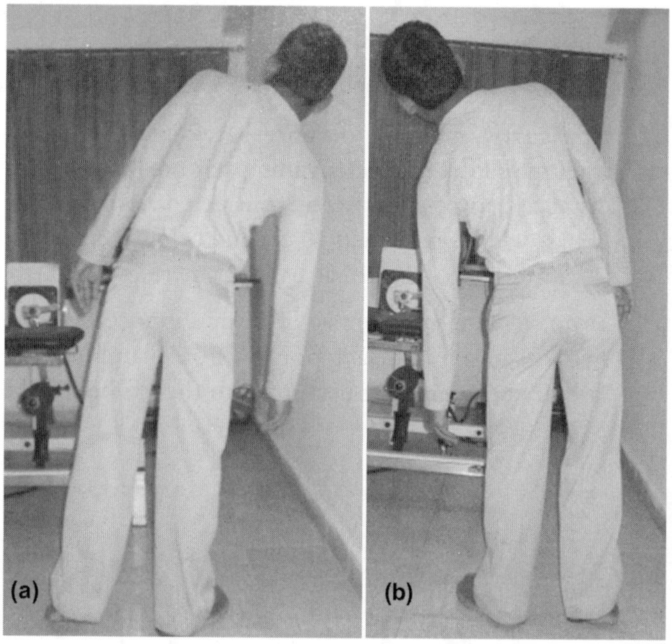

Figs. 5.59a and b: Waddling gait

Other possible causes of lateral trunk bending:

1. Hip dislocation, coxa vara and slipped capital femoral epiphysis.
2. Hip pain.
3. Involved limb relatively shorter-hip or knee flexion contracture.
4. Compensation for abducted gait.

2. *Circumductory gait*—Commonly seen in hemiplegic patients. Spasticity, decreased voluntary control, abnormal reflexes and abnormal synergy pattern are the common neurological manifestation of post cerebrovascular accident (CVA), which predispose the patient to circumductory gait. During swing phase normal person requires 30°-60° of knee flexion and 20°-30° of hip flexion while ankle joint remains in the neutral position. These movements allow the leg to swing forward. In hemiplegia no flexion occurs at the hip and knee joint and ankle joint remains plantar flexed which causes the limb to lengthen and patient finds difficult to swing the leg forward. To overcome this problem patient contracts the quadratus lumborum resulting in hip hiking which thrusts the limb in a circumductory manner and limb swings forward with or without dragging of the toes. Though hip hiking shortens the limb, still limb is longer and cannot swing beneath the body hence the patient

circumducts (pendular movement) the limb which further shortens the limb and swings it (Figs. 5.60a to e).

3. *Hip hiking*—Like circumductory gait patient contracts the quadratus lumborum of the affected side with lateral abdominals which causes hiking of the hip joint. Hiking swings the involved limb by increasing the rotation of the pelvis in the horizontal plane.

Possible causes of hip hiking:

- The involved limb either is relatively longer or cannot be shortened/flexed during swing phase:
  - Hip flexor weakness.
  - Extensor spasticity.
  - Mechanical lock at the hip joint.
  - Knee ankylosis.
  - Weakness of dorsiflexors.
- Shortening of contralateral limb (stance limb):
  - Hip or knee flexion contracture skeletal shortening.
  - Hamstrings weakness.

4. *Posterior trunk bending*—Weakness of hip extensors. Insufficient concentric contraction of gluteus maximus causes inability to extend the hip joint during stance phase. Therefore patient bends the trunk posteriorly causing extension at the hip joint (Fig. 5.61).

Sometimes patient places his or her hand over the gluteus maximus and pushes the buttock anteriorly which causes extension at the hip joint and trunk

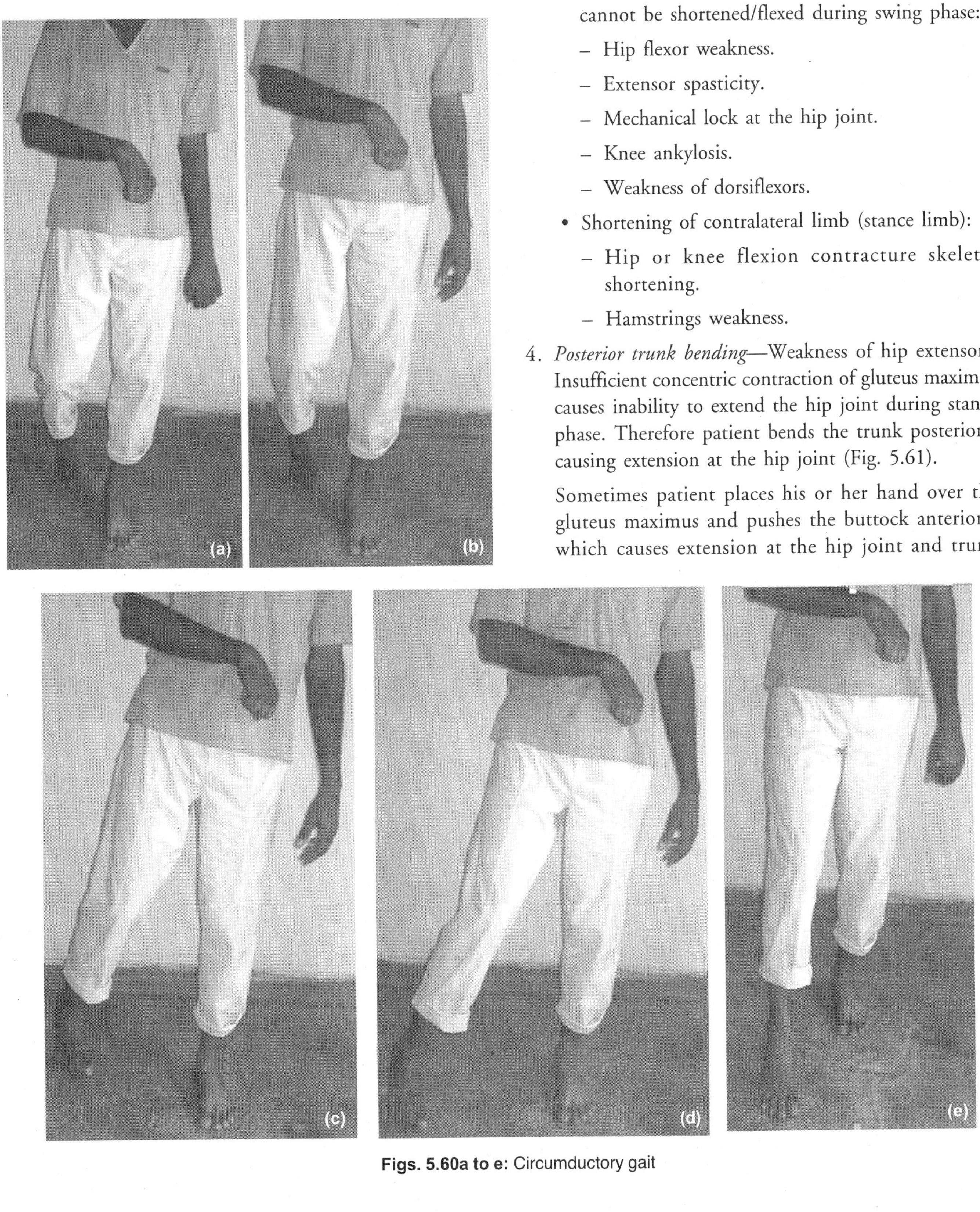

Figs. 5.60a to e: Circumductory gait

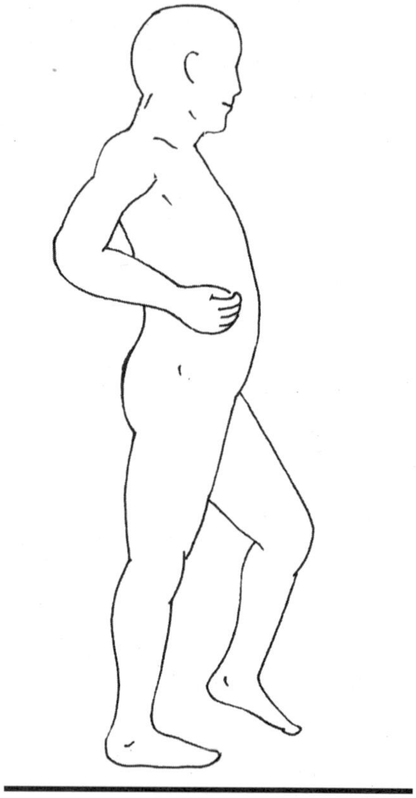

Fig. 5.61: Posterior trunk bending (Gluteus maximus gait)

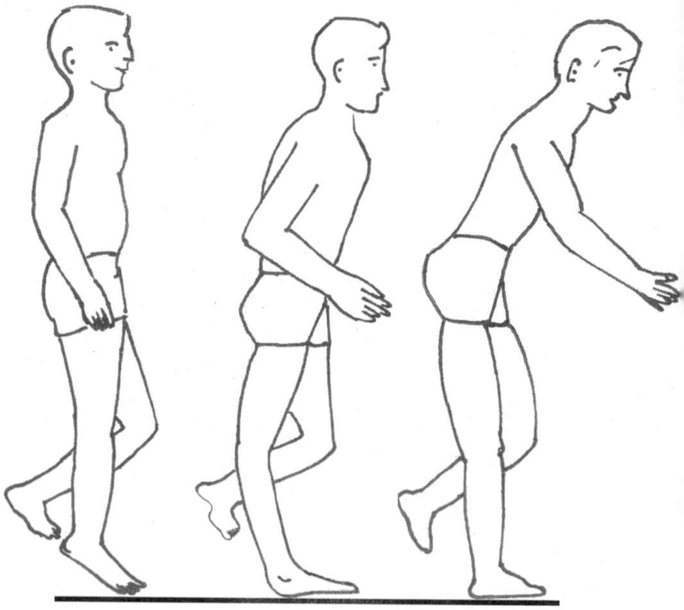

Fig. 5.62: Hyperextended knee (anterior trunk bending)

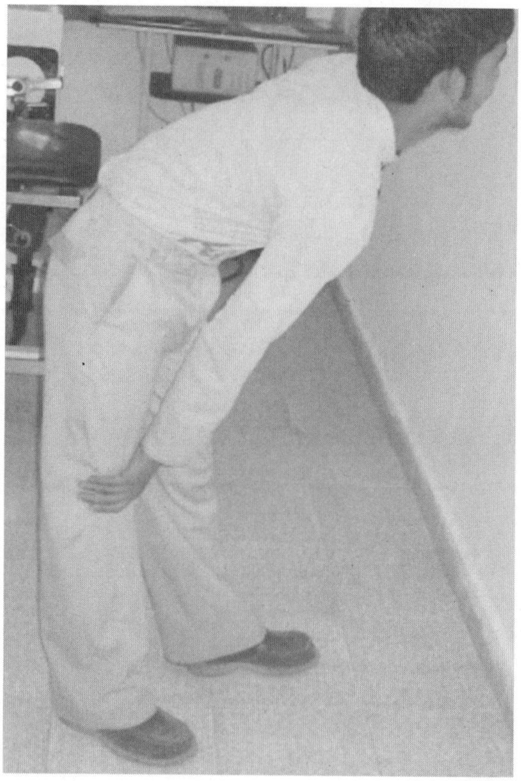

Fig. 5.63: Hand to knee gait

automatically bends posteriorly which is known as Jack knife gait.

5. *Anterior trunk bending*—Commonly seen in post polio residual paralysis (PPRP) in which paralysis of quadriceps is combined with weakness of gluteus maximus or gastrosoleus or both. During stance phase due to weakness of these muscles knee joint buckels. To avoid buckling patient bends the trunk anteriorly which places the centre of gravity anterior to the knee joint and prevents buckling of the knee joint during stance phase (Fig. 5.62).

   Some patients place their hand just above the knee joint, and walk with anterior trunk bending which is known as hand to knee gait (Fig. 5.63).

6. *Hyperextended knee*—Generally patient cannot walk if his quadriceps are zero (paralysed) without stabilising the knee joint by an external support or orthosis. But patient can walk without using an external stabilisers of the knee joint if his gluteus maximus and gastrosoleus are strong. The larger proximal portion and superficial fibres of distal portion of gluteus maximus muscle inserts into iliotibial tract of fascia lata. Deep fibres of distal portion insert into gluteal tuberosity of femur. The portion of gluteus maximus muscle which inserts into iliotibial band contract concentrically and pulls the femur posteriorly which creates extension moment arm (knee goes behind the centre of gravity). This action of gluteus maximus prevents buckling of knee joint during the stance phase and patient can walk without hand to knee. The gastrosoleus also do the same function (pull the tibia behind the centre of gravity which causes hyper-extension of the knee joint and prevent the buckling

of knee joint). If patient walks frequently with this gait after some time he develops genurecurvatum (Fig. 5.62).

Some patients also prefer to walk by creating equinus at ankle. Due to which the line of gravity (LOG) shifts anteriorly to the knee joint, causing increased extensor moment at the knee joint. This extensor moment is helpful in extending knee in spite of absent or weak quadriceps. In the beginning this equinus is flexible but later on it becomes a fixed deformity.

Some patients want to get this equinus corrected surgically. But surgery should be done cautiously, as correcting the deformity would definitely affect the functional performance (due to decrease in extensor moment at knee) of the patient. It is recommended not to achieve cosmetic outcome at the expense of functional one.

7. *Foot drop gait*—In normal human locomotion the ankle joint remains at neutral position through swing phase which is maintained by the contraction of dorsiflexors. Weakness of dorsiflexors prevents the patient from keeping the ankle joint in neutral position resulting into plantar flexion and toes drag during swing phase. To get rid of this problem patient flexes the hip joint beyond 30° and then strikes the ground with the toes (Fig. 5.64). This results in toe to heel pattern instead of normal heel to toe pattern.

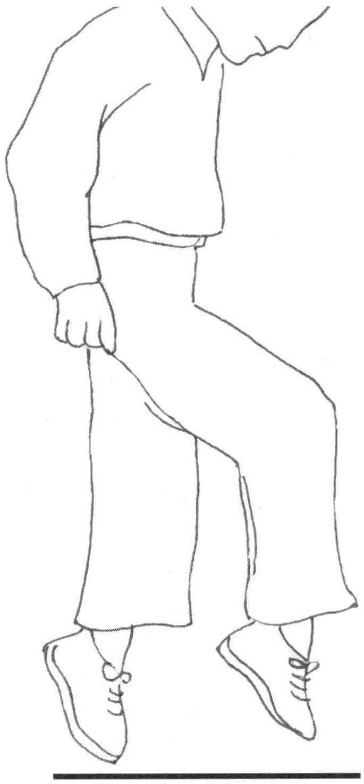

Fig. 5.64: Foot drop

8. *Calcaneal gait*—From foot flat to the end of stance phase plantar flexors (gastrosoleus, flexor digitorum longus and brevis, and flexor hallucis longus) contract and push the ground by foot which results in heel off. Insufficient contraction of plantar flexors causes muscular imbalance and ankle joint goes into dorsiflexion, forefoot does not make contact with the ground and whole weight of body is transferred only on the heel (calcaneum) during the stance phase so gait is known as calcaneal gait (Fig. 5.65).

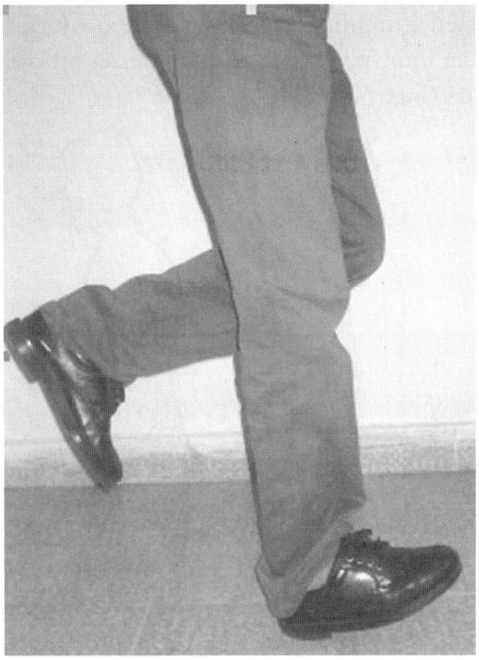

Fig. 5.65: Calcaneal

Other common causes of calcaneal gait:

- Rupture of the Achilles tendon or hammer toe.
- Pes calcaneus or pes varus or pes valgus.
- Metatarsalgia.
- Orthosis plantar stop.

9. *Vaulting*—The patient bobs up and down excessively as he walks, increasing the vertical displacement of centre of gravity by exaggerating plantar flexion of the contralateral ankle.

Possible causes:

- In all cases the involved limb is relatively longer:
  - Hip flexors weakness.
  - Ankylosis of hip in extension.
  - Extensor synergy.
  - Mechanical lock of hip joint.
  - Ankylosis of knee joint.
- Hamstring weakness in slow walking.

10. *Flexed knee gait*—Flexion contracture of the hamstring muscles does not allow the knee joint to extend during locomotion. Normally when heel strikes the ground, both knee joints remain fully extended. In knee flexion contracture as the heel strikes the ground the knee joint remains flexed which also deliberately forces the contralateral knee (normal knee) to flex at the same time and both knees during heel strike look flexed. The gait is characterised by flexion of the knees and excessive dorsiflexion during the late swing of the affected extremity which is followed by early stance on the uninvolved side and early heel off during mid stance (Fig. 5.66).

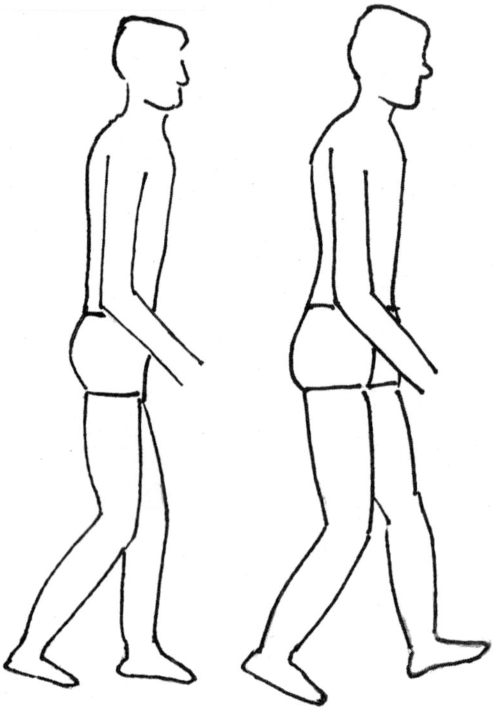

Fig. 5.66: Flexed knee gait

11. *Spastic diplegia gait*—The gait is characterised by excessive flexion at hip and knee joints during stance phase without significant heel strike. Child walks on forefeet.

12. *Lordotic gait*—Contracture of hip flexors can cause increase in lumbar lordotic curve during the stance phase. Normally after heel strike the hip joint goes into extension (from 30° flexion to 20° extension). The contracture does not allow hip joint to extend. Therefore, in stance phase if the hip joint remains flexed, the center of gravity moves anterior to the hip joint. The patient hyperextends lumbar spine to retain his head over his pelvis. This lordosis also increases the posterior excursion of the limb to permit a long stride (Fig. 5.67).

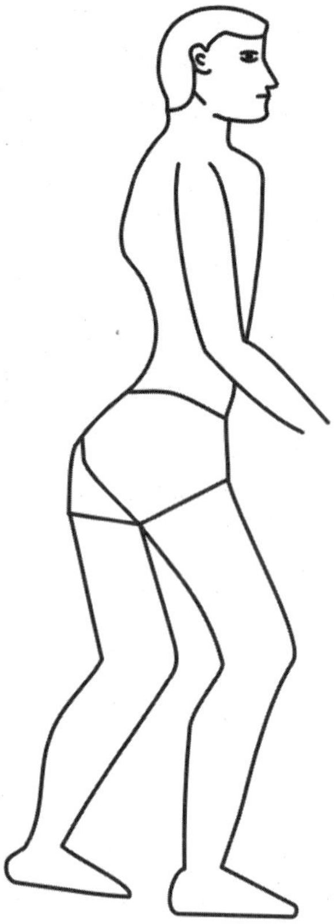

Fig. 5.67: Lordotic gait

Other possible causes:

- Weak hip extensors (posterior trunk bending).
- Weak abdominal wall.

12. *Antalgic gait*—It is also known as painful gait. During stance phase, to avoid pain patient attempts to remove weight from the affected leg as quickly as possible that results in short stance phase. Patient may also support affected limb with the same side's hand while opposite arm acts as a counter balance and is outstretched.

The patients with painful hip, bends the trunk toward the same side which minimises the external torque (hip abductors force) demand due to body weight on the painful side of the stance leg.

13. *Wide base gait (Ataxic gait)*—The patients with cerebellar ataxia have poor balance so they walks with broad base, and therefore lurche, stagger and exaggerate all movements (Fig. 5.68).

14. *Scissors gait*—Spasticity in the adductors of both hip joints causes great difficulty in swinging the leg forward. In swing phase, the non-weight bearing leg crosses the midline, draws the knees together and progresses forward by touching the middle thigh of the contralateral leg hence, both legs look like a pair of scissors (Fig. 5.69).

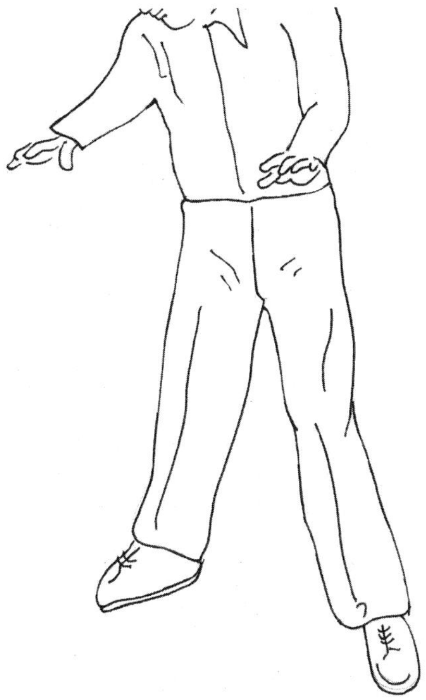

Fig. 5.68: Wide base gait (Ataxic gait)

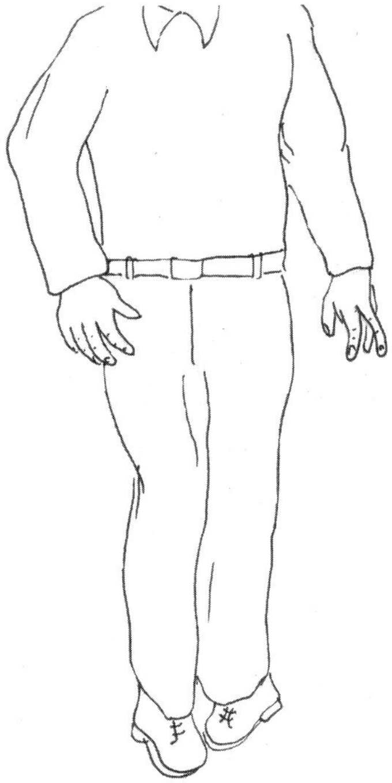

Fig. 5.69: Scissors gait

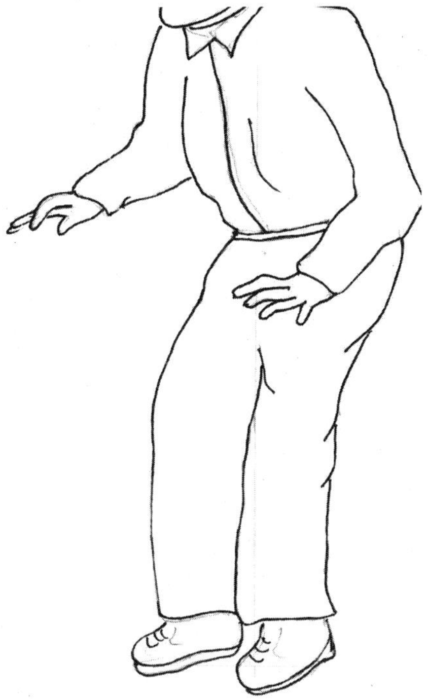

Fig. 5.70: Parkinson's gait

15. *Parkinson's gait (Shuffling in short step, festination gait)*—The gait Parkinsonism is highly stereotyped and characterised by an impoverishment of movement. Decreased generalised extension of lower limb joints (hip, knee and ankle), trunk and pelvic motions. So patient walks with flexed trunk, hip, knee and ankle joints with small steps. Persistent posturing of a forward head and trunk typically displaces the patient's center of gravity forward. The patient takes multiple short steps in order to avoid falling forward and eventually breaks into a run and looks like he is running to catch the center of gravity (Fig. 5.70).

Assessment of Gait

Impairment and disability in the broad context encompass physical, mental and social functions. Walking is largely a physical function. Gait assessment may not make a diagnosis but it helps to determine physical impairment deviation from normal. It has diagnostic value when it is combined and related with results from other clinical tests and the clinical examination, such as passive and active range of motion, muscle strength, muscle spasm, pain, tenderness, and sensory and motor functions.

Following movements should be observed carefully:

Head : Movement of head to right side during mid stance on the right foot.

Arm : Lateral arm swing to the left during entire stance phase on the right foot.

Trunk : Lateral movement of the trunk to the right during mid and late stance on the right foot.

Pelvis : Lateral movement of the pelvis to the right during mid stance on the right foot.

Hip : Adduction of hip during mid stance bilaterally. The opposite limb swings with 20° to 30° flexion during acceleration and mid swing.

Knee : Extension of knee during heel strike, 15° of flexion at foot flat and remain in extension in rest of stance phase. The opposite leg swings with 60°-30° flexion during acceleration and mid swing and neutral in deceleration.

Ankle : Neutral during heel strike and 15° of plantar flexion at foot flat.

General Energetic Consideration on Gait

The important energy-saving mechanism in walking is the transformation of kinetic into potential energy and vice versa. During each stride the transformation of both energies in each other is estimated to comprise 50% to 70% of the energy demand in walking at moderate speed. Muscular work required to cause energy transformation can reduce the mechanical efficiency of walking. The negative muscle work (eccentric contraction) often reduces the kinetic translation and rotational energy.

WALKING AIDS

INTRODUCTION

Crutch walking is a highly developed art which can be improved by training and practice. All the benefits of this art is similar to that of other therapeutic exercises. This aids not only make the subject independent in walking but also act as a type of exercise for them to improve their cardiovascular, pulmonary, renal and musculoskeletal system.

In essence a crutch or a cane is an extension of the upper extremity used to provide support, balance and weight bearing normally provided by an intact functioning of lower limb. One crutch (modulate or total loss) or one cane (little loss) should be prescribed for unilateral impairment (pain, weakness etc.) but clinically one crutch is rarely used.

Walking aids are assistive devices used for supportive walking. They are broadly divided into three categories:

i. Canes/walking sticks.
ii. Crutches.
iii. Walkers.

Indications

- Poor balance.
- Weakness of lower extremity muscles.
- Pain in weight bearing joints of the lower extremities.
- Joint instability.
- Fatigue.

Mechanism of Action

Walking aids eliminate weight bearing fully or partially from lower extremity. The unloading of the lower extremity is possible by transmission of weight bearing forces from the upper extremity to the ground by downward pressure on the aid.

I. CANES OR WALKING STICKS

Canes or walking sticks are used to increase base of support (Fig. 5.71a). These are used by holding in the hand opposite to affected lower extremity. The subject walks in a reciprocal gait pattern by moving the cane and affected leg together. Holding stick in contralateral upper extremity causes less later shift of centre of gravity. It reduces joint reaction force of abductor muscles at hip joint, therefore, it is important to hold the cane opposite to affected lower extremity. The implication of this concept is more in hip disorders such as arthroplasty, arthritis etc.

Standard Cane/Walking Stick

Conventionally it was made of wood, but now-a-days mainly of aluminium and has a half circle handle. It is a single piece with a distal rubber tip of approximately 1 inch in diameter. The handle may be covered by moulded rubber or plastic coating or wood (Figs. 5.71b and c). It is one of most light weighted and easy to carry assistive device for walking. The only disadvantage of this is that it is not adjustable and must be cut to fit the patient. Its point of support is anterior to hand and not directly beneath it.

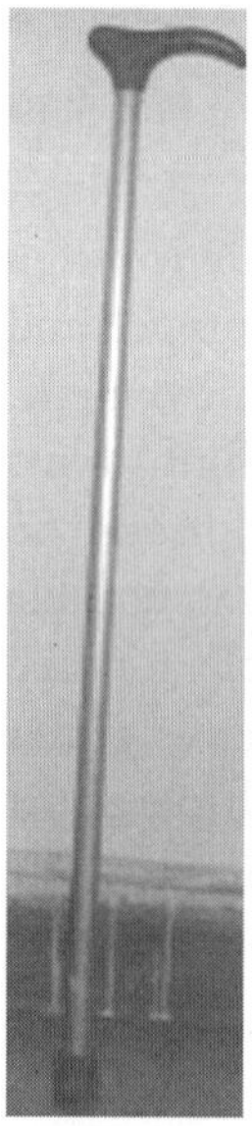

Fig. 5.71a: Walking stick

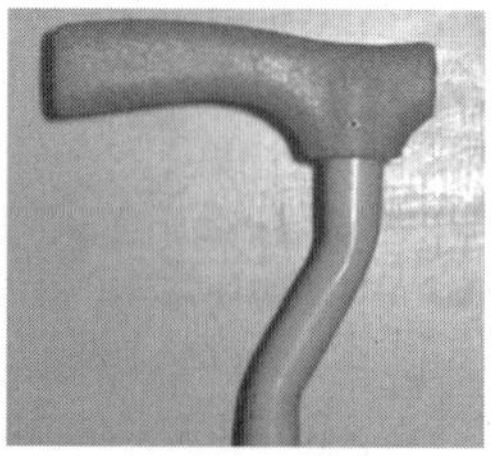

Fig. 5.71b: Hand grip with plastic coating

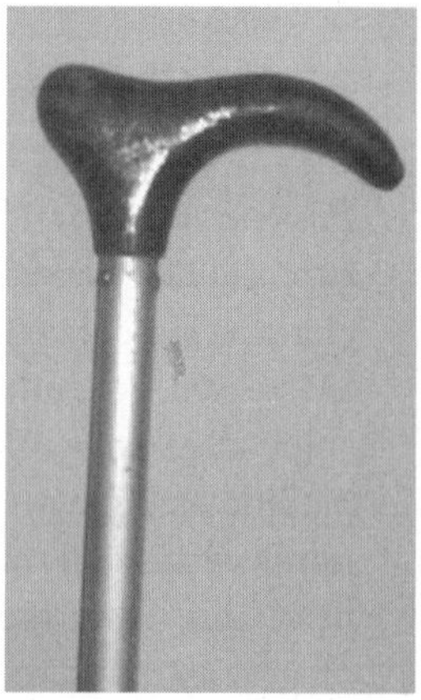

Fig. 5.71c: Wooden hand grip of a walking stick

Standard Adjustable Aluminium Cane/Stick

It has the same basic design as of the regular standard cane. It can be adjusted within the range of approximately 10 inches. It uses push button to alter height which can further be reinforced by a plastic metallic ring. Sometimes at this point the cane shows instability and make clicking sound during weight support, which does not give the feeling of adequate support to the user.

Offset Cane/Walking Stick

The proximal component of the body of the stick is offset anteriorly. This design allows weight to be borne over the center of the cane for greater stability. Most of them are adjustable and more costlier than standard cane.

Quadruped Cane or Walking Stick

The characteristic feature of this cane is that they have four points (legs) floor contact which gives broad base of support (Figs. 5.72a to c). All other aspects are same as in above-mentioned sticks. They may also be non-adjustable, adjustable or 3-points (legs)–Tripod (Fig. 5.72d).

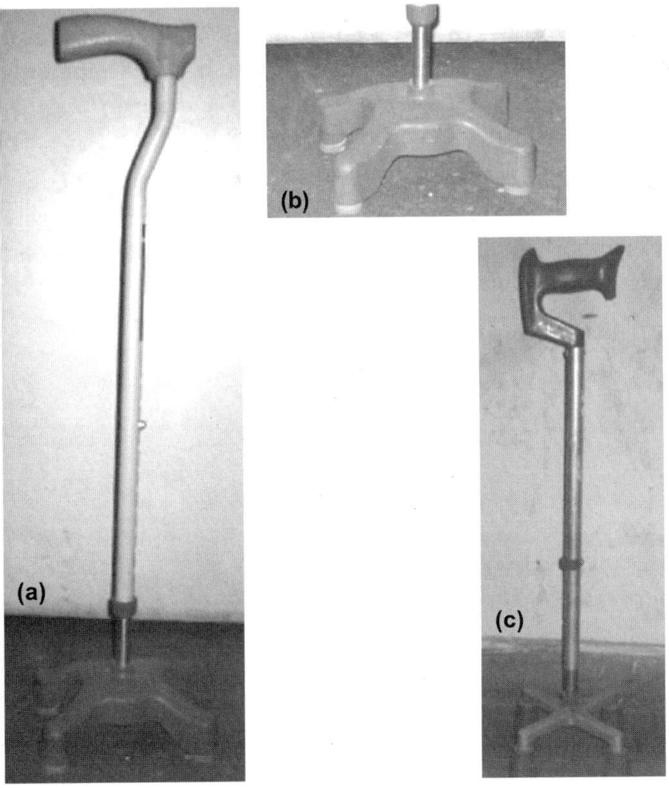

Figs. 5.72a to c: (a) Quadruped, (b) Base of quadruped, and (c) A small size quadruped

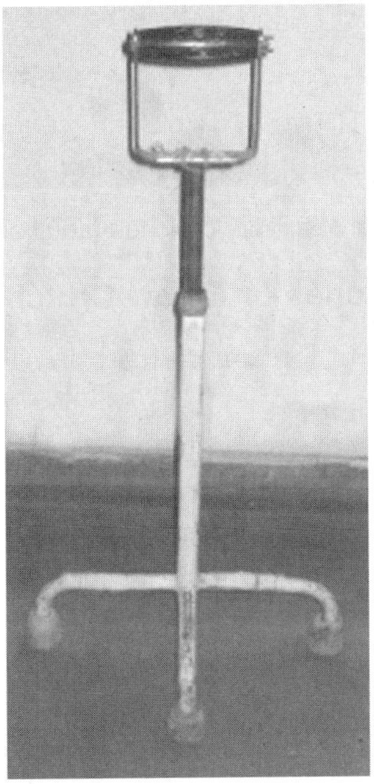

Fig. 5.72d: A tripod

These canes are not practical for stair activity because of broader base which cannot be adjusted on stair steps. Further the walking speed with this cane is slower as compared with others, as during walking the patient has to pick stick fully and place it back on the floor in such a manner that all its legs touches the floor simultaneously. Otherwise it would rock from rear legs to front leg and stability would be compromised.

They are also much costlier than other mentioned canes.

Other Considerations About Canes

- Measurement.
- Gait patterns.

Measurements for Canes

i. The cane should be placed approximately 6 inches from the lateral border of the toes.

ii. Take measurement for height of cane from greater trochanter of femur to the floor or from the hand (in gripping position) with elbow flexed to about 20° to 30° degrees to the floor.

   This is a more important indicator of correct cane height because of individual variation in body proportion and arm length.

iii. The cane should be assessed for client's comfort (Fig. 5.73).

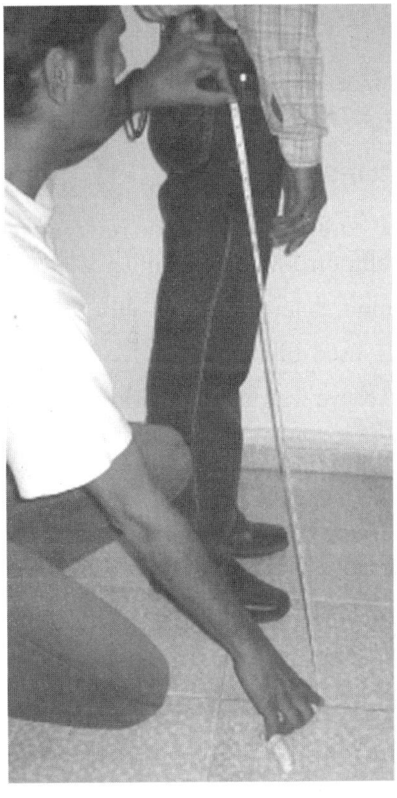

Fig. 5.73: Measurement for cane

Gait Pattern for Use of Canes

i. The cane should be close to the body (not to be placed ahead of the toe).

   As placing the cane far might cause threat to dynamic stability of the user.

ii. Gait pattern should be followed as shown in Figures 5.74a and b.
   - For bilateral involvement, the cane should be used on the side of comfort.
   - Or even two canes can be used in case more stability is required.

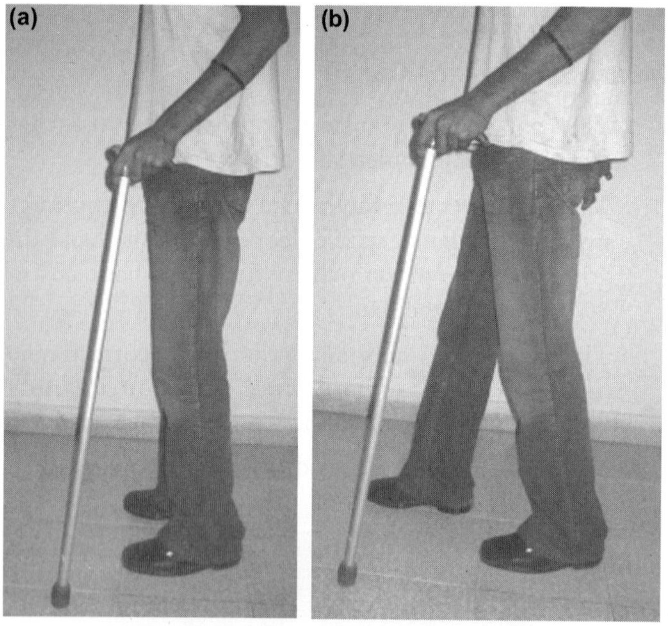

Figs. 5.74a and b: Gait pattern for cane use

II. CRUTCHES

Crutches are commonly used to relieve weight either partially or fully on lower extremities.

The common characteristics of this assistive device are:

i. Typically used bilaterally.
ii. Used to relieve weight either partially or fully on lower extremities.
iii. Used to improve balance.
iv. Increase the base of support.
v. Improve lateral stability.
vi. Allow upper extremity to transfer weight to the floor.
vi. The two commonly used types are: axillary and forearm or elbow crutches.

Axillary Crutches

These are regular crutches conventionally made of wood but now aluminium is the material of choice. The components of a standard axillary crutches are:

a. An axillary bar.
b. A hand piece.
c. Double upright joined distally by a single leg.
d. Rubber suction tip.

Most of crutches are adjustable at hand piece and at single leg to cater larger group of clients. In India commonly available in three sizes large, medium and small, wooden are quite cheaper than aluminium type.

Disadvantage of axillary crutches—Axillary crutches are difficult to use in crowded areas as they require larger base of support. They can cause compression of nervous and vascular structure in axilla if used improperly (Fig. 5.75).

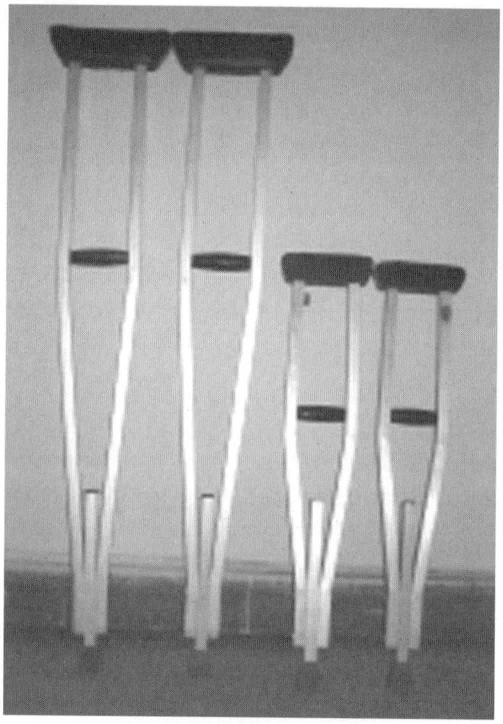

Fig. 5.75: Pair of axillary crutches (adult and small size)

Forearm Crutches or Elbow Crutches

The component of forearm crutches are (Figs. 5.76a to d):

a. A single upright.
b. A forearm cuff.
c. A hand grip.

The crutch is adjustable both proximally and distally to adjust the forearm cuff and height of crutch respectively.

They are also available in three different sizes as axillary crutch.

Significance of forearm cuff—it allows use of hands without the crutches becoming disengaged. The forearm

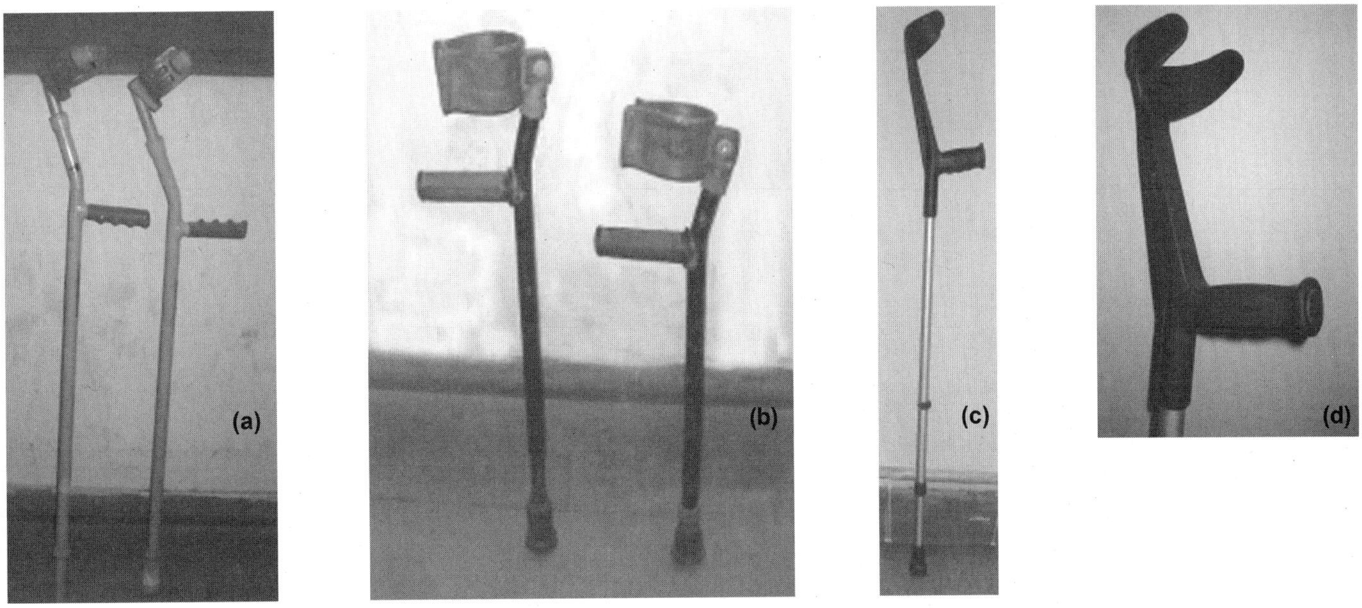

Figs. 5.76a to d: (a) A pair of adult elbow crutch, (b) A pair of small elbow crutch, (c) Elbow crutch without elbow strap and (d) Forearm part of elbow crutch without elbow strap

crutches are more practical to use on stairs, in buses/cars etc. Because of their smaller size client feels more comfortable with this type of crutch as compared to axillary crutch but they provide less lateral support due to absence of an axillary bar.

Other Consideration for Crutches

- Measurement.
- Gait patterns.

Measurement for Axillary Crutch

Measurement for axillary crutch can be done in any of the two positions, i.e., standing or supine. In standing position measurement is taken from 2 inches below the axilla to the point on floor 2 inches lateral and 6 inches anterior to the foot (Fig. 5.77).

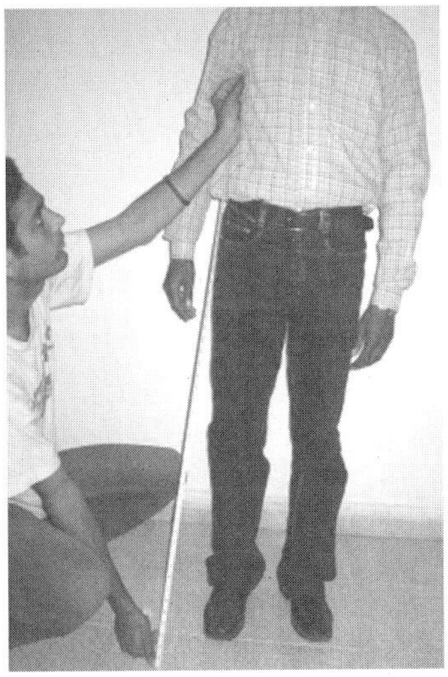

Fig. 5.77: Measurement for axillary crutch

In supine measurements are taken from axillary fold to a point on plinth 6 to 8 inches lateral to the heel.

Generally 16 inches may be subtracted from body height to measure crutch height. Hand grips can be adjusted by flexing the elbow at 20 to 30° of flexion.

Measurement for Forearm Crutches

Standing position in walker or parallel bar is preferred position for taking measurement. Measurements are taken from greater trochanter to a point on the floor 2 inches lateral and 6 inches anterior to the foot. Hand grip position can further be checked by creating 20-30 degree of elbow flexion. Cuff should be positioned approximately 2 to 1.5 inches below the elbow (Fig. 5.78).

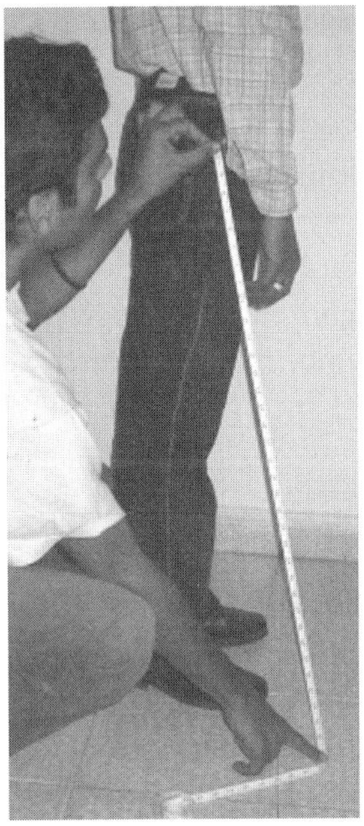

Fig. 5.78: Measurement for elbow crutch

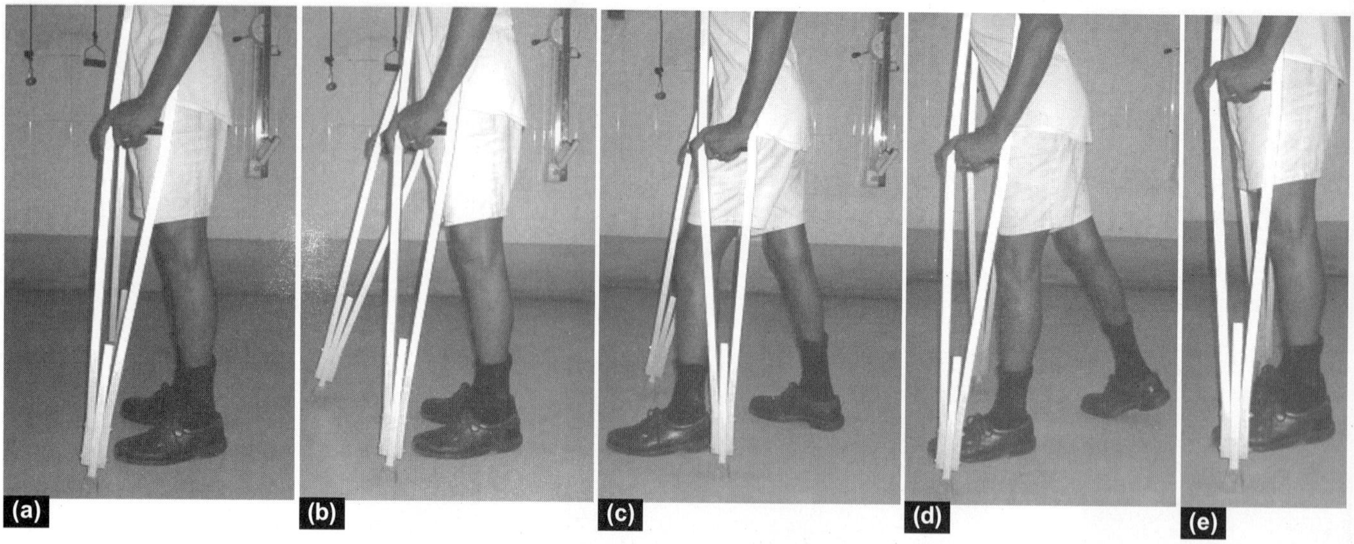

Figs. 5.79a to e: Four-point gait

General Instructions to Patient for Crutch Use:

1. In axillary crutches—Weight should be borne on the hands and not on the axillary bar to prevent pressure on vascular and neural structures. Axillary bars should be held near chest wall to improve lateral stability.
2. The patient should use maximum possible wide base of support (BOS) by keeping crutches at least 4 inches anterior and lateral to the foot.
3. The patient should maintain good posture while using crutch.

Gait Pattern for Crutch Use

Typically there are six gait patterns for crutch use which depends upon the patient's weight bearing condition, muscle strength, balance and coordination. All these gait patterns are different in terms of speed, base of support and energy requirement.

Four-point gait—In this gait weight is borne on four points (two crutches and both extremities). One crutch is placed forward which is followed by contralateral limb, then opposite crutch is placed forward and is followed by contralateral limb. For example—right crutch is progressed forward which is followed by left limb, then left crutch is progressed forward and is followed by right limb (Figs. 5.79a to e).

Two-point gait—Like four-point gait weight is borne on both crutches and lower limbs. In four points, progression of cructhes and limbs is one by one, but in two-point one crutch and opposite limb are progressed together. For example—right crutch and left limb is progressed forward together, and weight is taken/borne on these two (right crutch and left limb) then left crutch and right limb is progressed forward. Two-point gait is more faster than the four-point gait (Fig. 5.80).

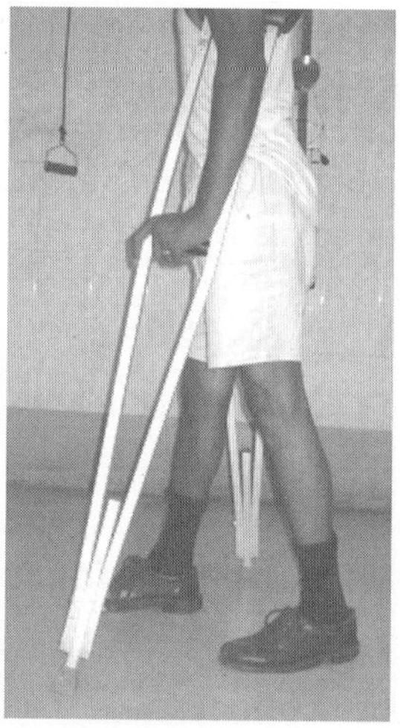

Fig. 5.80: Two-point gait

Three-point gait—In this gait both crutches are progressed forward weight is taken on these both crutches and then unaffected extremity is placed between the crutches or slightly forward. The affected extremity remain flexed at hip and knee joint and does not bear weight of the body. In the next step of this gait weight is taken on the unaffected extremity and both crutches are progressed forward (Figs. 5.81a and b).

Partial weight bearing gait—Like three-point gait two axillary

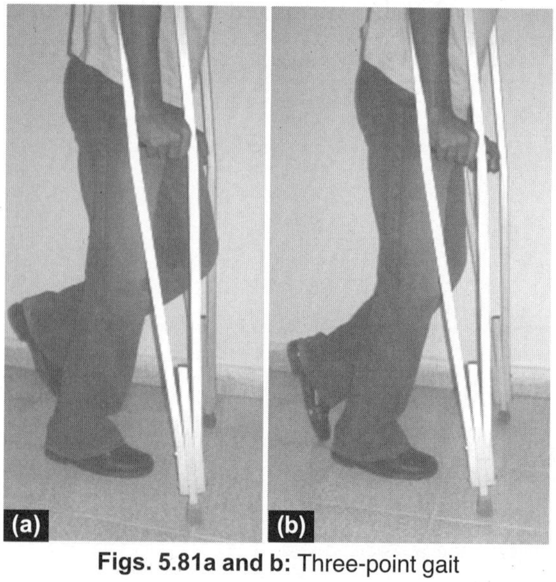

Figs. 5.81a and b: Three-point gait

crutches are used. Both crutches are placed forward with proper base of support then the affected limb is placed in the same line of the crutches. After placing the affected limb between the crutches the normal leg is placed forward to the crutches, with mild to moderate weight (light weight) bearing on affected leg (Figs. 5.82a and b).

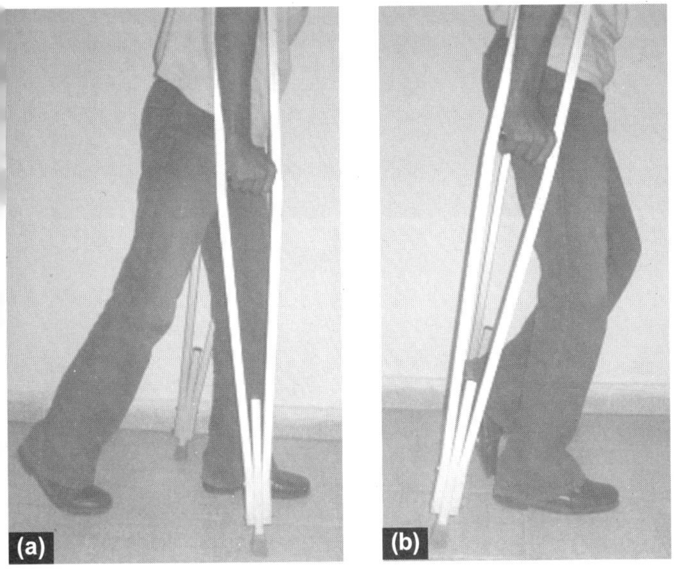

Figs. 5.82a and b: Partial weight bearing gait

Swing To and Swing Through

These gait patterns are commonly used by paraplegic patients (usually with lower extremity orthosis). In swing to both crutches are placed forward then both extremities swing with or without dragging of the feet which do not go beyond the crutches (Figs. 5.83a to c).

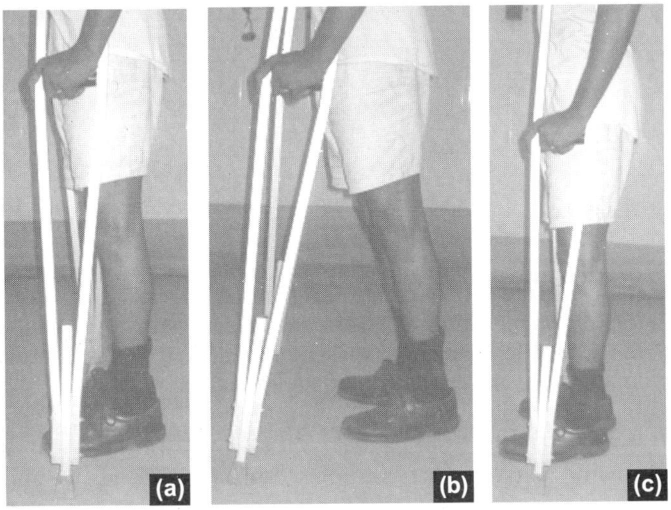

Figs. 5.83a to c: Swing to gait

In swing through, like swing to, both crutches move forward together then both extremities swing with or without draging of the feet but unlike swing to, this time extremities swing beyond the crutches (Figs. 5.84a to c).

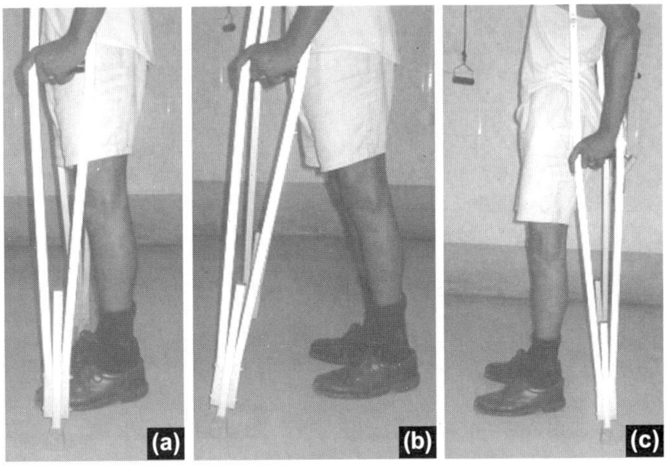

Figs. 5.84a to c: Swing through gait

Both types of crutches (axillary and elbow) can be used in swing to and swing through gait.

III. WALKERS

Among all the walking aids this is the most stable aid. Walkers provide better lateral and anterior posterior stability due to wider base of support.

They are used for:

i. Relieving weight partially or fully.
ii. Improve balance and stability.

They are typically made of tubular aluminium or iron frames. The hand grips are molded with rubber, foam or vinyl material. They are available in various forms such as (Figs. 5.85a to g):

- Adjustable/non-adjustable.
- Foldable/non foldable.
- Small/medium/large size.
- Rolator walker (Walker with front wheels).
- Anterior/posterior walker.

Each has some advantage over other. Like adjustable can be adjusted for taller population but are unstable and make clicking sound at the point of adjustment.

Foldable are easy to carry but same problem of instability is there. Rolator walker are helpful for those who can't lift the usual one. Other modifications such as carry bag, seat can be attached to the walker to make it more functional. Posterior walkers are used for children with cerebral palsy who have tendency to lean forward.

Disadvantage of walker—Stair activities are not possible, difficult to carry and to use in crowded places.

Measurement—Measurement for height are taken from greater trochanter to the floor. Further confirmation can

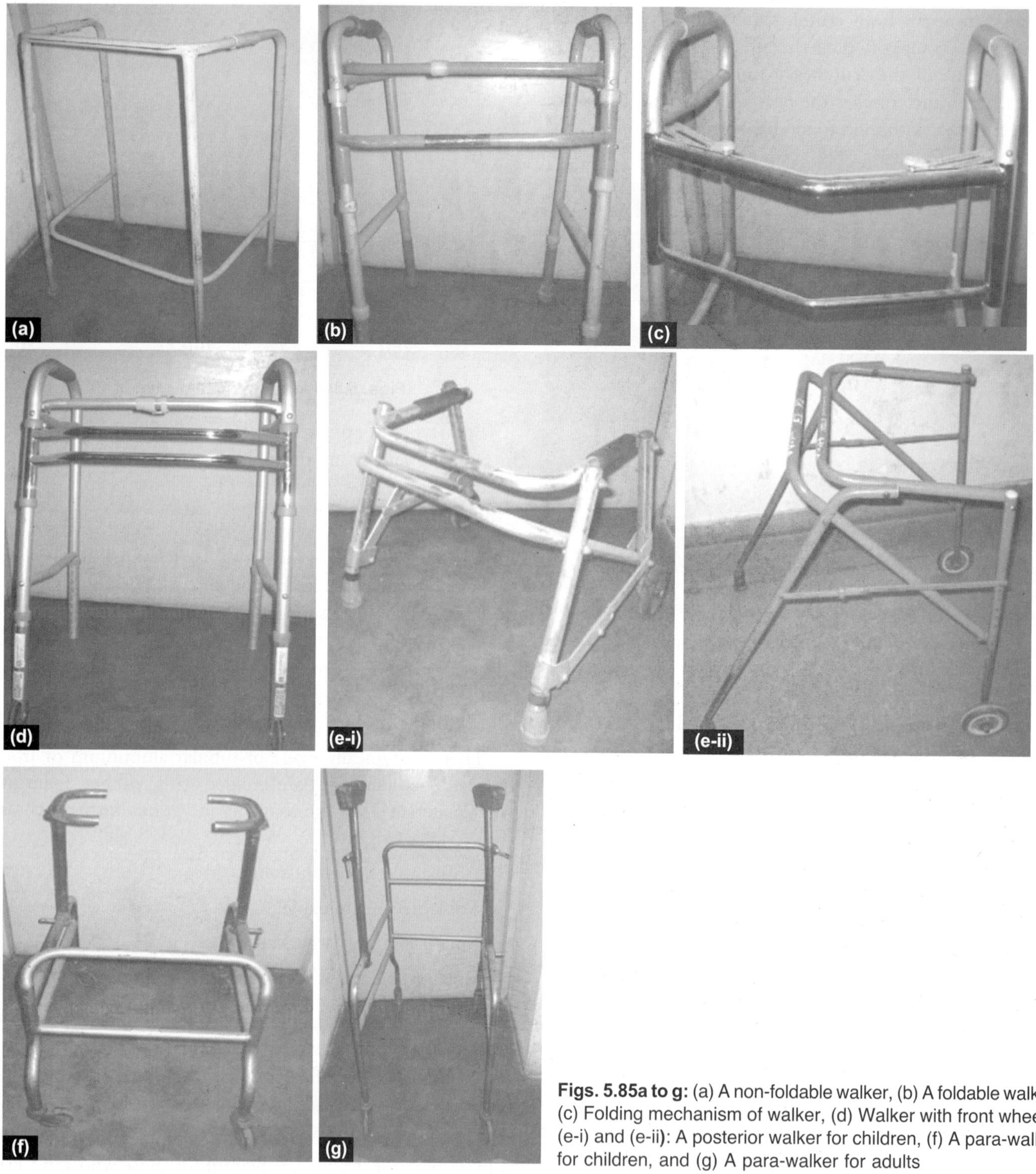

Figs. 5.85a to g: (a) A non-foldable walker, (b) A foldable walker, (c) Folding mechanism of walker, (d) Walker with front wheels, (e-i) and (e-ii): A posterior walker for children, (f) A para-walker for children, and (g) A para-walker for adults

be done by making the elbow flexed at 20° to 30° and the hands should reach comfortably to hand grip of the walker.

Gait Training with Walking Aids

Gait training should be started when the patient has achieved endurance and balance for standing with or without walking aids. Parallel bar may be used for this purpose. Therapist support, visual feedback, verbral clues, ball throwing activities etc. can be used to improve balance and stability in standing. Transfer from various positions seen as sit to stand, stand to sit with or without walking should be taught to the patient.

Note: Before actually starting walking with aids in various gait patterns (discussed earlier) patient may have some preliminary sessions of walking in parallel bars.

STAIR ACTIVITIES

1. *Cane:*

In stair ascending unaffected extremity goes up first followed by cane and affected extremity.

In stair descending affected extremity and cane lead down followed by unaffected lower extremity (as the leg which leads down later has to bear whole body weight by eccentric contraction of quadriceps) (Figs. 5.86a to f).

(Tips to remember "Sound leg takes to heaven, affected leg takes to hell").

2. *Crutches:*

a. *Three-point gait:* In stair ascending the patient stands close in front of step, giving some space for affected leg. Then he pushes down firmly on hand pieces of crutches and goes up with unaffected extremity. Which is followed by the crutches.

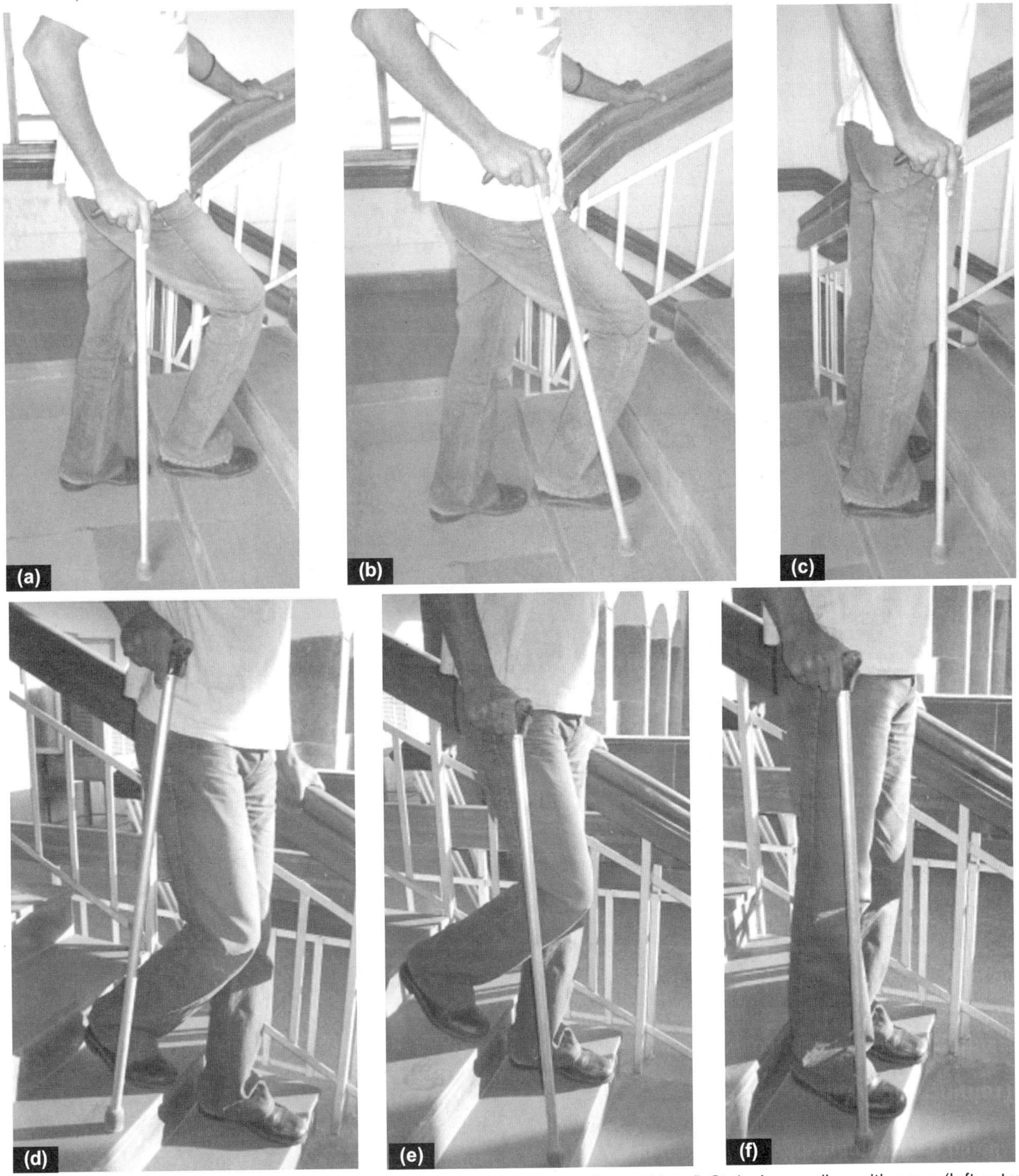

Figs. 5.86a to f: (a to c) Stair ascending with cane (left extremity–affected) and (d to f) Stair descending with cane (left extremity–affected)

While descending crutches are kept on the lower step (front half) then he pushes down on the hand piece of the crutches and moves downward. Crutches follows the unaffected leg (Figs. 5.87a to d).

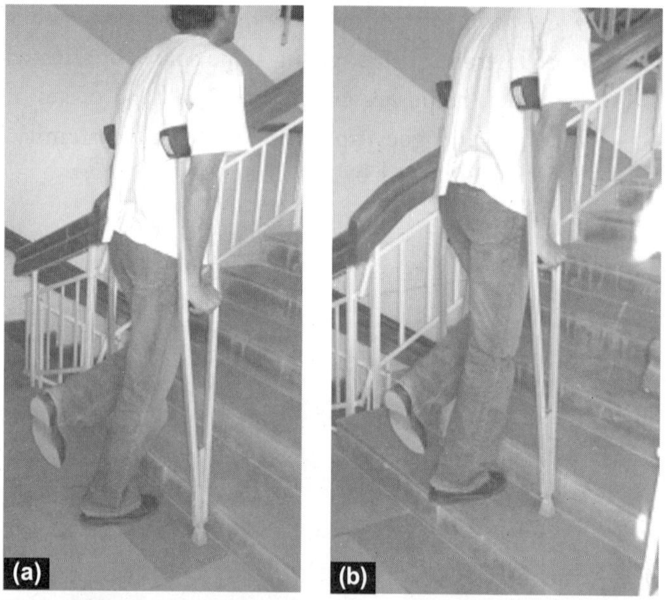

Figs. 5.87a and b: Stair ascending with crutches–three-point gait (left extremity–affected). Two crutches and one leg in contact with the ground

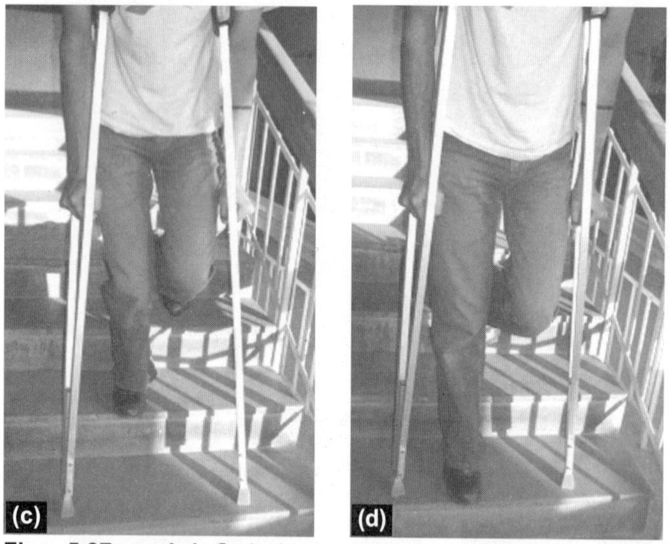

Figs. 5.87c and d: Stair descending with crutches–three-point gait (left extremity–affected). Two crutches and one leg in contact with the ground

b. *Partial weight bearing gait:* Pattern of ascending is same as with three-point gait, except that the involved extremity also bears some weight. The involved leg and crutches follow the unaffected leg.

c. *Four-point and two-point gait:* In ascending patient moves the left lower extremity first then the right. After that crutches may either follow one by one (i.e., first right crutch then the left) or together (Figs. 5.88a to j).

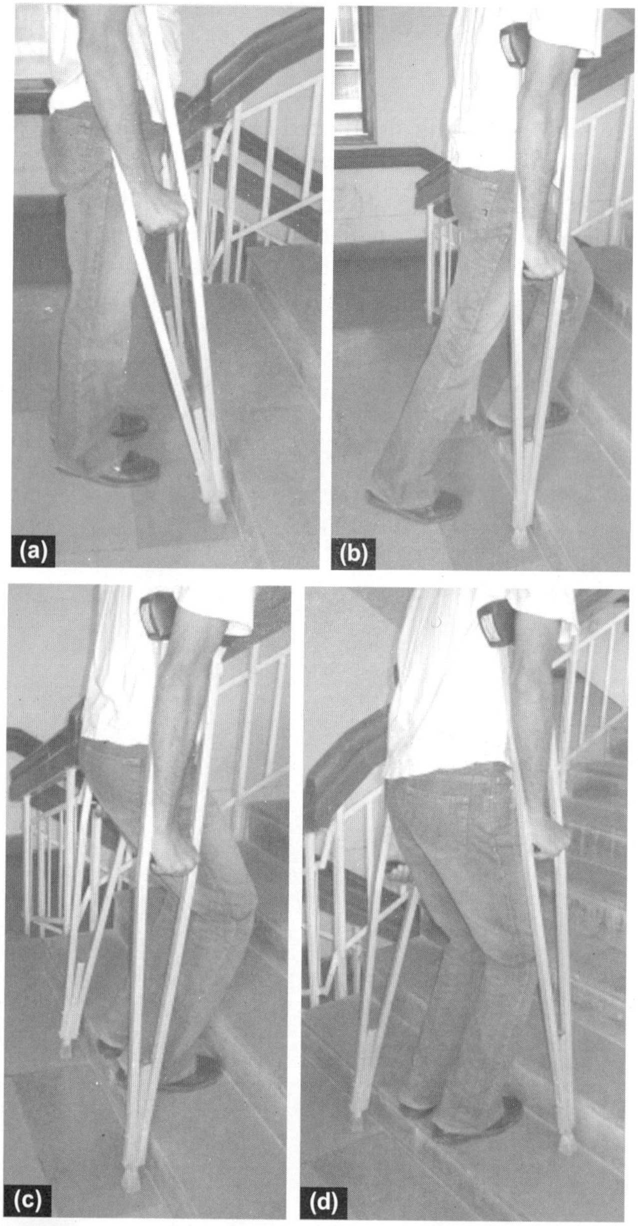

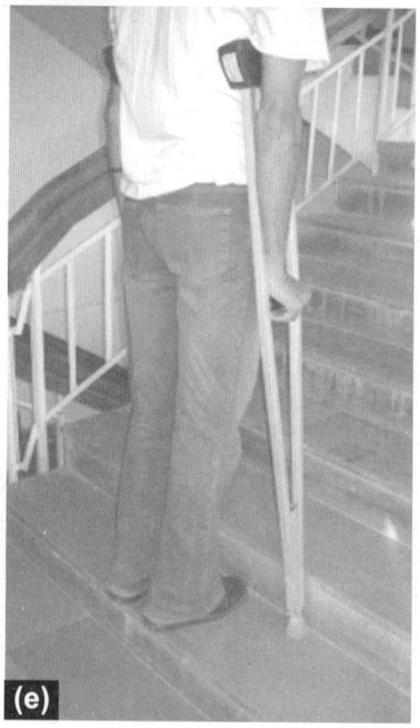

Figs. 5.88a to e: Stair ascending four-point gait

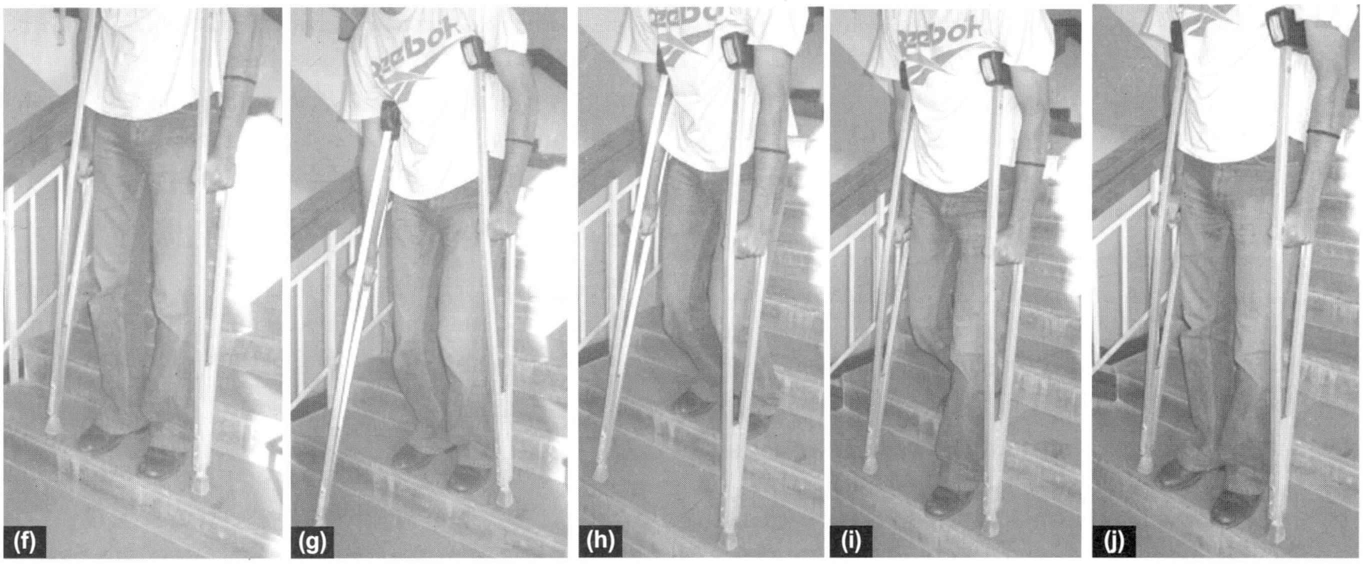

Figs. 5.88f to j: Stair descending four-point gait. f – both the legs and crutches are on the stair, g and h – right crutch is descended and then left, i and j – left leg is descended followed by right leg

In descending right crutch goes down then the left (may together also).

After that right lower extremity is moved down and then the left.

Note: If a railing is available it should always be used. Even the aid may be placed in other hand in which it is not normally used.

CRUTCH AND CANE EXERCISES

Muscles:

With their purpose required to perform crutch walking are:

i. *Scapular depressors (Latissimus dorsi, lower trapezius, pectoralis minor)*—To stabilise the upper limb and prevent hiking of the shoulder on weight bearing—Latissimus dorsi which is known as crutch walking muscle by virtue of its attachment with pelvis (origin point) helps in hiking of pelvis with or without quadratus lumborum to create ground clearance (Typically used by paraplegics).

ii. *Shoulder adductors (pectoralis major and latissimus dorsi)*—To hold the crutch close to the chest wall.

iii. *Shoulder flexors, extensors and abductor especially deltoid)*—For placement of the crutch forward, backward and sideward respectively.

iv. *Elbow extensors (Tricpes and anconeus)*—To stabilise elbow during weight bearing by preventing buckling.

v. *Wrist extensors (Extensor carpi radialis and ulnaris)*—To hold the wrist in proper position to bear weight on hand piece.

vi. *Finger and thumb flexors (Flexor digitorum superficial and profundus, flexor pollicis longus and brevis)*—To adequately grip the hand piece so that the crutch can be moved to the desired position.

(The use of muscles by the patients depends on the pattern of paresis or paralysis in all the extremities and trunk).

Strengthening of the abovementioned muscles should be started as early as possible in a view to use for crutch walking. The patient whose upper extremities are normal should be taught to do weight/resistive exercises as in crutch walking these muscles have to perform more work than usual.

Preparatory Exercises for Crutch Walking

I. Mat and Bed Exercises

i. *Pelvic tilter:* Patient in supine position on bed or mat, arms at side, legs extended, tries to flatten the lumbar spine. This movement is helpful during swing gait and getting up from seated position.

ii. *Hip hiker:* Patient in supine or prone position tries to lift the hip alternately to develop coordination and skills required for gait.

iii. *Sitter upper:* Patient tries to sit in long sitting position from supine position. This makes patient to use elbow and shoulder extensors, which are also important in crutch walking.

iv. *Sitting:* Push up—Patient does push up in long sitting position. Wooden block or push up handles may be used under hands to produce a greater lift.

v. *Trunk twister and hip raiser:* Patient in long sitting position turns on one side, places hands on mat/

bed then bearing weight on upper limbs tries to raise the hip.

vi. *Sitting hip hiker:* Hands on knee or hip, patient in long sitting position tries to approximate iliac crest to the lower hips on one side then the movement is repeated on other side.

vii. *Sitting swing through:* Patient in long sitting position, lifts buttocks on upper limbs by extending elbow then move buttocks backward and forward as much as possible. (These are prerequisite movements for swing through gait).

viii. *Prone push up:* Patient does push up in prone position by abducting the arm, elbow flexed and hands on the floor/mat or bed. (This exercise increases strength of almost all muscles used for crutch walking).

ix. *Tip swayer:* Patient is in quadruped position bears more weight on upper limbs, sways hip to one side then other (good for improving balance and coordination of the trunk and hips).

x. *Camel and Cat:* Patient in quadruped position, extends his neck and causes lordosis at lower trunk (camel), then flexes his neck, contracts abdominal causing rounding of back (cat).

xi. *Forward and backward reacher:* Patient in quadruped position lifts his one arm and tries to make it horizontal to the mat then repeats it with other extremity. In backward reacher exercise, everything is same except patient tries to reach back towards hips.

(**Note:** All exercise in quadruped position should be performed exclusively on mat).

II. Mat Exercises with Crutches and Benches

Mat exercise with crutches are done to improve balance, coordination and strength. These exercises are direct carry over of abovementioned mat and bed exercises (Mat crutches are smaller than usual crutches).

(*Crutch position:* Patient in long sitting mat crutches in the axilla, elbows flexed, wrist extended, hands grasping the hand pieces).

i. *Crutch raiser:* Patient raises the crutch on one side while bearing more weight on other, without displacing the crutch in the axilla. Repeat the same on other side.

ii. *Sitting crutch push up:* Patient pushes down on the hands raising the buttocks from the mat.

iii. *Sitting crutch swing through:* After pushing up on the crutches patient moves his buttocks backward and forward as much as possible.

III. Exercises with Kneeling Mat Crutches

Patient does weight shifts, crutch raising etc to improve balance and coordination in kneeling position. This may also be preceded by kneeling balance exercises along.

IV. Wheel Chair Exercises

Patient on wheel chair can do armrest push ups to improve strength of latissimus dorsi and triceps.

Sitting balance activities such as weight shifting, picking objects from (forward, side ward direction may also be performed.

V. Parallel Bar Exercises

Biomechanically due to bigger base of support parallel bar is the most stable among all the aids of walking. Parallel bar exercises start with standing endurance improvement. Patient stands in parallel bar, putting weight on bar through hand (level of parallel bar at the height of greater trochanter or to permit 20° to 30° of elbow flexion), with feet 4-6 inches apart. Visual feedback through mirror and verbal cues to improve posture is very important.

Patient perform following exercises in parallel bar which leads to independent and balanced walking:

- Weight shift.
- Arm raising alternately.
- Parallel bar push ups.
- Hip hiking and leg swing.
- 4-point gait (same discussed earlier with crutches). Patient shifts hands on the bar instead of crutches.
- Swing to and swing through gait (same as with crutches).
- Backward 4-point and swing gait.

The usual progression from the parallel bar is to one crutch and one bar and then to two crutches in a wide parallel bars. The final progression to 2 crutches with some passive support (wall or therapist etc.) then without any support.

6

MANUAL MUSCLE STRENGTH TESTING (MMST) AND GONIOMETRY

MANUAL MUSCLE STRENGTH TESTING (MMST)

INTRODUCTION

It is a diagnostic and prognostic approach in which the therapist tests the strength of the muscle by observing the contraction or movement or applying resistance against the action of agonist (prime mover) in the anatomical available range of motion (ROM). Examination of the strength of the muscle between two-time intervals provides information about the prognosis of the muscle which also helps to design the treatment.

Uses

Manual muscle testing is an important evaluative tool used to assess the strength of muscle or group of muscles; by the physical therapist, occupational therapist, chiropractors, physiological researchers, physical medicine and rehabilitation practitioners and orthopedicians.

Manual muscle testing is such an important tool of physical examination of patient that when performed appropriately can provide an accurate information of the strength of muscle which can assist the practitioner in planning an appropriate scheme of intervention or management.

Impairments in muscle function and strength may result from many of the conditions such as peripheral nerve injuries, spinal cord injuries, Guillain-Barré syndrome, cranial nerve dysfunctions, poliomyelitis, multiple sclerosis, amyotrophic lateral sclerosis, muscular dystrophy, myasthenia gravis, osteoarthritis, rheumatoid arthritis, and post fracture immobilization.

1. *Lower motor neuron diseases*–Such as peripheral nerve injuries, spinal cord injuries, Guillain-Bárre syndrome, cranial nerve dysfunctions, poliomyelitis, multiple sclerosis, amyotrophic lateral sclerosis.
2. *Primary muscle disease*–Muscular dystrophy, myasthenia gravis.
3. *Orthopaedic and other conditions*–In these conditions loss of muscle strength is caused by disuse and immobilization, rather than by a direct effect of the disease, such as–fractures, arthritis, amputation, burns.

Contraindications/Precautions

- Pain and inflammation.
- Healing wound.
- Subluxation and dislocation.
- Fracture.
- Hypermobility of a joint.
- Haemophilia.
- Cardiovascular conditions.
- Immediate after the surgery.
- Severe spasticity.
- Muscle fatigue.
- Osteoporosis.
- Osteomyelitis.
- Abdominal hernia.

Available Range of Motion

Normally the muscle strength is examined in full range of motion but due to some circumstances/abnormal conditions full range of motion cannot be achieved. Suppose a 45 years rheumatoid arthritic patient has 15° of flexion contracture of the knee joint, it means extension is restricted at the end of 15°. So the available range of motion of the extension is 135°-15° and muscle strength should be tested in this range only (135°-15°).

Make or Break Test

The break test is the manual resistance which is used to test the strength of the muscle. At the end of available range of motion or at a point in the range where the muscle is more challenged, the patient is asked to hold the limb at that point (by contracting the muscle), at the same time the therapist applies resistance to break the hold. For example to test the biceps brachii the patient is asked to flex the elbow joint with supination of the forearm and hold the elbow at end range and therapist tries to break the hold and move the limb downward into extension. This is called break test and it is the procedure most commonly used in manual muscle testing today.

Active Resistance Test

It is an alternative of break test in which manual active resistance is applied against the action of agonist muscle throughout available range of motion. During active resistance, an amount of resistance increases gradually until it reaches the maximum level the subject can tolerate and motion ceases. This kind of manual muscle test requires considerable skill and experience to perform and is so often equivocal that its use is not recommended. An active resistance test differs from break test for resistance is against concentric contraction of the agonist muscles action while in break test resistance is applied against eccentric contraction of the agonist muscles action.

The Grading System

The manual muscle strength testing are recorded as numerical scores or qualitative scores, which represent the strength of the muscle.

Numerical Score	*Qualitative Score*
0	Zero, No muscle contraction.
1	Trace or flicker muscle contraction.
2	Poor—Full range of motion in gravity minimized position.
3	Fair—Full range of motion against the gravity.
4	Good—Full range of motion against the gravity with moderate resistance.
5	Normal—Full range of motion against the gravity with maximum resistance.

(Each grading is described with illustration of quadriceps muscles).

Grade 0

"No muscle contraction" at all on palpation or visual inspection. Muscle is completely paralysed or quiescent (Figs. 6.1a and b).

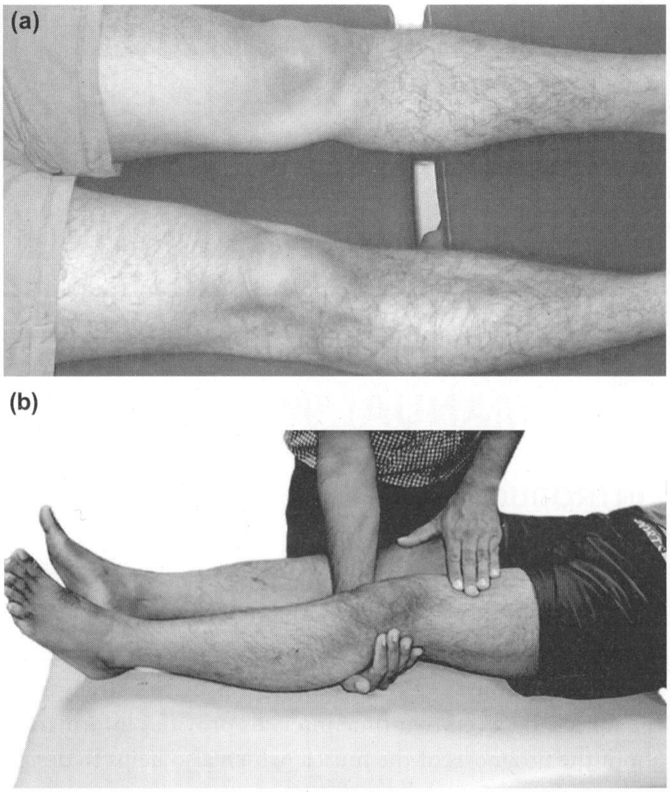

Figs. 6.1a and b: Grade-0 (No contraction—Quadriceps muscles)—(a) No visible contraction and (b) No palpable contraction

Grade 1

"Flicker muscle contraction" but no movement at all. The muscle contraction can be palpated by placing the hand over the muscle belly or therapist can also see or feel a tendon pop up or tense as the patient tries to perform the movement (Fig. 6.2).

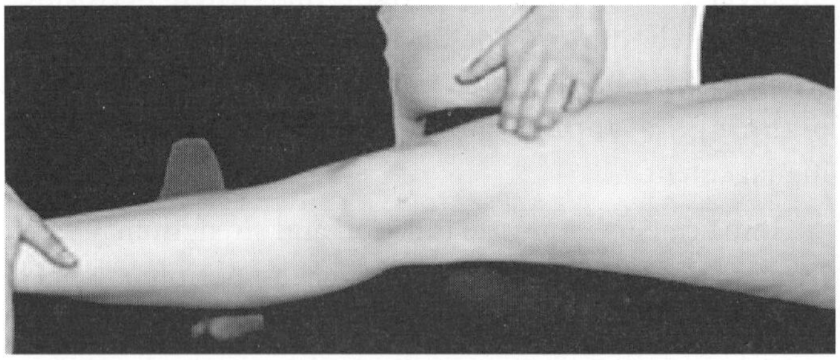

Fig. 6.2: Grade-1 (Flicker contraction—Quadriceps muscles)

Grade 2

"Poor" full range of motion (available range) in gravity minimized position. This position (gravity minimized) is often described as the horizontal plane of motion which minimises the force of gravity. The contraction of muscle is sufficient to perform the movement in gravity minimized position but not against the gravity (Fig. 6.3).

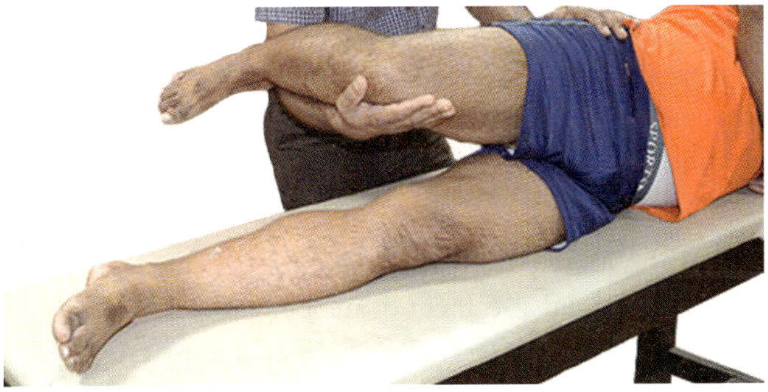

Fig. 6.3: Grade-2 (Gravity eliminated position for quadriceps muscles)

Grade 3

"Fair" full range of motion against the gravity.

The contraction of muscle is sufficient to perform the movement in full range of motion (available range of motion) against gravity, without an external resistance (by hand of therapist). The therapist observes the movement after stabilising the proximal part of the joint (Fig. 6.4).

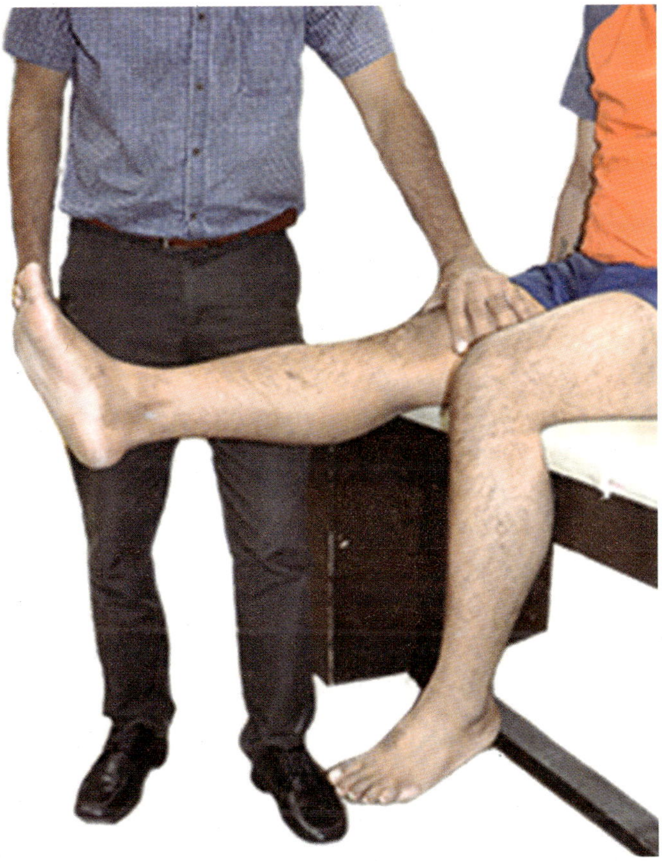

Fig. 6.4: Grade-3 (Against gravity for quadriceps muscles)

Grade 4

"Good"– Full range of motion against the gravity with moderate manual resistance by the hands of therapist. The contraction of muscle is sufficient to perform the movement in available range of motion against the gravity with moderate resistance which is applied by the hands of therapist.

Generally the therapist applies resistance just near the distal end of the segment to which the muscle attaches. There are two common exceptions of this rule are the gluteus medius, minimus and scapular muscles which do not follow the rule (Fig. 6.5).

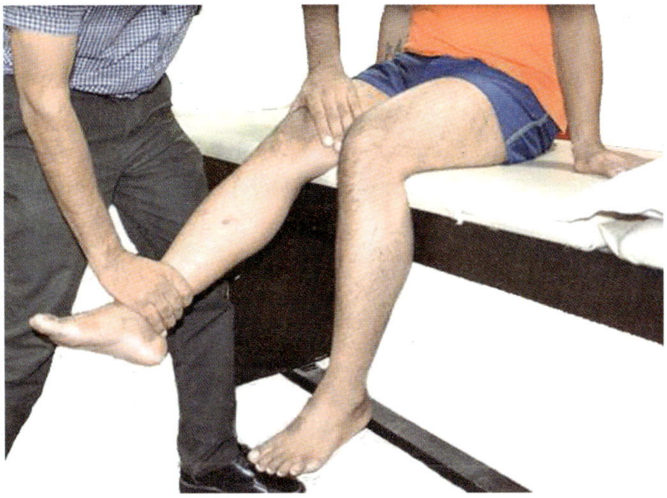

Fig. 6.5: Grade-4 (Against gravity with moderate resistance for quadriceps muscles)

Grade 5

"Normal" full range of motion, against the gravity with maximum resistance.

The resistance is applied gradually from initial range and at end range patient is asked to hold this position while therapist attempts to break the hold. In almost every instance when the therapist cannot break the hold position the muscle is rewarded grade 5.

While testing unilateral problem, the therapist can find out the difference in strength of the muscle by testing the sound limb. Though dominated side bears slightly more strength than the non-dominated side.

Therefore, to reward the grade 4 and grade 5 to an individual muscle, requires lot of experience and skills. Students should first practice on their classmates then on patients, which can make them perfect to differentiate the grade 4 from grade 5.

General Rules of MMST

- *Patient should be relaxed:* The procedure should be explained to the patient. MMST should be done on the sound limb first.

- *Position of patient* should be comfortable. Therapist should try to test all the suspected muscles strength in the same position and should not keep changing the position again and again which irritates the patient and can cause wrong muscle testing (for example to test the muscle strength of a post polio residual paralysis, therapist selects supine position to test the lower limb muscle strength, he tests the iliopsoas and changes the position of patient to prone lying and tests gluteus maximus, after that the position of patient is changed to the supine position for gluteus medius in grade 2. To avoid this the therapist should test all the suspected muscles in supine position—iliopsoas then gluteus medius in grade 2 and adductors in grade 2 and ankle muscles then change the position of patient for other muscles. Doing this is more convenient and does not irritate the patient.
- *Position of therapist* should be comfortable, which can be easiest to stabilise the proximal part of the joint as well as apply resistance against the agonist muscles in grade 4 and grade 5.

  To differentiate the grade 1 from grade 0 an examiner should have a knowledge of muscle anatomy (origin, insertion and muscle belly). To palpate the contraction of muscle therapist should place the hand over the muscle belly and ask the patient to contract the muscle, if therapist does not feel contraction of muscle, muscle should be rewarded grade 0, which is considered as a complete paralysis.
- *The movement should occur in anatomical range* (*For example*–When patient is asked to abduct the shoulder joint, patient lifts the shoulder between flexion and abduction that is in scapula plane and known as scaption plane which is neither flexion nor abduction) so therapist may demonstrate the movement prior to muscle strength testing.
- The proximal part of the joint which is being tested should be stabilised in three ways:
  1. By using the weight of the body.
  2. By one hand of the examiner; and
  3. By applying straps (applying tight straps can prevent the contraction of the muscle).

Trick Movements/Substitution/Vicarious Motions

The brain "thinks" in terms of movement and not contraction of an individual muscle. Thus a muscle or muscle group may attempt to compensate for the function of a weaker muscle to accomplish a movement. These movements are called Trick movements or substitutions or vicarious motions.

The other part of the body should also be observed during the muscle testing. Sometimes patient deliberately moves other joints, segment of the body to compensate the action of weakened muscle which is being tested. (*For example*–If abductors of shoulder joint, specially supraspinatus, is weak and as patient is asked to abduct the shoulder joint, the patient elevates the shoulder girdle of the same side and flexes the spine to the opposite side which gives thrust to arm and patient initiates the shoulder abduction. So patient is instructed prior to the test not to move other joints or segment of the body to avoid trick movements.

Classification of Trick Movements/Substitution/ Vicarious Motions

i. *Direct Substitution*: Direct substitution can be of two types. First type, which deceives the therapist. *For example*—Long extensors cause abduction of finger in a complete ulnar nerve injury.

   Second type, which successfully replace function lost by obvious paralysis. *For example*—Abduction and elevation of shoulder caused by long heads of biceps and triceps, the clavicular fibres of pectoralis major and the external rotators of the humerus in case of deltoid paralysis.

ii. *Accessory Insertion*: A very common example of this type is movement caused by abductor pollicis brevis and extensor pollicis brevis in case of paralysis of flexor pollicis longus due to radial nerve injury. This is because these muscles inserted at the extensor expansion of the thumb.

iii. *Tendon Action:* This is commonly known as tenodesis action. *For example*—When finger flexors are paralysed, wrist extension caused finger flexion as flexors are shorter than extensors.

iv. *Rebound Phenomenon*: It occurs when the antagonist of paralysed muscle contracts strongly and relaxes, it appears as if there is a contraction in the agonist. *For example*—Strong contraction of flexor hallucis longus and then relaxing it gives appearance of extension action of extensor hallucis longus.

v. *Anatomical Variation*: Almost one fifth of peripheral nerve injuries may have some anomaly of nerve supply.

For example—Presence of action of opponens and flexor pollicis brevis in complete median nerve injury (these muscles may be supplied by ulnar nerve).

vi. *Gravity*: Action of muscles like triceps can be performed by gravity as usually patient does in triceps paralysis by depressing the shoulder and allow gravity to cause extension.

Application of Resistance

The general rule of application of resistance is to apply it just near the distal end of the segment to which muscle is attached. There are two common exceptions of this rule– the gluteus medius and minimus and the scapular muscles. To test the abductors of hip joint resistance should be applied on the distal end of femur just above the knee joint. The abductor muscles are so strong, however, that most examiners, in testing a patient with normal knee strength and joint integrity, will choose to apply resistance at the lateral aspect of the ankle joint. To test the vertebroscapular muscles (e.g., rhomboids), the preferred point of resistance is on the arm rather than on the scapula where these muscles insert.

Generally, a muscle bears most resistance at the mid range because at this point lever arm is increased (e.g., in the case of biceps brachii, when the elbow is straight, the lever arm is short; leverage increases as an elbow flexes and becomes maximal at 90° flexion, but as flexion continues beyond that point, the lever arm again decreases in length and efficiency).

In manual muscle testing, the application of resistance at the end of the range in one joint muscles allows consistency of procedure rather than an attempt to select the estimated mid range position. In two joint muscles (e.g., medial or lateral hamstring muscles) the point of maximal resistance is generally at or near mid range.

The Plus (+) and Minus (–) Grades

Poor Minus (P^-) or 2^-

Poor Plus (P^+) or 2^+

Fair Minus (F^-) or 3^-

Fair Plus (F^+) or 3^+

Poor minus (P^-) or grade 2^-: The joint moves through incomplete range of motion in gravity minimized position. *For example:* The available range of motion of the elbow flexion) is 0° to 135° and when patient attempts to move the joint, he or she does not move the joint from 0°–135° in gravity minimized position, but moves from 0°–90° which is termed as grade 2^- or poor minus.

Poor plus or grade 2^+: Joint moves through incomplete range of motion (less than 50%) against gravity or joint moves through complete range of motion in gravity minimized position against slight resistance.

Fair minus (F^-) or grade 3^-: Joint moves through incomplete range of motion (less than 100% but more than 50%) against gravity.

Fair plus (F^+) or grade 3^+: Joint moves through complete range of motion, against gravity and slight resistance.

The plus/minus concept with grade 4 has been discarded.

MANUAL MUSCLE TESTING FOR UPPER EXTREMITY

Serratus Anterior – Scapular Abduction and Upward Rotation

Serratus anterior should always be tested in shoulder flexion to minimize the synergy with trapezius muscle. The deltoid muscles should be stronger enough to test the serratus anterior. If the deltoid muscles are weak, the lever for testing is gone; therefore, arm cannot be used for the resistance. Normally forward rotation of scapula from starting position to full flexion is about the breadth of two fingers. The testing of the serratus anterior for grading 1-5 depends on the position of scapula and movement of arm. Grade 3 to 5 is tested if the scapula rests on the thoracic wall in the starting position and rotates forward in a controlled and coordinated manner when the arm is raised above the shoulder. Grade 0 to 2 is tested if the patient is not able to raise the arm above the shoulder (Fig. 6.7).

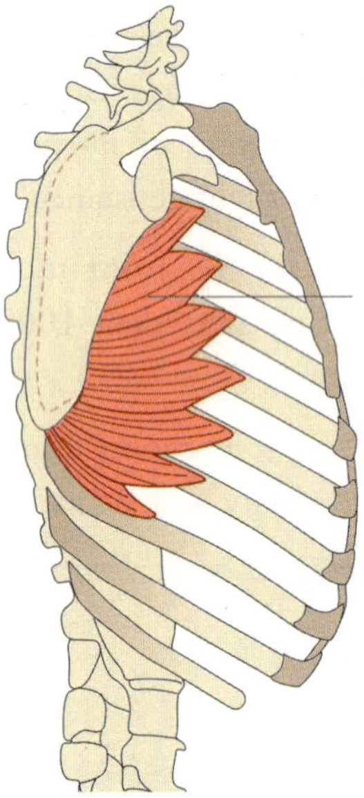

Fig. 6.7: Serratus anterior muscle origin and insertion

Origin: Outer surface and superior border of the upper eight or nine ribs.

Insertion: Costal surface of the medial border of the scapula.

Action: With the origin fixed, serratus anterior abducts the scapula, rotates the inferior angle laterally and the glenoid cavity cranially, and holds the medial border of the scapula firmly against the rib cage. The lower and upper fibers of serratus anterior depress and elevate the scapula slightly. The serratus may act in forced inspiration if the insertion is fixed in the adduction.

Nerve Supply: Long thoracic, $C_{5,6,7,8}$.

Grade 3 (Fair)

Position of Patient: Short sitting with both the hands on the edge of table.

Position of Examiner: Examiner stands at the side, which is being tested and may use his or her hand to support and maintain the arm above shoulder. The other hand is placed at the inferior angle of the scapula with the thumb positioned along the axillary border and the fingers along the vertebral border hence the hand makes a web.

Stabilization: Examiner stabilizes the trunk to prevent posterior and lateral bending (Fig. 6.8).

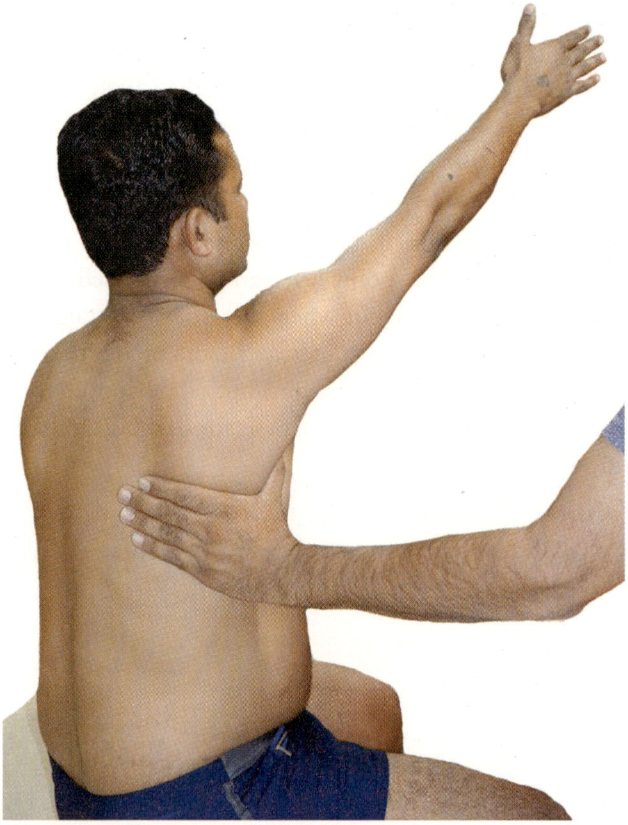

Fig. 6.8: Testing of serratus anterior for grade 3, examiner places the hand over the inferior angle of scapula to feel its movement during elevation

Test: Examiner instructs the patient to raise the arm above the shoulder around 130° and at the same time examiner feels the movement of the scapula. The scapula should rotate anteriorly in a smooth and coordinated manner without winging. The patient is instructed to hold the arm at the 130° and push it anteriorly towards the wall or ceiling. If the patient is able to do it without winging of the scapula it is considered grade 3.

Grade 4 and Grade 5 (Good and Normal)

Position of Patient: Short sitting with both the hands on the edge of table.

Position of Examiner: Examiner stands at the side, which is being tested and places one hand over the distal arm to apply resistance towards the shoulder joint and scapula. Examiner places other hand at the inferior angle of the scapula with the thumb positioned along the axillary border and the fingers along the vertebral border hence the hand makes a web.

Stabilization: Examiner stabilizes the trunk to prevent posterior and lateral bending (Fig. 6.9).

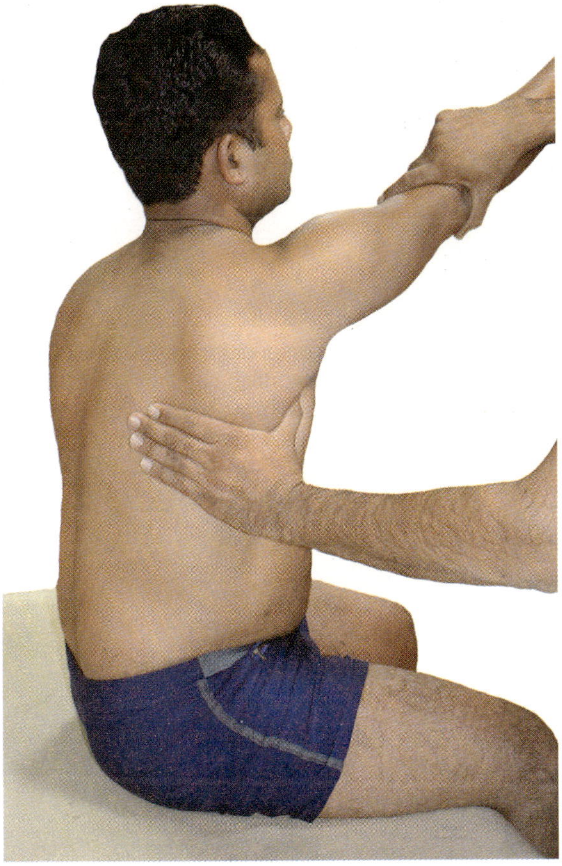

Fig. 6.9: Testing of serratus anterior for grade 4 and 5. Examiner stands at the side, which is being tested and places one hand over the distal arm to apply resistance towards the shoulder joint and scapula. Examiner places other hand at the inferior angle of the scapula with the thumb positioned along the axillary border and the fingers along the vertebral border hence the hand makes a web

Test: Examiner instructs the patient to raise the arm above the shoulder around 130° and at the same time examiner observes the movement of the scapula. The scapula should rotate anteriorly in a smooth and coordinated manner without winging.

Grade 4: The patient is instructed to hold the arm at the 130° and push it anteriorly towards the wall or ceiling against mild to moderate resistance applied by the examiner towards the scapula. If the patient is able to do it without winging of the scapula it is considered grade 4.

Grade 5: The patient is instructed to hold the arm at the 130° and push it anteriorly towards the wall or ceiling against maximum resistance applied by the examiner towards the scapula. If the patient is able to do it without winging of the scapula it is considered grade 5.

Grade 1 (Poor)

Position of Patient: Short sitting.

Position of Examiner: Examiner stands at the side, which is being tested. Examiner raises the arm above the shoulder and maintains this position with one hand. Examiner places his fingers of other hand just in front of the inferior angle along the axillary border for palpation.

Stabilization: Examiner stabilizes the trunk to prevent posterior and lateral bending (Figs. 6.10a and b).

(a)

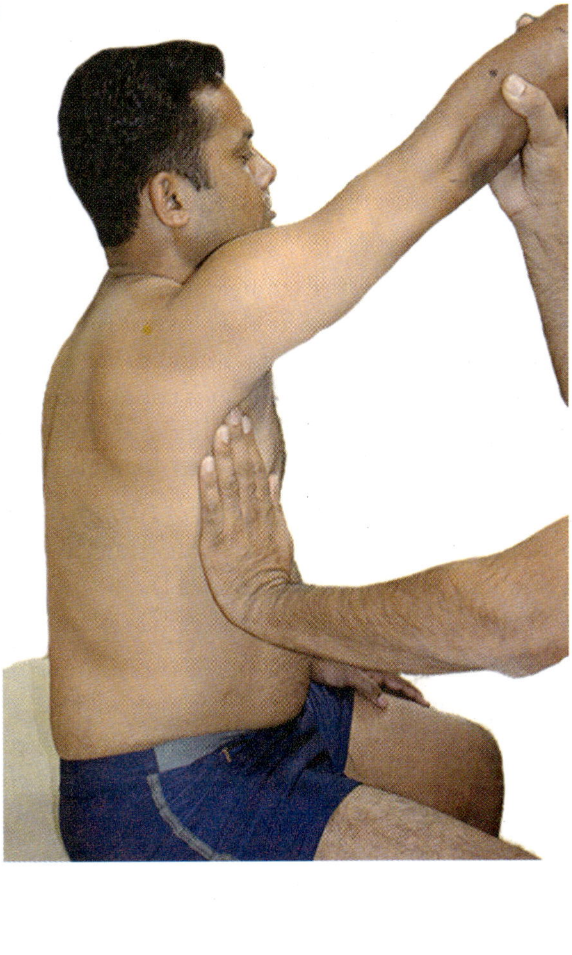

(b)

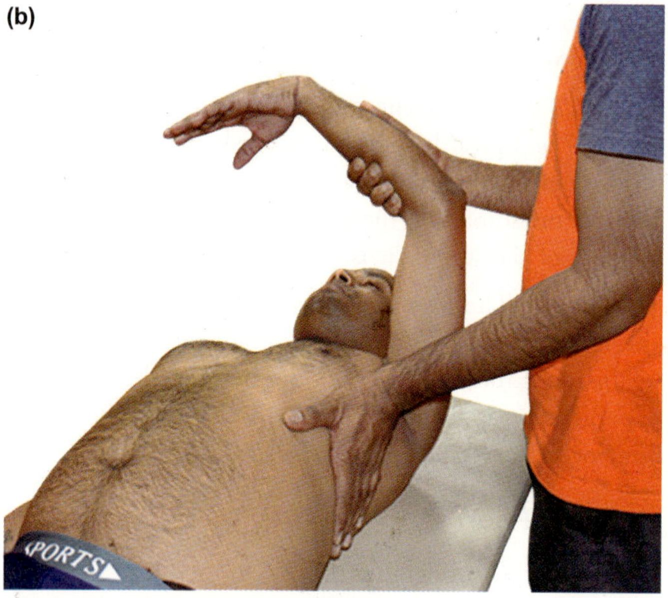

Figs. 6.10a and b: Palpating serratus anterior muscle over the rib cage for grade 1 testing. (a) Examiner stands at the side and places his fingers of other hand in front of the inferior angle along the axillary border for palpation. (b) Alternate position for palpating serratus anterior in supine lying

Test: Patient is instructed to try to hold the arm at this position while the examiner palpates the serratus anterior on axillary border. If examiner feels contraction on the axillary wall it is considered grade 1.

Grade 2 (Poor)

Position of Patient: Short sitting. Examiner should select the spot on wall or ceiling that can serve as target for the patient to reach toward in line with above the shoulder in sagittal plane.

Position of Examiner: Examiner stands at the side (or anteriorly to the side) which is being tested. Examiner uses his or her hand to support the arm and to maintain it in above shoulder position. The other hand is placed at the inferior angle of the scapula with the thumb positioned along the axillary border and the fingers along the vertebral border.

Stabilization: Examiner stabilizes the trunk to prevent posterior and lateral bending (Fig. 6.11).

Test: Examiner observes the position of the scapula during rest and the flexion at 90°. The patient is instructed to raise the arm above the shoulder and hold it in this position. Now hold your arm up again and let it go. If there is smooth coordinated movement of the scapula during the shoulder flexion and the scapula remains on the thoracic wall during the test it is considered grade 2.

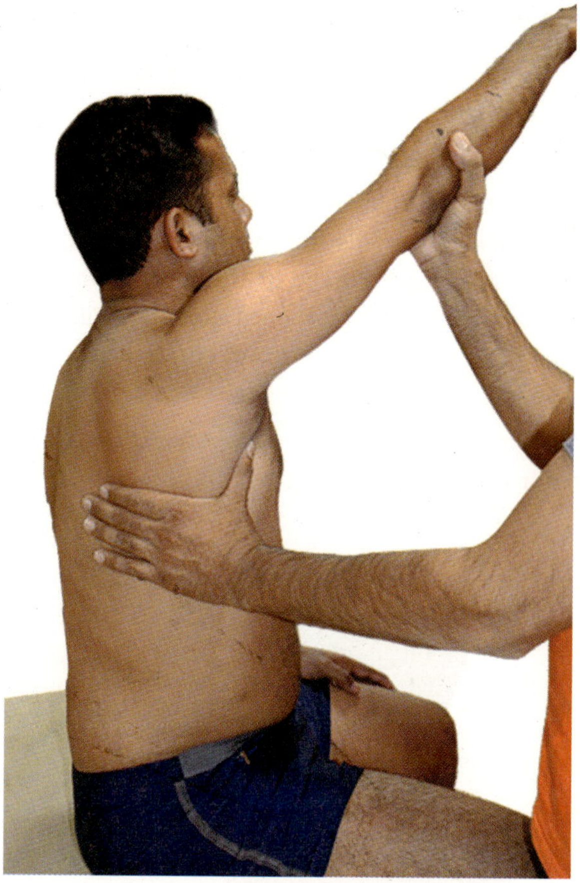

Fig. 6.11: Testing of serratus anterior for grade 2, examiner stands anterior to the patient and supports the arm at above the shoulder level and instructs the patient to push it upward to the wall or ceiling

TRAPEZIUS UPPER FIBERS – SCAPULAR ELEVATION

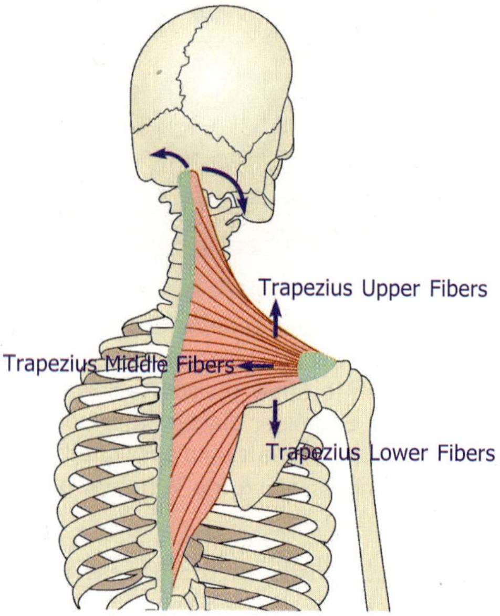

Fig. 6.12: Trapezius muscle fibers origin and insertion

Tapezius (Upper Fibers)

Origin: External occipital protuberance, medial 1/3rd of superior nuchal line, ligamentum nuchae, and spinous process of the seventh cervical vertebra.

Insertion: Lateral 1/3rd of the clavicle and acromion process of the scapula.

Action: Elevation of scapula. With the insertion fixed, the upper fibers extend, laterally flex, and rotate the head and joints of the cervical vertebrae so face turns toward the opposite side.

Nerve Supply: Spinal portion of cranial nerve XI (accessory) and ventral ramus, $C_{2,3,4}$.

Grade 3 (Fair)

Position of Patient: Short sitting, hands relaxed in lap.

Position of Examiner: Examiner stands behind the patient and observes the movement takes place in the shoulder girdle in the upward direction towards the ceiling.

Stabilization: Examiner should stabilize the trunk to prevent shoulder protraction, retraction and trunk bending (Fig. 6.13).

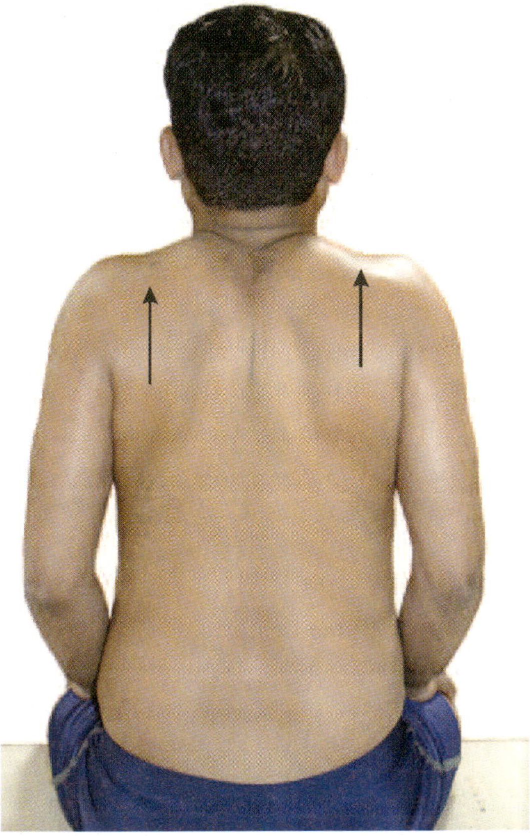

Fig. 6.13: Testing of trapezius upper fibers for grade 3, the examiner stands behind the patient and observes the elevation of the shoulder girdle

Test: Patient is instructed to raise the shoulders upward towards ceiling. Examiner must ensure erect sitting with no kyphosis and protraction of the shoulders.

Grade 4 and 5 (Good and Fair)

Position of Patient: Short sitting, hands relaxed in lap.

Position of Examiner: Examiner stands behind the patient and places both the hands on the top of the shoulder (fingers on the ventral surface and thenar on the top and dorsum of the shoulder girdle). The arms of examiner should be nearly straight to provide enough resistance.

Stabilization: Examiner should stabilize the trunk to prevent shoulder protraction, retraction and trunk bending (Fig. 6.14).

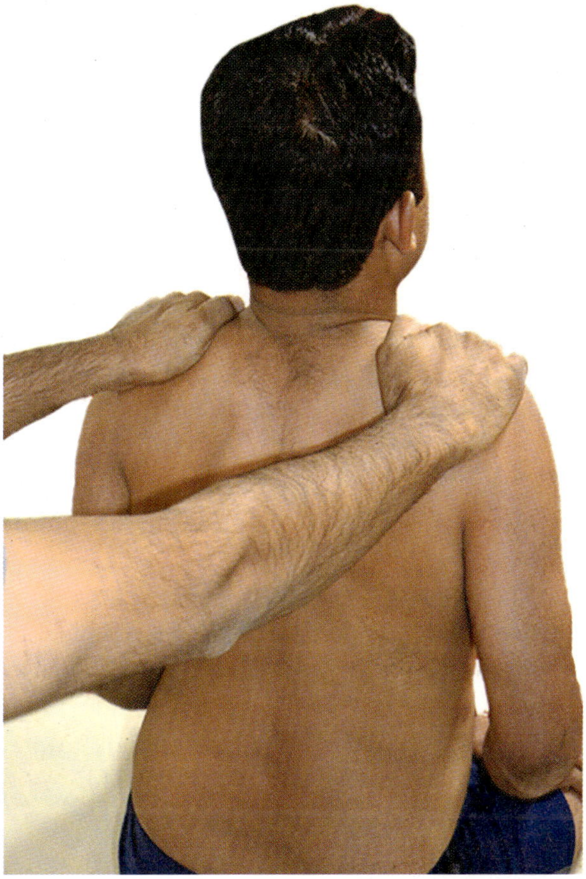

Fig. 6.14: Testing of trapezius upper fibers for grade 4 and 5, examiner places both the hands on the top of shoulders and applies resistance downward against the elevation

Test: Patient is instructed to raise the shoulders upward against the resistance in the available range of motion. Examiner must ensure erect sitting with no kyphosis and protraction of the shoulders or any trick movement.

Grade 4: Patient raises (shrugs) both the shoulders against minimal to moderate resistance in upward direction towards ceiling.

Grade 5: Patient raises (shrugs) both the shoulders against maximum resistance in upward direction towards ceiling.

Grade 1 (Trace)

Position of Patient: Supine lying with shoulders depression.

Position of Examiner: Examiner stands at the head of patient and places fingers of the hands on the top of patient's shoulders (Fig. 6.15).

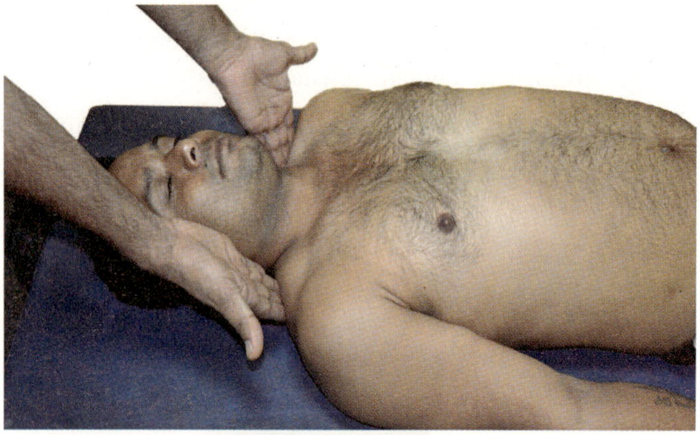

Fig. 6.15: Testing of trapezius upper fibers for grade 2

Test: Patient is instructed to shrug the shoulders upward towards the examiner waist. Examiner palpates the trapezius upper fibers for the contraction during elevation of the shoulders. If there is an appropriate contraction on the top of the shoulders, it is considered grade 1.

Grade 2 (Poor)

Position of Patient: Prone lying with the shoulders depression.

Position of Examiner: Examiner stands at the side of the patient and ensures comfortable lying. The examiner places one hand over the top of shoulder and other hand lateral to the arm.

Stabilization: Examiner stabilizes the trunk to prevent trunk bending and trunk extension (Fig. 6.16).

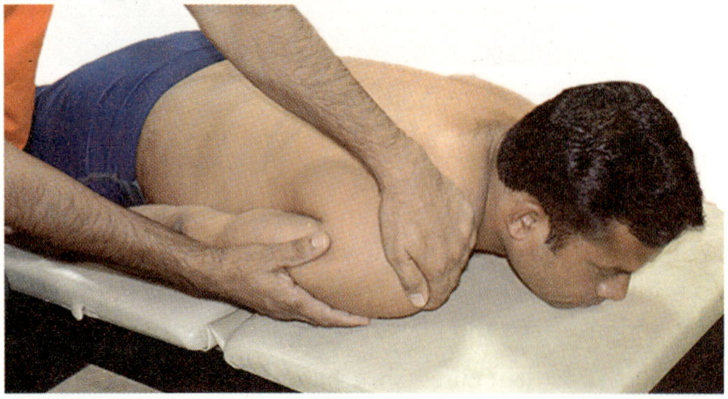

Fig. 6.16: Testing of trapezius upper fibers for grade 2. The examiner places one hand over the top of shoulder and other hand lateral to the arm

Test: Patient is instructed to shrug the shoulders upward. The friction between the anterior shoulder and plinth may offer some resistance against the shoulder elevation, which should carefully be avoided. If patient completes elevation in the available range of motion it is considered grade 2.

TRAPEZIUS MIDDLE FIBERS – SCAPULAR ADDUCTION

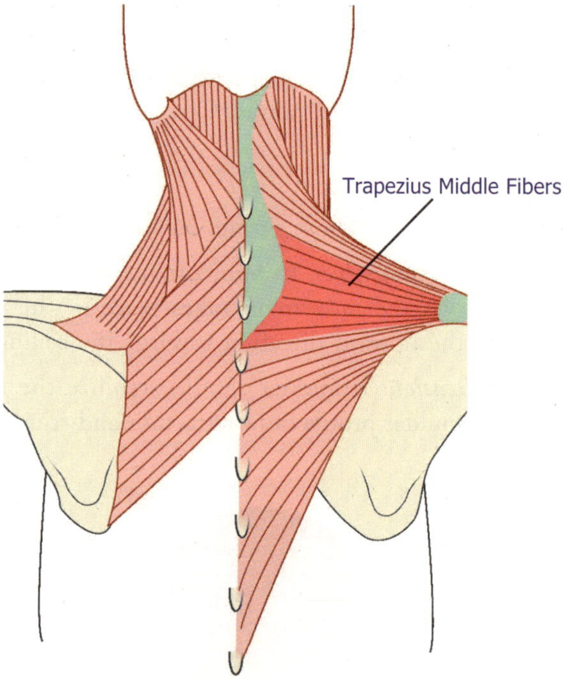

Fig. 6.17: Trapezius middle fibers origin and insertion

Origin: Spinous process of the first through fifth thoracic vertebrae.

Insertion: Medial margin of the acromion and superior lip of the spine of the scapula.

Action: With the origin fixed adduction of scapula.

Nerve Supply: Spinal portion of cranial nerve XI (accessory) and ventral ramus, $C_{2,3,4}$.

Grade 3 (Fair)

Position of Patient: Prone with shoulder abducted to 90° arm rests on the couch. Elbow is out at edge of table and flexed to 90° with the forearms hanging towards floor. Patient may turn the head to either side for comfort.

Position of Examiner: Examiner stands at the side, which is being tested and places one hand on the trunk. Examiner may place other hand on the distal arm to stabilize it.

Stabilization: Examiner stabilizes the trunk to prevent trunk rotation and bending (Fig. 6.18).

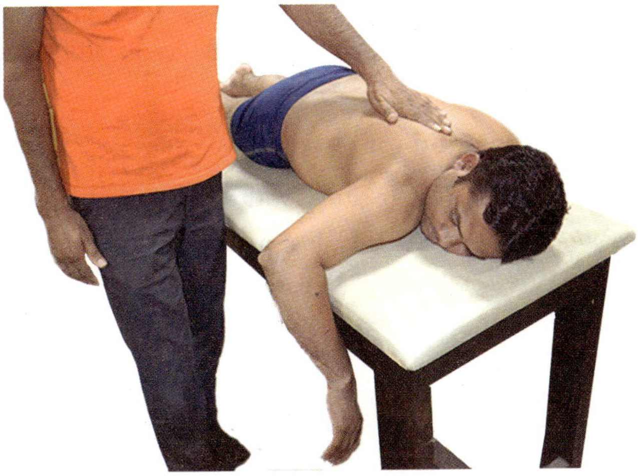

Fig. 6.18: Testing of trapezius middle fibers for grade 3, examiner stands at the side and places one hand over the trunk to stabilize it

Test: Examiner instructs the patient to "lift your elbow towards the ceiling".

Grade 4 and 5 (Good and Normal)

Position of Patient: Prone with shoulder abducted to 90°, arm rests on the plinth. Elbow is out at edge of table and flexed to 90° with the forearms hanging towards floor. Patient may turn the head to either side for comfort.

Position of Examiner: Examiner stands at the side, which is being tested and places one hand on the arm just proximal to the elbow to apply resistance and other hand on the contralateral scapular region to prevent trunk rotation. If the posterior deltoid muscle is weak or less than grade 3 then examiner should shift the hand from distal arm to the shoulder joint to apply resistance.

Stabilization: Examiner stabilizes the trunk to prevent trunk rotation and bending (Figs. 6.19a and b).

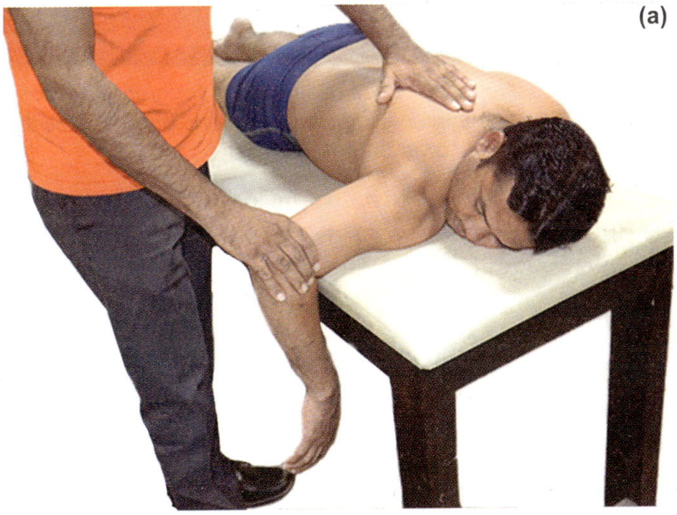

(a)

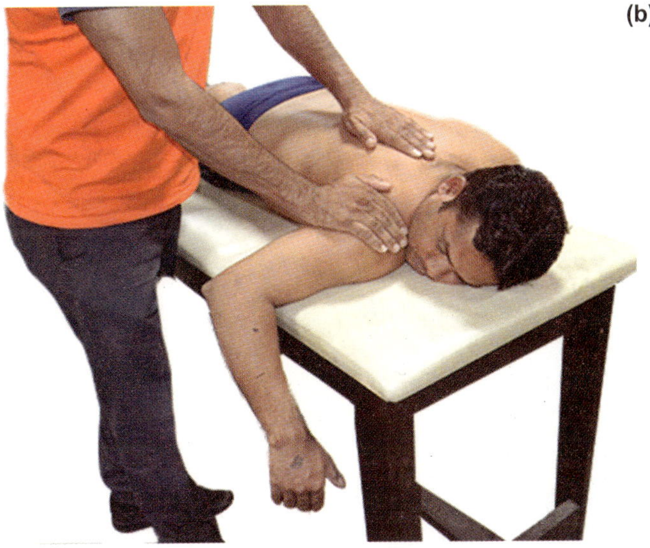

(b)

Figs. 6.19a and b: Testing of trapezius middle fibers for grade 4 and 5, examiner stands at the side of patient and stabilizes the trunk to prevent rotation and lateral bending of the trunk

Test: Examiner instructs the patient to "lift the elbow towards the ceiling" while stabilizing the trunk to prevent rotation and bending.

Grade 4: If patient is able to lift the arm or shoulder towards the ceiling against minimal to moderate resistance.

Grade 5: If patient is able to lift the arm or shoulder towards the ceiling against maximal resistance.

Grade 1 (Trace)

Position of Patient: Prone with shoulder abducted to 90° at edge of table. Elbow is flexed to 90° with the forearms hanging towards floor. Patient may turn the head to either side for comfort.

Position of Examiner: Examiner stands at the side, which is being tested and places his or her fingers on the vertebral border and root of spine to feel the contraction (Fig. 6.20).

Test: Examiner instructs the patient to "lift your elbow towards the ceiling" at the same time examiner palpates the muscle for contraction. If examiner feels contraction or observes movement of the scapula it is considered grade 1.

Grade 2 (Poor)

Position of Patient: Prone with shoulder abducted to 90° arm rests on the plinth. Elbow is out at edge of table and flexed to 90° with the forearms hanging towards floor. Patient may turn the head to either side for comfort.

Position of Examiner: Examiner stands at the side, which is being tested and supports the arm with one hand and places other hand on the contralateral scapular region to prevent trunk rotation.

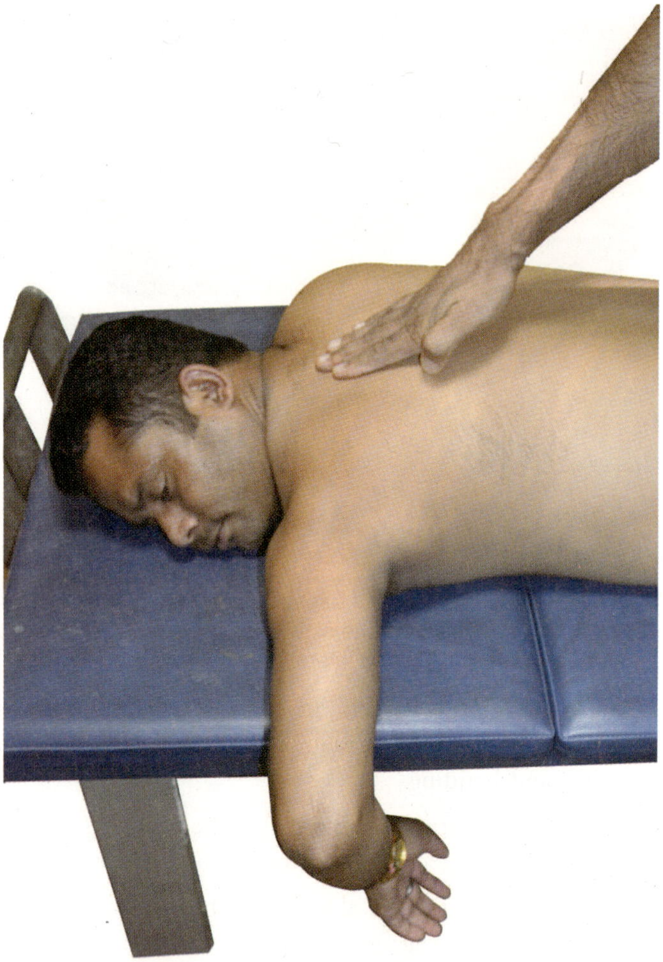

Fig. 6.20: Palpation of trapezius middle fibers for grade 1

Stabilization: Examiner stabilizes the trunk to prevent trunk rotation and bending (Fig. 6.21).

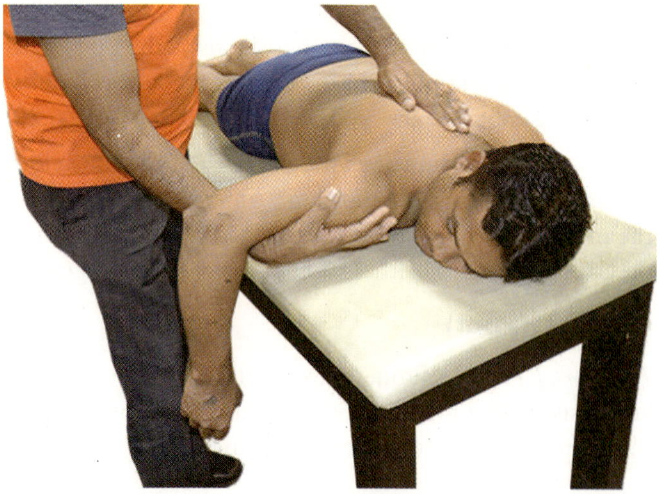

Fig. 6.21: Testing of trapezius middle fibers for grade 2, examiner stands at the side of the patient, supports the arm with one hand and places other hand on the contralateral scapular region to prevent trunk rotation

Test: Examiner instructs the patient to "lift your elbow towards the ceiling" and provides assistance in lifting the elbow and adducting the scapula.

Alternate Position for Grade 2

Position of Patient: Short sitting with the hands in lap.

Position of Examiner: Examiner stands behind the patient and observes scapula adduction.

Stabilization: Examiner stabilizes the trunk to prevent trunk rotation and bending (Fig. 6.22).

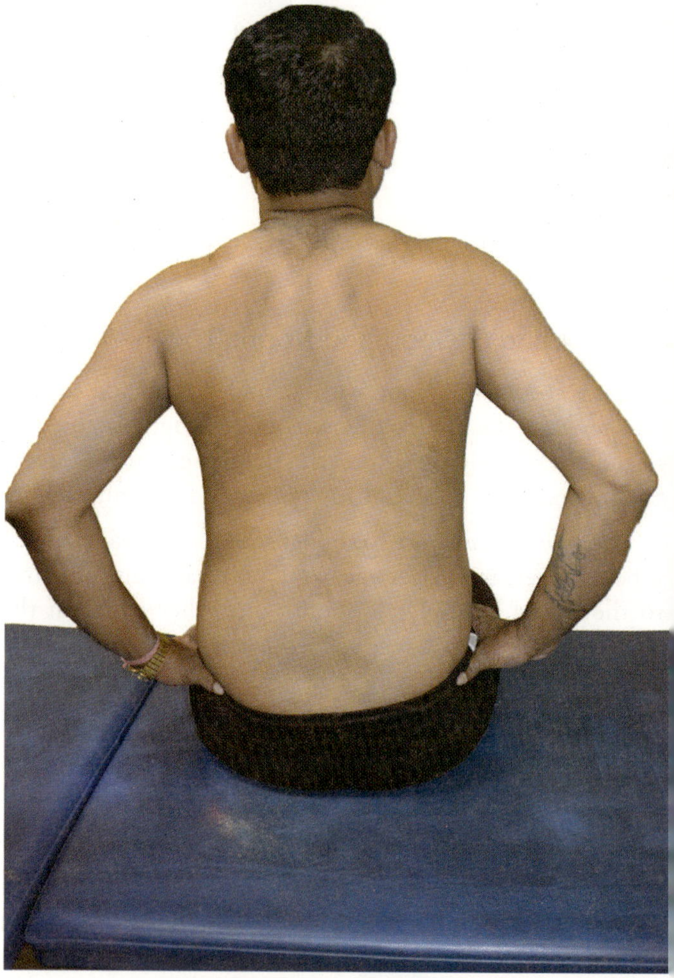

Fig. 6.22: Testing of trapezius middle fibers for grade 2 in short sitting, examiner stands behind the patient and patient takes the shoulder backward towards the examiner

Test: Examiner instructs the patient to bring the shoulder backwards towards the examiner. If patient completes adduction in the full range, it is considered grade 2.

TRAPEZIUS LOWER FIBERS–SCAPULAR DEPRESSION AND ADDUCTION

Origin: Spinous processes of the sixth through 12th thoracic vertebrae.

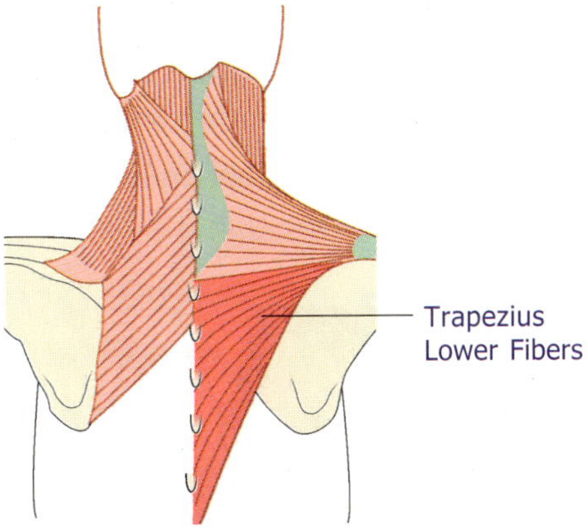

Fig. 6.23: Trapezius lower fibers origin and insertion

Insertion: Tubercle at the apex of the spine of the scapula.

Action: Depresses the scapula. Rotation of the scapula is produced by the action of both upper and lower fibers of the trapezius.

Nerve Supply: Spinal portion of cranial nerve XI (accessory) and ventral ramus, $C_{2,3,4}$.

Grade 3 (Fair)

Position of Patient: Prone, shoulder abducted to 145° and forearm in midprone with elbow extended and thumb pointing towards the ceiling. The arm rests on the plinth or couch.

Position of Examiner: Examiner stands at the side of patient, which is being tested and observes the movement of the arm and scapula.

Stabilization: Examiner stabilizes the trunk to prevent trunk rotation and bending (Fig. 6.24).

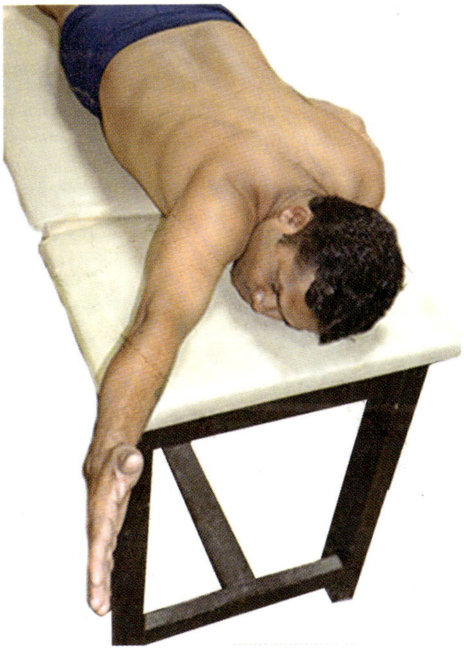

Fig. 6.24: Testing of trapezius lower fibers for grade 3

Test: Examiner instructs the patient to raise the arm in scaption plane from the table towards the ceiling and hold it. If patient raises the arm in the scaption plane against the gravity it is considered grade 3.

Grade 4 and 5 (Good and Normal)

Position of Patient: Prone, shoulder abducted to 145° and forearm in midprone with elbow extended and thumb pointing towards the ceiling. The arm rests on the plinth or couch.

Position of Examiner: Examiner stands at the side of patient, which is being tested and places one hand at the distal arm to apply resistance and other hand on the trunk to prevent rotation. The resistance is given straight downwards towards the floor.

Stabilization: Examiner stabilizes the trunk to prevent trunk rotation and bending (Fig. 6.25).

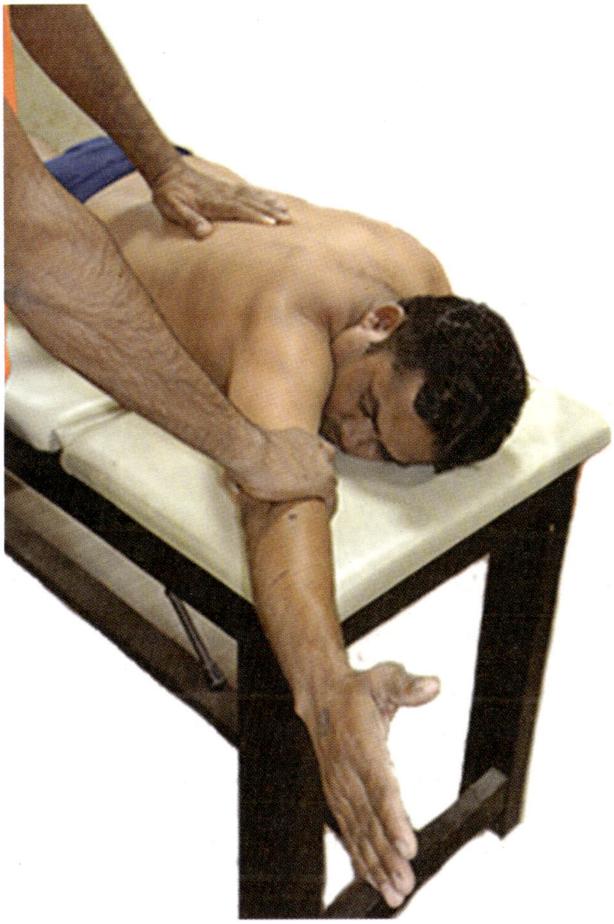

Fig. 6.25: Testing of trapezius lower fibers for grade 4 and 5, examiner stands at the side and places one hand on the distal arm to resist elevation in the scaption plane

Test: Examiner instructs the patient to raise the arm from the table as high as possible and to hold it against the resistance, do not let me push it down.

Grade 4: If patient raises the arm in the scaption plane against gravity against minimal to moderate resistance.

Grade 5: If patient raises the arm in the scaption plane against gravity against maximal resistance.

Grade 1 (Trace)

Position of Patient: Prone, shoulder abducted to 145° and forearm in midprone with elbow extended and thumb pointing towards the ceiling. The arm rests on the plinth or couch.

Position of Examiner: Examiner stands at the side of patient, which is being tested and places one hand between the spinous process of T6-T12 vertebrae and middle border of scapula.

Stabilization: Examiner stabilizes the trunk to prevent trunk rotation and bending (Fig. 6.26).

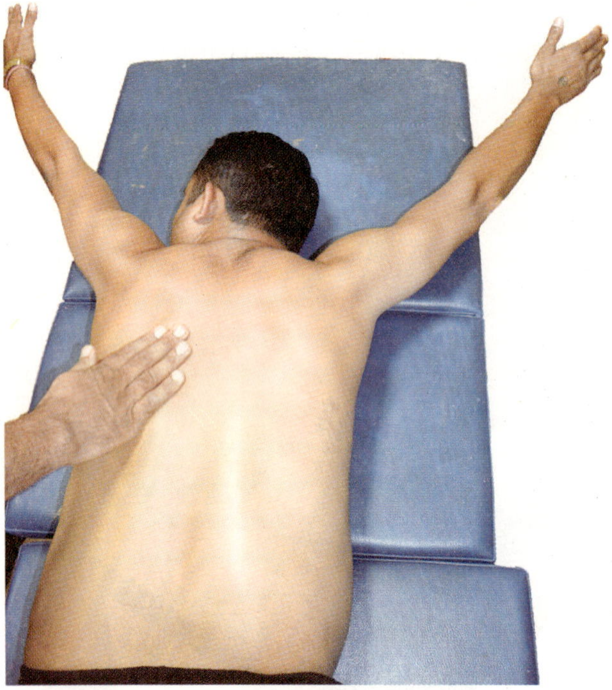

Fig. 6.26: Palpation of trapezius lower fibers for grade 1

Test: While maintaining the arm of the 145° the examiner instructs the patient to try to raise the arm and at the same time examiner palpates the muscle for any contraction. If examiner palpates the muscle while attempting the arm to raise from the table it is considered grade 1.

Grade 2 (Poor)

Position of Patient: Prone, shoulder abducted to 145° and forearm in midprone with elbow extended and thumb pointing towards the ceiling. The arm rests on the plinth or couch.

Position of Examiner: Examiner stands at the side of patient, which is being tested and supports the arm at the elbow joint and places other hand on the trunk.

Stabilization: Examiner stabilizes the trunk to prevent rotation and bending (Fig. 6.27).

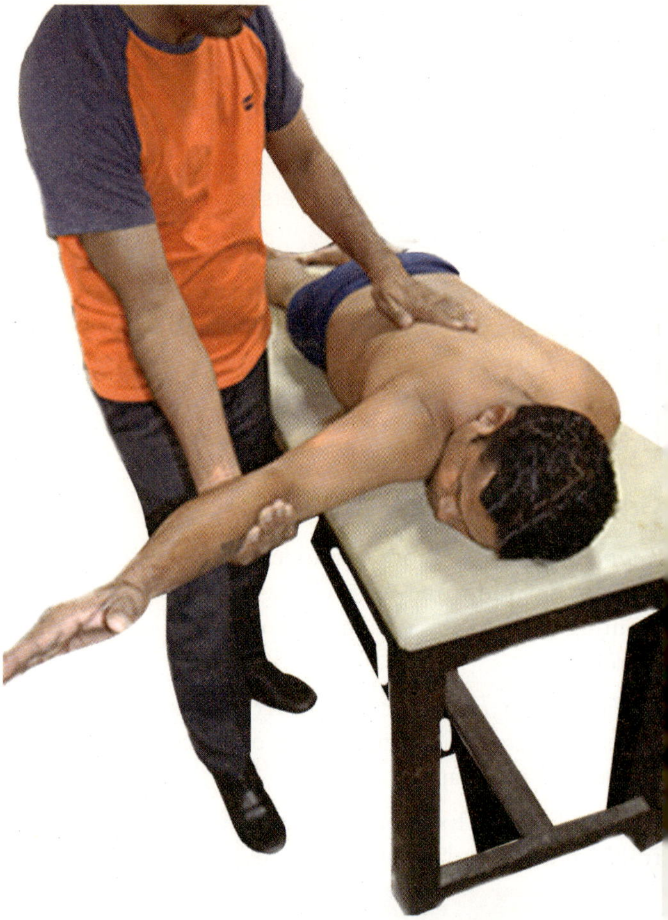

Fig. 6.27: Testing of trapezius lower fibers for grade 2, examiner stands at the side and supports the arm with one hand and stabilizes the trunk with other hand

Test: Examiner instructs the patient to raise the arm from the table and maintain at 145°, examiner provides minimal assistance.

Alternate Position for Grade 2

Position of Patient: Short sitting with the arm abducted to 145 degrees and forearm in midprone with elbow extended and finger pointing the ceiling diagonally.

Position of Examiner: Examiner stands behind the patient and observes the movement of the arm and scapula.

Stabilization: Examiner stabilizes the trunk to prevent trunk rotation and bending (Fig. 6.28), if patient attempts any trick movements.

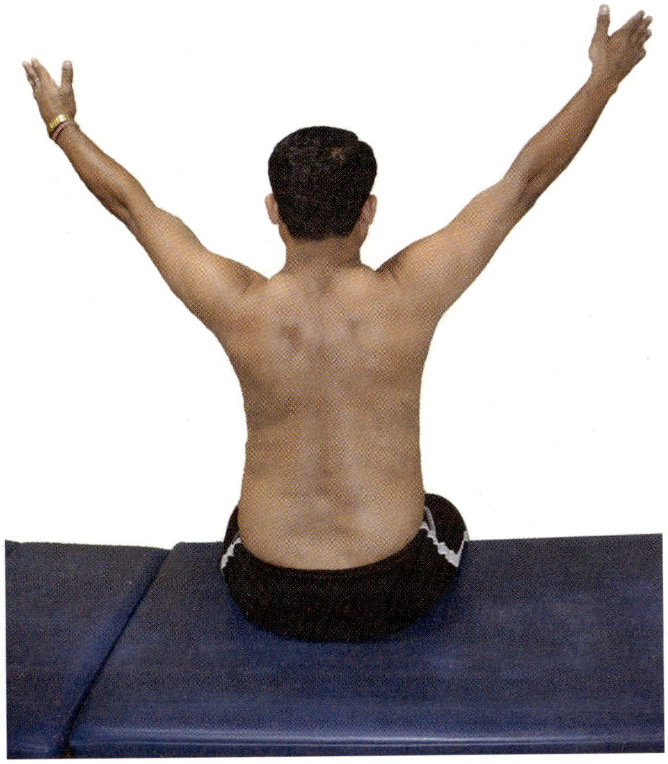

Fig. 6.28: Alternate testing position of trapezius lower fibers for grade 2

Test: Examiner instructs the patient to bring the arm and scapula backwards towards the examiner as much as possible. If examiner observes significant scapular adduction, it is considered grade 2.

RHOMBOIDS–SCAPULAR ADDUCTION AND DOWNWARD ROTATION

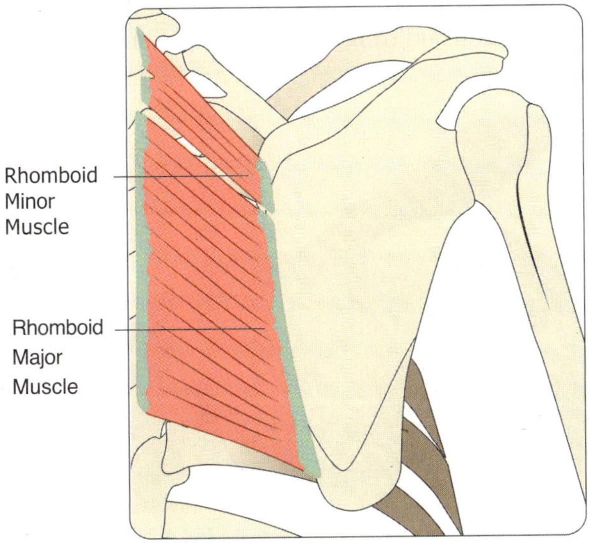

Fig. 6.29: Rhomboids (major and minor) origin and insertion

Origin: Rhomboid major originates from spinous processes of second through fifth thoracic vertebra. Rhomboid minor originates from ligamentum nuchae, spinous processes of seventh cervical and first thoracic vertebrae.

Insertion: Rhomboid major inserts on the fibrous attachment to medial border of the scapula between spine and inferior angle. Rhomboid minor inserts on the medial border at root of spine of the scapula.

Action: Rhomboid adducts and elevates the scapula, and rotates it so that the glenoid cavity faces caudally.

Nerve Supply: Dorsal scapular, $C_{4 \text{ and } 5}$.

Grade 3 (Fair)

Position of Patient: Prone, shoulder is adducted fully and rotated internally. Elbow is flexed to 90° and the dorsum of hand rests on the lower back of the patient (medial rotation of humerus).

Position of Examiner: Examiner stands at the side, which is being tested and places one hand on the scapula and observes the scapular adduction and downward rotation.

Stabilization: Examiner stabilizes the shoulder girdle to prevent elevation and trunk to prevent rotation and bending (Fig. 6.30).

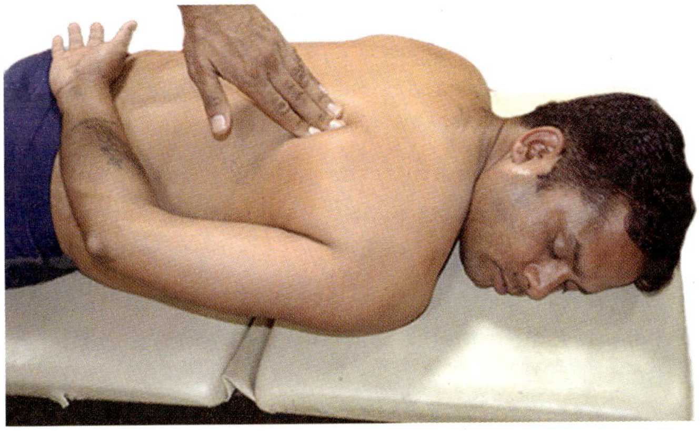

Fig. 6.30: Testing of rhomboid major for grade 3, examiner stands at the side and places one hand over the trunk to stabilize it

Test: Examiner instructs the patient to lift the hand off the back and elbow joint from the couch. If patient completes scapular adduction and downward rotation the fingers of examiner will pop out from under the edge of the scapular border.

Grade 4 and 5

Position of Patient: Prone, shoulder is adducted fully and rotated internally. Elbow is flexed to 90° and the dorsum of hand rests on the lower back of the patient.

Position of Examiner: Examiner stands at the side, which is being tested. He or she places resistance hand on the distal arm just above the elbow joint if the shoulder extensors are grade 3 or higher. If the extensors of the shoulders are less than grade 3 the resistance hand is placed on along the axillary border of the scapula. Resistance is applied in downward and outward direction.

Stabilization: Examiner stabilizes the shoulder girdle to prevent elevation and trunk to prevent rotation and bending (Fig. 6.31).

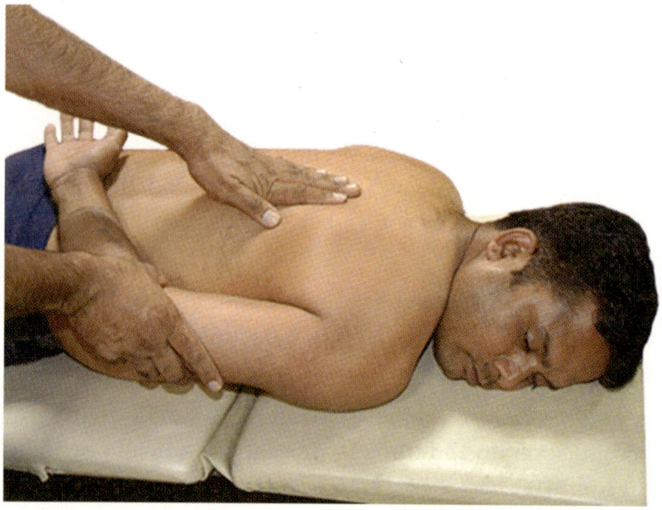

Fig. 6.31: Testing of rhomboid major for grade 4 and 5, examiner stands at the side and places one hand on the distal arm to offer resistance and other hand on the trunk to prevent rotation and bending and shoulder elevation

Test: Examiner instructs the patient to lift the hand off the back and the elbow joint from the couch and hold it. Do not let me push it down.

Grade 4: If patient is able to lift the hand off the back and elbow joint from the couch against strong to moderate resistance.

Grade 5: If patient is able to lift the hand off the back and elbow joint from the couch against maximal resistance.

Grade 1 (Poor)

Position of Patient: Prone, shoulder is adducted fully and rotated internally. Elbow is flexed to 90° and the dorsum of hand rests on the lower back of the patient. Head is turned to either side for comfortable.

Position of Examiner: Examiner stands at the side, which is being tested and places one hand between T2-T5 vertebrae and root of spine and inferior angle of the scapula.

Stabilization: Examiner stabilizes the shoulder girdle to prevent elevation and trunk to prevent rotation and bending (Fig. 6.32).

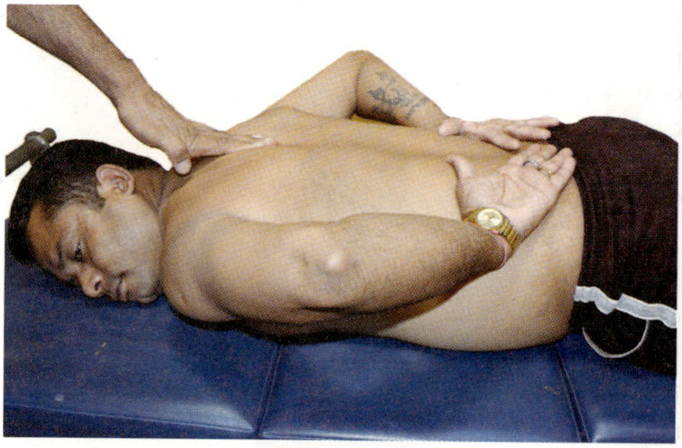

Fig. 6.32: Palpation of rhomboid muscles for grade 1, examiner stands at the side and places one hand between T2-T5 vertebrae and root of spine and inferior angle of the scapula to feel the contraction

Test: Examiner instructs the patient to try to lift the hand off the back. If examiner feels contraction it is considered grade 1.

Grade 2 (Poor)

Position of Patient: Prone, shoulder is adducted fully and rotated internally. Elbow is flexed to 90° and the dorsum of hand rests on the lower back of the patient.

Position of Examiner: Examiner stands at the side, which is being tested, and places one hand under the shoulder and arm and other hand on the inferior angle of scapula, observes the scapular adduction and downward rotation. Examiner provides minimal support to the arm in assisting the movement.

Stabilization: Examiner stabilizes the shoulder girdle to prevent elevation and trunk to prevent rotation and bending (Fig. 6.33).

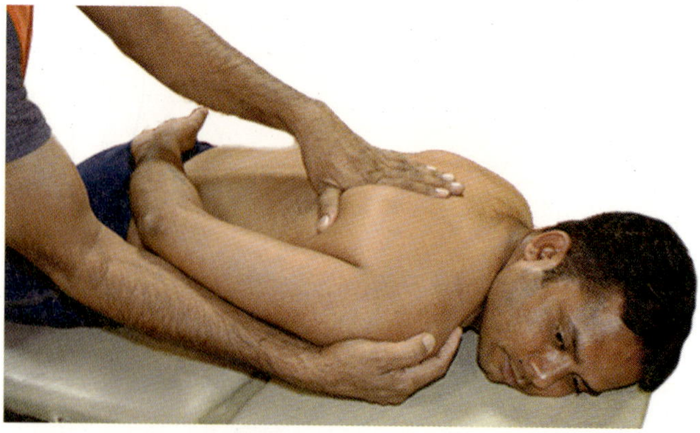

Fig. 6.33: Testing of rhomboid major for grade 2, examiner stands at the side and places one hand under the shoulder and arm and other hand on the inferior angle of the scapula to provide minimal support to the movement

Test: Examiner instructs the patient to lift the hand off the back and the elbow joint from the couch. If patient completes scapular adduction and downward rotation it is considered grade 2.

Alternate Position for Grade 2

Position of Patient: Short sitting, shoulder is adducted fully and rotated internally. Elbow is flexed to 90° and the dorsum of hand rests on the lower back of the patient.

Position of Examiner: Examiner stands at the side, which is being tested, places one hand under the inferior angle of the scapula, holds the distal forearm with the other hand, and observes the scapular adduction and downward rotation.

Stabilization: Examiner stabilizes the shoulder girdle to prevent elevation and trunk to prevent rotation and bending (Fig. 6.34a).

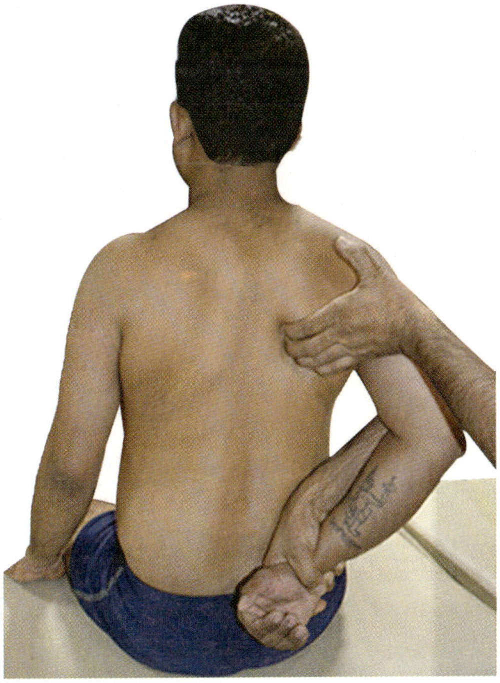

Fig. 6.34a: Alternate testing position of rhomboid major for grade 2, examiner stands at the side and grasps the distal arm with one hand and inferior angle with the other hand

Test: Examiner instructs the patient to lift the hand off the back and the elbow joint from the couch. If patient completes scapular adduction and downward rotation it is considered grade 2.

Alternate Test for Rhomboids (Kendall)

Position of Patient: Prone with head turned to the testing side. Non-testing side is abducted with elbow flexion. Testing shoulder is adducted and rotated externally with the elbow flexion. The arm and forearm rests on the couch close to the midaxillary line. This position brings the scapula in adduction, elevation, and downward rotation (glenoid down).

Position of Examiner: Examiner stands at the side, which is being tested. One hand is cupped around the flexed elbow. The resistance applied by this hand will be in the direction of scapular abduction and upward rotation (out and up). The other hand is also used to apply resistance simultaneously placed on the shoulder (fingers on superior and anterior aspect and thumb on the posterior aspect). The resistance is applied caudally in the direction of shoulder depression.

Stabilization: Examiner stabilizes the shoulder girdle to prevent elevation and trunk to prevent rotation and bending (Fig. 6.34b).

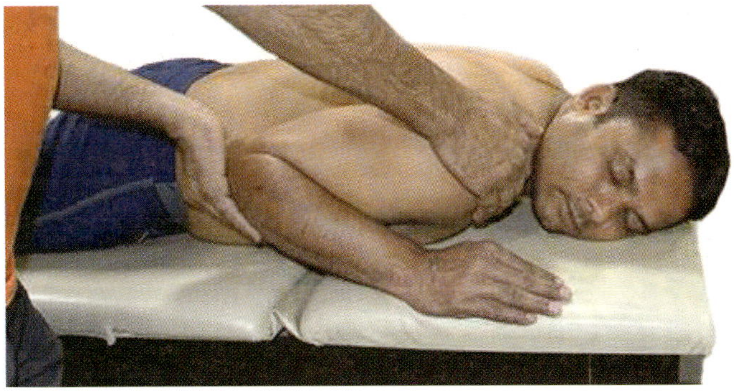

Fig. 6.34b: Alternate testing position for rhomboid after Kendal, examiner stands at the side and grasps elbow and shoulder to apply resistance against the movement in the direction of scapular abduction and shoulder girdle adduction

Test: Examiner instructs the patient to hold your arm as I have placed it. Do not let me pull your arm forward. OR "hold the position you are in; keep your shoulder blade against your spine as I try to pull it away.

WEAKNESS OF PARASCAPULAR MUSCLES

Serratus Anterior, Levator Scapulae, Trapezius All Fibers and Rhomboids

Scapular Dyskinesia: Scapular dyskinesia is considered any change in the scapulothoracic pace, which causes a change in the position, scapular movements or normal mobility of the scapula relative to the thorax. Kibler, 1991, observed consistent and abnormal scapular postural changes and altered scapular kinematics in overhead athletes with shoulder impingement syndrome, and coined the term scapular dyskinesia. The scapular changes such as downward rotation, prominent middle border and anterior tilting are the common manifestations of the scapular dyskinesia.

Kibler classified scapular dysfunction into three categories: Type I–The primary external visual feature is the prominence of the inferior angle as a result of anterior tilting of the scapula in the sagittal plane. This type of scapula dyskinesia results from the weakness of the middle and lower trapezius muscles. Type II–The primary external visual feature is the prominence of the entire middle scapular border. Type II is mainly due to the weakness of upper trapezius, middle trapezius, and serratus anterior muscles. These muscles act as scapula stabilizers on the thoracic wall. Type III–It is also called superior dysfunction of the scapula. It is characterized by excessive and early elevation of the scapula during upper extremity elevation. This type of dyskinesia has been referred as compensatory shoulder hiking or shrugging of the girdle (Figs. 6.35a).

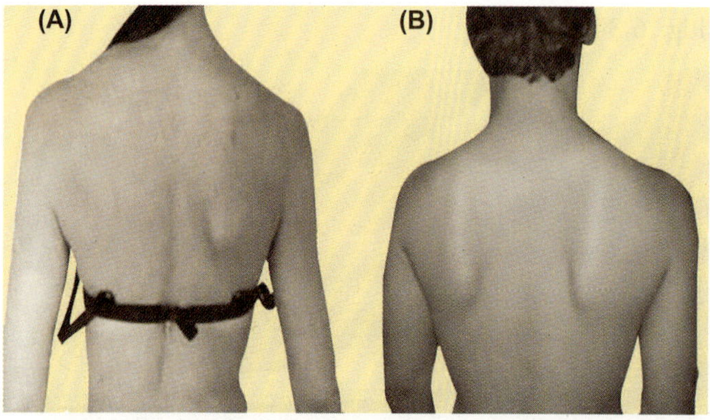

Figs. 6.35a: Scapular dyskinesia. A - Type I, patient shows right prominent inferior angle due to weakness of trapezius middle and lower fibers. Prominent inferior angle is associated with the anterior tipping of the scapula. B - Type II, Scapular dyskinesia, patient shows both the middle borders of scapula prominent (right more than the left) due to weakness of serratus anterior, trapezius middle and rhomboid muscles

Weakness of Scapula Force Couple Muscles and Deficient Scapulohumeral Rhythm: The scapula forms a stable base from which all shoulder movements occur and correct positioning of scapula is an essential for efficient and powerful glenohumeral joint movement. There is approximately 60 degree of external rotation of the scapula during elevation of the arm (Fig. 6.35b).

The external rotation of the scapula is provided by the two opposite forces of same magnitude acting on the scapula called scapula force couple. The upper portion of the force couple is formed by the trapezius upper fibers, levator scapulae and serratus anterior upper fibers. The lower portion of the scapula force couple is formed by the trapezius lower fibers and serratus anterior lower fibers (Fig. 6.35c).

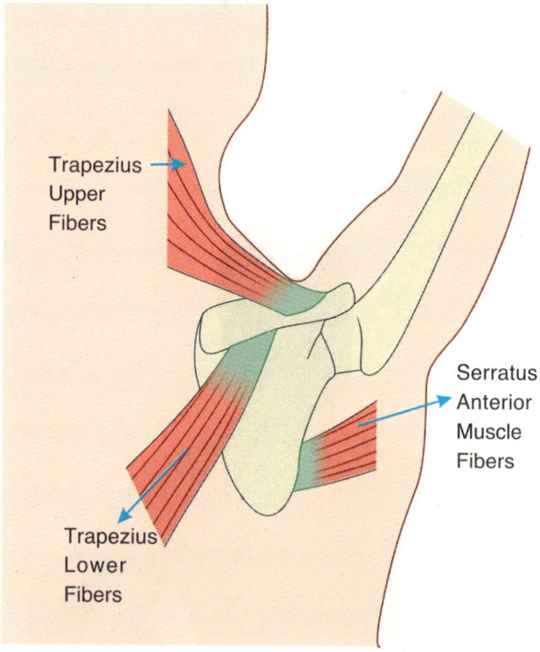

Fig. 6.35c: Scapula force couple. Arrows showing the direction of movement of scapula and contraction of the muscles

Simultaneous contraction of these two portions of muscles produces smooth, rhythmic and coordinated external rotation of the scapula along the posterior thorax

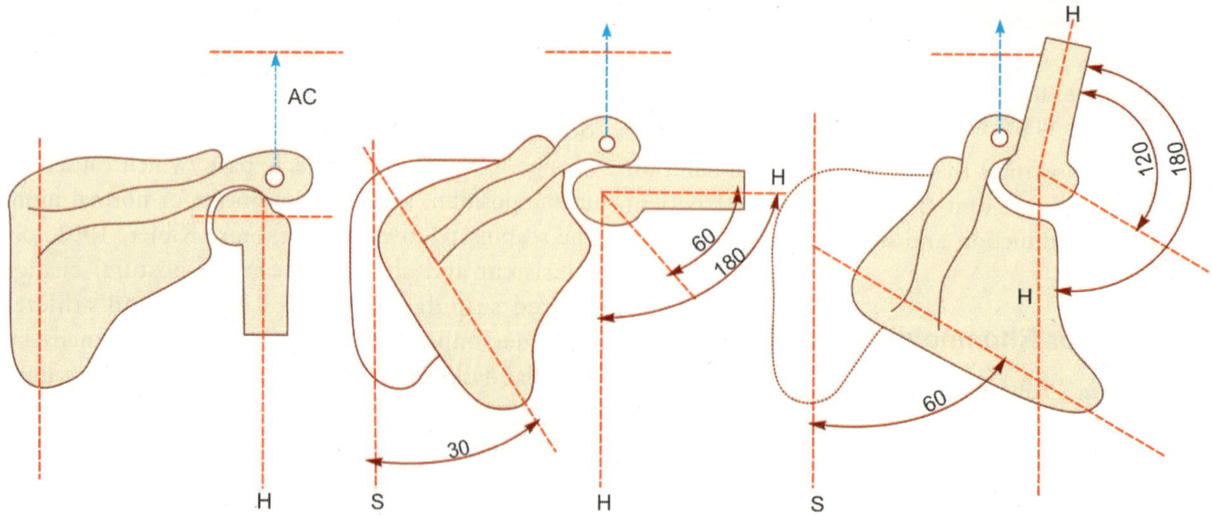

Fig. 6.35b: External rotation of scapula, at rest, 90° elevation arm and at 180° elevation of the arm

during elevation of the arm. The external rotation of the scapula functions to provide a stable base of support for the rotating humerus to allow the humeral head to maintain its normal pathway along the glenoid.

Weakness of any one portion of the force couple results in an inappropriate rotation of the scapula with rotating arm, that results in impingement of the head of humerus with the acromian arch. The soft tissues lie between the head of humerus and acromian arch such as subacromial bursa, tendon of supraspinatus and long head of biceps get compressed in the overhead activities.

LATISSIMUS DORSI–SCAPULAR DEPRESSION

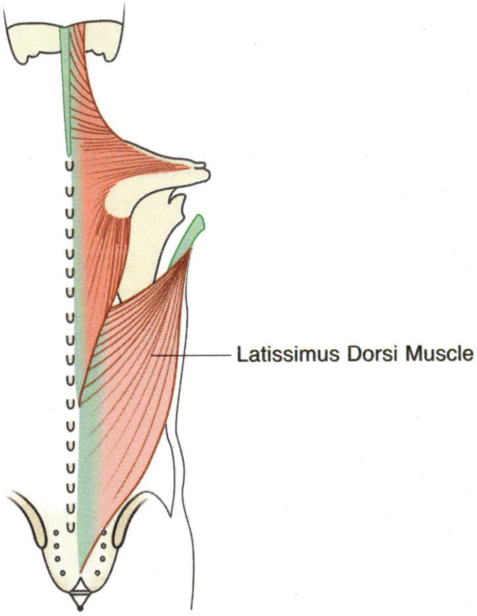

Fig. 6.36: Latissimus dorsi muscle origin and insertion

Origin: Latissimus dorsi originates from spinous processes of last six thoracic vertebrae, last three or four ribs, through the thoracolumbar fascia from the lumbar and sacral vertebrae and posterior 1/3rd of external lip of iliac crest, and a slip from the inferior angle of the scapula.

Insertion: Intertubercular grove of humerus.

Action: With the origin fixed, latissimus dorsi medially rotates, adducts and extends the shoulder and assists in lateral flexion of the trunk. With the insertion fixed, latissimus dorsi assists in tilting the pelvis both anteriorly and laterally. Simultaneous contraction of bilateral latissimus muscles causes hyperextension of the spine, and anterior tilting of the pelvis. Latissimus may also act as accessory muscles of respiration.

Nerve Supply: Thoracodorsal, $C_{6,\ 7,\ 8}$.

Grade 3 (Fair)

Position of Patient: Prone with both the shoulders, shrugged adducted and rotated internally palms facing upward. The testing side shoulder is raised to the level of chin. Head is rotated to either side for comfortable.

Position of Examiner: Examiner stands at the side of body and holds the forearms just distal to the elbow joint with both the hands.

Stabilization: Examiner instructs the patient to prevent rotation and bending of the trunk (Fig. 6.37).

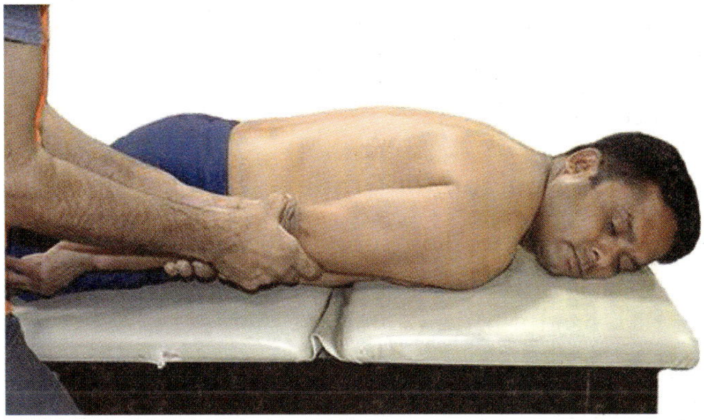

Fig. 6.37: Testing of latissimus dorsi muscle for grade 3, examiner stands at the side, grasps the arm at the elbow joint, and applies mild resistance against the shoulder depression

Test: Examiner instructs the patient to depress the shoulder or reach toward your feet. Examiner offers minimal resistance against the depression towards shoulder. If patient completes the shoulder depression against minimal resistance, it is considered grade 3.

Grade 4 and 5 (Good and Normal)

Position of Patient: Prone with both the shoulders, shrugged adducted and rotated internally palms facing upward. The testing side shoulder is raised to the level of chin. Head is rotated to either side for comfortable.

Position of Examiner: Examiner stands at the side of patient and holds the forearms just distal to the elbow joint with both the hands.

Stabilization: Examiner instructs the patient to prevent elevation and trunk to prevent rotation and bending (Fig. 6.38).

Test: Examiner instructs the patient to depress the shoulder or reach toward your feet. Examiner offers resistance against the depression towards shoulder.

Grade 4: If patient completes the shoulder depression against strong to moderate resistance.

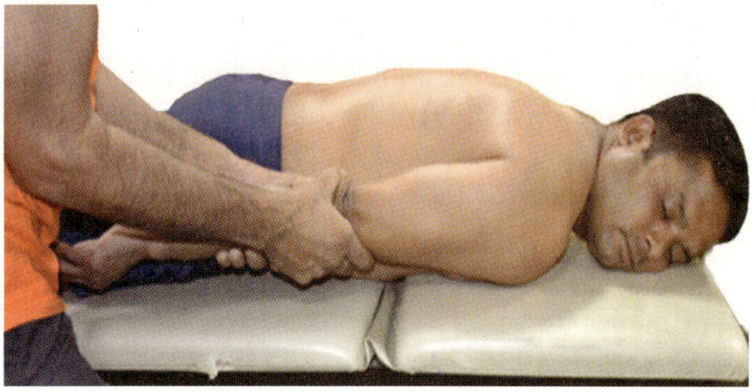

Fig. 6.38: Testing of latissimus dorsi muscle for grade 4 and 5, examiner stands at the side and grasps the arm at the elbow joint and resists the shoulder depression

Grade 5: If patient completes the shoulder depression against maximal resistance.

Alternate Position for Grade 5

Position of Patient: Short sitting with both the hands flat on the table adjacent to hips. Push up blocks are provided for each hand if patient's arms are short.

Position of Examiner: Examiner stands behind the patient and observes the movement of the shoulder girdle.

Stabilization: Examiner instructs the patient to prevent elevation and trunk rotation and bending (Fig. 6.39).

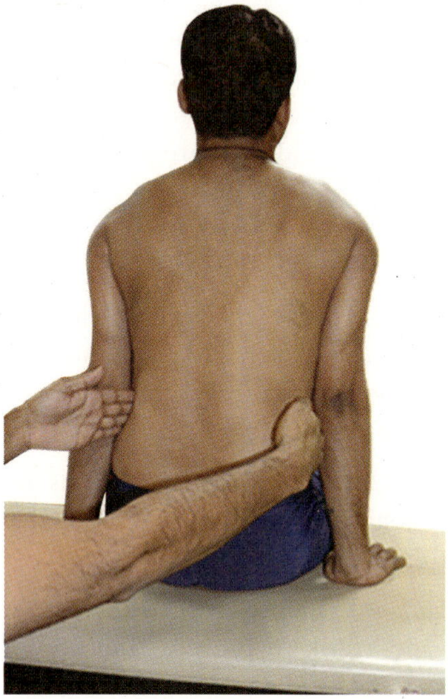

Fig. 6.39: Testing of latissimus dorsi muscle for grade 4 and 5, examiner stands behind the patient and places hands on either side of the waist above the pelvis

Test: Examiner instructs the patient to "lift your buttocks off the table". If patient is able to lift the buttocks off the table, it is considered grade 5 or normal.

Grade 1 (Trace)

Position of Patient: Prone with both the shoulders adducted and rotated internally palms facing upward. The testing side shoulder is raised to the level of chin. Head is rotated to either side for comfortable.

Position of Examiner: Examiner stands at the side anterior to the shoulder and places fingers over the lateral costal region (Fig. 6.40).

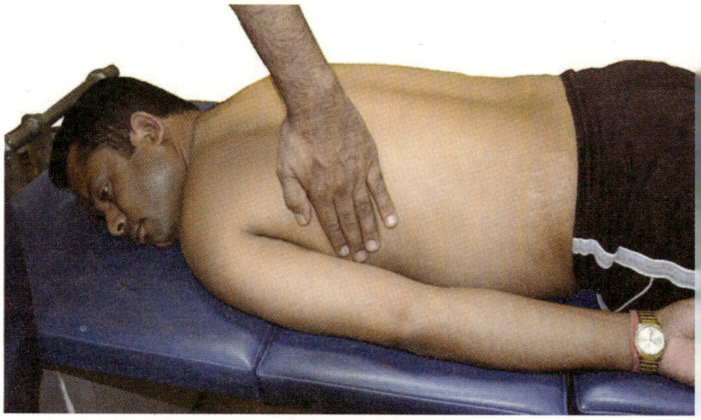

Fig. 6.40: Palpation of latissimus dorsi muscle for grade 1

Test: Examiner instructs the patient to try to depress the shoulder or reach toward your feet. If examiner feels the contraction over the lateral costal area while the patient attempts the movement it is considered grade 1.

Grade 2 (Poor)

Position of Patient: Prone with both the shoulders adducted and rotated internally palms facing upward. The testing side shoulder is raised to the level of chin. Head is rotated to either side for comfortable.

Position of Examiner: Examiner stands at the side of body and observes the movement, i.e., depression of the shoulder without retraction or protraction of the shoulder (Fig. 6.41).

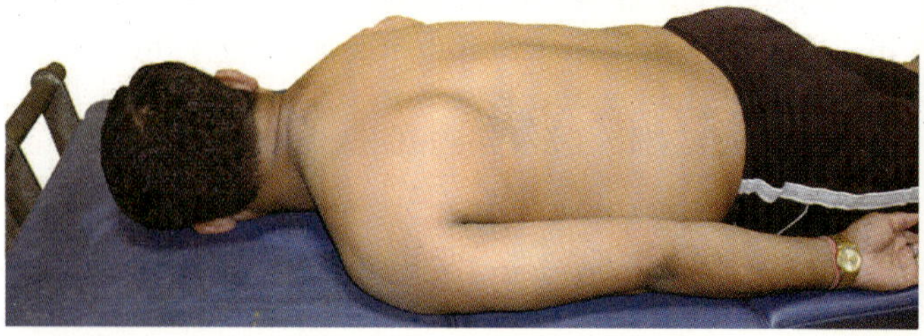

Fig. 6.41: Testing of latissimus dorsi muscle for grade 2, examiner stands at the side and observes the depression of the shoulder

Test: Examiner instructs the patient to depress the shoulder or reach toward your feet. If patient completes shoulder depression in the gravity eliminated position it is considered grade 2.

DELTOID (ANTERIOR FIBERS) – SHOULDER FLEXION

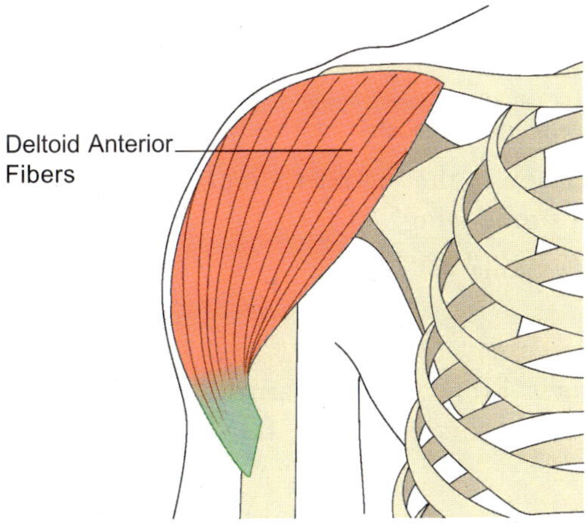

Fig. 6.42: Deltoid–Anterior muscle fibers origin and insertion

Origin: Anterior border, superior surface, and lateral 1/3rd of the clavicle.

Insertion: Deltoid tuberosity of the humerus.

Action: Flexion of the shoulder joint. Medially rotates the shoulder in supine lying.

Nerve Supply: Axillary, $C_{5 \text{ and } 6}$.

Grade 3 (Fair)

Position of Patient: Short sitting with arms at sides, elbow flexed slightly and forearm pronated.

Position of Examiner: Examiner stands behind the patient, places one hand on the top of the shoulder joint, and observes the flexion. There should not be elevation of the shoulder and trunk rotation during the flexion.

Stabilization: Examiner stabilizes the trunk rotation and bending and the shoulder elevation (Fig. 6.43).

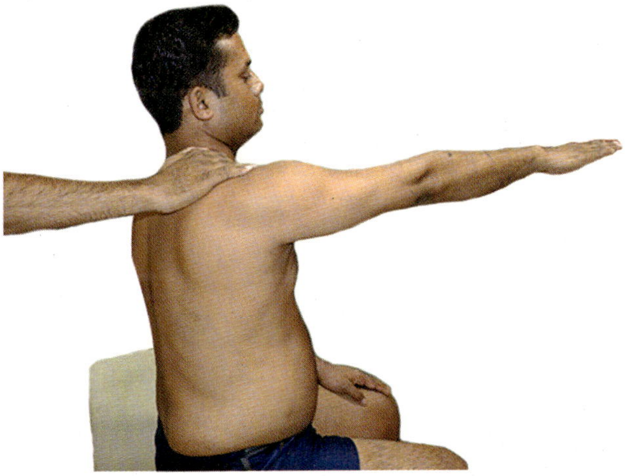

Fig. 6.43: Testing of deltoid muscle fibers for grade 3, examiner stands behind the patient and places one hand on the top of the shoulder to prevent trunk bending and rotation

Test: Examiner instructs the patient to raise the arm towards head. There should not be any rotation of the trunk and elevation of the shoulder during flexion. If patient completes full range of motion against the gravity it is considered grade 3.

Grade 4 (Good)

Position of Patient: Short sitting with arms at sides, elbow flexed slightly and forearm pronated.

Position of Examiner: Examiner stands behind the patient and places one hand on the top of the shoulder joint and other hand over the distal humerus just above the elbow joint. There should not be elevation of the shoulder and trunk rotation during the flexion.

Stabilization: Examiner stabilizes the trunk to prevent rotation and bending and the shoulder elevation (Fig. 6.44).

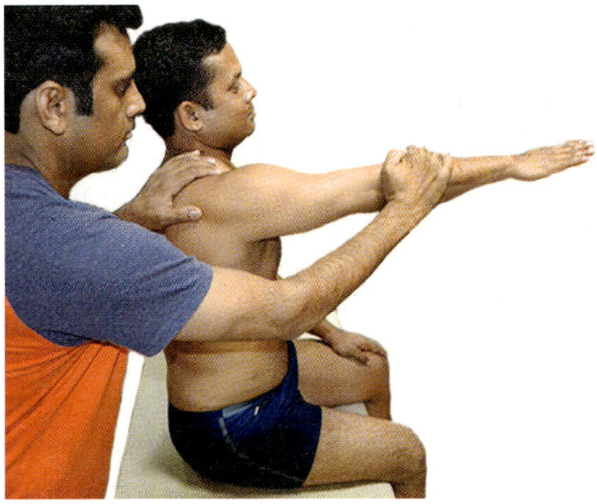

Fig. 6.44: Testing of deltoid muscle fibers for grade 4 and 5, examiner stands behind the patient and places one hand on the distal arm to resist the shoulder flexion and other hand on the top of the shoulder to prevent trunk rotation and bending

Test: Examiner instructs the patient to raise the arm towards head. There should not be any rotation of the trunk and elevation of the shoulder during flexion.

Grade 4: If patient completes full range of motion against strong to moderate resistance.

Grade 5: If patient completes full range of motion against maximal resistance.

Grade 1 (Flicker/Trace)

Position of Patient: Supine with both the shoulders at neutral position.

Position of Examiner: Examiner stands behind the patient and place one hand on the top of the shoulder, fingers over the lateral clavicle and head of humerus (anteriorly).

Stabilization: Examiner stabilizes the trunk to prevent rotation and bending and the shoulder elevation (Fig. 6.45).

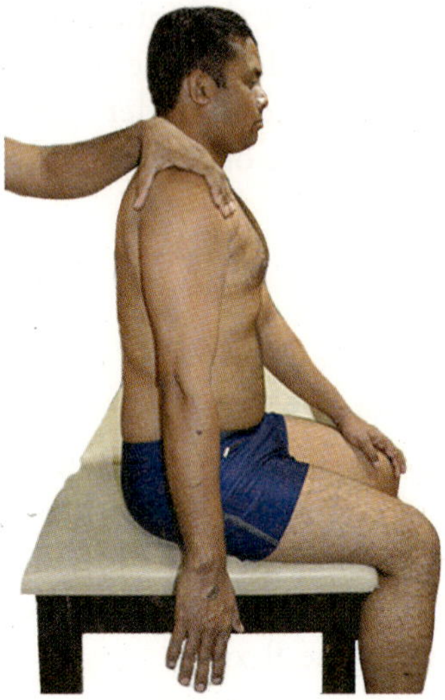

Fig. 6.45: Palpation of deltoid muscle fibers for grade 1, examiner stands behind the patient and places hand on the top of the shoulder, fingers on the anterior aspect of the shoulder to palpate the anterior fibers of the deltoid

Test: Examiner instructs the patient to raise the arm towards the ceiling. Examiner palpates the deltoid anterior fibers while the patient attempts to raise the arm. If examiner feels contraction on the anterior aspect of the shoulder while the patient attempts movement it is considered grade 1.

Grade 2 (Poor)

Position of Patient: Side lying with the testing arm uppermost. The patient places contralateral hand under the head for comfortable and flexes the lower knee and hip to stabilize the body.

Position of Examiner: Examiner stands behind the patient and may support the arm with one hand.

Stabilization: Examiner stabilizes the trunk rotation and bending and the shoulder elevation (Fig. 6.46).

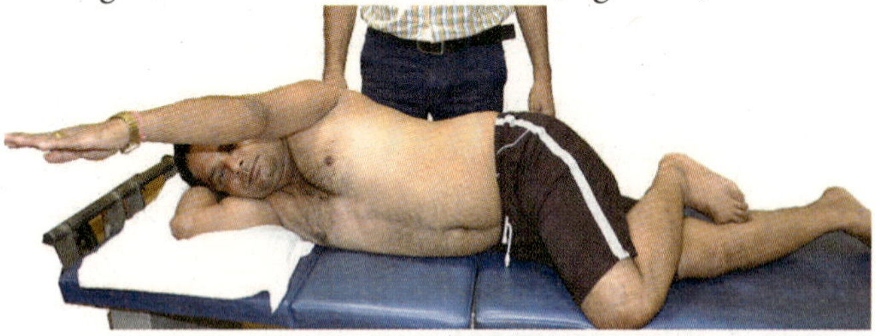

Fig. 6.46: Testing of anterior deltoid muscle fibers for grade 2

Test: Examiner instructs the patient to raise the arm towards head. There should not be any rotation of the trunk and elevation of the shoulder during flexion. Examiner should not assist the movement. If patient completes full range of motion in the gravity eliminated position it is considered grade 2.

Weakness: Loss of shoulder flexion in the sagittal plane.

DELTOID POSTERIOR FIBERS, LATISSIMUS DORSI – SHOULDER EXTENSION

Origin: Inferior lip of the posterior border of the spine of the scapula.

Insertion: Deltoid tuberosity of the humerus.

Action: Extension of the shoulder joint. Laterally rotates the shoulder in prone lying.

Nerve Supply: Axillary, $C_{5 \text{ and } 6}$.

Grade 3

Position of Patient: Prone with the arms at the sides and shoulders internally rotated. Palms face upwards to the ceiling.

Position of Examiner: Examiner stands at the side of the patient and observes the movement in the sagittal plane.

Stabilization: Examiner should not allow the patient to abduct the shoulder while extending the arm. There should not be trunk rotation and protraction of the shoulder (scapula) (Fig. 6.47).

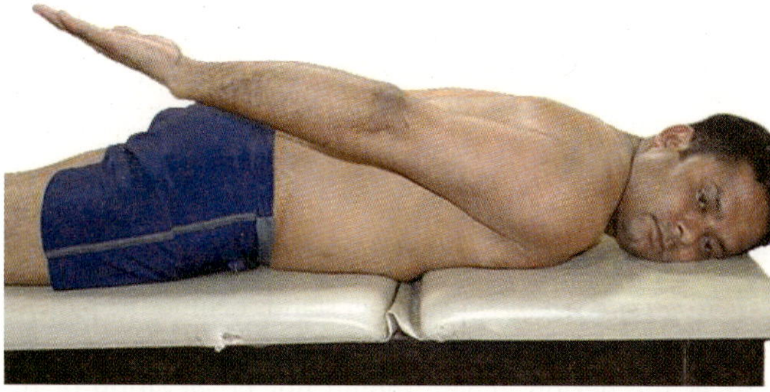

Fig. 6.47: Testing of posterior deltoid muscle fibers for grade 3, examiner stands at the side and observes the shoulder extension

Test: Examiner instructs the patient to try to lift the arm as high as he or she can do it against the gravity. If patient can complete the range of motion against the gravity in the sagittal plane, it is considered grade 3.

Grade 4 and 5 (Good and Fair)

Position of Patient: Prone with the arms at the sides and shoulders internally rotated. Palms face upwards to the ceiling.

Position of Examiner: Examiner stands at the side of the patient and places one hand over the posterior arm just above the elbow joint to apply resistance and other hand may be placed over the shoulder to prevent protraction and trunk rotation.

Stabilization: Examiner instructs the subject to prevent shoulder retraction and anterior tilting (Fig. 6.48).

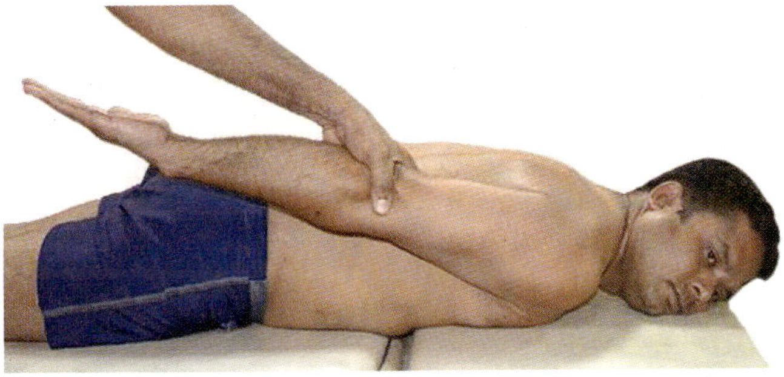

Fig. 6.48: Testing of posterior deltoid muscle fibers for grade 4 and 5, examiner stands at the side and places one hand over the elbow joint to resist the extension of shoulder joint

Test: Examiner instructs the patient to try to lift the arm as high as he or she can do it against the resistance. Examiner should not allow the patient to abduct the shoulder while extending the arm. There should not be trunk rotation and protraction of the shoulder joint.

Grade 4: If patient can complete the range of motion against strong to moderate resistance.

Grade 5: If patient can complete the range of motion against maximal resistance.

Grade 1 (Flicker/Trace)

Position of Patient: Prone with the arms at the sides and shoulders internally rotated. Palms face upwards to the ceiling.

Position of Examiner: Examiner stands at the opposite side of the patient and places one hand over the posterior deltoid (posterolateral scapula and posterior aspect of the head of humerus.

Stabilization: Examiner instructs the subject to prevent shoulder retraction anterior tilting (Fig. 6.49).

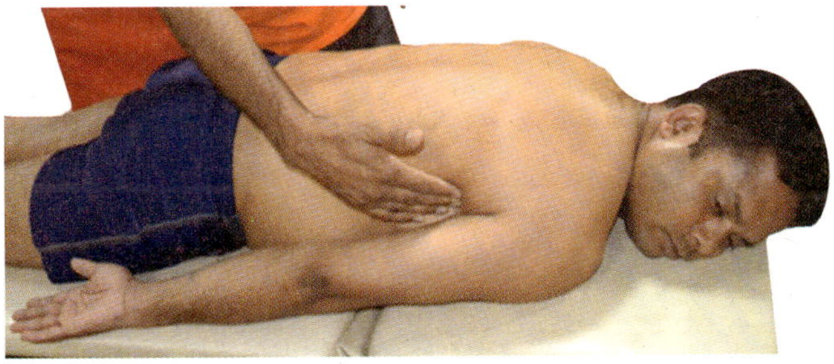

Fig. 6.49: Palpation of posterior deltoid fibers for grade 1

Test: Examiner instructs the patient to try to lift the arm. If examiner feels contraction while the patient attempts to lift the arm it is considered grade 1.

Grade 2 (Poor)

Position of Patient: Side lying with the extremity to be tested lies uppermost. Patient may place contralateral hand under the head for comfortable.

Position of Examiner: Examiner stands behind the patient and supports the arm for smooth movement.

Stabilization: Examiner instructs the subject to prevent shoulder retraction anterior tilting (Fig. 6.50).

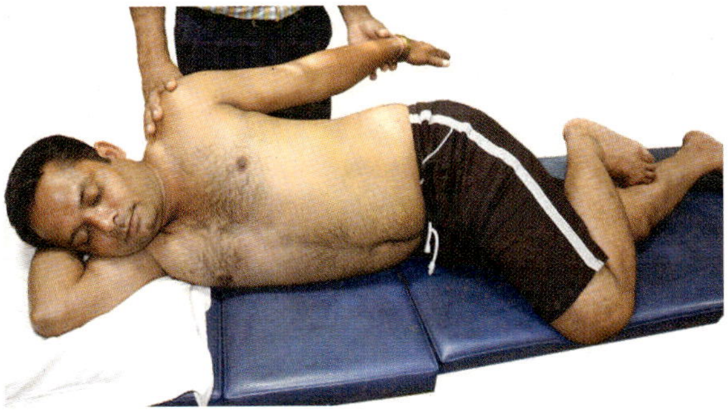

Fig. 6.50: Testing of posterior deltoid fibers for grade 2

Test: Examiner instructs the patient to bring the arm backward towards the examiner. The examiner should not assist the movement; however, support may be given for smooth movement of the shoulder. The examiner must ensure that the movement is taken place in the sagittal plane. Trunk rotation should be taken care of. If patient completes range of motion in the gravity eliminated position in the sagittal plane it is considered grade 2.

Weakness: Loss of extension of the shoulder joint in the sagittal plane.

DELTOID MIDDLE FIBERS AND SUPRA-SPINATUS–SHOULDER ABDUCTION

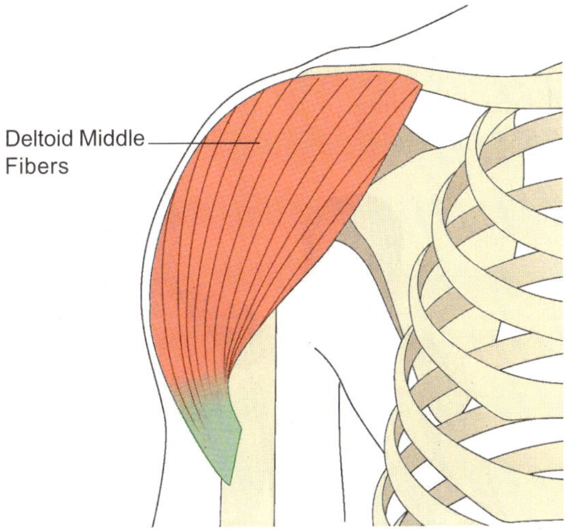

Fig. 6.51: Deltoid middle fibers origin and insertion

Origin: Lateral margin and posterior surface of the acromion.

Insertion: Deltoid tuberosity of the humerus.

Action: Abduction of the shoulder joint.

Nerve Supply: Axillary, $C_{5 \text{ and } 6}$ (Fig. 6.52).

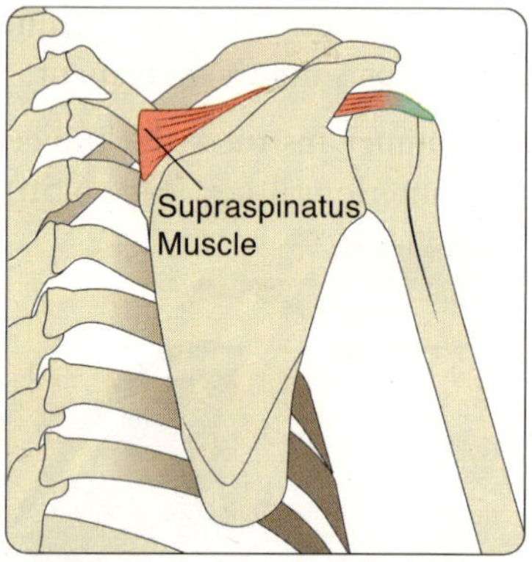

Fig. 6.52: Supraspinatus muscle origin and insertion

Origin: Supraspinatus fossa of the scapula.

Insertion: Superior facet of the greater tubercle of the humerus and shoulder joint capsule.

Action: Initiates abduction of the shoulder joint in first thirty degrees and stabilizes the head of humerus in the glenoid cavity during overhead activities of the shoulder joint.

Nerve Supply: Suprascapular, $C_{4,\ 5\ \text{and}\ 6}$.

Grade 3 (Fair)

Position of Patient: Short sitting with arms adducted and elbow flexed slightly.

Position of Examiner: Examiner stands behind the patient, places one hand over the top of the shoulder joint, and observe the movement that should take place in the frontal plane. Trunk rotation to the contralateral side should be taken care of.

Stabilization: Examiner stabilizes the trunk to prevent rotation and lateral bending of the trunk to the opposite side (Figs. 6.53a and b).

(a)

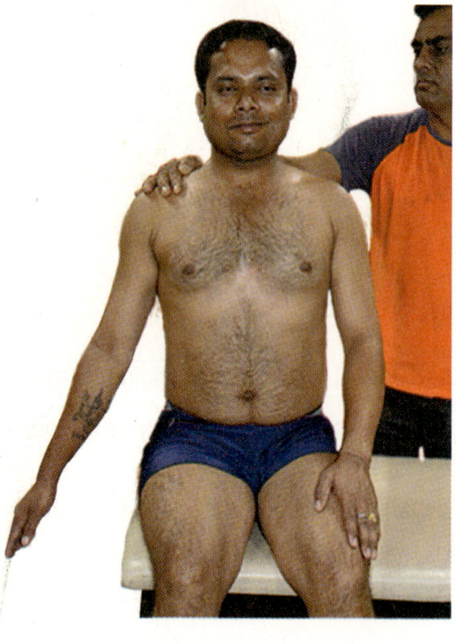

(b)

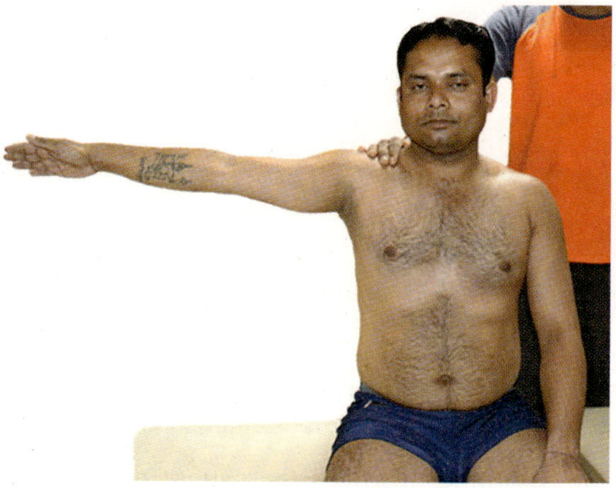

Figs. 6.53a and b: Testing of supraspinatus and middle fibers of deltoid muscle in grade 3, examiner stands behind the patient and places one hand on the top of shoulder to prevent lateral bending of the trunk to the opposite side

Test: Examiner instructs the patient to lift your arm out to the side to the shoulder level. If patient completes the movement in the available range against the gravity, it is considered grade 3. There should not be any trunk rotation.

Grade 4 and 5 (Good and Normal)

Position of Patient: Short sitting with arms adducted and elbow flexed slightly.

Position of Examiner: Examiner stands behind the patient and places one hand over the lateral arm just above the elbow joint and other hand is placed on the shoulder to stabilize it and prevent trunk rotation. Trunk rotation to the contralateral side should be taken care of.

Stabilization: Examiner stabilizes the trunk to prevent rotation and lateral bending of the trunk to the opposite side (Fig. 6.54).

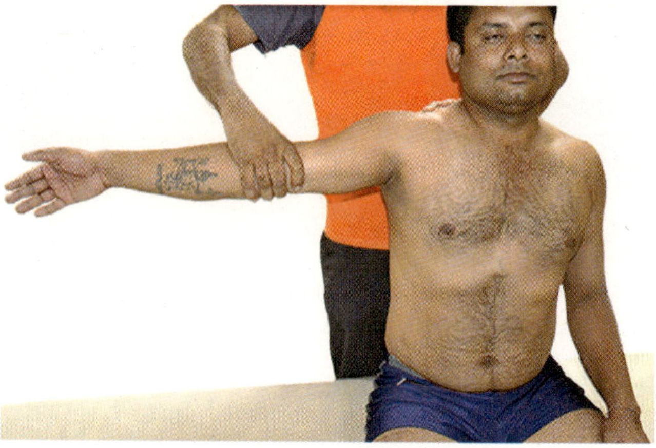

Fig. 6.54: Testing of middle fibers of deltoid for grade 4 and 5

Test: Examiner instructs the patient to lift the arm out to the side to the shoulder level without trunk rotation in the sagittal plane.

Grade 4: If patient completes the movement in the available range against strong to moderate resistance it is considered grade 4.

Grade 5: If patient completes the movement in the available range against maximal resistance, it is considered grade 5.

Grade 1 (Flicker/Trace)

Position of Patient: Short sitting with arms adducted.

Position of Examiner: Examiner stands behind the patient and places one hand on the lateral acromian and lateral aspects of head of humerus. Examiner supports the arm within abducted position with the other hand.

Stabilization: Examiner stabilizes the trunk to prevent rotation and lateral bending of the trunk to the opposite side (Fig. 6.55).

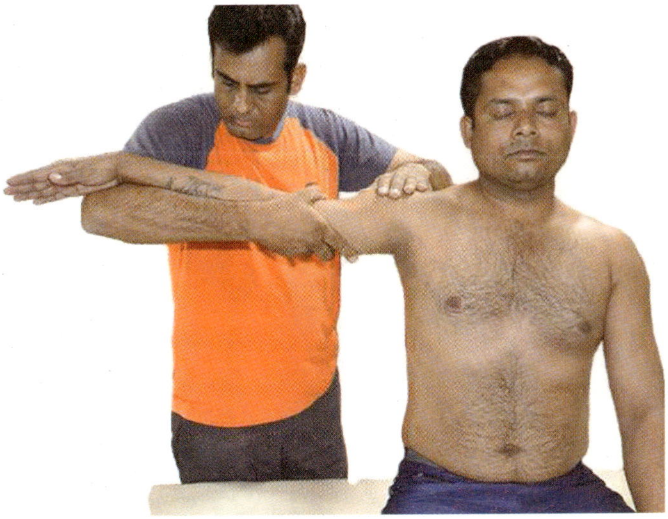

Fig. 6.55: Palpation of middle fibers of deltoid for grade 1

Test: Examiner instructs the patient to try to lift your arm out to the side to the shoulder. Examiner feels the contraction of the muscle while the patient attempts to lift the shoulder outwards. If examiner feels contraction, it is considered grade 1.

Grade 2 (Poor)

Position of Patient: Supine with the shoulders adducted and elbow extended.

Position of Examiner: Examiner stands at the top of the head and places one hand over the top of the shoulder joint to prevent elevation.

Stabilization: Examiner stabilizes the shoulder joint to prevent elevation and trunk bending (Fig. 6.56).

Weakness: Supraspinatus Muscle–Loss of initiation of the shoulder flexion in the first 30°. There is decreased

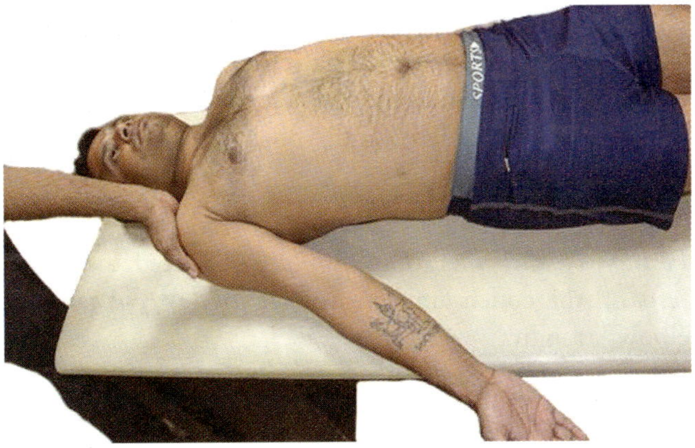

Fig. 6.56: Testing of supraspinatus and middle fibers of deltoid for grade 2, examiner stands at top of the shoulder joint to stabilize and prevent elevation and lateral trunk bending of the trunk and places hand on the middle fibers of deltoid

ability of the downward depression of the head of humerus during overhead activities, resulting the head of humerus migrated superiorly into the acromian arch, where it impinges subacromial bursa and long head of biceps tendon.

DELTOID POSTERIOR FIBERS–SHOULDER HORIZONTAL ABDUCTION

Grade 3 (Fair)

Position of Patient: Prone, shoulder abducted to 90°, arm rests on the couch and forearm off the edge of table with elbow flexed to 90°.

Position of Examiner: Examiner stands at the side of patient.

Stabilization: Examiner stands at the side and places one hand over the scapula to prevent rotation of the trunk (Fig. 6.57).

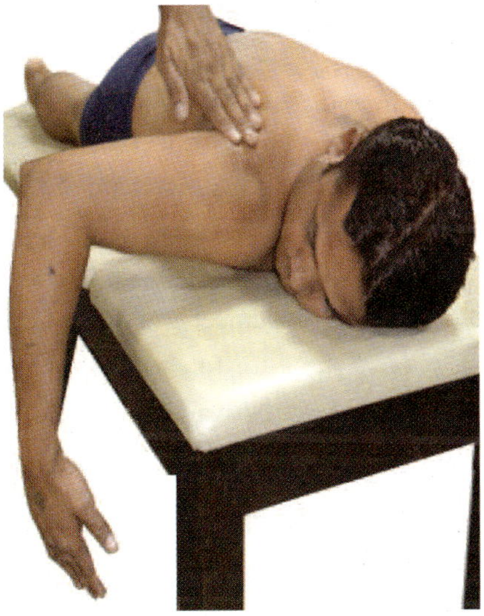

Fig. 6.57: Testing of posterior fibers of deltoid for grade 3, examiner stands at the side of the patient and places one hand over the posterior aspect of the shoulder girdle to prevent rotation of the trunk

Test: Examiner instructs the patient to "lift your elbow" up toward the ceiling. If patient completes shoulder, horizontal abduction in the available range of motion against the gravity is considered grade 3.

Grade 4 and Grade 5 (Good and Normal)

Position of Patient: Prone, shoulder abducted to 90°, arm rests on the couch and forearm off the edge of table with elbow straight.

Position of Examiner: Examiner stands at the side of patient places one hand on the posterior aspect of the elbow joint to apply resistance and other hand may be placed on the posterior aspect of the shoulder to stabilize it and to prevent rotation of the trunk.

Stabilization: Examiner instructs the patient to prevent rotation of the trunk (Fig. 6.58).

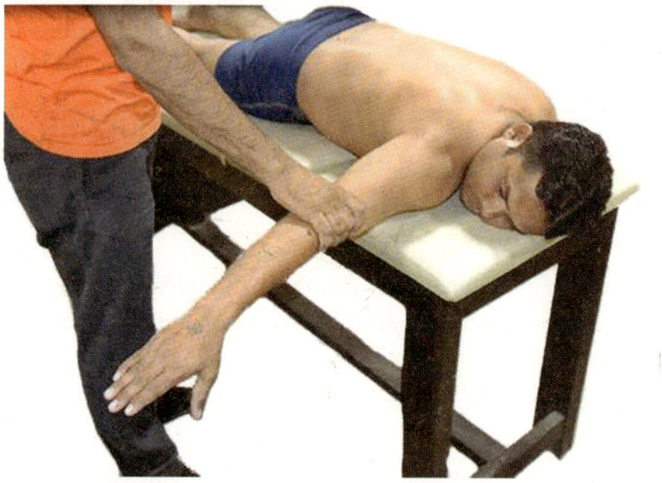

Fig. 6.58: Testing of posterior fibers of deltoid for grade 4 and 5, examiner stands at the side and places one hand on the dorsal aspect of distal arm to resist the horizontal abduction of the shoulder joint

Test: Examiner instructs the patient to "lift your elbow up toward the ceiling. Hold it; don't let me push it down." Examiner applies resistance downward into the floor.

Grade 4: If patient is able to complete the shoulder horizontal abduction in the available range of motion against strong to moderate resistance.

Grade 5: If patient is able to complete the shoulder horizontal abduction in the available range of motion against maximal resistance.

Grade 1 (Flicker/Trace)

Position of Patient: Sitting on a stool or over side of couch and abducts the shoulder to 90° with elbow flexed to 90° and forearm supinated, palm facing downward to the floor.

Position of Examiner: Examiner stands at the side of the patient, which is being tested and supports the arm at 90° abduction and 90° elbow flexion with one hand. Examiner places other hand over the posterior aspect of the deltoid to palpate the muscle for contraction.

Stabilization: Examiner stands at the side and places one hand over the scapula to prevent rotation of the trunk (Fig. 6.59).

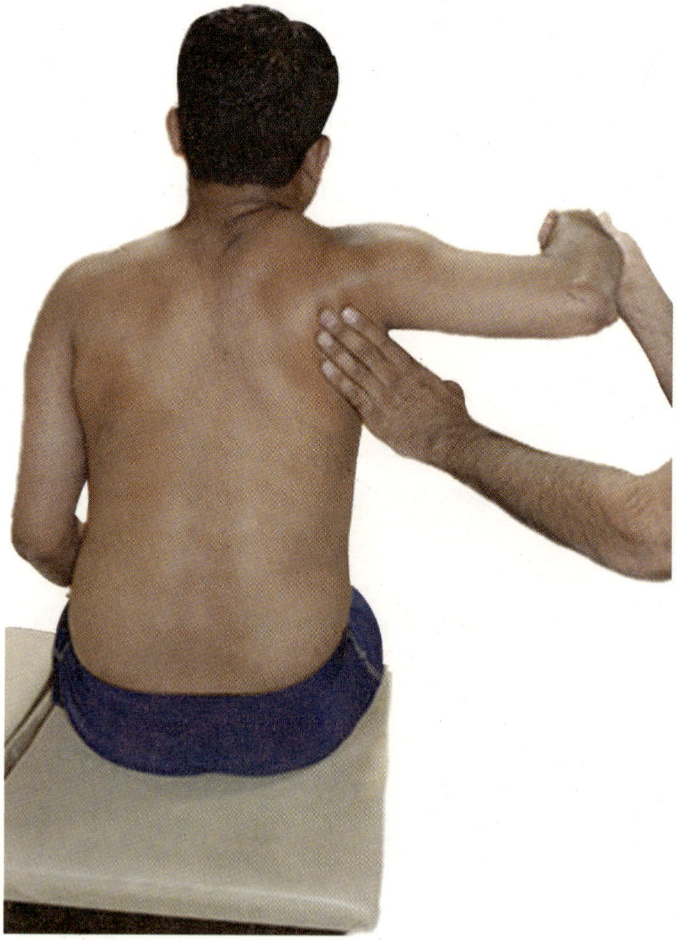

Fig. 6.59: Palpation of posterior fibers of deltoid for grade 1, examiner stands at the side and places other hand over the posterior aspect of the deltoid to palpate the muscle for contraction while supporting the arm of the patient with the other hand

Test: Examiner instructs the patient to try to move your arm backward while he or she palpates the muscle for the contraction. If examiner feels contraction, it is graded 1.

Grade 2 (Poor)

Position of Patient: Sitting on a stool or over side of couch and abducts the shoulder to 90° with elbow flexed to 90° and forearm supinated, palm facing downward to the floor.

Position of Examiner: Examiner stands at the side of the patient which is being tested and supports the arm at 90° abduction and 90° elbow flexion with one hand. Examiner places other hand on the shoulder joint to stabilize it and to prevent trunk rotation.

Stabilization: Examiner stands at the side and places one hand over the scapula to prevent rotation of the trunk (Figs. 6.60a and b).

(a)

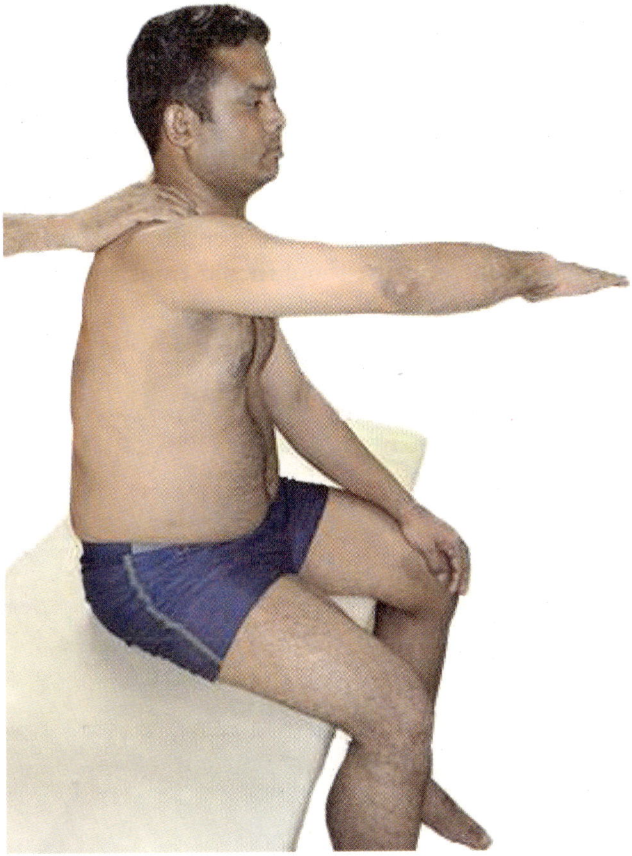

(b)

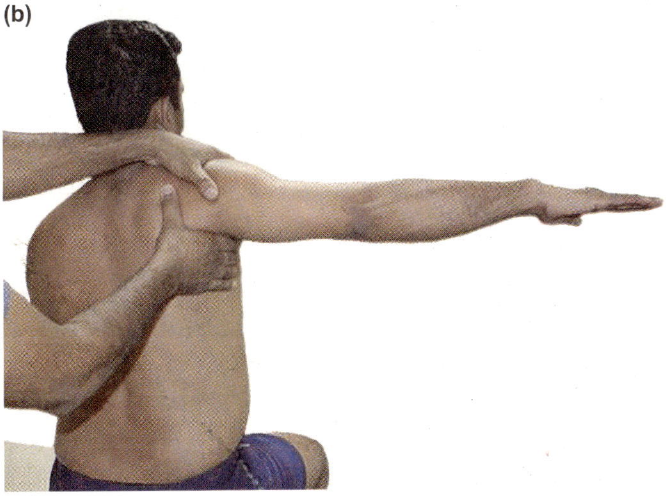

Figs. 6.60a and b: Testing of posterior fibers of deltoid for grade 2, examiner stands behind the patient and places one hand over the shoulder joint to stabilize it and prevent rotation and trunk bending. The examiner may stabilize the shoulder with both the hands

Test: Examiner instructs the patient to try to move your arm backward as far as possible without trunk rotation. If patient completes the range in the gravity eliminated position it is considered grade 2.

PECTORALIS MAJOR–SHOULDER HORIZONTAL ADDUCTION

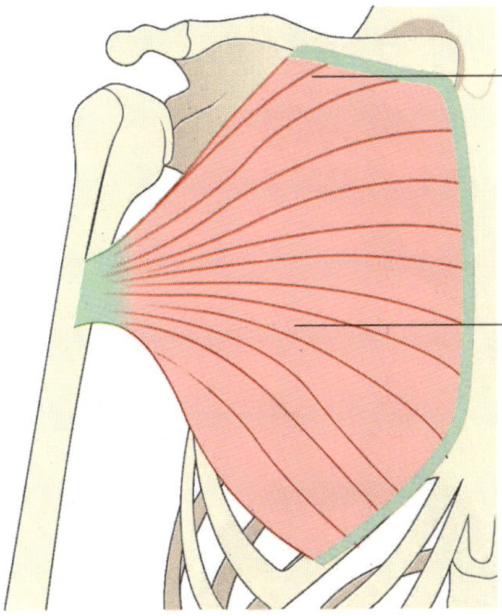

Fig. 6.61: Pectoralis major

Pectoralis Major (Clavicular Portion)

Origin: Anterior surface of the sternum ½ of the clavicle.

Insertion: Crest of greater tubercle (anteriorly and caudally) of the humerus.

Action: Clavicular portion of the pectoralis major flexes and medially rotates the shoulder joint, and horizontally adducts the humerus toward the opposite shoulder.

Nerve Supply: Lateral pectoral, $C_{5,\ 6\ \text{and}\ 7}$.

Pectoralis Major (Sternocostal)

Origin: Anterior surface of the sternum, cartilages of first six or seven ribs, and aponeurosis of the external oblique.

Insertion: Crest of greater tubercle (posteriorly and cranially) of the humerus.

Action: Depress the shoulder girdle by virtue of the attachment on the humerus, and obliquely adduct the humerus toward the opposite iliac crest.

Nerve Supply: Lateral and medial pectoral, $C_{6,\ 7,\ 8}$ and T_1.

Grade 3 (Fair)

Position of Patient: Supine with shoulder joint is abducted to 80° and elbow is flexed to 90°. The arm can be placed in three different positions – 80°, 90° and 120° of abduction with the elbow at 90° flexion for different fibers.

Position of Examiner: Examiner stands at the side of the patient, may support the forearm, and observes the movement. No assistance is given to facilitate the movement.

Stabilization: Examiner must ensure that movement should be there in the shoulder no trunk movement or rotation should take place (Fig. 6.62).

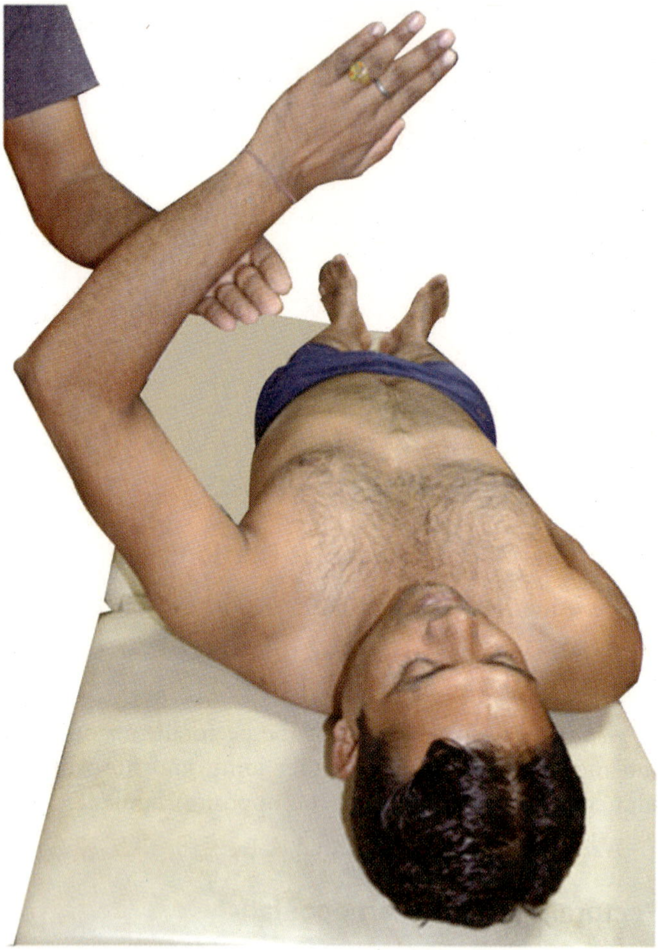

Fig. 6.62: Testing of pectoralis major muscle for grade 3, examiner stands at the side and guides the patient

Test: Examiner instructs the patient to move the arm according to the origin to insertion of the muscle or as per the action of muscle.

i. *For Clavicle Head:* Shoulder joint is abducted to 80° with elbow flexion. Patient is asked to adduct the shoulder joint diagonally towards the opposite shoulder.
ii. *For Sternal Head:* The pectoralis muscle is tested in the 120° abduction with the elbow joint flexion (90°). Patient is asked to adduct the shoulder joint diagonally towards the opposite shoulder joint.
iii. *Whole Muscle:* Shoulder joint is abducted to 90° with elbow flexion (90°). Patient is asked to bring the arm across the chest towards the opposite shoulder.

If patient completes horizontal abduction in the available range of motion against the gravity is considered grade 3.

Grade 4 and Grade 5 (Good and Normal)

Position of Patient: Supine with shoulder joint is abducted to 80° and elbow is flexed to 90°. The arm can be placed in three different positions – 80°, 90° and 120° of abduction.

Position of Examiner: Examiner stands at the side of the patient and places one hand over the anterior aspect of the shoulder joint to stabilize it and to prevent trunk rotation. Examiner grasps the elbow joint with the other hand to apply resistance.

Stabilization: Examiner must ensure that movement should be there in the shoulder, no trunk movement or rotation should take place (Fig. 6.63).

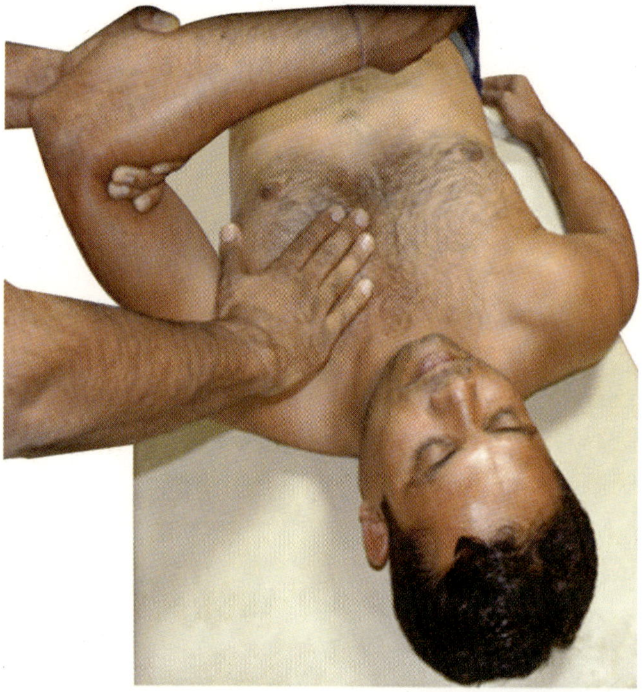

Fig. 6.63: Testing of pectoralis major muscle for grade 4 and 5, examiner stands at the side, places one hand on the anterior shoulder, and grasps the elbow joint with other hand to apply resistance

Test: Examiner instructs the patient to move the arm according to the origin to insertion of the muscle or as per the action of muscle.

i. *For Clavicle Head:* Shoulder joint is abducted to 80° with elbow flexion. Patient is asked to adduct the shoulder joint diagonally towards the opposite shoulder.
ii. *For Sternal Head:* The pectoralis muscle is tested in the 120° abduction with the elbow joint flexion (90°). patient is asked to adduct the shoulder joint diagonally towards the opposite shoulder joint.
iii. *Whole Muscle:* Shoulder joint is abducted to 90° with elbow flexion (90°). Patient is asked to bring the arm across the chest towards the opposite shoulder.

Grade 4: Patient is instructed to adduct the shoulder joint across the chest wall to the opposite shoulder as described above for different heads of the pectoralis against strong to moderate resistance. If patient is able to adduct the shoulder horizontally in the available range of motion it is considered grade 4.

Grade 5: Examiner instructs the patient to adduct the shoulder joint across the chest wall to the opposite shoulder as described above for different heads of the pectoralis against maximal resistance. If patient is able to adduct the shoulder horizontally against maximal resistance in the available range of motion it is considered grade 4.

Grade 1 (Fair/Flicker)

Position of Patient: Short sitting, shoulder is abducted to 90°, arm is supported on the examiner forearm and elbow is flexed to 90°.

Position of Examiner: Examiner stands behind the patient and places fingers of one hand on the medial clavicle up to the sternum.

Stabilization: Examiner stabilizes the trunk to prevent anterior rotation and bending (Fig. 6.64).

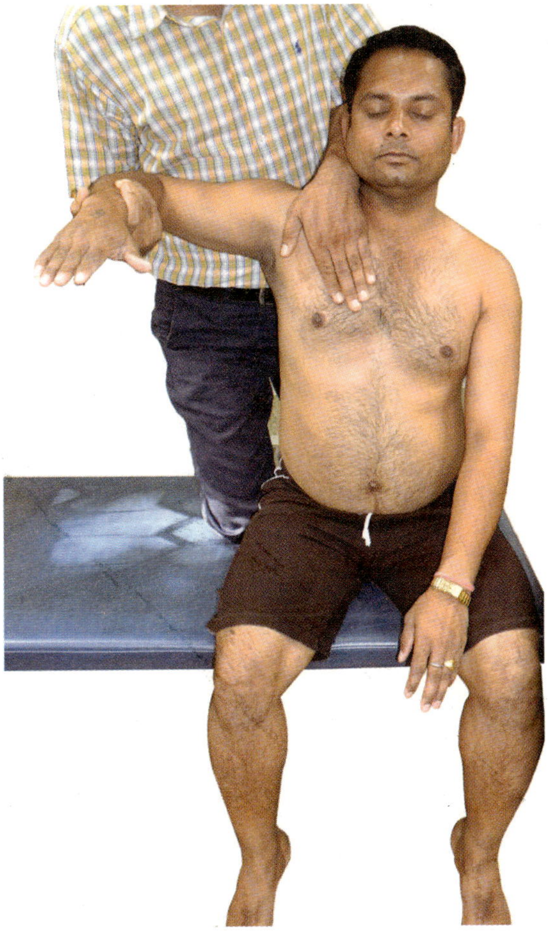

Fig. 6.64: Palpation of pectoralis major muscle for grade 1

Test: Examiner instructs the patient to try to move your arm across the chest to the opposite shoulder while he or she palpates the muscle for contraction. If examiner feels contraction of the pectoralis muscle, it is considered grade 1.

Grade 2 (Poor)

Position of Patient: Short sitting, shoulder is abducted to 90°, arm is supported on the couch and elbow is flexed to 90°.

Position of Examiner: Examiner stands behind the patient, places one hand on the top of the shoulder joint, and observes the movement of the arm. Examiner may support the arm at 90° abduction, if deltoid middle fibers are less than grade 3.

Stabilization: Examiner must ensure that movement should be there in the shoulder, no trunk movement or rotation should take place (Fig. 6.65).

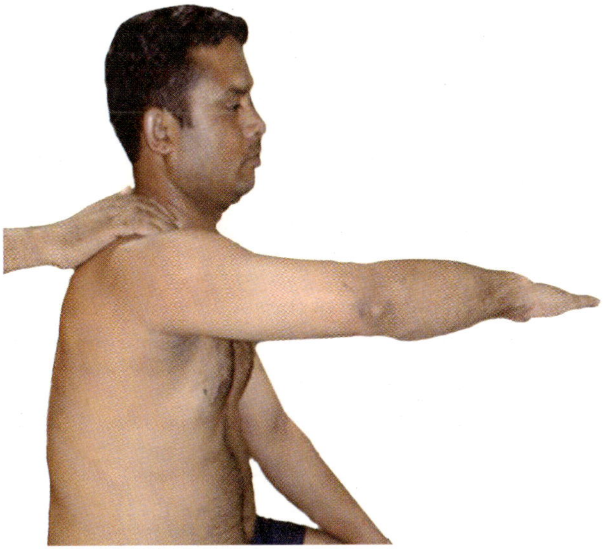

Fig. 6.65: Testing of pectoralis major muscle for grade 2, examiner stands behind the patient and stabilizes the shoulder to prevent rotation and lateral bending of the trunk

Test: Examiner instructs the patient to try to move your arm across the chest to the opposite shoulder without rotation of the trunk. If patient completes the movement across the chest towards opposite shoulder in the available range of motion in gravity eliminated position it is considered grade 2.

INFRASPINATUS AND TERES MINOR – SHOULDER EXTERNAL ROTATION

Infrapinatus

Origin: Medial 2/3rd of the infraspinatus fossa of the scapula.

Insertion: Middle facet of the greater tubercle of the humerus and shoulder joint.

Action: Lateral rotation of the shoulder joint and keeping the head of humerus in the glenoid fossa during overhead activities.

Nerve Supply: Suprascapular, $C_{4, 5, 6}$ (Fig. 6.66).

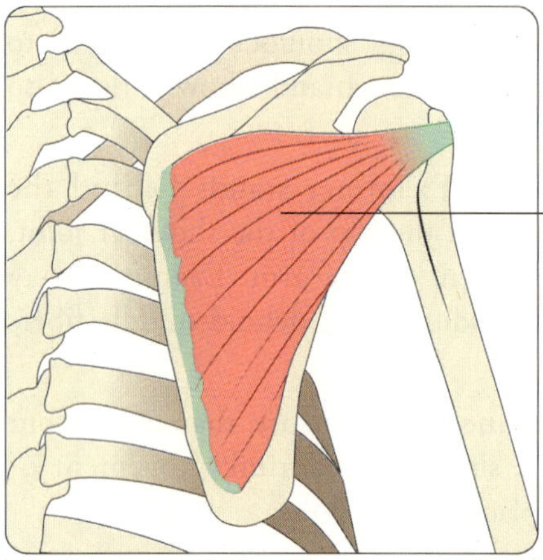

Fig. 6.66: Infraspinatus muscle origin and insertion

Teres Minor

Origin: Upper 2/3rd, dorsal surface of the lateral border of the scapula.

Insertion: Lowest facet of the greater tubercle of the humerus and shoulder joint (Fig. 6.67).

Action: Lateral rotation of the shoulder joint and keeping the head of humerus in the glenoid fossa during overhead activities.

Nerve Supply: Axillary, $C_{5, 6}$.

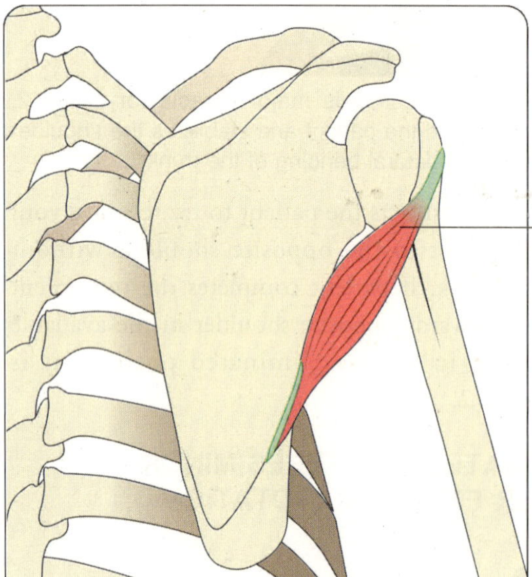

Fig. 6.67: Teres minor origin and insertion

Grade 3 (Fair)

Position of Patient: Prone, shoulder is abducted to 90°, elbow flexed to 90° and forearm in midprone position, with elbow out of the edge of couch. Arm rests on the couch whereas, forearm hangs vertically.

Position of Examiner: Examiner stands at the side of patient, places one hand on the posterior surface of the shoulder girdle, and observes the movement of the shoulder.

Stabilization: Examiner must ensure that movement should be there in the shoulder no retraction or elevation should take place in order to compensate external rotation (Fig. 6.68).

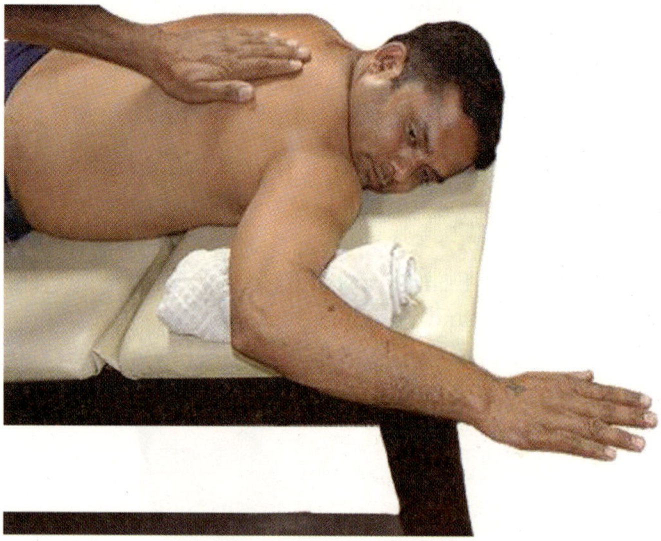

Fig. 6.68: Testing of infraspinatus and teres minor muscle for grade 3, examiner stands at the side and places one hand over the posterior surface of the scapula to prevent retraction and elevation of the shoulder girdle

Test: Examiner instructs the patient to "raise your arm to the level of the table". There should not be trunk rotation.

Grade 4 and 5 (Good and Normal)

Position of Patient: Prone, shoulder is abducted to 90°, elbow flexed to 90° and forearm in midprone position, with elbow out of the edge of couch. Arm rests on the couch whereas forearm hangs vertically.

Position of Examiner: Examiner stands at the side of patient and places one hand on the proximal forearm (dorsum) to apply resistance. Examiner may place other hand on the dorsal aspect of shoulder girdle to stabilize it.

Stabilization: Examiner must ensure that movement should be there in the shoulder no abduction or elevation should take place in order to compensate external rotation (Fig. 6.69).

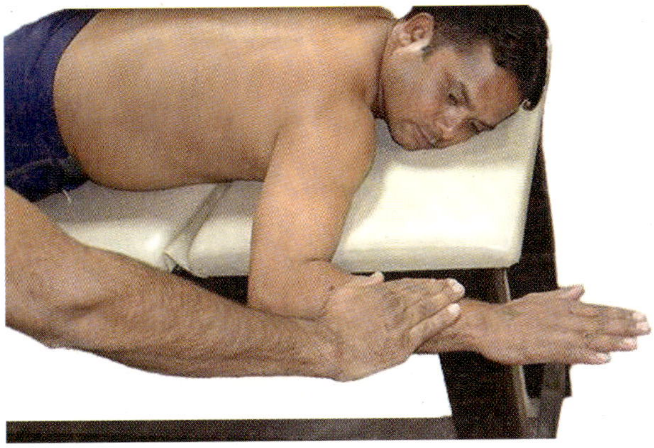

Fig. 6.69: Testing of infraspinatus and teres minor muscle for grade 4 and 5, examiner stands at the side and places one hand on the distal forearm to apply resistance against the external rotation. Examiner may place other hand on the dorsal aspect of shoulder girdle to stabilize the shoulder for retraction and elevation

Test: Examiner instructs the patient to "raise your forearm to the level of the table" against resistance. Hold it. Don't let me push down. There should not be trunk rotation.

Grade 4: If patient raises the forearm to the level of the table against strong to moderate resistance.

Grade 5: If patient raises the forearm to the level of the table against maximal resistance.

Alternate Position for Grade 4 and 5

Position of Patient: Short sitting on the couch, shoulder is adducted and elbow flexed to 90° with the forearm in mid prone position.

Position of Examiner: Examiner stands at the side of the patient and places one hand on the dorsum of distal forearm and other hand on the distal arm to stabilize and to prevent shoulder adduction.

Stabilization: Examiner must ensure that movement should be there in the shoulder no trunk movement or rotation should take place in order to compensate external rotation (Fig. 6.70).

Test: Examiner instructs the patient to move your forearm outwards as much as possible.

Grade 4: If patient is able to complete the movement in the available range against strong to moderate resistance.

Grade 5: If patient is able to complete the movement in the available range against maximal resistance.

Grade 1 (Trace)

Position of Patient: Short sitting, shoulder adducted, elbow flexed to 90° and forearm in midprone position. Forearm rests on the table.

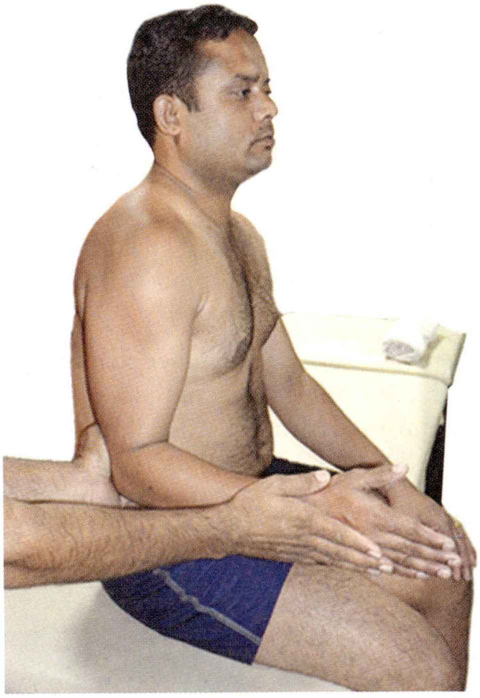

Fig. 6.70: Alternate testing position of infraspinatus and teres minor muscle for grade 4 and 5, examiner stands behind the patient and places one hand over the dorsum of the hand and grasps the elbow joint with the other hand to stabilize the shoulder joint

Position of Examiner: Examiner stands at the side of patient, which is being tested and places fingers on the infraspinatus fossa lateral border of scapula.

Stabilization: Retraction and elevation (Fig. 6.71).

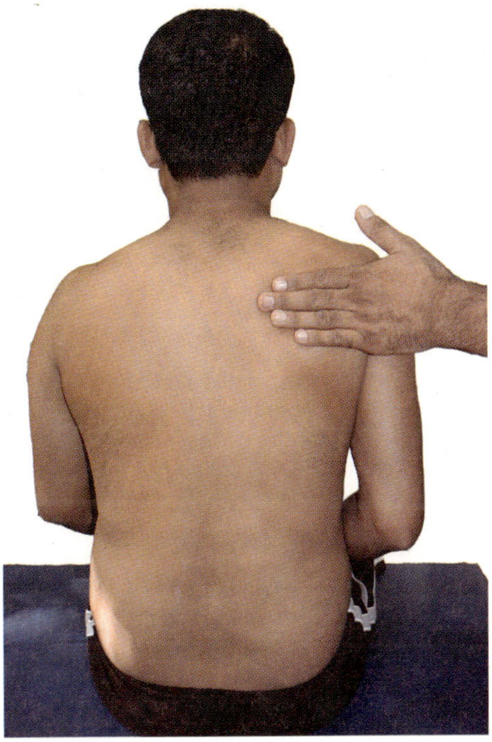

Fig. 6.71: Palpation of infraspinatus muscle for grade 1

Test: Examiner instructs the patient to try to move your forearm outwards while he or she palpates the muscle for contraction. If examiner feels contraction it is considered grade 1.

Grade 2 (Poor)

Position of Patient: Short sitting, shoulder adducted, elbow flexed to 90° and forearm in pronated position. Forearm rests on the table.

Position of Examiner: Examiner stands at the side of patient, which is being tested and places one hand under the forearm to avoid friction between the forearm and couch and observes the movement.

Stabilization: Examiner must ensure that movement should be there in the shoulder no adduction retraction or elevation should take place in order to compensate external rotation (Fig. 6.72).

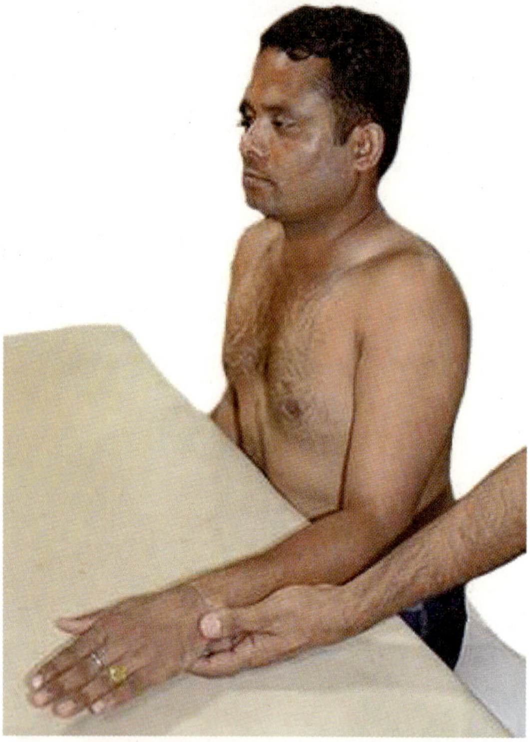

Fig. 6.72: Testing of infraspinatus and teres minor muscle for grade 2, examiner stands at the side of the patient and places one hand under the forearm of the patient to prevent friction between the forearm and the surface of the couch. Examiner must not help the patient in external rotation of the shoulder

Test: Examiner instructs the patient to move your forearm outwards as much as possible. Surface of couch offers some resistance to the movement due to friction, which can be minimized by pouring the powder on the surface or examiner may place hand under the forearm. If patient is able to rotate the shoulder externally in the available range of motion it is considered grade 2.

SUBSCAPULARIS – SHOULDER MEDIAL ROTATION

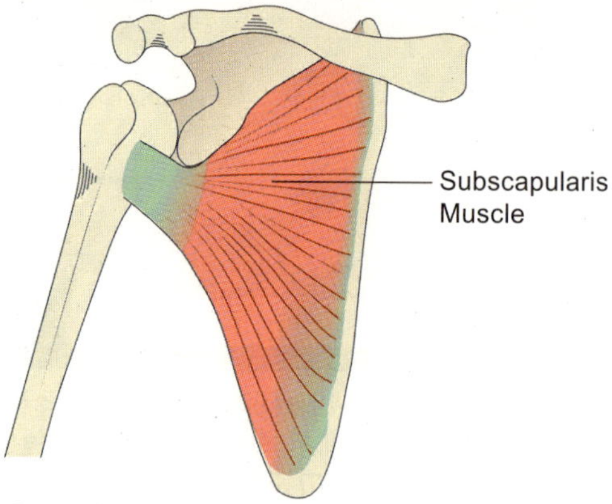

Fig. 6.73: Subscapularis muscle origin and insertion

Origin: Subscapular fossa of the scapula.

Insertion: Lesser tubercle of the humerus and shoulder joint capsule.

Action: Medially rotate the shoulder joint, and stabilizes the head of humerus in the glenoid fossa during overhead activities.

Nerve Supply: Upper and lower subscapular, $C_{5, 6, 7}$.

Grade 3 (Fair)

Position of Patient: Prone, shoulder is abducted to 90°, elbow flexed to 90° and forearm in midprone position, with elbow out of the edge of couch. Arm rests on the couch whereas, forearm hangs vertically.

Position of Examiner: Examiner stands at the same side of patient, places one hand on the posterior aspect of the shoulder and observes the movement of the shoulder.

Stabilization: Examiner must ensure that movement should be there in the shoulder, no elevation should take place in order to compensate internal rotation (Fig. 6.74).

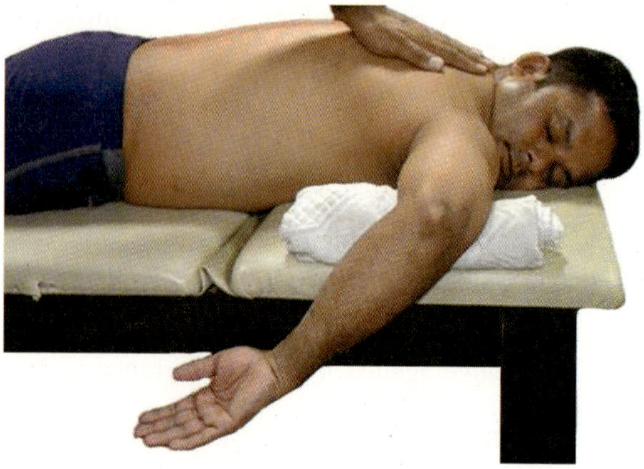

Fig. 6.74: Testing of subscapularis muscle for grade 3, examiner stands at the side of the patient and places one hand over the posterior surface of the shoulder to stabilize it

Test: Examiner instructs the patient to "move your forearm backward to the level of the table". There should not be trunk rotation. If patient completes movement in the available range is considered grade 3.

Grade 4 and 5 (Good and Normal)

Position of Patient: Prone, shoulder is abducted to 90°, elbow flexed to 90° and forearm midprone, with elbow out of the edge of couch. Arm rests on the couch whereas, forearm hangs vertically.

Position of Examiner: Examiner stands at the side of patient and places one hand on the distal forearm to apply resistance and other hand on the posterior surface of the shoulder joint to stabilize it.

Stabilization: Examiner must ensure that movement should be there in the shoulder no protraction or elevation should take place in order to compensate internal rotation (Fig. 6.75).

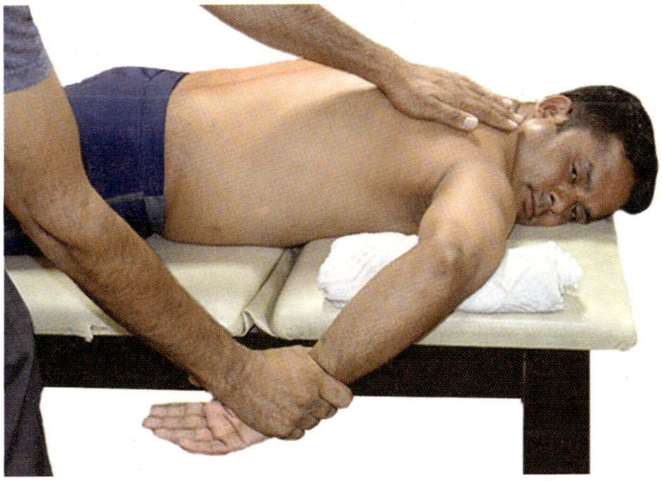

Fig. 6.75: Testing of subscapularis muscle for grade 4 and 5, examiner stands at the side and places one hand over the posterior surface of the shoulder girdle and grasps the distal forearm with the other hand to apply resistance against the internal rotation of the shoulder

Test: Examiner instructs the patient to "move your forearm backward to the level of the table" against resistance. Hold it. Don't let me push it down. There should not be trunk rotation.

Grade 4: If patient raises the forearm backward to the level of the table against strong to moderate resistance in available ROM.

Grade 5: If patient raises the forearm backward to the level of the table against maximal resistance in available ROM.

Alternate Position for Grade 4 and 5

Position of Patient: Short sitting on the couch, shoulder is adducted and elbow flexed to 90° with the forearm in midprone position.

Position of Examiner: Examiner stands at the side of patient and places one hand on the dorsum of distal forearm and other hand on the distal arm to stabilize to prevent shoulder abduction.

Stabilization: Examiner grasps the distal arm and stabilizes the shoulder to prevent abduction (Fig. 6.76).

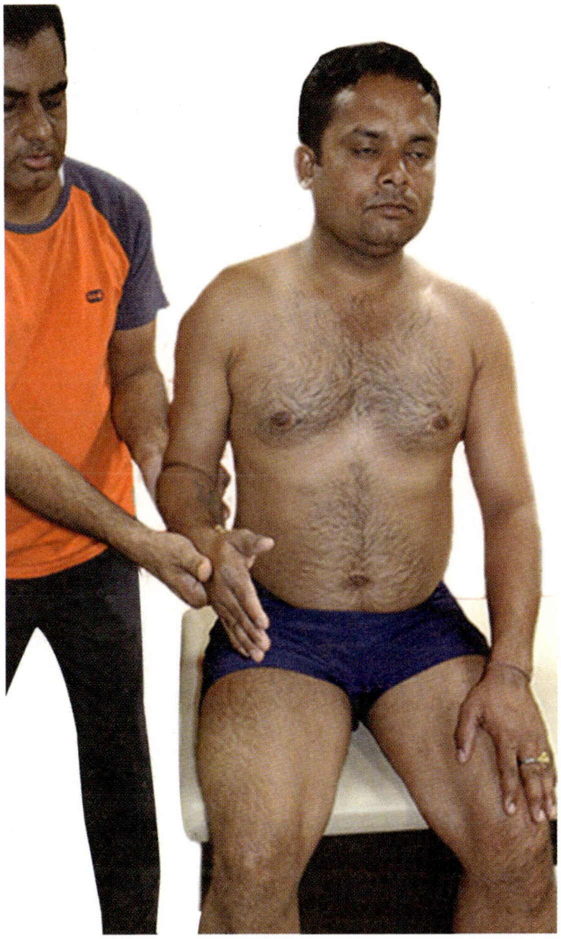

Fig. 6.76: Alternate testing position of subscapularis muscle for grade 4 and 5, examiner stands at the side and holds the distal forearm with one hand and stabilizes the distal arm with other hand to prevent abduction of the shoulder

Test: Examiner instructs the patient to move your forearm inwards towards the stomach or opposite shoulder.

Grade 4: If patient is able to complete the movement in the available range against strong to moderate resistance.

Grade 5: If patient is able to complete the movement in the available range against maximal resistance.

Grade 1 (Flicker/Trace)

Position of Patient: Short sitting, shoulder adducted, elbow flexed to 90° and forearm in midprone position. Forearm rests on the table.

Position of Examiner: Examiner stands at the side of patient, which is being tested and places fingers on medial to the lesser tubercle of the humerus.

Stabilization: Shoulder abduction and elevation (Fig. 6.77a).

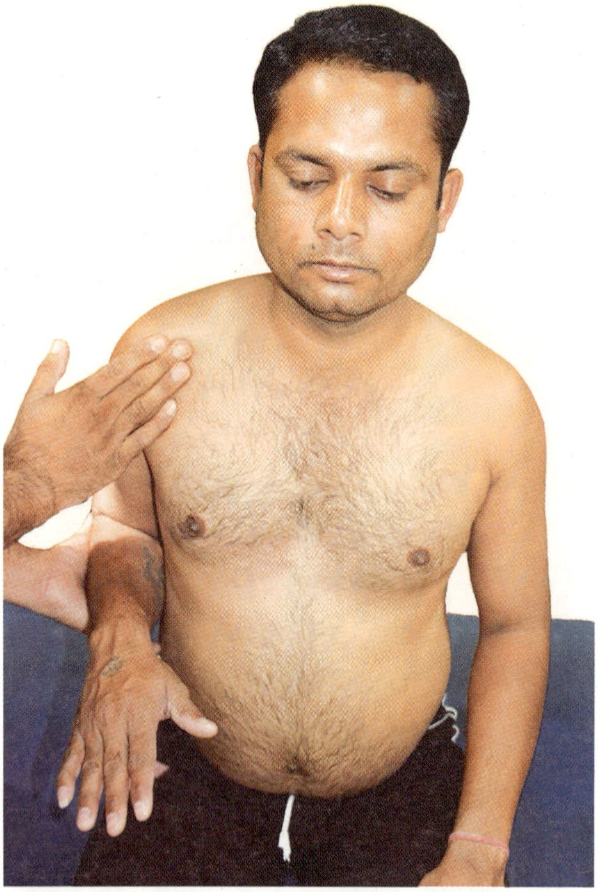

Fig. 6.77a: Palpation of subscapularis muscle for grade 1

Test: Examiner instructs the patient to try to move your forearm inwards towards your opposite hip joint while he or she palpates the muscle for contraction. If examiner feels contraction it is considered grade 1.

Grade 2 (Poor)

Position of Patient: Short sitting, shoulder adducted, elbow flexed to 90° and forearm in midprone position. Forearm rests on the table.

Position of Examiner: Examiner stands at the side of patient, which is being tested, places one hand on posterior aspect of the shoulder girdle and other under the forearm to prevent friction between the forearm and surface of the couch.

Stabilization: Examiner stabilizes the shoulder to prevent abduction, retraction and elevation of the shoulder girdle (Figs. 6.77b and c).

(b)

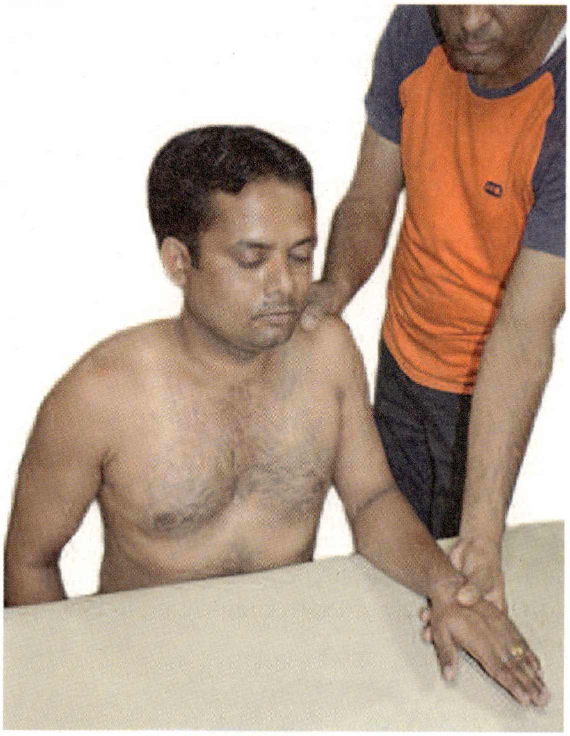

(c)

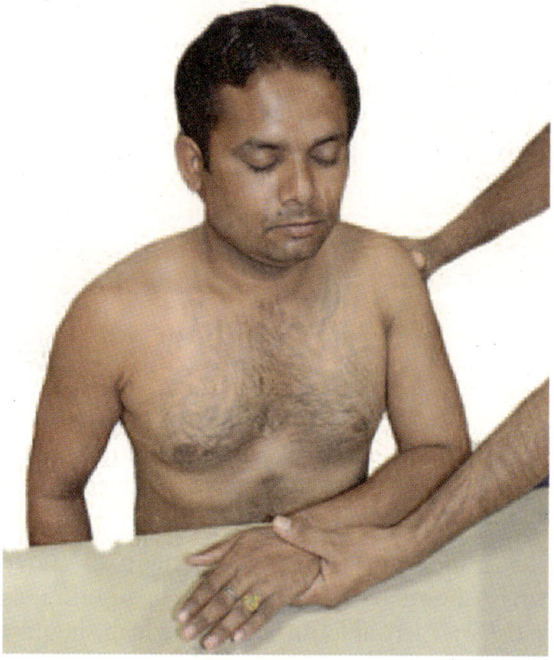

Figs. 6.77b and c: Testing of subscapularis muscle for grade 2, examiner stands behind the patient and places one hand on the shoulder and other under the forearm to prevent friction between the forearm and couch

Test: Examiner instructs the patient to move your forearm inwards to your stomach. Surface of couch offers some resistance to the movement due to friction, which can be minimized by pouring the powder on the surface. If patient is able to rotate the shoulder medially in the available range of motion is considered grade 2.

WEAKNESS OF SCAPULAR MUSCLES

Deltoid All Fibers and Rotators Cuff Muscles

Deficient Glenohumeral Rhythm and Shoulder Impingement Syndrome: The movement of the humerus on the glenoid is approximately 120 degree during the elevation of arm. Glenohumeral rhythm is produced by the two opposite forces of same magnitude acting on the humerus called glenohumeral force couple. The upper portion of the force couple is formed by the deltoid fibres and lower portion is formed by the supraspinatus muscle (Fig. 6.78a).

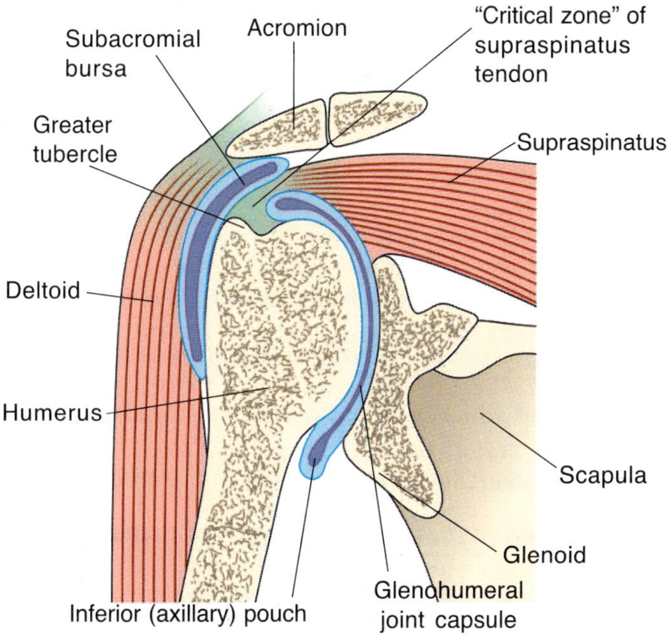

Fig. 6.78a: Glenohumeral force couple

Simultaneous contraction of the deltoid and supraspinatus muscles produces smooth and coordinated glenohumeral rhythm. The strong contraction of deltoid muscles pulls the head of humerus upward (superiorly), whereas, inferiorly and horizontally directed supraspinatus muscle force vectors maintain the humeral head within the glenoid and thereby resist the upward shear of the deltoid generated during active elevation of the arm. If the supraspinatus muscle functioning normally, the centre of the humeral head is restrained in a very small arc of motion usually less than 3 mm along the glenoid fossa. In the presence of supraspinatus muscle injury, tear, or pathology, the arc of motion of humeral head increases to 6 mm or greater. The weak supraspinatus muscle fails to counter the force generated by the deltoid muscle, that results in upward migration of the head of humerus. The structures lie between the head of humerus and acromian arch get impinged (Figs. 6.78b to d).

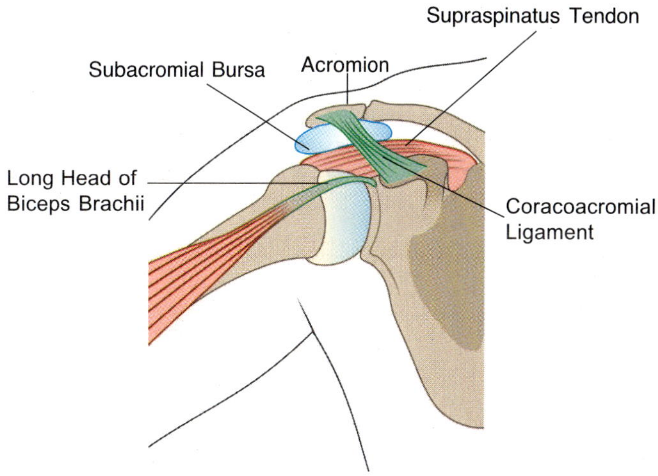

Fig. 6.78b: Normal suprahumeral space during elevation of arm

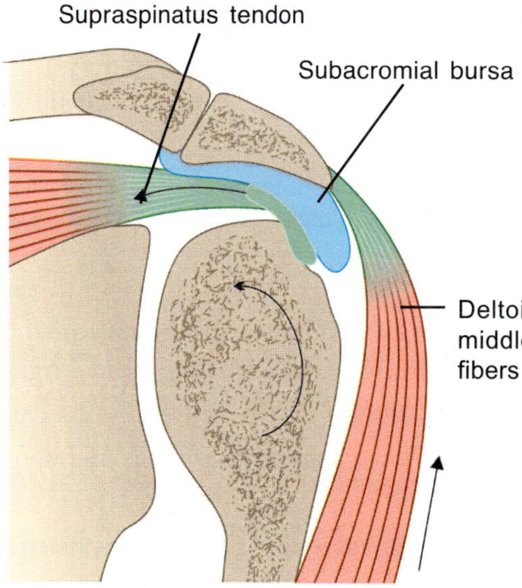

Fig. 6.78c: Normal suprahumeral space of neutral

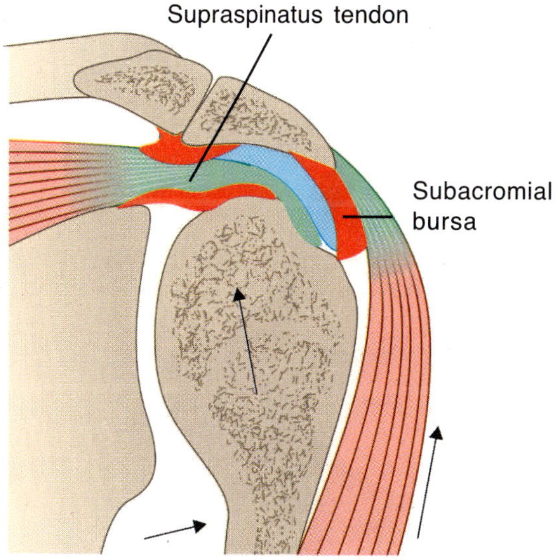

Fig. 6.78d: Deficient glenohumeral rhythm, compression of the soft tissues between head of humerus and acromion arch (shoulder impingement syndrome)

BICEPS BRACHII, BRACHIALIS AND BRACHIORADIALIS – ELBOW FLEXION

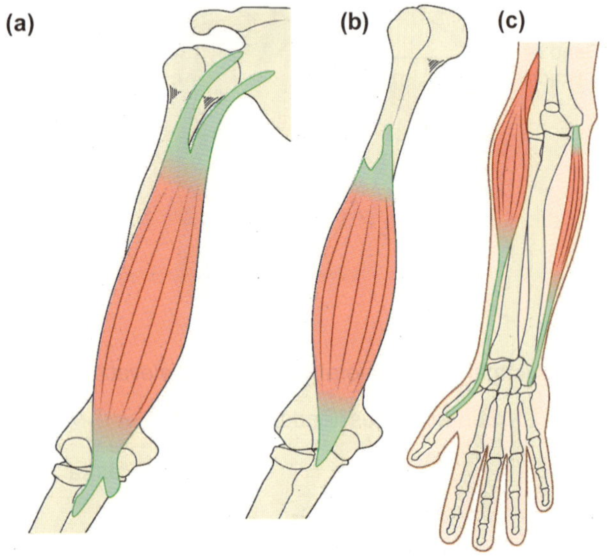

Figs. 6.79a, b and c: Biceps brachii, brachialis and brachioradialis muscles origin and insertion

Biceps Brachii

Origin: Short head originates from apex of the coracoids process of the scapula, and long head originates from supraglenoid tubercle of the scapula.

Insertion: Tuberosity of the radius and aponeurosis of the biceps brachii.

Action: With the origin fixed, biceps brachii flexes the elbow joint with supination of the forearm.

Brachialis

Origin: Distal ½ of the anterior surface of the humerus and both medial and lateral intermuscular septa.

Insertion: Tuberosity and coronoid process of the ulna.

Action: With the origin fixed, flexes the elbow joint with pronations.

Brachioradialis

Origin: Proximal 2/3rd of the lateral supracondylar ridge of the humerus and lateral intermuscular septum.

Insertion: Lateral side of the base of the styloid process of the radius.

Action: Flexes the elbow joint with forearm in midprone position.

Nerve Supply: $C_{5,\ 6}$.

Grade 3 (Fair)

Position of Patient: Short sitting on the edge of the couch so that patient can hang the hand vertically. Shoulder is adducted and elbow is extended.

Position of Examiner: Examiner stands at the side (posteriorly) which is being tested, may hold the elbow joint to stabilize it. Examiner also checks for if there is any trick movements in the shoulder joint.

Stabilization: Examiner must ensure that movement should be there in the elbow joint no flexion and no abduction of shoulder should take place in order to compensate elbow flexion (Figs. 6.80a, b and c).

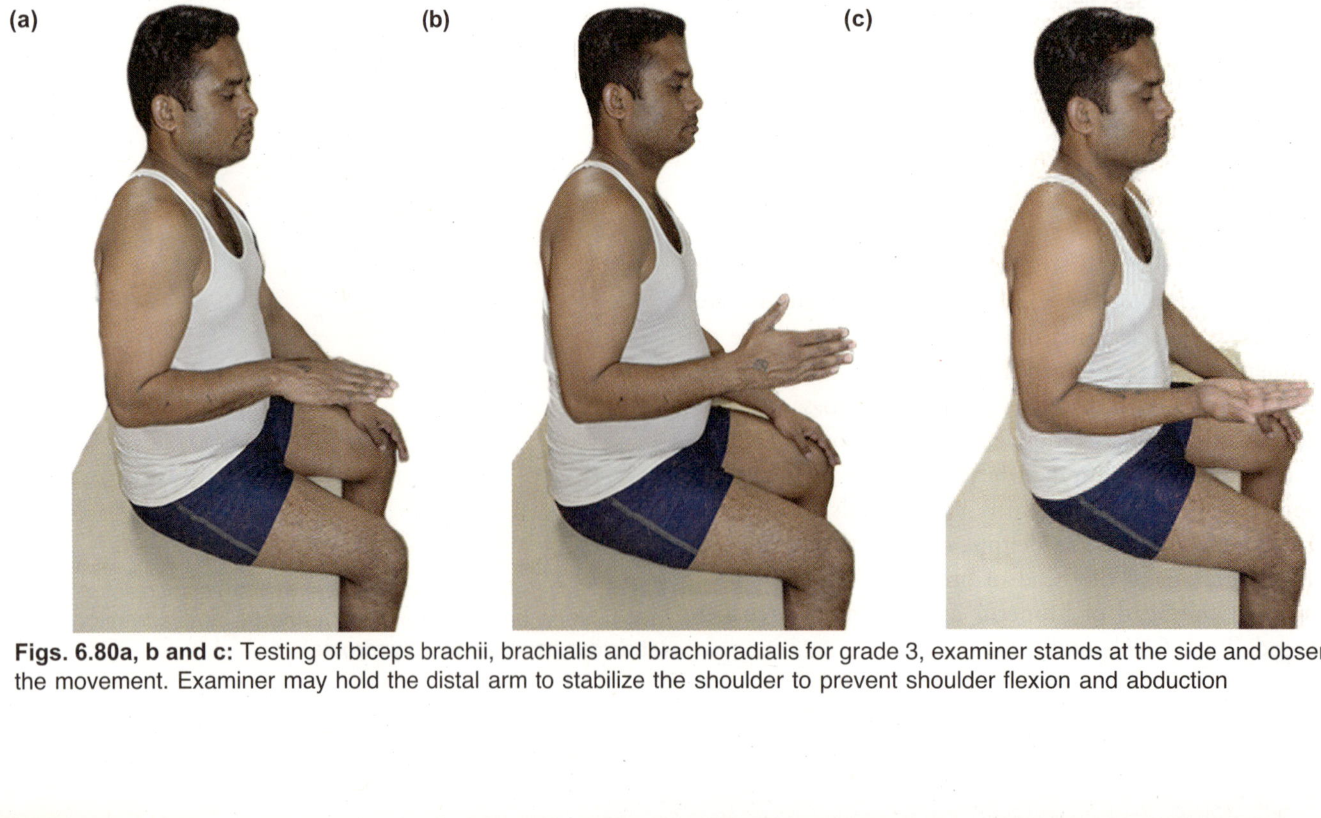

Figs. 6.80a, b and c: Testing of biceps brachii, brachialis and brachioradialis for grade 3, examiner stands at the side and observes the movement. Examiner may hold the distal arm to stabilize the shoulder to prevent shoulder flexion and abduction

Test: Examiner instructs the patient to bend the elbow or bring the hand to the shoulder joint.

i. If patient is able to flex the elbow joint with supination of forearm in the available range against the gravity it is considered grade 3 for biceps brachii.
ii. If patient is able to flex the elbow joint with pronation of forearm in the available range against the gravity it is considered grade 3 for brachialis.
iii. If patient is able to flex the elbow joint with forearm in midprone in the available range against the gravity it is considered grade 3 for brachioradialis.

Alternative Position for Grade 3

Position of Patient: Supine with arm at the side of body (mid axillary line), and elbow remains extended.

Position of Examiner: Examiner stands at the side of the patient and holds the distal arm to stabilize it. Examiner should check the trick movement at the shoulder joint.

Elbow flexion occurs against the gravity from 0° to 90°, however, gravity assists the movement from 90° to 140°, therefore, examiner may offer mild resistance from 90° to 140°.

Stabilization: Examiner stabilizes the shoulder to prevent flexion and elevation of the shoulder girdle.

Test: Examiner instructs the patient to bend the elbow as mentioned below:

i. If patient is able to flex the elbow joint with supination of forearm in the available range against the gravity it is considered grade 3 for biceps brachii.
ii. If patient is able to flex the elbow joint with pronation of forearm in the available range against the gravity it is considered grade 3 for brachialis.
iii. If patient is able to flex the elbow joint with forearm in midprone in the available range against the gravity it is considered grade 3 for biceps brachioradialis.

Grade 4 and Grade 5 (Good and Normal)

Position of Patient: Short sitting on the edge of the couch so that patient can hang the hand vertically. Shoulder is adducted and elbow is extended.

Position of Examiner: Examiner stands in front of the patient, holds the distal forearm with one hand, and stabilizes the shoulder joint with other hand.

Stabilization: Examiner must ensure that movement should be there in the elbow joint no flexion and no abduction of shoulder should take place in order to compensate flexion (Figs. 6.81a, b and c).

Test: Examiner instructs the patient to bend the elbow joint as mentioned under.

Grade 4 (Good)

i. If patient is able to flex the elbow joint with supination of forearm in the available range against strong to moderate resistance it is considered grade 4 for biceps brachii.
ii. If patient is able to flex the elbow joint with pronation of forearm in the available range against strong to moderate resistance it is considered grade 4 for brachialis.
iii. If patient is able to flex the elbow joint with forearm in midprone in the available range against strong to moderate resistance it is considered grade 4 for brachioradialis.

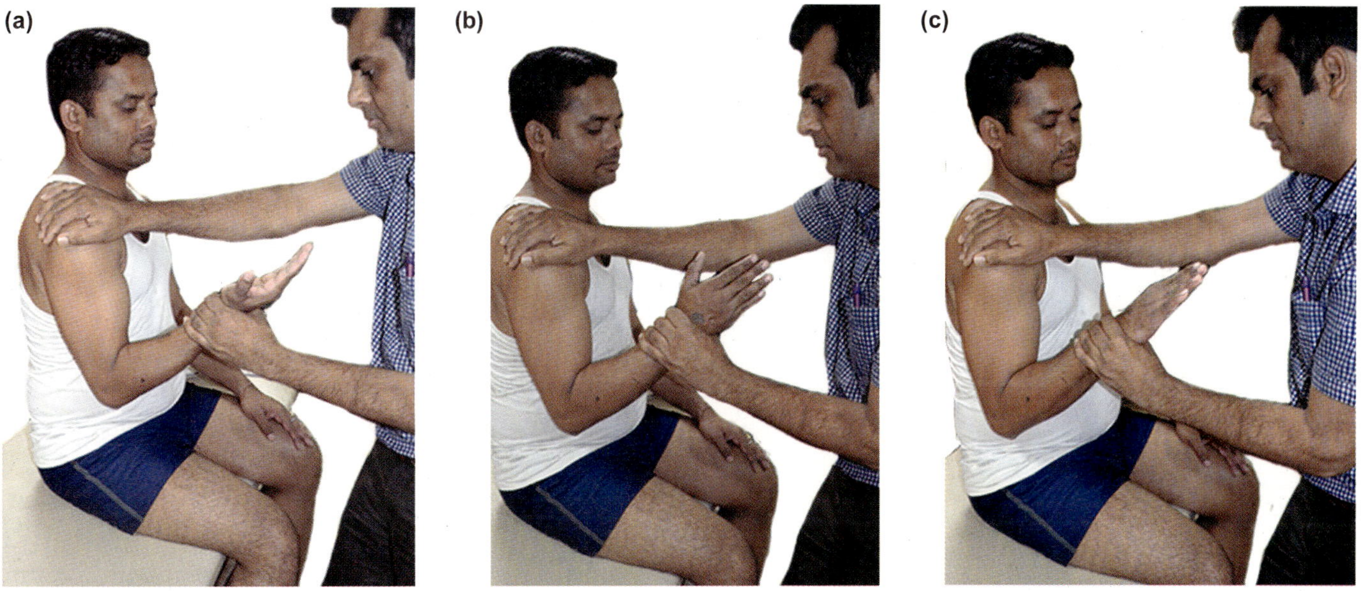

Figs. 6.81a, b and c: Testing of biceps brachii, brachialis and brachioradialis for grade 4 and 5. Examiner stands in front of the patient, places one hand on the shoulder and grasps the distal forearm to apply resistance against the elbow flexion

Grade 5 (Normal)

i. If patient is able to flex the elbow joint with supination of forearm in the available range against maximal resistance it is considered grade 5 for biceps brachii.

ii. If patient is able to flex the elbow joint with pronation of forearm in the available range against maximal resistance it is considered grade 5 for brachialis.

iii. If patient is able to flex the elbow joint with forearm in midprone in the available range against maximal, resistance it is considered grade 5 for brachioradialis.

Grade 1 (Flicker/Trace)

Position of Patient: Supine lying with elbow slightly flexed.

Position of Examiner: Examiner stands at the side, which is being tested and places one finger on the belly of muscle, which is being tested. There are three elbow flexors and all are palpated separatels for grade 1 (Figs. 6.82 to 6.84).

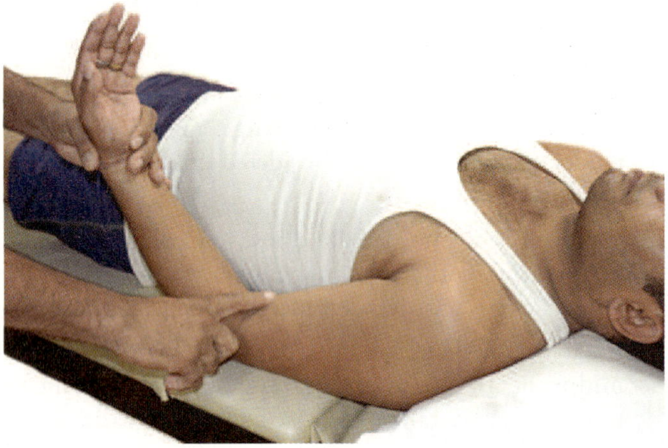

Fig. 6.82: Palpation of biceps brachii for grade 1, examiner stands at the side and places one index over the biceps brachii just above the cubital fossa to palpate it

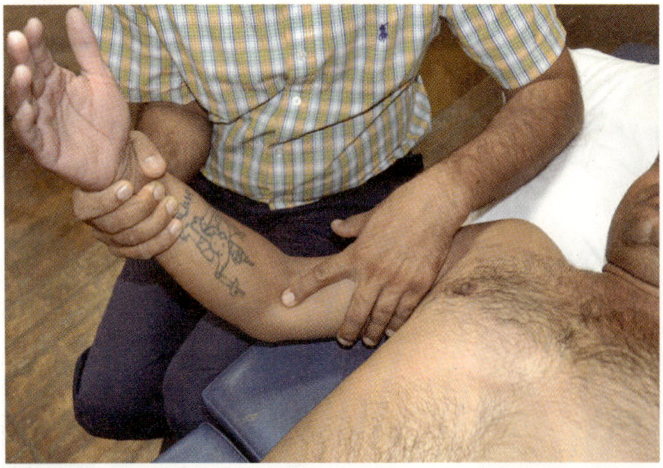

Fig. 6.83: Palpation of brachialis for grade 1, examiner stands at the side and places index finger over the brachialis on the medial aspect of the elbow joint

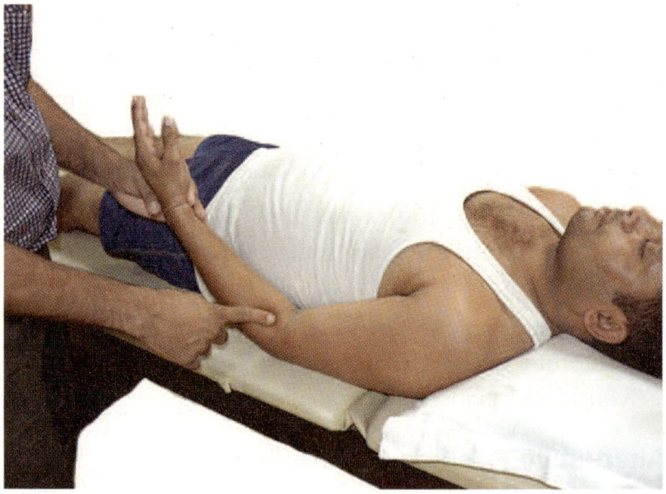

Fig. 6.84: Palpation of biceps brachioradialis for grade 1, examiner stands at the side and places one hand over the brachioradialis muscle belly on the proximal lateral surface of the forearm

Test: Examiner instructs the patient to try to bend the elbow. Examiner may place the fingers on the respective muscle belly as described below:

i. To palpate the contraction of biceps brachii examiner places fingers on the anterior surface of the middle two third with the short head lying medial to the long head.

ii. To palpate the contraction of brachialis examiner places fingers on the distal arm medial to the tendon of biceps brachii.

iii. To palpate the contraction of brachioradialis examiner places fingers on the lateral surface of the neutrally positioned forearm, where it forms the lateral border of the cubital fossa.

If examiner feels an appropriate contraction of the respective muscle belly, it is considered grade 1.

Grade 2 (Poor)

Position of Patient: Side lying with the contralateral hand is placed under the head and lower leg is flexed at hip and knee joint for base of support.

Position of Examiner: Examiner stands behind the patient and supports the arm and forearm. The arm is stabilized to prevent shoulder movements.

Stabilization: Examiner must ensure that movement should be there in the elbow joint no flexion and no abduction of shoulder should take place in order to compensate flexion (Fig. 6.85).

Test: Examiner instructs the patient to flex the elbow joint.

i. If patient is able to flex the elbow joint with forearm supination in the available range in gravity eliminated position it is considered grade 2 for biceps brachii.

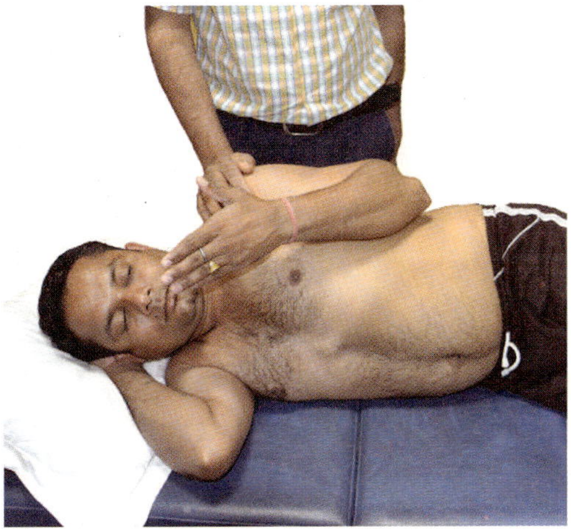

Fig. 6.85: Testing of elbow flexors in the side lying for grade 2

ii. If patient is able to flex the elbow joint with forearm pronation in the available range in gravity eliminated position it is considered grade 2 for brachialis.

iii. If patient is able to flex the elbow joint with forearm midprone in the available range in gravity eliminated position it is considered grade 2 for brachioradialis.

Alternative Position for Grade 2

Position of Patient: Short sitting with the shoulder abducted to 90 degrees and elbow is extended.

Position of Examiner: Examiner stands behind or in front of the patient and supports the arm at the elbow. Examiner also checks for any trick movement in the shoulder joint.

Stabilization: Examiner must ensure that movement should be there in the elbow joint no horizontal adduction of the shoulder should occur. Examiner should also check the trick movements such as trunk rotation and extension (Figs. 6.86a and b).

(a)

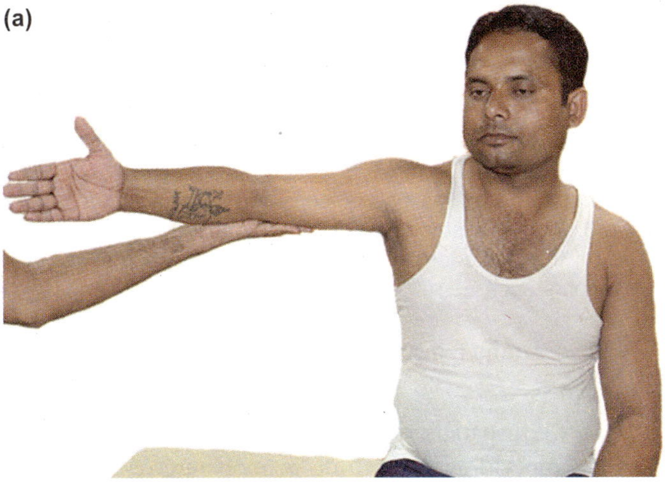

(b)

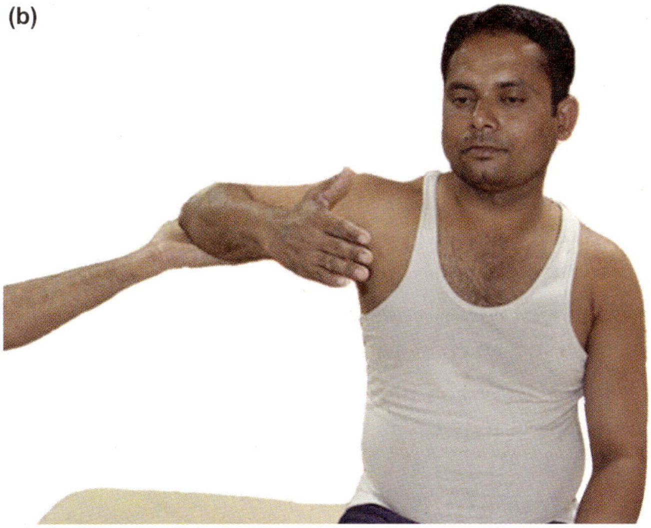

Figs. 6.86a and b: Testing of biceps brachii for grade 2, examiner stands in front of the patient and places one hand under the arm to support it

Test: Examiner instructs the patient to bend the elbow or bring the hand to the chest.

i. If patient is able to flex the elbow joint with forearm supination in the available range in gravity eliminated position it is considered grade 2 for biceps brachii.

ii. If patient is able to flex the elbow joint with forearm pronation in the available range in gravity eliminated position it is considered grade 2 for brachialis.

iii. If patient is able to flex the elbow joint with forearm midprone in the available range in gravity eliminated position it is considered grade 2 for brachioradialis.

TRICEPS BRACHII AND ANCONEUS–ELBOW EXTENSION

(a)

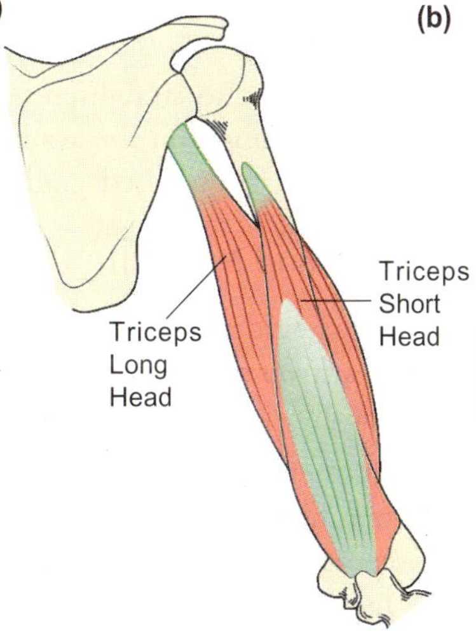

(b)

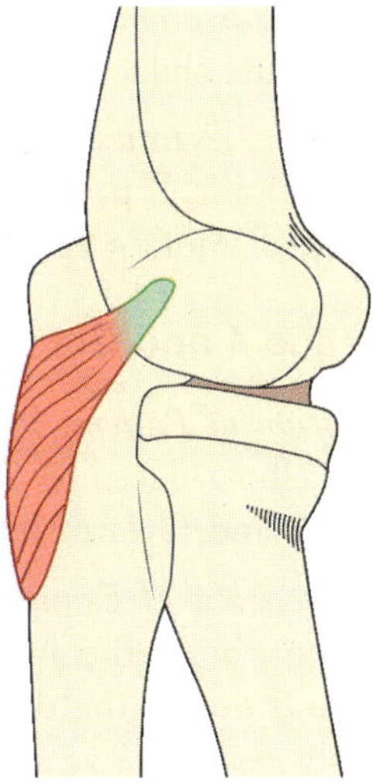

Figs. 6.87a and b: Triceps brachii and anconeus muscles origin and insertion

Triceps Brachii and Anconeus Muscles

Origin: Long head originates from infraglenoid tubercle of the scapula, and short head originates from lateral and posterior surfaces of the proximal ½ of the body of the humerus and lateral intermuscular septum. The medial head of triceps originates from distal 2/3rd of the medial and posterior surface of the humerus below the radial groove and from the medial intermuscular septum.

Insertion: Posterior surface of the olecranon process of the ulna and antebrachial fascia.

Action: Extension of the elbow joint. The long head of the triceps also assists in adduction and extension of the shoulder joint.

Nerve Supply: $C_{6, 7, 8}$ and T_1.

Anconeus

Origin: Posterior surface of lateral epicondyle of the humerus.

Insertion: Lateral side of the olecranon process and upper ¼th of the posterior surface of the body of the ulna.

Action: Extension of the elbow joint with stabilization of the ulna during supination and pronation.

Nerve Supply: $C_{7, 8}$.

Grade 3 (Fair)

Position of Patient: Prone with shoulder abducted to 90° and elbow flexed to 90°. The arm rests on the surface of couch and forearm hangs vertically.

Position of Examiner: Examiner stands at the side of patient and places one hand on the posterior aspect of the shoulder to prevent trick movements such as retraction and trunk rotation.

Stabilization: Examiner stabilizes the shoulder to prevent horizontal abduction and trunk rotation (Figs. 6.88a and b).

Test: Examiner instructs the patient to straighten your elbow joint. If patient completes movement in the available range of motion against the gravity is considered grade 3.

Grade 4 and Grade 5 (Good and Normal)

Position of Patient: Prone with shoulder abducted to 90° and elbow flexed to 90°. The arm rests on the surface of couch and forearm hangs vertically.

Position of Examiner: Examiner stands at the side of patient, holds the arm with one hand at distal to stabilize it, and grasps the distal forearm with the other hand to apply resistance against the movement.

Stabilization: Examiner stabilizes the shoulder to prevent horizontal abduction and trunk rotation (Figs. 6.89a and b).

(a)

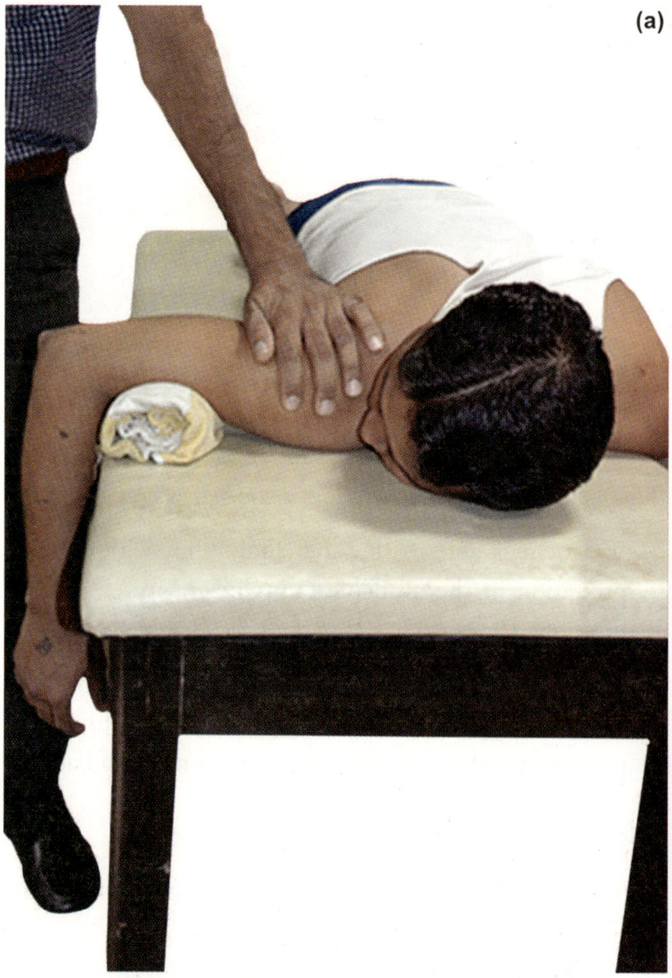

(b)

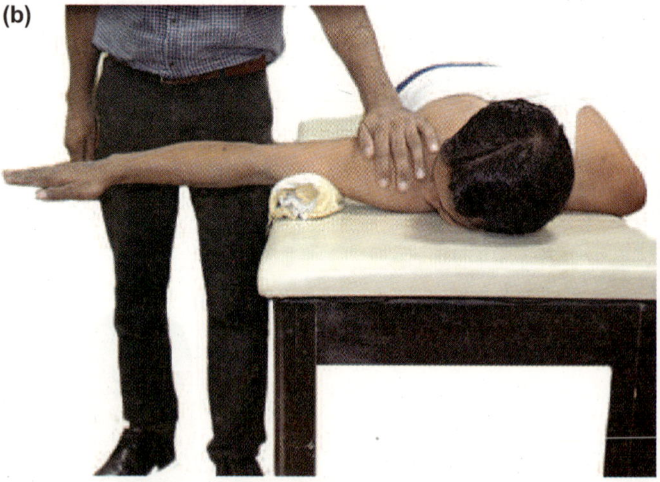

Figs. 6.88a and b: Testing of triceps and anconeus muscles for grade 3. Examiner stands at the side of patient and places one hand on the posterior aspect of the shoulder to prevent trick movements such as retraction and trunk rotation

Test: Examiner instructs the patient to straighten your elbow joint.

Grade 4: If patient completes movement in the available range of motion against strong to moderate resistance.

(a)

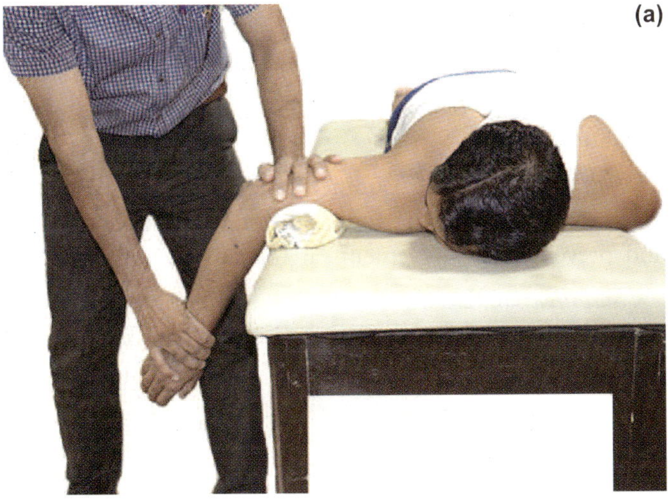

(b)

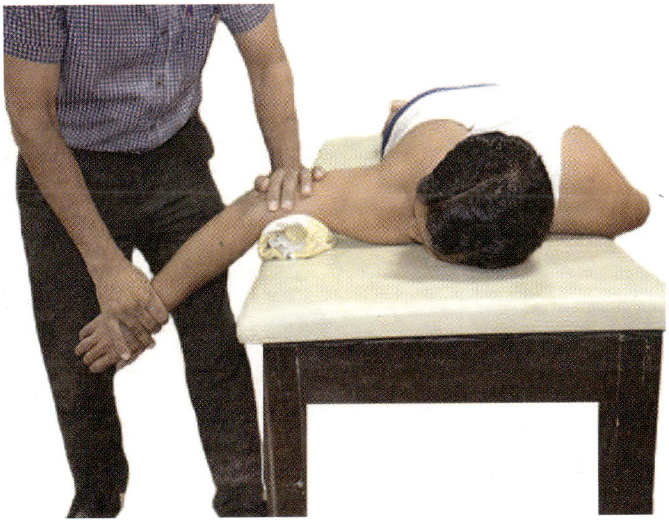

Figs. 6.89a and b: Testing of triceps and anconeus muscles for grade 4 and 5. Examiner stands at the side of patient, holds the arm with one hand at distal to stabilize it, and grasps the distal forearm with the other hand to apply resistance against the movement

Grade 5: If patient completes movement in the available range of motion against maximal resistance.

Grade 1 (Flicker/Trace)

Position of Patient: Short sitting with the shoulder abducted to 90 degrees and elbow is flexed to 45°.

Position of Examiner: Examiner stands at the side of patient and places fingers of one hand over the posterior aspect of mid arm for palpation of the contraction.

Stabilization: Does not require (Fig. 6.90).

Test: Examiner instructs the patient to try to straighten your elbow. If examiner feels contraction, it is considered grade 1.

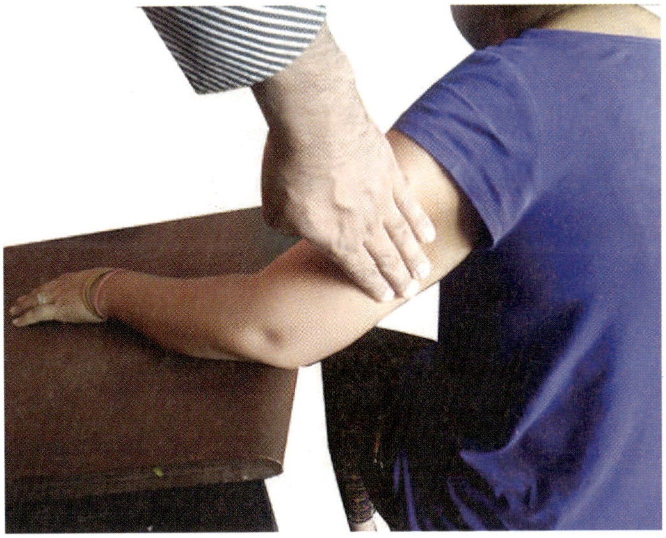

Fig. 6.90: Palpation of triceps brachii and anconeus muscle for grade 1

Grade 2 (Poor)

Position of Patient: Short sitting with the shoulder abducted to 90 degrees and elbow is fully flexed.

Position of Examiner: Examiner stands at the side of patient and places one hand under the distal arm to support it and other hand on the top of the shoulder to stabilize it and prevent horizontal abduction and trunk rotation.

Stabilization: Examiner stabilizes the shoulder to prevent horizontal abduction and trunk rotation (Figs. 6.91a and b).

(a)

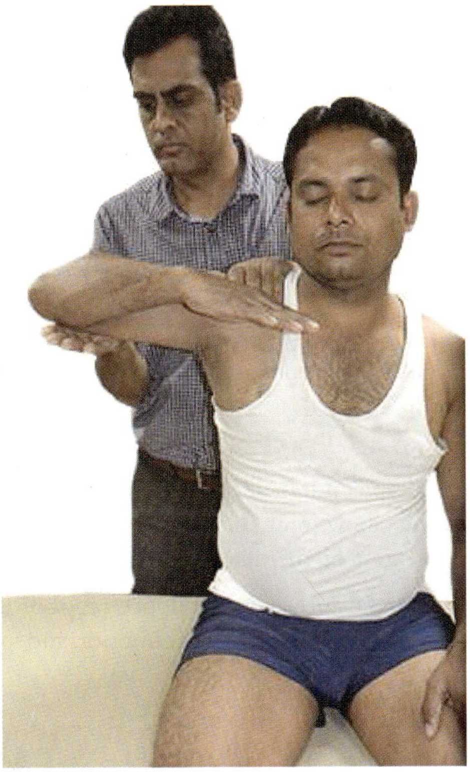

(b)

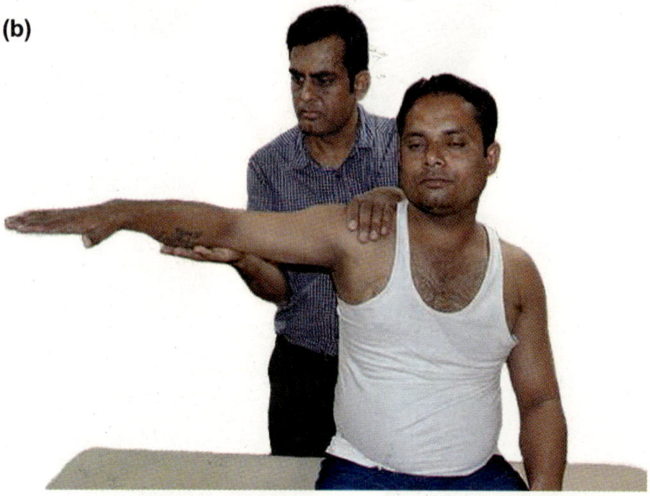

Figs. 6.91a and b: Testing of triceps and anconeus muscles for grade 2. Examiner stands at the side of patient and places one hand under the distal arm to support it and other hand on the top of the shoulder to stabilize it and prevent horizontal abduction and trunk rotation

Test: Examiner instructs the patient to try to straighten your elbow. If patient is able to straighten the elbow joint in gravity eliminated position it is considered grade 2.

SUPINATOR AND BICEPS BRACHII – FOREARM SUPINATION

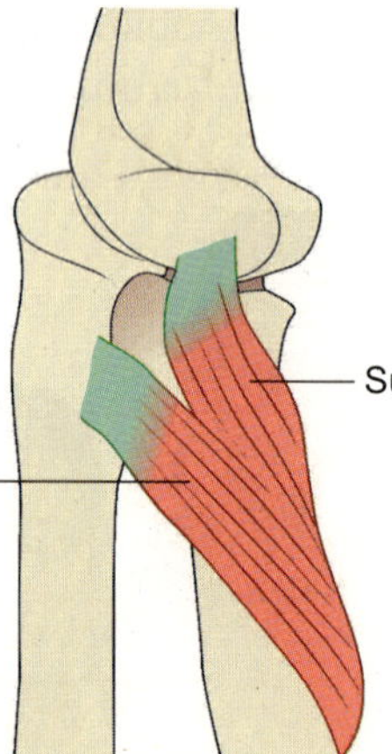

Fig. 6.92: Supinator muscle origin and insertion

Supinator

Origin: Lateral epicondule of the humerus, radial collateral ligament of the elbow joint, annular ligament of the radius and supinator crest of the ulna.

Insertion: Lateral surface of the upper 1/3rd of the body of the radius, covering part of the anterior and posterior surfaces.

Action: Supination of the forearm.

Nerve Supply: $C_{5, 6, 7}$.

Grade 3 (Fair)

Position of Patient: Short sitting with arm at the side of body and elbow flexed to 90°. Forearm is placed in full-pronated position.

Position of Patient: Examiner stands at the side of patient places one hand on the top of the shoulder to stabilize it and prevent trick movements at the shoulder joint.

Stabilization: Examiner stabilizes the shoulder to prevent adduction and external rotation (Figs. 6.93a and b).

(a)

(b)

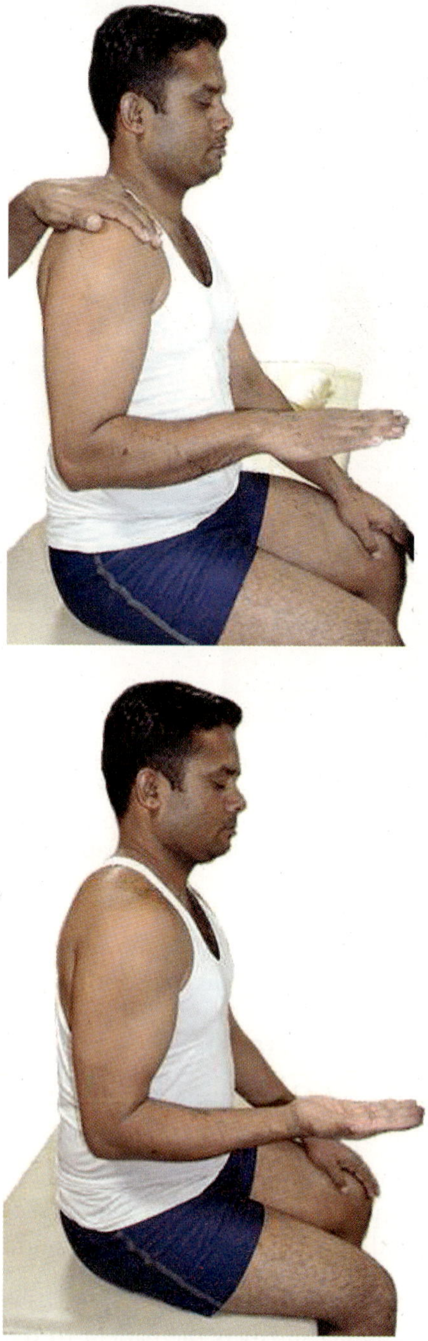

Figs. 6.93a and b: Testing of supinator muscle for grade 3, examiner stands behind the patient and stabilizes the shoulder joint to prevent abduction and external rotation

Test: Examiner instructs the patient to turn your palm up. If patient is able to turn the palm up against the gravity is considered grade 3.

Grade 4 and 5 (Good and Normal)

Position of Patient: Short sitting with arm at the side of body and elbow flexed to 90°. Forearm is placed in full-pronated position.

Position of Patient: Examiner stands behind the patient and places one hand at distal arm to stabilize it and prevent trick movements at the shoulder joint. Examiner grasps the forearm at distal to apply resistance.

Stabilization: Examiner stabilizes the shoulder to prevent adduction and external rotation (Figs. 6.94a and b).

Test: Examiner instructs the patient to turn your palm up.

Grade 4: If patient is able to turn the palm up against strong to moderate resistance.

Grade 5: If patient is able to turn the palm up against maximal resistance.

Grade 1 (Flicker/Trace)

Position of Patient: Short sitting with the shoulder adducted and elbow is flexed to 90°. Forearm is placed in full-pronated position.

Position of Examiner: Examiner stands at the side of patient and places fingers of one hand over the distal to the head of radius on the dorsal aspect of the forearm.

Stabilization: Shoulder adduction and external rotation (Fig. 6.95).

(a) (b)

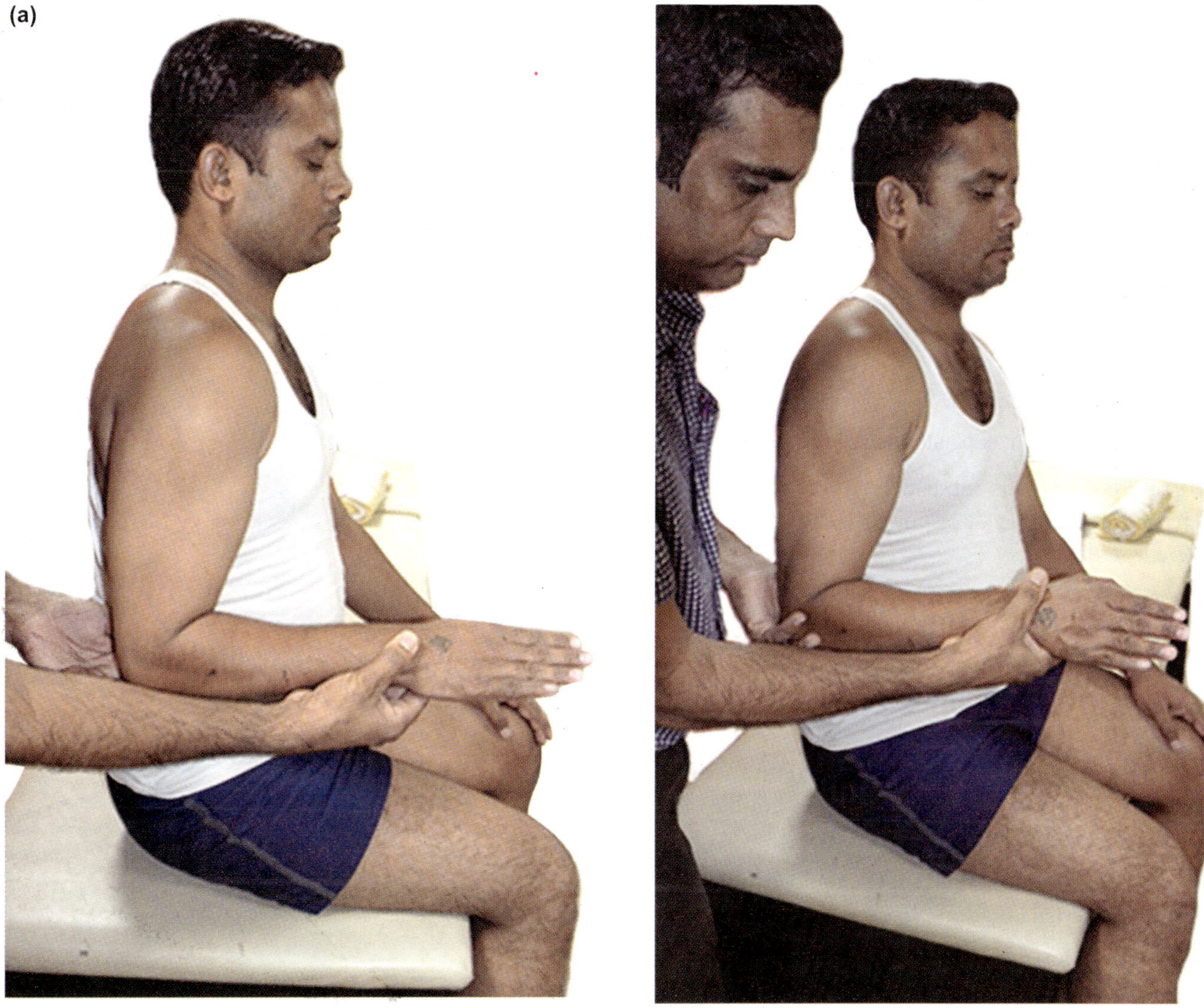

Figs. 6.94a and b: Testing of supinator muscle for grade 4 and 5, examiner stands behind the patient and grasps the distal forearm with the one hand to apply resistance against the supination movement

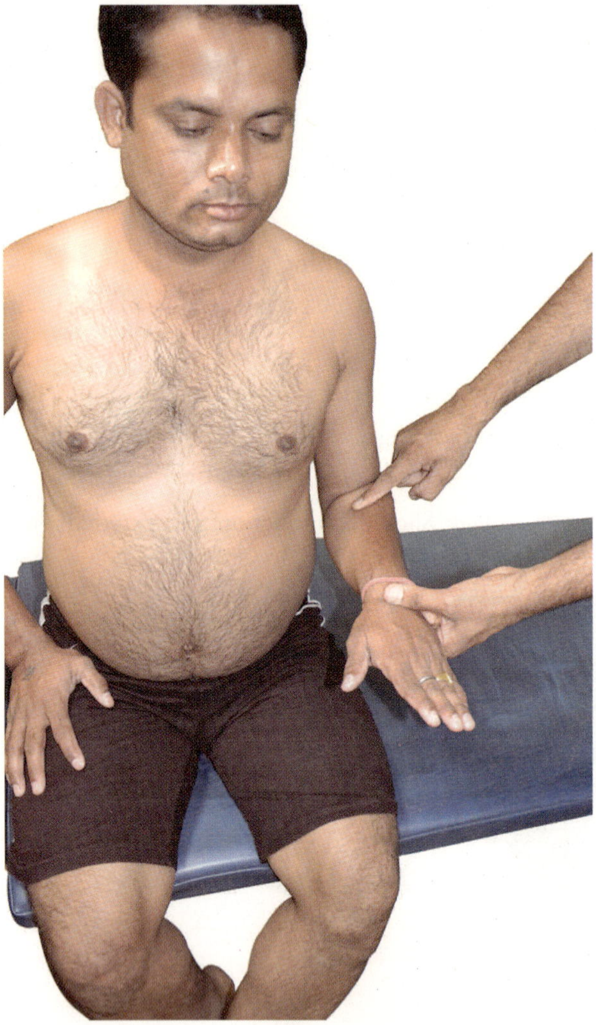

Fig. 6.95: Palpation of supinator muscle for grade 1

Test: Examiner instructs the patient to try to turn your palm so it faces the ceiling. If examiner feels contraction it is considered grade 1.

Grade 2 (Poor)

Position of Patient: Short sitting with shoulder flexed between 45° and 90° and elbow flexed to 90°. Forearm is placed in the fully pronated position.

Position of Examiner: Examiner stands at the side of patient and places one hand on the top of the shoulder and other hand at the elbow joint.

Stabilization: Examiner stabilizes the shoulder to prevent adduction and external rotation (Figs. 6.96a and b).

Test: Examiner instructs the patient to turn your arm towards your face. If patient completes movement in the available range of motion in the gravity, eliminated position is considered grade 2.

(a)

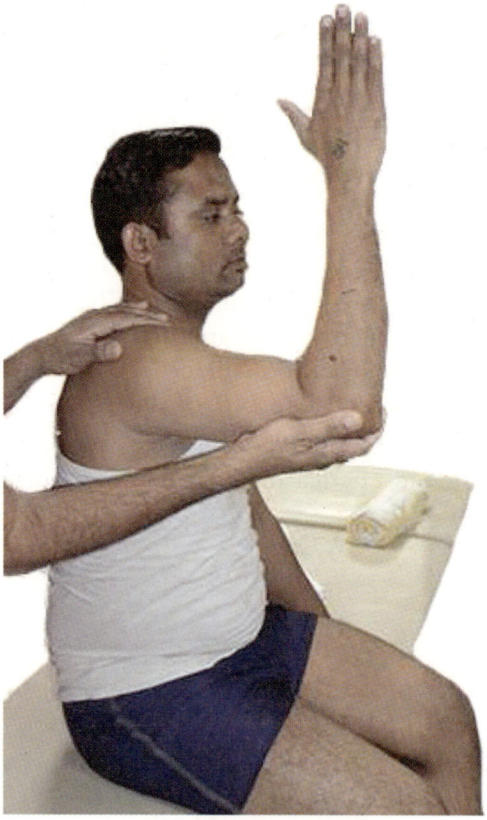

(b)

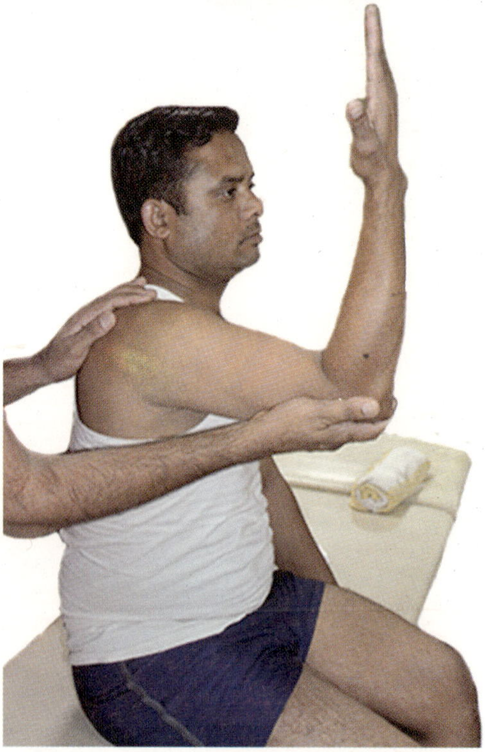

Figs. 6.96a and b: Testing of supinator muscle for grade 2, examiner stands behind the patient and stabilizes the shoulder with one hand and elbow joint with other hand

PRONATOR TERES AND PRONATOR QUADRATUS – FOREARM PRONATION

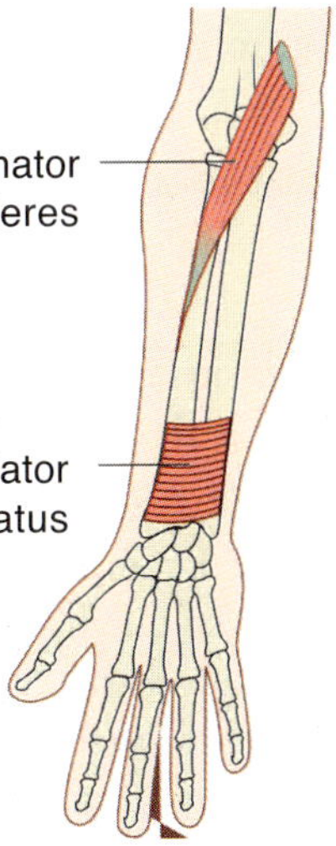

Fig. 6.97: Pronator teres and pronator quadratus muscle origin and insertion

Pronator Teres

Origin: Humeral head is originated immediately above the medial epicondyle of the humerus, common flexor tendon and deep antebrachial fascia. Ulnar head originates from medial side of the coronoid process of the ulna.

Insertion: Middle of the lateral surface of the radius.

Action: Pronation of the forearm with assistance in elbow flexion.

Nerve Supply: $C_{7,\,8,}\ T_1$.

Pronator Quadratus

Origin: Medial side, anterior surface of the distal ¼th of the ulna.

Insertion: Lateral side, anterior surface of the distal ¼th of the radius.

Action: Pronation of the forearm.

Nerve Supply: $C_{7,\,8,}\ T_1$.

Grade 3

Position of Patient: Short sitting with arm at the side of body and elbow flexed to 90°. Forearm is placed in full supinated position.

Position of Patient: Examiner stands behind the patient places one hand on the top of the shoulder to stabilize the trunk.

Stabilization: Examiner must instruct the patient to prevent abduction of the shoulder while pronating the forearm.

Substitution: Abduction of the shoulder compensates the pronation (Figs. 6.98a and b).

(a)

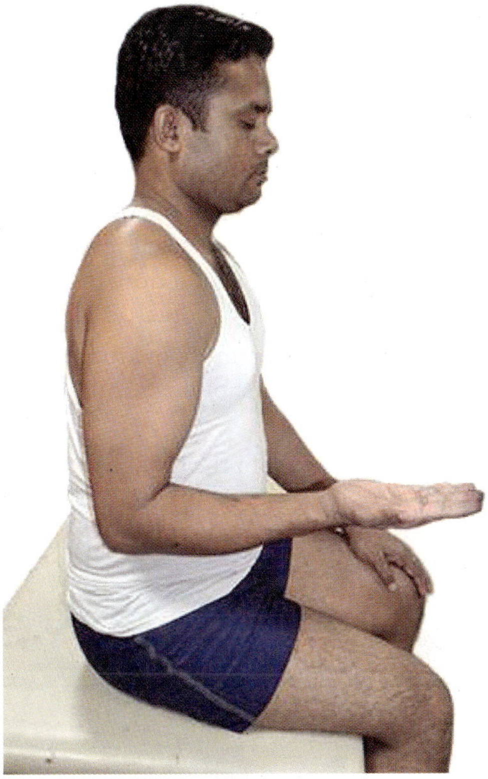

(b)

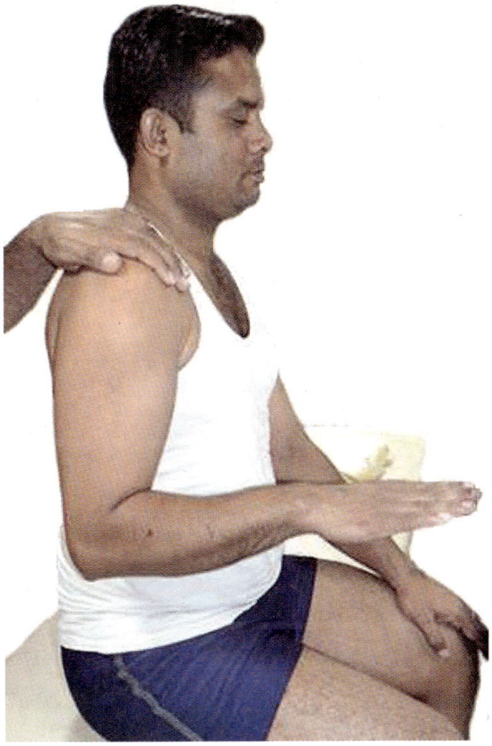

Figs. 6.98a and b: Testing of pronator teres and quadratus teres for grade 3, examiner stands behind the patient and places one hand on the top of the shoulder to prevent abduction. The last few degree movement occurs in the gravity assisted position which may be given mild resistance

Test: Examiner instructs the patient to turn your palm inwards. If patient is able to turn the palm inward against the gravity is considered grade 3.

Grade 4 and 5 (Good and Normal)

Position of Patient: Short sitting with arm at the side of body and elbow flexed to 90°. Forearm is placed in full supinated position.

Position of Examiner: Examiner stands behind the patient places one hand at distal arm to stabilize it and to prevent trick movements such as abduction of the shoulder. Examiner grasps the forearm at distal to apply resistance.

Stabilization: Examiner must instruct the patient to prevent abduction of the shoulder while pronating the forearm.

Substitution: Abduction of the shoulder compensates the pronation (Fig. 6.99).

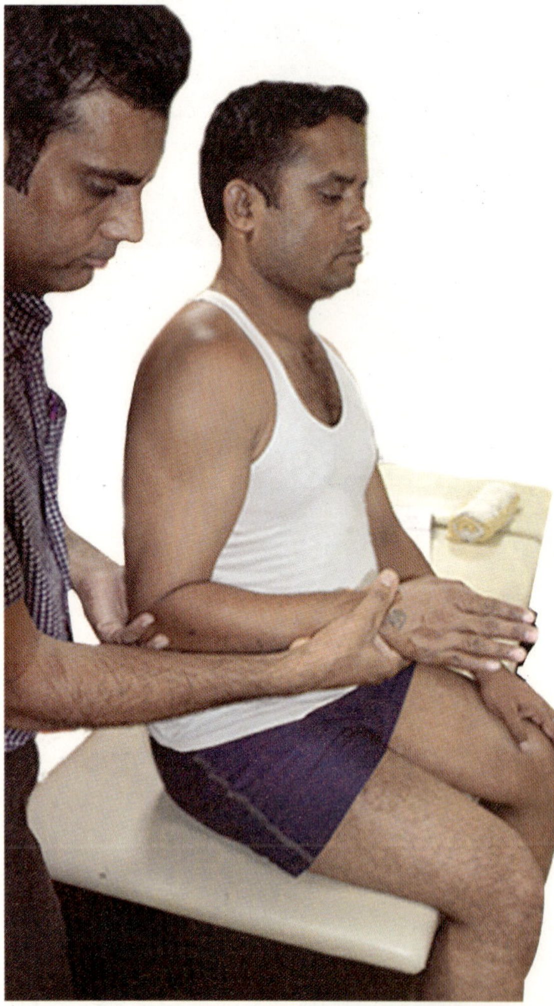

Fig. 6.99: Testing of pronator teres and quadratus teres for grade 4 and 5. Examiner stands behind the patient places one hand at distal arm to stabilize it and to prevent trick movements at such as abduction of the shoulder. Examiner grasps the forearm at distal to apply resistance

Test: Examiner instructs the patient to turn your palm up and inward.

Grade 4: If patient is able to turn the palm up and inwards against strong to moderate resistance.

Grade 5: If patient is able to turn the palm up and inward against maximal resistance.

Grade 1

Position of Patient: Short sitting with the shoulder adducted to 90 degrees and elbow is flexed to 90°. Forearm is placed in full supinated position.

Position of Examiner: Examiner stands at the side of patient and places fingers of one hand over the upper third of the volar surface of the forearm on a diagonal line from the medial condyle of the humerus to the lateral border of the radius.

Stabilization: Examiner instructs the patient to prevent abduction of the shoulder while pronating the forearm (Fig. 6.100).

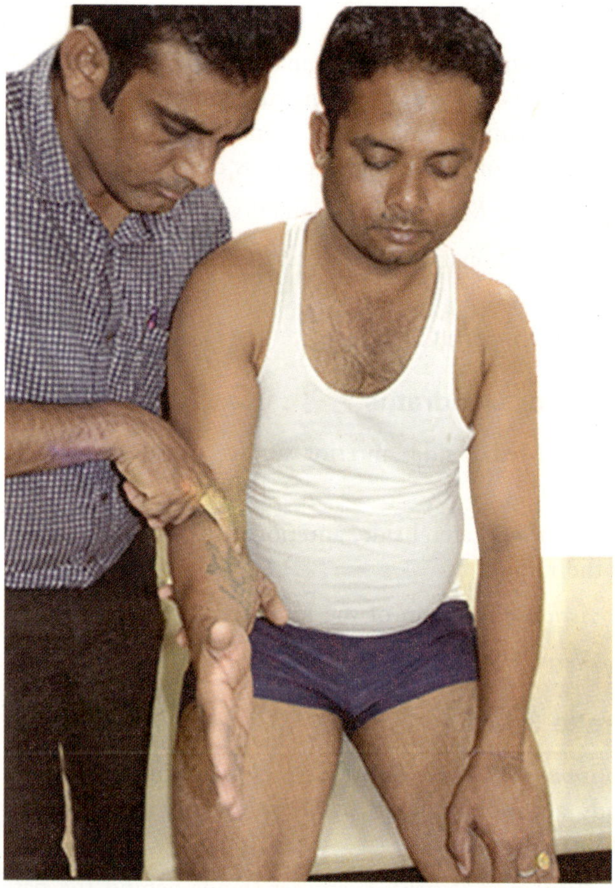

Fig. 6.100: Palpation of pronator teres and quadratus teres for grade 1, examiner stands at the side and palpates the muscle

Test: Examiner instructs the patient to try to turn your palm inwards to the body. If examiner feels contraction during pronation it is considered grade 1.

(a)

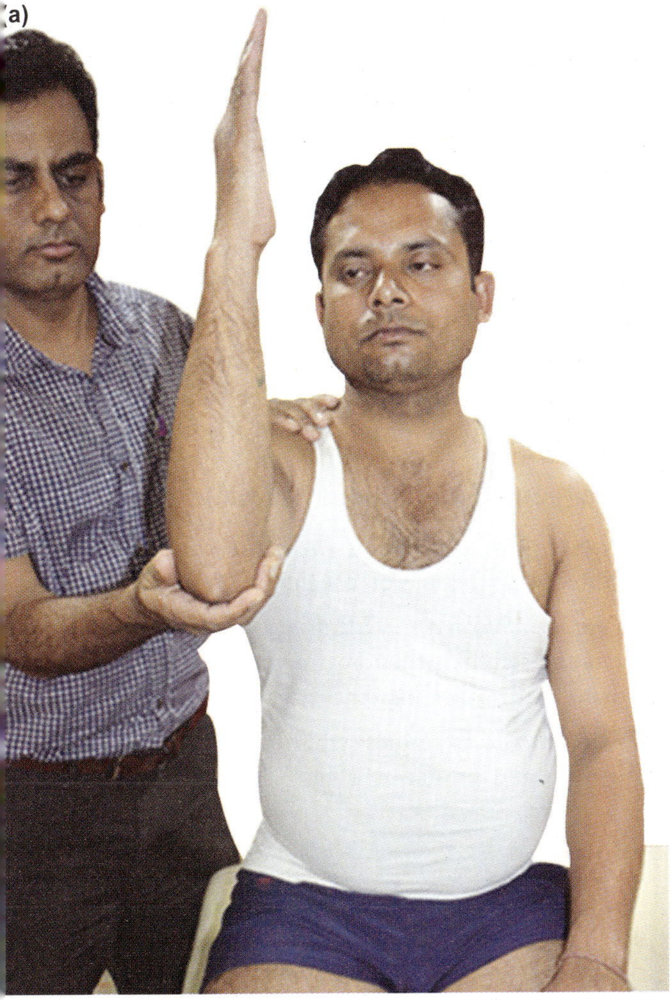

(b)

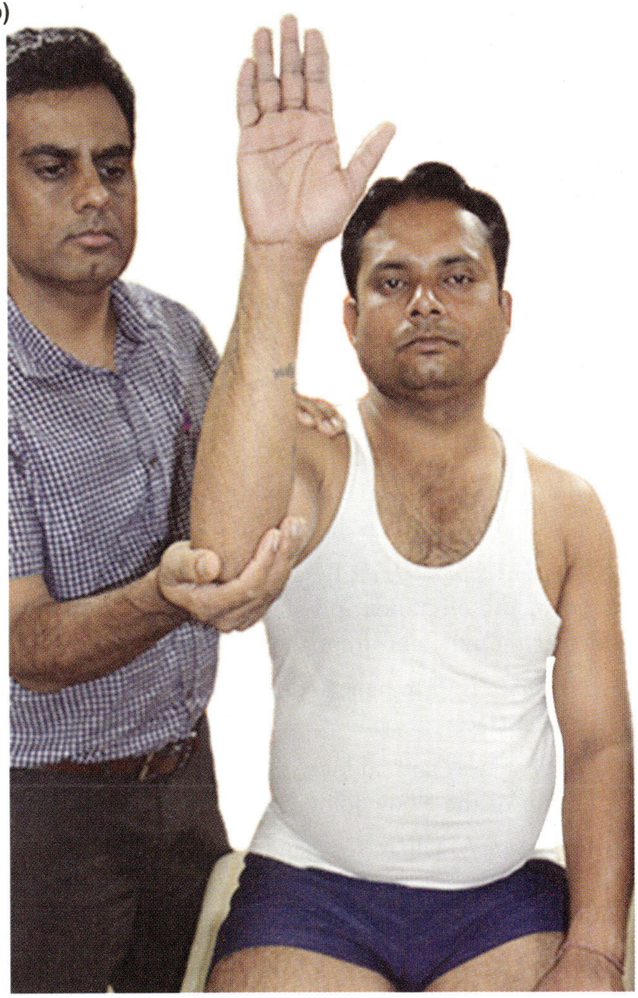

Figs. 6.101a and b: Testing of a pronator teres and pronator quadratus muscles for grade 2. Examiner stands at the side and supports the arm of the patient by holding it at the distal humerus

Grade 2

Position of Patient: Short sitting with shoulder flexed between 45° and 90° and elbow flexed to 90°. Forearm is placed in the midprone position.

Position of Examiner: Examiner stands at the side of patient and holds the arm at distal to stabilize it and prevent trick movements at the shoulder joint.

Stabilization: Examiner must instruct the patient to prevent abduction of the shoulder while pronating the forearm.

Substitution: Abduction of the shoulder compensates the pronation (Figs. 6.101a and b).

Test: Examiner instructs the patient to turn your forearm inwards. If patient completes movement in the available range of motion in the gravity eliminated position is considered grade 2.

Weakness: Loss of pronation at superior and inferior radioulnar joint.

FLEXOR CARPI RADIALIS AND FLEXOR CARPI ULNARIS – WRIST FLEXION

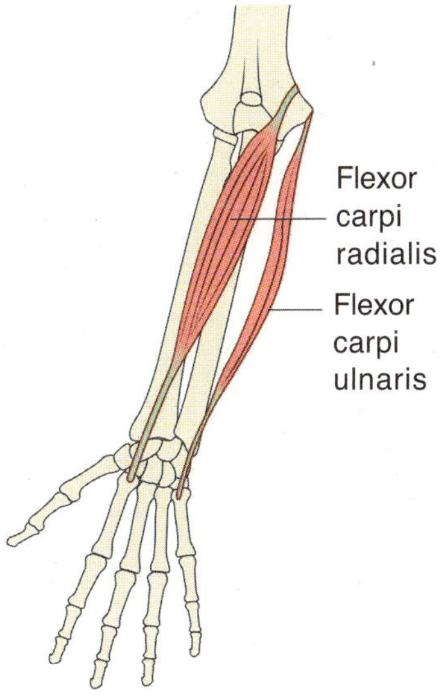

Fig. 6.102: Flexor carpi radialis and flexor carpi ulnaris origin and insertion

Flexor Carpi Radialis

Origin: Common flexor tendon from the medial epicondyle of the humerus and deep antebrachial fascia.

Insertion: Flexor carpi radialis inserts on the base of the second metacarpal bone and a slip to the base of the third metacarpal bone.

Action: Flexor carpi radialis flexes and abducts the wrist, and may assist in pronation of the forearm and flexion of the elbow joint.

Nerve Supply: Median nerve: $C_{6,\ 7\ \text{and}\ 8}$.

Flexor Carpi Ulnaris

Origin of Humeral Head: Common flexor tendon from the medial epicondyle of the humerus.

Origin of Ulnar Head: By aponeurosis from the medial margin of the olecranon, proximal 2/3rd of the posterior border of the ulna and from the deep antebrachial fascia.

Insertion: Pisiform bone and by ligaments to the hamate and fifth metacarpal bone.

Action: Flexes and adducts the wrist and may assist in the flexion of the elbow joint.

Nerve Supply: Ulnar, $C_{7,\ 8}$ and T_1.

Grade 3 (Fair)

Position of Patient: Sitting with forearm supinated and supported on the table or couch.

Position of Examiner: Examiner stands at the side of the patient which is being tested and stabilizes the forearm with one hand.

Stabilization: Forearm is stabilized to prevent supination and pronation (Figs. 103a and b).

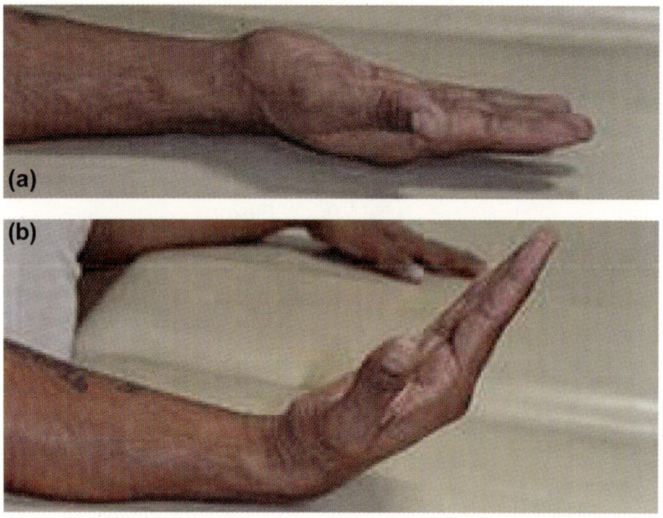

Figs. 6.103a and b: Testing of flexor carpi radialis and flexor carpi ulnaris for grade 3

Test: Examiner instructs the patient to bend your wrist with the fingers relaxed or slightly flexed. Excessive flexion of the DIP and PIP can limit the wrist flexion.

i. If patient completes wrist flexion with radial deviation against the gravity is considered grade 3 for the flexor carpi radialis.
ii. If patient completes wrist flexion with ulnar deviation against the gravity is considered grade 3 for flexor carpi ulnaris.
iii. If patient completes wrist flexion without ulnar or radial deviation against the gravity is considered grade 3 for both the flexor carpi ulnaris and flexor carpi radialis.

Grade 4 and 5 (Good and Normal)

Position of Patient: Sitting with forearm supinated and supported on the table or couch.

Position of Examiner: Examiner stands in front of the patient and stabilizes the forearm with one hand and grasps the hand with other hand.

Stabilization: Examiner stabilizes the forearm to prevent supination and pronation (Fig. 6.104).

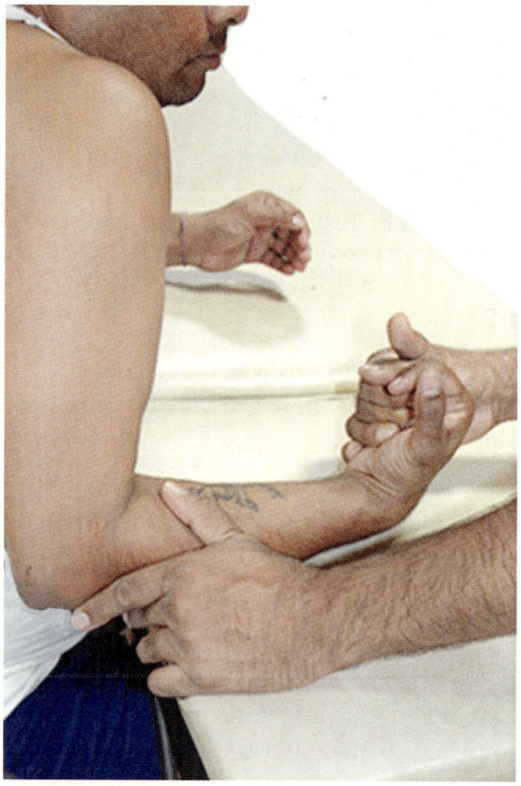

Fig. 6.104: Testing of flexor carpi radialis and flexor carpi ulnaris for grade 4 and 5, examiner grasps the hand of the patient and resist the wrist flexion

Test: Examiner instructs the patient to bend your wrist with the fingers relaxed or slightly flexed. Excessive flexion of the DIP and PIP can limit the wrist flexion.

i. If patient completes wrist flexion with radial deviation against strong to moderate resistance is considered grade 4 for the flexor carpi radialis.

ii. If patient completes wrist flexion with ulnar deviation against strong to moderate resistance is considered grade 4 for flexor carpi ulnaris.

iii. If patient completes wrist flexion without ulnar or radial deviation against strong to moderate resistance is considered grade 4 for both the flexor carpi ulnaris and flexor carpi radialis.

Grade 5: If patient completes wrist flexion against maximal resistance is considered grade 5.

Grade 1 (Trace)

Position of Patient: Sitting, forearms supinated and supported on the table or couch.

Position of Examiner: Examiner stands at the side which is being tested and places index finger of one hand on the respective tendon of the muscle. For flexor carpi radialis–finger is placed on the lateral palmar aspect of the wrist lateral to the palmaris longus. For flexor carpi ulnaris–finger is placed on the medial palmar aspect of the wrist, at the base of 5th metacarpal bone.

Stabilization: Does not require (Figs. 6.105a and b).

(a)

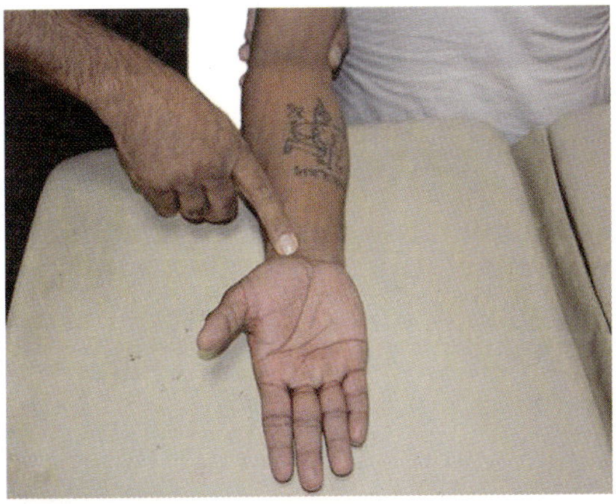

(b)

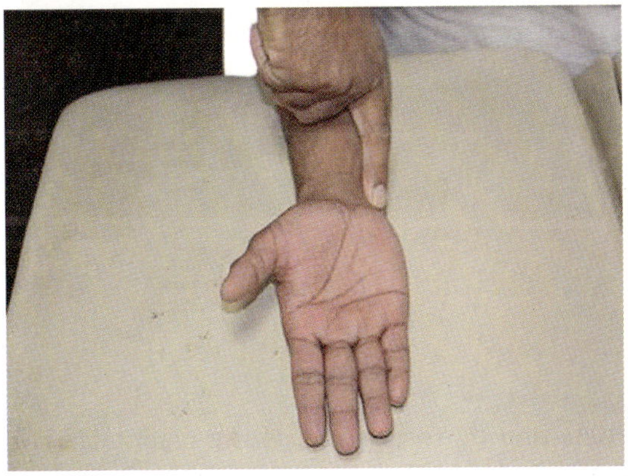

Figs. 6.105a and b: Palpation of flexor carpi radialis and flexor carpi ulnaris for grade 1

Test: Examiner instructs the patient to try to bend your wrist while he or she palpates the tendon of the corresponding muscle. If examiner feels contraction it is considered grade 1.

Grade 2 (Poor)

Position of Patient: Sitting, forearm in midprone position and supported on the table or couch.

Position of Examiner: Examiner stands at the side of the patient and supports the forearm to prevent supination and pronation. A towel roll can be placed under the forearm up to the wrist to keep the hand slightly over the table.

Stabilization: Examiner stabilizes the forearm to prevent supination and pronation (Figs. 106a and b).

(a)

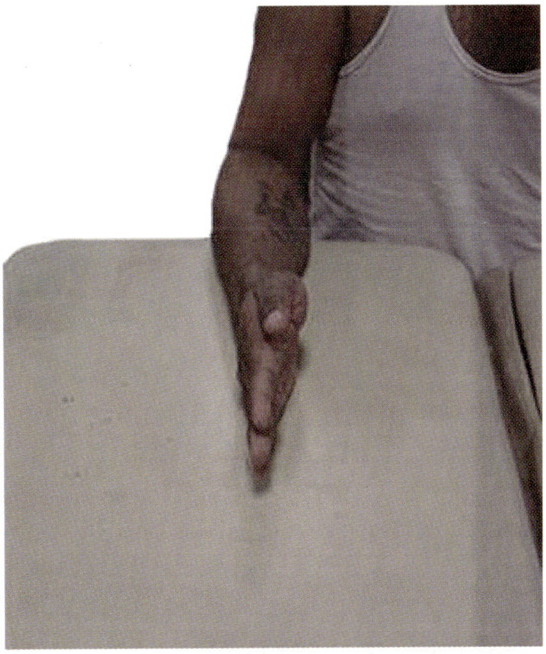

(b)

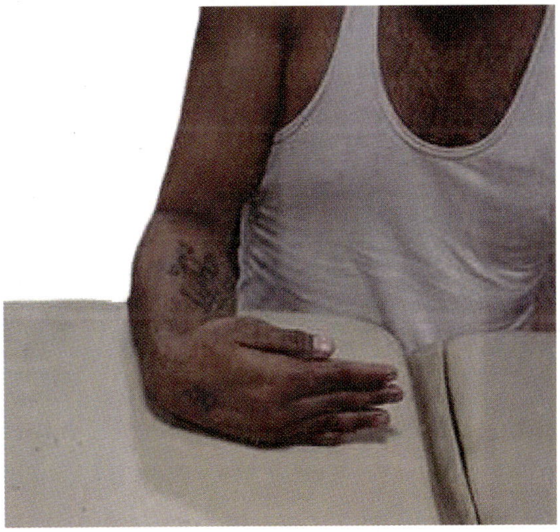

Figs. 6.106a and b: Testing of flexor carpi radialis and flexor carpi ulnaris for grade 2

Test: Examiner instructs the patient to bend your wrist with the fingers slightly flexed. Excessive flexion of the PIP and DIP can limit the wrist flexion. If patient completes wrist flexion with radial deviation in the gravity eliminated position it is considered grade 2 for flexor carpi radialis. If patient completes wrist flexion with ulnar deviation in the gravity eliminated position it is considered grade 2 for flexor carpi ulnaris.

Weakness: Loss of flexion with radial deviation of the wrist.

EXTENSOR CARPI RADIALIS LONGUS, EXTENSOR CARPI RADIALIS BREVIS AND EXTENSOR CARPI ULNARIS – WRIST EXTENSION

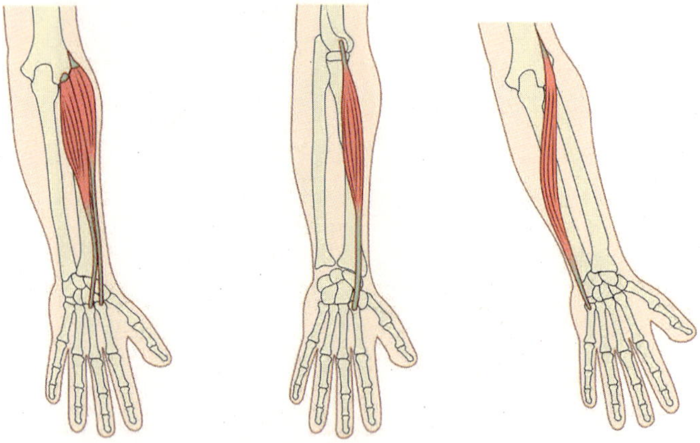

(a) (b) (c)

Figs. 6.107a to c: Extensor carpi radialis longus, extensor carpi radialis brevis and extensor carpi ulnaris muscles origin and insertion

Extensor Carpi Radialis Longus

Origin: Distal 1/3rd of the lateral supracondylar ridge of the humerus and lateral intermuscular septum.

Insertion: Dorsal surface of the base of second metacarpal bone, radial side.

Action: Extension and radial deviation of the wrist.

Nerve Supply: Radial, $C_{5,\ 6,7 \text{ and } 8}$.

Extensor Carpi Radialis Brevis

Origin: Common extensor tendon from the lateral epicondyle of the humerus, radial collateral ligament of elbow joint and deep antebrachial fascia.

Insertion: Dorsal surface of the base of the third metacarpal bone.

Action: Extension of the wrist with assistance in the radial deviation.

Nerve Supply: Radial, $C_{6,\ 7 \text{ and } 8}$.

Extensor Carpi Ulnaris

Origin: Common extensor tendon from the lateral epicondyle of the humerus, by the aponeurosis from the posterior border of the ulna and deep antebrachial fascia.

Insertion: Base of the fifth metacarpal bone, ulnar side.

Action: Extension of the wrist and assistance in the ulnar deviation of the wrist.

Nerve Supply: Radial, $C_{6,\ 7 \text{ and } 8}$.

Grade 3

Position of Patient: Sitting, elbow flexed slightly, forearm fully pronated and supported on the table or couch.

Position of Examiner: Examiner stands at the side of the patient and stabilizes the forearm with one hand to prevent supination, pronation and movement at the elbow joint.

Stabilization: Examiner stabilizes the elbow joint to prevent flexion of the elbow joint and abduction of the shoulder joint. No supination should take place (Figs. 108a and b).

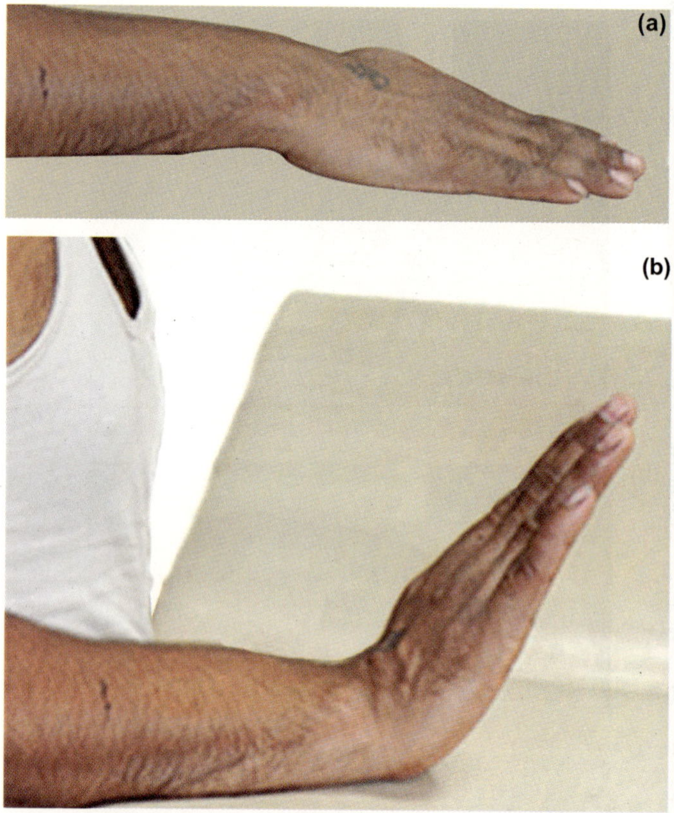

Figs. 6.108a and b: Testing of extensor carpi radialis longus, extensor carpi radialis brevis and extensor carpi ulnaris muscles for grade 3

Test: Examiner instructs the patient to bring your wrist up. The PIP and DIP joints are kept slightly flexed to allow full extension of the wrist joint. Examiner should test all the wrist extensors separately.

i. *Extensor carpi radialis longus and extensor carpi radialis brevis*: Patient extends the wrist joint with radial deviation against the gravity.

ii. *Extensor carpi ulnaris:* Patient extends the wrist joint with the ulnar deviation against the gravity.

iii. *All three extensors (combined):* Patient extends the wrist joint in the sagittal plane without ulnar or radial deviation.

Grade 4 and 5 (Good and Normal)

Position of Patient: Sitting, elbow flexed slightly, forearm fully pronated and supported on the table or couch.

Position of Examiner: Examiner stands at the side of the patient and stabilizes the forearm with one hand to prevent supination, pronation and movement at the elbow joint. Places the other hand at the dorsum surface of metacarpal bones to apply resistance.

Stabilization: Examiner stabilizes the elbow joint to prevent flexion of the elbow joint and abduction of the shoulder joint (Fig. 6.109).

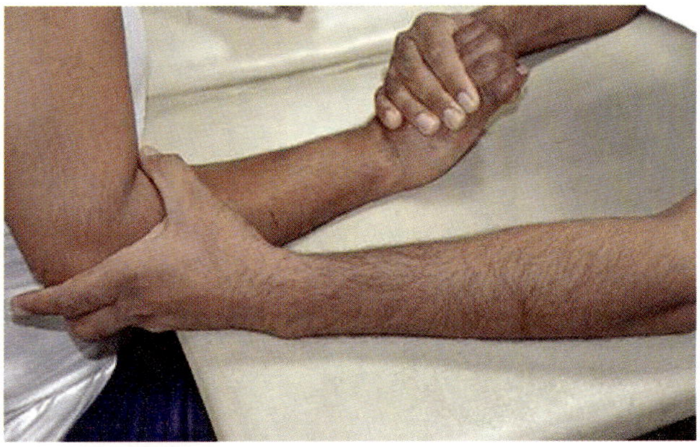

Fig. 6.109: Testing of extensor carpi radialis longus, extensor carpi radialis brevis and extensor carpi ulnaris muscles for grade 4 and 5

Test: Examiner instructs the patient to bring your wrist up against the resistance. Examiner should test all the wrist extensors separately.

Grade 4

i. *Extensor carpi radialis longus and extensor carpi radialis brevis:* Patient extends the wrist joint with radial deviation against strong to moderate resistance.

ii. *Extensor carpi ulnaris:* Patient extends the wrist joint with the ulnar deviation against strong to moderate resistance.

iii. *All three extensors (combined):* Patient extends the wrist joint in the sagittal plane without ulnar or radial deviation against strong to moderate resistance.

Grade 5

i. *Extensor carpi radialis longus and extensor carpi radialis brevis:* Patient extends the wrist joint with radial deviation against maximal resistance.

ii. *Extensor carpi ulnaris:* Patient extends the wrist joint with the ulnar deviation against maximal resistance.

iii. *All three extensors (combined):* Patient extends the wrist joint in the sagittal plane without ulnar or radial deviation against maximal resistance.

Grade 1

Position of Patient: Sitting with forearm fully pronated and supported on the table or couch.

Position of Examiner: Examiner stands at the side of patient and places index finger on the respective tendon of the muscle.

Stabilization: Elbow joint is stabilized to prevent flexion.

i. *Extensor carpi radialis longus:* On the dorsum of the wrist in line with the second metacarpal.

ii. *Extensor carpi radialis brevis:* On the dorsal surface of the wrist in line with the third metatarsal bone.

iii. *Extensor carpi ulnaris:* On the dorsal wrist surface proximal to the fifth metacarpal and just distal to the ulnar styloid process (Fig. 6.110).

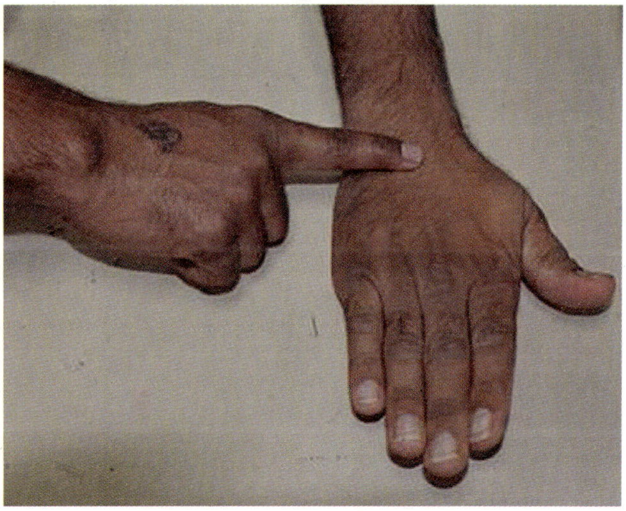

Fig. 6.110: Palpation of extensor carpi radialis brevis muscles for grade 1

Test: Examiner instructs the patient to try to bend the wrist back to the dorsal aspect. If examiner feels the contraction on the respective tendon of the muscle is considered grade 1 for that muscle.

Grade 2 (Poor)

Position of Patient: Sitting, forearm in midprone position and supported on the table or couch.

Position of Examiner: Examiner stands at the side of the patient and holds the forearm to prevent supination and pronation. A towel roll can be placed under the forearm up to the wrist to keep the hand slightly over the table.

Stabilization: Examiner stabilizes the elbow joint to prevent flexion, and supination and pronation of the forearm (Figs. 6.111a and b).

(a)

(b)

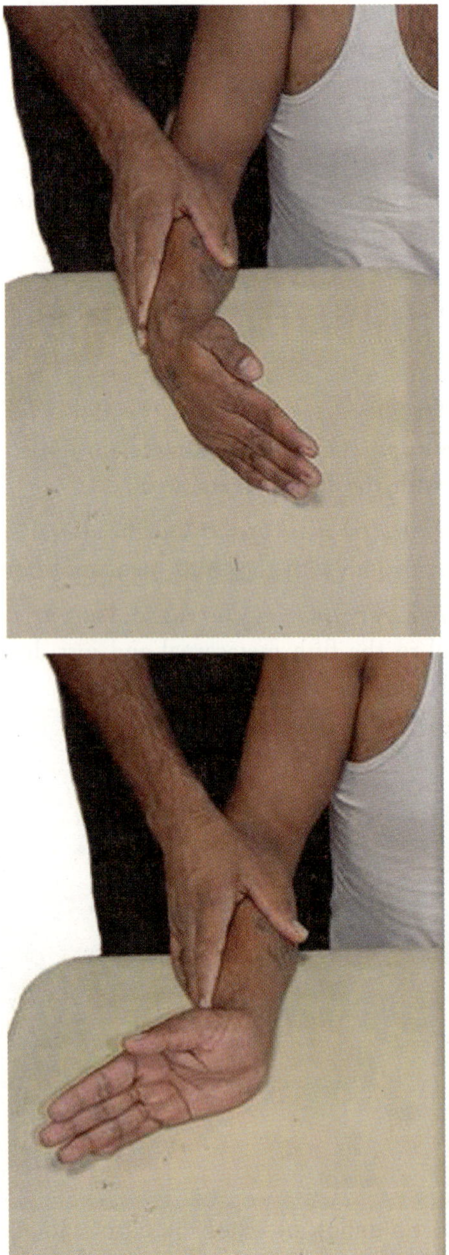

Figs. 6.111a and b: Testing of extensor carpi radialis longus, extensor carpi radialis brevis and extensor carpi ulnaris muscles for grade 2

Test: Examiner instructs the patient to bend your wrist back. If patient completes wrist extension in the gravity eliminated position it is considered grade 2.

Weakness of extensor group of muscles innervated by radial nerve: Weakness of extensors of the wrist are usually the result of the radial nerve injury or palsy. Radial nerve palsy involves paralysis of extensors of wrist as well as abductor pollicis longus. The classic biomechanical consequence of the radial nerve paralysis is the inability to extend the wrist, loss of extension of the fingers in the metacarpophalangeal joints and inability to extend and abduct the thumb. Also known as "wrist drop", the deformity that is established after a radial nerve injury represents a significant functional damage to the hand, since the inability to extend and stabilize the wrist prevents proper use of extrinsic flexors for hand closing, thus, weakening and lowering the hold and diminishing coordination.

The motor component of the radial nerve also innervates the triceps, anconeus, brachialis, brachioradialis, supinator, thereby enabling elbow extension, part of elbow flexion and forearm supination.

PALMAR INTEROSSEI – METACARPOPHALANGEAL JOINT ADDUCTION

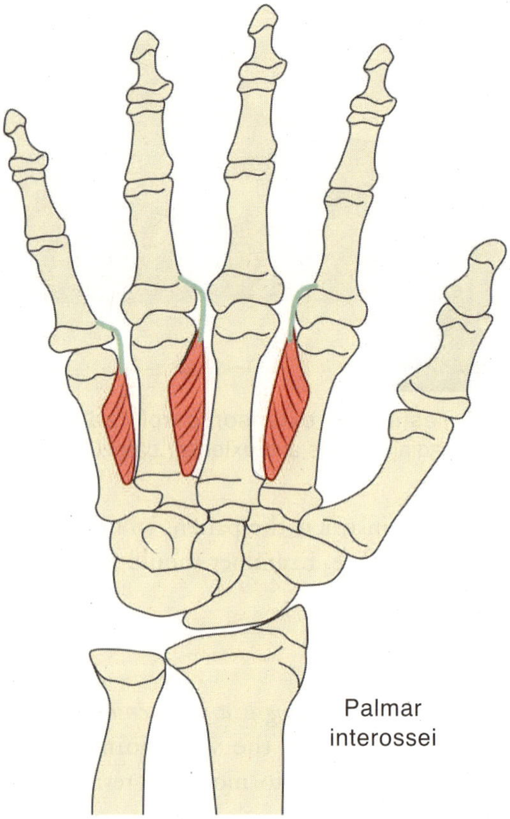

Fig. 6.112: Palmar interossei muscles origin and insertion

Palmar Interossei

Origin and Insertion

First: From ulnar side of base of first metacarpal bone with insertion on the ulnar side of the base of proximal phalanx of thumb.

Second: From length of the second metacarpal bone (ulnar side) with insertion on the base of proximal phalanx of index finger on the ulnar side.

Third: From length of the fourth metacarpal bone (radial side) with insertion on the base of proximal phalanx of ring finger on the radial side.

Fourth: From length of the fifth metacarpal bone (radial side) with insertion on the radial side of the proximal phalanx of little finger.

Action: Adduction of thumb, index, ring and little finger towards the axial line through the third digit. Palmar interossei assists in the flexion of the metacapophalangeal joints and extension of the interphalangeal joint of the three fingers.

Nerve Supply: Ulnar Nerve, C_8, T_1.

Grade 3 (Fair)

Position of Patient: Sitting, forearm pronated, wrist be at neutral no ulnar or radial deviation, MCP joints should be abducted, PIP and DIP should be at neutral.

Position of Examiner: Examiner stands at the side of the patient and grasps middle finger with one hand and testing finger with other hand.

Stabilization: Examiner stabilizes the forearm and wrist to prevent motions at the wrist and forearm.

Substitution: Flexor digitorum superficialis and profundus flexes the PIP and DIP which may contribute to the adduction of the MCP joints (Fig. 6.113).

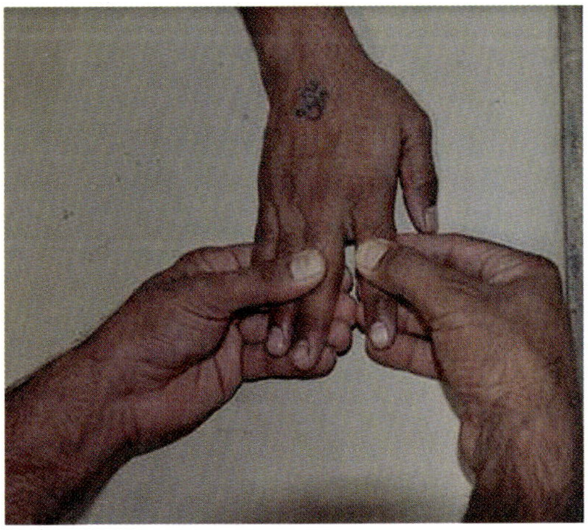

Fig. 6.113: Testing of palmar interossei muscles for grade 3

Test: Examiner instructs the patient to bring the fingers towards middle finger. If patient is able to adduct the fingers in the available range of motion but cannot hold against resistance is considered grade 3. Examiner should ensure that no flexion should occur at the PIP and DIP joints as it may contribute to the adduction.

Grade 4 and 5 (Good and Fair)

Position of Patient: Sitting, forearm pronated, wrist at neutral no ulnar or radial deviation, MCP joints should be abducted, PIP and DIP should be at neutral.

Position of Examiner: Examiner stands at the side of the patient and grasps the middle phalanx of each of two adjoining fingers. Resistance is given in the direction of abduction for each finger tested.

Stabilization: Examiner ensures PIP and DIP at extended position and wrist at neutral and with no supination and pronation during the testing.

Substitution: Flexor digitorum superficialis and profundus flexes the PIP and DIP which may contribute to the adduction of the MCP joints (Figs. 6.114a and b).

(a)

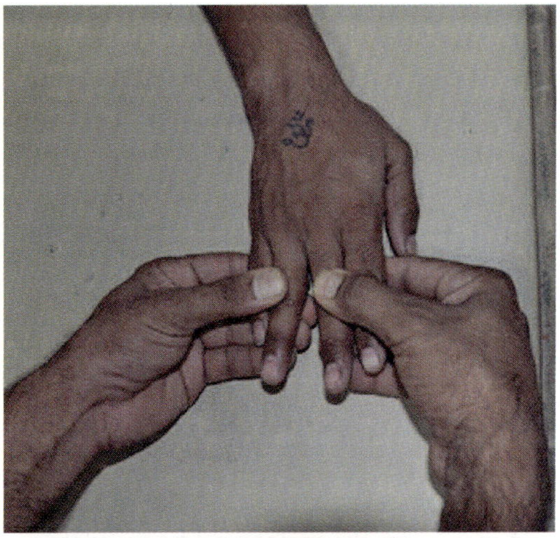

(b)

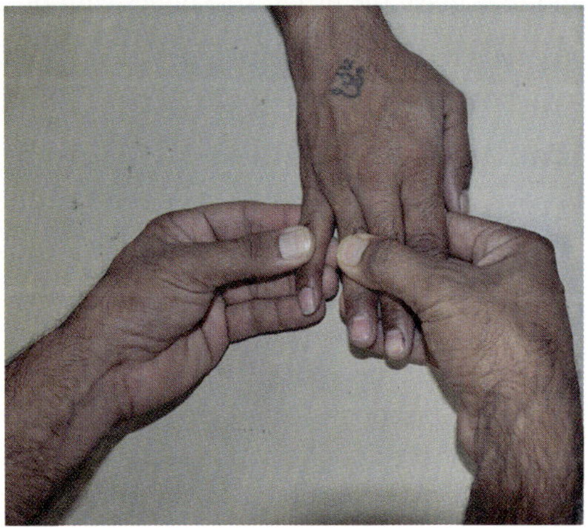

Figs. 6.114a and b: Testing of palmar interossei muscles for grade 4 and 5

Test: Examiner instructs the patient to bring the finger towards middle finger. Examiner tries to pull the finger apart (abduction). Examiner should ensure that no flexion should occur at the PIP and DIP joints as it may contribute to the adduction. Palmar interossei are the small muscles, which cannot take much resistance, therefore, examiner, offers moderate resistance for grade 4 and 5. Distinguishing between grade 4 and 5 depends on the experience of the examiner. Students should practice testing of palmar interossei on maximum number of subjects to distinguish grade 4 and 5.

Grade 1 (Trace)

Position of Patient: Sitting, forearm pronated, wrist at neutral no ulnar or radial deviation, MCP joints should be abducted, PIP and DIP should be at neutral.

Position of Examiner: Examiner stands at the side of the patient and places index finger on the side of the finger which is being tested.

Stabilization: Wrist and CMC joints.

Test: Examiner instructs the patient to try to adduct the MCP joints and palpates the contraction. Palpation of palmar interossei is rarely possible; therefore, examiner can grade 2 if there is a minimal adduction of the concerned finger. Examiner should ensure that no flexion should occur at the PIP and DIP joints which may contribute to the adduction.

Grade 2 (Poor)

Position of Patient: Sitting, forearm pronated, wrist should be at neutral no ulnar or radial deviation, MCP joints should be abducted, PIP and DIP should be at neutral.

Position of Examiner: Examiner stands at the side of the patient and may grasp the metacarpal bones with one hand.

Stabilization: Examiner instructs the patient to maintain the wrist at neutral position.

Substitution: Flexor digitorum superficialis and profundus flexes the PIP and DIP which may contribute to the adduction of the MCP joints (Figs. 6.115a and b).

Test: Examiner instructs the patient to bring the fingers towards each other, and hold them. If patient is able to adduct the fingers in the available range of motion in the gravity eliminated position is considered grade 2. Examiner should ensure that no flexion should occur at the PIP and DIP joints which may contribute to the adduction.

Weakness: Loss of adduction of the metacarpophalangeal joints.

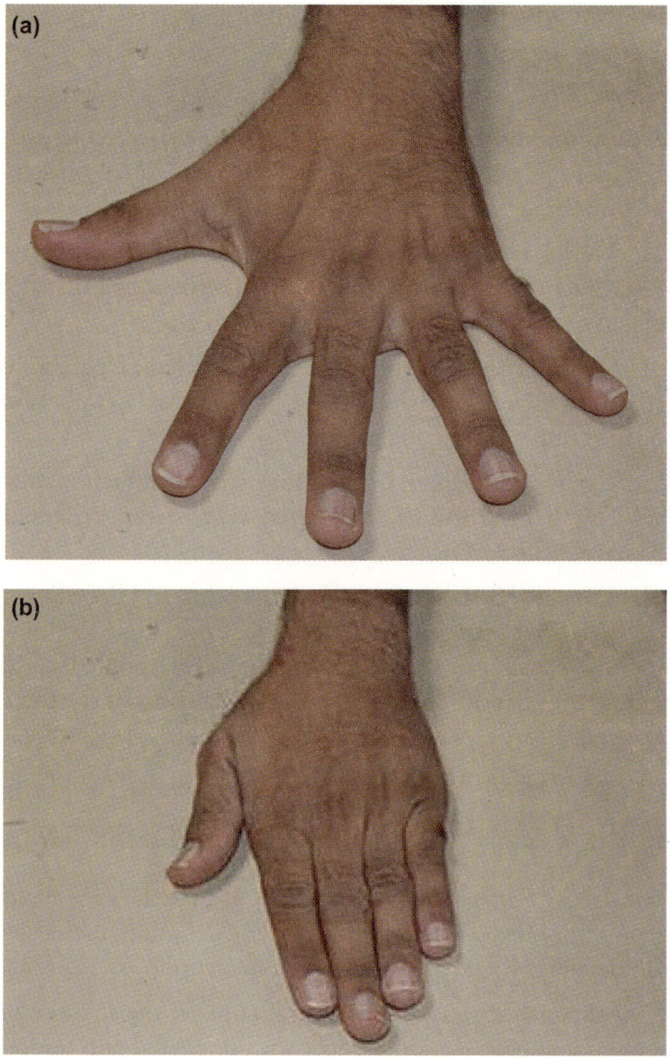

Figs. 6.115a and b: Testing of palmar interossei muscles for grade 2

DORSAL INTEROSSEI – 2nd to 5th METACARPOPHALANGEAL JOINT ABDUCTION

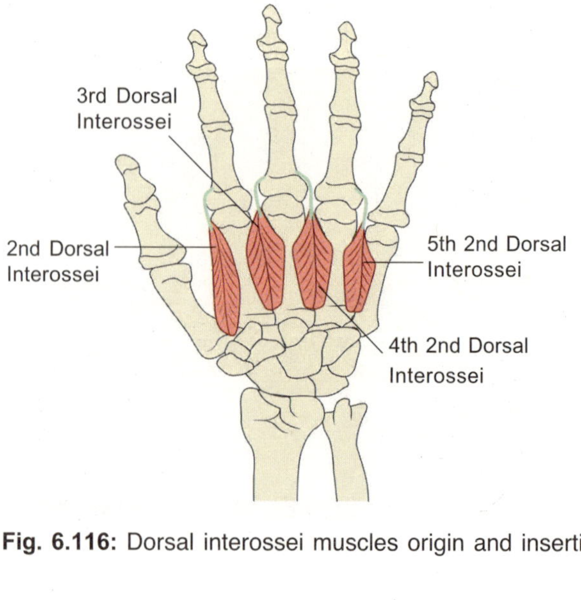

Fig. 6.116: Dorsal interossei muscles origin and insertion

Origin: First dorsal interossei has two heads medial and lateral. Lateral head originates from proximal ½ of the ulnar border of the first metacarpal bone. The medial head originates from radial border of the second metacarpal bone. Second, third and fourth dorsal interossei originate from adjacent side of the metacarpal bones in each interspace.

Insertion: First dorsal interossei inserts on the base of proximal phalanx of the index finger on the radial side. Second dorsal interossei inserts on the base of proximal phalanx of middle finger on the radial side. Third dorsal interossei inserts on the ulnar side of the middle finger, chiefly into extensor expansion. Fourth dorsal interossei inserts on the ulnar side of the ring finger.

Action: Abduction of the index, middle and ring fingers from the axial line through the third digit. Assist in flexion of the metacarpophalangeal joint and extension of the interphalangeal joint of the same fingers.

Nerve Supply: Ulnar, C_8, T_1.

Grade 3

Position of Patient: Sitting, forearm pronated, wrist, MCP, DIP and PIP at neutral.

Position of Examiner: Examiner stands at the side which is being tested and holds the wrist joint to maintain it in the neutral position.

Stabilization: Examiner stabilizes the wrist joint to maintain it at the neutral position.

Test: Examiner instructs the patient to "spread your fingers outwards". If patient is able to abduct the fingers in the available range of motion but cannot hold against resistance is considered grade 3 (Fig. 6.117).

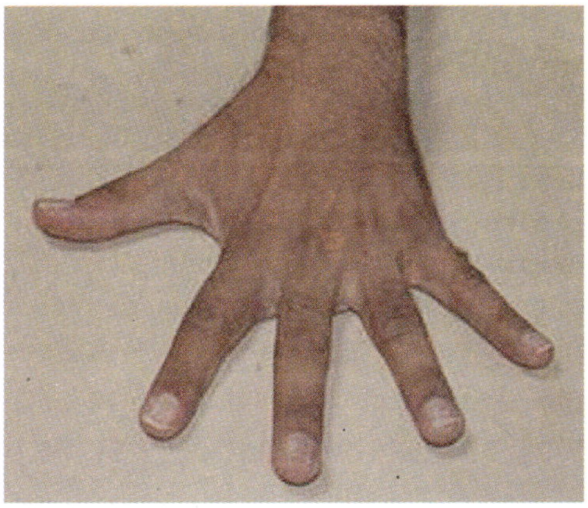

Fig. 6.117: Testing of dorsal interossei for grade 3

Grade 4 and 5 (Good and Normal)

Position of Patient: Sitting, forearm pronated, wrist, MCP, DIP and PIP at neutral.

Position of Examiner: Examiner stands at the side which is being tested and holds the wrist joint to maintain it in the neutral position and places fingers on the patient fingers to offer resistance.

Stabilization: Examiner stabilizes the wrist joint to maintain it at the neutral position. The fingers of other hand are placed on the ulnar and radial side of the patient's fingers to apply resistance.

Test: Examiner instructs the patient to "spread your fingers outwards".

Grade 4: If patient completes movement in the available range of motion against strong to moderate resistance.

Grade 5: If patient completes movement in the available range of motion against maximal resistance (Fig. 6.118).

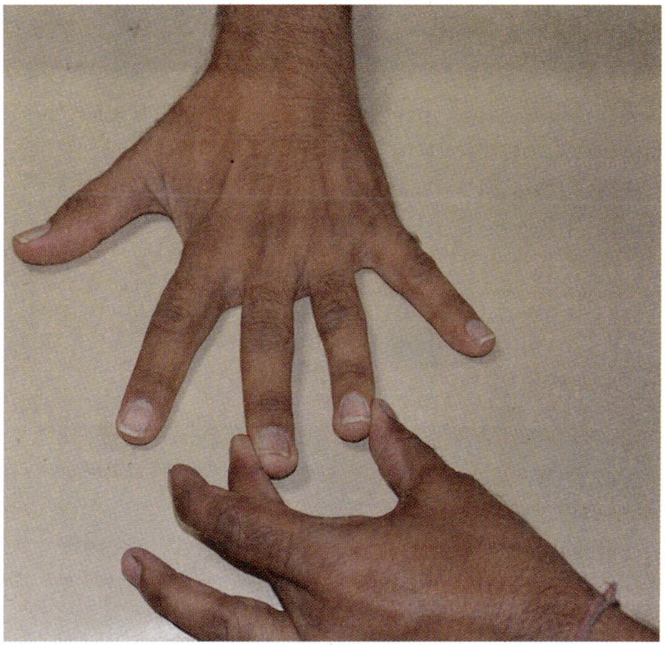

Fig. 6.118: Testing of dorsal interossei muscles for grade 4 and 5

Grade 1 (Flicker)

Position of Patient: Sitting, forearm pronated, wrist, MCP, DIP and PIP at neutral.

Position of Examiner: Examiner stands at the side which is being tested and places finger on the base of radial side of the index finger.

Stabilization: Examiner may stabilize the wrist joint to maintain it at the neutral position.

Test: Examiner instructs the patient to "try to spread your fingers outwards" at the same time the examiner palpates the dorsal interossei for contraction. If examiner finds contraction it is considered grade 1 (Fig. 6.119).

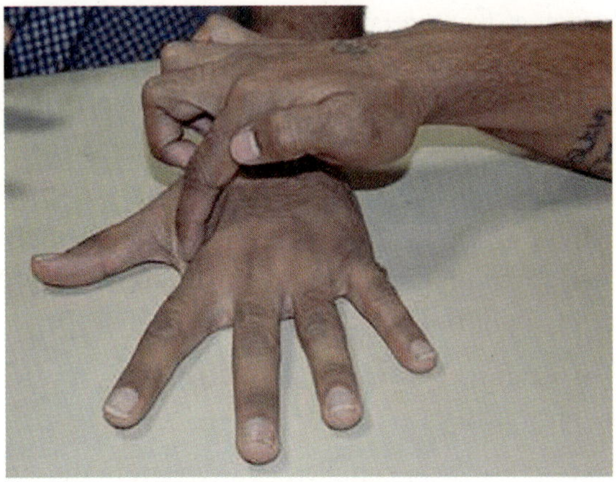

Fig. 6.119: Palpation of dorsal interossei for grade 1

Grade 2

Position of Patient: Sitting, forearm pronated, wrist, MCP, DIP and PIP at neutral.

Position of Examiner: Examiner stands at the side which is being tested and may hold the wrist joint to maintain it in the neutral position.

Stabilization: Examiner stabilizes the wrist joint to maintain it at the neutral position.

Test: Examiner instructs the patient to "spread your fingers outwards". If patient completes movement in the available range of motion it is considered grade 2 (Figs. 6.120a and b).

(a)

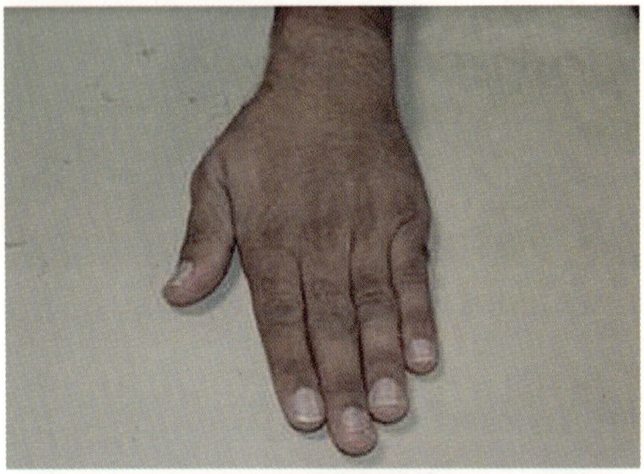

(b)

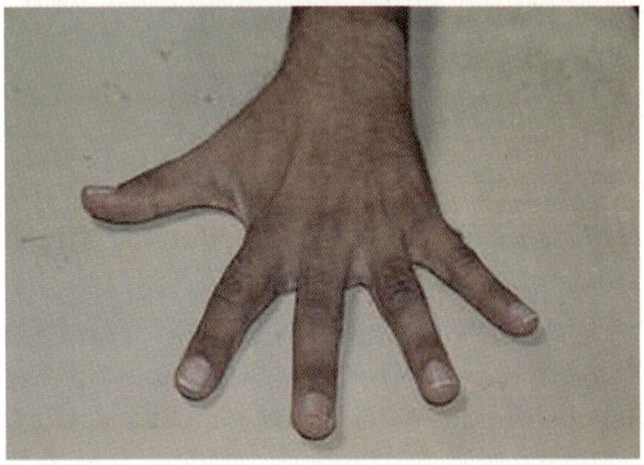

Figs. 6.120a and b: Testing of dorsal interossei for grade 2

Weakness: Loss of abduction of the metacarpophalangeal joints. **Klumpke's Paralysis** – Klumpke's paralysis is a form of paralysis involving the muscles of the forearm and hand, resulting from a brachial plexus injury in which the eighth cervical (C8) and first thoracic (T1) nerves are injured either before or after they have joined to form the lower trunk. The subsequent paralysis affects, principally, the intrinsic muscles of the hand (notably the interossei, thenar and hypothenar muscles) and the flexors of the wrist and fingers (notably flexor carpi ulnaris and ulnar half of the flexor digitorum profundus). Forearm pronators and wrist flexors may be involved, as may dilators of the iris and elevators of the eyelid (both of which may be seen in the case of associated Horner's syndrome). The classic presentation of Klumpke's palsy is the "claw hand" where the forearm is supinated and the wrist and fingers are flexed.

LUMBRICALS – METACARPOPHALANGEAL FLEXION

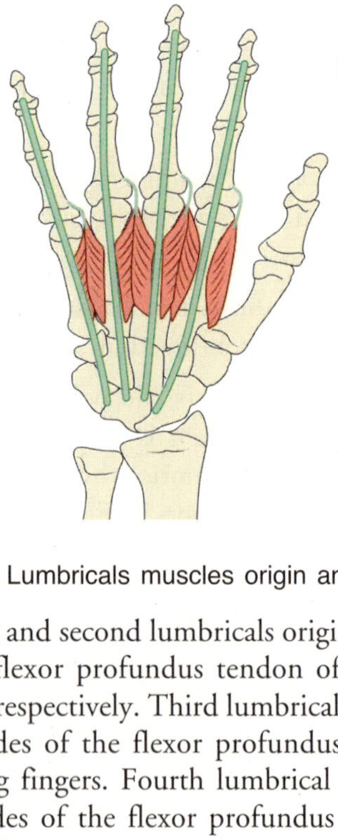

Fig. 6.121: Lumbricals muscles origin and insertion

Origin: First and second lumbricals originate from radial surface of the flexor profundus tendon of the index and middle fingers, respectively. Third lumbrical originates from the adjacent sides of the flexor profundus tendon of the middle and ring fingers. Fourth lumbrical originates from the adjacent sides of the flexor profundus tendons of the ring and little fingers.

Insertion: Lumbricals insert into the radial border of the extensor expansion on the dorsum of the respective digits.

Action: Lumbricals flex the metacarpophalangeal joints and extend the interphalangeal joints simultaneously.

Nerve Supply: First and second lumbricals: Median nerve, $C_{6, 7, 8}$ and T_1.

Third and fourth: Ulnar, $C_{7, 8}$ and T_1.

Grade 3 (Fair)

Position of Patient: Sitting, wrist at neural with no deviation, forearm supinated and supported on the table or couch. Metacarpophalangeal joints should be at neutral and interphalangeal joints are extended.

Position of Examiner: Examiner stands at the side which is being tested and holds the forearm at the distal end with one hand and metacarpal bones with other hand to prevent flexion, radial and ulnar deviations at the wrist joint.

Stabilization: Examiner instructs the patient to maintain the PIP joints in the neutral and forearm in the supinatied position.

Substitution: Flexor digitorum superficialis and profundus flexes the PIP and DIP which may contribute to the adduction of the MCP joints. To avoid substitution the PIP joints should be at neutral during the MCP flexion (Fig. 6.122).

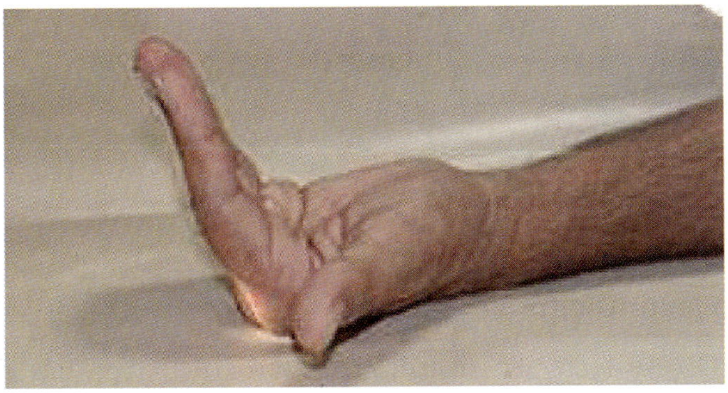

Fig. 6.122: Testing of lumbricals muscles for grade 3

Test: Patient is instructed to bend the knuckles (flexion of MCP joints) and straighten the fingers (extension of PIP and DIP joints) simultaneously. If patient is able to flex the metacarpophalangeal joints with extension of PIP and DIP simultaneously against the gravity in the available range of motion is considered grade 3.

Grade 4 and 5 (Good and Normal)

Position of Patient: Sitting, wrist at neural with no deviation, forearm supinated and supported on the table or couch. Metacarpophalangeal joints should be at neutral and interphalangeal joints are flexed.

Position of Examiner: Examiner stands at the side, which is being tested and holds the forearm at the distal end with one hand to prevent flexion, radial and ulnar deviations at the wrist joint and holds the proximal phalanges with other hand to apply resistance.

Substitution: Flexor digitorum superficialis and profundus flexes the PIP and DIP which may contribute to the adduction of the MCP joints. To avoid substitution the PIP joints should be at neutral during the MCP flexion (Figs. 6.123 and 6.124).

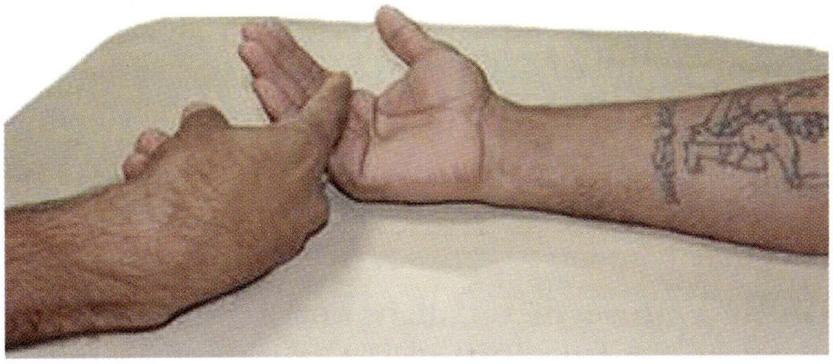

Fig. 6.123: Testing of lumbricals for grade 4 and 5 against finger resistance

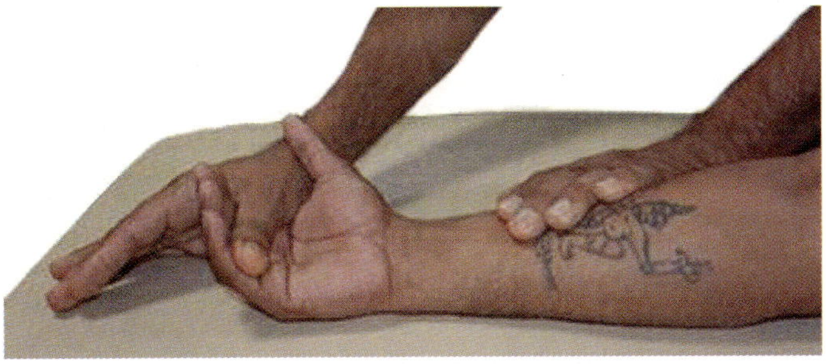

Fig. 6.124: Testing of lumbricals against resistance with thumb

Test: Patient is instructed to bend the knuckles (flexion of MCP joints) and straighten the fingers (extension of PIP and DIP joints) simultaneously.

Grade 4: If patient is able to flex the metacarpophalangeal joints with extension of the PIP and DIP simultaneously against strong to moderate resistance.

Grade 5: If patient is able to flex the metacarpophalangeal joints with extension of the PIP and DIP simultaneously against maximal resistance.

Grade 1

Position of Patient: Sitting, forearm in midprone position, supported on the table or couch. Metacarpophalangeal joints fully extended with IP and DIP flexion.

Position of Examiner: Examiner stands at the side which is being examined and grasps the forearm to prevent supination and pronation.

Stabilization: CMC and wrist joint.

Test: Examiner instructs the patient to try to bend the knuckles (flexion of MCP joints) and straighten the fingers (extension of PIP and DIP joints). Palpation of interossei and lumbricals is difficult, therefore, minimal flexion of metacarpal joints in the gravity eliminated position is considered grade 1.

Grade 2 (Poor)

Position of Patient: Sitting, forearm in midprone position, supported on the table or couch. Metacarpophalangeal joints fully extended with IP and DIP.

Position of Examiner: Examiner stands at the side which is being examined and grasps the forearm to prevent supination and pronation. There should not be any trick movements at the elbow joints also.

Stabilization: Examiner maintains the forearm in the midprone position.

Substitution: Flexor digitorum superficialis and profundus flexes the PIP and DIP which may contribute to the flexion of the MCP joints. To avoid substitution the PIP joints should be at neutral during the MCP flexion (Figs. 6.125a and b).

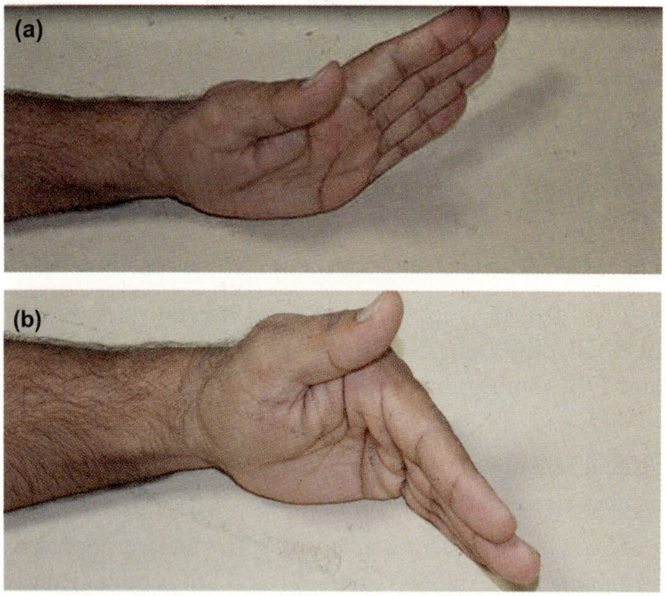

Figs. 6.125a and b: Testing of lumbricals for grade 2

Test: Examiner instructs the patient to try to bend the knuckles (flexion of MCP joints) and straighten the fingers (extension of PIP and DIP joints) simultaneously. If patient is able to flex the metacarpophalangeal joints with extension of the PIP and DIP simultaneously in the gravity eliminated position is considered grade 2.

Weakness: The weakness of fourth and fifth lumbricals and flexor digitorum profundus is represented by a **Claw Hand Deformity**: It is the deformity of hand which occurs due to injury to the ulnar nerve. The fourth and fifth lumbricals are innervated by the ulnar nerve. There is loss of flexion at the fourth and fifth metacarpophalangeal joints and loss of extension of the fourth and fifth interphalangeal joints. Paralysis of lumbricals is associated with paralysis of flexor digitorum profundus due to ulnar nerve injury results in hyperextension at the metacarpophalangeal joints and flexion at the PIP joints. This presentation gives a claw like appearance. The patients with claw hand can make a full fist but they extend their fingers at the MCP joints. Claw hand is also referred to Spinster's claw.

FLEXOR DIGITORUM SUPERFICIALIS – PROXIMAL INTERPHALANGEAL FLEXION

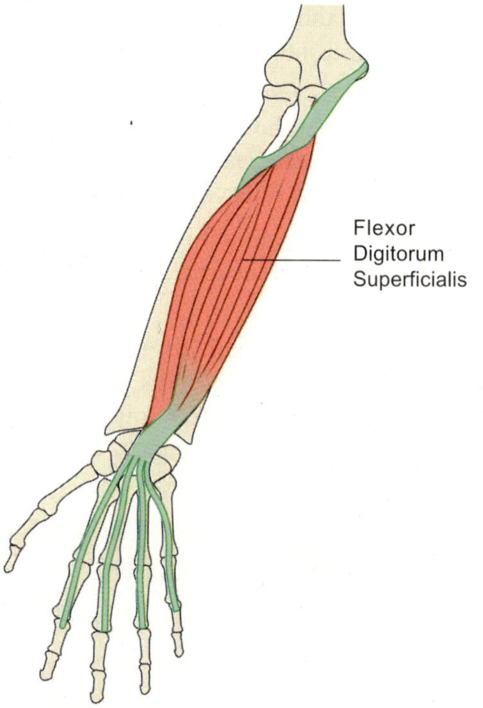

Fig. 6.126: Flexor digitorum superficialis origin and insertion

Flexor Digitorum Superficialis

Origin: Humeral head originates from common flexor tendon from the medial epicondyle of the humerus, ulnar collateral ligament of the elbow joint and deep antebrachial fascia. Ulnar head originates from medial side of the coronoid process and radial side originates from the oblique line of the radius.

Insertion: By four tendons into the sides of the middle phalanges of the second through fifth digits.

Action: Flexion of the proximal interphalangeal joints of the second through fifth digits, and assists in flexion of the metacarpophalangeal joints and in flexion of the wrist

Nerve Supply: Median, $C_{7,\,8}$ and T_1.

Grade 3 (Fair)

Position of Patient: Sitting, wrist at neural with no deviation, forearm supinated and supported on the table or couch. Metacarpophalangeal joints and interphalangeal joints should be at neutral.

Position of Examiner: Examiner stands at the side which is being tested and holds metacarpal bones and proximal phalanx with one hand.

Stabilization: Examiner stabilizes the forearm to prevent pronation and keeps the wrist joint at the neutral position.

The flexor digitorum profundus substitutes the action of flexor digitorum superficialis, which can be prevented by keeping the DIP joint in the extended position. The wrist joint should be maintained in the neutral position as the wrist extension produces tension in the long flexors that results in flexion of the PIP joint (Fig. 6.127).

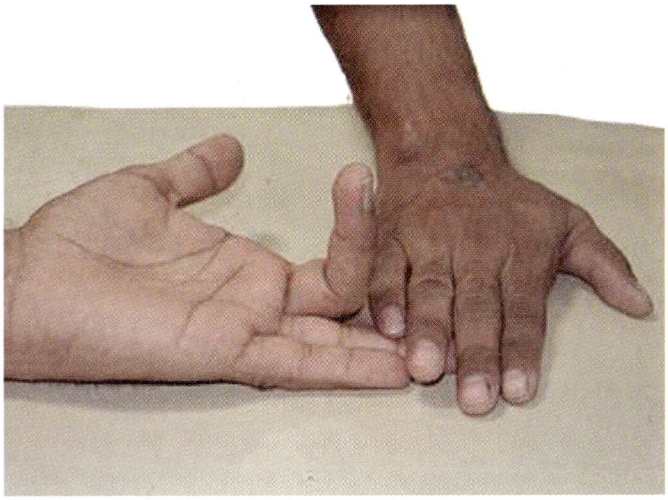

Fig. 6.127: Testing of flexor digitorum superficialis muscle for grade 3

Test: Examiner instructs the patient to bend your proximal interphalangeal joint. All the tendons of flexor digitorum superficialis are tested separately. It is important to demonstrate the movement of PIP joint as some patients find it difficult to understand. If patient is able to flex proximal the interphalangeal joint against the gravity is considered grade 2.

Grade 4 and 5 (Good and Normal)

Position of Patient: Sitting, wrist at neural with no deviation, forearm supinated and supported on the table or couch. Metacarpophalangeal joints and interphalangeal joints should be at neutral.

Position of Examiner: Examiner stands at the side which is being tested and holds metacarpal bones with one hand to stabilize MCP joints and places other hand on the middle phalanx to apply resistance.

Stabilization: Examiner stabilizes the forearm to prevent pronation and keeps the wrist joint at the neutral position.

The flexor digitorum profundus substitutes the action of flexor digitorum superficialis, which can be prevented by keeping the DIP joint in the extended position. The wrist joint should be maintained in the neutral position as the wrist extension produces tension in the long flexors that results in flexion of the PIP joint (Fig. 6.128).

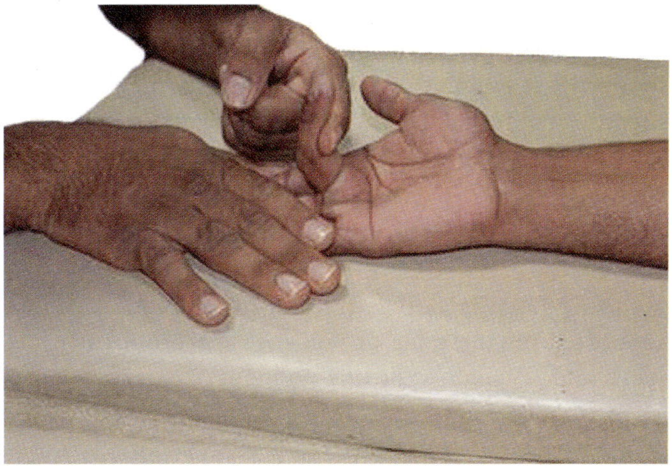

Fig. 6.128: Testing of flexor digitorum superficialis for grade 4 and 5

Test: Examiner instructs the patient to bend your proximal interphalangeal joint. Each PIP joint is flexed separately to test all the tendons of flexor digitorum superficialis. It is important to demonstrate the movements of PIP joint as some patients find it difficult to understand.

Grade 4: If patient is able to flex the interphalangeal joint against mild resistance.

Grade 5: If patient is able to flex the interphalangeal joint against maximal level of resistance.

Grade 1 (Trace)

Position of Patient: Sitting, forearm supinated, supported on the table or couch. Metacarpophalangeal joints, IP and DIP at neutral.

Position of Examiner: Examiner stands at the side which is being examined and places tip of index finger on the palmar surface of the wrist between the palmaris longus and the flexor carpi ulnaris.

Stabilization: Examiner stabilizes the forearm to prevent pronation and keeps the wrist joint at the neutral position (Fig. 6.129).

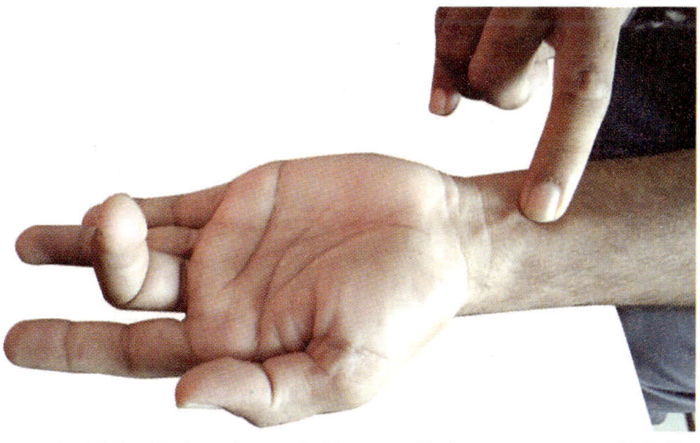

Fig. 6.129: Palpation of flexor digitorum superficialis muscle for grade 1

Test: Examiner instructs the patient to try to bend the middle finger. Patient is instructed to flex each PIP joint separately. If examiner feels contraction on the tendon of superficialis on palmar surface of the wrist between the palmaris longus and the flexor carpi ulnaris is considered grade 1.

Grade 2 (Fair)

Position of Patient: Sitting, forearm in midprone position, supported on the table or couch. Metacarpophalangeal joints and IP joints at neutral position.

Position of Examiner: Examiner stands at the side which is being tested and grasps metacarpal and proximal phalanges to prevent flexion at the metacarpophalangeal joints.

Stabilization: Examiner stabilizes the forearm to prevent pronation and keeps the wrist joint at the neutral position.

The flexor digitorum profundus substitutes the action of flexor digitorum superficialis, which can be prevented by keeping the DIP joint in the extended position. The wrist joint should be maintained in the neutral position as the wrist extension produces tension in the long flexors that results in flexion of the PIP joint (Fig. 6.130).

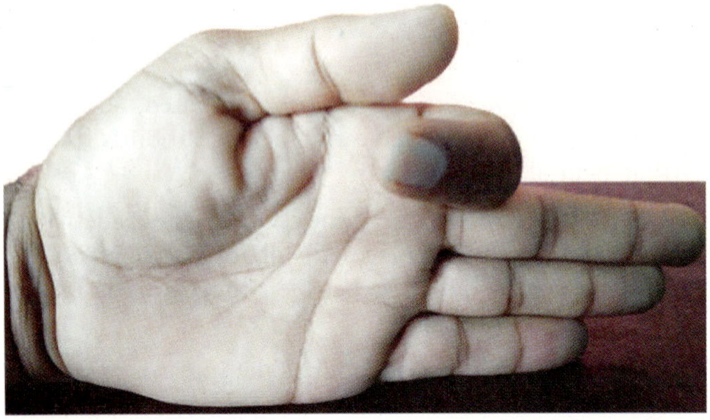

Fig. 6.130: Testing of flexor digitorum superficialis for grade 2

Test: Examiner instructs the patient to try to bend your proximal interphalangeal joint. Each PIP joint is tested separately for all the tendons of flexor digitorum superficialis. If patient is able to flex the proximal interphalangeal joint in the gravity eliminated position is considered grade 2.

Weakness: Loss of flexion of the proximal interphalangeal joints from second to fifth is the common consequence following weakness of flexor digitorum superficialis. **Swan Neck Deformity**–Weakness of flexor digitorum superficialis leads to muscular imbalance, the antagonistic extensors, pull the PIP joint into the hyperextension. The hyperextension at the PIP joint produces tension in the flexor digitorum profundus which pulls the DIP joint into the flexion. The hyperextension at the PIP and flexion at the DIP predisposes to swan neck deformity. It is very common in the rheumatoid arthritis, where the flexor digitorum superficialis gets ruptured or torned in the process of inflammation.

FLEXOR DIGITORUM PROFUNDUS – DISTAL INTERPHALANGEAL JOINT FLEXION

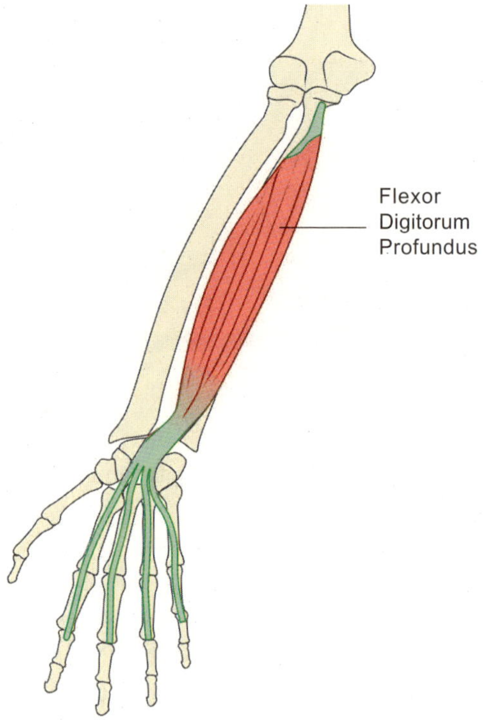

Fig. 6.131: Flexor digitorum profundus origin and insertion

Flexor Digitorum Profundus

Origin: Anterior and medial surface of the proximal ¾th of the ulna, interosseous membrane and deep antebrachial fascia.

Insertion: By four tendon into the bases of the distal phalanges, anterior surface.

Action: Flexion of the distal interphalangeal joints of the index, middle, ring, and little fingers and assists in flexion of the proximal interphalangeal and metacarpophalangeal joints. May assist in flexion of the wrist.

Nerve Supply: First and second: Median, $C_{7,\,8}$ and T_1. Third and fourth: Ulnar, C_7, $_8$, T.

Grade 3 (Fair)

Position of Patient: Sitting, wrist at neural with no deviation, forearm supinated and supported on the table or couch.

Metacarpophalangeal, proximal and distal interphalangeal joints should be at neutral.

Position of Examiner: Examiner stands at the side which is being tested and holds metacarpal bones, proximal and middle phalanges with one hand.

Stabilization: Examiner stabilizes the forearm to prevent pronation and keeps the wrist and metacarpal joints at the neutral position.

Substitution: The patient may extend the wrist joint to substitute the action of flexor digitorum profundus. To avoid substitution, wrist joint should be in a neutral position during the testing of FDP (Fig. 6.132).

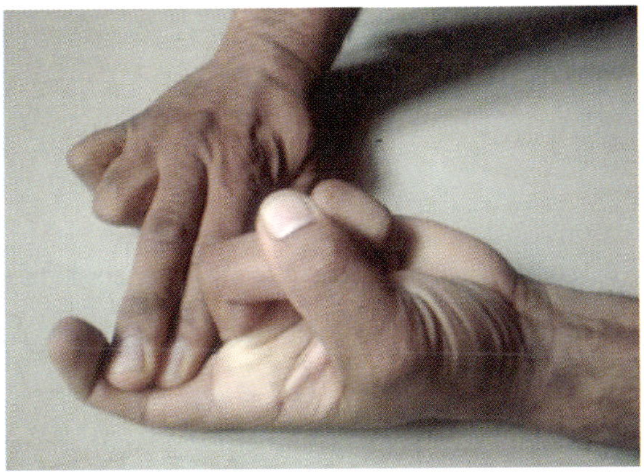

Fig. 6.132: Testing of flexor digitorum profundus for grade 3

Test: Examiner instructs the patient to bend your distal interphalangeal joint. Each DIP joint is tested separately for all the tendons of flexor digitorum superficialis. It is important to demonstrate the movement of DIP joint as some patients find it difficult to understand. If patient is able to flex the distal interphalangeal joint in the available range against the gravity is considered grade 3.

Grade 4 and 5 (Good and Normal)

Position of Patient: Sitting, wrist at neural with no deviation, forearm supinated and supported on the table or couch. Metacarpophalangeal joints, proximal and distal interphalangeal joints should be at neutral.

Position of Examiner: Examiner stands at the side which is being tested and holds metacarpal bones, proximal and distal phalanges with one hand to stabilize them and prevent flexion at PIP and places other hand on the distal phalanx to apply resistance.

Stabilization: Examiner stabilizes the forearm to prevent pronation and keeps the wrist and metacarpal joints at the neutral position.

Substitution: The patient may extend the wrist joint to substitute the action of flexor digitorum profundus. To avoid substitution, wrist joint should be in a neutral position during the testing of FDP (Fig. 6.133).

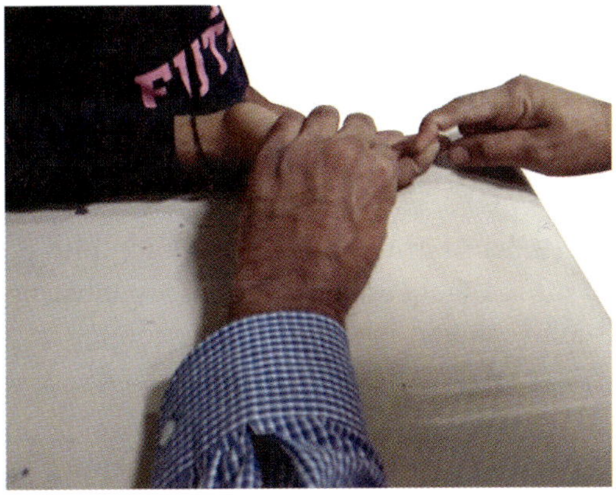

Fig. 6.133: Testing of flexor digitorum profundus muscle for grade 4 and 5

Test: Examiner instructs the patient to bend your distal interphalangeal joint. Each DIP joint is flexed separately to test all the tendons of flexor digitorum profundus. It is important to demonstrate the movements of DIP joint as some patients find it difficult to understand.

Grade 4: If patient is able to flex the distal interphalangeal joint in the available range of motion against some resistance.

Grade 5: If patient is able to flex the distal interphalangeal joint in the available range of motion against maximal level of resistance.

Grade 1 (Trace)

Position of Patient: Sitting, forearm in midprone position, supported on the table or couch. Metacarpophalangeal joints, IP and DIP at neutral.

Position of Examiner: Examiner stands at the side which is being tested and places tip of index finger on the palmar surface of the wrist medial to the flexor digitorum superficialis (Fig. 6.134).

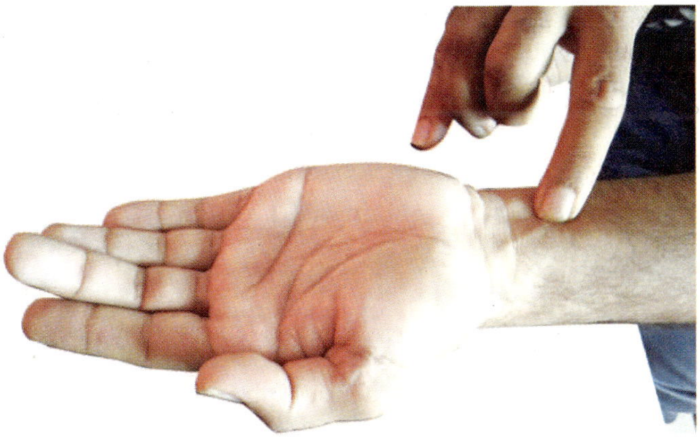

Fig. 6.134: Palpation of flexor digitorum profundus for grade 1

Test: Examiner instructs the patient to try to bend the distal interphalangeal joint. Patient is instructed to flex each PIP joint separately for all the tendons of flexor digitorum profundus. If examiner feels contraction on the tendon of profundus on palmar surface of the wrist to the ulnar side is considered grade 1.

Grade 2 (Fair)

Position of Patient: Sitting, forearm in midprone position, supported on the table or couch. Metacarpophalangeal, IP and DIP joints should be at neutral position.

Position of Examiner: Examiner stands at the side which is being tested and grasps metacarpal, proximal and middle phalanx to prevent flexion at the PIP joint.

Stabilization: Examiner stabilizes the forearm to prevent pronation and keeps the wrist and metacarpal joints at the neutral position.

Substitution: The patient may extend the wrist joint to substitute the action of flexor digitorum profundus. To avoid substitution, wrist joint should be in a neutral position during the testing of FDP (Fig. 6.135).

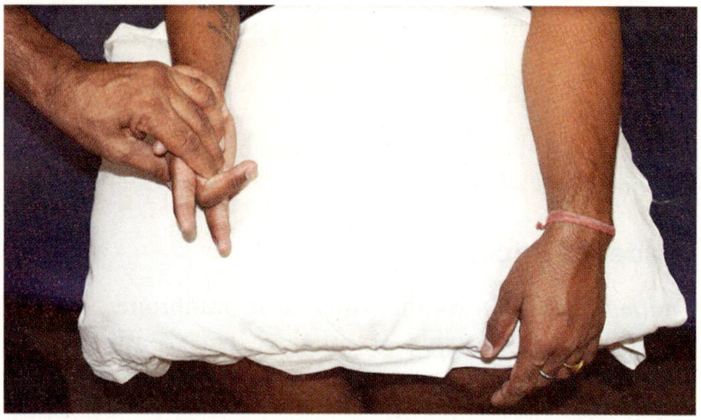

Fig. 6.135: Testing of flexor digitorum profundus muscle for grade 2

Test: Examiner instructs the patient to try to bend your distal interphalangeal joint. Each DIP joint is flexed separately for all the tendons of flexor digitorum profundus. It is important to demonstrate the movement of PIP joint as some patients find it difficult to understand. If patient is able to flex the distal interphalangeal joint in the available range in the gravity eliminated position is considered grade 2.

Weakness: Weakness of flexor digitorum profundus allows antagonistic muscles to pull the distal interphalangeal joint into the hyperextension. The hyperextension at the DIP forces the flexor digitorum to pull the PIP joint into the flexion. Hence, weakness of flexor digitorum produces hyperextension at the DIP and flexion at the PIP joint. Such presentation is known as boutonnier deformity.

EXTENSOR DIGITORUM, EXTENSOR INDICIS, EXTENSOR DIGITI MINIMI – 2nd to 5th METACARPOPHALANGEAL JOINT EXTENSION

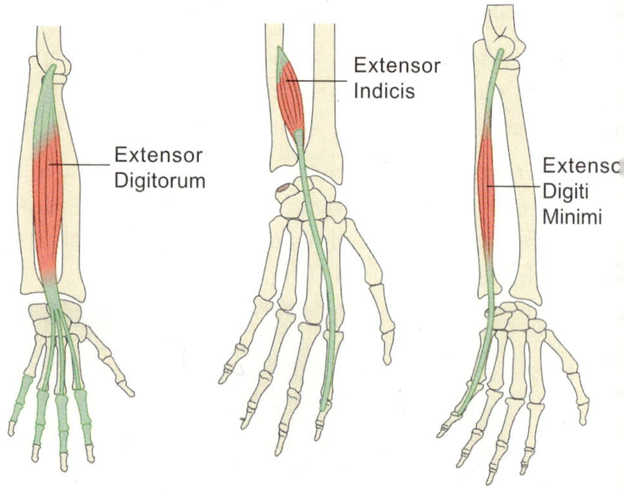

Figs. 6.136a to c: Extensor digitorum, extensor indicis and extensor digiti minimi–origin and insertion

Extensor Digitorum

Origin: Lateral epicondyle of humerus by common tendon and deep antebrachial fascia.

Insertion: By four tendons, each penetrating a membranous expansion on the dorsum of the second through fifth digits and dividing over the proximal phalanx into a medial and two lateral bands. The medial band inserts into the base of the middle phalanx; the lateral band reunite over the middle phalanx and inserts into the base of the distal phalanx.

Action: Extension of the metacarpophalangeal joints. Assist in extension of interphalangeal joints in association with lumbricals and interossei. Also assist in abduction of the index, ring and little fingers and in extension and abduction of the wrist.

Nerve Supply: Radial, $C_{6, 7, 8}$.

Extensor Indicis

Origin: Posterior or dorsal surface of the ulna below origin of extensor pollicis longus.

Insertion: Extensor indicis inserts into extensor expansion of the index finger with the extensor digitorum longus tendon.

Action: Extension of the metacarpophalangeal joint. Extension of the interphalangeal joints of the index finger in association with the lumbricals and interossei.

Nerve Supply: Radial, $C_{6, 7, 8}$.

Extensor Digiti Minimi

Origin: Common extensor tendon from lateral epicondyle of humerus.

Insertion: Extension expansion of the little finger with he extensor digitorum tendon.

Action: Extension of the metacarpophalangeal joint. Extension of the interphalangeal joints of the little finger n association with the lumbricals and interossei. Assist in bduction of the little finger.

Nerve Supply: Radial, $C_{6,\,7,\,8}$.

Grade 3 (Fair)

Position of Patient: Sitting, wrist at neural with no deviation, orearm pronated and supported on the table or couch. Metacarpophalangeal, proximal and distal interphalangeal oints should be flexed.

Position of Examiner: Examiner stands at the side which s being tested and holds metacarpal to stabilize them and prevent wrist extension.

Stabilization: Examiner ensures forearm pronation, wrist, PIP and DIP joint at neutral position.

Substitution: Wrist flexion may produce IP extension hrough a tenodesis action (Figs. 6.137 and 6.138).

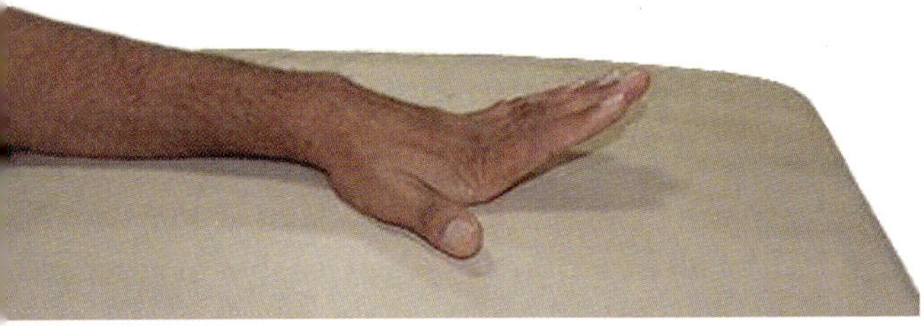

Fig. 6.137: Testing of extensor digitorum, extensor indicis and extensor digiti minimi for grade 3

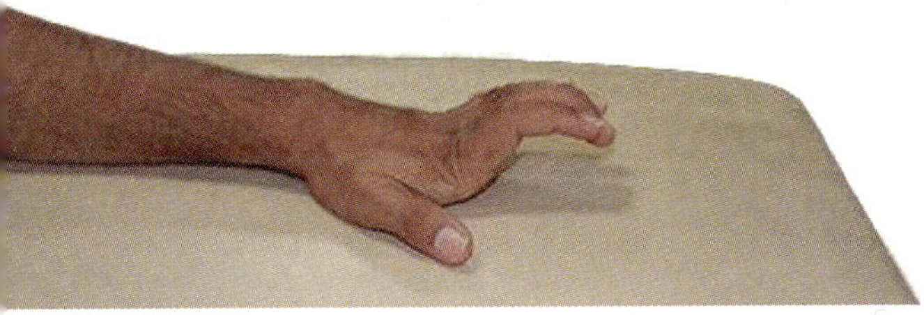

Fig. 6.138: Testing of extensor digitorum, extensor indicis and extensor digiti minimi for grade 3 with slight flexion of PIP and DIP to eliminate tension in the FDS and FDP as it may imit the terminal of the MCP joints

Test: Examiner instructs the patient to bend your knuckles back. Each MCP joint is tested separately. It is mportant to demonstrate the movement of MCP joint as some patients find it difficult to do. If patient is able to extend the MCP joint in the available range against the gravity is considered grade 3.

Grade 4 and 5 (Good and Normal)

Position of Patient: Sitting, wrist at neural with no deviation, forearm pronated and supported on the table or couch. Metacarpophalangeal joints, proximal and distal interphalangeal joints should be in flexion. A towel roll is placed under the metacarpal bones to allow flexion at MCP, PIP and DIP.

Position of Examiner: Examiner stands at the side which is being tested and holds metacarpal bones to stabilize them and prevent extension at the wrist joint. Examiner places other hand on the proximal phalanx of the finger which is being tested to apply resistance.

Stabilization: Examiner ensures forearm pronation, wrist PIP and DIP joint at neutral position.

Substitution: Wrist flexion may produce IP extension through a tenodesis action (Figs. 6.139 to 6.141).

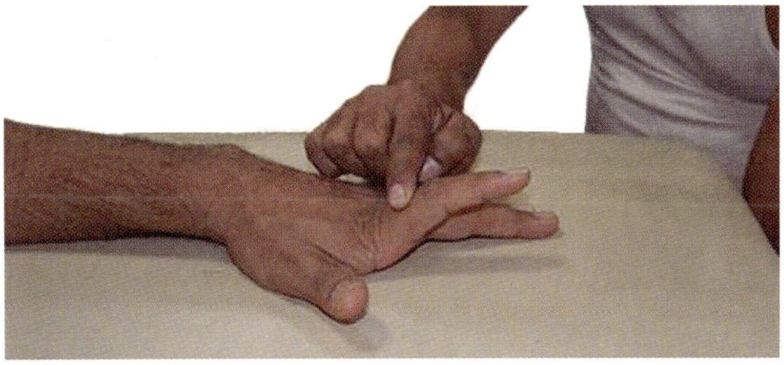

Fig. 6.139: Testing of extensor indicis for grade 4 and 5

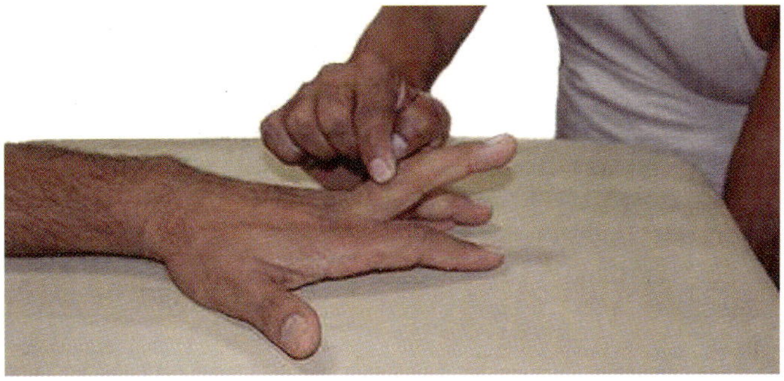

Fig. 6.140: Testing of extensor digitorum, extensor indicis and extensor digiti minimi for grade 4 and 5

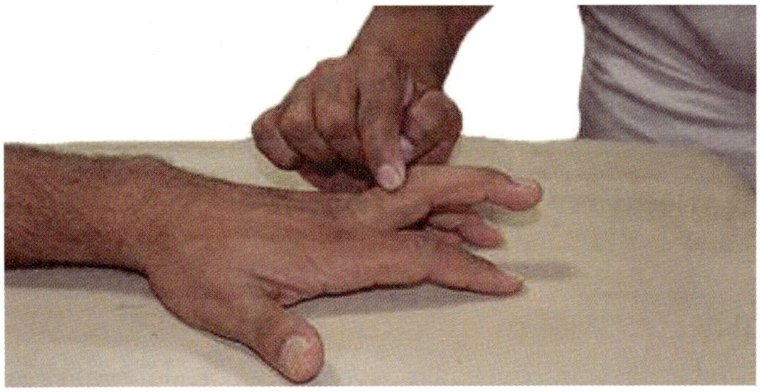

Fig. 6.141: Testing of extensor digiti minimi for grade 4 and 5

Test: Examiner instructs the patient to bend the knuckles back. Each MCP joint is extended separately to test all the extensors. It is important to demonstrate the movements of MCP joint as some patients find it difficult to do it. PIP and DIP joint may be kept slightly flexed to eliminate tension in the FDS and FDF as it may limit extension at MCP.

Grade 4: If patient is able to extend the MCP joint against minimum resistance in the available range of motion.

Grade 5: If patient is able to extend the MCP joint against maximal level of resistance in the available range of motion against maximal level of resistance.

Grade 1 (Trace)

Position of Patient: Sitting, forearm pronated and supported on the table or couch. Metacarpophalangeal joints, IP and DIP may be in the flexion.

Position of Examiner: Examiner stands at the side which is being tested and places tip of index finger on the dorsum surface of mid forearm (Fig. 6.142).

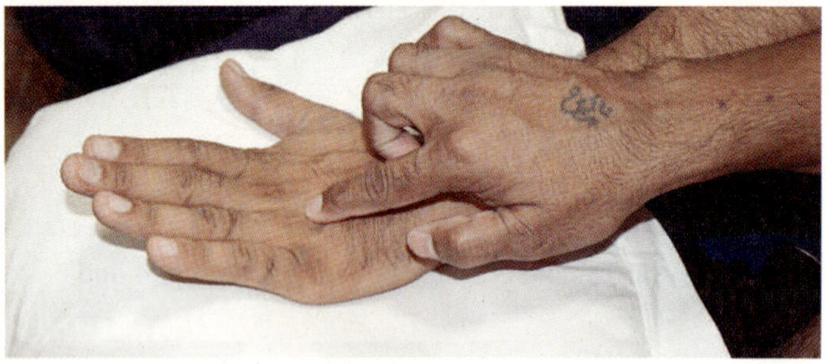

Fig. 6.142: Palpation of extensor digitorum

Test: Examiner instructs the patient to try to bend metacarpophalangeal joint back. Patient is instructed to try to extend each MCP joint separately to test all the extensors. If examiner feels contraction on the dorsum of mid forearm side on respective extensor is considered grade 1.

Grade 2 (Fair)

Position of Patient: Sitting, forearm in midprone position, supported on the table or couch. Metacarpophalangeal, IP and DIP joints should be in the flexion.

Position of Examiner: Examiner stands at the side which is being tested and may grasp metacarpal bones to stabilize them.

Stabilization: Examiner instructs the patient to maintain the wrist, PIP and DIP joints in the neutral position.

Substitution: Wrist flexion may produce IP extension through a tenodesis action (Figs. 6.143 to 6.145).

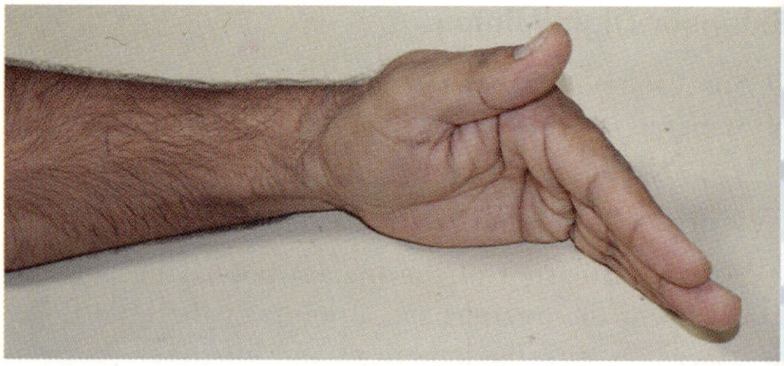

Fig. 6.143: Testing of extensor digitorum, extensor indicis anc extensor digiti minimi for grade 2, starting position

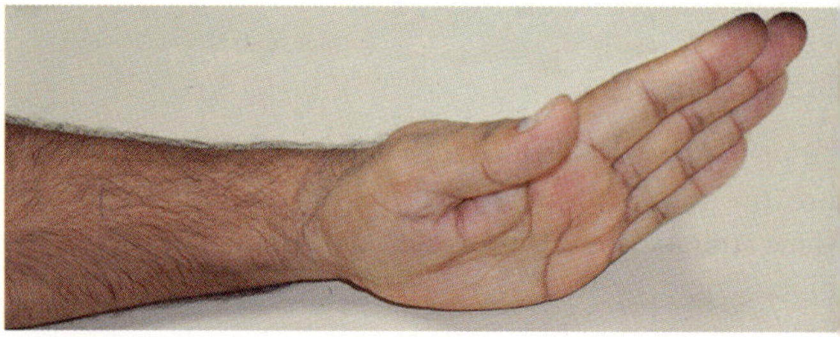

Fig. 6.144: Testing of extensor digitorum, extensor indicis an extensor digiti minimi for grade 2 with PIP and DIP neutral

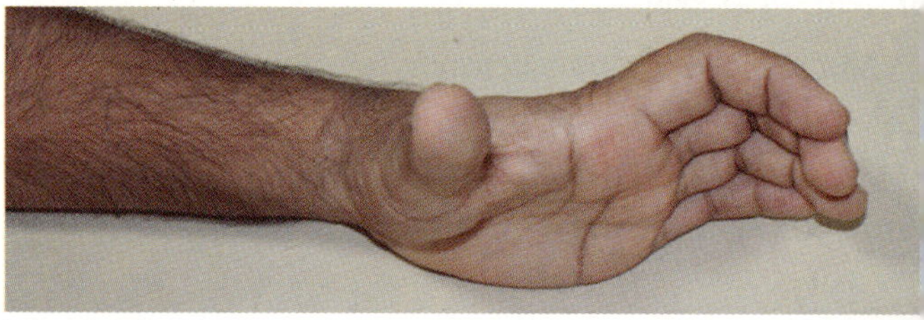

Fig. 6.145: Testing of extensor digitorum, extensor indicis anc extensor digiti minimi for grade 2 with PIP and DIP flexion

Test: Examiner instructs the patient to bend the knuckles back in the available range. Each MCP joint is extended separately to test all the extensors. It is important t demonstrate the movement of MCP joint as some patient find it difficult to do it. If patient is able to extend th metacarpophalangeal joint in the available range in th gravity eliminated position is considered grade 2.

PALMARIS LONGUS AND PALMARIS BREVIS–WRIST FLEXION AND TENSING PALMAR FASCIA

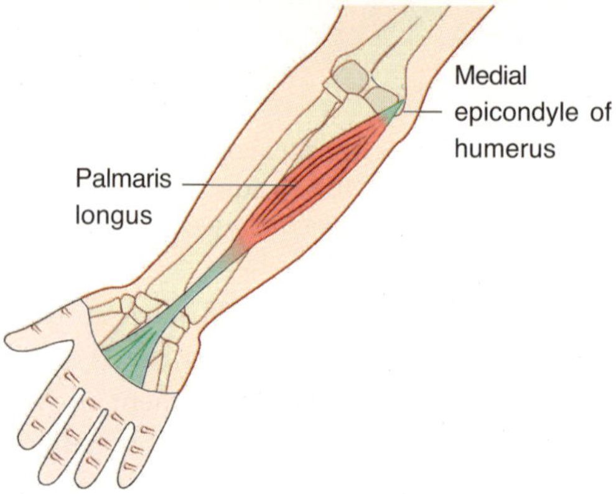

Fig. 6.146: Palmaris longus and brevis

Origin: Palmaris longus originates from the common flexor tendon at the medial epicondyle of the humerus and the deep antebrachial fascia.

Insertion: Palmaris longus inserts on the flexor retinaculum and palmar aponeurosis.

Action: Increase tension in the palmar fascia. Flexion of the wrist and assists in elbow flexion.

Nerve Supply: Median Nerve, $C_{6, 7, 8,}$ and T_1.

Palmaris Brevis

Origin: Palmaris brevis originates from the ulnar border of the palmar aponeurosis and palmar surface of the flexor retanaculum.

Insertion: Palmaris brevis inserts on the skin on the ulnar border of the flexor retanaculum.

Action: Corrugates the skin on the ulnar side of the hand.

Nerve Supply: Ulnar Nerve, $C_{7, 8,}$ T_1.

Grade 3 (Fair)

Position of Patient: Sitting, with the forearm supinated and wrist at neutral position. No ulnar or radial deviation.

Position of Examiner: Examiner stands or sits comfortably at the side of the patient which is being tested and grasps the forearm to stabilize it and prevent pronation.

Stabilization: Examiner grasps the distal forearm to prevent pronation of the forearm and deviations at the wrist.

Test: Examiner instructs the patient to tense the forearm and flex the wrist joint. If patient can corrugate the skin on ulnar side of the hand with wrist flexion it is considered grade 3 (Fig. 6.147).

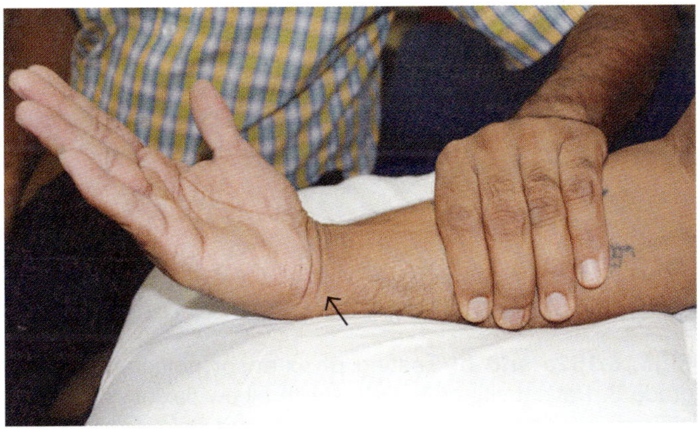

Fig. 6.147: Testing of palmaris longus and brevis

Grade 4 and 5 (Good and Normal)

Position of Patient: Supine, with the forearm supinated and wrist at neutral position. No ulnar or radial deviation.

Position of Examiner: Examiner stands at the side of the patient which is being tested and grasps the forearm to stabilize it and prevent pronation.

Stabilization: Examiner grasps the distal forearm to prevent pronation of the forearm and deviations at the wrist.

Test: Examiner instructs the patient to tense the forearm and flex the wrist joint.

Grade 4: If patient can corrugate the skin on ulnar side of the hand with wrist flexion against strong to moderate resistance.

Grade 4: If patient can corrugate the skin on ulnar side of the hand with wrist flexion against strong to moderate resistance (Fig. 6.148).

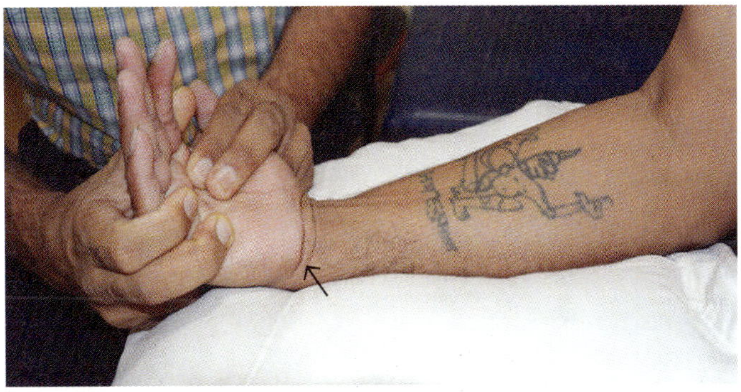

Fig. 6.148: Testing of palmaris longus and brevis

Grade 2 (Poor)

Position of Patient: Sitting, with the forearm in midprone and wrist at neutral position. No ulnar or radial deviation.

Position of Examiner: Examiner stands or sits at the side of the patient which is being tested and grasps the forearm to stabilize it and prevent supination and pronation.

Stabilization: Examiner grasps the distal forearm to prevent pronation of the forearm and deviations at the wrist.

Test: Examiner instructs the patient to tense the forearm and flex the wrist joint. If patient can corrugate the skin on ulnar side of the hand with wrist flexion it is considered grade 3 (Fig. 6.149).

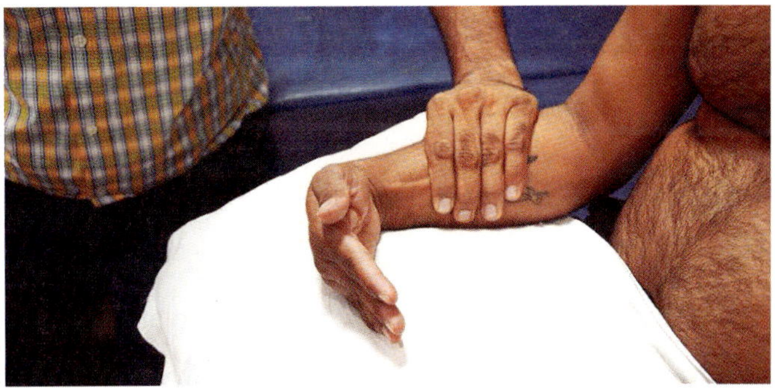

Fig. 6.149: Testing of palmaris longus and brevis

Grade 1 (Flicker)

Position of Patient: Sitting, with the forearm in midprone and wrist at neutral position. No ulnar or radial deviation.

Position of Examiner: Examiner stands or sits at the side of the patient which is being tested and grasps the forearm to stabilize it and prevent supination and pronation.

Stabilization: Examiner grasps the distal forearm to prevent pronation of the forearm and deviations at the wrist.

Test: Examiner instructs the patient to try to tense the forearm and flex the wrist joint. If examiner observes the tension in the skin of ulnar side of the hand is considered grade 1 (Fig. 6.150).

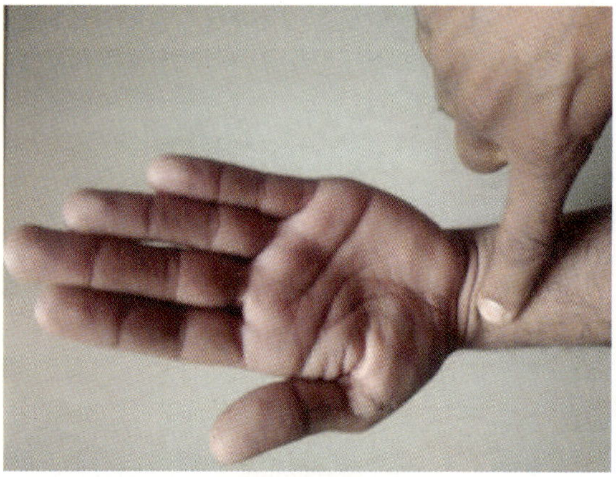

Fig. 6.150

EXTENSOR POLLICIS BREVIS – FIRST METACARPOPHALANGEAL JOINT EXTENSION

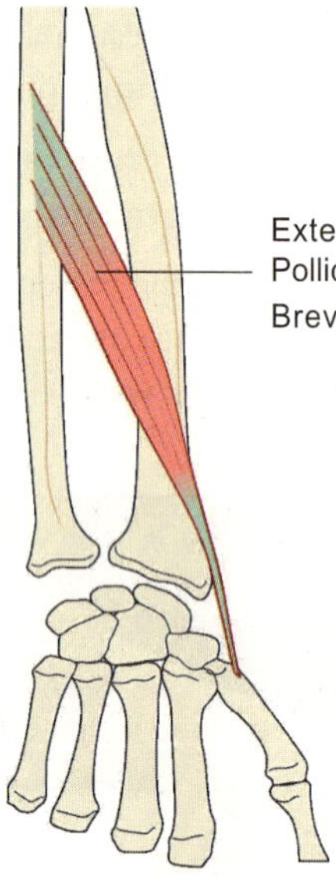

Fig. 6.151: Extensor pollicis brevis muscle origin and insertion

Origin: Extensor pollicis brevis originates from posterior surface of the radius adjacent to the interosseous membrane.

Insertion: Dorsolateral surface of the base of proximal phalanx of thumb.

Action: Extension of the metacarpophalangeal joint of the thumb and extension and abduction of the carpometacarpal joint, assists in radial deviation of the wrist.

Nerve Supply: Radial nerve, $C_{6, 7, 8}$.

Grade 3

Position of Patient: Sitting on stool with elbow flexion, forearm in midprone, wrist, carpometacarpal and interphalangeal joints at neutral. Metacarpophalangeal joint of the thumb in the abduction and flexion.

Position of Examiner: Examiner stands at the side of the patient which is being tested.

Stabilization: Examiner grasps the first metacarpal bone with one hand and stabilizes it to prevent movement at the carpometacarpal joint and forearm.

Substitution: The muscles of thenar eminence such as abductor pollicis brevis, flexor pollicis brevis, and adductor pollicis can extend metacarpophalangeal joint of the thumb (Figs. 6.152a and b).

(a)

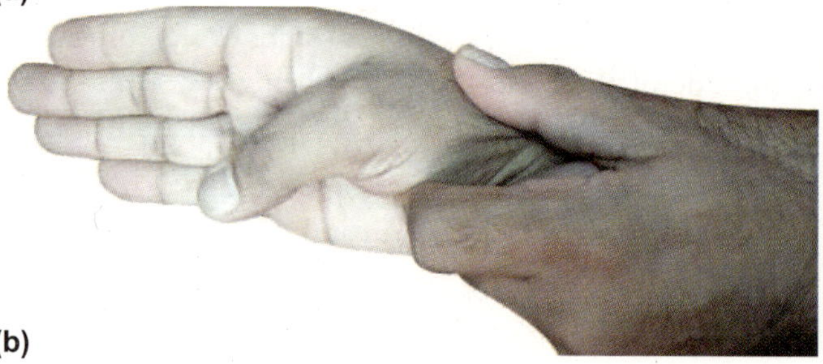

(b)

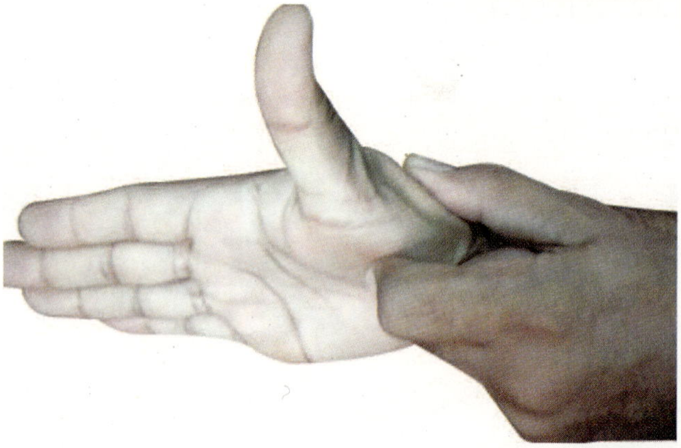

Figs. 6.152a and b: Testing of extensor pollicis brevis for grade 3. Patient sits on the stool with elbow flexion, forearm in midprone, wrist, carpometacarpal and interphalangeal joints at neutral. Metacarpophalangeal joint of the thumb in the abduction and flexion. Examiner stands at the side of the patient which is being tested. Examiner grasps the first metacarpal bone with one hand and stabilizes it to prevent movement at the carpometacarpal joint and forearm. If patient completes movement in the available range of motion it is considered grade 3

Test: Examiner asks the patient to extend the netacarpophalangeal joint. Examiner may demonstrate the novement to the patient if patient finds difficulty in performing the movement. If patient completes movement n the available range of motion it is considered grade 3.

Grade 4 and 5

Position of Patient: Sitting on stool with elbow flexion, orearm in midprone, wrist, carpometacarpal and nterphalangeal joints at neutral. Metacarpophalangeal joint of the thumb in the abduction and flexion.

Position of Examiner: Examiner stands at the side of the patient which is being tested and places thumb on the lorsum of proximal phalanx to apply resistane.

Stabilization: Examiner grasps the first metacarpal bone with one hand to prevent movement at the carpometacarpal joint and also grasps the proximal phalanx with the other hand for the resistance.

Substitution: The muscles of thenar eminence such as abductor pollicis brevis, flexor pollicis brevis, and adductor pollicis can extend metacarpophalangeal joint of the thumb Fig. 6.153).

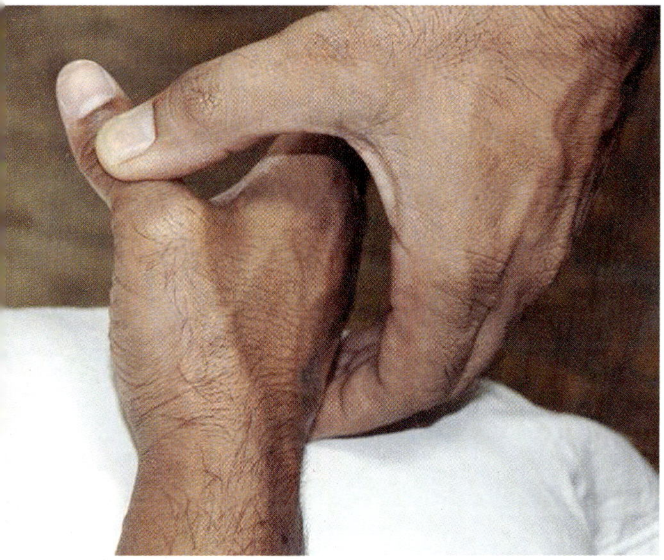

Fig. 6.153: Testing of extensor pollicis brevis for grade 4 and 5. Patient sits on the stool with elbow flexion, forearm in midprone, wrist, carpometacarpal and interphalangeal joints at neutral. Metacarpophalangeal joint of the thumb in the abduction and flexion. Examiner stands at the side of the patient which is being tested. Examiner grasps the first metacarpal bone with one hand to prevent movement at the carpometacarpal joint and also grasps the proximal phalanx with the other hand for the resistance. If patient completes movement in the available range of motion against the resistance it is considered grade 4 and 5

Test: Examiner asks the patient to extend the first netacarpophalangeal joint against the resistance.

Grade 4: If patient completes range of motion against strong to moderate resistance.

Grade 5: If patient completes movement in the available range of motion against the maximal resistance.

Grade 2

Position of Patient: Sitting on stool with elbow flexion, forearm in supination, wrist, carpometacarpal and interphalangeal joints at neutral. Metacarpophalangeal joint of the thumb in the adduction and flexion.

Position of Examiner: Examiner stands at the side of the patient which is being tested.

Stabilization: Examiner grasps the first metacarpal bone with one hand to stabilize it to prevent movement at the carpometacarpal joint and forearm.

Substitution: The muscles of thenar eminence such as abductor pollicis brevis, flexor pollicis brevis, and adductor pollicis can extend metacarpophalangeal joint of the thumb. Examiner should distinguish the action of extensor pollicis brevis from the thenar muscles (Figs. 6.154a and b).

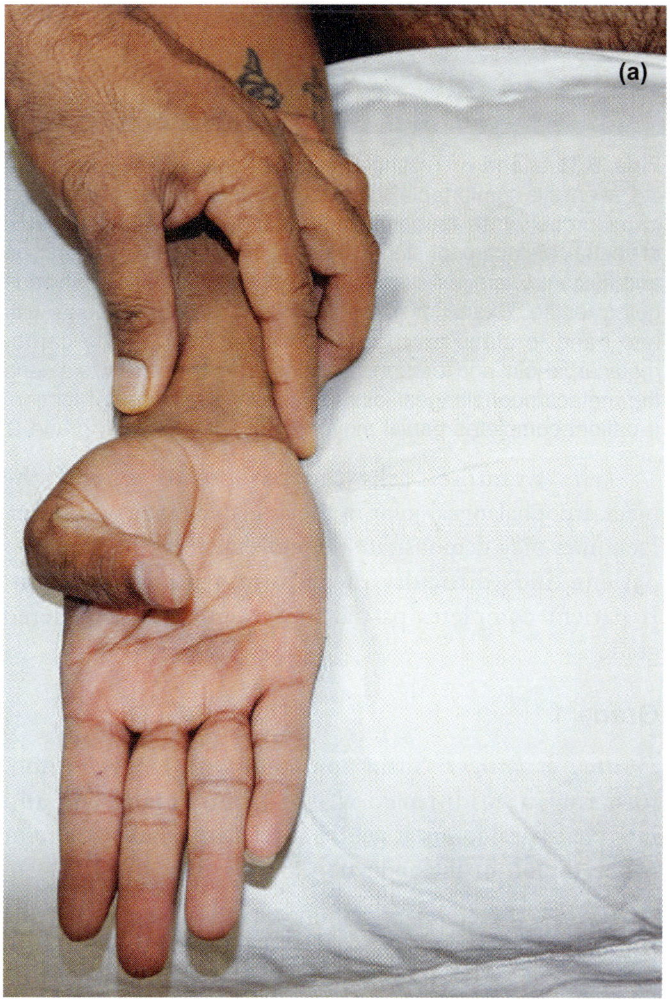

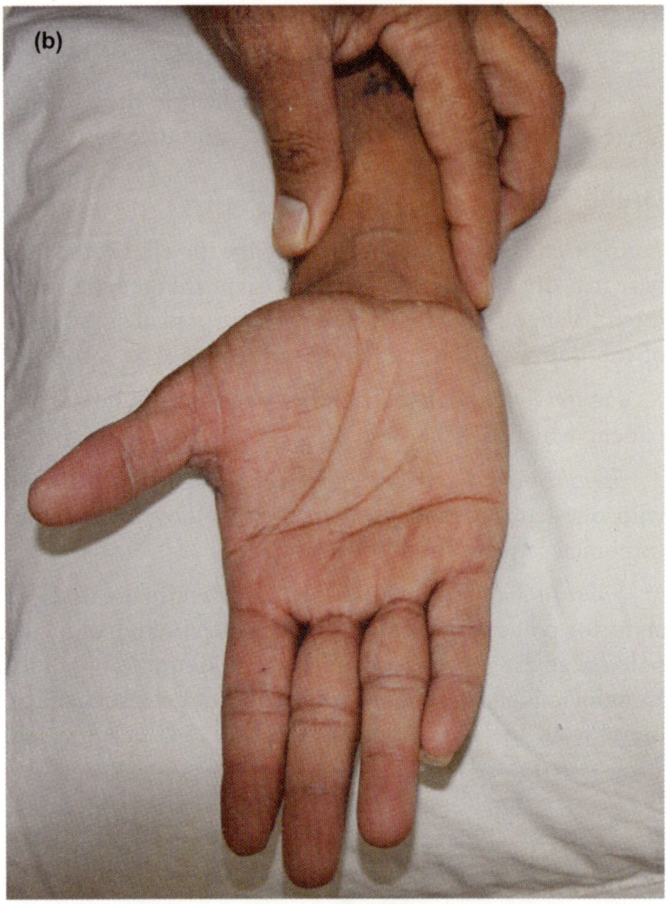

Figs. 6.154a and b: Testing of extensor pollicis brevis for grade 2. Patient sits comfortable on the stool with elbow flexion, forearm in midprone, wrist, carpometacarpal and interphalangeal joints at neutral. Metacarpophalangeal joint of the thumb in the abduction and flexion. Examiner stands at the side of the patient which is being tested. Examiner grasps the first metacarpal bone with one hand to stabilize it to prevent movement at the carpometacarpal joint and forearm. Examiner asks the patient to extend the metacarpophalangeal joint in the available range of motion. If patient completes partial movement it is considered grade 2

Test: Examiner asks the patient to extend the metacarpophalangeal joint in the available range of motion. Examiner may demonstrate the movement to the patient if patient finds difficulty in performing the movement. If patient completes partial movement it is considered grade 2.

Grade 1

Position of Patient: Sitting on stool with elbow flexion, forearm in midprone, wrist, carpometacarpal and interphalangeal joints at neutral. Metacarpophalangeal joint of the thumb in the abduction and flexion.

Position of Examiner: Examiner stands at the side of the patient which is being tested and palpates the extensor pollicis brevis at the base of the first metacarpal (Fig. 6.155).

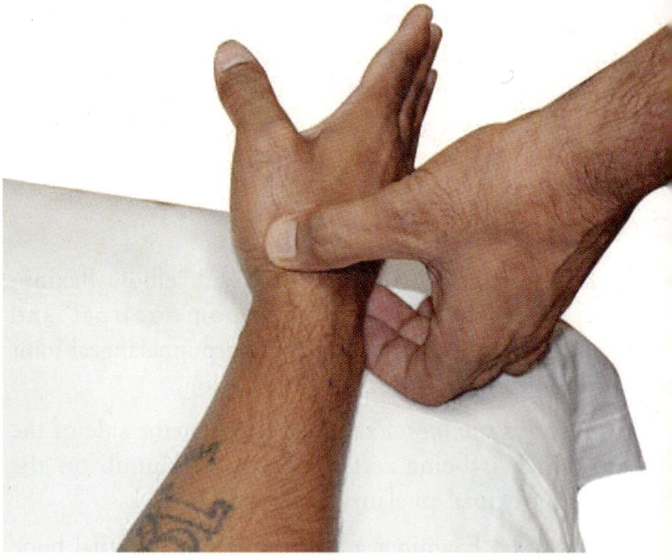

Fig. 6.155: Testing of extensor pollicis brevis for grade 1. Patient sits comfortable on the stool with elbow flexion, forearm in midprone, wrist, carpometacarpal and interphalangeal joints at neutral. Metacarpophalangeal joint of the thumb in the abduction and flexion. Examiner stands at the side of the patient which is being tested and palpates the extensor pollicis brevis at the base of the first metacarpal. Examiner asks the patient to extend the metacarpophalangeal joint in the available range of motion. If examiner feels contraction at the base of first metacarpal bone it is considered grade 1

Test: Examiner asks the patient to extend the metacarpophalangeal joint in the available range of motion. If examiner feels contraction at the base of first metacarpal bone it is considered grade 1.

EXTENSOR POLLICIS LONGUS (FIRST THUMB) INTERPHALANGEAL JOINT EXTENSION

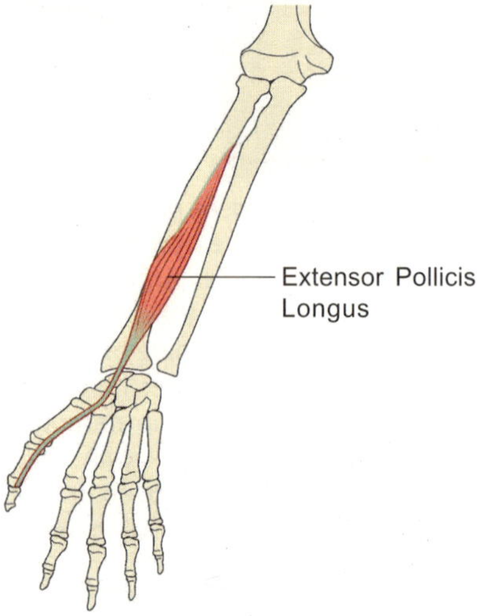

Fig. 6.156: Extensor pollicis longus origin and insertion

Extensor Pollicis Longus

Origin: Middle 1/3rd of the posterior surface of the ulna distal to origin of the abductor pollicis longus and to the interosseous membrane.

Insertion: Extensor pollicis longus inserts on the base of distal phalanx of the thumb.

Action: Extension of interphalangeal joint of the thumb. Assists in extension of the metacarpophalangeal and carpometacarpal joints of the thumb. Also assists in radial deviation and extension of the wrist joint.

Grade 3

Position of Patient: Sitting on stool with elbow flexion, forearm in midprone, wrist, carpometacarpal and interphalangeal joints at neutral. Metacarpophalangeal joint of the thumb in the abduction and flexion. IP joint of thumb should be in the extended position.

Position of Examiner: Examiner stands at the side of the patient which is being tested, and stabilizes the first metacarpal bone.

Stabilization: Examiner grasps the proximal phalanx of the thumb with one hand to stabilize and to prevent movement at the carpometacarpal joint and forearm.

Substitution: The muscles of thenar eminence such as abductor pollicis brevis, flexor pollicis brevis, and adductor pollicis can extend metacarpophalangeal joint of the thumb. Examiner should distinguish the action of extensor pollicis brevis from the thenar muscles (Fig. 6.157).

Test: Examiner asks the patient to extend the proximal interphalangeal joint. Examiner may demonstrate the movement to the patient if patient finds difficulty in performing the movement. If patient completes movement in the available range of motion is considered grade 1.

Grade 4 and 5

Position of Patient: Sitting on stool with elbow flexion, forearm in midprone, wrist, carpometacarpal and interphalangeal joints at neutral. Metacarpophalangeal joint of the thumb in the abduction and flexion.

Position of Examiner: Examiner stands at the side of the patient which is being tested.

Stabilization: Examiner grasps the first proximal phalanx with one hand to prevent movement at the metacarpophalangeal joint and also grasps the distal phalanx with the other hand for the resistance.

Substitution: The muscles of thenar eminence such as abductor pollicis brevis, flexor pollicis brevis, and adductor pollicis can extend metacarpophalangeal joint of the thumb. Examiner should distinguish the action of extensor pollicis brevis from the thenar muscles (Fig. 6.158).

Test: Examiner asks the patient to extend the interphalangeal joint of thumb against the resistance.

Grade 4: If patient completes range of motion against strong to moderate resistance.

Grade 5: If patient completes movement in the available range of motion against the maximal resistance.

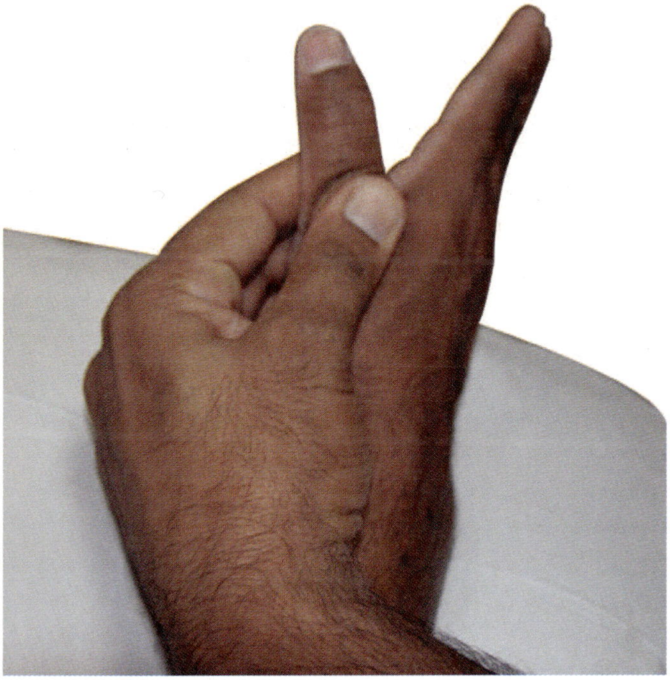

Fig. 6.157: Testing of extensor pollicis longus for grade 3

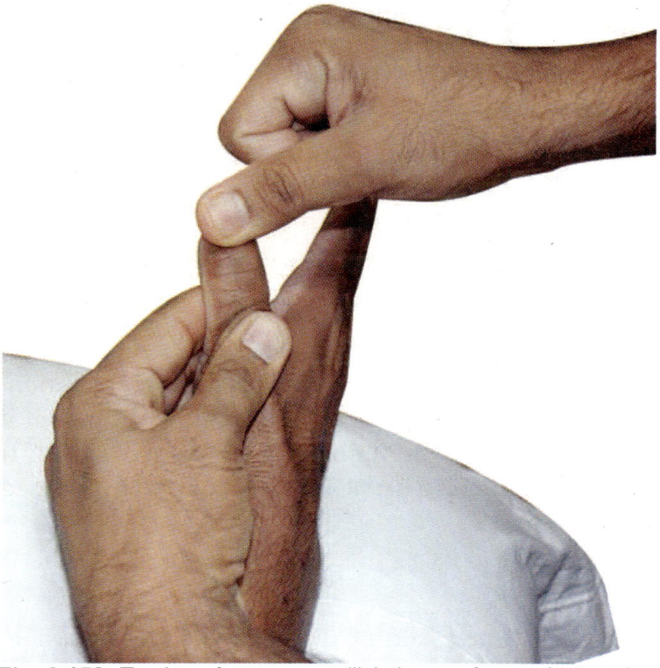

Fig. 6.158: Testing of extensor pollicis longus for grade 4 and 5

Grade 2

Position of Patient: Sitting on stool with elbow flexion, forearm in midprone, wrist, carpometacarpal and interphalangeal joints at neutral. Metacarpophalangeal joint of the thumb in the abduction and flexion. IP flexed.

Position of Examiner: Examiner stands at the side of the patient which is being tested.

Stabilization: Examiner grasps the proximal phalanx bone with one hand to stabilize and to prevent movement at the metacarpophalangeal joint.

Substitution: The muscles of thenar eminence such as abductor pollicis brevis, flexor pollicis brevis and adductor pollicis can extend metacarpophalangeal joint of the thumb. Examiner should distinguish the action of extensor pollicis brevis from the thenar muscles (Fig. 6.159).

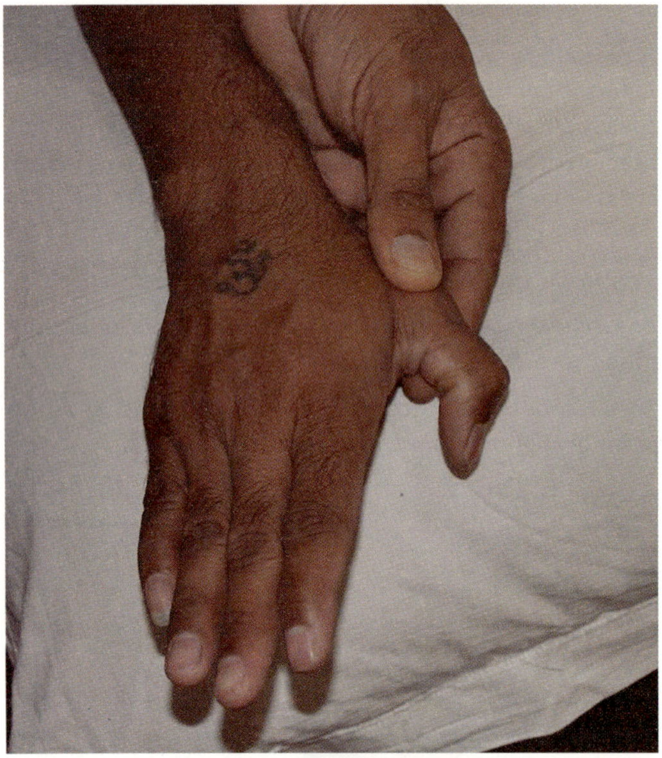

Fig. 6.159: Testing of extensor pollicis longus for grade 2

Test: Examiner asks the patient to extend the first interphalangeal joint in the available range of motion. Examiner may demonstrate the movement to the patient if patient finds difficulty in performing the movement. If patient completes partial movement it is considered grade 2.

Grade 1

Position of Patient: Sitting on stool with elbow flexion, forearm in midprone, wrist, carpometacarpal and interphalangeal joints at neutral. Metacarpophalangeal joint of the thumb should be in the abduction and flexion.

Position of Examiner: Examiner stands at the side of the patient which is being tested and palpates the extensor pollicis longus at the base of the first metacarpal (Fig. 6.160).

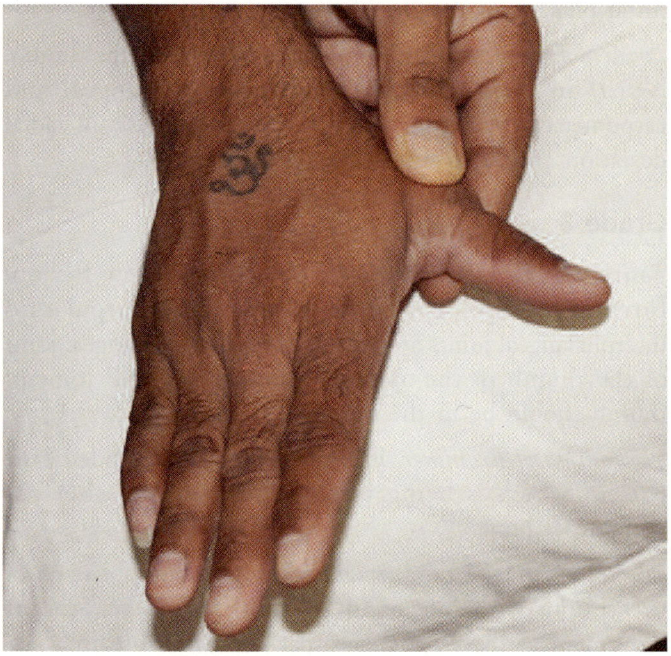

Fig. 6.160: Palpation of extensor pollicis longus for grade 1

Test: Examiner asks the patient to try to extend the first interphalangeal joint in the available range of motion. If examiner feels contraction at the base of first metcarpal bone it is considered grade 1.

FLEXOR POLLICIS BREVIS – FIRST METACARPOPHALANGEAL JOINT FLEXION

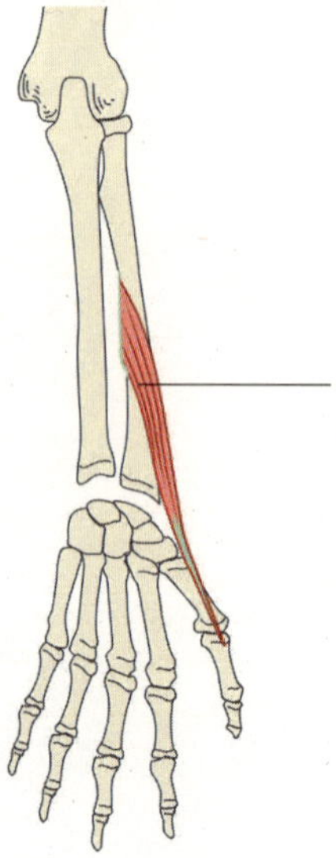

Fig. 6.161: Flexor pollicis brevis origin and insertion

Origin: Superficial head originates from the flexor retinaculum and trapezium bone. Deep head originates from trapezoid and capitates bones.

Insertion: Flexor pollicis brevis inserts on the base of the proximal phalanx of the thumb, radial side and extension expansion.

Action: Flexion of the metacarpophalangeal and carpometacarpal joints of the thumb and assists in opposition of the thumb towards the little finger.

Nerve Supply: Superficial head is supplied by C6,7,8, T1 and deep head is supplied by ulnar nerve, C8,T1.

Grade 3 (Fair)

Position of Patient: Sitting, forearm supination, wrist neutral, carpometacarpal and interphalangeal joints in the neutral.

Position of Examiner: Examiner stands or sits at the side which is being tested and grasps the first metacarpal bone to stabilize it and prevent motion at wrist and first CMC joint.

Stabilization: Examiner stabilizes the first carpometacarpal joint and the wrist to maintain them at the neutral position during the testing.

Substitution: Flexor pollicis longus can substitute the action of flexor pollicis brevis which can be prevented by keeping the first interphalangeal joint extended (Fig. 6.162).

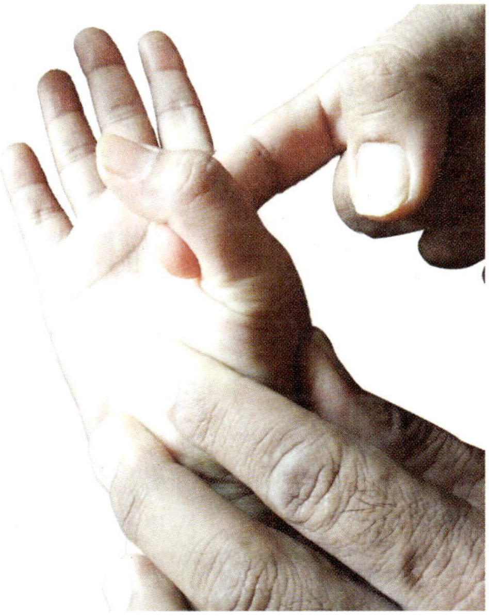

Fig. 6.162: Testing of flexor pollicis brevis for grade 3

Test: Examiner instructs the patient to bring your thumb across the palm of your hand. If patient is able to flex the first MCP joint in the available range is considered grade 3.

Grade 4 and 5 (Good and Normal)

Position of Patient: Sitting, forearm supination, wrist neutral, carpometacarpal and interphalangeal joints in the neutral.

Position of Examiner: Examiner stands or sits at the side which is being tested and grasps the first metacarpal bone with one hand to stabilize it and prevent motion at wrist and first CMC joint. Examiner grasps the proximal phalanx to apply resistance in the extension direction.

Stabilization: Examiner stabilizes the first carpometacarpal joint and the wrist to maintain them at the neutral position during the testing.

Substitution: Flexor pollicis longus can substitute the action of flexor pollicis brevis which can be prevented by keeping the first interphalangeal joint extended (Fig. 6.163).

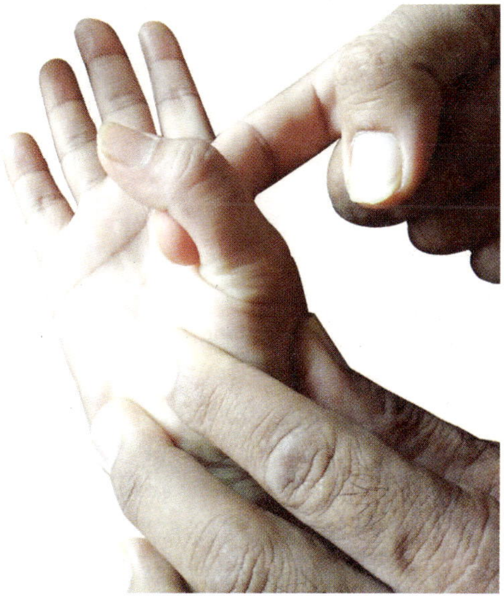

Fig. 6.163: Testing of flexor pollicis brevis (FPB) for grade 4 and 5

Test: Examiner instructs the patient to bring your thumb across the palm of your hand.

Grade 4: If patient is able to flex the first MCP joint in the available range against strong to moderate resistance.

Grade 5: If patient is able to flex the first MCP joint in the available range against maximal resistance.

Grade 2 (Poor)

Position of Patient: Sitting, forearm supination, wrist neutral, carpometacarpal and interphalangeal joints in the neutral.

Position of Examiner: Examiner stands at the side which is being tested and grasps the first metacarpal bone to stabilize it and prevent flexion motion at wrist and first CMC joint.

Stabilization: Examiner stabilizes the first metacarpal bone and the wrist to maintain them at the neutral position during the testing.

Substitution: Flexor pollicis longus can substitute the action of flexor pollicis brevis which can be prevented by keeping the first interphalangeal joint extended (Fig. 6.164).

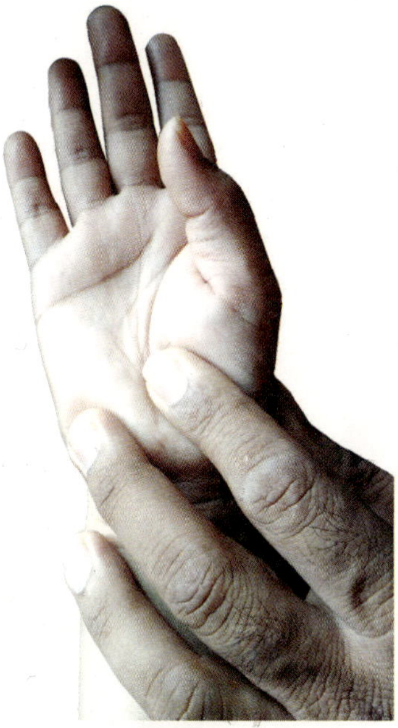

Fig. 6.164: Manual muscle testing of flexor pollicis brevis for grade 2

Test: Examiner instructs the patient to try to bring your thumb across the palm of your hand. If patient is able to flex the first MCP joint in the available range in gravity eliminated position is considered grade 2.

Grade 1 (Trace)

Position of Patient: Sitting, forearm supination, wrist neutral, carpometacarpal and interphalangeal joints in the neutral.

Position of Examiner: Examiner stands at the side which is being tested and places index finger on the ulnar side of the flexor pollicis longus tendon in the thenar eminence (Fig. 6.165).

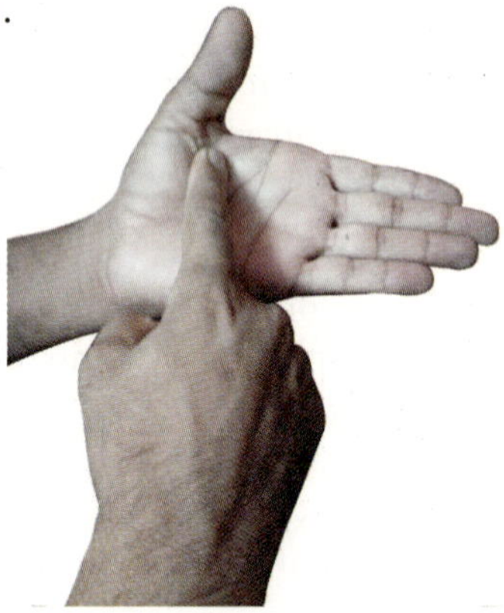

Fig. 6.165: Palpation of flexor pollicis brevis for grade 1

Test: Examiner instructs the patient to try to bring your thumb across the palm of your hand while examiner palpates the contraction of the muscle. If examiner feels contraction it is considered grade 1.

FLEXOR POLLICIS LONGUS – INTERPHALANGEAL JOINT FLEXION (THUMB)

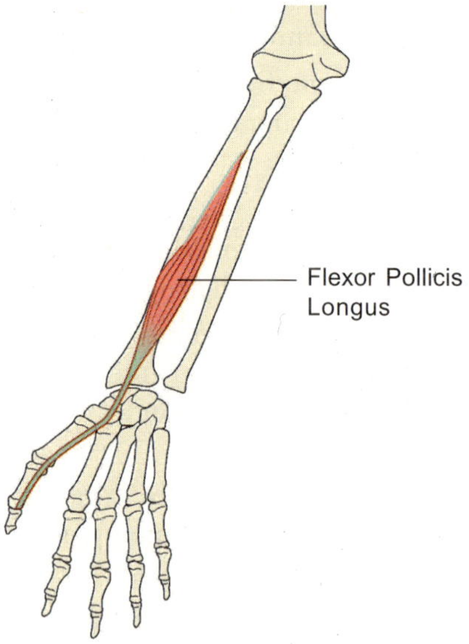

Fig. 6.166: Flexor pollicis longus origin and insertion

Origin: Anterior surface of the body of the radius below the tuberosity, interosseous membrane, medial border of the coronoid process of the ulna, and or the medial epicondyle of the humerus.

Insertion: Base of the distal phalanx of the thumb, palmar surface.

Action: Flexion of the interphalangeal joint of the thumb and assists in flexion of the metacarpophalangeal and carpometacarpal joint, and may assist in flexion of the wrist.

Nerve Supply: $C_{6,7,8,}T_1$.

Grade 3 (Fair)

Position of Patient: Sitting, forearm supination, wrist neutral, carpometacarpal and interphalangeal joints in the neutral.

Position of Examiner: Examiner stands at the side which is being tested and grasps the first metacarpal and proximal phalanx to stabilize it and prevent flexion motion at wrist, first CMC and MCP joints.

Stabilization: Metacarpophalangeal joint to prevent movement at the wrist and MCP joint (Fig. 6.167).

Test: Examiner instructs the patient to bend your thumb as much as possible. If patient is able to flex the first MCP joint in the available range against minimal resistance is considered grade 3.

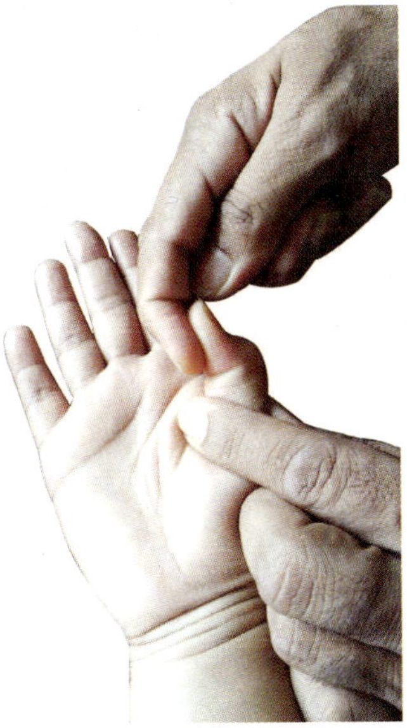

Fig. 6.167: Testing of flexor pollicis longus for grade 3

Grade 4 and 5 (Good and Normal)

Position of Patient: Sitting, forearm supination, wrist neutral, carpometacarpal and interphalangeal joints in the neutral.

Position of Examiner: Examiner stands or sits at the side which is being tested and grasps the first metacarpal and proximal phalanx with one hand to stabilize it and prevent motion at wrist, first CMC and MCP joint. Examiner grasps the distal phalanx to apply resistance in the extension direction (Fig. 6.168).

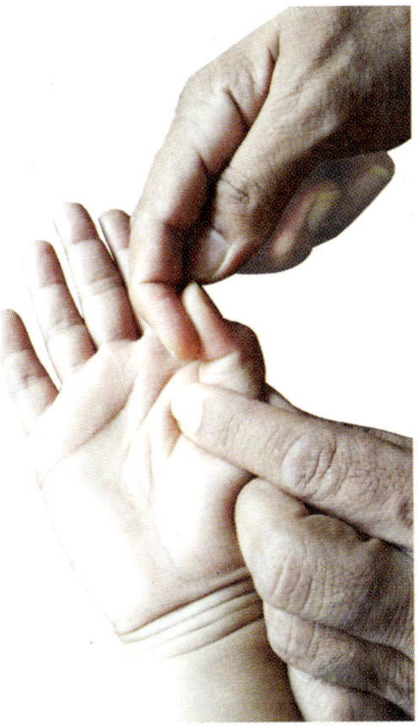

Fig. 6.168: Testing of flexor pollicis longus for grade 4 and 5

Test: Examiner instructs the patient to bring end of your thumb towards the palm.

Grade 4: If patient is able to flex the first interphalangeal joint in the available range against strong to moderate resistance.

Grade 5: If patient is able to flex the first DIP joint in the available range against maximal resistance.

Grade 2 (Poor)

Position of Patient: Sitting, forearm supination, wrist neutral, carpometacarpal and interphalangeal joints in the neutral.

Position of Examiner: Examiner stands at the side which is being tested and grasps the first metacarpal and proximal phalanx to stabilize it and prevent flexion motion at wrist, first CMC and MCP joints.

Test: Examiner instructs the patient to try to bend your thumb as much as possible. If patient is able to flex the first MCP joint in the available range in gravity eliminated position is considered grade 2 (Fig. 6.169).

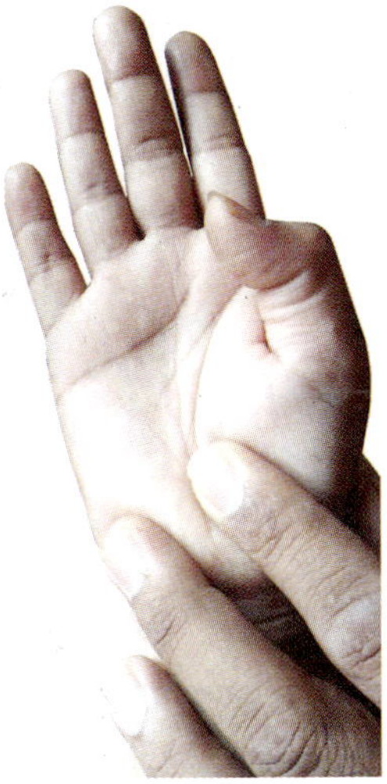

Fig. 6.169: Testing of flexor pollicis longus for grade 2

Grade 1 (Trace)

Position of Patient: Sitting, forearm supination, wrist neutral, carpometacarpal and interphalangeal joints in the neutral.

Position of Examiner: Examiner stands at the side which is being tested and places index finger on the palmar surface of thenar eminence (Fig. 6.170).

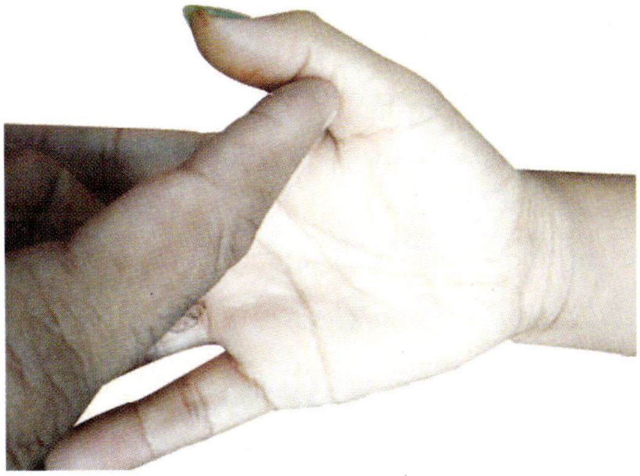

Fig. 6.170: Testing of flexor pollicis longus for grade 1

Test: Examiner instructs the patient to try to bend the end of your thumb while examiner palpates the contraction of the muscle. If examiner feels contraction it is considered grade 1.

ABDUCTOR POLLICIS LONGUS

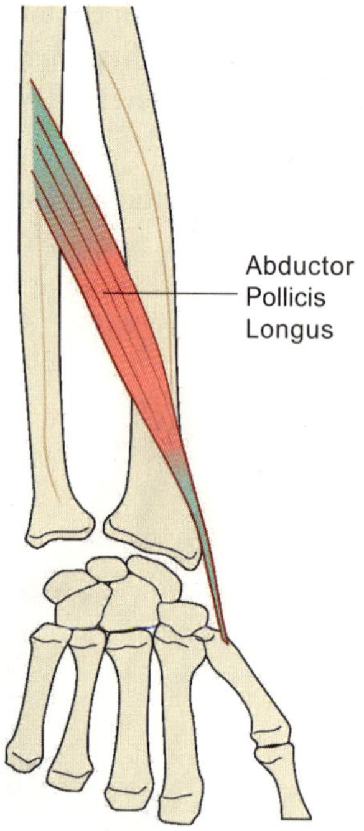

Fig. 6.171: Abductor pollicis longus origin and insertion

Origin: Abductor pollicis longus originates from flexor retinaculum, tubercle of the trapezium bone and tubercle of the scaphoid bone.

Insertion: Base of the proximal phalanx of the thumb, on the radial side and extensor expansion.

Action: Abduction and extension of the carpometacarpal joint of the thumb in a plane parallel to the finger metacarpals and assists in radial deviation and flexion of the wrist.

Nerve Supply: Median Nerve, $C_{6,\ 7,\ 8}$ T_1.

Grade 3 (Fair)

Position of Patient: Sitting, forearm midprone and wrist in neutral, thumb in adducted position.

Position of Examiner: Sitting comfortably at the side of the patient and holds the hand.

Stabilization: Examiner grasps the hand and stabilizes the metacarpals of the fingers to maintain the fingers at the neutral position.

Substitution: Extensor pollicis brevis can work as an abductor pollicis brevis (Figs. 6.172a and b).

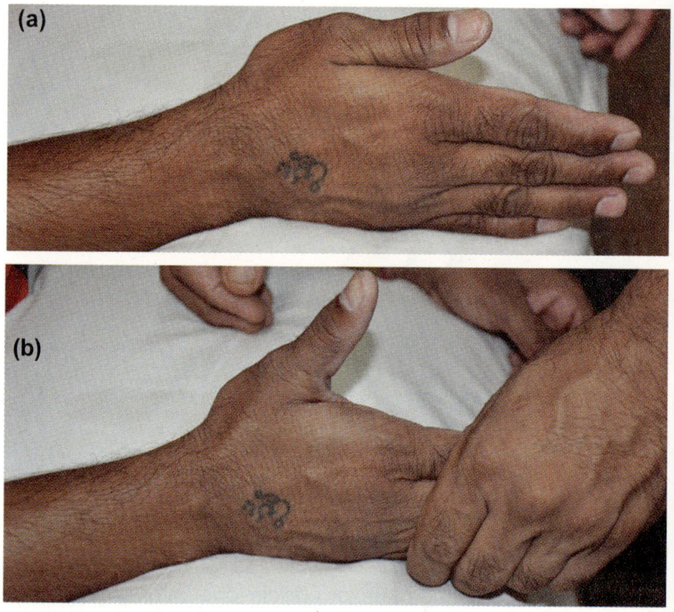

Figs. 6.172a and b: Testing of abductor pollicis longus (APL) for grade 3

Test: Examiner instructs the patient to take the thumb away from the hand in a plane parallel to the finger metacarpals. If patient is able to complete the range of motion against the gravity in the available range of motion it is considered grade 3.

Grade 4 and 5 (Good and Normal)

Position of Patient: Sitting, forearm midprone and wrist in neutral, thumb in adducted position.

Position of Examiner: Sitting comfortably at the side of the patient and holds the hand with one hand and places thumb on the first metacarpal bone for resistance.

Stabilization: Examiner grasps the hand and stabilizes the metacarpals of the fingers to maintain them at the neutral position.

Substitution: Extensor pollicis brevis can work as an abductor pollicis brevis (Fig. 6.173).

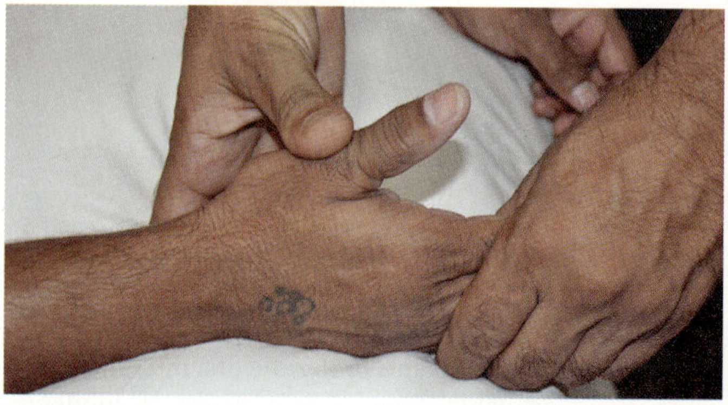

Fig. 6.173: Testing of abductor pollicis longus for grade for 4 and 5

Test: Examiner instructs the patient to take the thumb away from the hand in a plane parallel to the finger metacarpals.

Grade 4: If patient is able to complete the range of motion against moderate resistance in the available range of motion.

Grade 5: If patient is able to complete the range of motion against maximal resistance in the available range of motion.

Grade 2 (Poor)

Position of Patient: Sitting, forearm supinated and wrist in neutral, thumb in adducted position.

Position of Examiner: Sitting comfortably at the side of the patient and holds the fingers.

Stabilization: Examiner grasps the hand and stabilizes the metacarpals of the fingers to maintain them at the neutral position.

Substitution: Extensor pollicis brevis can work as an abductor pollicis brevis (Figs. 6.174a and b).

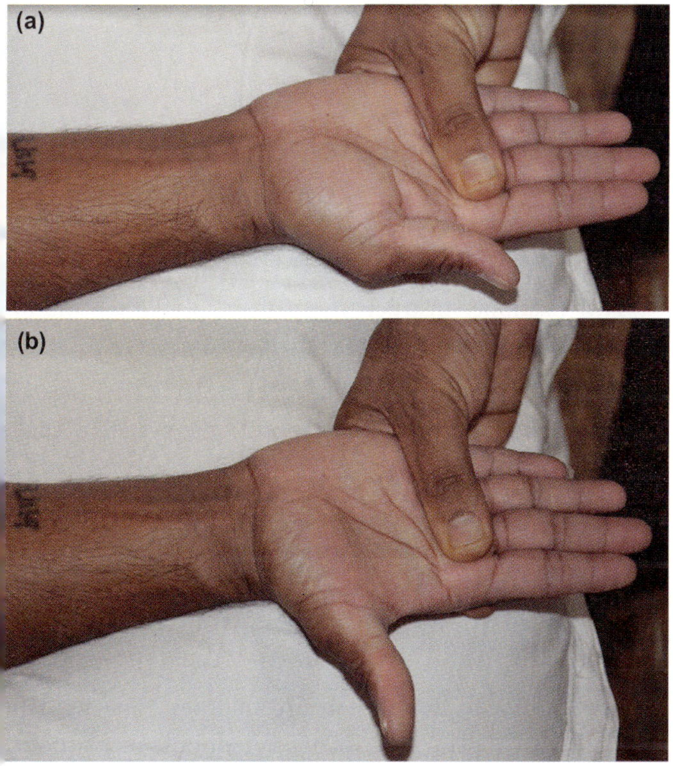

Figs. 6.174a and b: Testing of abductor pollicis longus (APL) for grade 2

Test: Examiner instructs the patient to take the thumb away from the hand in a plane parallel to the finger metacarpals. If patient is able to complete the range of motion in the available range of motion it is considered grade 2.

Grade 1 (Flicker)

Position of Patient: Sitting, forearm supinated and wrist in neutral, thumb in adducted position.

Position of Examiner: Sitting comfortably at the side of the patient and holds the hand.

Stabilization: Examiner may grasp the hand and stabilizes the metacarpals of the fingers with one hand and places the index finger of the other hand on the radial side of the distal forearm for palpating the tendon (Fig. 6.175).

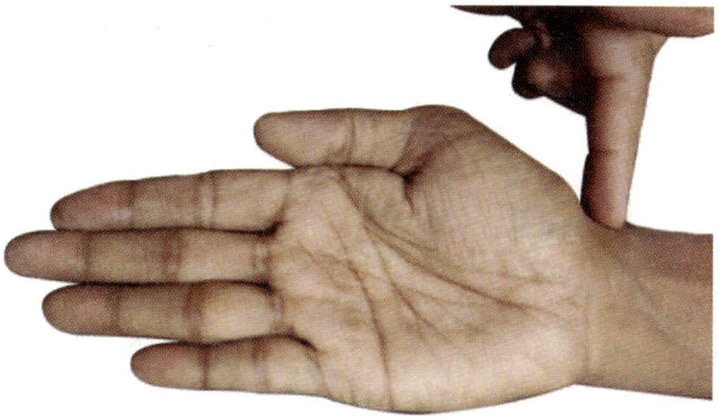

Fig. 6.175: Testing of abductor pollicis longus for grade 1

Test: Examiner instructs the patient to try to take the thumb away from the hand in a plane parallel to the finger metacarpals while examiner palpates the contraction. If examiner finds contraction it is considered grade 1.

ABDUCTOR POLLICIS BREVIS

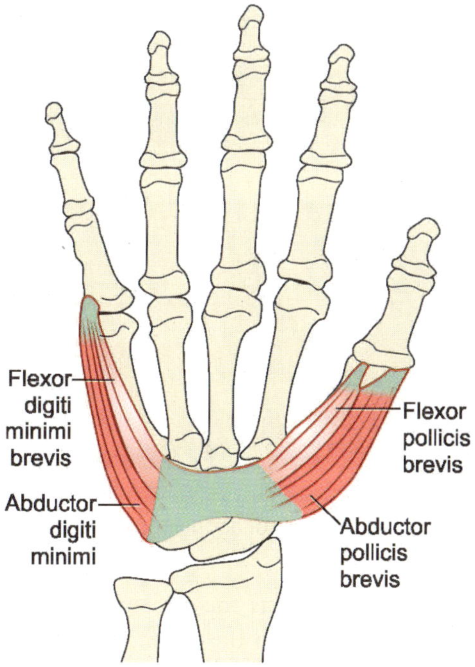

Fig. 6.176: Abductor pollicis brevis origin and insertion

Origin: Flexor retanaculum, tubercle of scaphoid bone, tubercle of trapezium bone and tendon of abductor pollicis longus.

Insertion: On the radial side of base of proximal phalanx and dorsal extensor expansion of thumb.

Action: Abduction of carpometacarpal and metacarpophalangeal joint. Assists in extension and opposition of thumb.

Nerve Supply: C_8, T_1.

Grade 3 (Fair)

Position of Patient: Sitting, forearm supinated and wrist in neutral, MCP, PIP, DIP in neutral and thumb in an adducted position.

Position of Examiner: Sitting comfortably at the side of the patient and holds the hand.

Stabilization: Examiner grasps the hand and stabilizes the metacarpals of the fingers to maintain them at the neutral position.

Substitution: Abductor pollicis longus may substitute the action of abductor pollicis brevis if the abduction is parallel to the fingers and not perpendicular to the fingers (Figs. 6.177a and b).

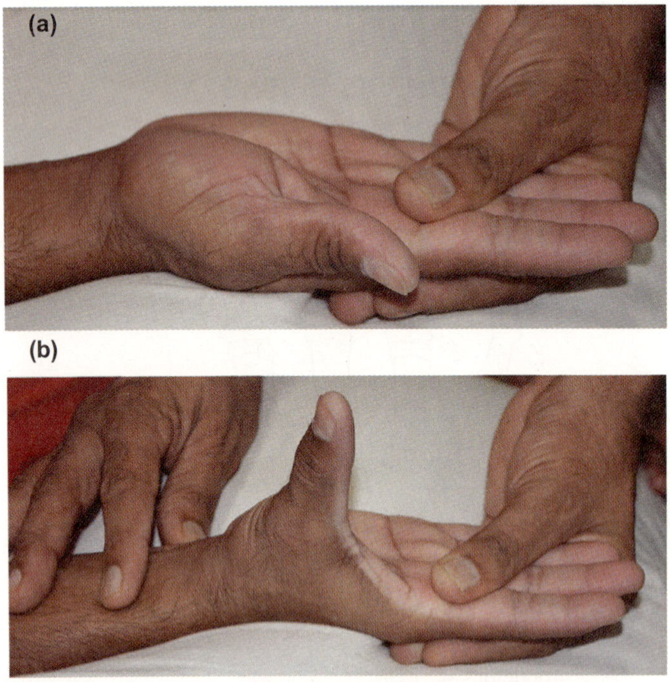

Figs. 6.177a and b: Testing of abductor pollicis brevis (APB) for grade 3

Test: Examiner instructs the patient to lift the thumb in a plane perpendicular to the palm. If patient is able to complete the range of motion against the gravity in the available range of motion it is considered grade 3.

Grade 4 and 5 (Good and Normal)

Position of Patient: Sitting, forearm supinated and wrist in neutral, MCP, PIP, DIP in neutral and thumb in an adducted position.

Position of Examiner: Sitting comfortably at the side of the patient and holds the metacarpals of the fingers with the one hand and places thumb on the thenar aspect of the first metacarpal bone for resistance.

Stabilization: Examiner grasps the hand and stabilizes the metacarpals of the fingers to maintain the MCP, PIP, DIP at the neutral position.

Substitution: Abductor pollicis longus may substitute the action of abductor pollicis brevis if the abduction is parallel to the fingers and not perpendicular to the fingers (Fig. 6.178).

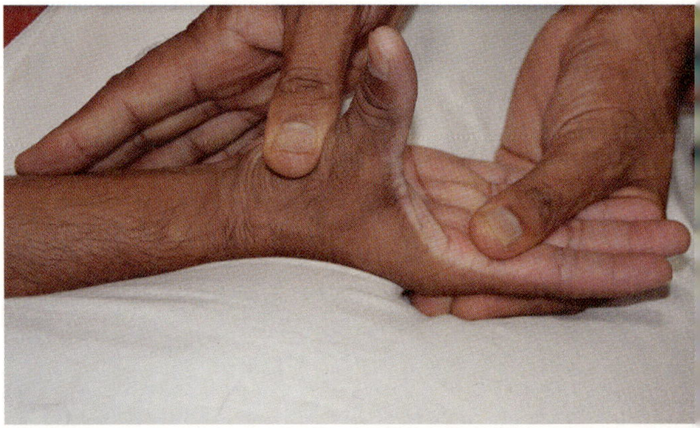

Fig. 6.178: Testing of abductor pollicis brevis for grade 4 and 5

Test: Examiner instructs the patient to take the thumb away in a plane perpendicular to the palm.

Grade 4: If patient is able to complete the range of motion against moderate resistance in the available range of motion.

Grade 5: If patient is able to complete the range of motion against maximal resistance in the available range of motion.

Grade 2 (Poor)

Position of Patient: Sitting, forearm midprone and wrist in neutral, MCP, PIP, DIP in neutral thumb in adducted position.

Position of Examiner: Sitting comfortably at the side of the patient and holds the hand.

Stabilization: Examiner grasps the hand and stabilizes the metacarpals of the fingers to maintain them at the neutral position (Fig. 6.179).

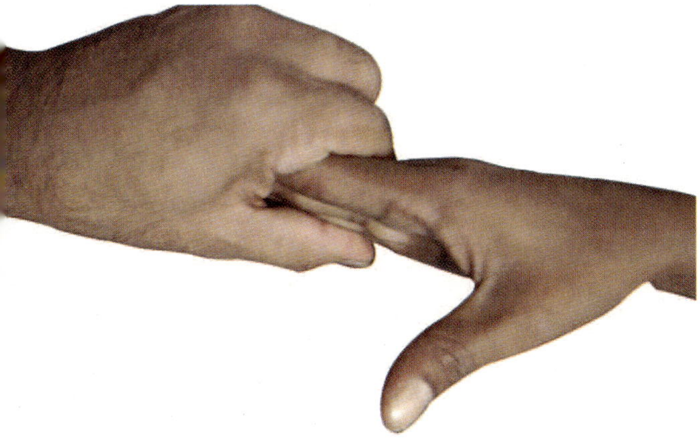

Fig. 6.179: Testing of abductor pollicis brevis for grade 2

Test: Examiner instructs the patient to take the thumb away from the hand in a plane perpendicular to the palm. If patient is able to complete the range of motion in the available range of motion it is considered grade 2.

Grade 1 (Flicker)

Position of Patient: Sitting, forearm midprone and wrist in neutral, thumb in adducted position.

Position of Examiner: Sitting comfortably at the side of the patient and holds the hand.

Stabilization: Examiner may grasp the hand and stabilizes the metacarpals of the fingers with one hand and places the index finger of the other hand on the thenar aspect of the first metacarpal bone to palpate the contraction of the muscle (Fig. 6.180).

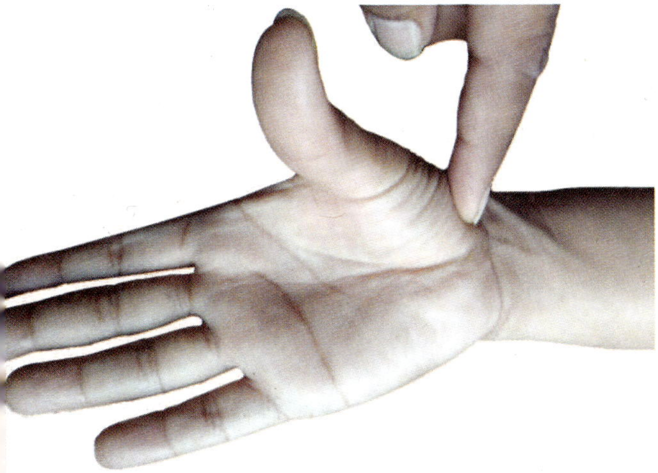

Fig. 6.180: Palpation of abductor pollicis brevis for grade 1

Test: Examiner instructs the patient to try to take the thumb away from the hand in a plane perpendicular to the palm while examiner palpates the contraction. If examiner finds contraction it is considered grade 1.

ADDUCTOR POLLICIS

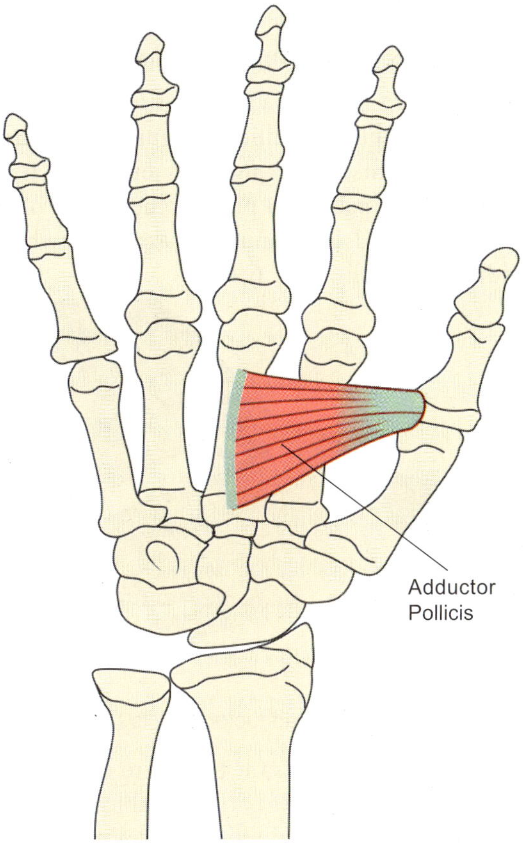

Fig. 6.181: Adductor pollicis origin and insertion

Adductor Pollicis

Adductor pollicis has two variation of fibers, oblique fibers and transverse fibers.

Origin: Oblique fibers originate from capitates bone and base of the second and third metacarpal bones. Transverse fibers originate from palmar surface of the third metacarpal bone.

Insertion: Oblique head inserts into the extensor expansion and transverse fibers insert at the base of the proximal phalanx of the thumb on the ulnar side.

Action: Adduction of the carpometacarpal joint. Assists in flexion of the metacarpophalangeal joint in the plane of palm and extension of the interphalangeal joints. Also assists in the opposition of the thumb towards the little finger.

Nerve Supply: Ulnar Nerve, C_8, T_1.

Grade 3 (Fair)

Position of Patient: Sitting, forearm pronated and wrist in neutral, MCP, PIP, DIP in neutral and thumb in an abducted position.

Position of Examiner: Sitting comfortably at the side of the patient and grasps the metacarpal bones of the finger.

Stabilization: Examiner grasps the hand and stabilizes the metacarpals of the fingers to maintain them at the neutral position.

Substitution: Flexor pollicis longus and flexor pollicis brevis flexes the first MCP and PIP joints which draw the thumb across the palm. To prevent the action of FPL and FPB the MCP and PIP should be extended while testing the adductor pollicis (Fig. 6.182).

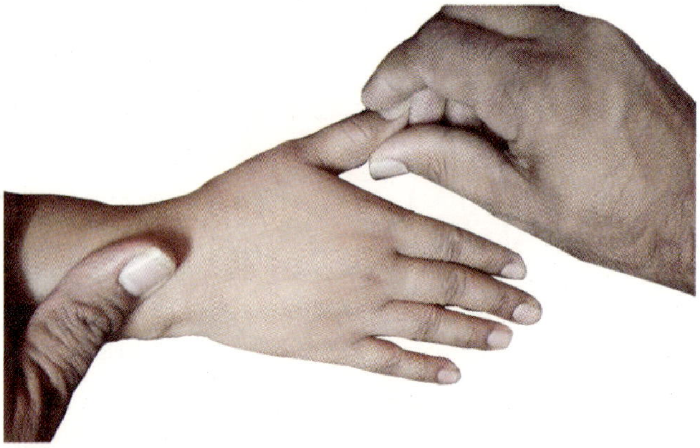

Fig. 6.182: Testing of adductor pollicis (AP) for grade 3

Test: Examiner instructs the patient to bring your thumb up to your index finger. If patient is able to complete the range of motion against minimal resistance in the available range of motion it is considered grade 3.

Grade 4 and 5 (Good and Normal)

Position of Patient: Sitting, forearm pronated and wrist in neutral, MCP, PIP, DIP in neutral and thumb in an abducted position.

Position of Examiner: Sitting comfortably at the side of the patient and grasps the metacarpal bones of the finger with one hand and places index finger of other hand on the ventral surface of the thumb for the resistance.

Stabilization: Examiner grasps the hand and stabilizes the metacarpals of the fingers to maintain them at the neutral position.

Substitution: Flexor pollicis longus and flexor pollicis brevis flexes the first MCP and PIP joints which draw the thumb across the palm. To prevent the action of FPL and FPB the MCP and PIP should be extended while testing the adductor pollicis (Fig. 6.183).

Test: Examiner instructs the patient to bring your thumb toward your index finger.

Grade 4: If patient is able to complete the range of motion against moderate resistance in the available range of motion.

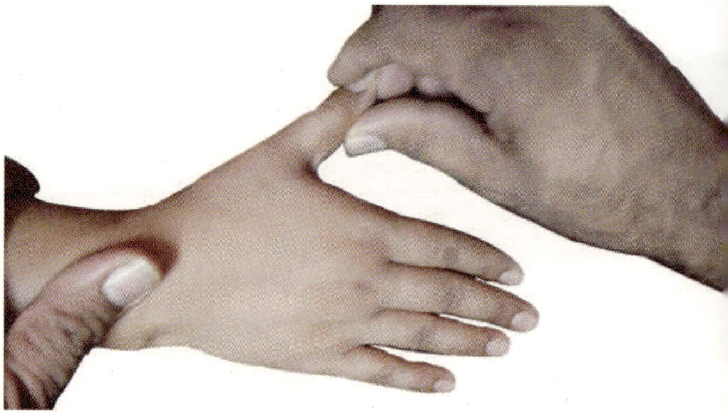

Fig. 6.183: Testing of adductor pollicis for grade 4 and 5

Grade 5: If patient is able to complete the range of motion against maximal resistance in the available range of motion.

Grade 2 (Poor)

Position of Patient: Sitting, forearm pronated and wrist in neutral, MCP, PIP, DIP in neutral, thumb in an abducted position.

Position of Examiner: Sitting comfortably at the side of the patient and may hold the hand.

Stabilization: Examiner grasps the hand and stabilizes the metacarpals of the fingers to maintain them at the neutral position.

Substitution: Flexor pollicis longus and flexor pollicis brevis flexes the first MCP and PIP joints which draw the thumb across the palm. To prevent the action of FPL and FPB the MCP and PIP should be extended while testing the adductor pollicis (Figs. 6.184a and b).

Test: Examiner instructs the patient to take the thumb towards the index finger. If patient is able to complete the movement in the available range of motion it is considered grade 2.

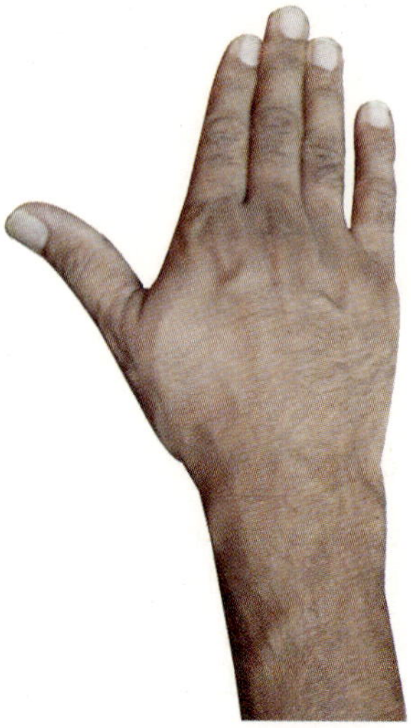

(a)

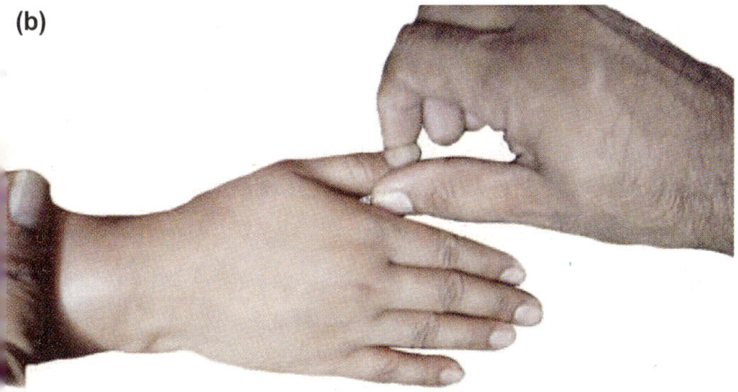

Figs. 6.184a and b: Testing of adductor pollicis for grade 2

Grade 1 (Flicker)

Position of Patient: Sitting, forearm midprone and wrist in neutral, thumb in abducted position.

Position of Examiner: Sitting comfortably at the side of the patient and palpate the adductor pollicis on the palmar side of the web space of the thumb by grasping the web between the index finger and thumb (Fig. 6.185).

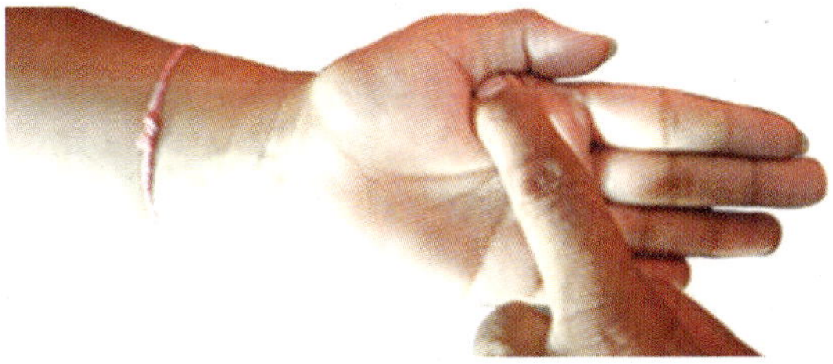

Fig. 6.185: Testing of adductor pollicis for grade 1

Test: Examiner instructs the patient to try to take the thumb towards the index finger while examiner palpates the contraction. If examiner finds contraction it is considered grade 1.

OPPONENS POLLICIS

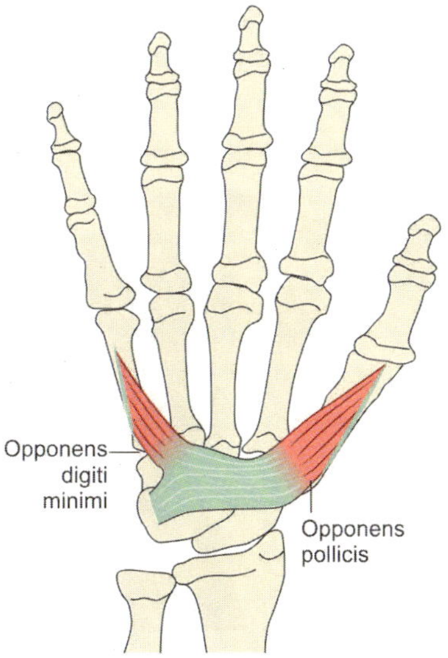

Fig. 6.186: Opponens pollicis origin and insertion

Origin: From tubercle of trapezium bone and flexor retanaculum.

Insertion: Opponens pollicis inserts on first metacarpal bone (along entire length of radial side of shaft).

Action: flexion of carpometacarpal joint medially across the palm, abduction of carpometacarpal joint and medial rotation of carpometacarpal joint.

Nerve Supply: $C_{6, 7, 8,}$ T_1.

Grade 3 (Fair)

Position of Patient: Sitting, forearm supinated, wrist, MCP, PIP, DIP at neutral and thumb adducted.

Position of Examiner: Sitting, grasps the metacarpals of the fingers to maintain them in the neutral position.

Stabilization: Examiner grasps the metacarpals of the fingers to maintain them in the neutral position.

Substitution: Flexor pollicis longus and flexor pollicis brevis flexes the first MCP and PIP joints which draw the thumb across the palm toward the little finger. The flexion at the MCP and PIP should be distinguishes from the opposition (Figs. 6.187a and b).

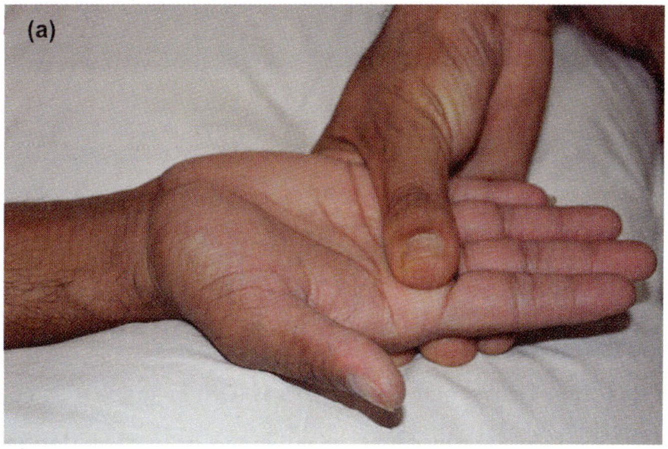

(b)

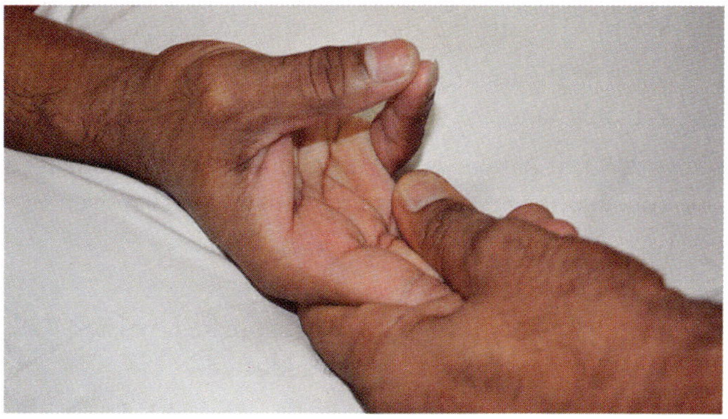

Figs. 6.187a and b: Testing of opponens pollicis (OP) for grade 3

Test: Examiner instructs the patient to bring your thumb towards your little finger and touch the two pads, forming the letter "O" with the thumb and little finger. If patient is able to bring the thumb towards the little finger against minimal resistance and forms the letter "O" it is considered grade 3.

Grade 4 and 5 (Good and Normal)

Position of Patient: Sitting, forearm supinated, wrist, MCP, PIP, DIP at neutral and thumb adducted.

Position of Examiner: Sitting, grasps the metacarpals of the fingers to maintain them in the neutral position and places the thumb of other hand on the head of the first metacarpal for resistance in the direction of lateral rotation, extension and adduction.

Stabilization: Examiner grasps the metacarpals of the fingers to maintain them in the neutral position.

Substitution: Flexor pollicis longus and flexor pollicis brevis flexes the first MCP and PIP joints which draw the thumb across the palm toward the little finger. The flexion at the MCP and PIP should be distinguishes from the opposition (Fig. 6.188).

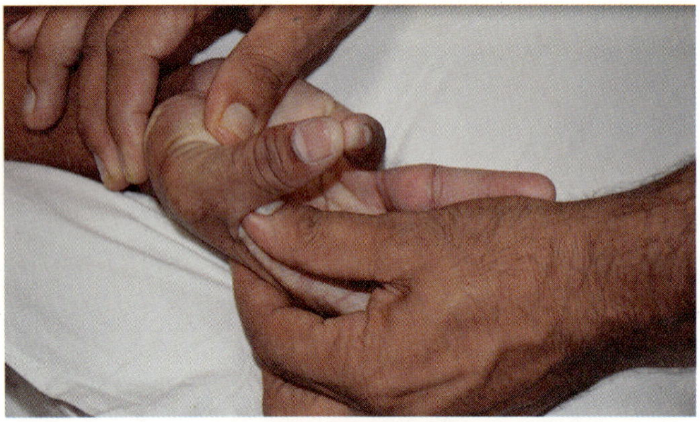

Fig. 6.188: Testing of opponens pollicis (OP) for grade 4 and 5

Test: Examiner instructs the patient to bring your thumb towards your little finger and touch the two pads, forming the letter "O" with the thumb and little finger.

Grade 4: If patient is able to complete the movement in the available range of motion against moderate resistance.

Grade 5: If patient is able to complete the movement in the available range of motion against maximal resistance.

Grade 2 (Poor)

Position of Patient: Sitting, forearm supinated, wrist, MCP, PIP, DIP at neutral and thumb adducted.

Position of Examiner: Sitting, grasps the fingers to maintain them in the neutral position.

Stabilization: Examiner grasps the fingers to maintain them in the neutral position.

Substitution: Flexor pollicis longus and flexor pollicis brevis flexes the first MCP and PIP joints which draw the thumb across the palm toward the little finger. The flexion at the MCP and PIP should be distinguished from the opposition (Fig. 6.189).

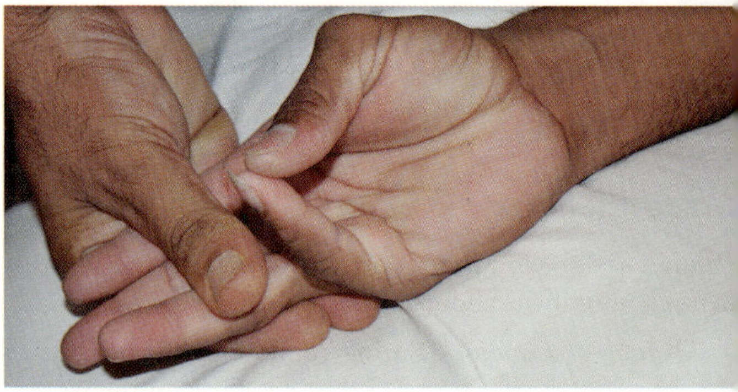

Fig. 6.189: Testing of opponens pollicis for grade 2

Test: Examiner instructs the patient to bring your thumb towards your little finger and touch the two pads, forming the letter "O" with the thumb and little finger. If patient is able to bring the thumb towards the little finger and forms the letter "O" it is considered grade 3.

Grade 1 (Flicker)

Position of Patient: Sitting, forearm supinated, wrist, MCP, PIP, DIP at neutral and thumb adducted.

Position of Examiner: Sitting, grasps the metacarpals of the fingers to maintain them in the neutral position. Examiner places his or her index finger on the radial shaft of the first metacarpal for palpation of the contraction. The opponens pollicis lies lateral to the abductor pollicis brevis.

Stabilization: Examiner grasps the metacarpals of the fingers to maintain them in the neutral position (Fig. 6.190).

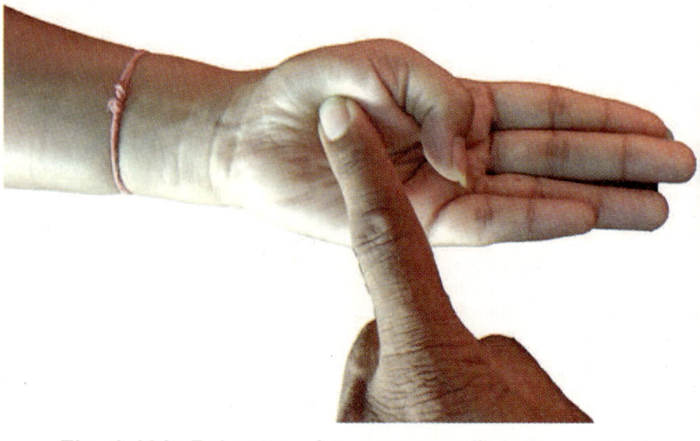

Fig. 6.190: Palpation of opponens pollicis for grade 1

Test: Examiner instructs the patient to try to bring your thumb towards your little finger and touch the two pads, while palpating the muscle for contraction. If examiner feels contraction it is considered grade 1.

OPPONENS DIGITI MINIMI

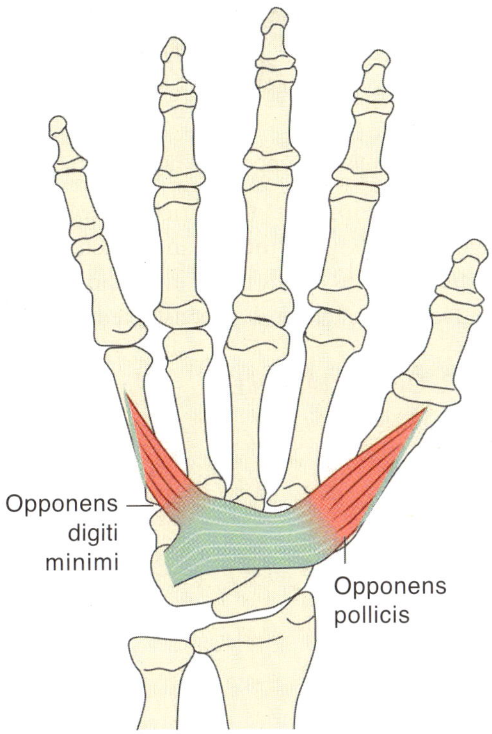

Fig. 6.191: Opponens digiti minimi

Opponens Digiti Minimi

Origin: Hook of the hamate bone and the flexor retanaculum.

Insertion: Entire length of the fifth metacarpal bone on the ulnar side.

Action: Opposition of the carpometacarpal joint of the little finger, i.e., flexion with slight rotation of the fifth, carpometacarpal joint in which little finger is opposed to the thumb.

Nerve Supply: Ulnar nerve, $C_{7,\ 8,}$ T_1.

Grade 3 (Fair)

Position of Patient: Sitting, forearm supinated, wrist, MCP, PIP, DIP at neutral and little finger adducted.

Position of Examiner: Sitting, grasps first three metacarpals of the fingers to maintain them in the neutral position.

Stabilization: Examiner grasps the metacarpals of the fingers to maintain them in the neutral position (Figs. 6.192a and b).

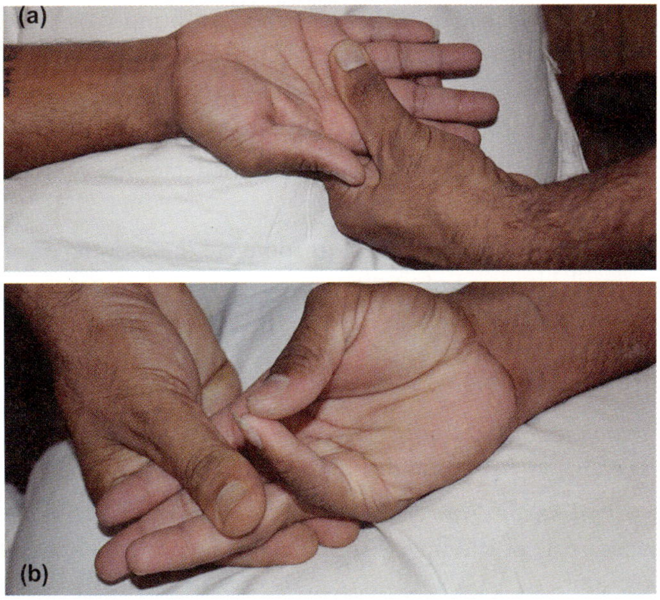

Figs. 6.192a and b: Testing of opponens digiti minimi for grade 3

Test: Examiner instructs the patient to bring your little finger towards your thumb and touch the two pads, forming the letter "O" with the thumb and little finger. If patient is able to bring the little finger towards the thumb and forms the letter "O" it is considered grade 3.

Grade 4 and 5 (Good and Normal)

Position of Patient: Sitting, forearm supinated, wrist, MCP, PIP, DIP at neutral and thumb adducted.

Position of Examiner: Sitting, grasps first three metacarpals of the fingers to maintain them in the neutral position and places the thumb of other hand on the head of the fifth metacarpal for resistance.

Stabilization: Examiner grasps the metacarpals of the fingers to maintain them in the neutral position (Fig. 6.193).

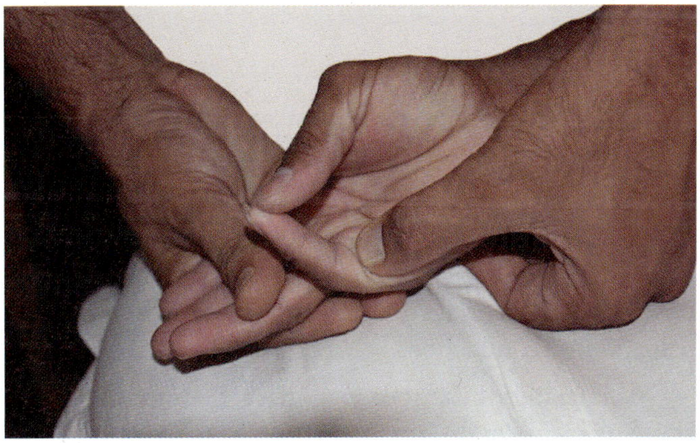

Fig. 6.193: Testing of opponens digiti minimi for grade 4 and 5

Test: Examiner instructs the patient to bring your little finger towards your thumb and touch the two pads, forming the letter "O" with the thumb and little finger.

Grade 4: If patient is able to complete the movement in the available range of motion against moderate resistance it is considered grade 4.

Grade 5: If patient is able to complete the movement in the available range of motion against maximal resistance it is considered grade 5.

Grade 2 (Poor)

Position of Patient: Sitting, forearm supinated, wrist, MCP, PIP, DIP at neutral and thumb adducted.

Position of Examiner: Sitting, grasps the first three metacarpals of the fingers to maintain them in the neutral position.

Stabilization: Examiner grasps the metacarpals of the fingers to maintain them in the neutral position (Fig. 6.194).

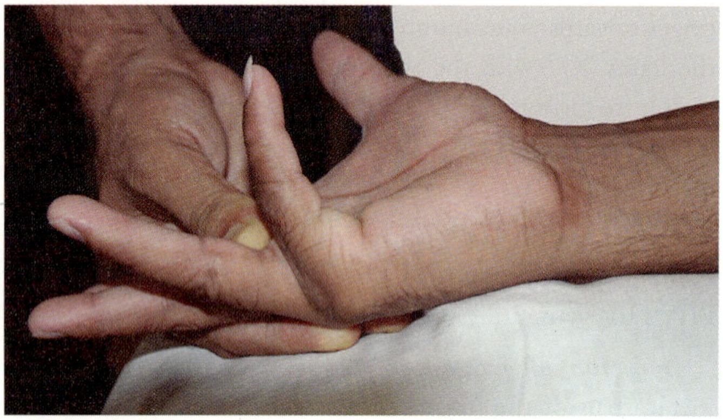

Fig. 6.194: Testing of opponens digiti minimi for grade 2

Test: Examiner instructs the patient to bring your little finger towards your thumb and touch the two pads, forming the letter "O" with the thumb and little finger. If patient is able to bring the little finger towards the thumb and forms the letter "O" it is considered grade 2.

Grade 1 (Flicker)

Position of Patient: Sitting, forearm supinated, wrist, MCP, PIP, DIP at neutral and thumb adducted.

Position of Examiner: Sitting, grasps the thumb and first three metacarpals of the fingers to maintain them in the neutral position. Examiner places his or her index finger on the palmar surface of the fifth metacarpal bone for palpation of contraction.

Stabilization: Examiner may grasp the metacarpals of the fingers to maintain them in the neutral position (Fig. 6.195).

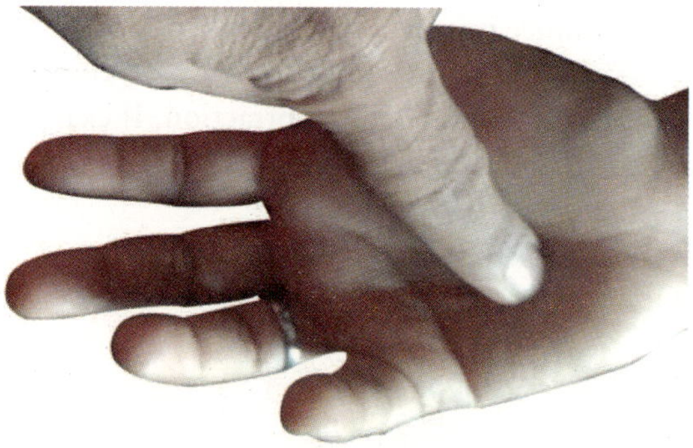

Fig. 6.195: Palpation of opponens digiti minimi for grade 1

Test: Examiner instructs the patient to try to bring your little finger towards your thumb and touch the two pads, forming the letter "O" with the thumb and little finger. If examiner feels contraction it is considered grade 1.

FLEXOR DIGITI MINIMI

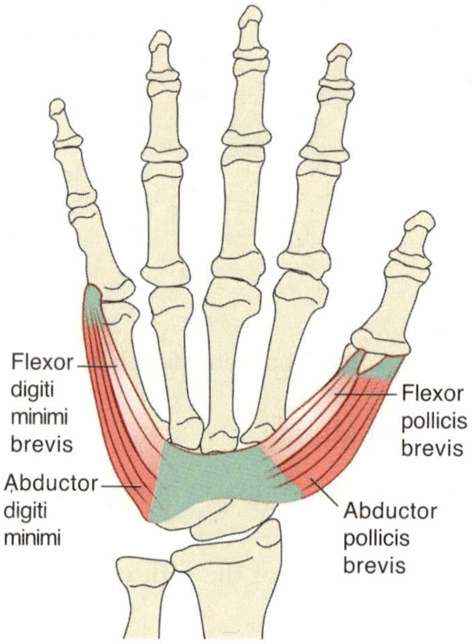

Fig. 6.196: Flexor digiti minimi origin and insertion

Flexor Digiti Minimi

Origin: Hook of the hamate bone and the flexor retanaculum.

Insertion: Base of the proximal phalanx of the little finger on the ulnar side.

Action: Flexion of the metacarpophalangeal joint of the little finger. Assists in opposition of the little finger.

Nerve Supply: Ulnar Nerve, $C_{7,\,8,}$ and T_1.

Grade 3 (Fair)

Position of Patient: Sitting, forearm supinated, wrist, MCP, PIP, DIP at neutral and thumb adducted.

Position of Examiner: Sitting, grasps first three metacarpals of the fingers to maintain them in the neutral position.

Stabilization: Examiner grasps the metacarpals of the fingers to maintain them in the neutral position.

Substitution: Flexion at PIP and DIP joints may substitute the action of flexor digiti minimi (Figs. 6.197a and b).

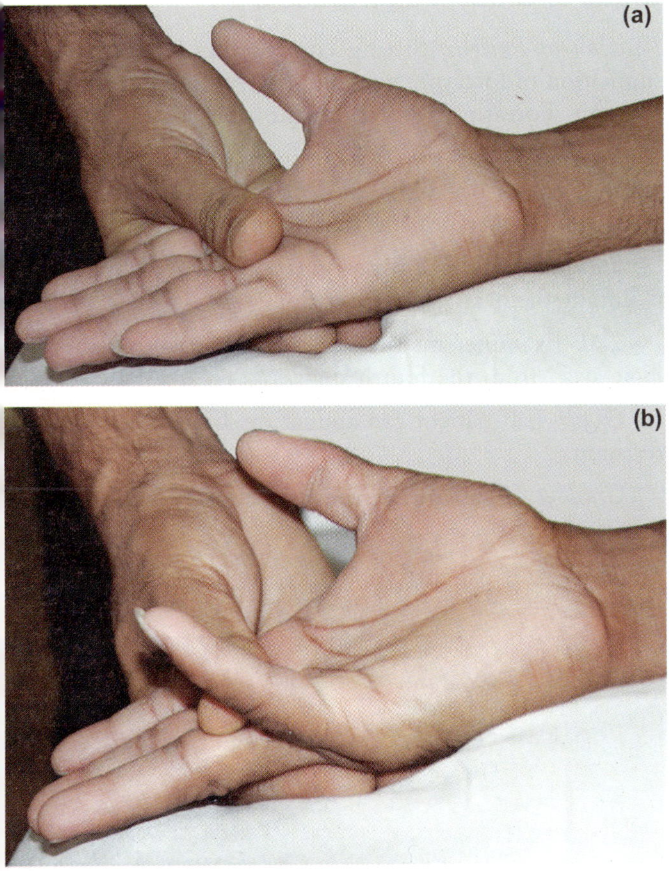

Figs. 6.197a and b: Testing of a flexor digiti minimi for grade 3

Test: Examiner instructs the patient to bring your little finger towards wrist joint. If patient is able to bring the little finger towards the ulnar side of the wrist joint it is considered grade 3.

Grade 4 and 5 (Good and Normal)

Position of Patient: Sitting, forearm supinated, wrist, MCP, PIP, DIP at neutral and thumb adducted.

Position of Examiner: Sitting, grasps first three metacarpals of the fingers with one hand to maintain them in the neutral position and places the index finger of other hand on the head of the fifth metacarpal bone for resistance.

Stabilization: Examiner grasps the metacarpals of the fingers to maintain them in the neutral position.

Substitution: Flexion at PIP and DIP joints may substitute the action of flexor digiti minimi (Fig. 6.198).

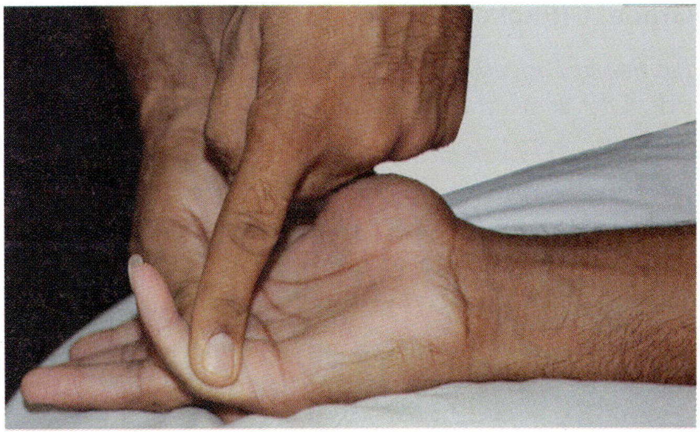

Fig. 6.198: Testing of flexor digiti minimi for grade 4 and 5

Test: Examiner instructs the patient to bring your little finger towards wrist joint.

Grade 4: If patient is able to complete the movement in the available range of motion against moderate resistance.

Grade 5: If patient is able to complete the movement in the available range of motion against maximal resistance.

Grade 2 (Poor)

Position of Patient: Sitting, forearm in midprone position, wrist, MCP, PIP, DIP at neutral and thumb adducted.

Position of Examiner: Sitting, grasps the first three metacarpals of the fingers to maintain them in the neutral position.

Stabilization: Examiner grasps the metacarpals of the fingers to maintain them in the neutral position.

Substitution: Flexion at PIP and DIP joints may substitute the action of flexor digiti minimi (Fig. 6.199).

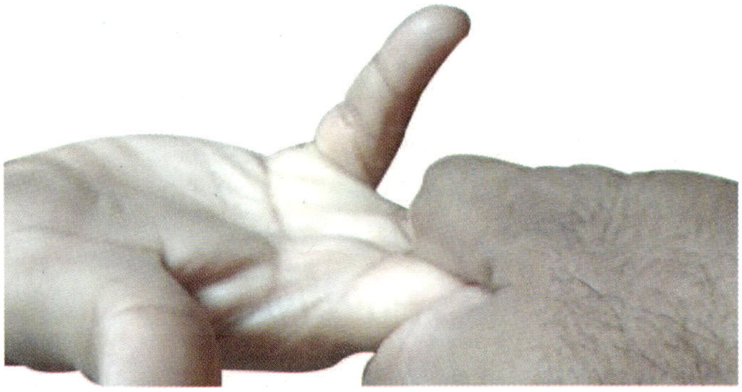

Fig. 6.199: Testing of flexor digiti minimi for grade 2

Test: Examiner instructs the patient to bring your little finger towards wrist joint. If patient is able to bring the little finger towards the ulnar side of the wrist joint it is considered grade 3.

Grade 1 (Flicker)

Position of Patient: Sitting, forearm supinated, wrist, MCP, PIP, DIP at neutral and thumb adducted.

Position of Examiner: Sitting, grasps the thumb and first three metacarpals of the fingers to maintain them in the neutral position. Examiner places his or her index finger on the palmar surface of the fifth metacarpal bone for palpation of contraction.

Stabilization: Examiner grasps the metacarpals of the fingers to maintain them in the neutral position (Fig. 6.200).

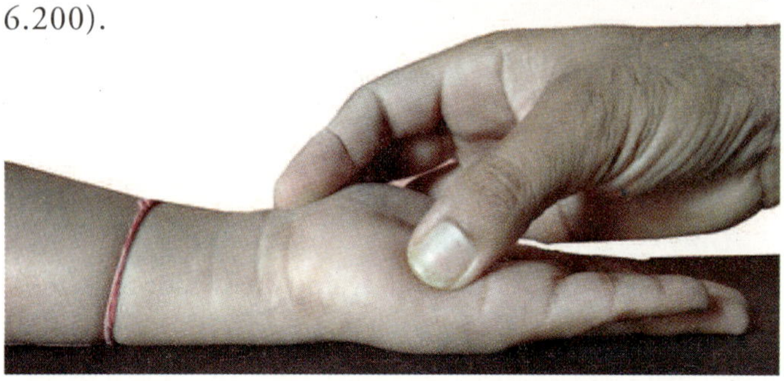

Fig. 6.200: Testing of a flexor digiti minimi for grade 1

Test: Examiner instructs the patient to try to bring your little finger towards your ulnar side of the wrist joint. If examiner feels contraction it is considered grade 1.

ABDUCTOR DIGITI MINIMI

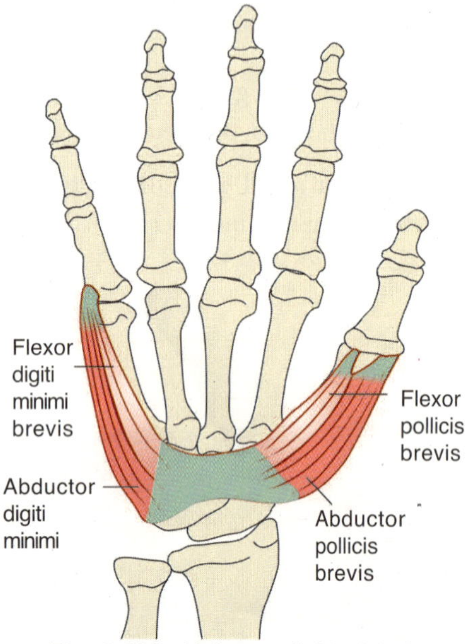

Fig. 6.201: Abductor digiti minimi

Abductor Digiti Minimi

Origin: Tendon of the flexor carpi ulnaris and the pisiform bone.

Insertion: There are two slips of the tendon. One slip inserts into the base of proximal phalanx of little finger on the ulnar side. The other slip inserts into the ulnar border of the extensor expansion.

Action: Abduction of the fifth metacarpophalangeal joint, assists in flexion of the fifth metacarpophalangeal joint.

Nerve Supply: Ulnar nerve, $C_{7,\ 8,}$ T_1 (Figs. 6.202 to 6.205).

Grade 3, Grade 4 and Grade 5

Position of Patient: Sitting comfortably in a chair with supination of forearm, wrist and MCP should be at neutral position. Forearm is placed on the table.

Position of Examiner: Examiner sits comfortably and grasps 2nd to 4th digits, and places index finger on the ulnar side of the fifth metacarpal bone for resistance.

Stabilization: Examiner grasps 2nd to 4th digits to maintain them at neutral position.

Test: Examiner instructs the patient to bring the fifth digit away from the fourth digit.

Grade 3: If patient can abduct the finger with minimal resistance.

Grade 4: If patient can abduct the finger with moderate resistance.

Grade 5: If patient can abduct the finger with maximal resistance.

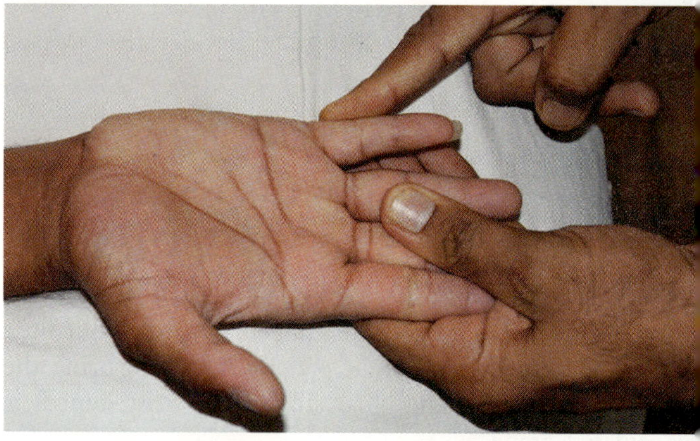

Fig. 6.202: Testing of abductor digiti minimi for grade 3

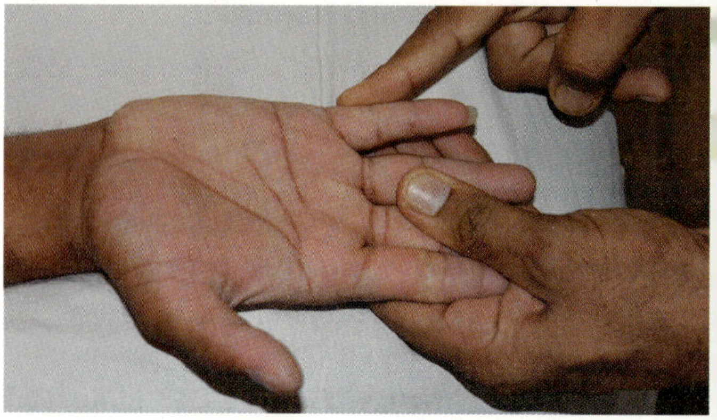

Fig. 6.203: Testing of abductor digiti minimi for grade 4 and 5

Grade 2

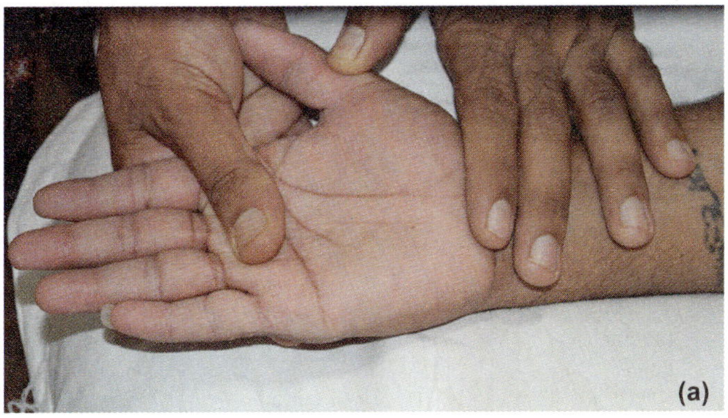

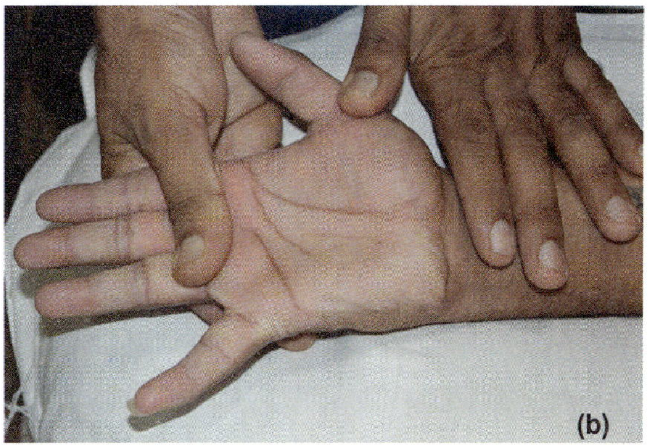

Figs. 6.204a and b: Testing of abductor digiti minimi for grade 2. Patient is placed in a sitting position with an appropriate back support. Forearm is placed on the table with pronation. The wrist and MCP joints should be at neutral. Examiner grasps the 2nd to 4th digits to stabilize and maintain them at neutral position and instructs the patient to bring the fifth digit away from the fourth digit in the gravity eliminated plane

Grade 3

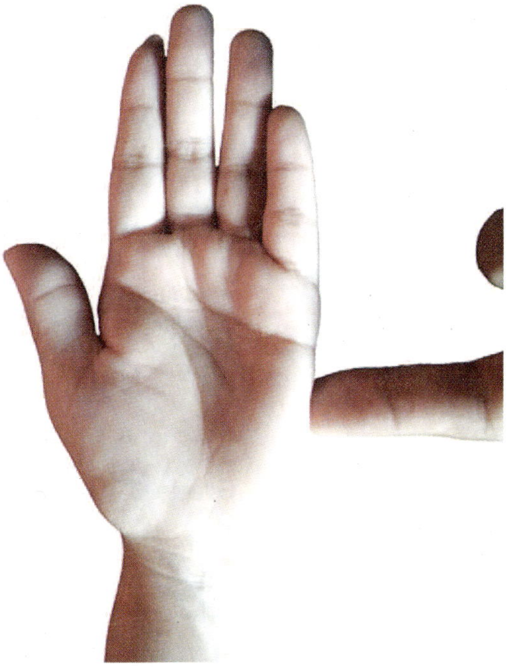

Fig. 6.205: Testing of abductor digiti minimi for grade 1. Patient sits comfortably in a chair and places dorsum of hand on the table with forearm pronated. Examiner places tip of index finger on the ulnar side of middle of fifth metacarpal bone for palpation of muscle. Examiner instructs the patient to try to bring the fifth digit away from fourth digit. Grade 1 is considered if examiner feels contraction

MANUAL MUSCLE TESTING FOR LOWER EXTREMITY

TESTING OF HIP FLEXORS – ILIACUS AND PSOAS MAJOR

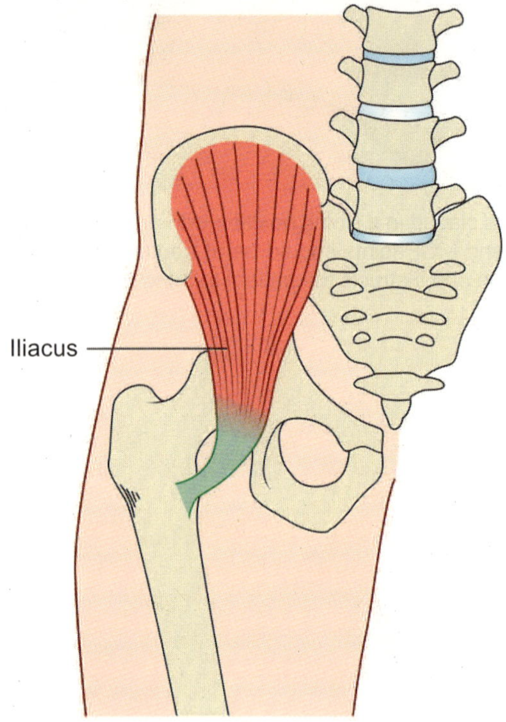

Fig. 6.206: Iliacus muscle origin and insertion

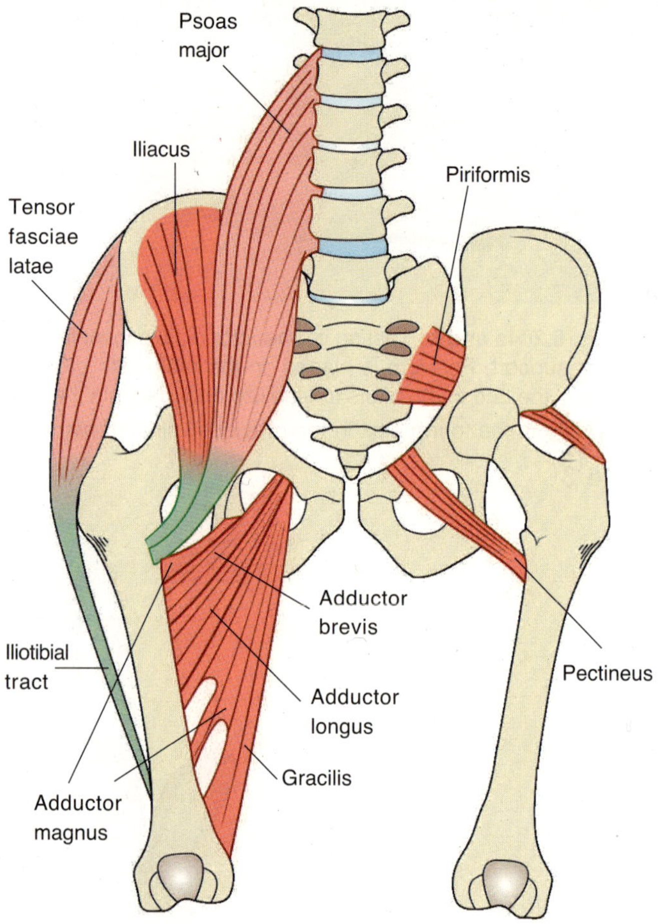

Fig. 6.207: Psoas major muscle origin and insertion

Iliacus

Origin: Superior two third of the iliac fossa, internal lip of the iliac crest, iliolumbar and ventral sacroiliac ligaments and ala of the sacrum.

Insertion: Lateral side of the tendon of psoas major and dust distal to the lesser trochanter.

Action: Flexion of the hip joint.

Nerve Supply: L_1, L_2, L_3 and L_4.

Psoas Major

Origin: Ventral surface of the transverse process of all lumbar vertebrae, side of the bodies and corresponding intervertebral disks of the last thoracic and all lumbar vertebrae, and the membranous arches that extend over the sides of the bodies of the lumbar vertebrae.

Insertion: Lesser trochanter of the femur.

Nerve Supply: Lumbar plexus, L1, L2, L3 and L4.

Action: Flexion of hip joint.

Grade 3

Position of Patient: High sitting with an appropriate back support to prevent backward leaning. Patient may be asked to hold the edges of the couch to prevent backward leaning.

Position of Examiner: The examiner stands at the side of the patient and places one hand on the top of the iliac crest to prevent trunk movements. The patient is asked to flex the hip joint with the knee flexion upto the chest.

Stabilization: Examiner places his or her hand on to the same side of the pelvis to prevent trunk movements. The focus is also made on the hip joint movement that should occur in the sagittal plane. The tight tensor fascia lata and Sartorius may pull the thigh towards the scaption during the flexion (Figs. 6.208a and b).

Test: The patient is instructed to lift the knee joint up towards the chest. The complete range of motion of hip without any external support is considered as grade 3. If

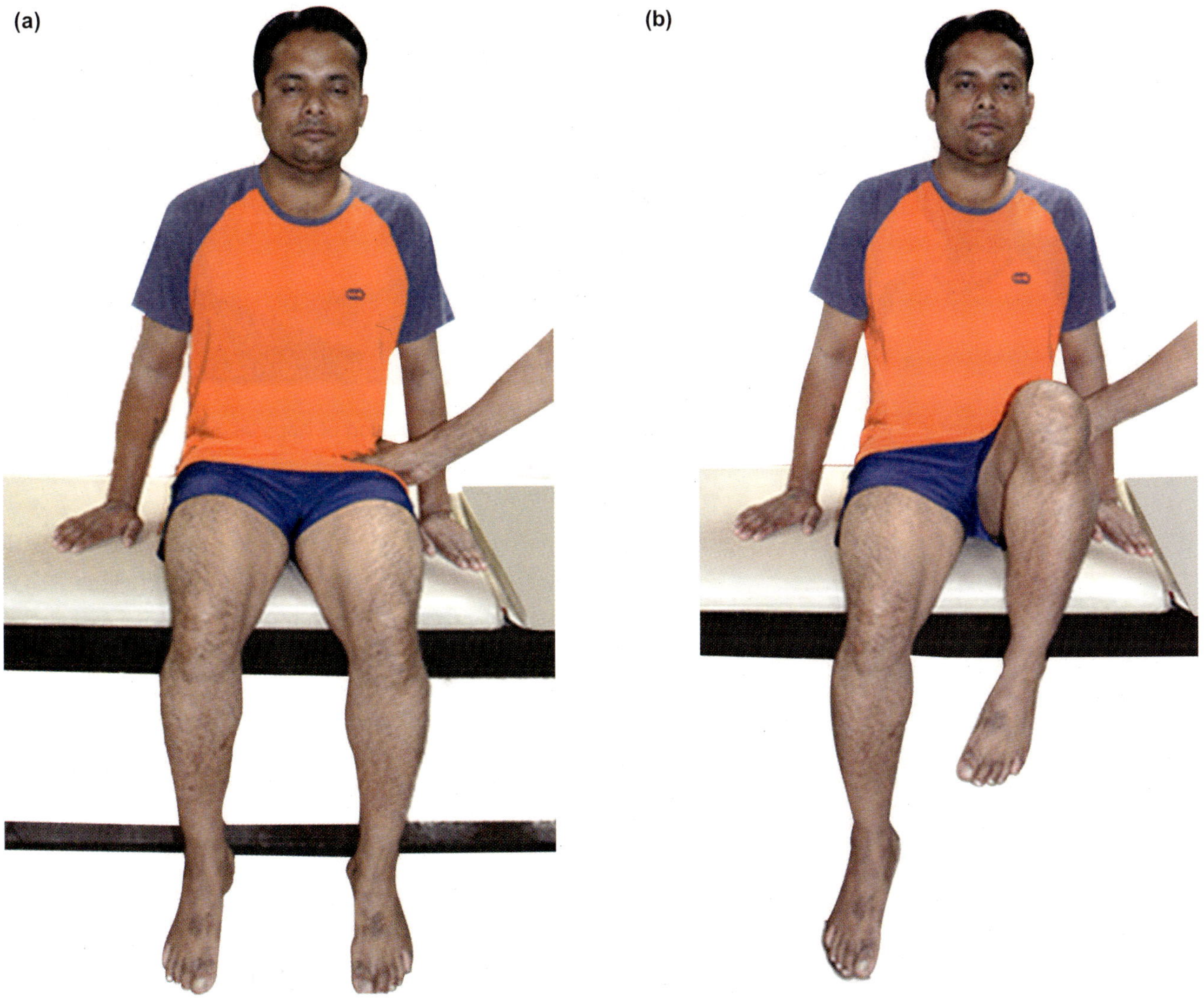

Figs. 6.208a and b: Testing of iliopsoas muscles for grade 3. Patient is placed in a high sitting. He may hold the edges of the couch to prevent backward leaning. Examiner stands at the side of the patient and places one hand on the top of the iliac crest to prevent trunk movements

patient initiates the movement and flexes the hip joint upto mid range may be considered as grade 3^{-} (three minus). If patient completes the range upto the chest against the gravity is considered grade 3.

Grade 4 and 5

Position of Patient: High sitting with an appropriate back support to prevent backward leaning. Patient may be asked to hold the edges of the couch to prevent backward leaning and to stabilize the trunk.

Position of Examiner: Examiner stands at the side of the patient and places one hand on the top of the iliac crest to prevent trunk movements. The examiner places other hand on the suprapatellar region (distal thigh) of the same side which is being tested to apply resistance during the hip flexion.

Stabilization: Examiner places his or her hand on to the same side of the iliac crest to prevent trunk movements. The focus is also made on the hip joint movement that should occur in the sagittal plane. The tight tensor fascia lata and Sartorius may pull the thigh towards the scaption during the flexion (Fig. 6.209).

Test: Patient is instructed to flex the hip joint with the knee flexion upto the chest.

Grade 4: If patient completes full hip flexion upto the chest against strong to moderate resistance is considered grade 4.

Grade 5: If patient completes movement in the available range of motion against the maximal resistance in the sagittal plane is considered grade 5.

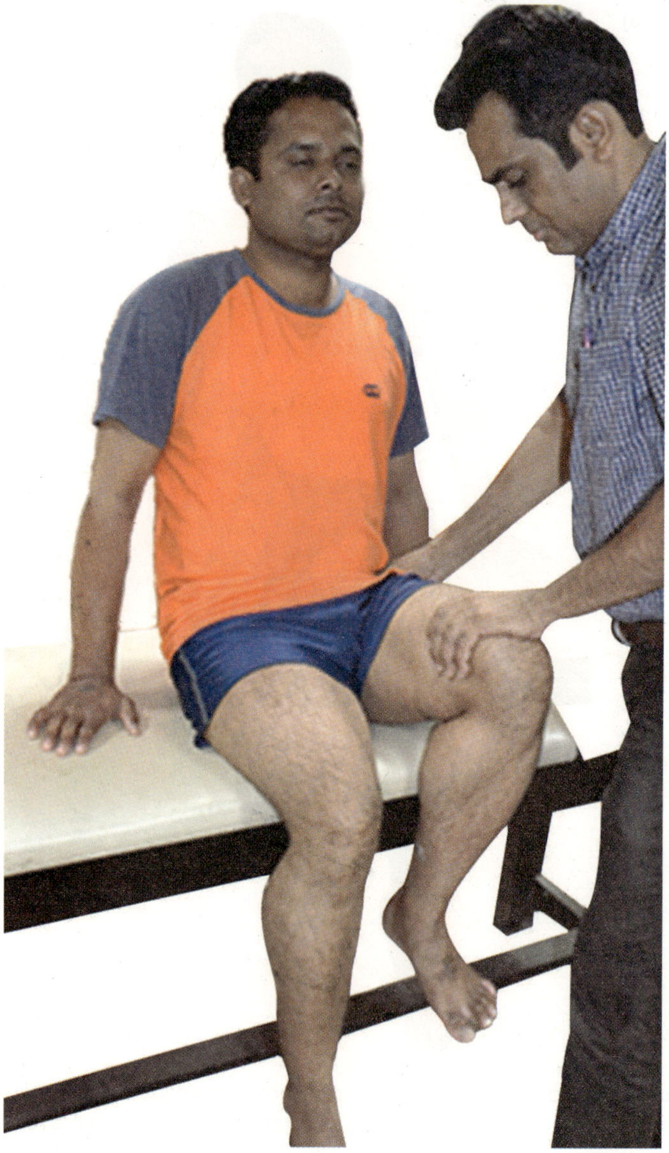

Fig. 6.209: Testing of iliopsoas muscles for grade 4 and 5. High sitting with an appropriate back support to prevent backward leaning. Patient may be asked to hold the edges of the couch to prevent backward leaning and stabilize the trunk. Examiner stands at the side of the patient and places one hand on the top of the iliac crest to prevent trunk movements. Examiner places other hand on the supra-patellar region (just above the knee joint) of the same side which is being tested to apply resistance

Grade 1

Position of Patient: Side lying or supine examiner stands behind the patient or at the side and places thumb just below the superior two third of the iliac fossa. The patient is asked to take the knee towards the chest. Attempt to flex the hip joint or taking the knee towards the chest would cause contraction and examiner would appreciate a contraction (Fig. 6.210).

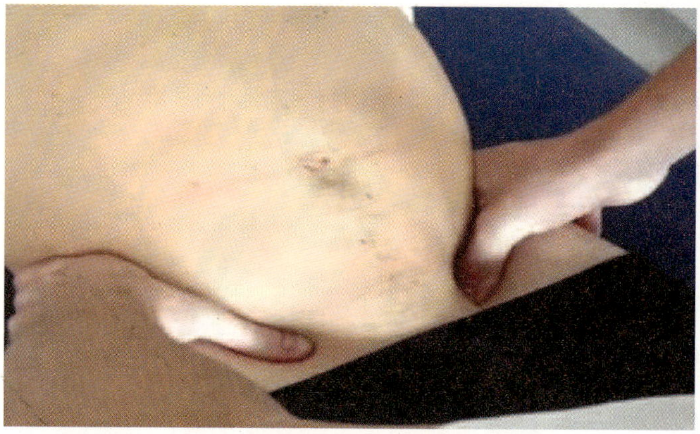

Fig. 6.210: Palpation of iliopsoas muscle for grade 1

Grade 2

Position of Patient: Side lying, with one hand under the head. The lower leg is flexed for the base of support.

Position of Examiner: Stands behind the patient and places left hand at the lateral pelvis and the right hand under the medial aspect of leg and knee joint. Patient is asked to flex the hip with knee flexion while the examiner's right hand keeps the leg above the opposite leg (left) to avoid friction or movement direct over the left leg. The examiner's right hand must not help in flexing the leg.

Stabilization: The placement of examiner's left hand on the patient's lateral iliac crest should prevent trunk rotation, anterior, posterior and lateral movement of the pelvis (Fig. 6.211).

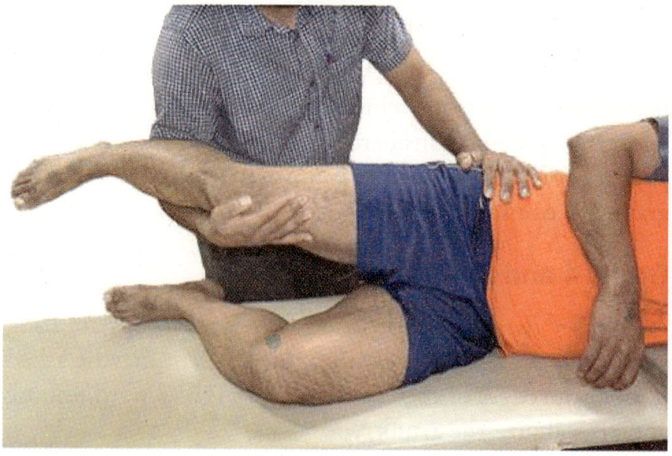

Fig. 6.211: Testing of iliopsoas muscles for grade 2. Position of patient – Side lying, with one hand under the head. Lower leg is flexed for the base of the support. Stands behind the patient and places left hand at the lateral pelvis and the right hand under the medial aspect of leg and knee joint

Test: The subject is instructed to bring the knee joint anterior parallel to the floor. Completion of flexion in full range in gravity eliminated position is considered grade 2. Attempting flexion upto mid range should be considered less than grade 2 which may be stated as 2^- (two minus).

ISOLATED TESTING OF RIGHT HIP FLEXORS – PSOAS MAJOR

Grade 3

Position of Patient: Supine.

Position of Examiner: The examiner stands at the opposite side of the leg and places one hand on the left pelvis to stabilize and prevent trunk movements.

Stabilization: Examiner stabilizes the pelvis to prevent trunk rotation.

Test: Patient is asked to flex the hip joint while keeping the knee at the full extension. Complete range of motion in the sagittal plane is considered grade three and incomplete range upto the mid range is considered grade 3^- (Three minus) (Fig. 6.212).

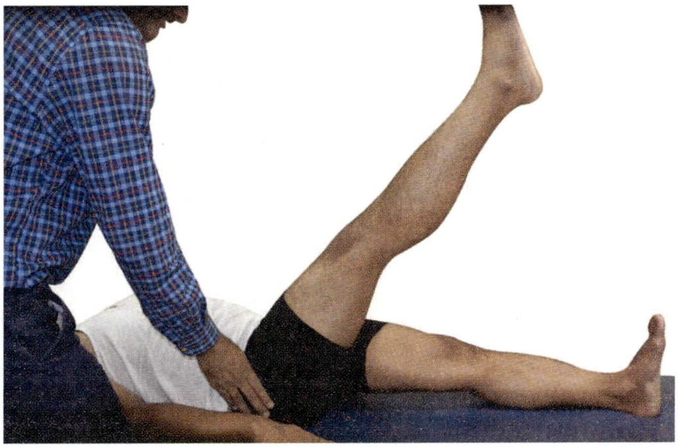

Fig. 6.212: Testing of psoas major muscles for grade 3

Grade 4 and 5

Position of Patient: Supine.

Position of Examiner: The examiner stands at the opposite side of leg which is being tested. Examiner places right hand on the left side of pelvis and left hand over the suprapatellar region of the right knee joint (distal thigh).

Stabilization: Examiner stabilizes the pelvis with the right hand to prevent trunk rotation.

Test: Patient is asked to flex the hip joint as much as possible while the knee remains extended (Fig. 6.213).

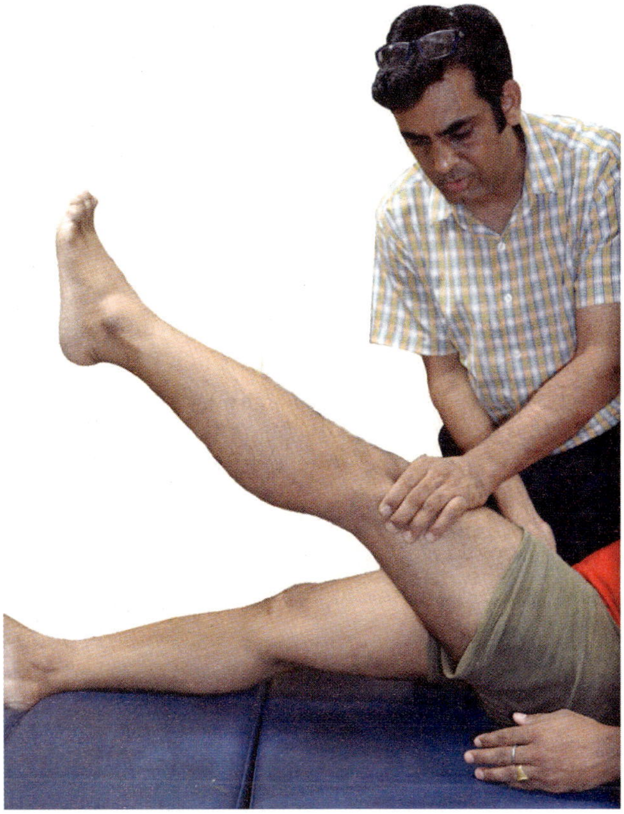

Fig. 6.213: Testing of psoas major muscles for grade 4 and 5

Grade 4: If patient completes movement in the available range of motion against strong to moderate resistance is considered grade 4.

Grade 5: If patient completes movement in the available range of motion against the maximal resistance it is considered grade 5.

Grade 1

The position of patient and therapist for the grade 1 (psoas major) remains same as mentioned for the iliopsoas.

Grade 2

Position of Patient: Side lying with the knee extended.

Position of Examiner: The examiner stands behind the patient and places left hand on the iliac crest and right hand under the medial surface of the leg and knee.

Stabilization: The pelvis is stabilized to prevent trunk movements.

Test: Patient is instructed to flex the hip joint with knee extension in the available range of motion towards the chest. The examiner should keep the leg above the left extremity but should not facilitate the movement.

Weakness: The weakness of the iliopsoas is not very common as it is a tonic muscle, however; injury to the lumbar plexus can cause paralysis or weakness of the muscle that result severe disability. The patient with iliopsoas weakness find difficulty in stair climbing, walking up an incline, getting up from a reclining position, and bringing the trunk forward in the sitting position preliminary to rising from chair.

Shortening: The shortening of the iliopsoas is very common that results in increasing lordosis of the lumbar spine and anterior tilting of the pelvis. Shortening is often bilateral. The shortening of the iliopsoas is also associated with the tightness of the quadriceps muscles and lengthening of the gluteus maximus and hamstrings muscles. The patients with iliopsoas and quadriceps shortening or contracture complaint pain in the knee joint as the patella moves slightly superior to the trochlear groove that puts excessive pressure on the suprapatellar region.

The patients with short iliopsoas walk with the lumbar lordosis. Normally after heel strike the hip joint goes into extension from 30° flexion to 20° extension. The short iliopsoas does not allow hip joint to extend, therefore, the hip joint remains flexed. The patient hyperextends the lumbar spine to retain his head over the pelvis. The lordosis increases the posterior excursion on the limb to permit a long stride. Patients with bilateral hip flexors often exhibit lower crossed syndrome (Figs. 6.214a and b).

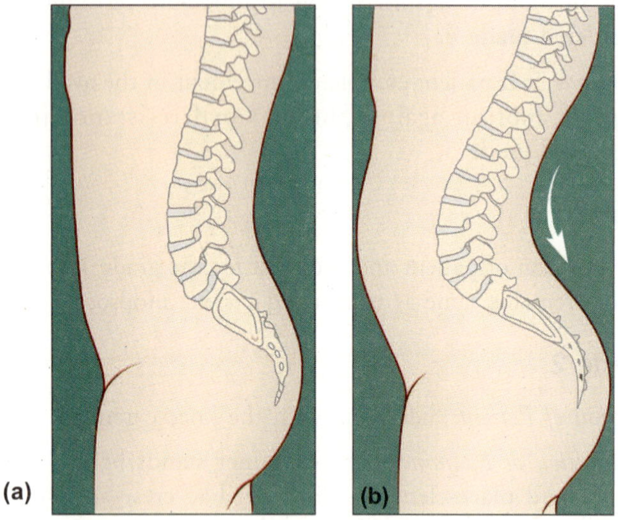

Figs. 6.214a and b: (a) Normal lumbar spine lordosis, (b) Excessive lumbar spine lordosis due to shortening of iliopsoas muscles

Iliopsoas Length Testing

To test the iliopsoas muscle the physical therapist often do Thomas test. To test the shortening or flexibility of the left iliopsoas muscles the patient is placed on supine position with the knees flexed to 90 degrees which hang at the end of the tables or couch. The examiner may stand at the side of the leg which is being tested. Patient is asked to flex the hip and knee joints of the contralateral side passively, i.e., right hip and knee. The flexion of the hip joint flattens the lumbar spine and sacrum on the couch. Normally when the right hip joint is flexed with the knee joint, the right innominate rotates posteriorly and the left innominate remains neutral therefore, the left hip joint should remain neutral and the thigh remains on the couch or on the edge of the table (Fig. 6.215a). If the left thigh goes off the table it indicates shortening of the iliopsoas muscles (Fig. 6.215b).

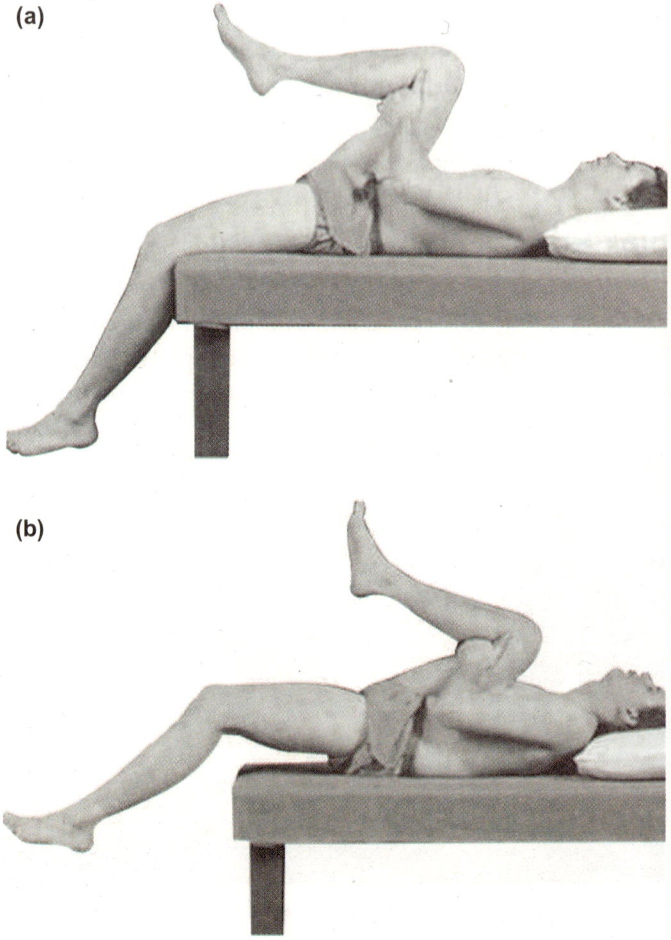

Figs. 6.215a and b: Testing of right hip flexors (Thomas test) (a) Normal iliopsoas, (b) Shortening of left iliopsoas–thigh raises from couch. Positive Thomas test

When hip is flexed with knee flexion, the sacrum of the patients with excessive back flexibility no longer remains flats on the table. The result is that the one joint hip flexors, which are normal in length, appear to be tight.

SARTORIUS MUSCLE TESTING

Origin: Anterosuperior iliac spine and superior half of the notch just distal to the spine.

Insertion: Proximal part of the medial surface of the tibia near the anterior border.

Nerve Supply: Femoral nerve (L_2–L_4).

Action: Flexion, abduction and lateral rotation of the hip joint (Fig. 6.216).

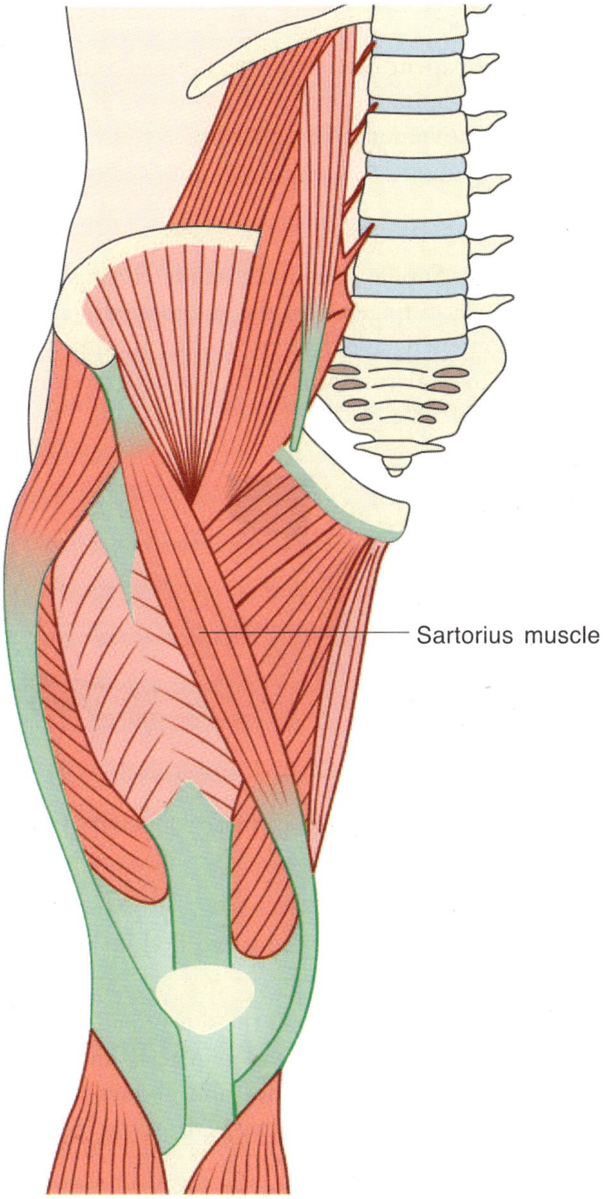

Fig. 6.216: Sartorius muscle origin and insertion

Grade 3 (Fair)

Position of Patient: Short sitting, with thighs on the couch and legs hang freely on the edge. The hands are placed on the table to provide support and stabilization. The back may be supported.

Position of the Examiner: The examiner may stand at the side of the patient which is being tested.

Stabilization: Trunk to prevent posterior or lateral bending and rotation (Fig. 6.217).

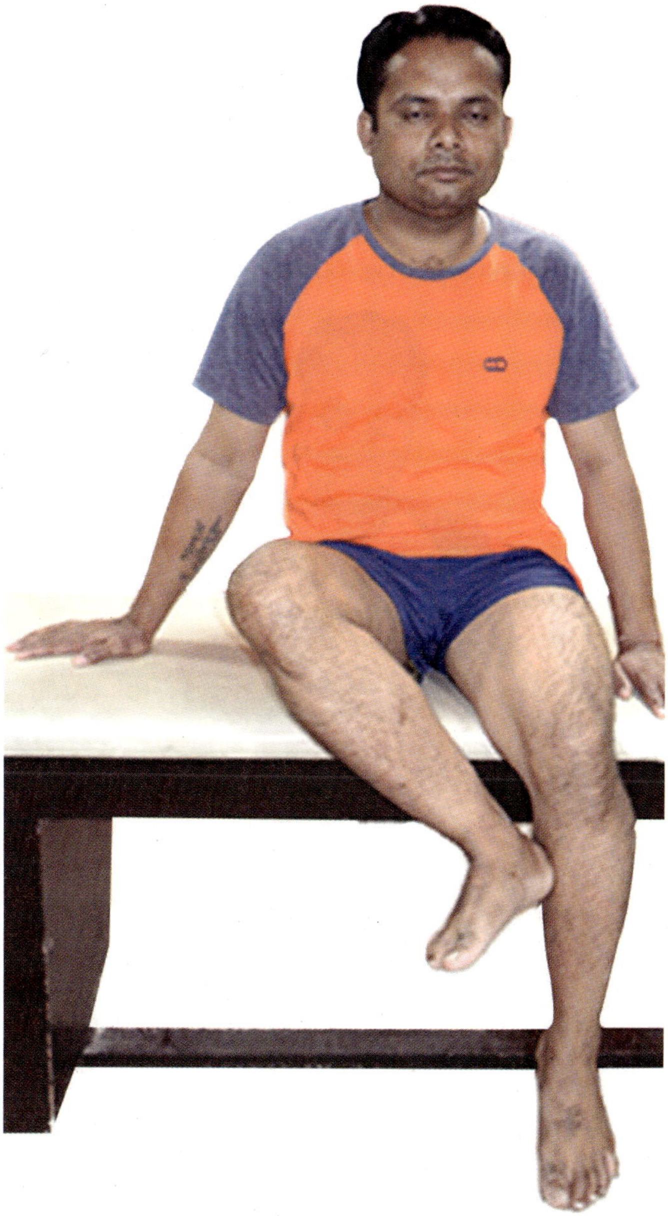

Fig. 6.217: Testing of sartorius muscle for grade 3. Position of patient – Short sitting, with thighs on the couch and knees hangs freely on the edge. The hands are placed on the table to provide support and stabilization

Test: The examiner demonstrates the direction of movement to the patient before testing it. The patient is instructed to flex, abduct, and externally rotate the hip joint. If patient completes movement in the available range of motion is considered grade 3.

Grade 4 and 5 (Good and Normal)

Position of Patient: Short sitting, with thighs on the couch and legs hang freely on the edge. Hands are placed on the table to provide support and stabilization. The back should be supported.

Position of Examiner: The examiner either stands or sits at the side of the leg which is being tested. Examiner demonstrates the movements to the patient before testing the muscle. Examiner places one hand on the anterolateral aspect of the knee joint and other hand is placed on the anteromedial aspect of the distal leg.

Stabilization: Trunk to prevent posterior or lateral bending and rotation (Fig. 6.218).

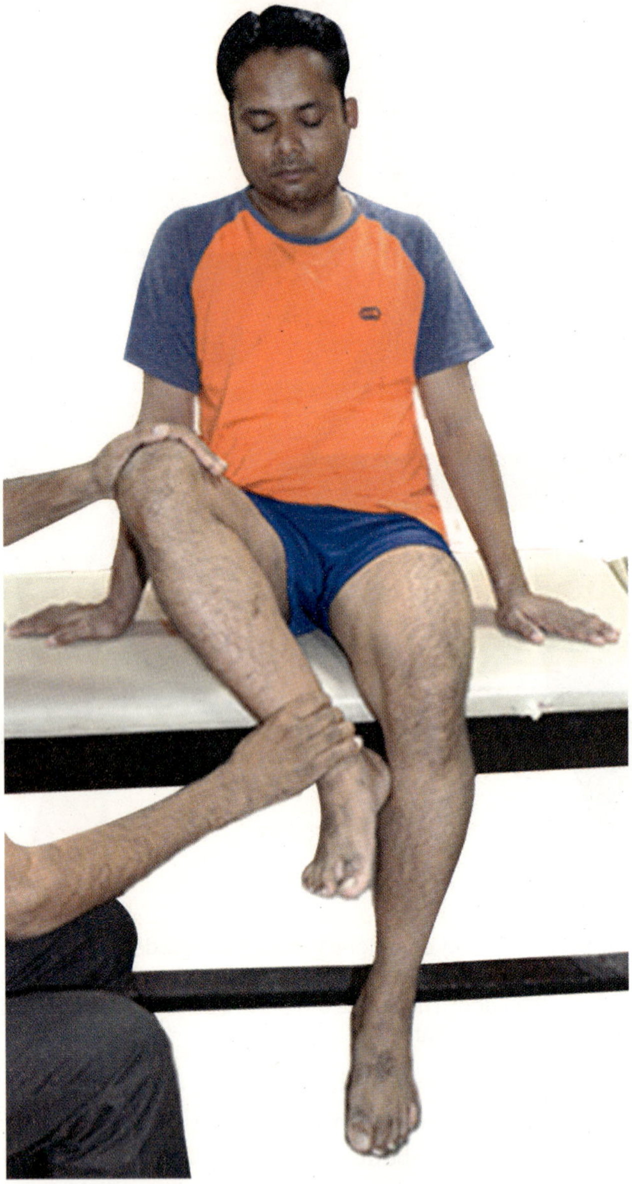

Fig. 6.218: Testing of sartorius muscle for grade 4 and 5. Position of patient – Short sitting, with thighs on the couch and legs hang freely on the edge. Hands are placed on the table to provide support and stabilization. The examiner sits comfortably on the stool at the side of the leg which is being tested and places one hand on the top of the knee joint and grasps the distal leg with other hand

Test: Examiner instructs the patient to raise the knee joint up and outwards with the knee bending.

Grade 4: Patient is asked to flex, abduct and laterally rotate the hip joint against the moderate to heavy resistance for the grade 4. If the patient completes the range of motions against strong to moderate resistance is considered grade 4.

Grade 5: The patient is asked to flex, abduct and rotate the hip laterally against the maximal resistance. If patient completes the movements in full range is considered grade 5.

Grade 1

Position of Patient: Supine. Examiner stands at the side of the patient and places fingers over the antero medial aspect of the thigh. Patient is asked to try to flex the hip with abduction and lateral rotation. A flicker contraction is considered grade 1 (Fig. 6.219).

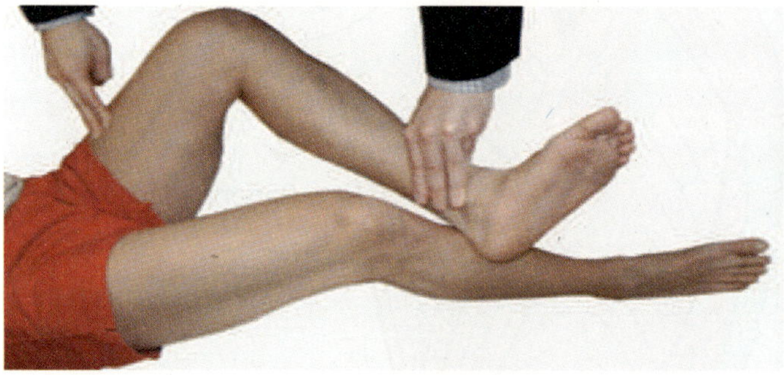

Fig. 6.219: Palpation of sartorius muscle for grade 1

Grade 2

Position of Patient: Supine with the tested heel on the shin of contralateral leg.

Position of Therapist: Standing at the side of patient with leaning slightly forward. One hand is placed under the knee joint and proximal calf to flex and abduct the hip joint. Other hand of the examiner grasps the distal leg (Fig. 6.220).

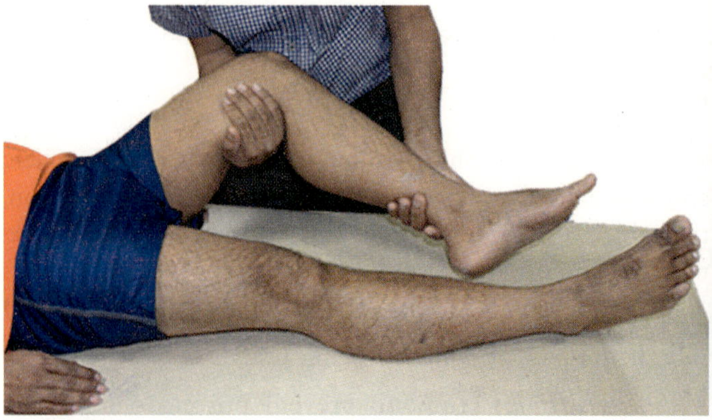

Fig. 6.220: Testing of sartorius muscle for grade 2

Test: Patient is asked to slide the heel up towards the knee and hip of the tested side on the contralateral leg. If examiner ables to feel the contraction of the muscle it is graded 01. If there is no contraction it is graded zero.

TENSOR FASCIA LATA STRENGTH TESTING

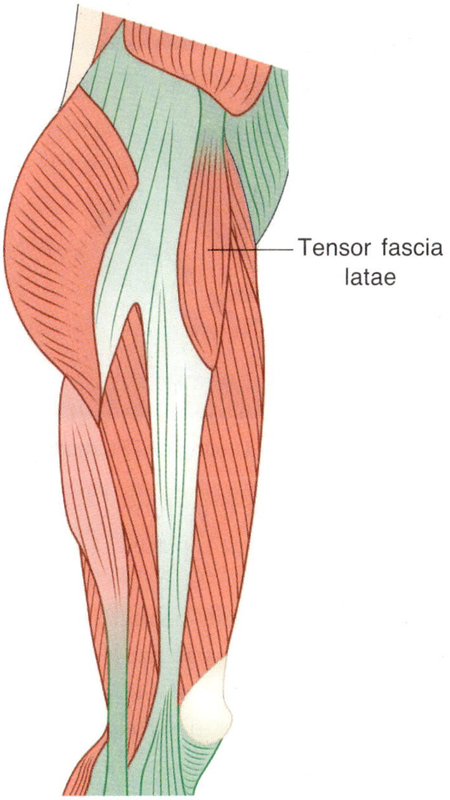

Fig. 6.221: Tensor fascia lata muscle origin and insertion

Grade 3 (Good)

Position of Patient: Short sitting with thighs on the couch and legs hang freely on the edge. The hands hold the couch for stabilization and support.

Position of Examiner: Examiner stands at the side of the leg which is being tested and demonstrates the movements to the patient (Fig. 6.222).

Test: Patient is asked to take the knee away from midline with flexion and abduction of hip joint. If patient completes the range of motion is considered grade 3.

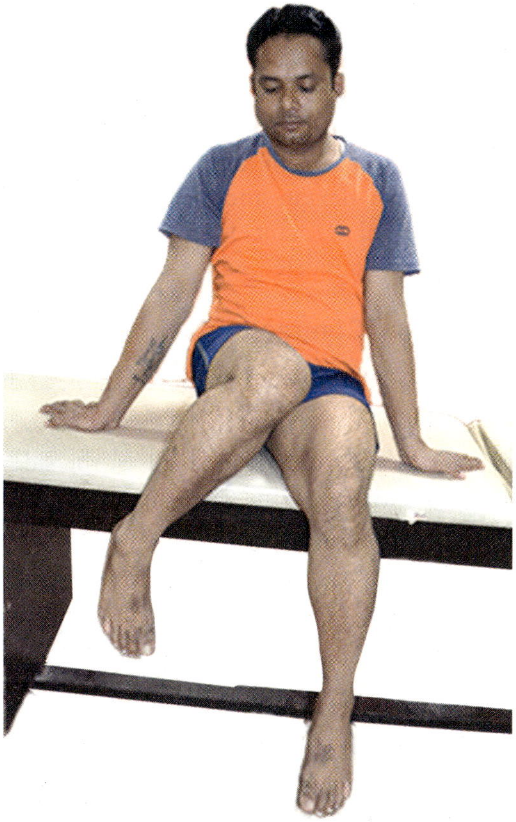

Fig. 6.222: Testing of TFL for grade 3

Grade 4 and 5 (Good and Normal)

Position of Patient: Short sitting with thighs on the couch and legs hang freely on the edge. The hands hold the couch for stabilization and support.

Position of Examiner: Examiner stands at the side which is being tested and places one hand on the anterolateral aspect of the knee joint and other hand on the anterolateral aspect of the distal leg (Fig. 6.223).

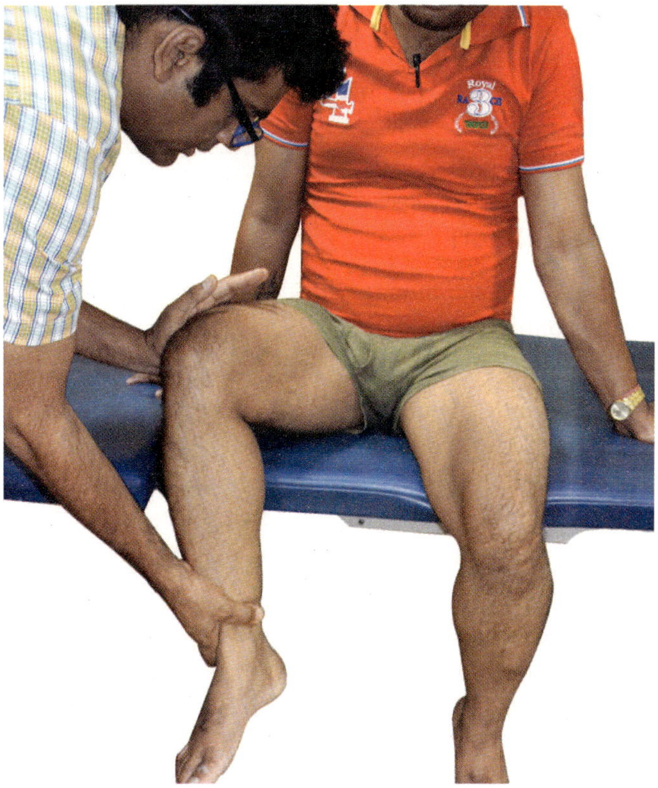

Fig. 6.223: Testing of TFL for grade 4 and 5

Grade 4: Patient is asked to take the lower leg away from midline with flexion and abduction of hip joint. If patient completes the range of motion against moderate resistance is considered grade 4.

Grade 5: The patient is asked to take the lower leg away from midline with flexion and abduction of hip joint against the maximal resistance. If patient completes the range of motion is considered grade 5.

Grade 1 (Flicker Contraction)

Position of Patient: Supine with slight flexion, abduction and medial rotation.

Position of Therapist: Examiner stands at the side which is being tested and places one hand on the anterolateral aspect of the knee and other hand over the muscle just below the origin of it. The patient is asked to try to flex, abduct and medially rotate the hip joint while the examiner palpates the contraction of the muscle just below its origin. If examiner ables to palpate the contraction it is considered grade 1. If examiner feels no contraction it is considered grade zero (Fig. 6.224).

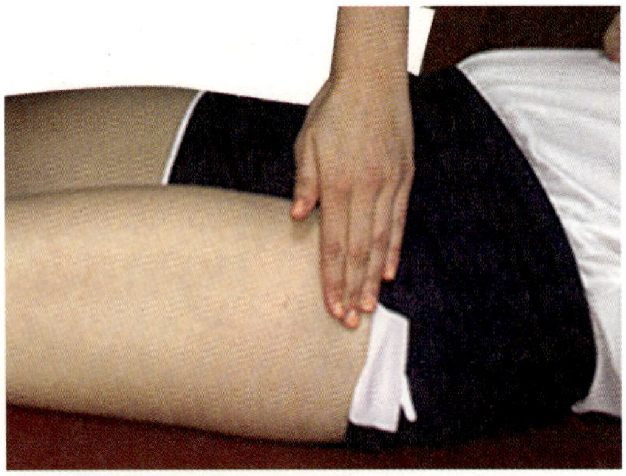

Fig. 6.224: Palpation of TFL muscle for grade 1

Grade 2 (Poor)

Position of Patient: Supine with the tested leg over the shin of the contralateral leg.

Position of Examiner: The examiner stands at the side of the leg which is being tested. Examiner demonstrates the movements before testing the muscle. Patient is asked to slide the heel over the shin of the contralateral leg with the knee away from midline. If patient completes the range of motion is considered grade 2 (Figs. 6.225a and b).

Shortening: Tensor fascia lata flexes, abducts and rotates the hip joint internally. Shortening of TFL produces flexion and abduction of the hip joint. Any attempt to bring the leg into adduction or extension produces anterior tilting of the pelvis. In a long standing cases there is a marked anterior tilting of the pelvis in standing and in supine position.

(a)

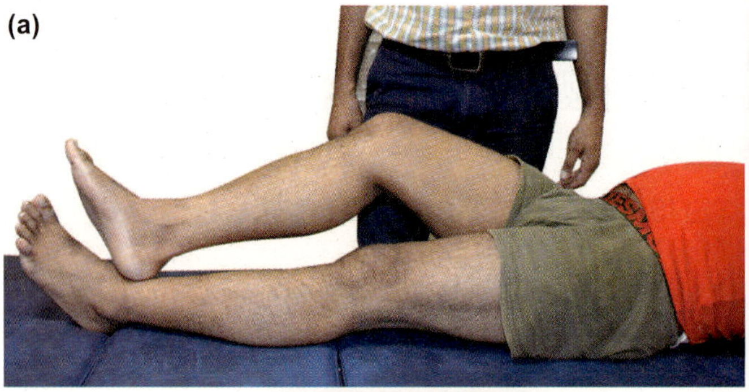

(b)

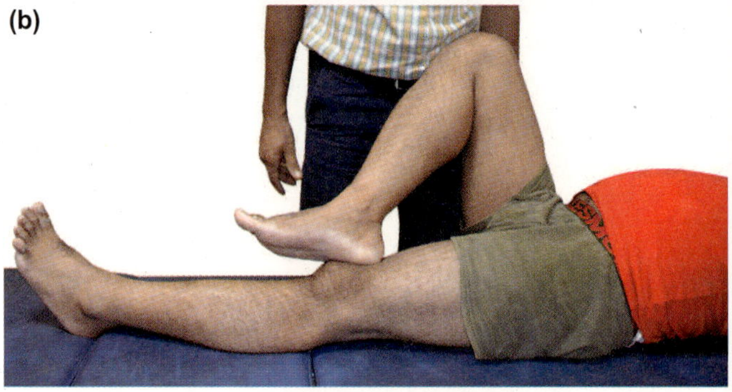

Figs. 6.225a and b: Testing of TFL muscle for grade 2

Ober's Sign: The test is performed to test the flexibility of the TFL muscle. Patient is placed in a side lying position. The affected side which is being examined is placed uppermost. Examiner stands behind the patient and places one hand over the pelvis to stabilize it and other hand grasps the knee joint while the leg of the patient remains on the examiner hand. Examiner passively abducts and extends the hip joint. Examiner removes the hand from the knee while lower leg remain in the hand of examiner to maintain hip flexion and abduction and allows the knee to drop downward. The knee joint drops on the contralateral knee joint in the normal cases, however, it remains suspended in the air if the tensor fascia latae is contracted or tight. Weakness of TFL is not common unless and until there is a nerve injury (Fig. 6.226).

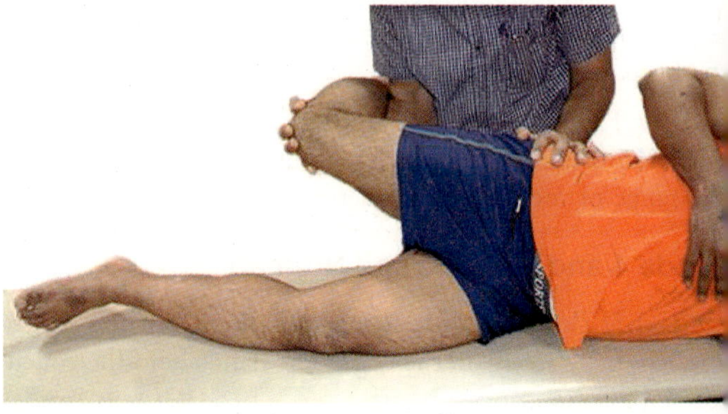

Fig. 6.226: Testing the length of TFL (Ober's sign)

GLUTEUS MAXIMUS STRENGTH TESTING WITH HAMSTRING MUSCLES

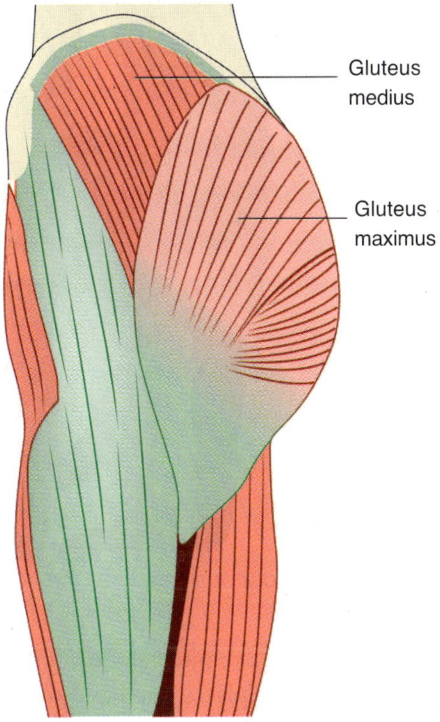

Fig. 6.227: Gluteus maximus muscle origin and insertion

Origin: Posterior gluteal line of the ilium and portion of the bone superior and posterior to it, posterior surface of the sacrum, side of the coccyx, aponeurosis of the erector spinae, sacrotuberous ligament and gluteal aponeurosis.

Insertion: Larger proximal portion and superficial fibers of the distal portion of the muscles into the iliotibial tract of the fascia lata. Deep fibers of the distal portion into the gluteal tuberosity of the femur.

Action: Extension and external rotation of the hip joint. Lower fibers assist in adduction of the hip joint; upper fibers assist in abduction. The attachment of the gluteus muscle fibers with the tensor fascia lata helps in stabilizing the knee joint in extension.

Grade 3

Position of Patient: Prone with the knees extended.

Position of Examiner: Examiner stands opposite to the side which is being tested and places one hand on the pelvis to stabilize and prevent trunk movements. Patient is asked to extend the hip joint against the gravity in the sagittal plane. If patient completes full range of motion in the sagittal place it is considered grade 3 (Fig. 6.228).

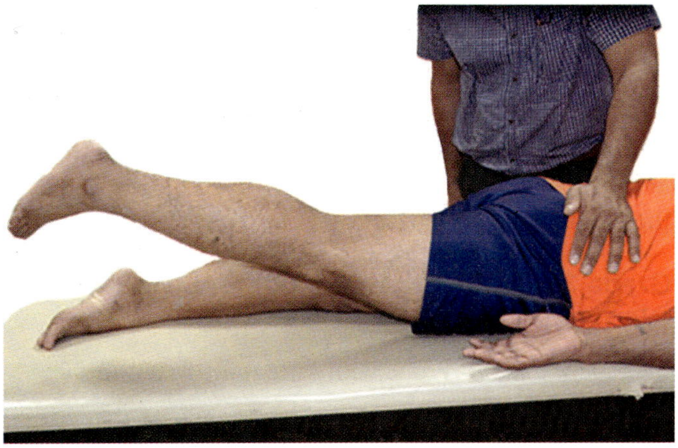

Fig. 6.228: Testing of gluteus maximus muscle for grade 3

Grade 4 (Good) and Grade 5 (Normal)

Position of Patient: Prone with the knees extended.

Position of Examiner: Examiner stands opposite the side which is being tested and places one hand over the pelvis to stabilize and prevent trunk movements, the other hand is placed on the posterior aspect of distal thigh for resistance. Patient is asked to extend the hip joint with the knee extended while the therapist stabilizes the pelvis and applies strong to moderate resistance against the movement at the posterior distal thigh (Fig. 6.229).

Grade 4: If patient completes the movement against the gravity with strong to moderate resistance is considered grade 4.

Grade 5: If patient completes movement against gravity with maximal resistance is considered grade 5.

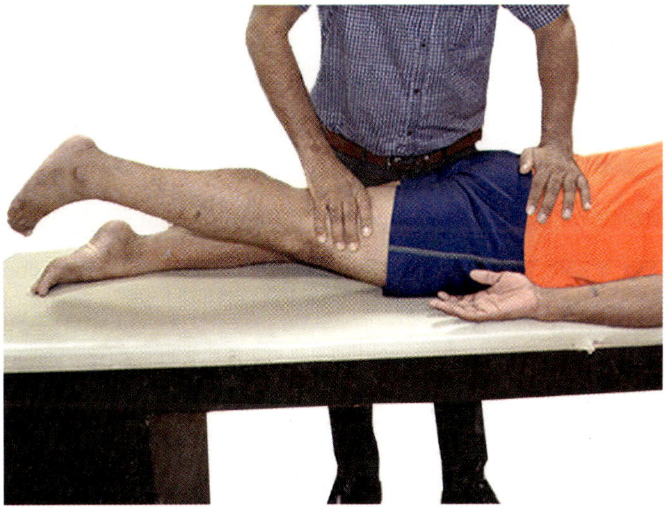

Fig. 6.229: Testing of gluteus maximus muscle for grade 4 and 5

ISOLATE GLUTEUS MAXIMUS STRENGTH TEST

Gluteus maximus muscle is tested isolated with the knee joint flexed to 90 degrees to eliminate the action of hamstring muscles. The flexion of knee joint eliminates the action of hamstring muscles.

Grade 3 (Fair), Grade 4 (Good) and Grade 5 (Normal)

Position of Patient: Prone with knee joint flexed to 90°.

Position of Examiner: Examiner stands at the side of patient which is being tested, and places one hand on the pelvis to stabilize and prevent trunk movement and places other hand on the posterior distal thigh to apply resistance.

Grade 3: Patient is asked to extend the hip joint with the knee flexion up to full range against the gravity in sagittal plane. If patient completes full range against the gravity is considered grade 3.

Grade 4: If patient completes the movement against the gravity with strong to moderate resistance is considered grade 4.

Grade 5: If patient completes movement against gravity with maximal resistance is considered grade 5 (Fig. 6.230).

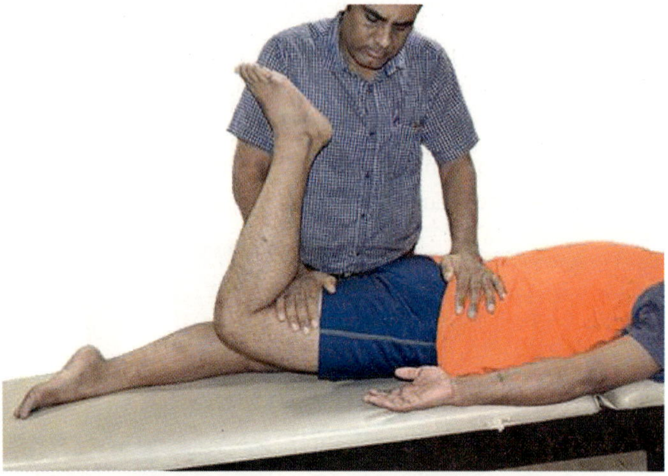

Fig. 6.230: Testing of gluteus maximus muscle with knee flexion for grade 4 and 5. Flexion of knee joint eliminates the action of hamstring muscles

Alternate Position for Grade 4 and 5

The head and trunk of the patient remains on the couch, and hip and legs out of the couch, so there is flexion at the hip joints. The position eliminates action of hamstrings. Patient is instructed to extend the hip against the resistance (Fig. 6.231).

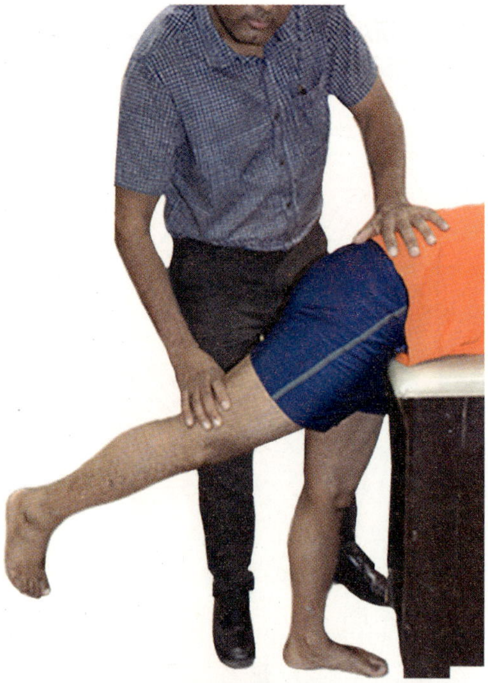

Fig. 6.231: Testing of gluteus maximus muscle for grade 4 and 5

Grade 1 (Trace)

Position of Patient: Prone with the knees extended.

Position of Examiner: Examiner stands opposite the side which is being tested and places one hand over the belly of the gluteus maximus muscle (upper and lower fibers). The patient is asked to extend the hip joint with the knee extension. If examiner feels a contraction over the upper and lower fibers of gluteus maximus it is considered grade 1 (Figs. 6.232a and b).

(a)

(b)

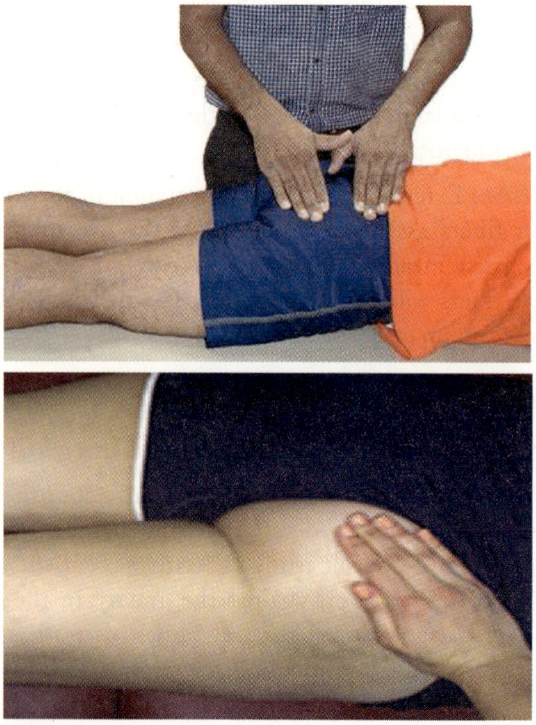

Figs. 6.232a and b: Palpation of gluteus maximus muscle for grade 1

Grade 2 (Poor)

Position of Patient: Side lying with the knees flexion.

Position of Examiner: Examiner stands behind the patient and stabilizes the pelvis with one hand and supports the leg at the distal knee joint with other hand. The patient is asked to extend the knee joint up to the full range in the gravity eliminated plane. If patient completes movement in the gravity eliminated position, is considered grade 2 (Figs. 6.233 and 6.234).

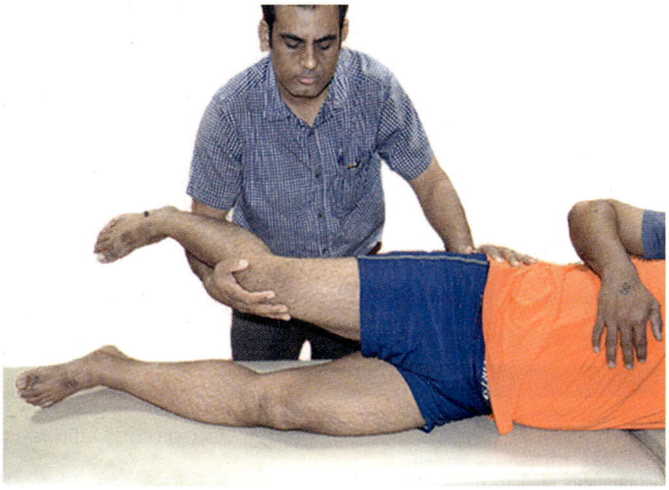

Fig. 6.233: Testing of gluteus maximus muscle for grade 2 with knee flexion

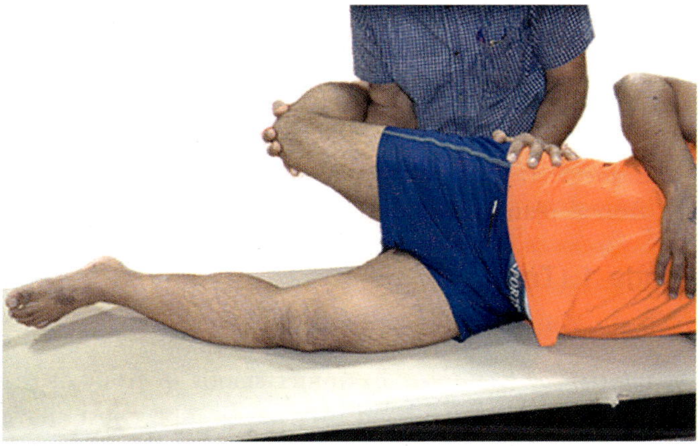

Fig. 6.234: Testing of gluteus maximus muscle for grade 2 with knee flexion

Weakness of Gluteus Maximus: The patients with weak hip extensors unable to walk upright. There is posterior and lateral bending of the trunk to compensate the action of gluteus maximus during the stance phase. Some patients put the ipsilateral hand on the glutei to push the hip joint anterior to the center of gravity to stabilize the hip in stance phase. Such gate is known as Jack Knife Gait. Shortening of gluteus maximus is uncommon unless and until there is a marked antagonistic muscle weakness. Patients with weak gluteus maximus usually exhibit hyperlordosis and anterior tilting of pelvis.

GLUTEUS MEDIUS MUSCLE STRENGTH TESTING

(a)

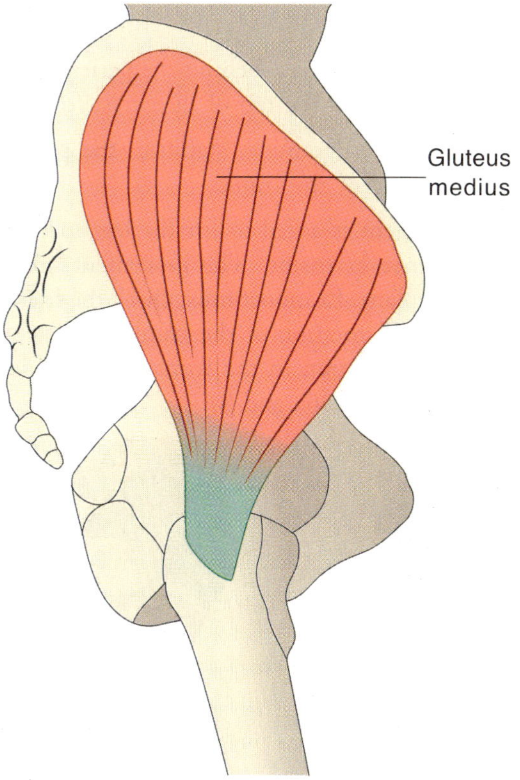

(b)

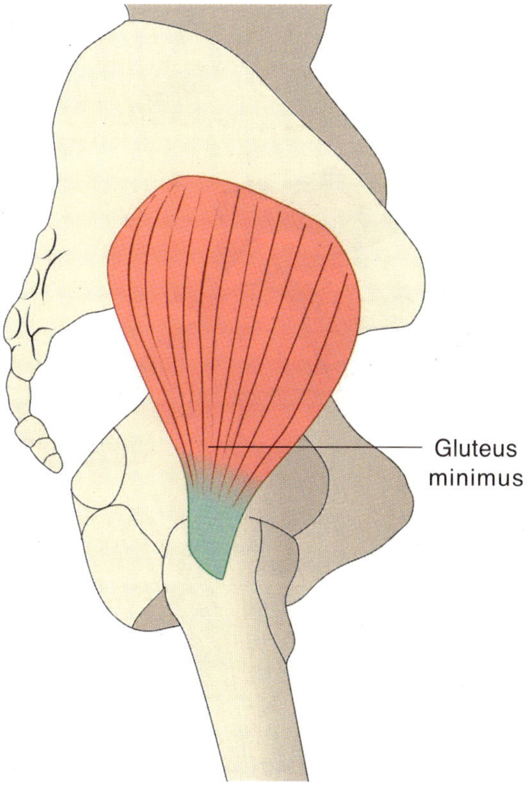

Figs. 6.235a and b: Gluteus medius and gluteus minimus muscles origin and insertion

Grade 3 (Fair)

Position of Patient: Opposite side lying. Patient places one hand under the head (lateral) and other hand on the lateral chest wall.

Position of Examiner: Behind the patient. Examiner may place one hand on the top of iliac crest for stabilization.

Stabilization: Examiner stabilizes the pelvis to prevent lateral banding of the trunk.

Test: Patient is asked to lift the leg up towards ceiling with the knee extension. The movement should occur in the frontal plane. Examiner must check the trick movements such as lateral rotation of the trunk. If patient completes full range of motion in the frontal plane it is considered grade 3 (Figs. 6.236a and b).

(a)

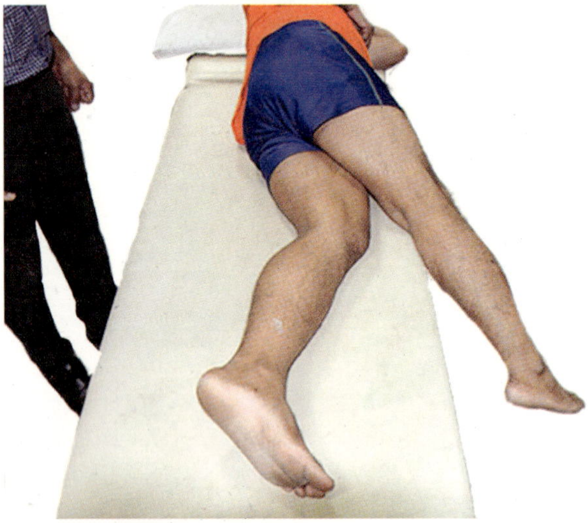

(b)

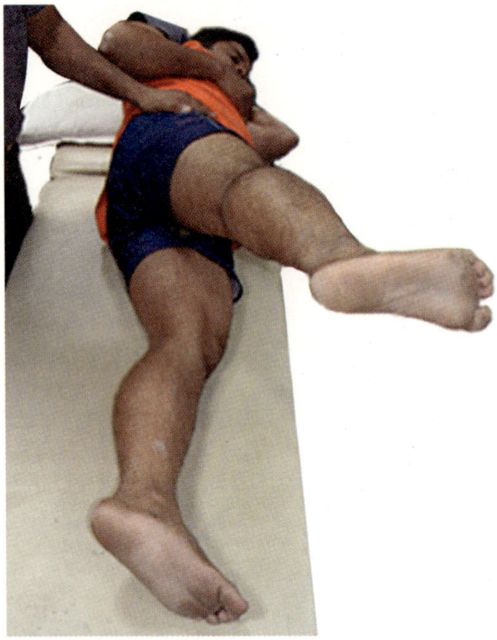

Figs. 6.236a and b: Testing of gluteus medius and gluteus minimus muscles for grade 3

Grade 4 and Grade 5 (Good and Normal)

Position of Patient: Opposite side lying. Patient places one hand under the head (lateral aspect) and other hand on the lateral chest wall.

Position of Examiner: Behind the patient. Examiner places one hand on the top of iliac crest and other hand on the distal lateral leg (Fig. 6.237).

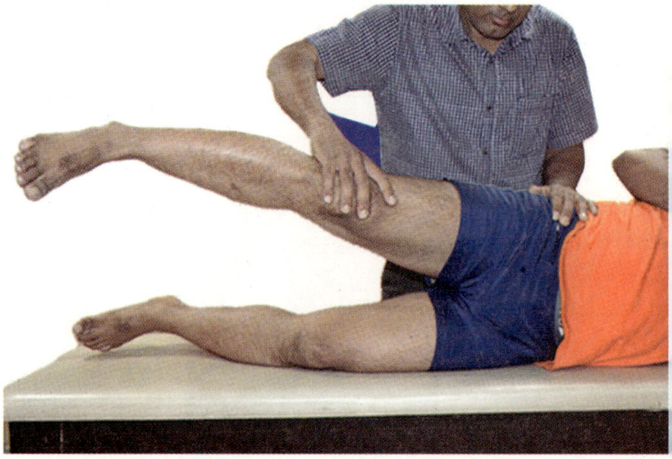

Fig. 6.237: Testing of gluteus medius and gluteus minimus muscles for grade 4 and 5

Test: Patient is asked to abduct the hip joint with the knee extension. The movement should occur in the frontal plane. Examiner must check the trick movements such as lateral bending of the trunk.

Grade 4: If patient completes full range of motion in the frontal plane against moderate resistance.

Grade 5: If patient completes full range of motion in the frontal plane against maximal resistance.

Grade 1 (Trace)

Position of Patient: Side lying, with the knees extended.

Position of Examiner: Examiner stands in front of the patient and places one hand over lateral aspect just above the greater trochanter (Fig. 6.238).

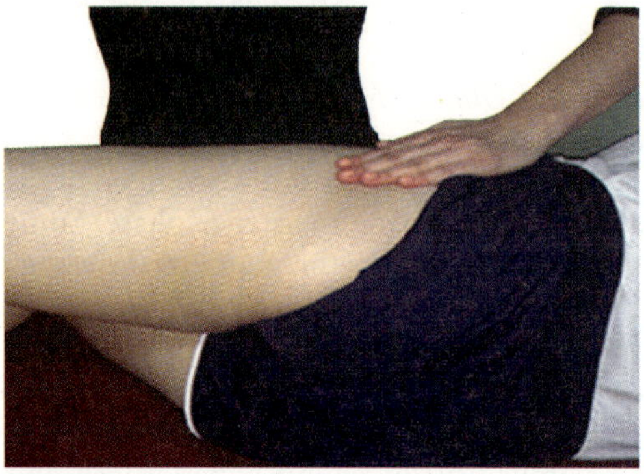

Fig. 6.238: Palpation of gluteus medius and gluteus minimus muscles for grade 1

Test: Patient is asked to try to bring leg out to the side. If examiner feels contraction at the lateral aspect of the thigh just above greater trochanter, it is considered grade 1. If examiner feels no contraction despite of patients fair attempt it is considered grade zero.

Grade 2 (Poor)

Position of Patient: Supine with knees extended.

Position of Examiner: Examiner stands at the side which is being tested and places one hand on the pelvis to prevent trunk rotation while other hand grasps the leg at distal to support it during the movement (Figs. 239a and b).

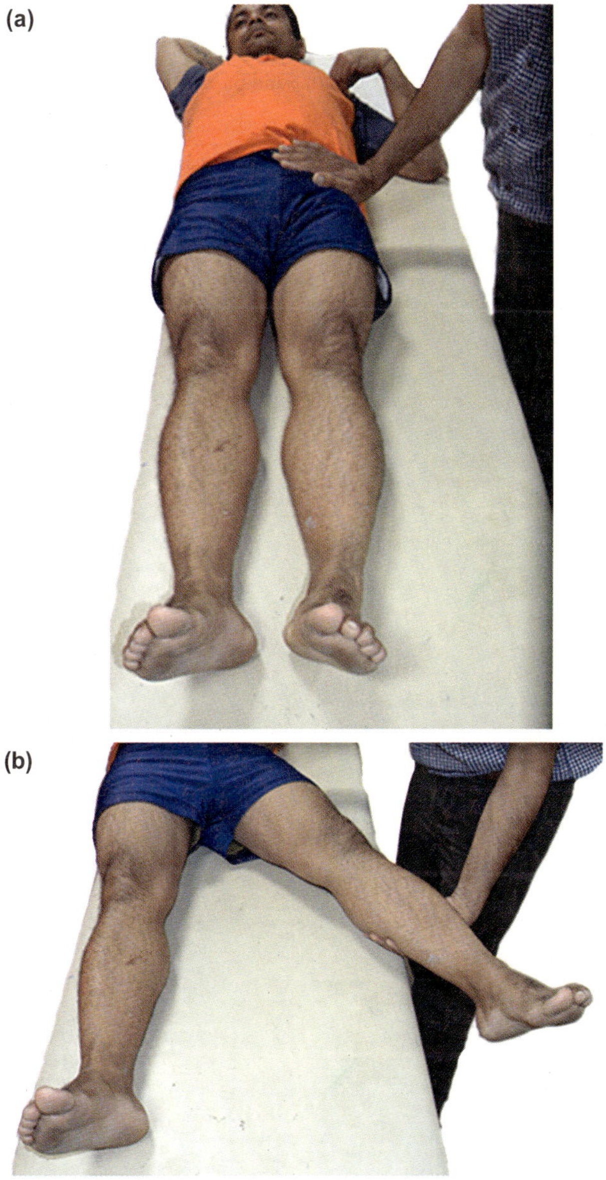

Figs. 6.239a and b: Testing of gluteus medius and gluteus minimus muscles for grade 2

Test: Patient is asked to abduct or take the leg out away from midline. Examiner must ensure that no assistance or resistance is offered to the leg during the movement. The movement should occur in the frontal plane.

Weakness: Gluteus medius and minimus contract eccentrically to maintain the trunk upright on the hip joint in mid stance. The resultant force across the hip is about three times body weight because the force of abductors acts on the greater trochanter to offset body weight and levels the pelvis in single stance. Weak gluteus medius and minimus unable to level the pelvis in single stance, hence the pelvis drops to the side contralateral to the stance. The patients with weak gluteus medius and minimus find difficulty in clearing the ground due to lengthening of the leg (due to drop of the contralateral side pelvis). Hence, patient bends the trunk to the ipsilateral side to clear the ground. It is known as Trendelenburg sign. If the bending of trunk to both the sides is present due to bilateral weakness of the gluteus medius and minimus, such gait is known as Trendelenburg gait. Shortening of gluteus medius is not common unless and until there is gross loss of mobility of the patient (Figs. 6.240a and b).

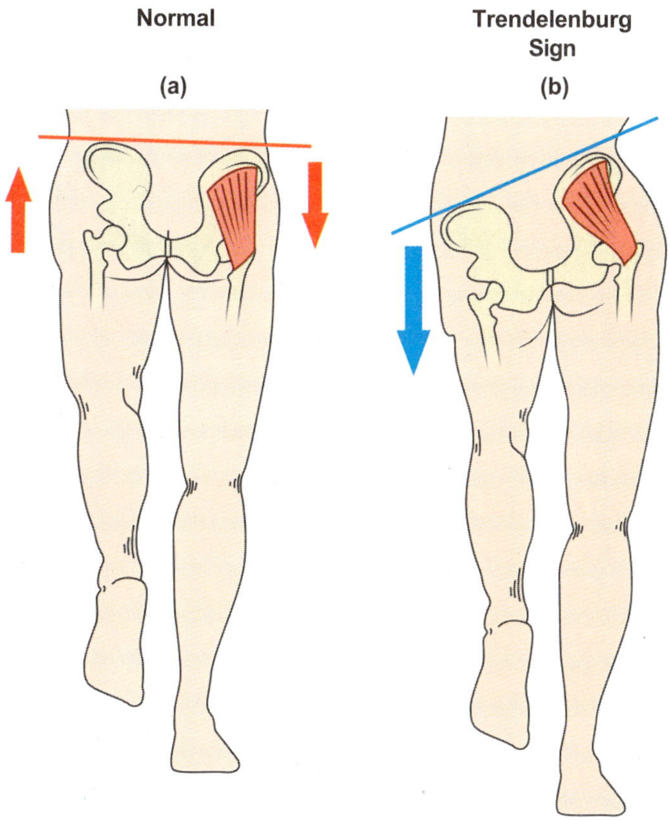

Figs. 6.240a and b: Trendelenburg sign (if unilateral involvement) and trendelenburg gait if both the sides are involved

HIP ADDUCTORS TESTING

Table 6.1

Name of muscle	*Origin*	*Insertion*
Pectineus	Surface of the superior ramus of the pubis, ventral to the pectin, between the iliopectineal eminence and the pubic tubercle.	Pectineal line of the femur.
Adductor magnus	Inferior pubis ramus, ramus of the ischium (anterior fibers) and ischial tuberosity (posterior fibers).	Medial to the gluteal tuberosity, middle of the linea aspera, medial supracondylar line and adductor tubercle of the medial condyle of the femur.
Gracilis	Inferior half of the symphysis pubis and medial margin of the inferior ramus of the pubic bone.	Medial surface of the body of the tibia, distal to the condyle, proximal to the insertion of the semitendinosus and lateral to the insertion of the sartorius.
Adductor brevis	Outer surface of the inferior ramus of the pubis.	Distal $^{2}/_{3}$rd of the pectineal line and proximal half of the medial lip of the linea aspera.
Adductor longus	Anterior surface of the pubis at the junction of the crest and the symphysis.	Middle $^{1}/_{3}$rd of the medial lip of the linea aspera.

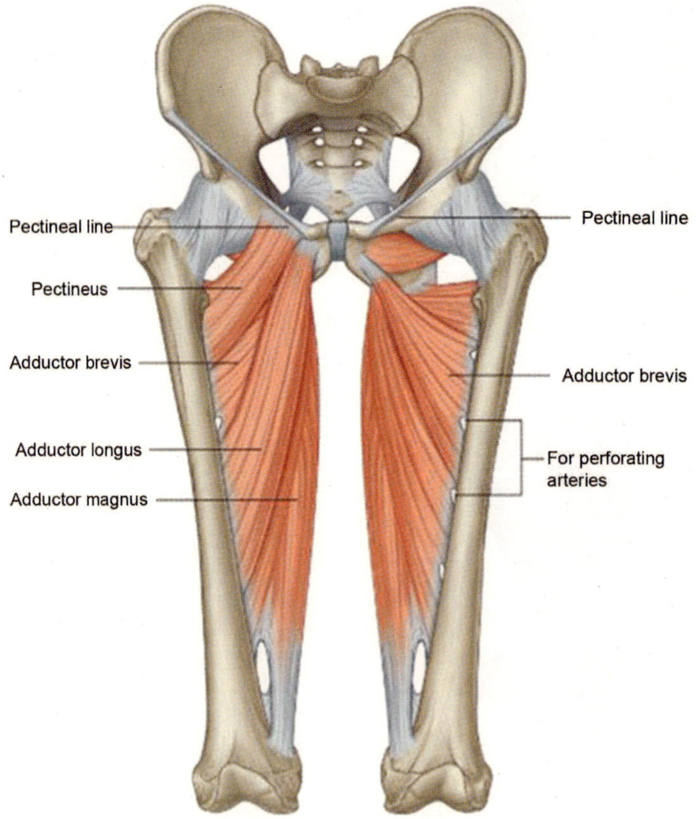

Fig. 6.241: Origin and insertion of adductors of hip joint

Grade 3

Position of Patient: Same side lying, hip joint which is being tested should the lower most.

Position of Examiner: Stands behind the patient places one hand on the lateral iliac crest and other hand grasps the contralateral leg to keep it in abducted position to provide the space for the adduction (Figs. 6.242 and 6.243).

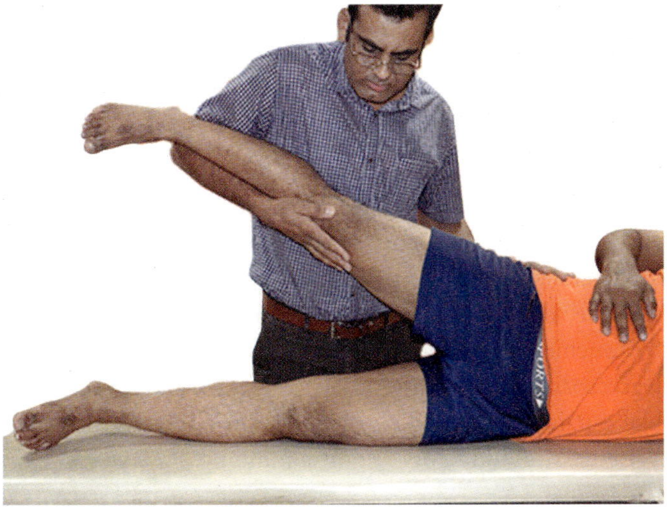

Fig. 6.242: Testing of adductors of lower most leg for grade 3 starting position

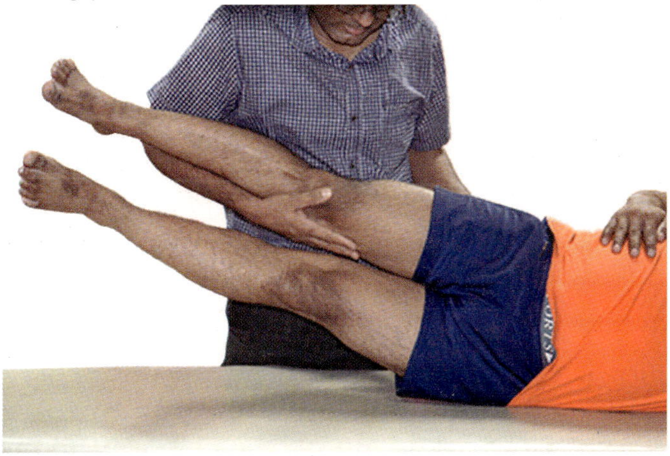

Fig. 6.243: Testing of adductors of lower most leg for grade 3

Test: The examiner asks the patient to adduct the hip joint in the frontal plane across the midline. If patient completes range of motion and touches the upper most leg it is considered grade 3.

Grade 4 and Grade 5 (Good and Normal)

Position of Patient: Side lying. The side which is being tested should be the lower most.

Position of Examiner: Examiner stands behind the patient and grasps the upper most leg (non testing side) at the knee joint to abduct it for 25° so that the space can be made for the adduction of lower most leg. The leg should be close to the chest of the examiner for the stabilization. Examiner places other hand on the medial aspect of knee joint of the leg which is being tested (lower most) for the resistance.

Test: Examiner asks the patient to adduct the testing hip joint in the frontal plane across the midline. While maintaining the uppermost leg in the abducted position the examiner applies strong to moderate resistance against the adduction with other hand (Fig. 6.244).

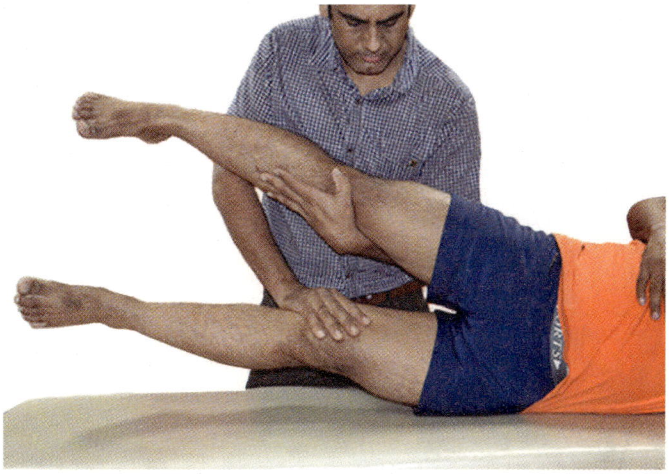

Fig. 6.244: Testing of adductors of lower most leg for grade 4 and 5

Grade 4: If patient can hold the leg in adduction against strong to moderate resistance.

Grade 5: If patient can hold the leg in adduction against maximal resistance.

Grade 1 (Trace)

Position of Patient: Supine with slight abduction.

Position of Examiner: Standing at the side which is being tested. Examiner places one hand on the proximal medial thigh to palpate the muscles and other hand is placed on the distal thigh to stabilize the hip joint (Fig. 6.245).

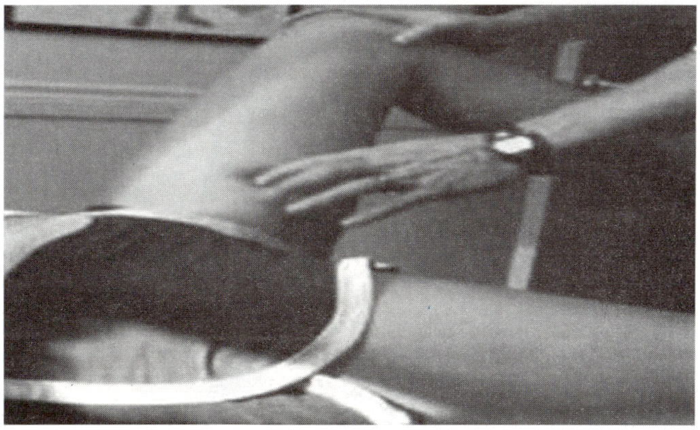

Fig. 6.245: Palpation of adductors for grade 1

Test: Examiner asks the patient to try to adduct the hip joint in the frontal plane across the midline while palpating the muscle on the proximal medial thigh. If examiner feels contraction on the proximal medial thigh it is considered grade 1.

Grade 2 (Poor)

Position of Patient: Supine with the contralateral hip joint in abducted position to provide space for the adduction.

Position of Examiner: Standing at the side which is being tested. Examiner places one hand on the iliac crest to stabilize the pelvis and other hand may be placed under the distal leg for support (Figs. 6.246a and b).

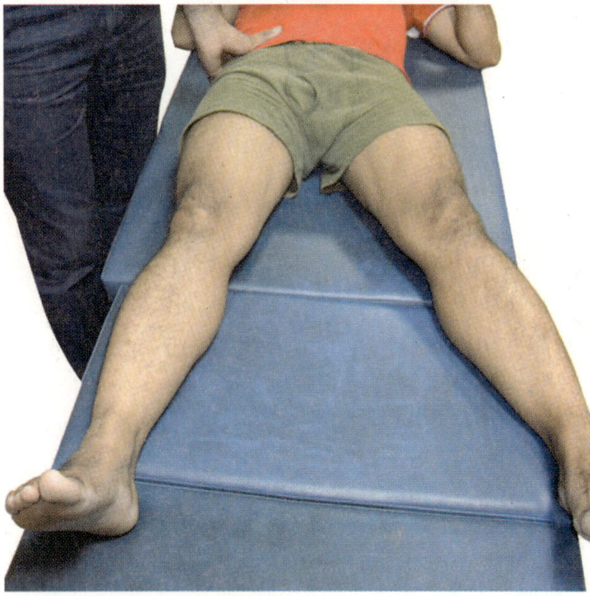

(a)

(b)

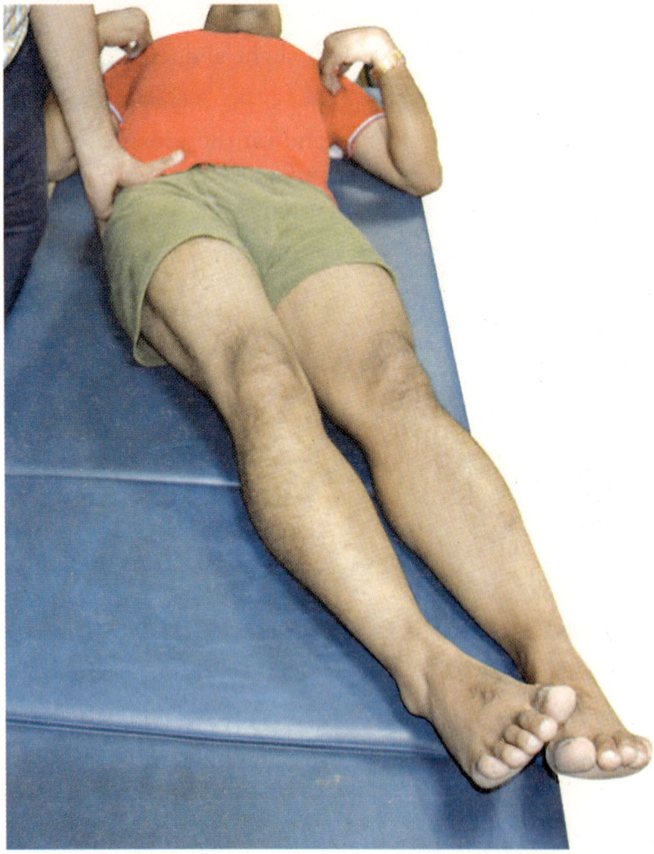

Figs. 6.246a and b: Testing of adductors for grade 2

Test: The examiner asks the patient to adduct the hip joint in the frontal plane across the midline while the extremity is supported on the examiner's hand. Examiner must not provide assistance or resistance to the extremity. If patient completes full range of motion in the frontal plane without assistance it is considered grade 2.

Shortening: Shortening of adductors limits the abduction range. Mild shortening does not affect the gait. Marked shortening of the adductors causes great difficulty in swing as well as in stance as the leg crosses the midline. If there is a bilateral shortening of the adductors, the legs crosses the midline, draws the knee together and progresses forward by touching the middle thigh of the contralateral leg. The legs crosses the midline alternately in walking and look like a pair of scissor. This gait is known as Scissoring gait. Weakness of adductors is not common.

EXTERNAL ROTATORS TESTING

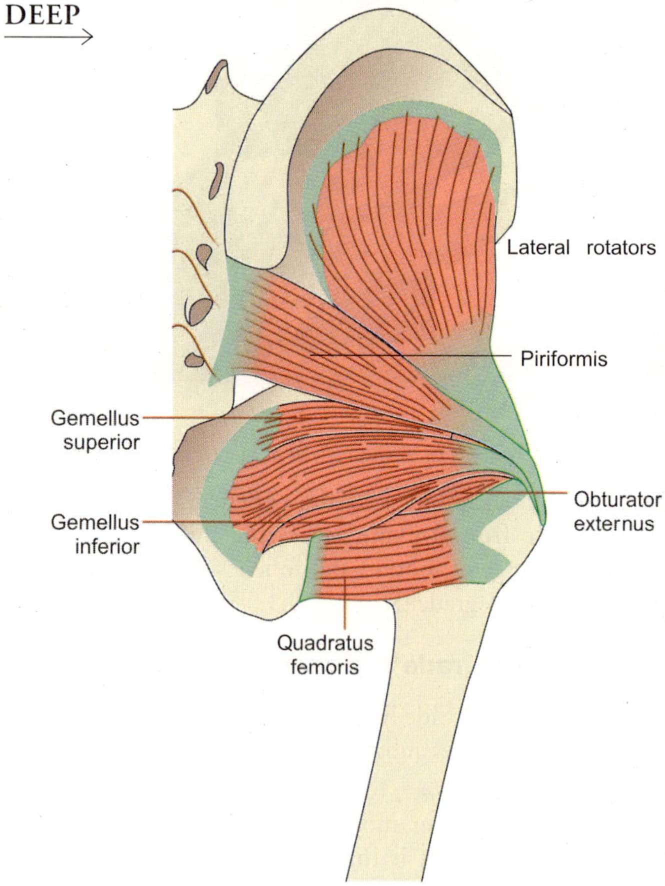

Fig. 6.247: Origin and insertion of hip external rotators

Grade 3 (Fair)

Position of Patient: Short sitting with both the hands grasp the edge of the couch.

Position of Examiner: Stands at the side which is being tested and places one hand on the pelvis to stabilize it (Fig. 6.248).

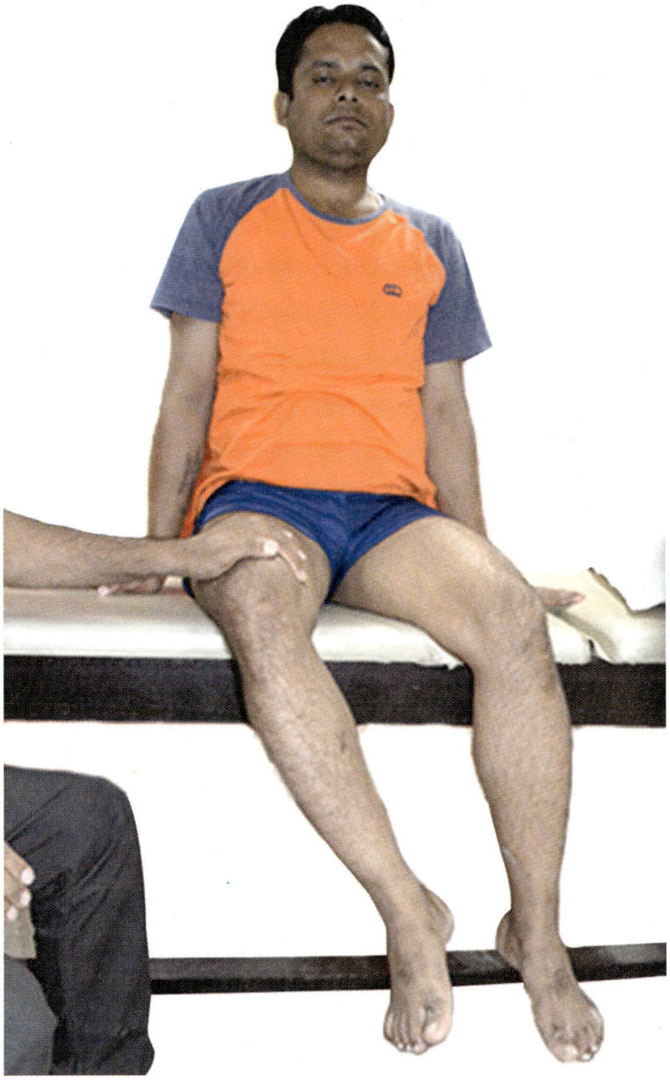

Fig. 6.248: Testing of external rotators for grade 3

Test: Examiner asks the patient to bring the ankle towards other leg. If the patient completes range of motion against the gravity it is considered grade 3.

Grade 4 and Grade 5 (Fair and Normal)

Position of Patient: Short sitting with both hands grasp the edge of the couch.

Position of Examiner: Sits comfortably at the side which is being tested and places one hand on anterior aspect of the distal thigh and other hand grasps the leg above the ankle (Fig. 6.249).

Tests: Examiner asks the patient to bring the ankle joint towards the opposite leg against the resistance.

Grade 4: If patient completes range of motion against strong to moderate resistance.

Grade 5: If patient completes range of motion against maximal resistance.

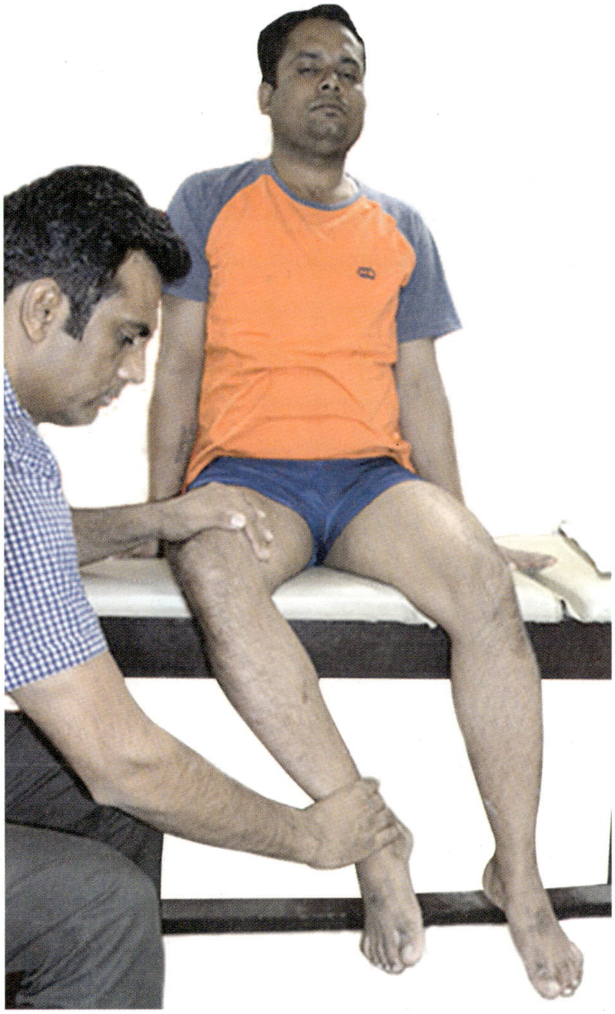

Fig. 6.249: Testing of external rotators for grade 4 and 5

Grade 1

Position of Patient: Supine with the hip joint at neutral position.

Position of Examiner: Examiner stands at side of the patient and places one hand on the anterolateral aspect of the hip joint (Fig. 6.250).

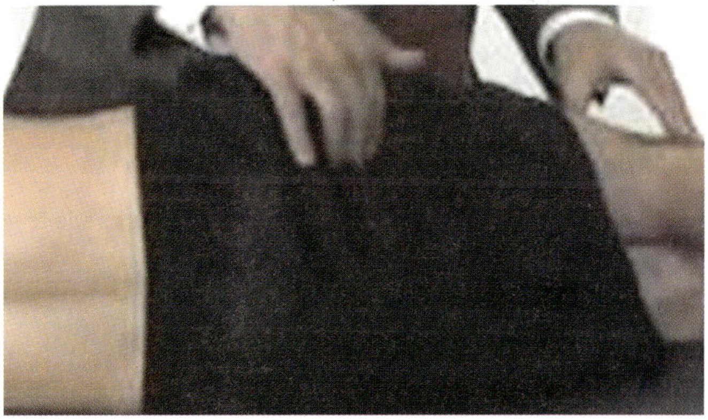

Fig. 6.250: Palpation of external rotators for grade 1

Test: Examiner asks the patient to roll the leg out. The external rotators are the deep situated muscles and cannot be palpated except of gluteus maximus which is a secondary mover. If examiner feels any discernible movement or contraction it may be graded 1.

Grade 2

Position of Patient: Supine with the hip joint in full internal rotation.

Position of Examiner: Examiner stands to the opposite side which is being tested and places one hand on the iliac crest to stabilize the pelvis (Figs. 6.251a and b).

(a)

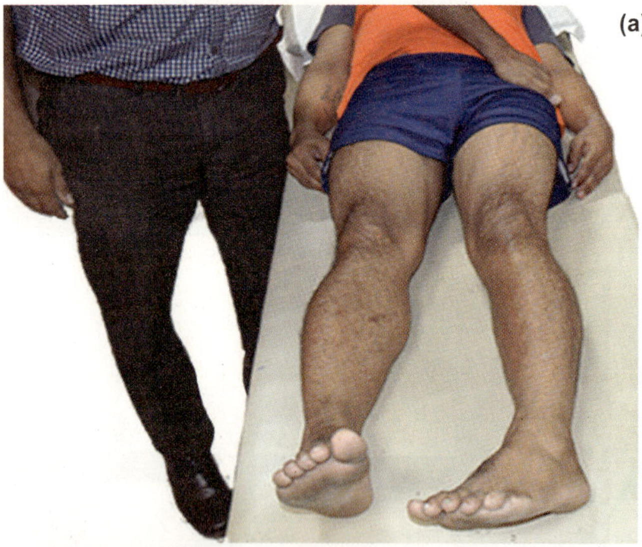

(b)

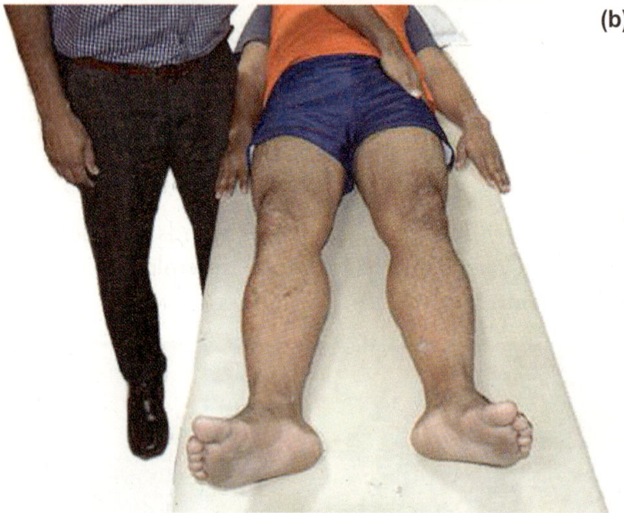

Figs. 6.251a and b: Testing of external rotators for grade 2

Test: Rotation of hip joint occurs in the transverse plane, therefore, full range of motion does not occur in gravity eliminated position. Some part of the movement occurs in the gravity assisted position, and other part of movement occurs against the gravity. The therapist may assist and resist the movement in according to the position of the leg with respect to the gravity to test the external rotators in grade 2. Examiner instructs the patient to rotate the hip joint from full internal rotation to the full external rotation. Initially examiner assists the movement as the movement occurs against the gravity and resists the movement to test the external rotators. The assistance and resistance should be an appropriate.

Weakness: Weakness of external rotators results in anteversion (excessive internal rotation) of the femur, which also forces the tibia to rotate internally. The internal rotation is associated with the excessive pronation of the foot. Patients with femur anteversion offen complaint pain in knee and ankle joint.

Shortening: Shortening of the external rotators of the hip joint limit the internal rotation. The patients find difficulty in taking sharp turns.

INTERNAL ROTATORS TESTING

Grade 3

Position of Patient: Short sitting with both hands grasp the edge of the table for stabilization.

Position of Examiner: Examiner stands at the side which is being tested and places one hand on anterior surface of the distal thigh for stabilization (Figs. 6.252a and b).

(a)

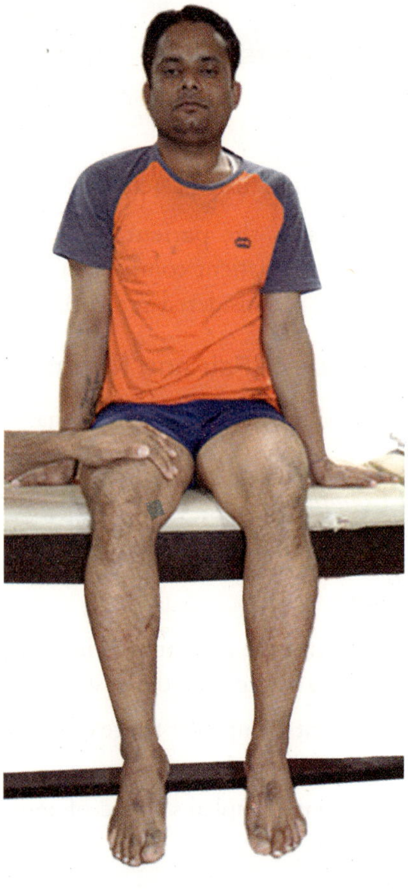

(b)

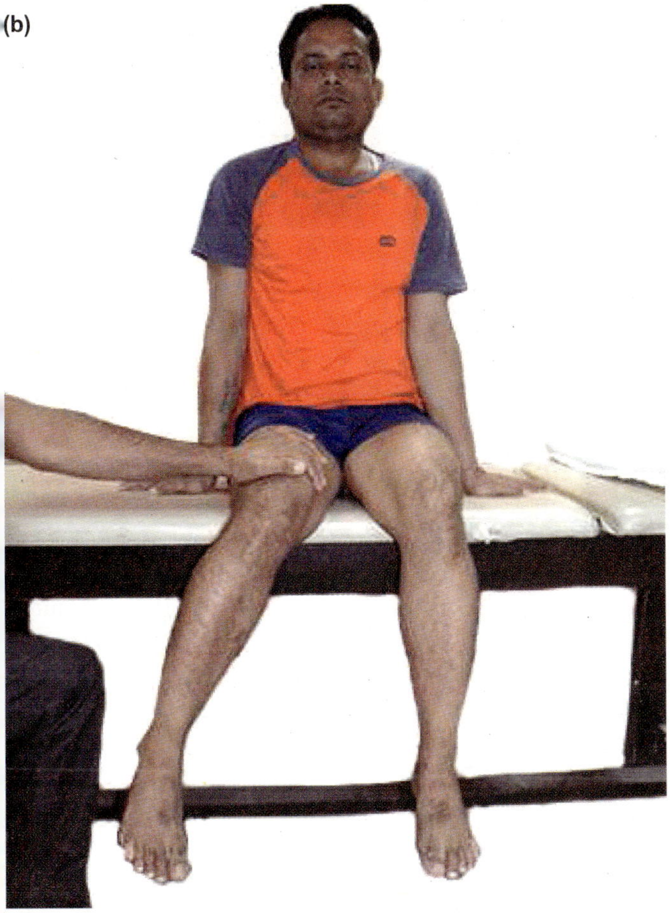

Figs. 6.252a and b: Testing of internal rotators of hip joint for grade 3

Test: Examiner instructs the patient to take the leg outwards away from the midline. If patient completes range of motion it is considered grade 3.

Grade 4 and Grade 5 (Fair and Normal)

Position of Patient: Short sitting with both the hands grasp the edge of the table for stabilization.

Position of Examiner: Examiner stands at the side which is being tested and places one hand on the anterior surface of the distal thigh and other hand grasps the leg just above the ankle joint (Fig. 6.253).

Test: Examiner instructs the patient to take the leg outwards away from the midline while the examiner resists the movement.

Grade 4: If patient completes range of motion against strong to moderate resistance.

Grade 5: If patient completes range of motion against maximal resistance.

Grade 1

Position of Patient: Supine with the external rotation of the hip joint (testing side).

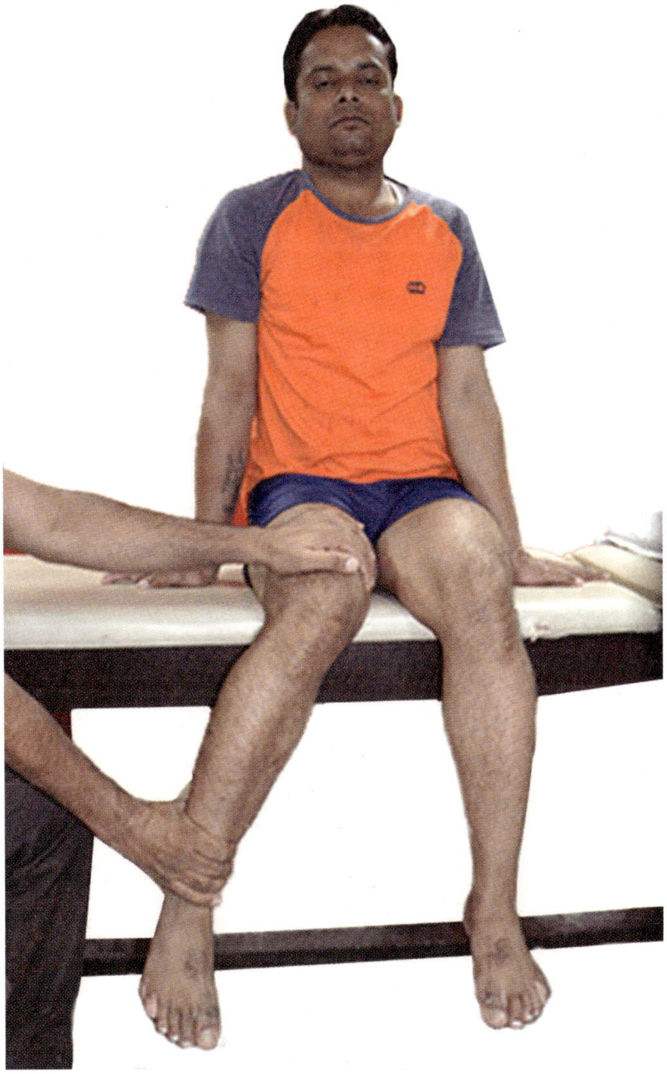

Fig. 6.253: Testing of internal rotators of hip joint for grade 4 and 5

Position of Examiner: The examiner stands at the side which is being tested and places one hand on the posterolateral surface of the hip above the greater trochanter (Fig. 6.254).

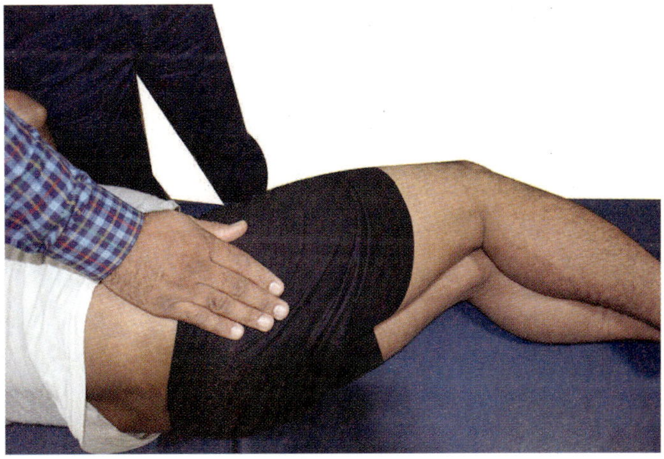

Fig. 6.254: Palpation of internal rotators of hip joint for grade 1

Test: Examiner asks the patient to try to roll your leg inward (internal rotation) while one hand of the examiner remains on the posterolateral surface of the hip above the greater trochanter of femur. If examiner feels contraction over the aforesaid area it is considered grade 1.

Grade 2

Position of Patient: Supine with external rotation of the hip joint (testing side).

Position of Examiner: The examiner stands at the side which is being tested and places one hand on the posterolateral surface of the hip above the greater trochanter to stabilize the pelvis (Figs. 6.255a and b).

Test: Rotation of hip joint occurs in the transverse plane, therefore, full range of motion does not occur in gravity eliminated position. Some part of the movement occurs in the gravity assisted position, and other part of movement occurs against the gravity. The therapist may assist and resist the movement according to the position of the leg with respect to the gravity to test the internal rotators for grade 2. Examiner instructs the patient to rotate the hip joint from full external rotation to the full internal rotation. Initially examiner assists the movement as the movement occurs against the gravity and then after resists the movement to test the internal rotators. The assistance and resistance should be an appropriate. The rotators may also be tested from the neutral position.

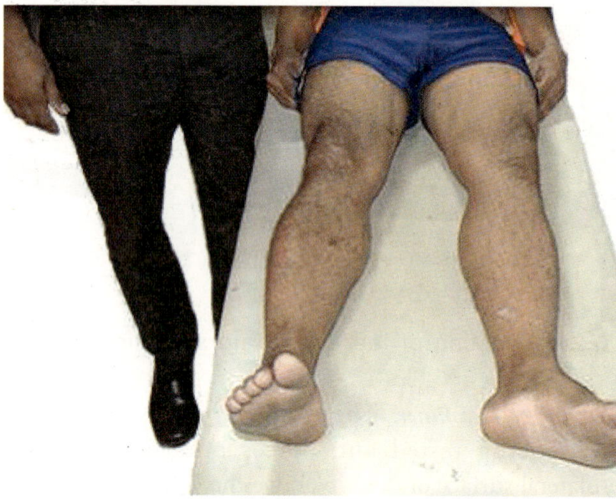
(a)

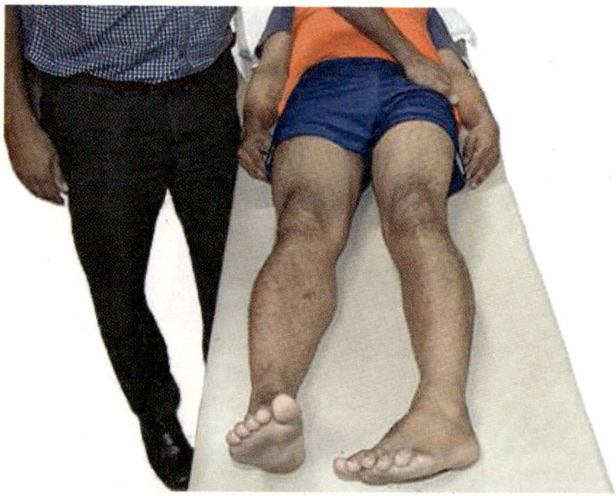
(b)

Figs. 6.255a and b: Testing of internal rotators of hip joint for grade 2

Alternative position for the grade 2. The patient is placed in the short sitting with the hands grasps the edge of the table for stabilization. Examiner places one hand on the anterior surface of the distal thigh and other hand grasps the leg above the ankle joint. Patient is instructed to take the leg away from the midline while the examiner assists the movement as it occurs against the gravity. If patient completes full range of motion against the gravity with little assistance it is considered grade 2.

Shortening: The shortening produces excessive external rotation of the hip that results in decrease quadriceps angle. The excessive external rotation of hip may disrupt the screw home mechanism and can produce impingement of soft tissues in the knee joint at the terminal extension.

KNEE JOINT MUSCLE TESTING

HAMSTRINGS – KNEE FLEXION

Semitendinosus

Origin: Tuberosity of ischium by the tendon common with the long head of biceps femoris.

Insertion: Proximal part of medial surface of the body of the tibia and deep fascia of the leg.

Nerve Supply: Sciatic $L_{4,5}$, $S_{1,2}$.

Semimembranosus

Origin: Tuberosity of the ischium, proximal and lateral to the biceps femoris and semitendinosus.

Insertion: Posteromedial aspect of the medial condyle of the tibia.

Nerve Supply: Sciatic (tibial branch) $L_{4,5}$, $S_{1,2}$.

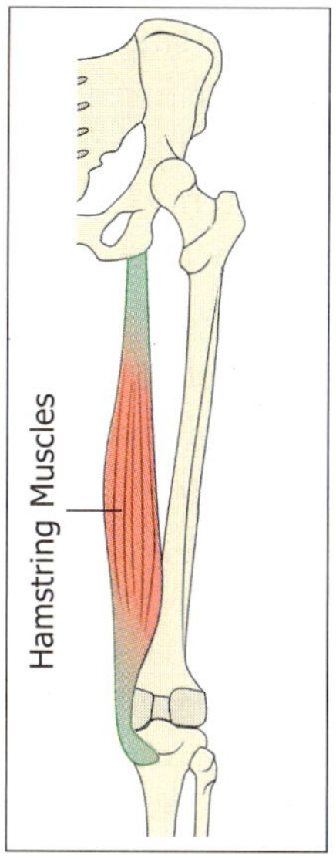

Fig. 6.256: Hamstring muscles origin and insertion

Biceps Femoris

Origin: Long head originates from distal part of the sacrotuberous ligament and posterior part of the ischium.

Nerve Supply: Long head–Sciatic (tibial branch) L_5, $S_{1,2,3}$.

Short Head: Peroneal branch L_5, $S_{1,2}$.

Action: Semimebranosus and semitendinosus flexes and medially rotates the knee joint. Assist in extending and medially rotating the hip joint.

Biceps femoris flexes and laterally rotates the hip joint. Assists in extending and laterally rotating the hip joint.

Grade 3

Position of Patient: Prone lying with both the knees extended.

Position of Examiner: Examiner stands at the side which is being tested and places his or her hand on the posterior aspect of the distal thigh to stabilize it (Figs. 6.257 and 6.258).

Test: Examiner instructs the patient to bend the knee joint in the available range of motion against the gravity. The flexion after 90° occurs in the gravity assisted position, therefore; examiner may resist the movement. If patient completes movement against the gravity it is considered grade 3.

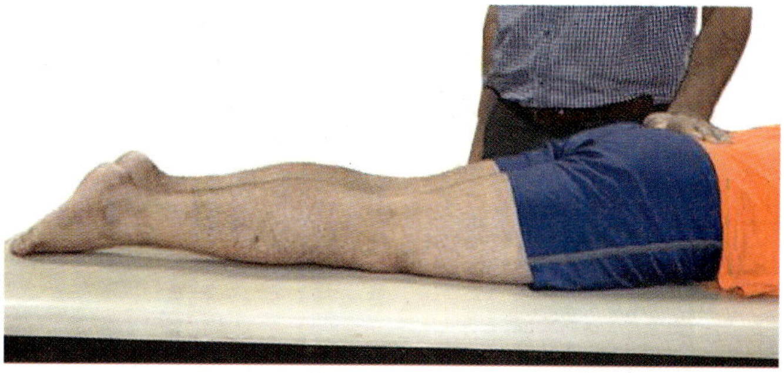

Fig. 6.257: Testing of hamstring muscles for grade 3–Starting position

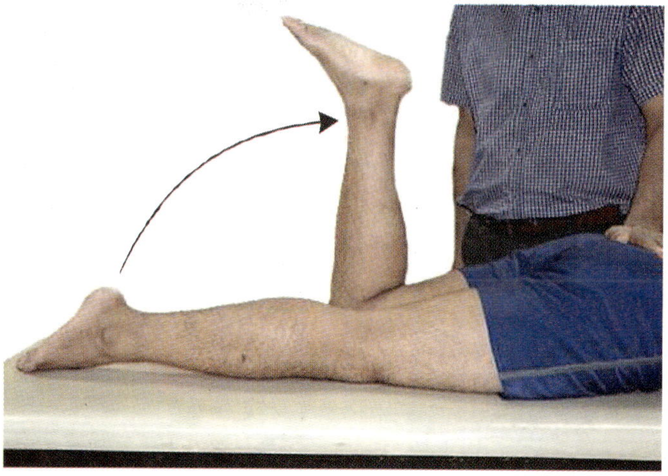

Fig. 6.258: Testing of hamstring muscles for grade 3

Grade 4 and Grade 5 (Good and Normal)

Position of Patient: Prone lying with both the knees extended.

Position of Examiner: Examiner stands at the side which is being tested and grasps the leg just above the ankle joint and places other hand on the posterior aspect of the distal thigh to stabilize it (Figs. 6.259, 6.260a and b).

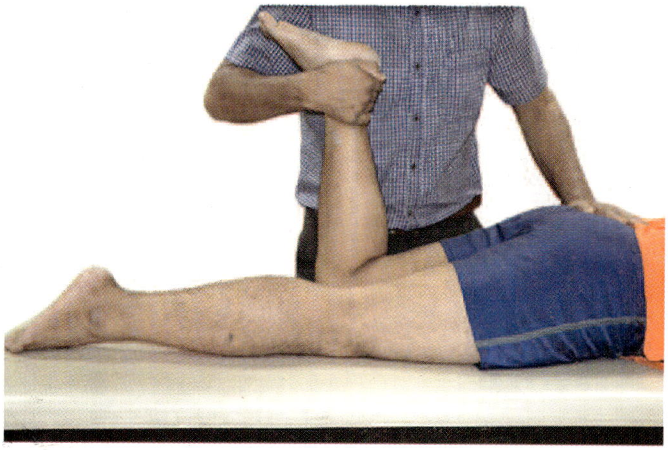

Fig. 6.259: Testing of hamstring muscles for grade 4 and 5

(a)

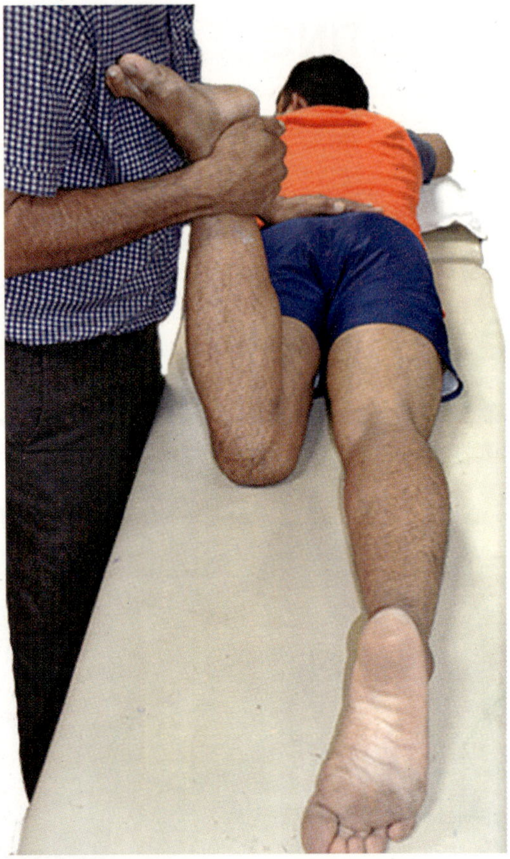

(b)

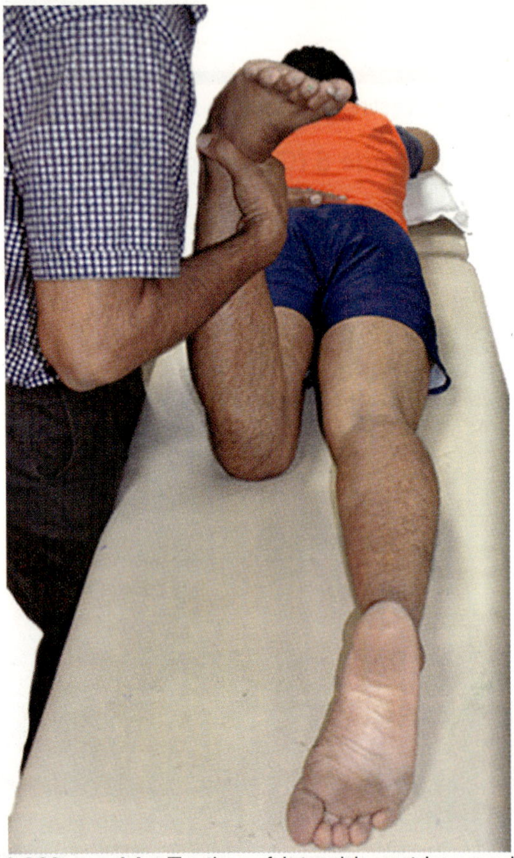

Figs. 6.260a and b: Testing of lateral hamstrings and medial hamstrings for grade 4 and 5

Test: Examiner instructs the patient to bend the knee joint in the available range of motion against the gravity.

Grade 4: If patient completes range of motion against strong to moderate resistance it is considered grade 4 for all three hamstring muscles. To test the biceps femoris muscle (lateral hamstring) examiner rotates the leg laterally and then instructs the patient to bend the knee joint against the strong to moderate resistance. To test the medial hamstrings (semimembranosus and semitendinosus) examiner rotates the leg medially and instructs the patient to bend the knee joint against strong to moderate resistance.

Grade 5: If patient completes range of motion against maximal resistance it is considered grade 5 for all three hamstring muscles. To test the biceps femoris muscle (lateral hamstring) examiner rotates the leg laterally and then instructs the patient to bend the knee joint against maximal resistance. To test the medial hamstrings (semimembranosus and semitendinosus) examiner rotates the leg medially and instructs the patient to bend the knee joint against maximal resistance.

Grade 1 (Trace)

Position of Patient: Prone with both the knees extended.

Position of Examiner: The examiner stands at the side which is being tested and places index of one hand on the medial or lateral hamstrings tendon to palpate and other hand grasps the leg just above the ankle joint (Figs. 6.261 and 6.262).

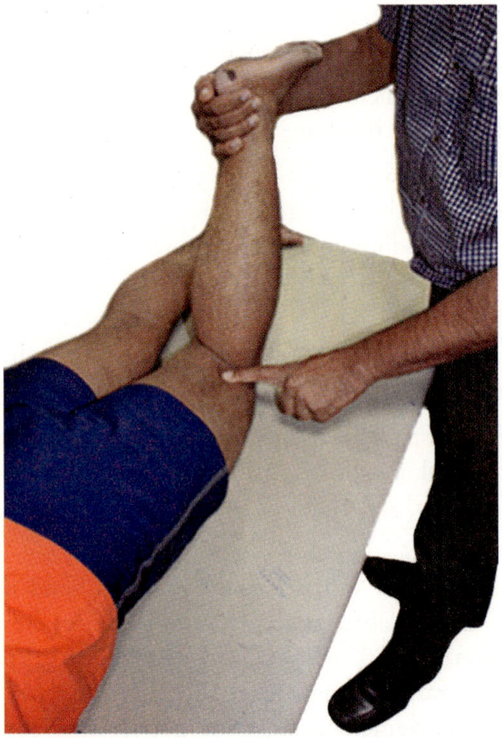

Fig. 6.261: Palpation of lateral hamstrings for grade 1

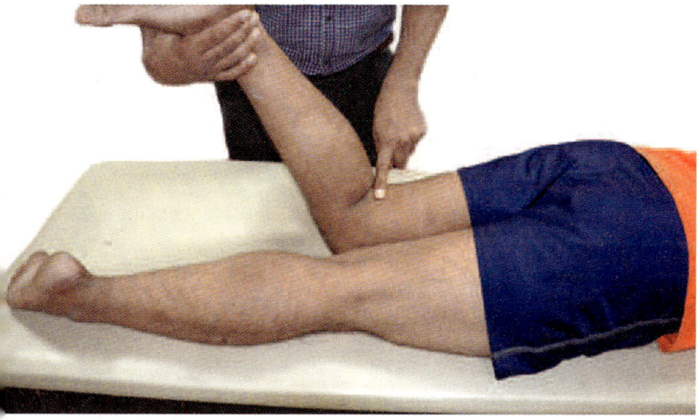

Fig. 6.262: Palpation of medial hamstrings for grade 1

Test: Examiner flexes the knee joint about 30° and instructs the patient to bend the knee joint. If examiner feels contraction on the medial or lateral tendons of the hamstrings it is considered grade 1.

Grade 2

Position of Patient: Side lying with the testing leg uppermost. The lower non testing leg is flexed to 45° at hip and knee joint.

Position of Examiner: Examiner stands behind the patient and places one hand under the medial surface of the leg just above the ankle joint and arm of the examiner is used to cradle thigh to support at the medial side of knee joint (Figs. 6.263 and 6.264).

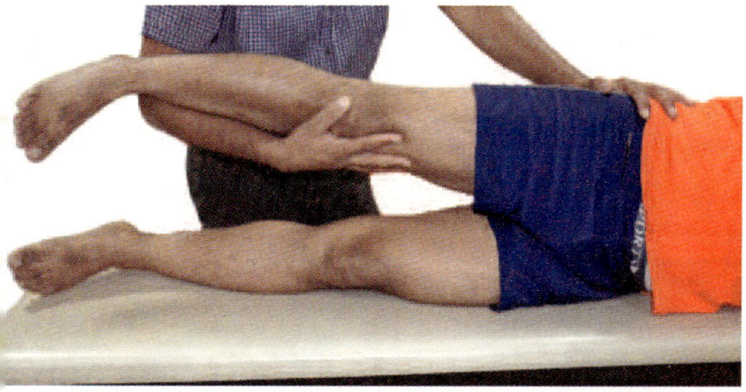

Fig. 6.263: Testing of hamstring muscles for grade 2–Starting position

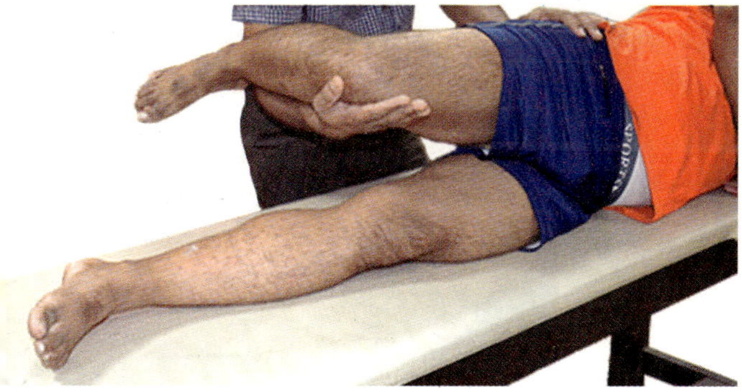

Fig. 6.264: Testing of hamstrings for grade 2 in the available range of motion

Test: Examiner supports the leg and keeps it slightly above the lower leg. Patient is instructed to bend the knee joint in the available range of motion. If patient completes range of motion it is considered grade 2.

Shortening: Hamstrings are the two joint muscles. The shortening affects both the hip and knee joints. Pelvis rotates posteriorly that results in decrease lumbar lordosis. However, mild shortening of hamstrings observed in many of individuals, does not affect the normal posture very much.

Test: Patient is placed in the supine position and the examiner stands at the side of the patient. Examiner holds the leg and raises it with the knee extension. An angle of approximately 80° between the table and the raised leg is considered to be a normal range of hamstrings length. The examiner must observe the lumbar lordosis while raising the leg. Normally the lordosis should decrease while raising the leg. Loss of lumbar flexion while raising the leg shows the shortening of hamstring muscles length. If there is hip flexors tightness, a towel roll is placed under the knees and then leg is held firmly. If the leg is raised with the lumbar lordosis and anterior tilting of the pelvis positions, hamstring normal length would appear short. Hence the flattening of lumbar spine must be ensured for the correct testing of the hamstrings length by placing the towel roll under the contralateral leg and holding it firmly.

Weakness: Weakness of hamstrings is common in patients with the anterior tilting of the pelvis and excessive lordosis of the lumbar spine. The hamstrings get strained repeatedly if the strength is below the normal. The individuals find difficulty in prolong walking.

QUADRICEPS MUSCLES–KNEE EXTENSORS

Rectus Femoris

Origin: Anteroinferior iliac spine.

Vastus Lateralis

Origin: Proximal part of intertrochanteric line, anterior and inferior border of greater trochanter, lateral tip of gluteal tuberosity and proximal half of tip of linea aspera.

Vastus Intermedius

Origin: Anterior and lateral surface of the proximal 2/3rd of the body of femur and distal half of the linea aspera.

Vastus Medialis

Origin: Distal half of the intertrochanteric line, medial tip of the linea aspera and proximal part of the medial supracondylar line.

Insertion: All four quadriceps muscles insert on the proximal border of patella and through the patella ligament to the tuberosity of the tibia.

Action: All four quadriceps muscles extend the knee joint. Rectus femoris assists in flexion of hip joint.

Nerve Supply: $L_{2,3,4}$.

Grade 3 (Fair)

Position of Patient: Short sitting with both the hands hold the edge of table for stability. A wedge or towel roll can be placed under the knee joint to level the femur.

Position of Examiner: Examiner stands at the side which is being tested and places one hand on the anterior aspect of the distal thigh (Figs. 6.265a and b).

Test: Examiner instructs the patient to straighten the knee joint against the gravity. If patient completes extension in full range of motion it is considered grade 3.

Grade 4 and Grade 5 (Good and Normal)

Position of Patient: Short sitting with both the hands hold the edge of table for stability. A wedge or towel roll can be placed under the knee joint to level the femur or thigh.

(a)

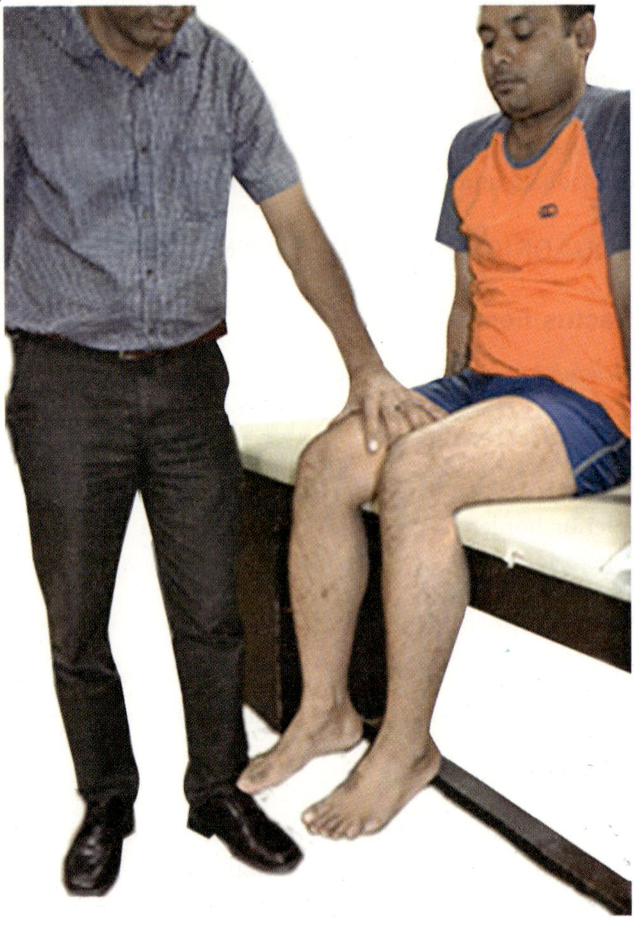

(b)

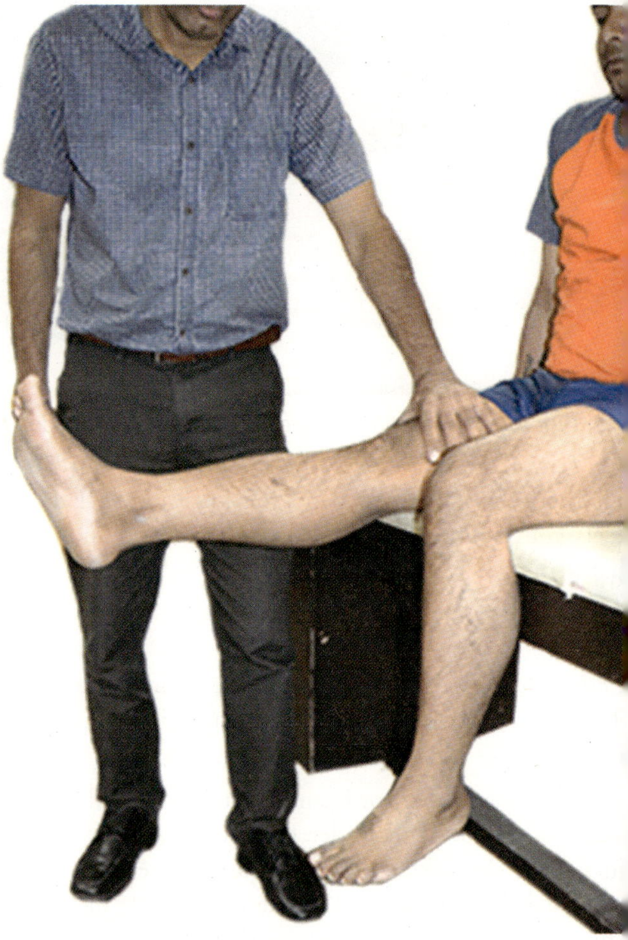

Figs. 6.265a and b: Testing of right side quadriceps muscles for grade 3 from 90 degrees to the available range of motion

Position of Examiner: Examiner stands at the side which is being tested and places one hand on the anterior aspect of the distal thigh and other hand grasps the distal leg just above the ankle joint (Fig. 6.266).

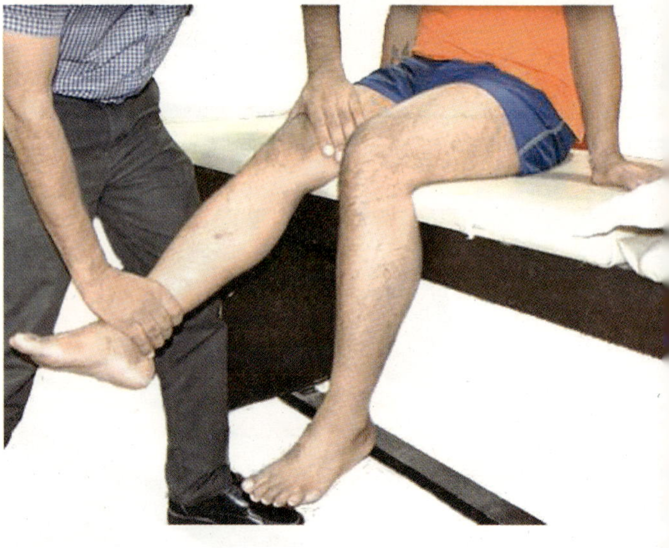

Fig. 6.266: Testing of right side quadricep muscles for grade 4 and 5

Test: Examiner instructs the patient to straighten the knee joint against the gravity.

Grade 4: If patient completes extension against strong to moderate resistance. The examiner must check for trick movement such as leaning backward and lifting the buttocks from the couch during testing.

Grade 5: If patient completes extension against maximal resistance. The examiner must check for trick movement such as leaning backward and lifting the buttocks from the couch during testing.

Grade 1 (Trace)

Position of Patient: Supine with both the knees extended.

Position of Examiner: Examiner stands at the side which is being tested and places fingers of one hand on the quadriceps tendon just above the patella (Figs. 6.267a and b).

(a)

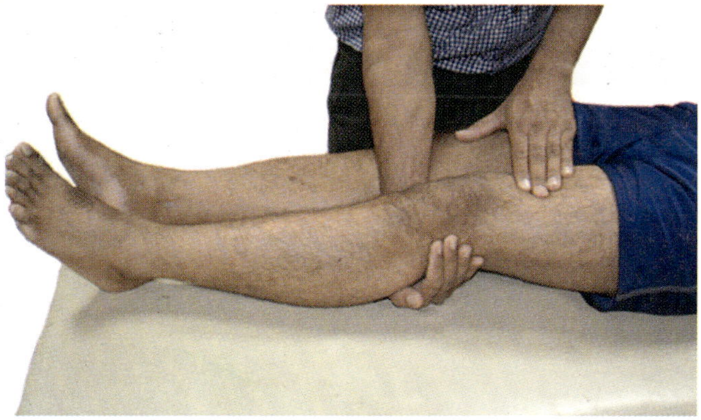

(b)

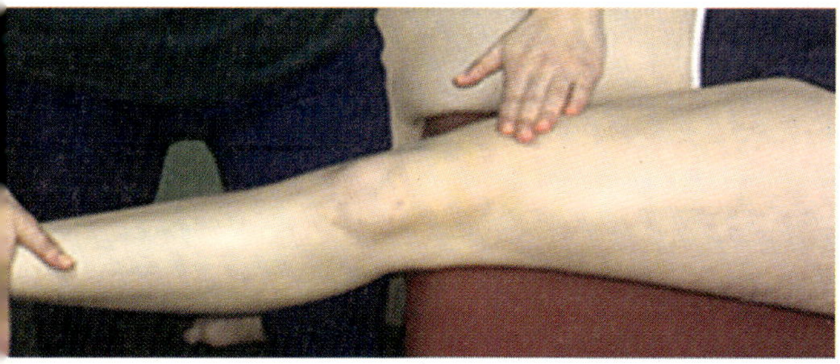

Figs. 6.267a and b: (a) Palpation of left side rectus femoris (quadriceps) muscle above the patella for grade 1, (b) Palpation of vastus medialis (quadriceps) muscles

Test: Examiner asks the patient to press the knee joint downward or contract the quadriceps muscles. For the alternate position therapist may place his or her other hand under the knee joint that allows little flexion of the knee joint. Examiner instructs the patient to try to straighten the knee joint. An attempt would cause contraction of the quadriceps.

Grade 2 (Poor)

Position of Patient: Side lying with the testing leg on the upper most. The lower leg (non testing) is flexed 45° at hip and knee joint for stability.

Position of Examiner: Examiner stands behind the patient and stabilizes the pelvis and supports distal leg with the forearm (Figs. 6.268 and 6.269).

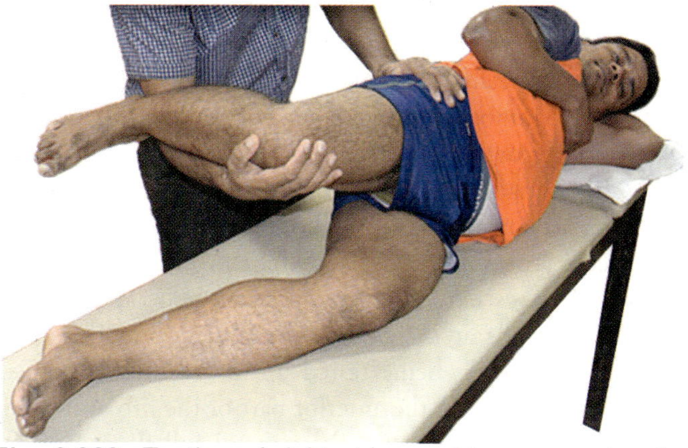

Fig. 6.268: Testing of right side quadriceps muscles for grade 2–Starting position

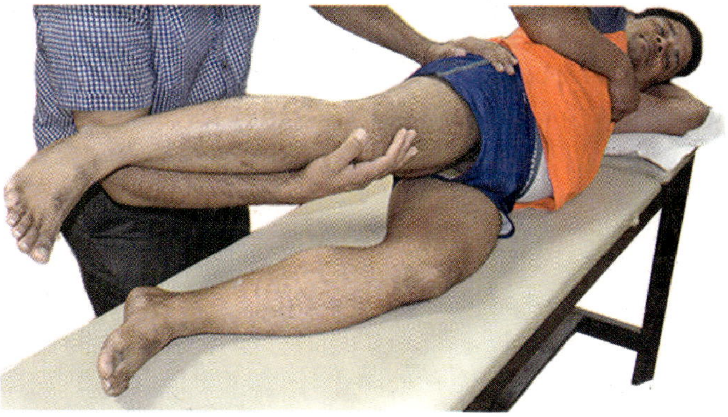

Fig. 6.269: Testing of right side quadriceps muscles for grade 2 in the available range of motion

Test: Examiner instructs the patient to band the knee in the available range without rotating the trunk and hip joint. Examiner suppose to support the leg and should not offer resistance or assistance to the movement. If patient completes extension in the full range in gravity eliminated position it is considered grade 2.

Weakness of Quadriceps: Like hamstrings, the quadriceps muscles are also two joint muscles, therefore, weakness or shortening affects both the joints. The weak quadriceps inables the patella to keep on the trochlear groove in walking. The patella may shift medially or laterally. Quadriceps helps in maintaining the pelvis at neutral. Weakness of quadriceps may cause posterior tilt of the pelvis with flattening of the lumbar spine. The patients with paralysis of quadriceps muscles especially below grade 3 cannot walk without substituting the other muscles. These patients bring the knee joint behind the center of gravity by hyperextending the knee joint, either by using the gluteus maximus or gastrosoleus muscle with anterior tilting of the trunk. Such gait is known as anterior trunk bending gait. Some patients walk by placing the ipsilateral hand over the knee joint. This is known as hand to knee gait.

Shortening of Quadriceps: Shortening of quadriceps muscles is associated with anterior tilting of the pelvis and exaggerated lumbar lordosis. The short quadriceps pull the patella superior to the trochlear groove. The individuals with short quadriceps complaint pain in the suprapatellar region and anterior thigh. To test the shortening of quadriceps, the subject is placed in a prone position with both the knees extended and hips at neutral position. Examiner stands at the side of the subject and flexes the knee joint which is being tested up to the full range, i.e., 0° to 135°. Normally the anterior part of the hip and pelvis remains on the surface of the couch till full flexion of the knee joint. If hip joint flexion occurs and it gets off of the surface of couch when knee is flexed, a tightness in the rectus femoris is considered. The test is known as Ely's test or prone knee bending test for rectus femoris tightness (Figs. 6.270 and 6.271).

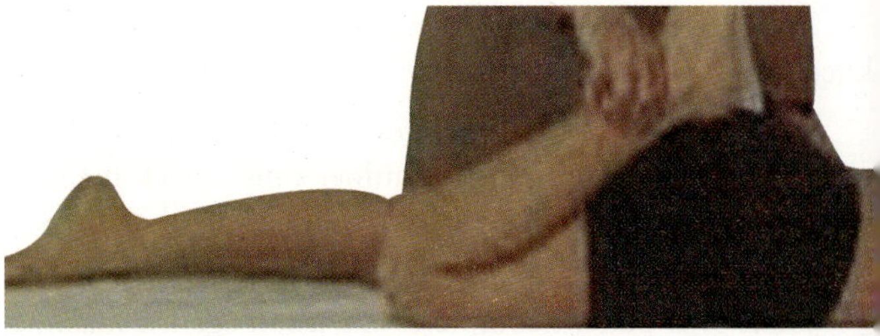

Fig. 6.270: Prone knee bending test for testing the length of the quadriceps. Hips are at neutral with knee bending shows normal length of quadriceps muscles. Examiner may stand opposite side for convenience

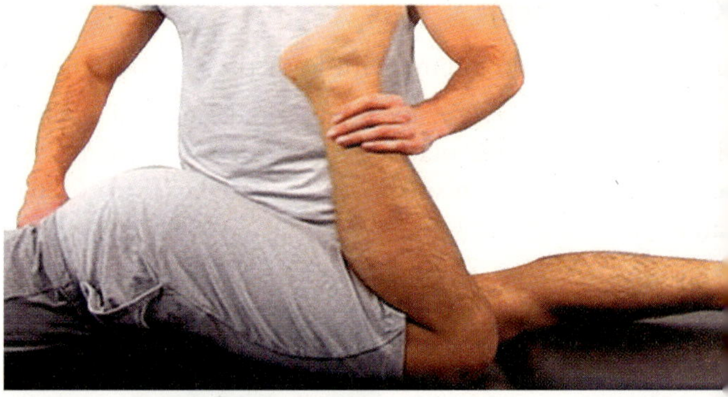

Fig. 6.271: Positive Ely's test or prone knee bending test for testing the length of the quadriceps. Increase flexion at the hip joint with knee bending shows shortening of quadriceps muscles

ANKLE AND FOOT MUSCLES TESTING

GASTROCNEMIUS AND SOLEUS – ANKLE PLANTAR FLEXORS

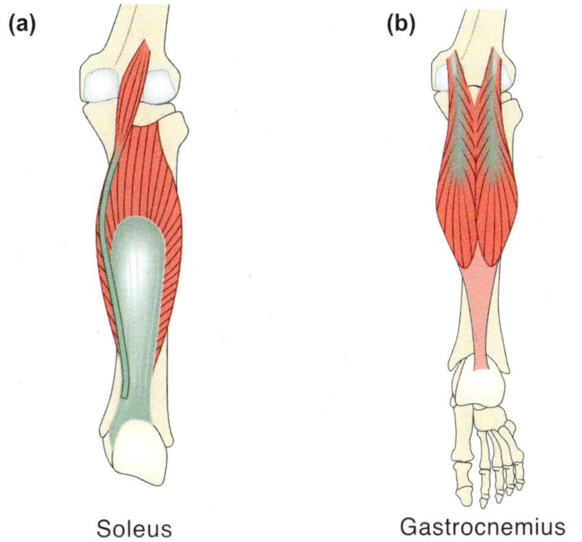

Figs. 6.272a and b: Origin and insertion of gastrocnemius and soleus muscles

Soleus

Origin: Posterior surface of the head of the fibula and proximal 1/3rd of its body, soleal line and middle 1/3rd of the medial border of the tibia, and tendinous arch between the tibia and fibula.

Insertion: Posterior surface of the calcaneum.

Action: Plantar flexion of the ankle joint.

Nerve Supply: Tibial L_5, S_1 and S_2.

Gastrocnemius

Origin of Medial Head: Proximal and posterior part of the medial condyle and adjacent part of the femur, capsule of the knee joint.

Origin of Lateral Head: Lateral condyle and posterior surface of the femur, capsule of the knee joint.

Insertion: Middle part of the posterior surface of the calcaneus.

Action: Plantar flexion of the ankle joint.

Nerve Supply: Tibial nerve S_1 and S_2.

Grade 3, Grade 4 and Grade 5 (Fair, Good and Normal)

Position of Patient: Patient stands on the foot, which is being tested with support of two fingers on the couch. The other leg remains unloaded (flexed at hip and knee joints to 45°).

Position of Examiner: Examiner may stand at the side, which is being tested (Figs. 6.273a and b).

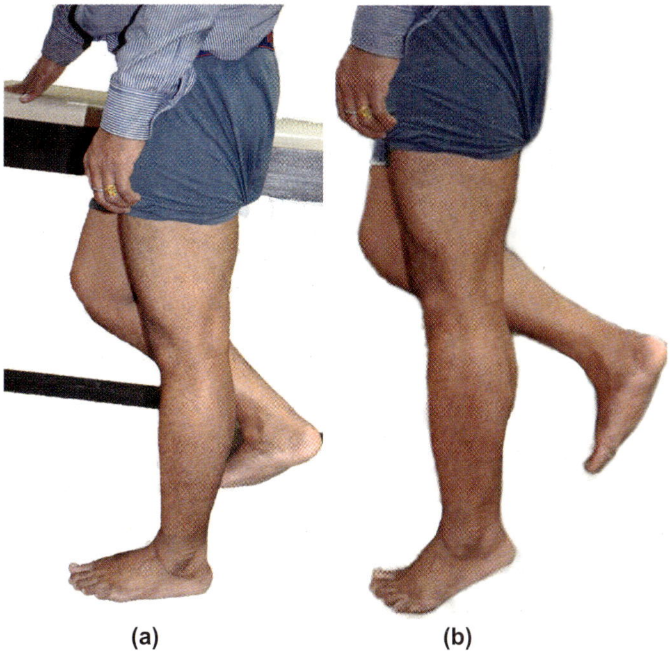

Figs. 6.273a and b: Testing of gastrocnemius and soleus for grade 3, 4 and 5

Test: Examiner instructs the patient to raise the heel in the full range of motion.

Grade 3: Patient must complete one heel raise in full range. If patient fails to complete the one heel raise in the full range it should be graded less than grade 3.

Grade 4: If patient completes between 2 and 24 heel rises at a consistent rate of one rise every 2 seconds using correct form in all repetitions.

Grade 5: Patient must complete minimum of 25 heel rises successfully through full range of motion without a rest between rise and without fatigue.

Grade 1 (Trace)

Position of Patient: Prone with the ankle joint out of edge of the couch.

Position of Examiner: Examiner stands at side, which is being tested and places fingers on gastrosoleus muscle to palpate it (Figs. 6.274a and b).

Test: Examiner instructs the patients to point your ankle and toes up towards the ceiling while examiner palpates the tendoachillis. If examiner finds contraction it is considered grade 1.

(a) (b)

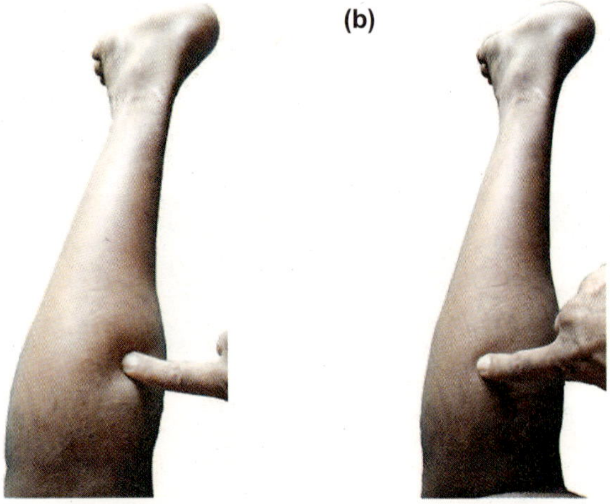

Figs. 6.274a and b: Palpation of gastrocnemius and soleus for grade 1

Grade 2 (Poor)

Position of Patient: Side lying with the testing leg upper most and lower leg (non testing) is flexed to 45° at hip and knee joint.

Position of Examiner: Examiner stands at the side, which is being tested and places one hand at the medial surface of the distal thigh and other hand grasps the distal leg just above the ankle joint to support the leg (Figs. 6.275a and b).

(a)

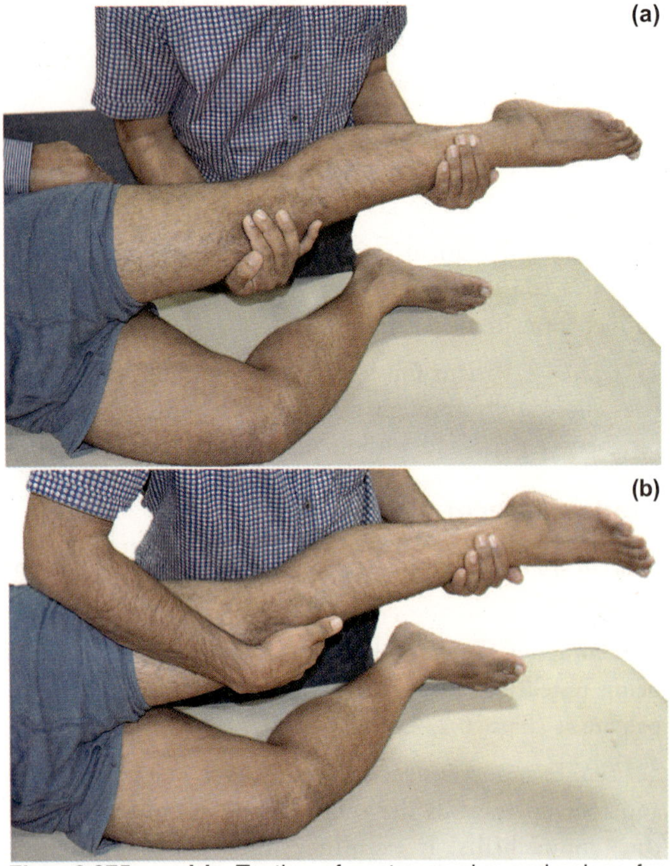

(b)

Figs. 6.275a and b: Testing of gastrocnemius and soleus for grade 2

Test: Examiner instructs the patient to point the toes towards heel (plantar flexion). The examiner must not offer the resistance or assistance to the movement but support the leg for smooth movement. If patient completes plantar flexion in full range it is considered grade 2.

Gastrosoleus Weakness: Weakness of gastrocnemius soleus muscles may occur following tibial nerve injury. The individuals find difficulty in push off, and show decrease step length, delay in heel off, and reduction in a forward progression of the hip to avoid collapse of the foot into dorsiflexion.

Gastrosoleus Shortening: Contracture of the gastrosoleus usually occurs if the antagonistic muscles are weak. There is loss of heel strike, and patients walk on the toes. This is known as equines gait.

ISOLATED STRENGTH TESTING OF GASTROCNEMIUS MUSCLES

Position of Patient: Prone with knee flexion.

Position of Examiner: Standing at the side which is being tested.

Stabilization: Examiner stabilizes the leg to prevent flexion and extension of knee joint.

Test: If patient completes plantar flexion against gravity (Figs. 6.276a, b and Figs. 6.277a, b).

(a)

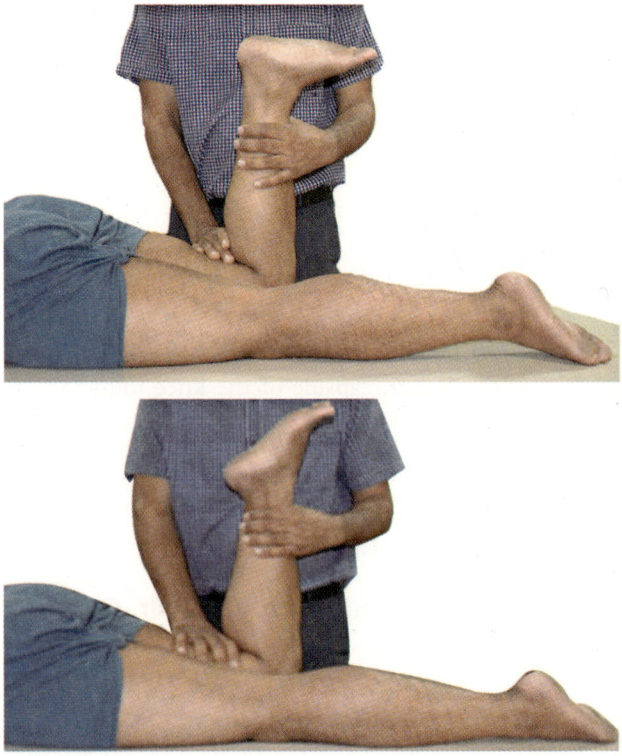

(b)

Figs. 6.276a and b: Testing of gatrocnemius for grade 3

(a)

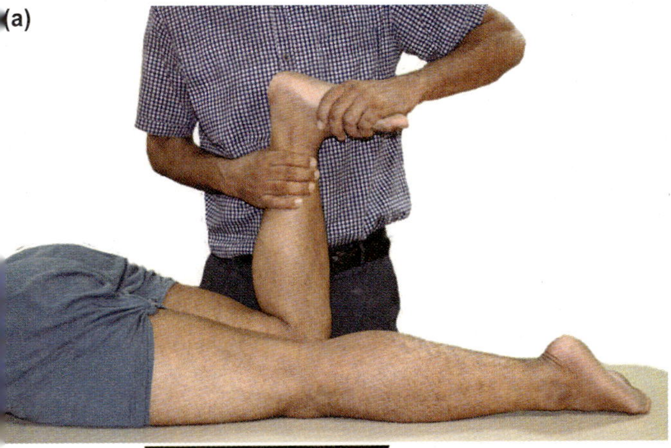

(b)

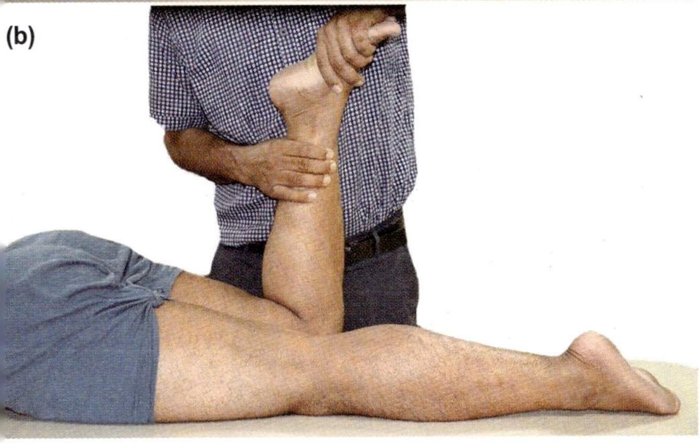

Figs. 6.277a and b: Testing of gatrocnemius for grade 4 and 5

Grade 4: If patient completes plantar flexion against strong to moderate resistance.

Grade 5: If patient completes plantar flexion against maximal resistance.

TIBIALIS POSTERIOR – ANKLE PLANTAR FLEXOR

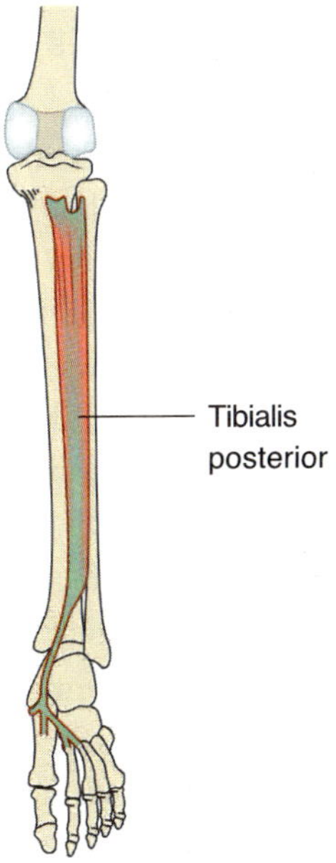

Fig. 6.278: Origin and insertion of tibialis posterior muscle

Origin: Interosseous membrane, lateral portion of the posterior surface of the tibia, proximal 2/3rd of the medial surface of the fibula, adjacent intermuscular septa and deep fascia.

Insertion: Tuberosity of the navicular bone and by fibrous expansion to the sustentaculum tali, three cuneiforms, cuboid, and bases of the second through fourth metatarsal bones.

Action: Plantar flexion of the ankle joint with inversion of the foot.

Nerve Supply: Tibial Nerve $L_{4,5}$ and S_1.

Grade 3, Grade 4 and Grade 5

Position of Patient: Prone with testing side knee flexed to 90°.

Position of Examiner: Examiner stands at the side of leg, which is being tested and holds the leg just above the ankle joint to stabilize it.

Test: Examiner instructs the patient to bring the foot up and outwards. Examiner must ensure that movement is taking place at the ankle and not at the MTP joints. Trick movements such as rotation at the hip joint and flexion and extension at the knee joint should be taken care of.

Grade 3: If patient completes plantar flexion with inversion against the gravity, it is considered grade 3 (Figs. 6.279a and b).

(a)

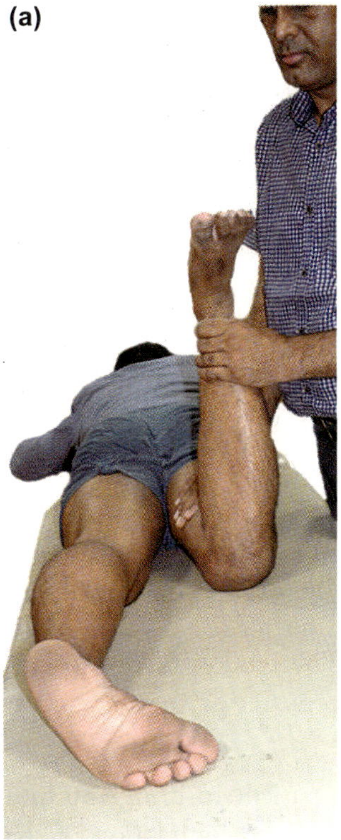

(b)

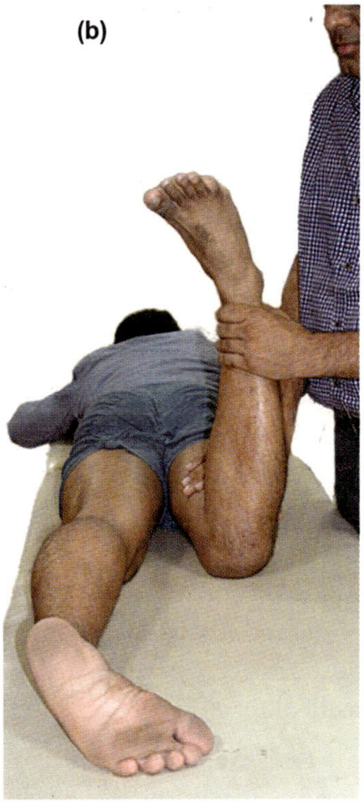

Figs. 6.279a and b: Testing of tibialis posterior muscle for grade 3

Grade 4: If patient completes plantar flexion with inversion against strong to moderate resistance, it is considered grade 4 (Fig. 6.280).

Grade 5: If patient completes plantar flexion with inversion against maximal resistance, it is considered grade 5 (Fig. 6.280).

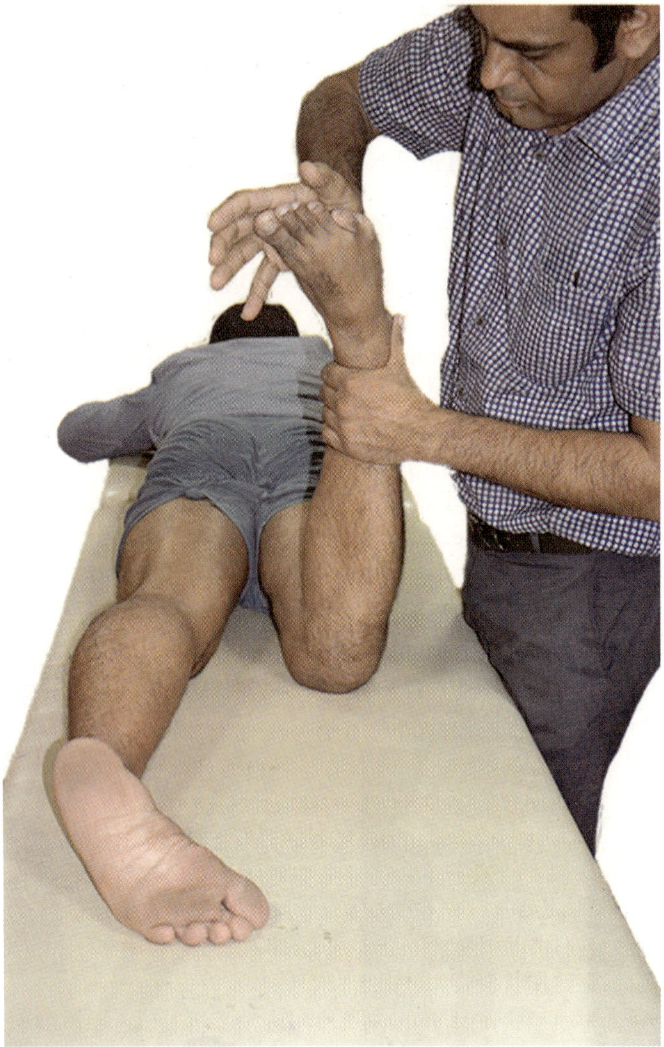

Fig. 6.280: Testing of tibialis posterior muscle for grade 4 and 5

Grade 1

Position of Patient: Supine lying.

Position of Examiner: Examiner stands at the side, which is being tested and grasps the leg just above the ankle joint and places fingers of other hand on medial portion of the posterior surface of the tibia. The tendon of the tibialis posterior can be palpated just posterior to the medial malleolus.

Test: Examiner instructs the patient to bring the foot down and inwards while palpating the contraction of the muscles. If examiner feels contraction during the attempt of movement, it is considered grade 1.

Grade 2

Position of Patient: Side lying with the non-testing leg lowermost and the leg which is being tested, remains uppermost. The non-testing leg is flexed to 45° at hip and knee joint for stabilization.

Position of Examiner: Examiner may stand behind the patient and cradles the leg at the knee joint and grasps the distal leg just above the ankle joint (Fig. 6.281).

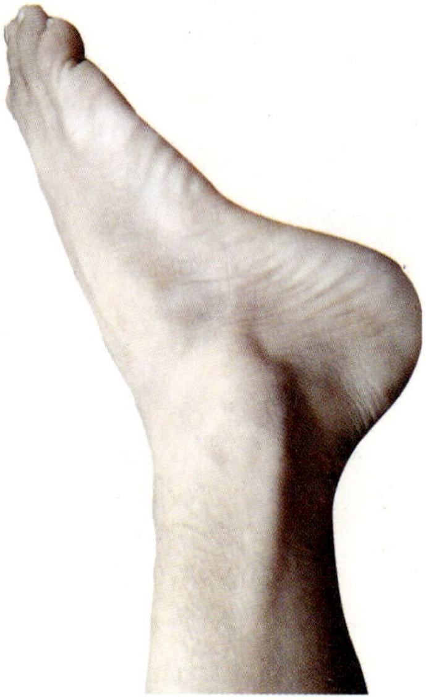

Fig. 6.281: Testing of tibialis posterior muscle for grade 2

Test: Examiner instructs the patient to bring the foot down and inwards. If patient completes plantar flexion with inversion in full range of motion it is considered grade 2. It is noted that the inversion is taken place in the gravity assisted position, therefore, examiner may resist the inversion. The tibialis posterior may also be tested in the short sitting position with the testing leg is placed on the knee joint of the non testing leg.

Weakness: Tibialis posterior acts as the primary dynamic stabilizer of the medial longitudinal arch and main inverter of the midfoot. Its contraction also elevates the medial longitudinal arch, causing the hind foot and midfoot to become a rigid structure. This allows the gastrocnemius to act with greater efficiency during the gait cycle. As the muscle loses function, the medial longitudinal arch of the foot collapses, which causes a relative internal rotation of the tibia and talus. There is eversion of the subtalar joint, which forces the heel into valgus alignment, and abduction at the talonavicular joint. Varus alignment of the heel causes a lateral shift in the normal axis of the achilles tendon, which in time will lead to a contracture. As the deformity gets worsen, the distal fibula comes into contact with the lateral calcaneus, causing lateral hind foot pain.

TIBIALIS ANTERIOR – ANKLE DORSIFLEXORS

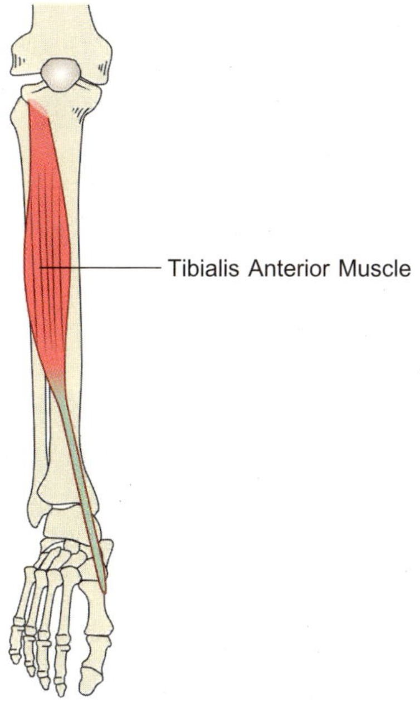

Fig. 6.282: Origin and insertion of tibialis anterior muscle

Origin: Lateral condyle of the tibia, proximal ½ -2/3rd.

Insertion: Medial and plantar surfaces of first cuneiform and on base of first metatarsal bone.

Action: Dorsiflexion of ankle joint with inversion.

Nerve Supply: Deep peroneal nerve L_4, L_5 and S_1.

Grade 3, Grade 4 and Grade 5

Position of Patient: Short sitting with both the hands hold the edges of the table.

Position of Examiner: Examiner sits at the side of leg, which is being tested and holds the leg at knee joint and just above the ankle to stabilize it (Figs. 283a and b, Fig. 284).

Stabilization: Examiner holds the leg and thigh to prevent knee flexion and hip rotations.

Test: Examiner instructs the patient to bring the foot up and in. Examiner must ensure that the movement is taking place at the ankle and not at the MTP joints.

Grade 3: If patient completes dorsiflexion with inversion against the gravity it is considered grade 3.

Grade 4: If patient completes dorsiflexion with inversion against strong to moderate resistance, it is considered grade 4.

Grade 5: If patient completes dorsiflexion with inversion against maximal resistance, it is considered grade 5.

(a)

(b)

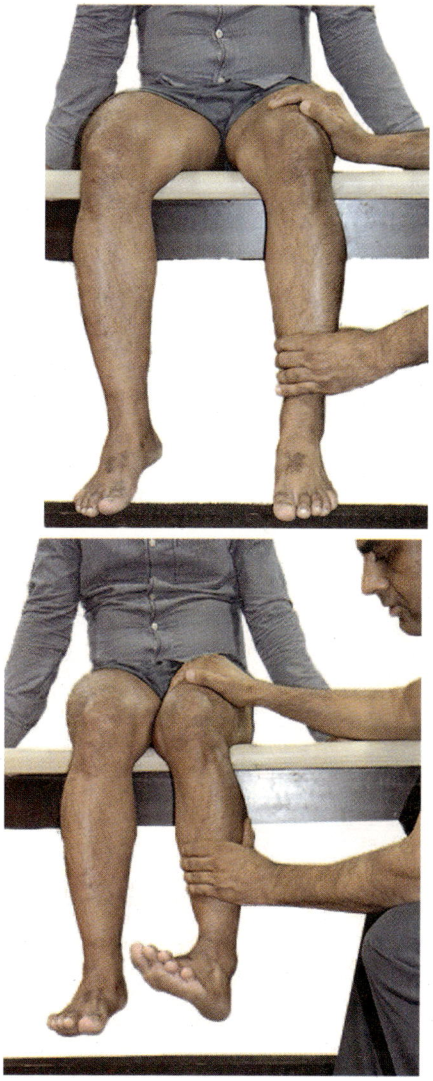

Figs. 6.283a and b: Testing of tibialis anterior for grade 3

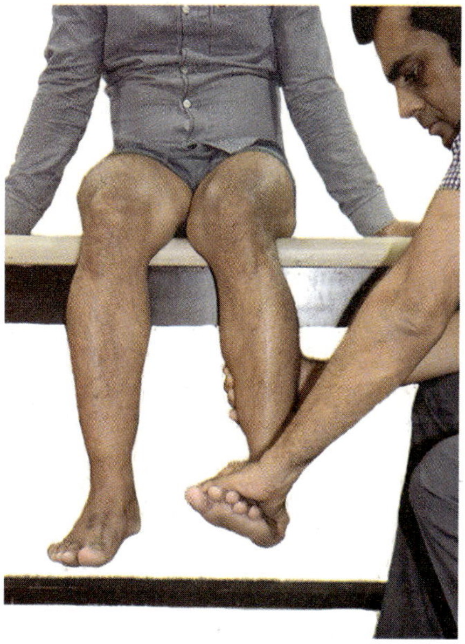

Fig. 6.284: Testing of tibialis anterior muscle for grade 4 and 5

Grade 1

Position of Patient: Supine or short sitting with both the hands hold the edge of table.

Position of Examiner: Sitting on stool and places the heel of the patient on the thigh. Examiner places finger of other hand on the lateral to the shin of tibia just below the knee joint.

Test: Examiner instructs the patient to bring the foot up and inwards while palpating the contraction of the tibialis anterior muscle. If examiner feels contraction during the attempt of movement, it is considered grade 1 (Fig. 6.285).

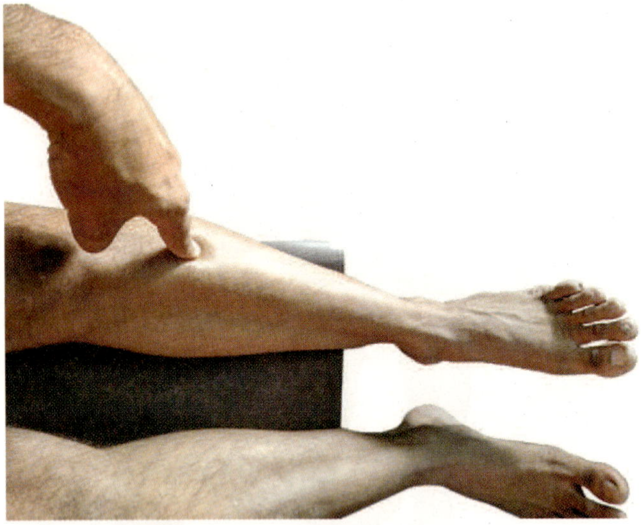

Fig. 6.285: Palpation of tibialis anterior muscle for grade 1

Grade 2

Position of Patient: Short sitting with the testing leg is on the contralateral thigh.

Position of Examiner: Examiner stands at the side, which leg is being tested and holds the knee joint to stabilize the leg.

Stabilization: Examiner stabilizes the knee to prevent flexion and hip to prevent rotation.

Test: Examiner instructs the patient to bring the foot up toward knee joint and in. If patient completes dorsiflexion with inversion in full range it is considered grade 2. It is to be noted that the inversion movement is taken place against the gravity, therefore; examiner may apply little resistance to inversion to test it.

The alternate position for grade 2 is side lying with the testing leg uppermost. Examiner stands at the side, which is being tested and hold the leg at the knee joint and just above the ankle to support it. The patient is instructed to bring the ankle joint up and inwards in the full range of motion (Figs. 286a and b).

(a)

(b)

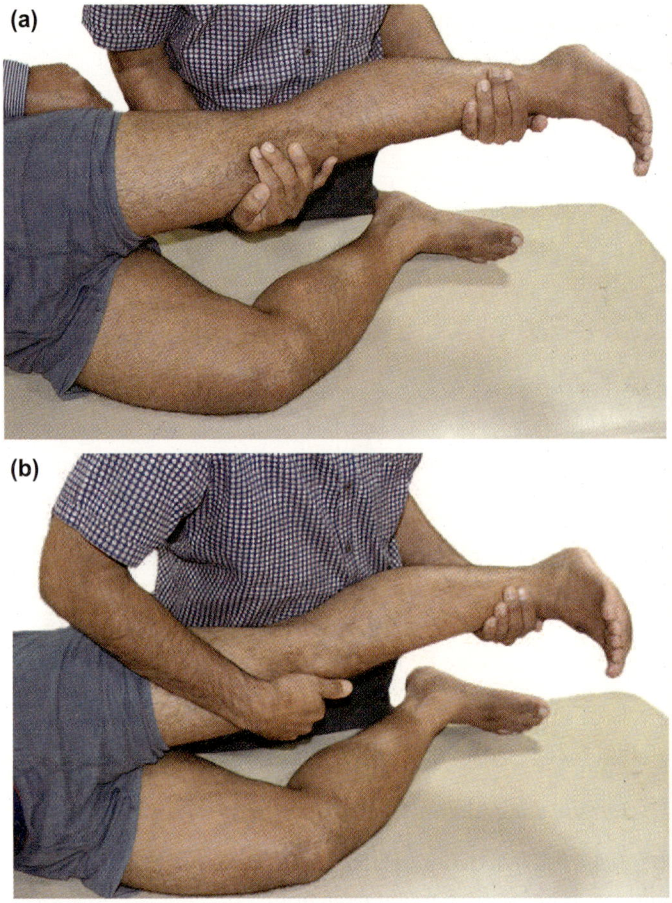

Figs. 286a and b: Testing of tibialis anterior muscle for grade 2

Weakness: Weakness of tibialis anterior muscles results in an equinovarus deformity. Foot drop can result if there is injury to the dorsiflexors or to any point along the neural pathways that supply them. The patient with weak tibialis anterior finds difficulty in dorsiflexion of the ankle joint. There is loss of heel strike and toes contact with the ground first than with the heel in the stance phase. The toes drag on the ground in swing phase. To clear the ground patient walks with the exaggerated flexion of the hip and knee joints. This sometimes referred to as steppage gait. During gait, the force of heel strike exceeds body weight, and the direction of the ground reaction vector passes behind the ankle and knee center (Fig. 6.287).

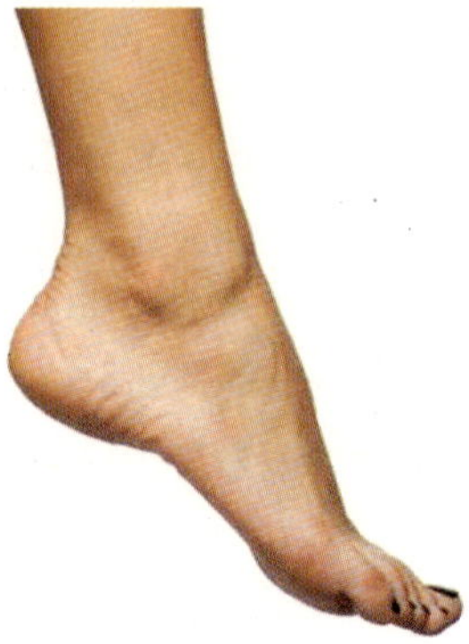

Fig. 6.287: Foot drop

PERONEUS LONGUS AND BREVIS – ANKLE PLANTAR FLEXION WITH EVERSION

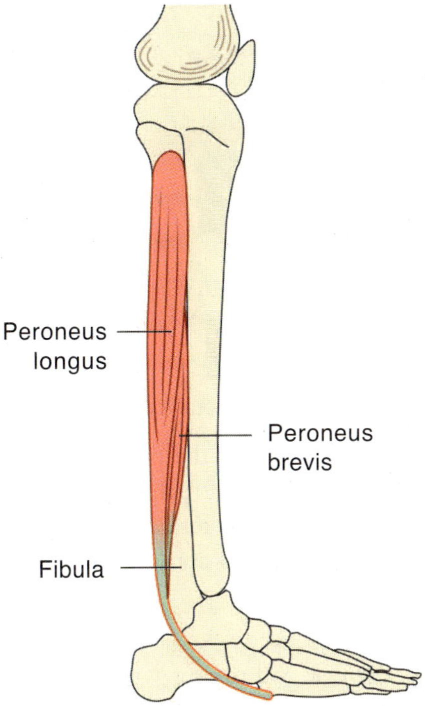

Fig. 6.288: Origin and insertion of peroneus longus and peroneus brevis muscles

Peroneus Longus

Origin: Lateral condyle of the tibia, head and proximal 2/3rd of the lateral surface of the fibula, intermuscular septa and adjacent deep fascia.

Insertion: Lateral side of the base of the first metatarsal and of the medial cuneiform bone.

Peroneus Brevis

Origin: Distal 2/3rd of the lateral surface of the fibula and adjacent intermuscular septa.

Insertion: Tuberosity at the base of the fifth metatarsal bone, lateral side.

Action: Eversion of the foot, lateral flexion of the ankle joint and helps in depressing the first metatarsal head.

Nerve Supply of Peroneus longus and bravis: $L_{4, 5}$ and S_1.

Grade 3, Grade 4 and Grade 5

Position of Patient: Prone with knee flexion.

Position of Examiner: Examiners stands at the side of leg which is being tested and holds the leg just above the ankle joint to stabilize it.

Stabilization: Examiner stabilizes the ankle to prevent flexion and extension and hip joint to prevent rotations.

Test: Examiner instructs the patient to bring the foot up and outwards. Examiner must ensure that movement is taking place at the ankle and not at the MTP joints. Trick movements such as rotation at the hip joint and flexion and extension at the knee joint should be taken care of.

Grade 3: If patient completes plantar flexion with eversion against the gravity, it is considered grade 3 (Figs. 6.289a and b).

(a)

(b)

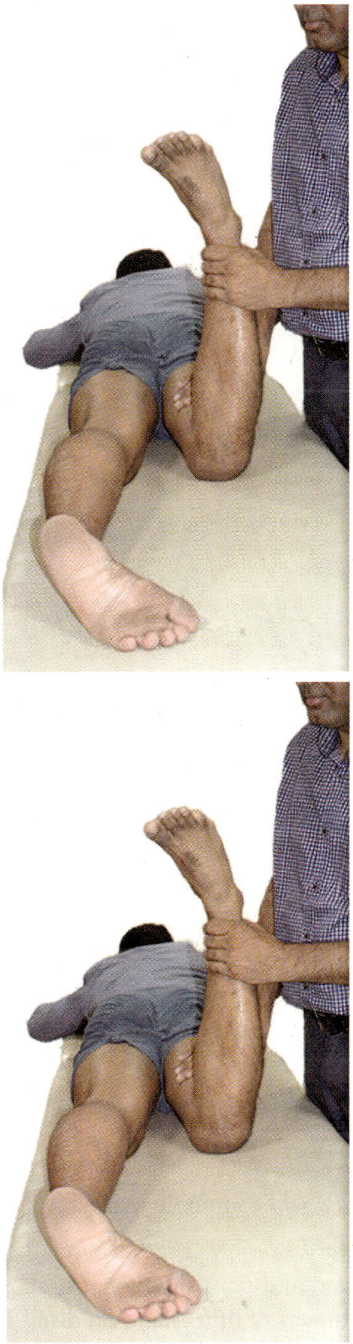

Figs. 6.289a and b: Testing of peroneus longus and brevis for grade 3

Grade 4: If patient completes plantar flexion with eversion against strong to moderate resistance, it is considered grade 4.

Grade 5: If patient completes plantar flexion with eversion against maximal resistance, it is considered grade 5 (Fig. 6.290).

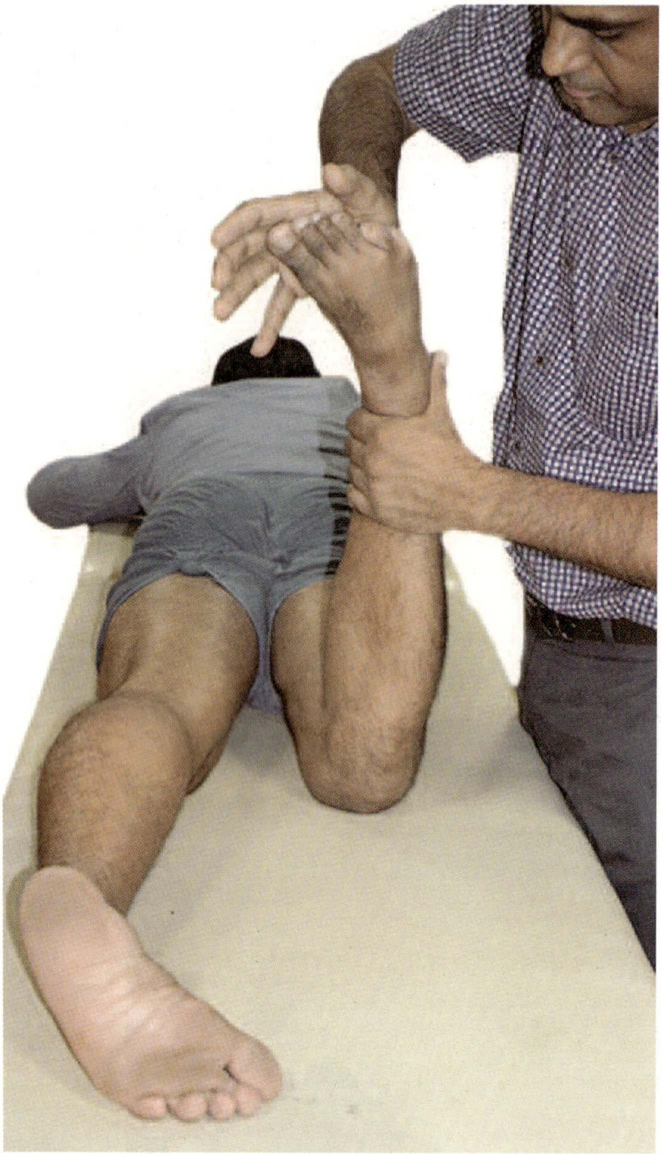

Fig. 6.290: Testing of peroneus longus and brevis for grade 4 and 5

Grade 1

Position of Patient: Supine lying.

Position of Examiner: Examiner stands at the side, which is being tested and grasps the leg just above the ankle joint and places fingers of other hand on distal 1/3rd of the fibula (Fig. 6.291).

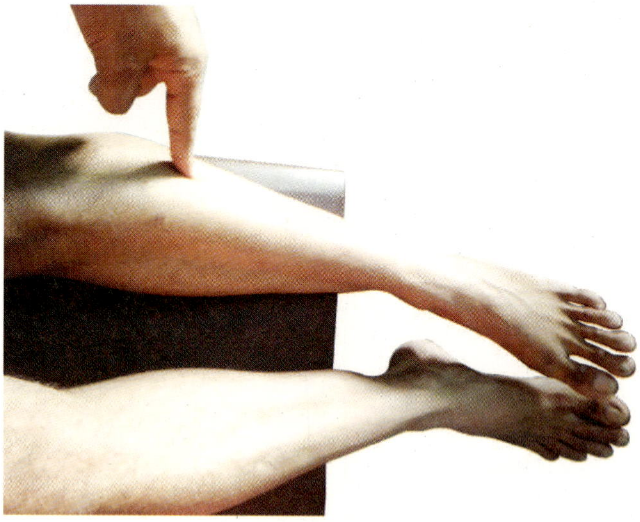

Fig. 6.291: Palpation of peroneus longus and brevis for grade 1

Test: Examiner instructs the patient to try to bring the foot up and outwards while palpating the contraction of the muscles. If examiner feels contraction during the attempt of movement, it is considered grade 1.

Grade 2

Position of Patient: Side lying with the non-testing leg lowermost and the leg which is being tested, remains on the non-testing leg The non-testing leg is flexed to 50° at hip and knee joint for stabilization.

Position of Examiner: Examiner stands behind the patient and cradles the leg at the knee joint and grasps the distal leg just above the ankle joint (Fig. 6.292).

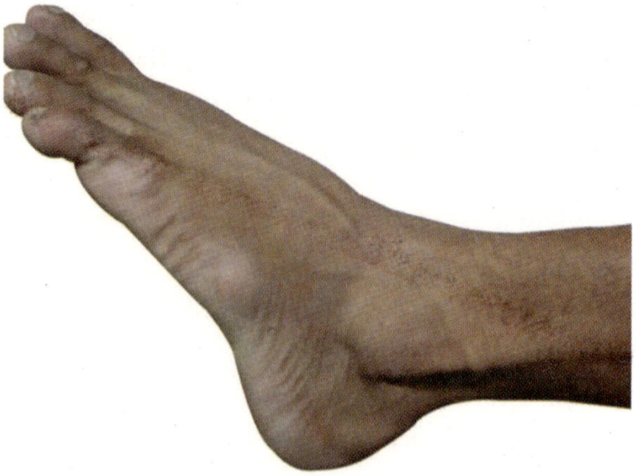

Fig. 6.292: Testing of peroneus longus and peroneus brevis for grade 2

Test: Examiner instructs the patient to bring the foot down and outwards. If patient completes plantar flexion with eversion in full range of motion it is considered grade 2. It is to note that the eversion movement is taken place in the gravity-assisted position, therefore, examiner may resist.

PERONEUS TERTIUS – ANKLE DORSIFLEXION

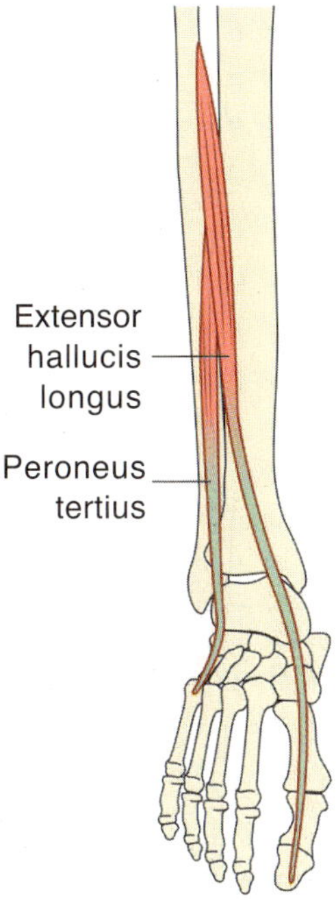

Fig. 6.293: Origin and insertion of peroneus tertius muscle

Origin: Distal 1/3rd of the anterior surface of the fibula, interosseous membrane and adjacent intermuscular septum.

Insertion: Dorsal surface of the fifth metatarsal.

Action: Dorsiflexion with eversion of the foot.

Nerve Supply: Deep Peroneal Nerve–L_4, L_5 and S_1.

Grade 3, Grade 4 and Grade 5

Position of Patient: Short sitting with both the hands hold the edge of the table.

Position of Examiner: Examiner sits at the side of leg, which is being tested and holds the leg at knee joint to stabilize it (Figs. 6.294a, b and Fig. 6.295).

Test: Examiner instructs the patient to bring the foot up and outwards. Examiner must ensure that movement is taking place at the ankle and not at the MTP joints.

Grade 3: If patient completes dorsiflexion with eversion against the gravity.

Grade 4: If patient completes dorsiflexion with eversion against strong to moderate resistance.

Grade 5: If patient completes dorsiflexion with eversion against maximal resistance.

Grade 1

Position of Patient: Supine lying with both the hands hold the edge of the table.

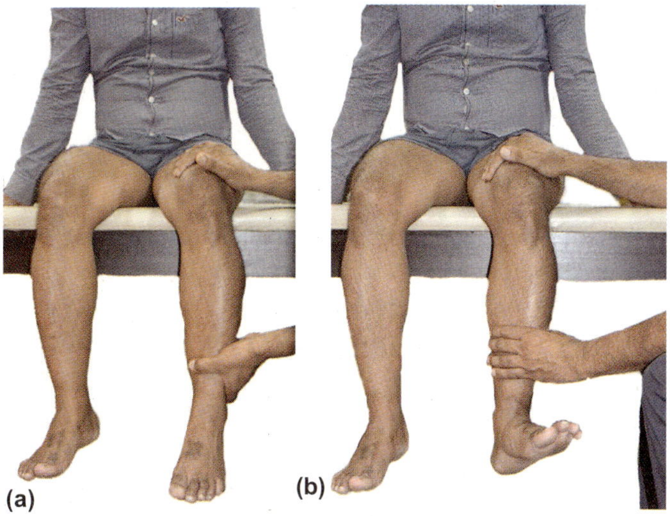

Figs. 6.294a and b: Testing of peroneus tertius muscle for grade 3

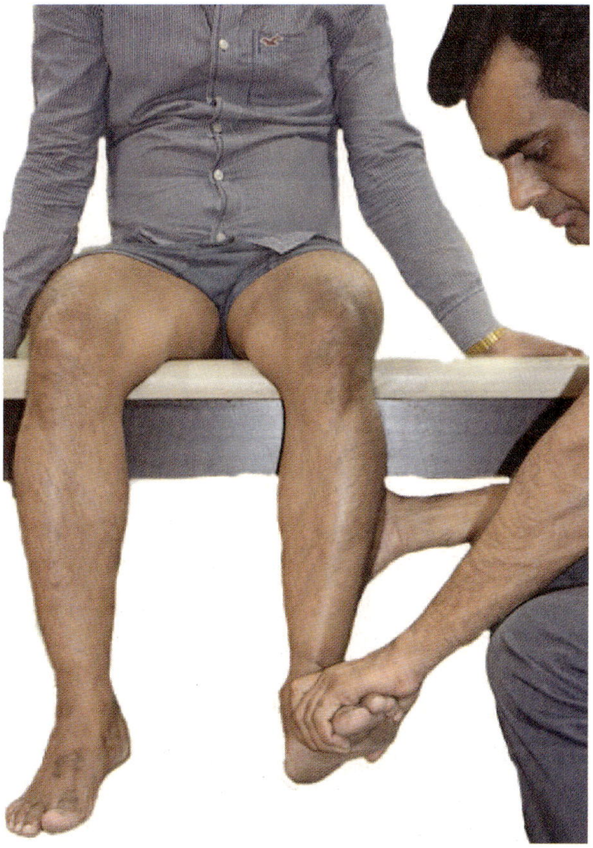

Fig. 6.295: Testing of peroneus muscle for grade 4 and 5

Position of Examiner: Examiner stands at the side, which is being tested. Examiner grasps the ankle joint and places fingers of other hand on the lateral aspect of leg just below the head of fibula.

Test: Examiner instructs the patient to bring the foot up and outwards while palpating the contraction of the muscles. If examiner feels contraction during the attempt of movement, it is considered grade 1.

Grade 2

Position of Patient: Short sitting with the testing leg is on the contralateral thigh.

Position of Examiner: Examiner stands at the side, which is being tested and holds the knee joint to stabilize the leg.

Test: Examiner instructs the patient to bring the foot up towards knee joint and outwards. If patient completes dorsiflexion with eversion in full range it is considered grade 2. It is noted that the eversion movement is taken place in the gravity-assisted position, therefore, examiner may apply little resistance to the eversion to test it correctly.

The alternate position for grade 2 is side lying with the testing leg upper most. Examiner stands at the side, which is being tested and holds the leg at the knee joint and just above the leg for support of the leg. The patient is instructed to bring the ankle joint up and inwards in the full range of motion (Figs. 6.296a and b).

(a)

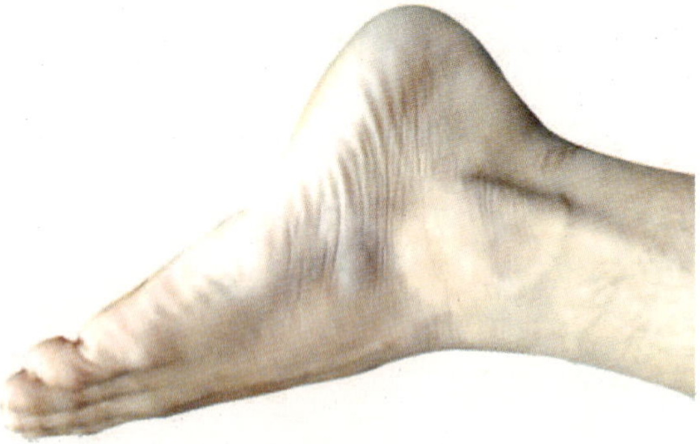

(b)

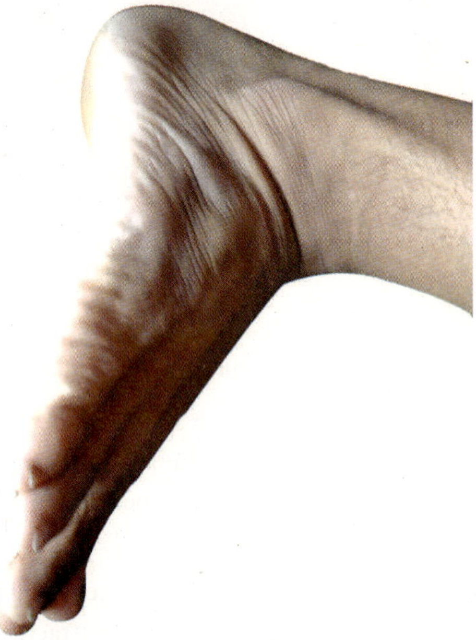

Figs. 6.296a and b: Testing of peroneus tertius muscle for grade 4 and 5

EXTENSOR HALLUCIS LONGUS – ANKLE DORSIFLEXION

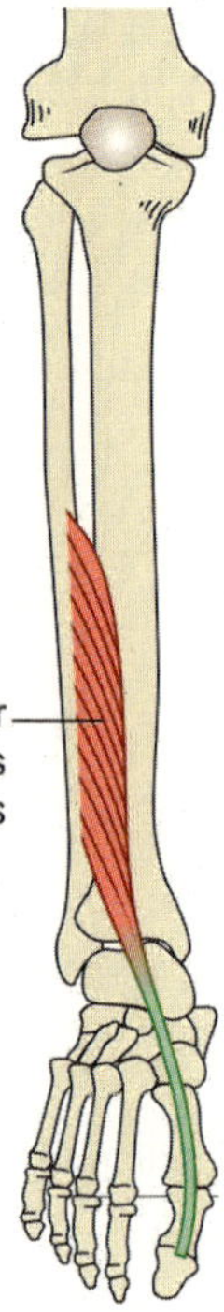

Fig. 6.297: Origin and insertion of extensor hallucis longus muscle

Extensor Hallucis Longus

Origin: Middle two quarters of the anterior surface of the fibula and adjacent interosseous membrane.

Insertion: Base of the distal phalanx of the great toe.

Action: Extensor hallucis longus extends the metatarsophalangeal and interphalangeal joints of the great toe, and assists in inversion of the foot and dorsiflexion of the ankle.

Nerve Supply: L_4, L_5, S_1.

Grade 3, Grade 4 and Grade 5 (Fair, Good and Normal)

Position of Patient: High sitting with the leg hanging freely on the floor.

Position of Examiner: The examiner stands at the side of the leg, which is being tested and grasps the hind foot with one hand.

Stabilization: Examiner grasps the distal leg at the ankle joint to stabilize and prevent knee flexion and extension, and also to maintain ankle joint at neutral.

Test: Patient is instructed to bring the great toe up towards the ceiling.

Grade 3: If patient completes extension of the great toe in full range against the gravity without assistance (Fig. 6.298).

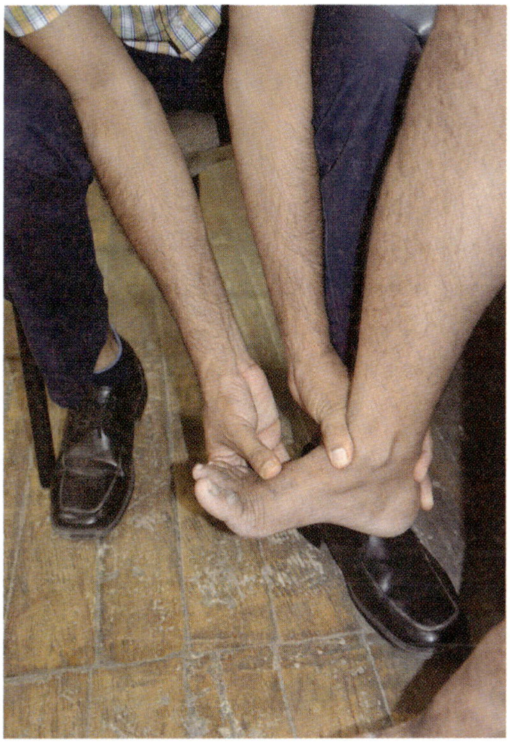

Fig. 6.298

Grade 4: If patient completes extension of the great toe in full range against the moderate resistance (Fig. 6.299).

Grade 5: If patient completes extension of the great toe in full range against maximum resistance.

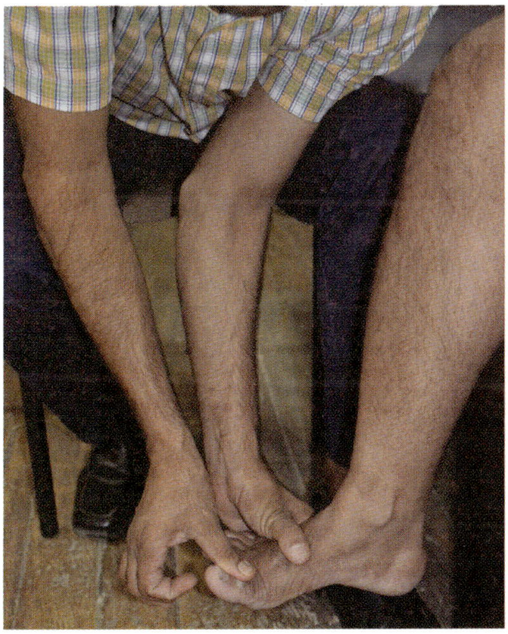

Fig. 6.299

Grade 1

Position of Patient: Supine.

Position of Examiner: Examiner stands at the side of the leg which is being tested and places the fingers on the distal part of the extensor hallucis longus muscle over the dorms of the foot (Fig. 6.300).

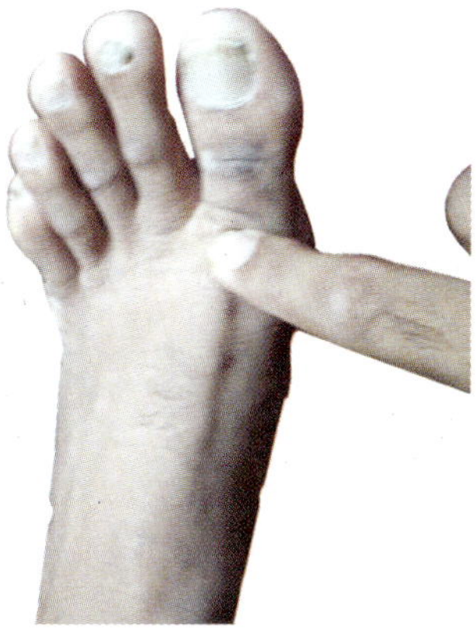

Fig. 6.300: Palpation of EHL for grade 1

Test: Examiner asks the patient to take the thumb up towards the dorsum of foot. If there is a palpable contraction over the dorsum of foot, it is considered grade 1.

Grade 2

Position of Patient: Side lying with the testing leg upper most. The lower leg is flexed for the good base of support.

Position of Examiner: The examiner stands at the side of the leg which is being tested and grasps the leg and ankle joint and maintains it above the other leg (Figs. 6.301a and b).

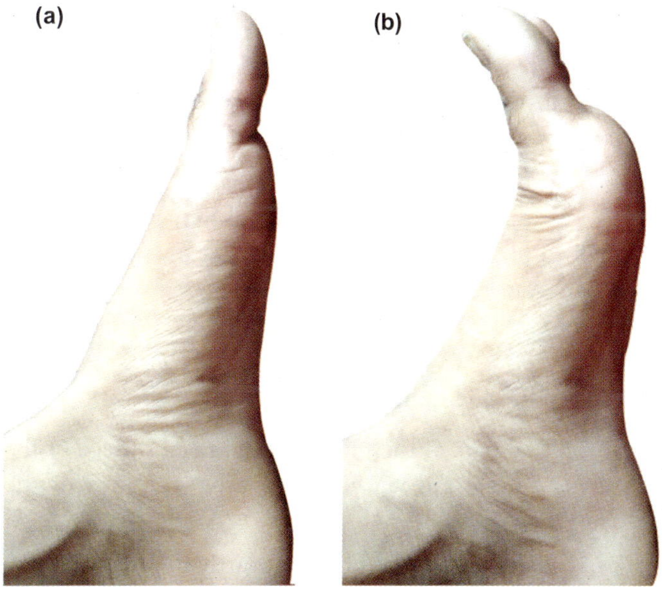

Figs. 6.301a and b: Testing of extensor hallucis longus for grade 2

Test: The examiner instructs the patient to bring the toe up towards the dorsum of foot. If the patient completes movement in full range, it is considered grade 2.

EXTENSOR DIGITORUM LONGUS AND BREVIS AND EXTENSOR HALLUCIS LONGUS–MTP JOINT EXTENSION

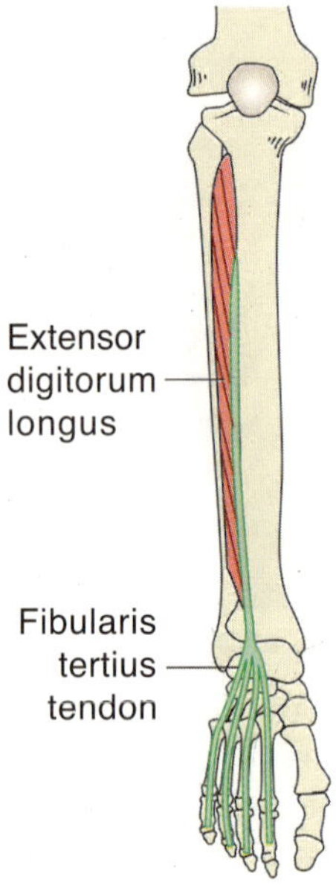

Fig. 6.302: Origin and insertion of EDL and EDB

Extensor Digitorum Longus (EDL)

Origin: Latearal condyle of tibia, proximal of the anterior surface of the body of the fibula, proximal part of the interosseous membrane, adjacent intermuscular septa and deep fascia.

Insertion: The tendon of the extensor digitorum divides into four tendons slip to dorsum of foot that forms an expansion over each toe (2nd to 5th). Intermediate slip attached to the base of the middle phalanx, and into two lateral slips attached to the base of the distal phalanx.

Action: EDL extends metatarsophalangeal joints, and assists in extending the interphalangeal joint of the second through fifth digits, also assists in dorsiflexion of the ankle joint and eversion of foot.

Nerve Supply: $L_{4,\,5}$ and S_1.

Extensor Digitorum Brevis

Origin: Distal part of the superior and lateral surface of the calcaneus, lateral talocalcaneal ligament and apex of the inferior retinaculum.

Insertion: First digit through fourth digit. The most medial slip, also known as the extensor hallucis brevis inserts into the dorsal surface of the base of the proximal phalanx of the great toe. The other three tendons join the lateral sides of the tendons of the extensor digitorum longus to the second, third and fourth digits.

Action: Extensor digitorum brevis extends metatarsophalangeal joint of the first through fourth digit, and assists in extending the interphalangeal joints of the second through fourth digits.

Nerve Supply: $L_{4,5}$ and S_1.

Origin: Middle two quarters of the anterior surface of the fibula and adjacent interosseous membrane.

Insertion: Base of the distal phalanx of the great toe.

Action: Extensor hallucis longus extends the metatarsophalangeal and interphalangeal joints of the great toe, and assists in inversion of the foot and dorsiflexion of the ankle joint.

Grade 3, Grade 4 and Grade 5 (Fair, Good and Normal)

Position of Patient: Short sitting with both the hands grasp the edge of the table.

Position of Examiner: Examiner sits on the stool and grasps the ankle joint for stabilization and foot in slight plantar flexion.

Test: Examiner instructs the patient to raise the toes from 2nd through 5th against the gravity, there should not be any movement at the ankle and knee joint.

Grade 3: If patient completes extension of the toes from 2nd to 5th against the gravity (Fig. 6.303).

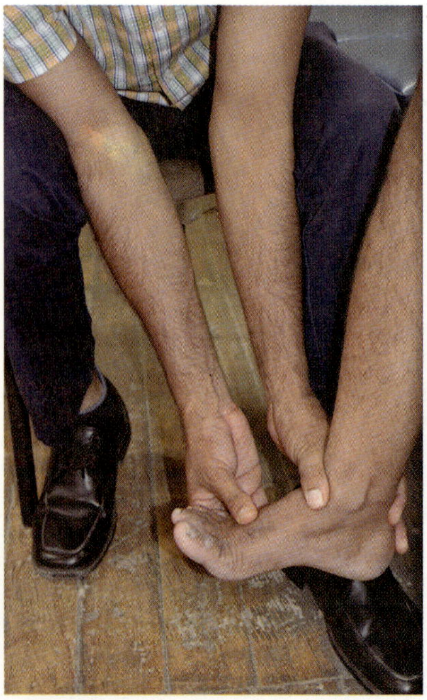

Fig. 6.303

Grade 4: If patient completes extension of the toes from 2nd to 5th against moderate to strong resistance against the gravity (Fig. 6.304).

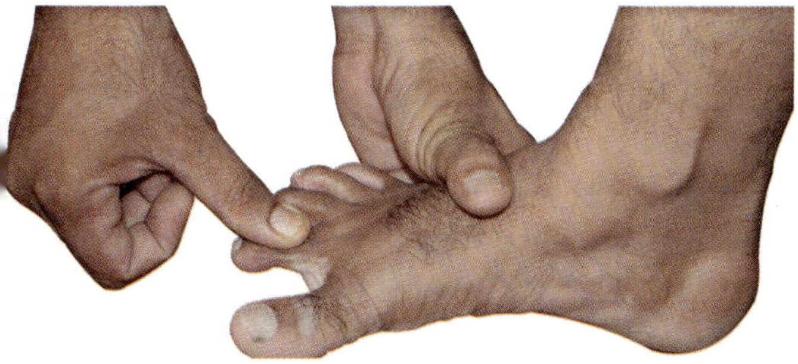

Fig. 6.304

Grade 5: If patient completes extension of the toes from 2nd to 5th against the maximal resistance against gravity (Fig. 6.305).

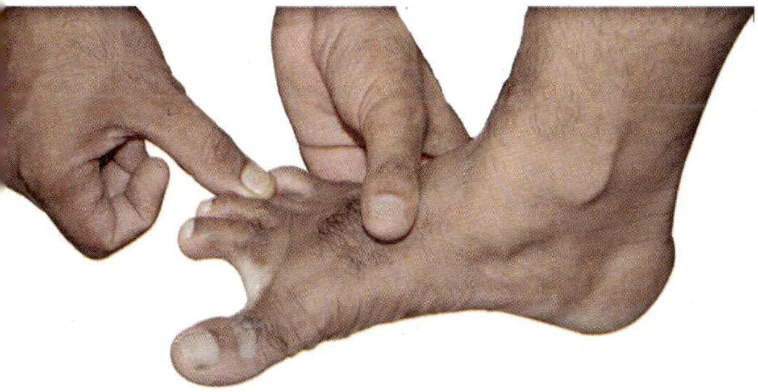

Fig. 6.305

Extensor Hallucis Longus, Grade 3 to 5: Extensor hallucis longus is tested separately by stabilizing the first metatarsal head. Position of patient, therapist, direction of movement and resistance remain same as for digits (2nd to 5th) (Fig. 6.306).

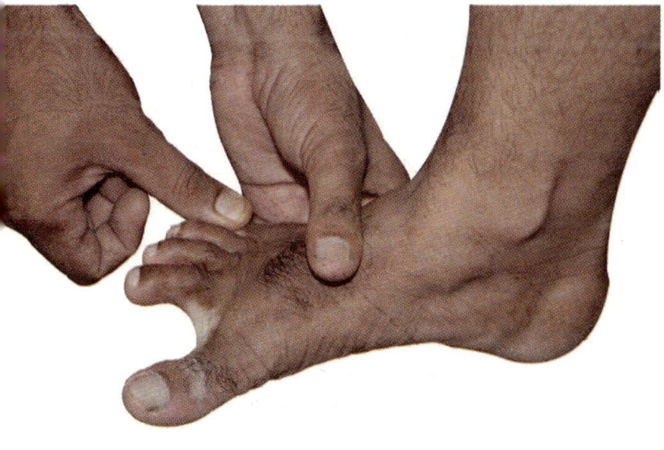

Fig. 6.306

Grade 1

Position of Patient: Supine lying with both the knees extended and the ankle joint in neutral position.

Position of Examiner: Examiner stands at the side of the leg, which is being tested and places the fingers on the proximal lateral leg and grasps the ankle joint with other hand (Fig. 6.307).

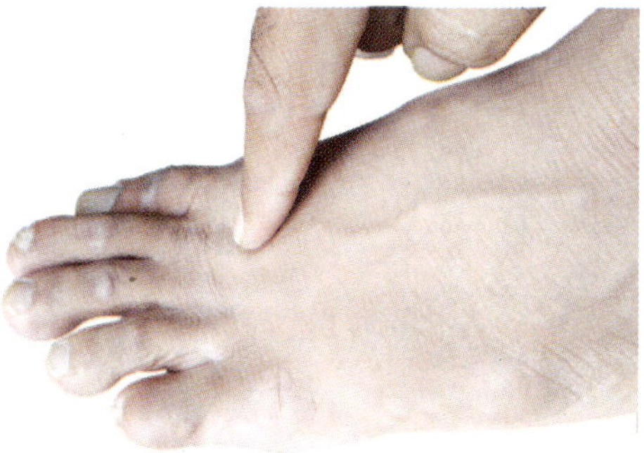

Fig. 6.307

Test: Examiner instructs the patient to bring the toes up towards the knee joint. If examiner finds contraction it is graded 1. The examiner must ensure that the patient is attempting to extend the toes from 2nd to 5th.

Grade 2

Position of Patient: Side lying with the testing leg upper most. The lower leg is flexed to 45° at hip and knee joint for the stabilization.

Position of Examiner: Examiner stands at the side of the patient, cradles the knee joint with the arm, and grasps the ankle joint for stabilization (Fig. 6.308).

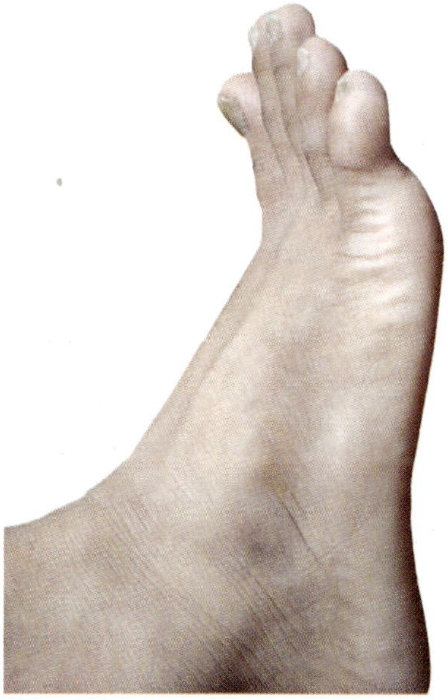

Fig. 6.308

Test: The patient is instructed to curl toes separately from 1st to 5th upwards. If examiner finds movement of the MTP joints from 2nd to 5th in full range in gravity assisted position it is given grade 2.

FLEXOR DIGITORUM LONGUS, FLEXOR DIGITORUM BREVIS AND FLEXOR HALLUCIS LONGUS – MTP FLEXION

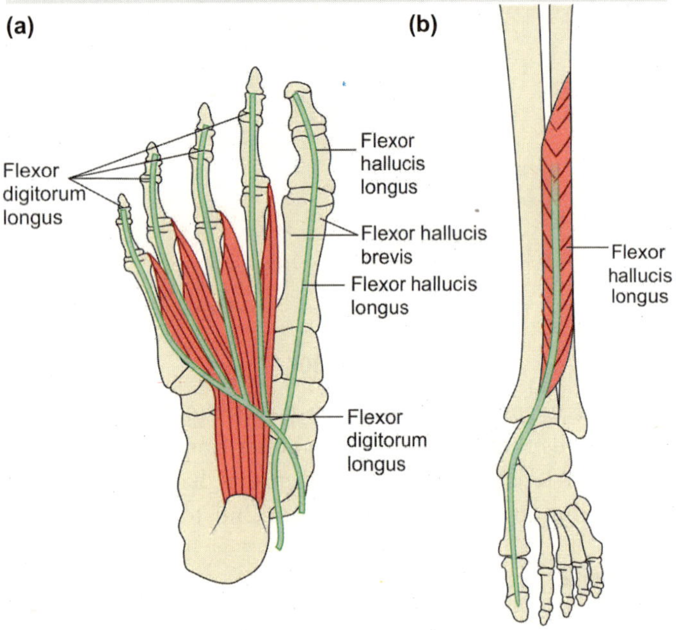

Figs. 6.309a and b: Origin and insertion of FDL, FDB and FHL

Flexor Digitorum Longus

Origin: Posterior surface of the tibia, just below the soleal line to within 7 or 8 cm of the distal end of the bone, and to the medial part of the fascia covering the tibialis posterior.

Insertion: Plantar surface of the bases of the distal phalanges of the four lateral toes.

Action: Flexion of the four lateral toes, assists with plantar flexion of the foot at the ankle.

Nerve Supply: Tibial nerve ($L_5 - S_{1\text{-}2}$).

Flexor Digitorum Brevis

Origin: Medial process of the calcaneal tuberosity, the central part of the plantar aponeurosis, and the intramuscular septa between it and adjacent muscles.

Insertion: By four tendons, each attaching to the medial and lateral borders and plantar surface of the middle phalanx of each of the four lateral toes.

Action: Flexion of the four lateral toes.

Innervation: Medial plantar nerve ($S_{1,2}$).

Flexor Hallucis Longus

Origin: Posterior surface of the distal 2/3rd of the fibula, interosseous membrane, and adjacent intermuscular septa and fascia.

Insertion: Base of the distal phalanx of the great toe, plantar surface.

Action: Flexor hallucis flexes the interphalangeal joint of the great toe, and assists in flexion of the metatarsal joint, plantar flexion of the ankle joint, and inversion of the joint.

Nerve Supply: L_5, S_1 and S_1.

Grade 1 (2nd to 5th)

Position of Patient: Supine with both the knees extended.

Position of Examiner: Examiner stands at the side, which is being tested and places the fingers on the palmar surface of the mid foot and grasps the ankle joint with the other hand.

Test: Patient is instructed to curl the toes down to the floor while the examiner palpates the muscles for contraction. If examiner feels contraction during the attempt of the movement of 2nd to 5th toes is given grade 1 (Fig. 6.310).

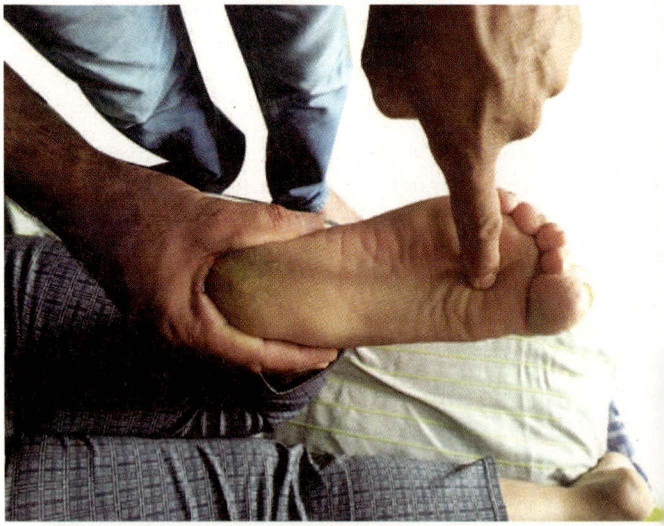

Fig. 6.310: Palpation of FDL for grade 1

Grade 1 (Trace) for Flexor Hallucis Longus

Position of Patient: Supine with ankle joint at neutral position.

Position of Examiner: Examiner stands at the side of the leg which is being tested and places fingers on the tendon of the flexor hallucis longus (plantar surface of the first metatarsal bone).

Stabilization: Examiner grasps the mid foot and stabilizes the metatarsophalangeal joints to prevent trick movement to occur (Fig. 6.311).

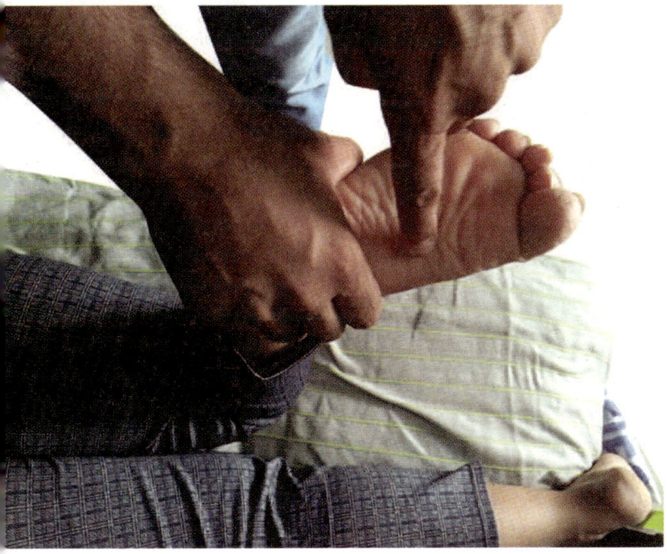

Fig. 6.311: Palpation of FHL for grade 1

Test: Examiner instructs the patient to curl the big toe. If examiner feels contraction at the plantar aspect of the first metatarsal bone, it is considered grade 1.

Grade 2

Position of Patient: Side lying with the testing leg uppermost. The non-testing leg is flexed to 45° at hip and knee joint for the stabilization.

Position of Examiner: Examiner stands behind the patient and cradles the leg at the knee joint and grasps the ankle joint with the other hand (Fig. 6.312).

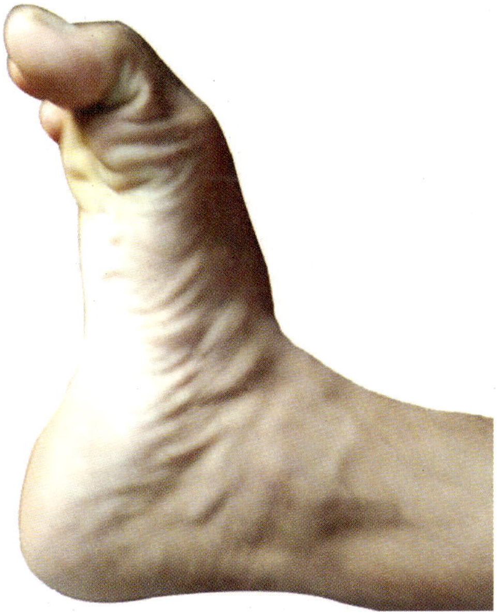

Fig. 6.312: Testing of FDL and FHL for grade 2

Test: Examiner instructs the patient to curl the toes downwards towards palmar surface. If patient completes range of motion in the gravity eliminated position it is considered grade 2.

Grade 2 (Poor) for Great Toe

Position of Patient: Short sitting with ankle joint is placed on the non-testing knee joint.

Position of Examiner: Examiner stands at the non-testing leg and stabilizes the ankle joint to prevent plantar flexion and metatarsophalangeal flexion.

Test: Examiner instructs the patient to curl your big toe. If patient finds no difficulty in flexing the great toe without assistance in the gravity eliminated position, it is considered grade 2.

Grade 3, Grade 4 and Grade 5 (Fair, Good and Normal)

Position of Patient: Prone with knee joint flexed to 90°.

Position of Examiner: Examiner stands at the side of testing leg and stabilizes the knee and ankle joint to prevent movements at the knee and ankle joint.

Test: Examiner instructs the patient to curl your big toe.

Grade 3: If patient completes plantar flexion of first metatarsophalangeal against the gravity, it is considered grade 3.

Grade 4 and 5: If patient completes plantar flexion of first metatarsophalangeal joint against moderate to maximal resistance, it is considered grade 4 and 5, repectively.

Grade 3, Grade 4 and Grade 5

Position of Patient: Prone with the knee flexion to 90° and ankle joint at neutral position.

Position of Examiner: Examiner stands at the side of the leg, which is being tested and grasps the ankle joint.

Test: Patient is instructed to make a fist with the toes from 2nd to 5th.

Grade 3: If patient makes a fist with the toes against the gravity (Fig. 6.313).

Grade 4: Examiner grasps the toes of the patient and asks the patient to make a fist against moderate to strong resistance (Fig. 6.314).

Grade 5: Examiner grasps the toes of the patient and asks the patient to make a fist against maximal resistance.

Flexor Hallucis Longus, Grade 3 to 5: Flexor hallucis longus is tested separately by stabilizing the first metatarsal

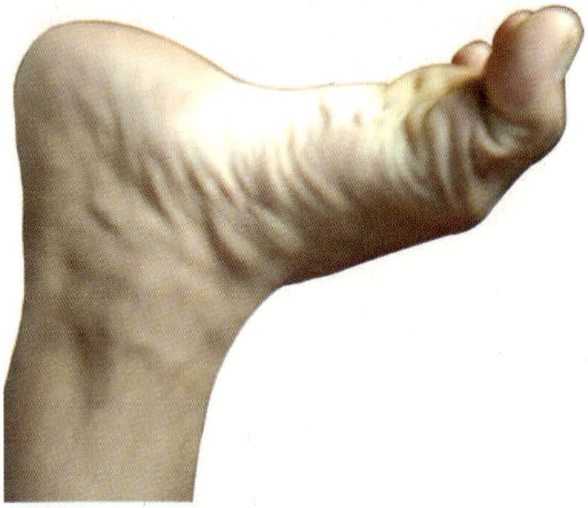

Fig. 6.313: Testing of FDL for grade 3

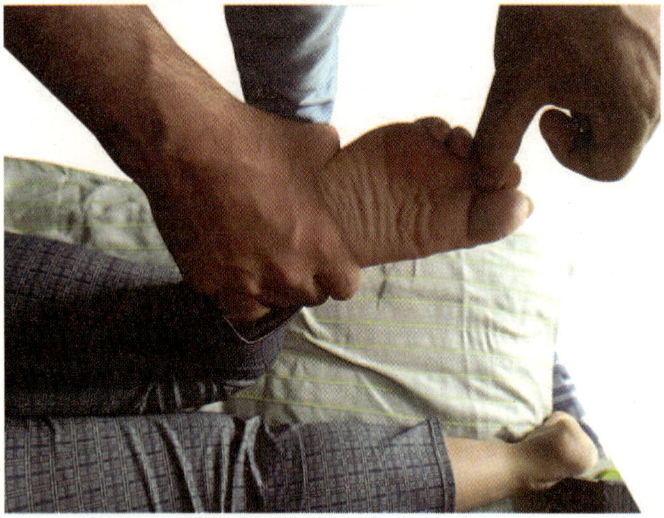

Fig. 6.314: Testing of FDL for grade 4 and 5

bone. Position of patient, therapist, direction of movement and resistance remain same as for 2nd to 5th toes (Figs. 6.315a and b).

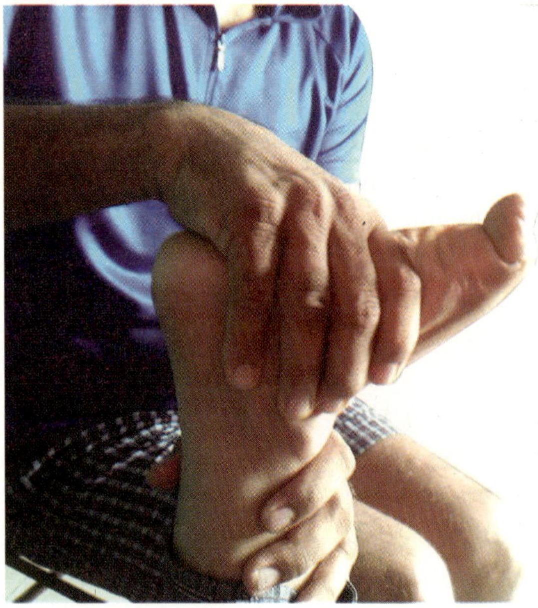

(a)

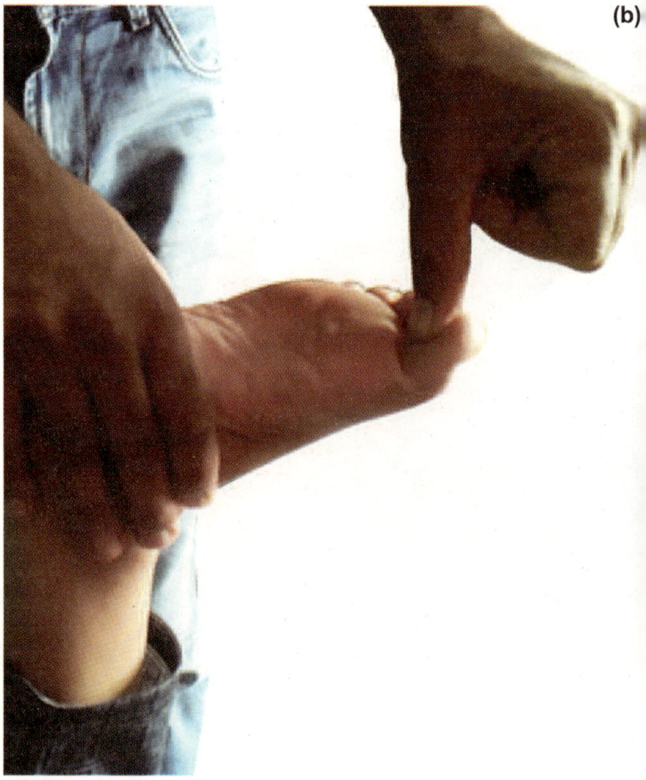

(b)

Figs. 6.315a and b: Testing of FHL for grade 3, 4 and 5

ABDUCTOR HALLUCIS – GREAT TOE ABDUCTION AND ASSISTS IN FLEXION

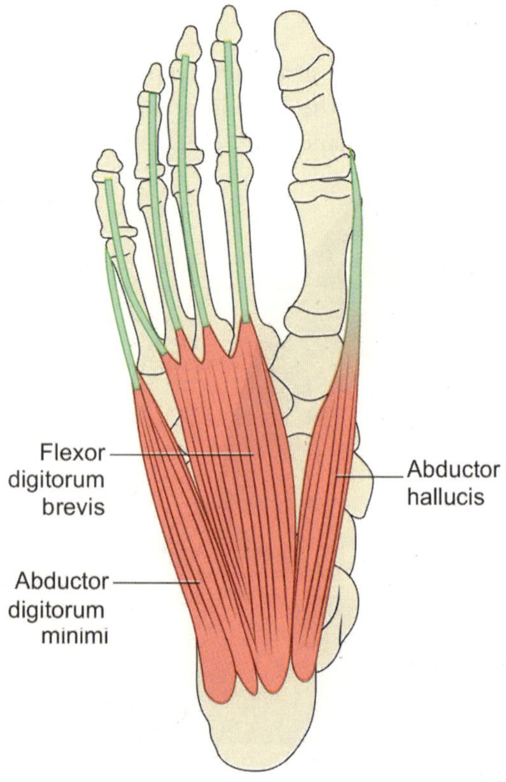

Fig. 6.316: Origin and insertion of abductor hallucis

Origin: Medial process of tuberosity of the calcaneus, flexor retanaculum, plantar aponeurosis, and adjacent intermuscular septum.

Insertion: Medial side of the base of the proximal phalanx of the great toe. Some fibers are attached to the medial sesamoid bone, and a tendinous slip may extend to the base of the proximal phalanx of the great toe.

Action: Abductor hallucis longus abducts and assists in flexion of the metatarsophalangeal joint of the great toe and assists with adduction of the forefoot.

Nerve Supply: Tibial nerve, L_4, L_5 and S_1.

Grade 2 to 5

Position of Patient: Short sitting.

Position of Examiner: Stands at the side of the patient and grasps the ankle joint to stabilize it.

Test: Examiner instructs the patient to move the great toe away from the second toe towards midline.

Grade 2: If patient completes range of motion in the gravity eliminated position it is considered grade 2 (Figs. 6.317a and b).

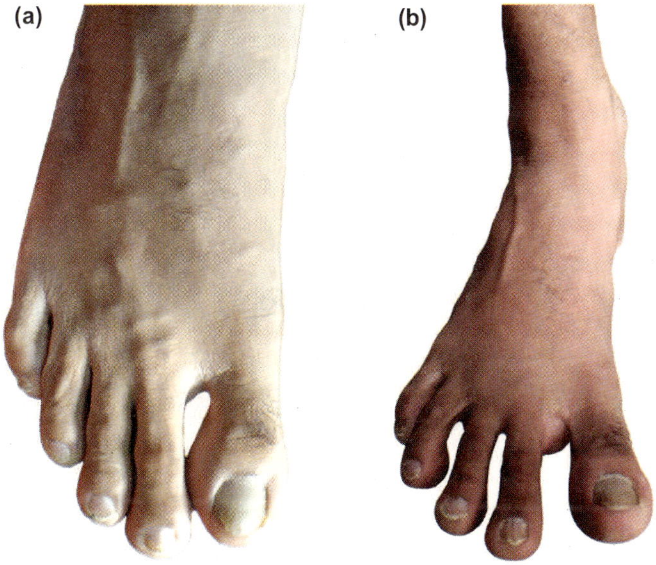

Figs. 6.317a and b: Testing of abductor pollicis for grade 2

Grade 3: If patient completes range of motion against the minimal resistance it is considered grade 3.

For grade 3, 4 and 5 patient can be placed in the side lying so that the movement takes place against the gravity (Fig. 6.318).

Grade 4: If patient completes range of motion against moderate resistance it is considered grade 4 (Fig. 6.319).

Grade 5: If patient completes range of motion against maximal resistance it is considered grade 5.

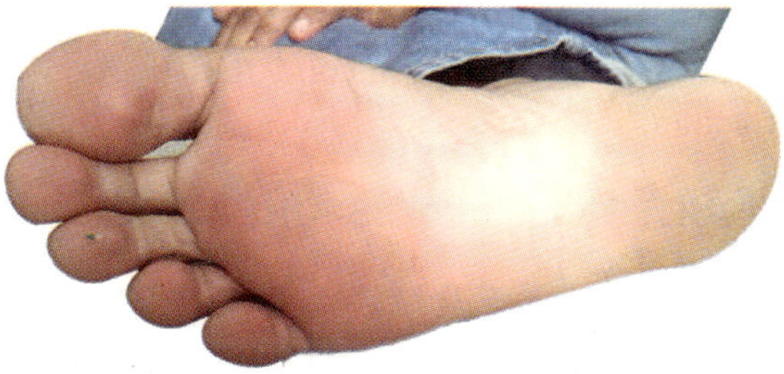

Fig. 6.318: Testing of abductor pollicis for grade 3

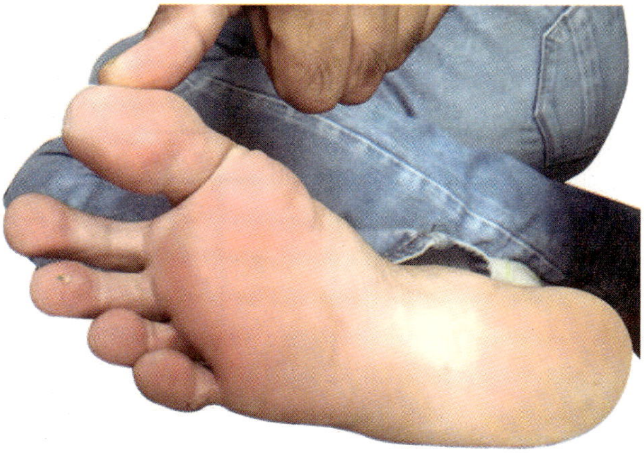

Fig. 6.319: Testing of abductor pollicis for grade 4 and 5

Grade 1

Position of Patient: Short sitting.

Position of Examiner: Stands at the side of the patient and grasps the ankle joint to stabilize it. Examiner places fingers on the calcaneum and palmar surface of the first metatarsal bone (Fig. 6.320).

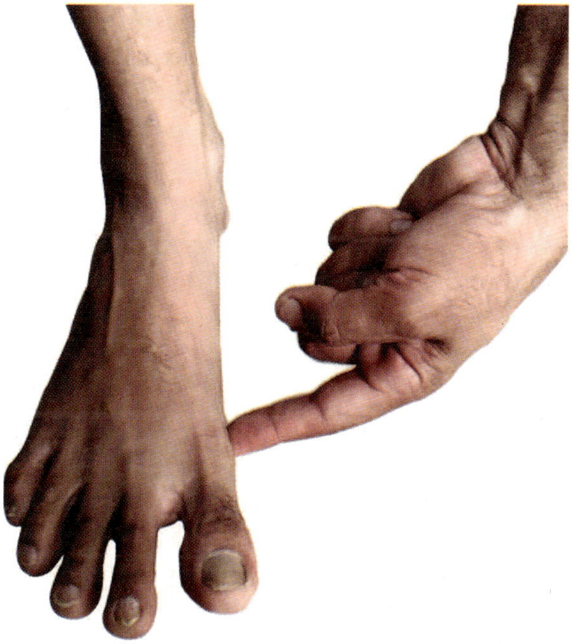

Fig. 6.320: Testing of abductor hallucis for grade 1

Test: Examiner instructs the patient to try to take the great toe out away from second toe. If examiner feels contraction, it is considered grade 1.

ADDUCTOR HALLUCIS–GREAT TOE ADDUCTION

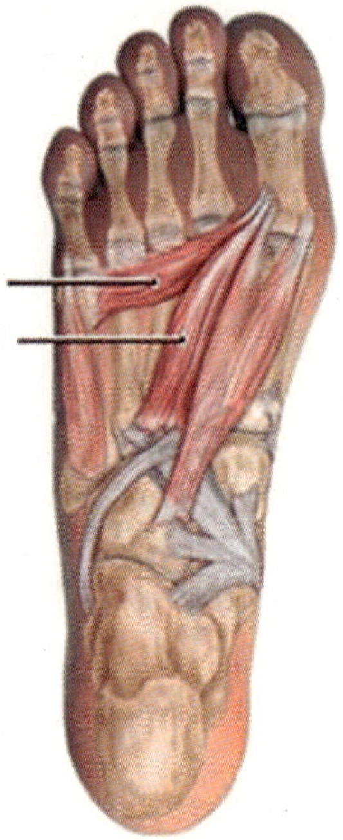

Fig. 6.321: Origin and insertion of adductor hallucis

Origin: **Oblique head** of adductor hallucis originates from the base of the second through fourth metatarsal bones and the sheath of the tendon of the peroneus longus. **The transverse head** of adductor longus originates from the plantar metatarsophalangeal ligament of the third through fifth digits and the deep transverse metatarsal ligament.

Insertion: Adductor hallucis inserts at the lateral side of the base of the proximal phalanx of the great toe.

Action: Adductor hallucis adducts and assists in flexing the metatarsophalangeal joint of the great toe.

Grade 2 to 5

Position of Patient: Short sitting.

Position of Examiner: Stands at the side of the patient and grasps the ankle joint to stabilize it. Examiner places fingers on the palmar surface of the second metatarsal bone for resistance.

Test: Examiner instructs the patient to take the great toe towards second toe.

Grade 2: If patient completes range of motion in the gravity eliminated position it is considered grade 2 (Figs. 6.322 and 6.323).

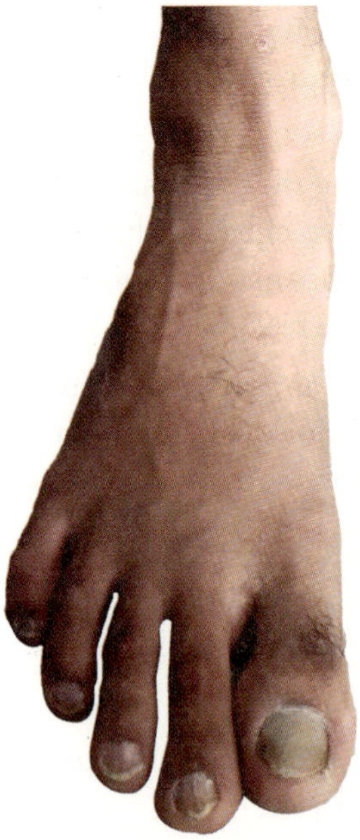

Fig. 6.322: Testing of adductor hallucis for grade 2

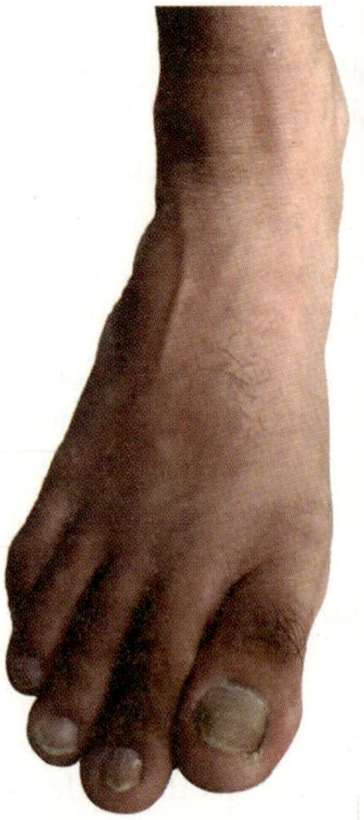

Fig. 6.323: Testing of adductor hallucis for grade 2

Grade 3: If patient completes range of motion against the minimal resistance it is considered grade 3 (Fig. 6.324).

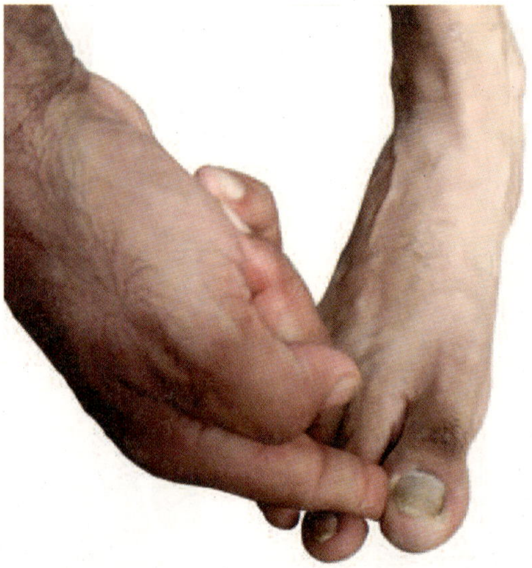

Fig. 6.324: Testing of adductor hallucis for grade 3, 4 and 5

Grade 4: If patient completes range of motion against moderate resistance it is considered grade 4.

Grade 5: If patient completes range of motion against maximal resistance it is considered grade 5.

Grade 1

Position of Patient: Short sitting.

Position of Examiner: Stands at the side of the patient and grasps the ankle joint to stabilize it. Examiner places fingers on the palmar surface of the second metatarsal bone.

Test: Examiner instructs the patient to take the great toe towards second toe. If examiner feels contraction it is considered grade 1 (Fig. 6.325).

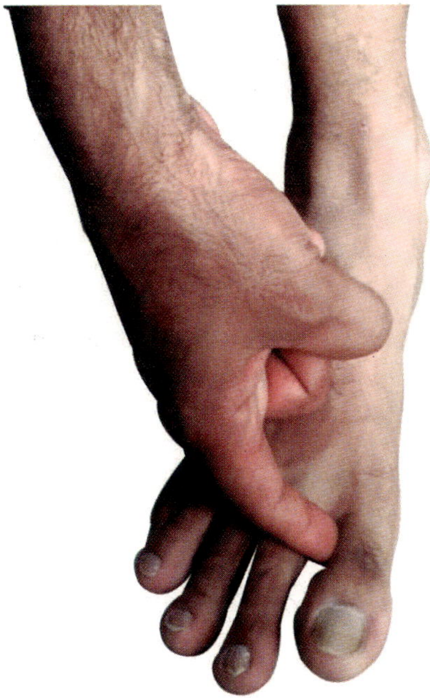

Fig. 6.325: Palpation of adductor hallucis for grade 1

LUMBRICALS – METATARSOPHALANGEAL JOINT FLEXION

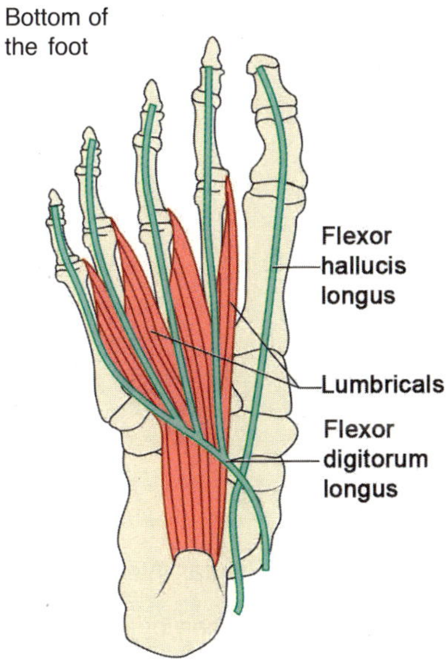

Fig. 6.326: Origin and insertion of lumbricals

Origin: First lumbricals originate from the medial side of the first flexor digitorum longus tendon. Second originates from the adjacent sides of the first and second flexor digitorum longus tendon third lumbrical originates from the adjacent sides of the second and third flexor digitorum longus tendon. And fourth lumbrical originated from the adjacent sides of third and fourth flexor digitorum longus tendons.

Insertion: Medial side of the proximal phalanx and dorsal expansion of the extensor digitorum longus tendon of the second through fifth digits.

Action: The lumbricals flexes the metatarsophangeal joints and assists in extending the interphalangeal joints of the second through fifth.

Nerve Supply: Tibial L_4, L_5 and S_1.

Grade 2 to 5

Position of Patient: Supine lying with knee and ankle at neutral position. MTP joints should be dorsi flexed. The patient is placed in prone position with knee flexion to 90° for grade 3, 4 and 5.

Position of Examiner: Stands at the side of the patient and grasps the ankle joint to stabilize it.

Test: Examiner instructs the patient to bend the toes from 2nd to 5th.

Grade 2: If patient completes range of motion in the gravity eliminated position it is considered grade 2 (Fig. 6.327).

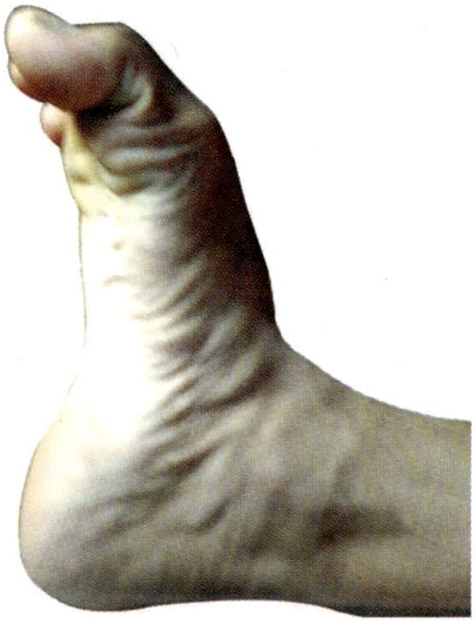

Fig. 6.327: Testing of lumbricals for grade 2

Grade 3: If patient completes range of motion against the minimal resistance it is considered grade 3 (Fig. 6.328).

Grade 4: Examiner places the fingers under the toes and instructs the patient to bend your toes over my fingers. If patient completes range of motion against moderate resistance it is considered grade 4 (Fig. 6.329).

Grade 5: Examiner places the fingers under the toes and instructs the patient to bend your toes over my fingers. If patient completes range of motion against maximal resistance it is considered grade 5.

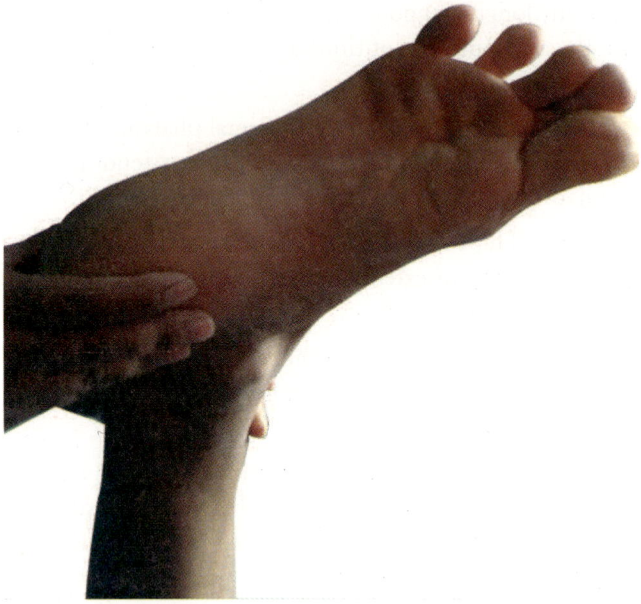

Fig. 6.328: Testing of lumbricals for grade 3

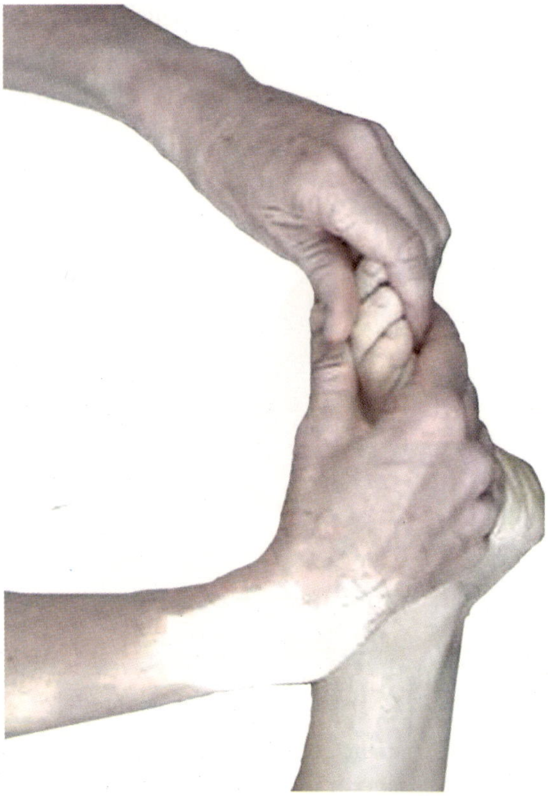

Fig. 6.329: Testing of lumbricals for grade 4 and 5

Grade 1

Position of Patient: Long sitting.

Position of Examiner: Stands at the side of the patient and grasps the ankle joint to stabilize it. Examiner places fingers on the palmar surface of the second to fifth metatarsal bone (Fig. 6.330).

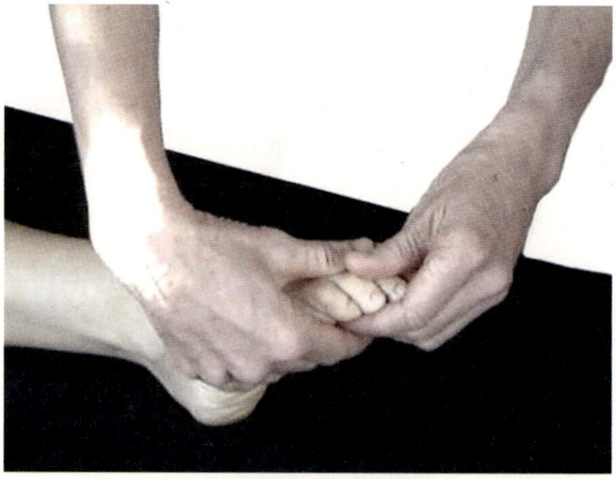

Fig. 6.330

Test: Examiner instructs the patient to curl the toes from 2nd to 5th towards palmar side. If examiner feels contraction during the movement it is considered grade 1.

PLANTAR INTEROSSEI (2nd to 5th)

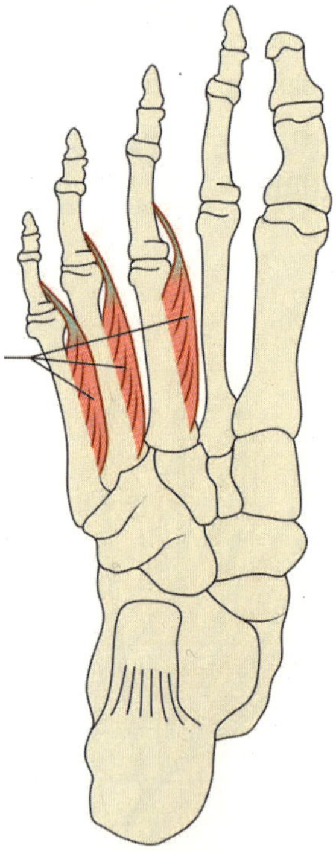

Fourth layer: Plantar interossei

Fig. 6.331: Origin and insertion of plantar interossei

Origin: Bases and medial sides of the bodies of the third through fifth metatarsal bones.

Insertion: Medial sides of the base of the proximal phalanges of the same digit.

Action: The plantar interossei adducts their corresponding third, fourth and fifth digits towards the axial line through the second digits. Plantar interossei assist in flexion of the metatarsophalangeal joints, and may assist in extension of interphalangeal joints of the third, fourth and fifth digits.

Nerve Supply: First lumbrical–Tibial Nerve, L_4, L_5 and S_1 and 2nd to 4th plantar interossei–Tibial Nerve, L_4, L_5, S_1 and S_2 (Figs. 6.332a,b and 6.333a,b).

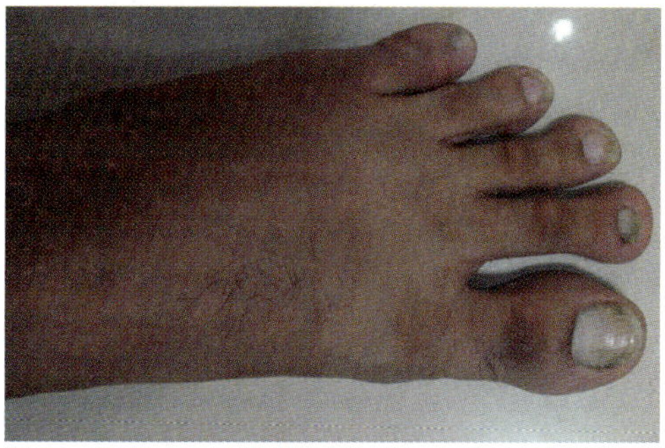

Fig. 6.332a: Testing of plantar interossei for grade 2. Patient sits comfortably on a stool or chair. Foot remains on the ground or slightly raised. All toes are in the abducted position. Examiner instructs the patient to bring the third, fourth and fifth toe towards second toe

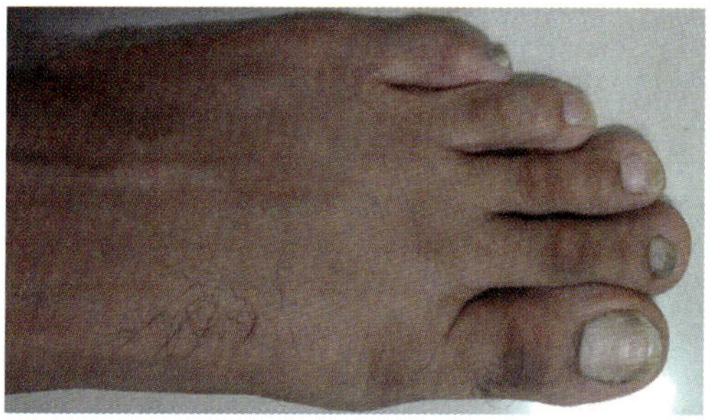

Fig. 6.332b: Testing of interossei for grade 2. Patient adducts the toes towards the axial line through the second digit

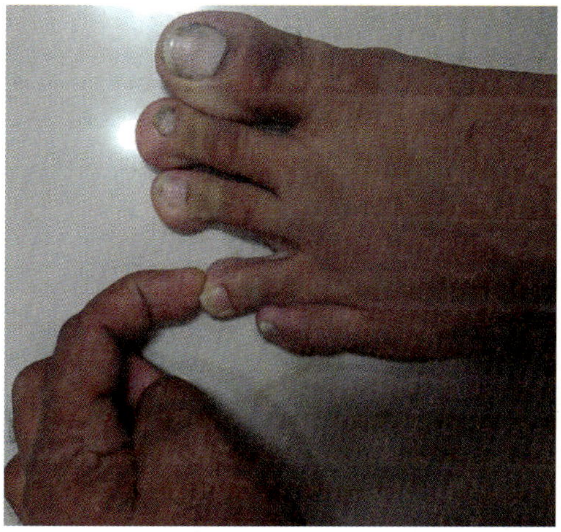

Fig. 6.333a: Testing of interossei for grade 3. Position of patient remains same as for grade 2. Examiner applies minimal resistance against the adduction

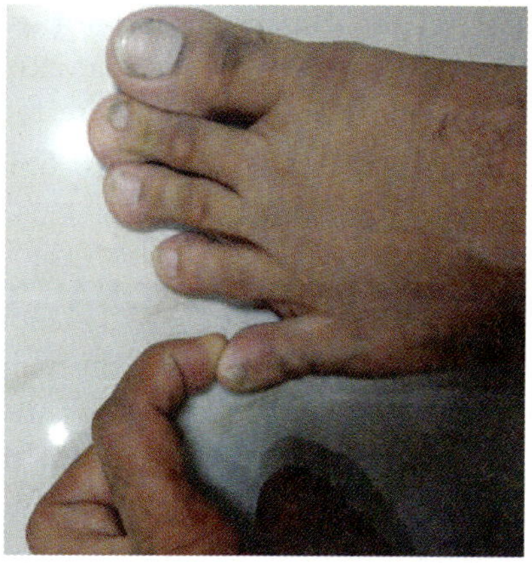

Fig. 6.333b: Testing of interossei for grade 4 and 5. Position of patient remains same as for grade 2. Examiner applies strong for 4 and maximal resistance for grade 5 against the adduction of little toe and other toes

DORSAL INTEROSSEI (2nd to 5th)

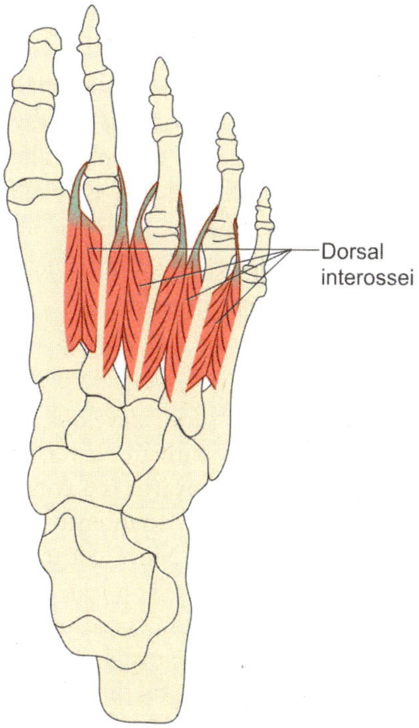

Fourth layer: Dorsal interossei

Fig. 6.334: Origin and insertion of dorsal interossei

Origin: Each head of dorsal interossei originates from the adjacent sides of their corresponding metatarsal bones.

Insertions: The dorsal interossei inset at the side of the proximal phalanx and capsule of the metatarsophalangeal joint. First dorsal interossei inserts to the medial side of the second digit. Second through fourth dorsal interossei inserts to the lateral sides of the second through fourth digits.

Action: The dorsal interossei abducts the second through fourth digits from the axial line through the second digit.

The dorsal interossei also assist in flexion of the metatarsophalangeal joints, and may assist in extension of interphalangeal joints, of the second through fourth digits.

Nerve Supply: Tibial, S_1 and S_2 (Figs. 6.335a,b and 6.336a,b).

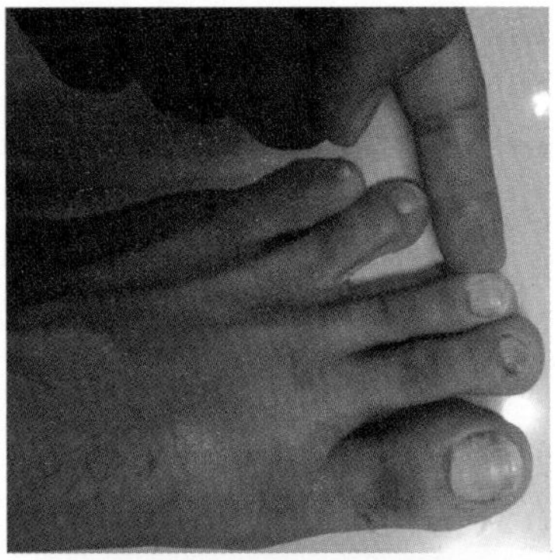

Fig. 6.335a: Testing of dorsal interossei for 3. Examiner applies minimal resistance against the abduction of toe

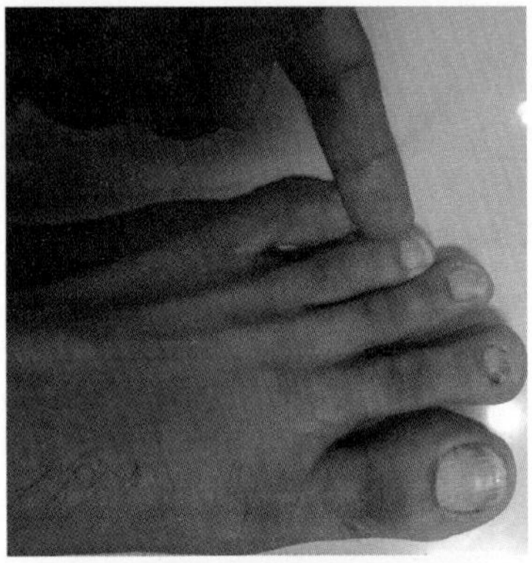

Fig. 6.335b: Testing of dorsal interossei for grade 4 and 5. Examiner applies strong resistance for grade 4 and maximal for grade 5 against the abduction of toe

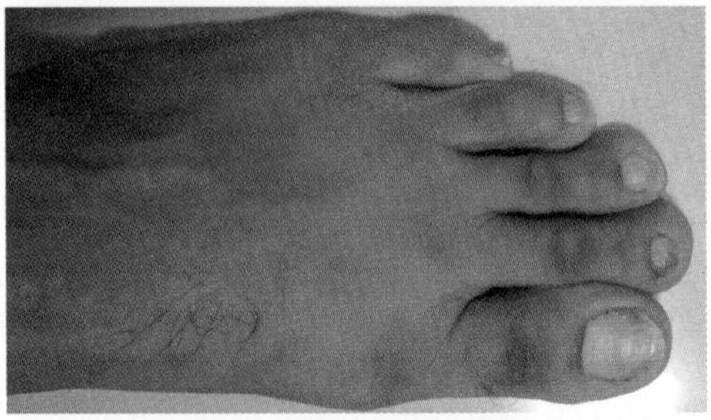

Fig. 6.336a: Testing of dorsal interossei for grade 2. Position of patient high sitting foot rests on the ground or slightly above the ground. Toes remain adducted (Starting position)

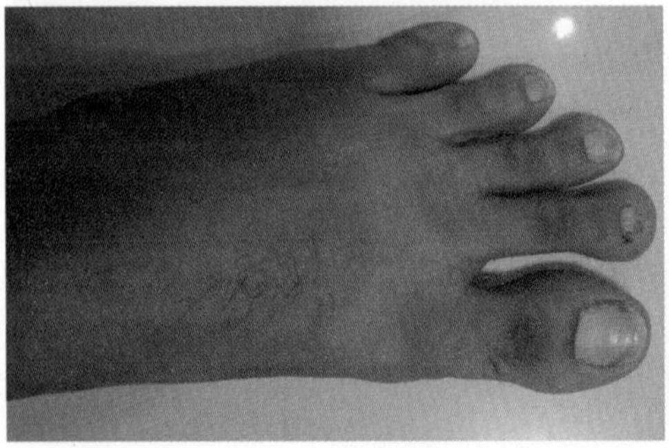

Fig. 6.336b: Testing of dorsal interossei for grade 2. Examiner instructs the patient to take the second, third and fourth toes away from the axial line

INTRINSIC MUSCLES FUNCTIONAL TESTING

The intrinsic foot muscles are presented in their anatomic orientation within the four plantar layers and the dorsal intrinsic muscle. The numbers correspond to the muscles as follows: (1) abductor hallucis, (2) flexor digitorum brevis, (3) abductor digiti minimi, (4) quadratus plantar, (5) lumbricals, (6) flexor digiti minimi, (7) adductor hallucis oblique, (a) transverse, (b) heads, (8) flexor hallucis brevis, (9) plantar interossei, (10) dorsal interossei, and (11) extensor digitorum brevis.

The intrinsic foot muscle test has been proposed as a functional assessment of a patient's ability to maintain a neutral foot posture and medial longitudinal arch height during single limb stance. To perform this test, the clinician sets the patient's test foot in subtalar neutral with the calcaneus and all the metatarsal heads on the ground, and asks the patient to fully extend the toes. The patient then lowers their toes to the ground and is asked to maintain the foot position in single limb stance for 30 seconds. The clinician observes for gross changes in navicular height and overactivity of the extrinsic muscles.

PES CAVUS

Cavus is condition in which foot develops excessively high arch. If the cavus is present with the inversion of the foot, it is called cavovarus. The cavovarus is a complex deformity of the forefoot and hind foot, frequently associated with the neuropathologic etiology. More commonly, however, it is the result of Charcot-Marie Tooth disease, a hereditary disorder in which the conduction speed of nerves slow over time and causes weakness of the distal muscles of the hands and feet. The cavus deformity of the forefoot consists of plantar flexion of the metatarsals, which is generally more pronounced in the medial column, especially in the first ray. *(Aminian A, Sangeorzan BJ. The anatomy of cavus foot deformity. Foot Ankle Clin 2008;13(2):191-198).*

The critical point of this change is that it causes secondary hind foot varus. *(Coleman SS, Chesnut WJ. Simple test for hind foot flexibility in cavovarus foot Clin Orthop Relat Res 1977; 123 :60-62).*

In the early stages of deformity, although muscular forces maintain the deformity, the foot is flexible because the soft parts are still elastic and there are no associated bone or joint deformity. In this circumstances, the subtalar joint compensates for the promotion of the forefoot and varus does not develop. With disease progression, flexible structures such as the plantar fascia, joint capsule, and interosseous ligaments become contracted and the deformity is structured (Figs. 6.337a and b).

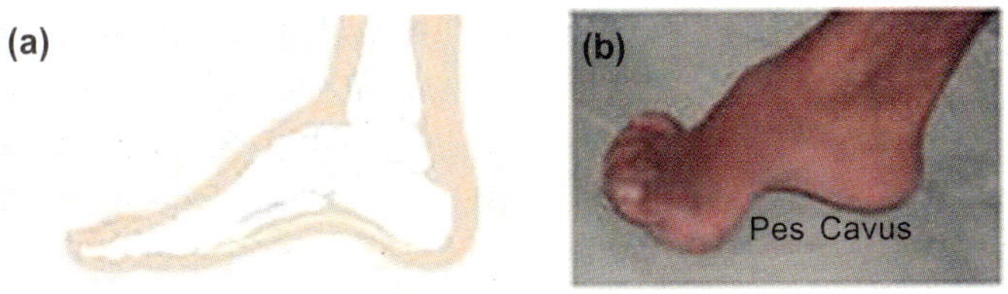

Figs. 6.337a and b: Pes cavus

The muscular imbalance results from the action of peroneus longus muscle not being counterbalanced by the tibialis anterior muscle, which is weakened. *(Mann RA, Missirian J. Pathophysiology of Charcot-Marie tooth disease. Clin Orthop Relat Res 1988;(234):221-228),* thus the peroneus longus muscle flexes the first metatarsal plantarly, causes forefoot pronation, and thus produces cavus. However, the lateral column remains unchanged. When unloading weight, the foot as a whole is forced to supinate to accommodate the equinus deformity of the first ray, which leads to hind foot varus. *(Paulos L, Coleman SS, Samuelson KM. Pes cavovarus–review of a surgical approach using selective soft tissue procedures. J Bone Joint Surg AM 1980;62(6):942-953).*

HAMMER TOE

It is the deformity, particularly affects second metatarsophalangeal joint, that results in pain in the forefoot. There is dorsiflexion at the metatarsophalangeal joint, and plantar flexion at the proximal interphalangeal joint *(Tollafild DR, Merriman LM, assessment of the locomotor system. Churchill Livingstone 1995; pp 139-191),* the distal interphalangeal joint may remain at neutral or dorsiflexed. Weakness of flexor digitorum longus, interosseus and intrinsic muscles (lumbricals) fail the balance the force of extensor digitorum longus and extensor digitorum brevis. The strong extension forces generated by EDL and EDB pull the metatarsophalangeal joint into dorsiflexion. There is tension in the flexors of proximal interphalangeal (PIP) joint, which pull the PIP joints into flexion, which results hammer toe (Figs. 6.338 and 6.339).

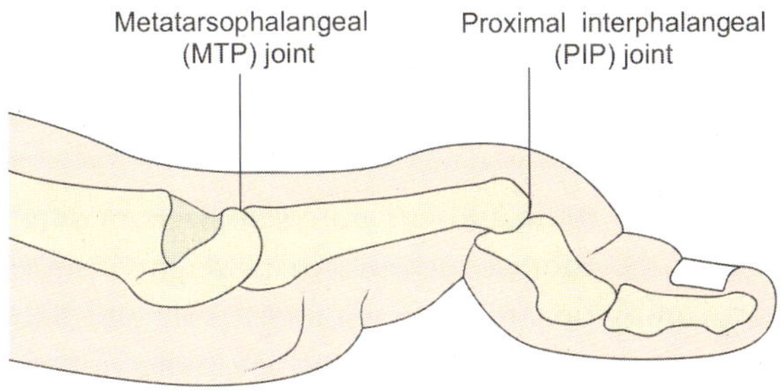

Fig. 6.338: Hammer toes

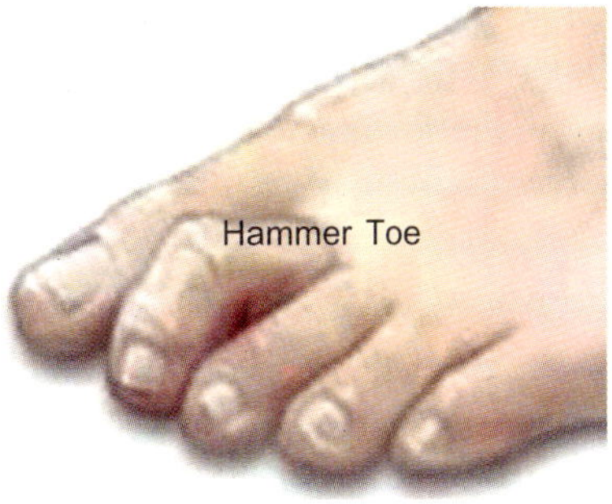

Fig. 6.339: Hammer toes

An overactivity of extensor digitorum longus (EDL), in attempt to produce dorsiflexion of the ankle joint, may lead to shortening of the EDL and lengthening (weakness) of the intrinsic muscles, can also produce hammer toe deformity. *(Bus SA, Maas M, Michels RP, Levi M. The role of muscle atrophy in the etiology of claw toe deformity in diabetes may not be as straight forward as widely believed. Diabetes Care 2009 E pub ahead of print, OY Kwon, LJ Tuttle, JE Johnson, MJ Mueller. Muscle imbalance and reduced ankle joint motion in people with hammer toe deformity, Clinical Biomech (Bristol, Avon), 2009 October 24(8):670-675).*

CLAW TOES

It is the deformity of forefoot in which there is hyperextension at the metatarsophalangeal joint and flexion at the proximal interphalangeal and distal interphalangeal joints. The most common cause of claw deformity, reported in the literatures is the weakness and atrophy of interossei and lumbrical (intrinsic) muscles due to pathology or injury leading to an imbalance between intrinsic and extrinsic muscles across the metatarsophalangeal and interphalangeal joints (Fig. 6.340).

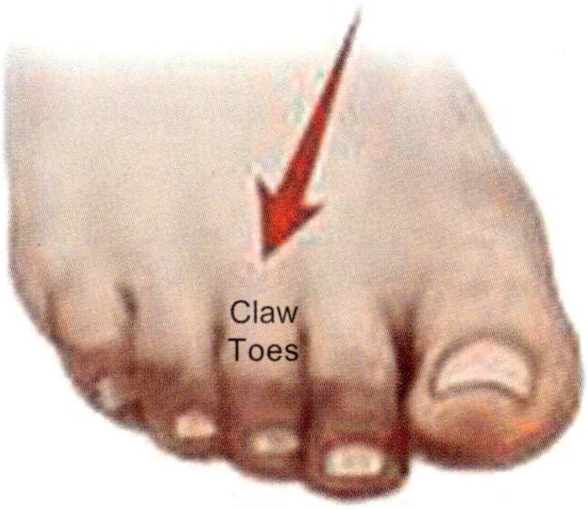

Fig. 6.340: Claw toes

The long extrinsic flexors have a greater mechanical advantage over the extensors at the interphalangeal joints, whereas, the extensors have a greater mechanical advantage over the flexors at the metatarsophalangeal joints. This, mechanical advantage is compensated by the intrinsic muscles; interossei and lumbricals by flexing the MTP joints while extending the interphalangeal joints. However, this, stabilizing action is lost when there is weakness of the intrinsic muscles. The action of the intrinsic muscles is overpowered by the strong extrinsic muscles (EDL and EDB) which eventually may result in clawing of the toes.

FLAT FEET

Flat foot is the loss of medial longitudinal arch with excessive pronation and larger plantar contact with the floor. Flat foot can either be physiological (flexible) or pathological (rigid). Physiologicval flat feet are very common, flexible, benign and a normal varient. This type of flat feet may be developmental or static. Developmental flat foot appears when the child starts to walk and disappears spontaneously at around the age of 3-5 years. Static flat feet are associated with generalised laxity and often other family members have the history of flat feet. The pathological flat feet show some degree of stiffness, such as loss of subtalar movement or tightness of the achilles tendon (Fig. 6.341).

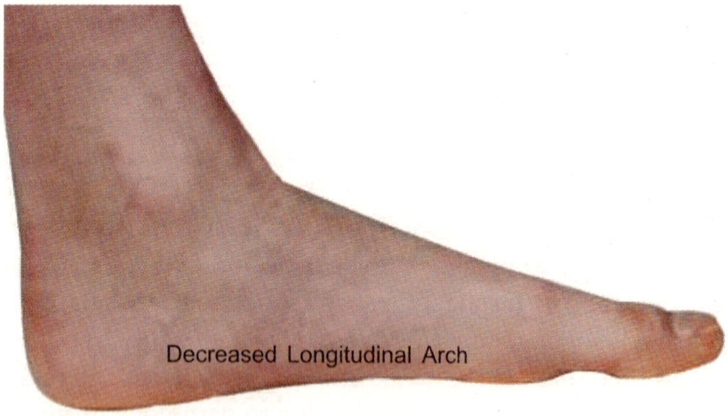

Fig. 6.341: Flat feet

The arch is supported by the small joints, ligaments, plantar aponeurosis, intrinsic muscles in the sole of foot, and the extrinsic muscles. The muscles which originate and insert in the foot are generally called intrinsic muscles whereas, muscles such as tibialis posterior, tibialis anterior and peroneoi which originate from leg and insert in the foot are called extrinsic muscles. The intrinsic muscles of the foot not only support and maintain the medial arch but also compress the joints of the foot that allows the muscles of the lower leg (extrinsic muscles) to effectively raise the arch. The chief characteristic of the medial arch is its elasticity, due to its height and to the number of small joints between its component parts.

The layout of the intrinsic muscles in the foot is very similar to the structure of hand. These muscles of the foot are arranged in the four layers. The flexor digitorum brevis flanked by abductor hallucis and abductor digiti minimi forms the first layer of the foot just below the plantar aponeurosis. The second layer is formed by the quadratus plantae, located below flexor digitorum brevis, inserts into the tendon of flexor digitorum longus on which the lumbricals originate. In the third layer, the oblique head of adductor hallucis joins the muscle's transversal head on the lateral side of the big toe. Medially to adductor hallucis are the two heads of flexor hallucis brevis, deep to the tendon of flexor hallucis longus. The considerably smaller flexor digiti minimi brevis on the lateral side can be mistaken for one of the interossei. In the fourth layer the dorsal and plantar interossei are located between and below the metatarsal bones and act as antagonists (Figs. 6.342a,b,c and Figs. 6.343a,b,c).

Proper Alternation of Attitude

The foot is progressed almost in the line of the walk with but slight eversion, so that the weight, falling momentarily on the heel, follows the outer or strong side o the foot around to the great toe. The outer border of the foot from heel to the head of the fifth metatarsal bone, is shorter than the corresponding inner border. In stance phase, when the body weight is directly on the foot, the forefoot turns in or adducts mechanically or involuntarily to throw off the weight to the shorter outer border at the moment of greater strain. Simultaneously, the muscles passing behind the medial malleoulus, working to advantage, give the final push or spring to the step. This attitude of normal foot to best absorb the forces of impacts from walking or running is part of the normal gait cycle, allowing the foot to absorb shock and adjust to uneven surfaces.

The function of the foot is to bear the weight of the body and to serve as a lever for its work. Normally, this weight and strain fall through the centre of the foot and are balanced there by muscular activity. Hence it is important, for the normal foot to have its component parts in normal condition and held in a proper relation to one another, the muscular power must be sufficient, and the strain and weight must not be too great for the strength of the mechanism. If any one of these conditions is lacking, the foot becomes unbalanced and ineffective as a lever; in other words, it loses its spring and elasticity, the ability to raise and propel the body. *Royal Whitman, The Classic: A Study of the Weak Foot, with Reference to its Causes, its Diagnosis, and its Cure; with an Analysis of a Thousand Cases of So-Called Flat-Foot Clin Orthop Relat Res. 2010 Apr; 468(4): 925–939. Published online 2009 Oct 24.*

The various static and dynamic stabilizers maintain the stability of the foot at rest and in a weight bearing. All work in conjusction to keep the arch stable and allow for ideal fuction, invesion and push off. Weakness of intrinsic muscles fails to maintain the medial arch. There is decrease

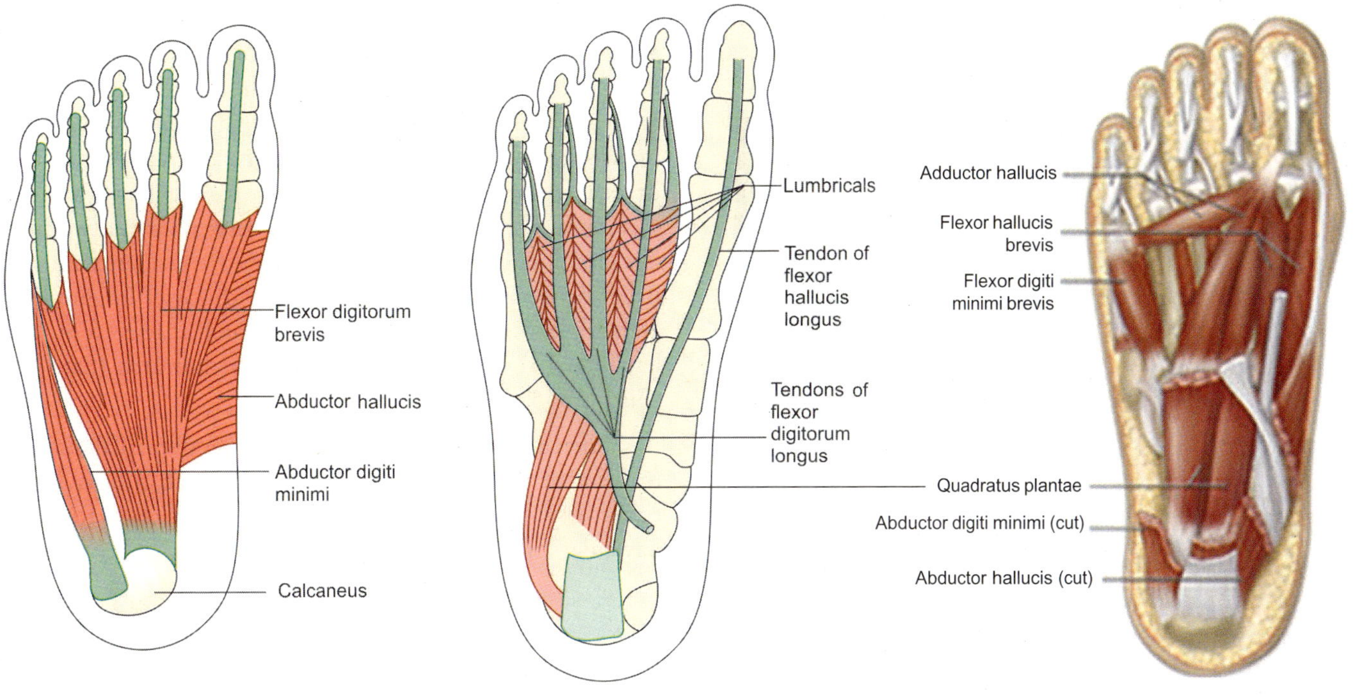

(a) Layer 1 (superficial) (b) Layer 2 (deep) (c) Layer 3 (deeper)

Figs. 6.342a, b and c: Intrinsic muscles of foot

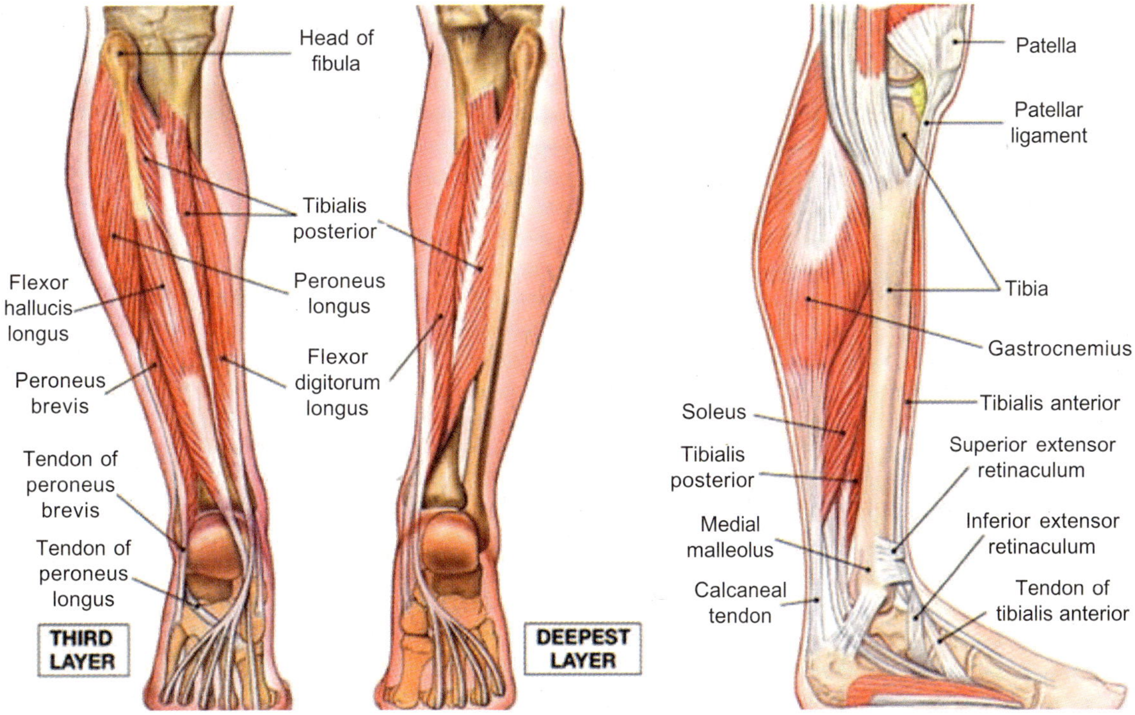

(a) (b) (c)

Fig. 6.343a, b and c: Extrinsic muscles of the foot

or loss of medial arch with excessive pronation of the foot. The achilles tendon insertion moves more laterally, and the gastosoleus complex becomes more deforming force, pulling the heel into more valgus. There is shifting of the load into the extrinsic muscles of the foot especially, tibialis posterior, tibialis anterior and peronei. Flat foot, when fully developed, is practically a dislocation in which the astragalus has slipped downward and inward from the remainder of the foot to which the muscles are attached, this causes the bulging on the inner side, the most noticeable and characteristic sign of the affection (Fig. 6.344).

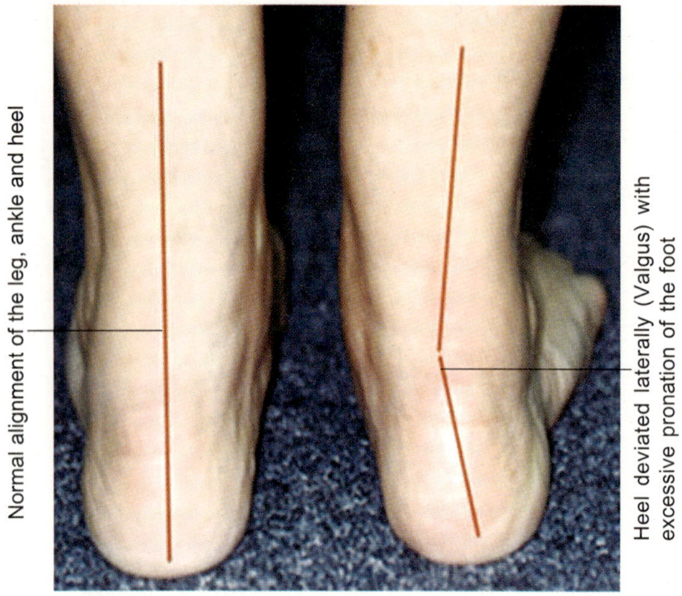

Fig. 6.344: Flat foot with bulging on the inner side, the most noticeable and characteristic sign of the affection

Medial Longitudinal Arch Angle (MLAA)

The MLAA is robust uni-planar measure with a higher level of reliability, good agreement within measure for foot classification and broader foot classification boundaries. *Langley B, Cramp M, Morrison SC. Clinical measures of static foot posture do not agree. Journal of Foot and Ankle Research. 2016 Dec. 1;9(1):45.* To measure the medial longitudinal arch angle one line is drawn from the center of medial malleolus to the navicular tuberosity and another line is drawn from navicular tuberosity to the head of first metatarsal bone. The angle formed between these two lines is called longitudinal arch angle and is considered normal if lies between 131° to 152°. Foot with lower longitudinal arch angle is considered to be high arch (cavus) foot, and less than 131 degree is considered to be low arch (flat foot) (Fig. 6.345).

When a Feiss line is drawn from center of medial malleoli to head of 1st metatarsal. If it is high arch the navicular tuberosity is above the line and in low-arched foot the navicular tuberosity is below the line.

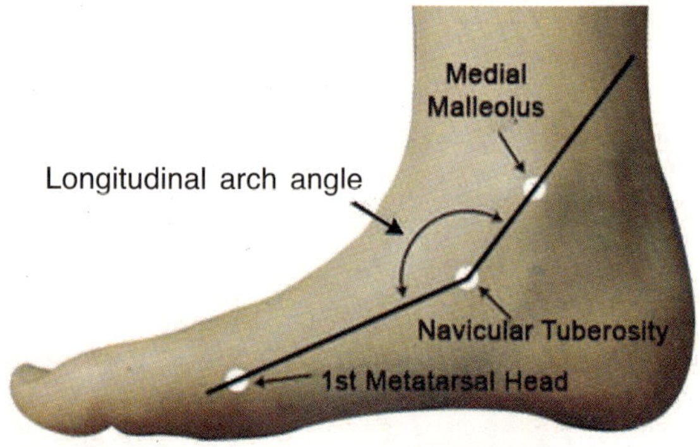

Fig. 6.345: Medial longitudinal arch angle (MLAA)

ABDOMINALS

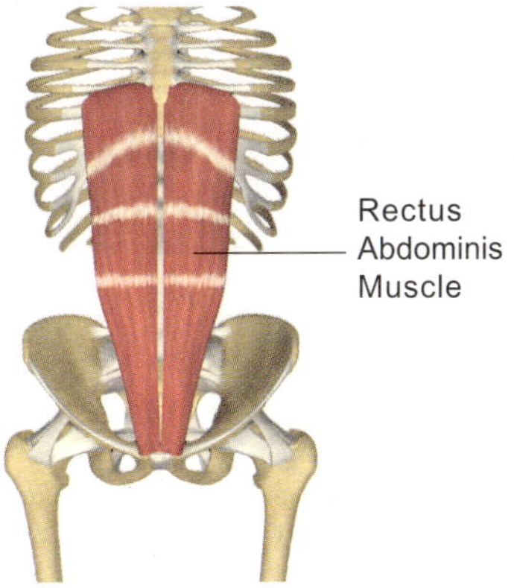

Fig. 6.346: Origin and insertion of abdominals

RECTUS FEMORIS

Origin: Pubic crest and pubic symphysis.

Insertion: Costal cartilage of fifth through seventh ribs and xiphoid process of the sternum.

Action: With the pelvis fixed, the thorax will move towards the pelvis and with the thorax fixed, the pelvis will move towards the thorax.

Grade 3 (Fair)

Position of Patient: Supine with arms outstretched in full extension above plane of body.

Position of Examiner: Standing at the side of the body.

Stabilization: Examiner stabilizes the trunk to prevent rotation (Figs. 6.347a,b and c).

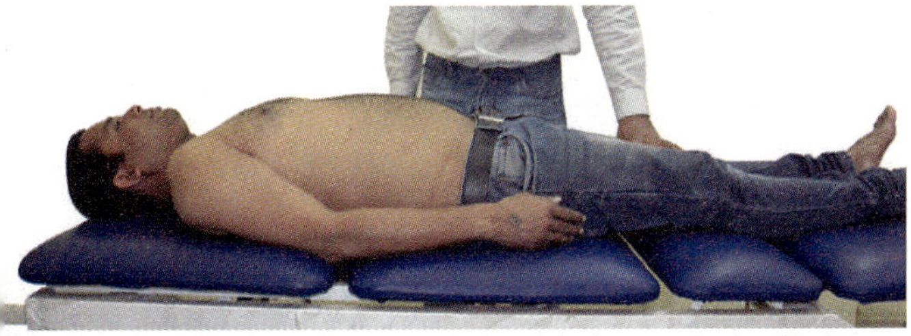

Fig. 6.347a: Testing of rectus abdominis for grade 3 with knees extended (starting position)

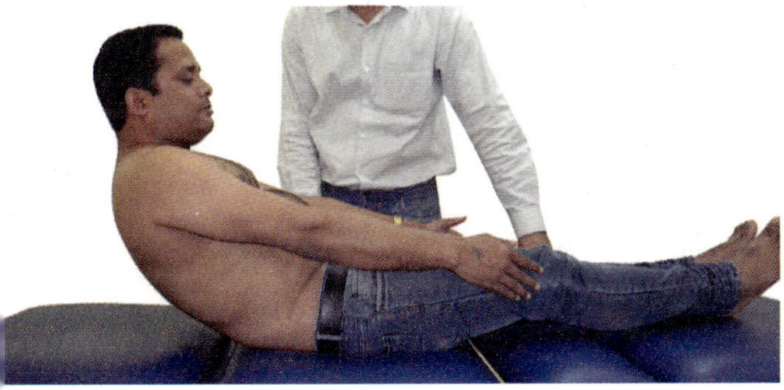

Fig. 6.347b: Testing of rectus abdominis for grade 3 with knees extended

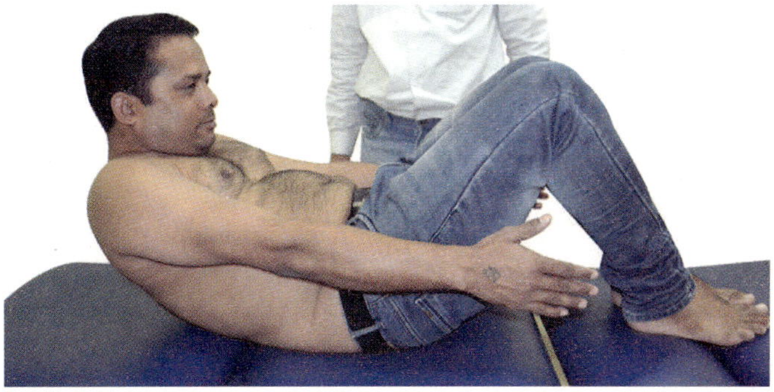

Fig. 6.347c: Testing of rectus abdominis for grade 3 with knees flexed

Test: Examiner instructs the patient to keep the chin tucked in and lift the head, shoulders and arms off the table. The patient completes full range and lifts the head, and shoulders up to the inferior angle of scapula.

Grade 4 (Good) and Grade 5 (Normal)

Position of Patient: Supine with arms crossed over the chest.

Position of Examiner: Standing at the side of patient and grasps the legs.

Stabilization: Examiner stabilizes the pelvis if hip flexors are weak (Figs. 6.348a and b).

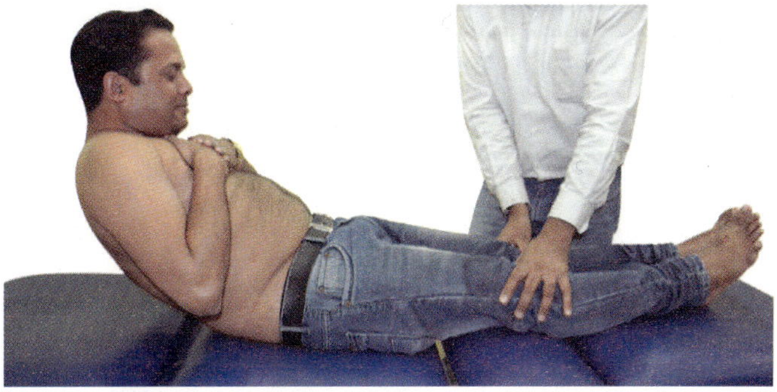

Fig. 6.348a: Testing of rectus abdominis for grade 4 with knees extended

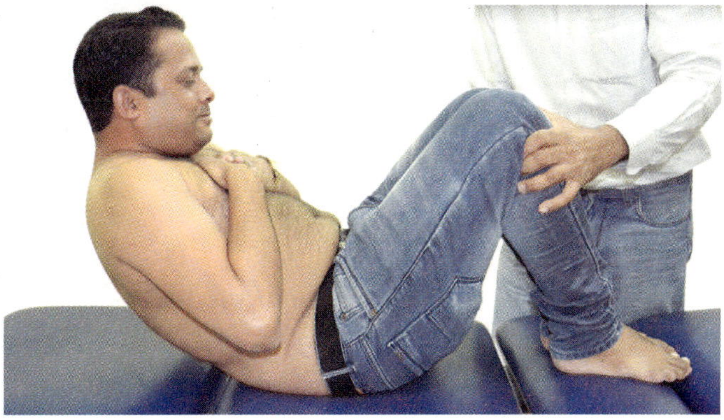

Fig. 6.348b: Testing of rectus abdominis for grade 4 with knees flexed

Test: Examiner instructs the patient to keep the chin tucked in and lift the head, shoulders and arms off the table. The patient completes full range and lifts the head, and shoulders up to the inferior angle of scapula.

Grade 5 (Normal)

Position of Patient: Supine with hands clasped behind the head.

Position of Examiner: Standing at the side of patient and grasps the legs.

Stabilization: Examiner stabilizes the pelvis if hip flexors are weak.

Test: Examiner instructs the patient to keep the chin tucked in and lift the head, shoulders and arms off the table. The patient completes full range and lifts the head, and shoulders up to the inferior angle of scapula (Figs. 6.349a and b).

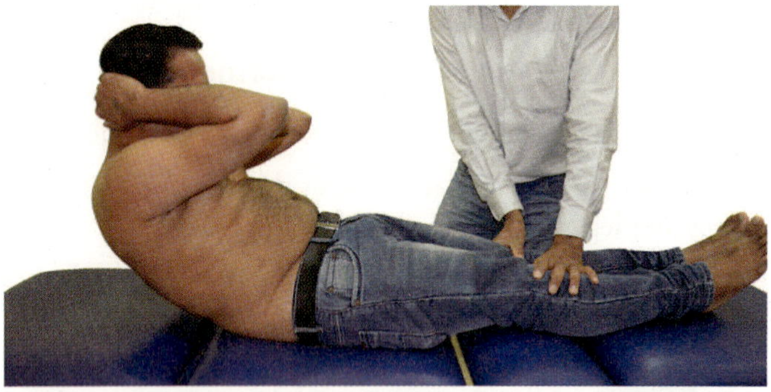

Fig. 6.349a: A testing of rectus abdominis for grade 5 with knees extended

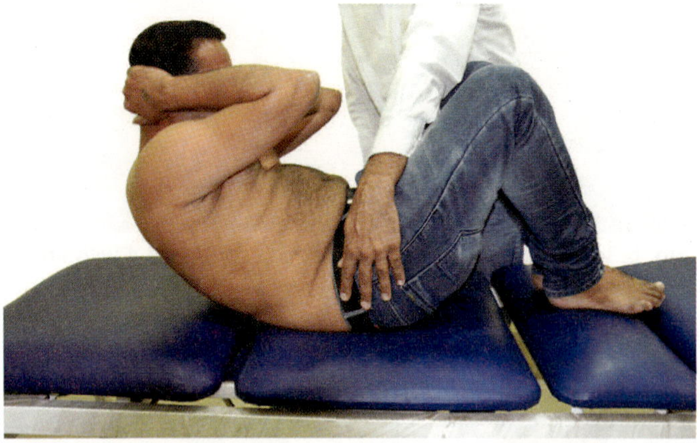

Fig. 6.349b: Testing of rectus abdominis for grade 5 with knees flexed

Grade 2 (Poor)

Position of patient: Supine with both the knees flexed or extended.

Position of Examiner: Standing at the side of patient.

Stabilization: Examiner stabilizes the trunk to prevent rotation and knees to keep flexed (Fig. 6.350).

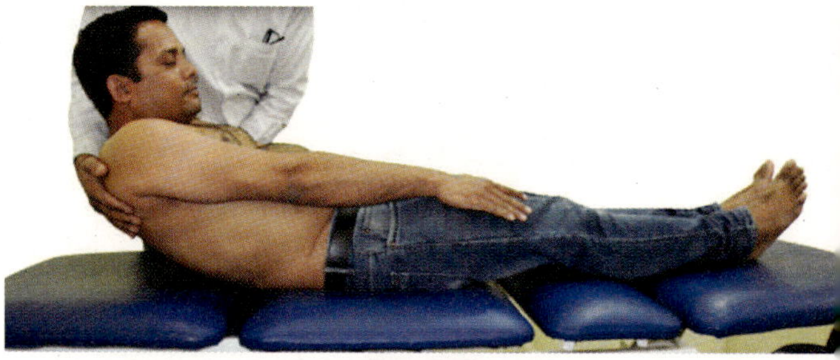

Fig. 6.350: Testing of rectus abdominis or grade 2

Test 1: Examiner instructs the patient to lift the head off the table. If patient lifts the head off the table without clearing the scapula is given grade 2.

Test 2: Examiner cradles the upper trunk and lifts it off the table and instructs the patient to lean forward. if there is depression of the rib cage is given grade 2.

Grade 1

Position of Patient: Supine with both the knees flexed or extended.

Position of Examiner: Standing at the side of patient. Examiner places hand on the midline of thorax over the linea alba, and fingers on the rectus abdominis.

Stabilization: Examiner stabilizes the trunk to prevent rotation and knees to keep flexed (Fig. 6.351).

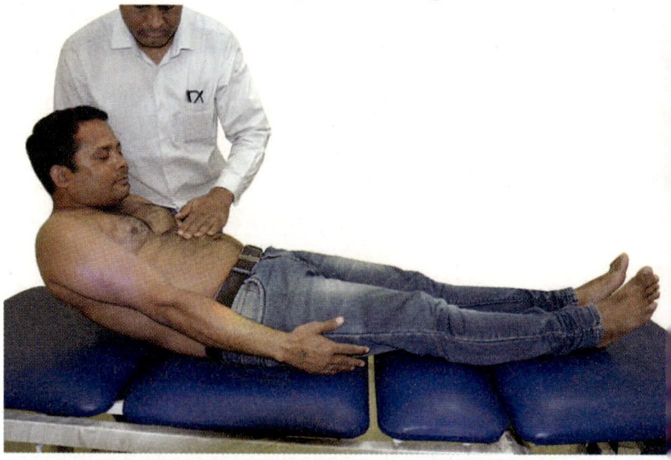

Fig. 6.351: Palpation of rectus abdominis or grade 1

Test: Examiner cradles the upper trunk and lifts it off the table and instructs the patient to lean forward. If examiner feels contraction at the midline of thorax on the linea alba is given grade 1. If there is no contraction it is given grade 0.

BACK EXTENSORS

Grade 3 (Fair)

Position of Patient: Prone, with hands at the side of the body.

Position of Therapist: Standing at the side of patient, and grasps the legs.

Stabilization: Examiner stabilizes the legs firmly on the table.

Test: Examiner instructs the patient to raise your head, shoulders, and chest off the table as high as possible. If patient is able to lift the head, shoulders, and chest off the table it is given grade 3 (Figs. 6.352a and b).

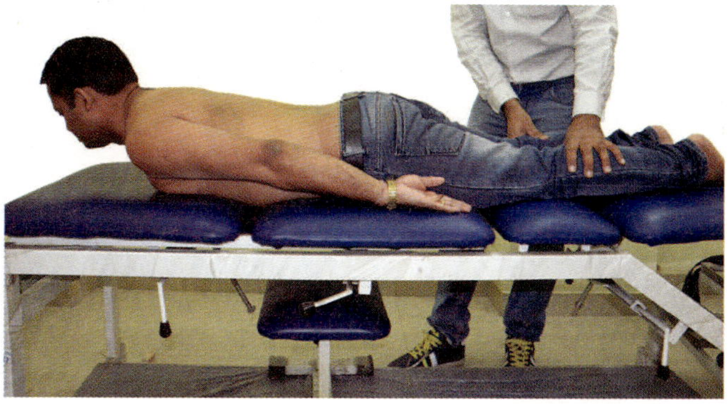

Fig. 6.352a: Testing of back extensors for grade 3 (Starting)

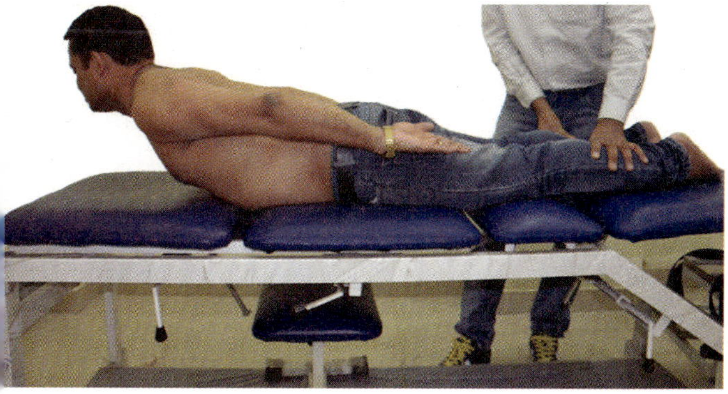

Fig. 6.352b: Testing of back extensors for grade 3

Grade 4 (Good) and 5 (Normal)

Position of Patient: Prone, with hands clasped behind the head.

Position of Therapist: Standing at the side of patient, and grasps the legs.

Stabilization: Examiner stabilizes the legs firmly on the table.

Test: Examiner instructs the patient to raise your head, shoulders, and chest off the table as high as possible (Fig. 6.353).

Grade 4: If patient is able to lift the head, shoulders, and chest off the table quickly and hold that position with an additional significant efforts.

Grade 5: If patient is able to lift the head, shoulders, and chest off the table without any of additional efforts.

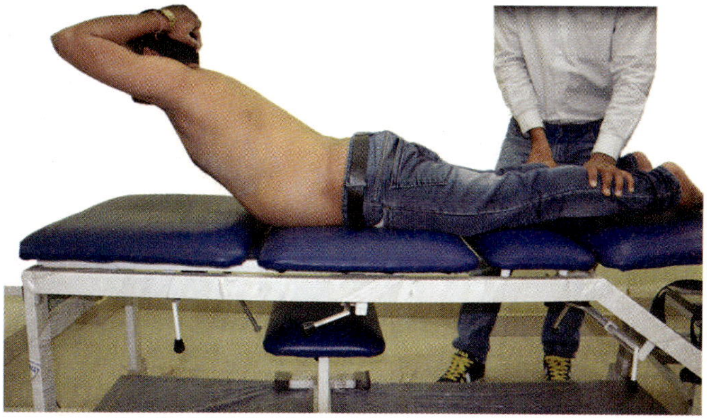

Fig. 6.353: Testing of back extensors for grade 4 and 5

Note: Normally, extension of hip and lumbar spine are initiated simultaneously, not as two separate movements.

i. The patients with strong back extensors and hip extensors can raise the head, shoulders, and chest off the table.
ii. The patients with weak gluteal muscles but strong back extensors will hyperextend the lumbar spine and fail to lift the trunk high from the couch.
iii. The patients with weak back extensors and strong gluteal muscles cannot raise the trunk off the table. The pelvis rotates posteriorly and lumbar spine lexes to the efforts of trunk extension.
iv. Tight hip flexors will not allow the hip to move into the extension. All the movement in the direction of raising the leg backward is accomplished by lumbar spine hyperextension and pelvic tilt.

Biering-Sorensen Lumbar Spine Extension Endurance Test

An alternative position for Grade 5

Position of Patient: Prone with the trunk flexed off the end of the table at a level between the anterior superior iliac spine and umbilicus. The arms are folded across the chest.

Position of Examiner: Examiner kneels on the couch and grasps the legs at just above the ankle joints.

Stabilization: Examiner stabilizes the legs by kneeling on the table and grasping the distal legs (Fig. 6.354).

Test: Examiner instructs the patient to raise your head, shoulders, chest, and trunk from the table and hold the position for 113±46 seconds. Women and elderly individuals will hold for less time than the adult men (Fig. 6.354).

Weakness: Weakness of bilateral back extensor muscles results in lumbar flattening and increase dorsal kyphosis.

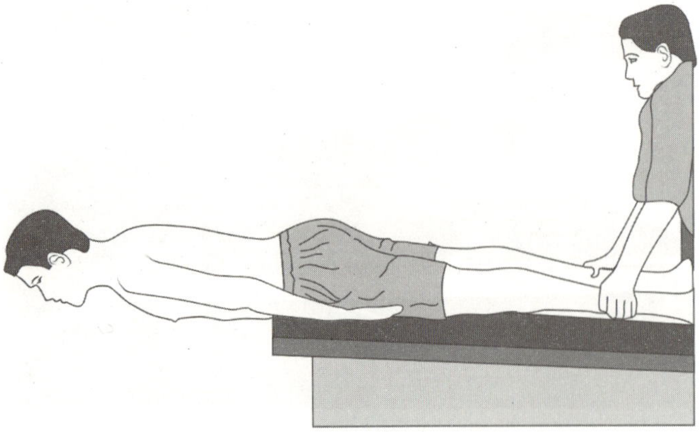

Fig. 6.354: Extensor endurance test

Unilateral weakness results in a lateral bending of the trunk with convexity towards the weaker or same side.

Contracture: Contracture of bilateral back extensors results in hyperlordosis of the lumbar spine. Unilateral contracture results in a scoliosis with convexity towards the opposite side.

LATERAL FLEXORS

Grade 3 (Fair, Grade 4(Good) and Grade 5 (Normal)

Position of Patient: Side lying, with a pillow between the thighs and legs and with the head, upper trunk, pelvis and lower extremities in a straight line. The underarm is forward across the chest, with the hand holding the upper shoulder to rule out assistance by pushing up with the elbow. The uppermost arm is extended down along the side, and the fingers are closed so that the patient will not hold onto the thigh and attempt to assist with the hand.

Position of Examiner: Examiner stands behind the patient and places one hand over the pelvis and other on the uppermost leg.

Stabilization: Examiner stabilizes the pelvis and legs to counter balance the weight of the trunk. The stabilization should not prevent the downward movement of the pelvis and leg essential during the lateral bending. Examiner should not push the pelvis upward as it may block the downward movement (Figs. 6.355a,b and c).

Test: Examiner instructs the patient to lift the head, shoulders, and trunk off the table or couch.

Grade 3: If patient can raise the head and shoulder approximately two inches up from the table.

Grade 4: If patient can raise head and shoulder approximately four inches up from the table.

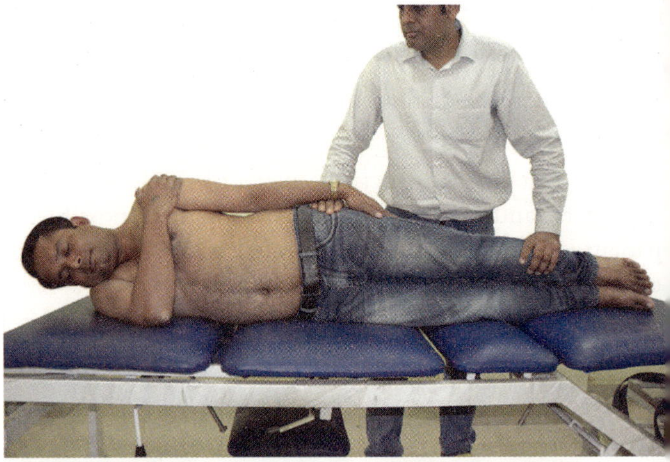

Fig. 6.355a: Testing of trunk lateral flexors for grade 3

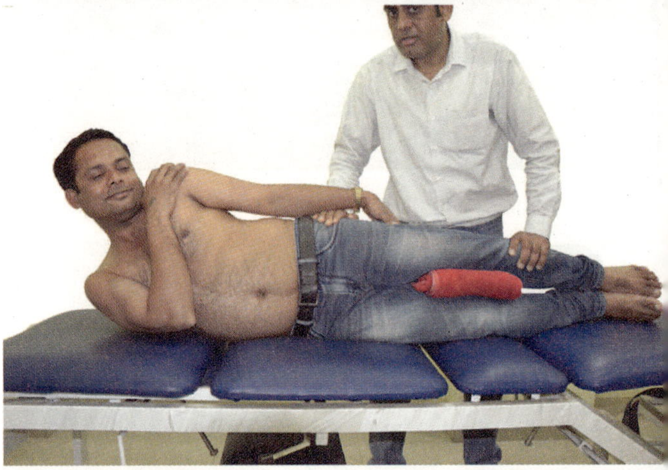

Fig. 6.355b: Testing of trunk lateral flexors for grade 4

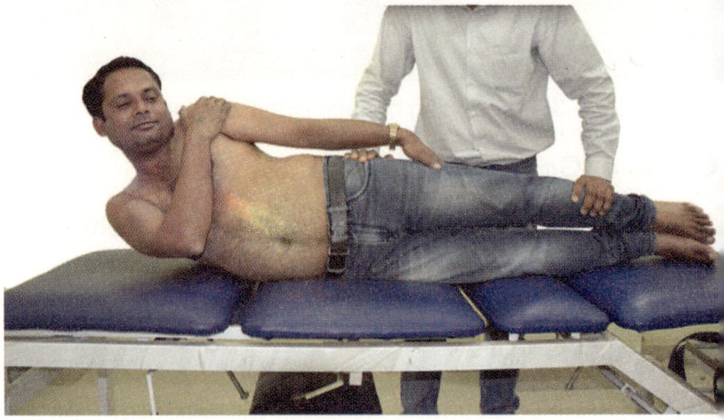

Fig. 6.355c: Testing of trunk lateral flexors for grade 5

Grade 5: If patient can raise the trunk laterally from a side lying position to a point of maximum lateral flexion.

Grade 2 (Poor) and Grade 1 (Flicker)

Position of Patient: Supine, with both the hands at the side of body.

Position of Examiner: Examiner stands at the side of the patient. Places one hand on the lateral flexors between the iliac crest and rib cage for palpation for grade 1.

Stabilization: Does not need (Fig. 6.356).

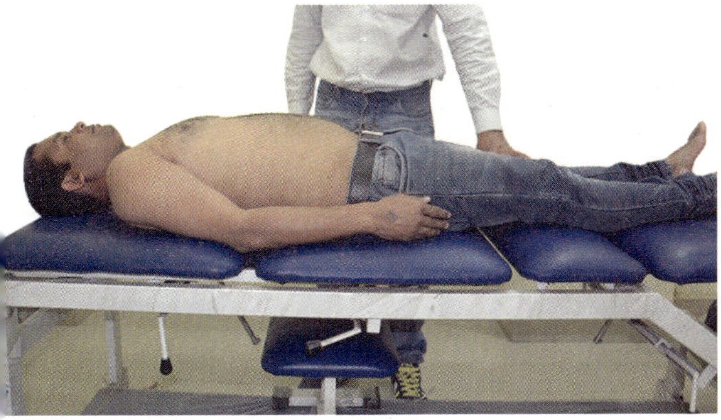

Fig. 6.356: Testing of trunk lateral flexors for grade 2

Test: Examiner instructs the patient to bring the head, shoulders and trunk towards the testing side. If patient can complete range of motion it is graded 2. If patient fails to bend the trunk toward testing side but shows the contraction while attempting the movement it is graded 1.

OBLIQUUS EXTERNUS AND OBLIQUUS INTERNUS TRUNK ROTATION

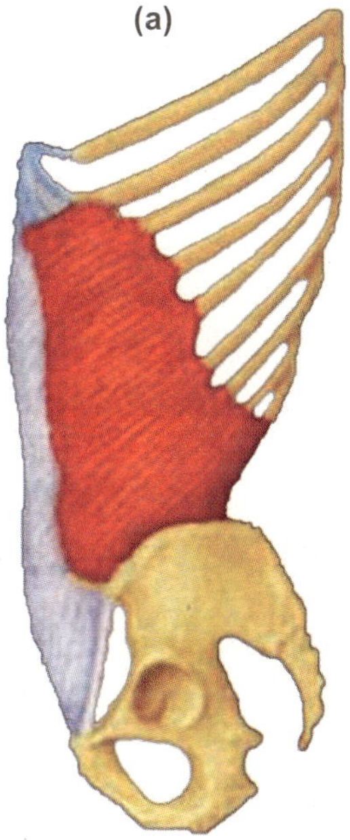

Fig. 6.357a: Obliqus externus

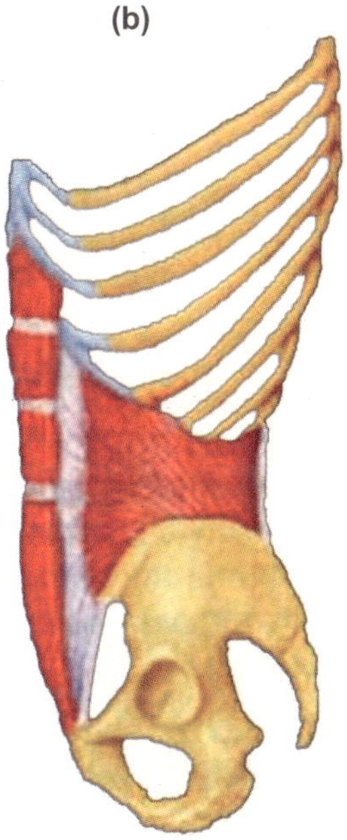

Fig. 6.357b: Obliqus internus

Grade 3 (Fair)

Position of Patient: Supine with arms outstretched above plane of body.

Position of Examiner: Standing at the side of patient at the level of pelvis.

Stabilization: Examiner may stabilize the legs (Figs. 6.358a,b and c).

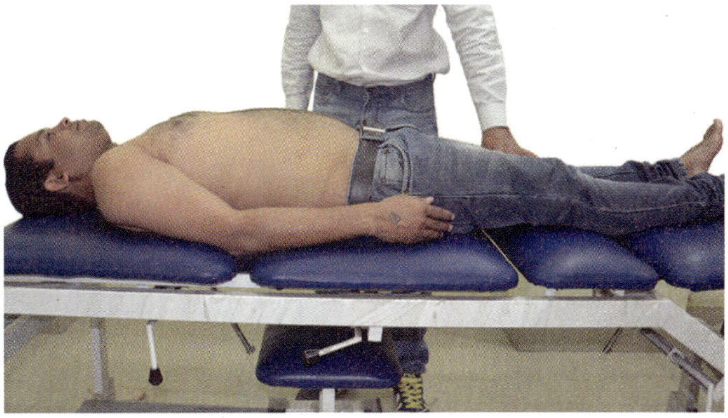

Fig. 6.358a: Testing of obliqus externus and obliqus internus for grade 3 (Starting)

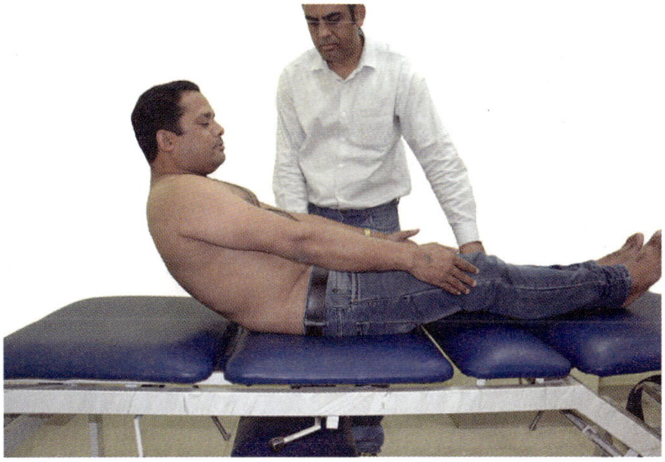

Fig. 6.358b: Testing of obliqus externus and obliquus internus for grade 3 (Mid range)

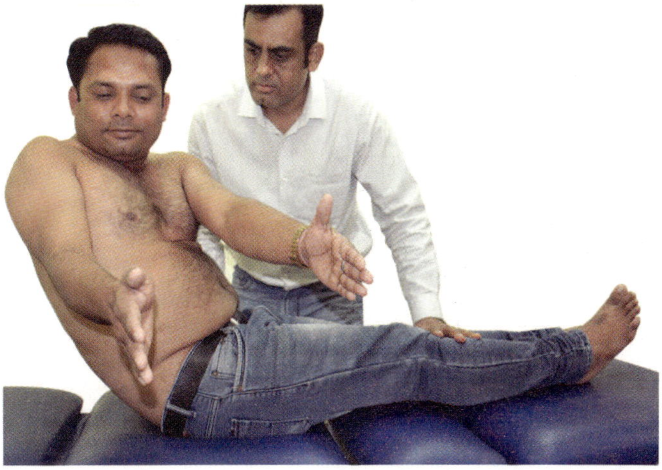

Fig. 6.358c: Testing of right obliqus externus and left obliqus internus for grade 3 (End range)

Test: Examiner instructs the patient to lift the head and scapula off the table and turn to the left side for testing of left obliquus externus and right obliquus internus. If patient can lift the scapulae and can rotate the trunk to the left side it is given grade 3 for left obliquus externus and right obliquus internus. If patient can lift the scapulae off the table and can rotate to the right side it is given grade 3 for the right obliquus externus and left obliquus internus.

Grade 4 (Good)

Position of Patient: Supine with arm crossed over chest.

Position of Examiner: Standing at the side of patient at the level of pelvis.

Stabilization: An assistant may stabilize the legs as the examiner assists the patient in placing the testing position.

Test: Examiner instructs the patient to lift the head and scapulae off the table and turn to the left side. Examiner assists in lifting the head and scapulae off the table. If patient can rotate the trunk to the left side while maintaining the head and scapulae lifted off the table it is given grade 4 for left obliquus externus and right obliqus internus. If patient can rotate the trunk to the right side with arms crossed over the chest while maintaining head and scapulae off the table is given grade 4 for right obliqus externus and left obliqus internus (Figs. 6.359a,b and c).

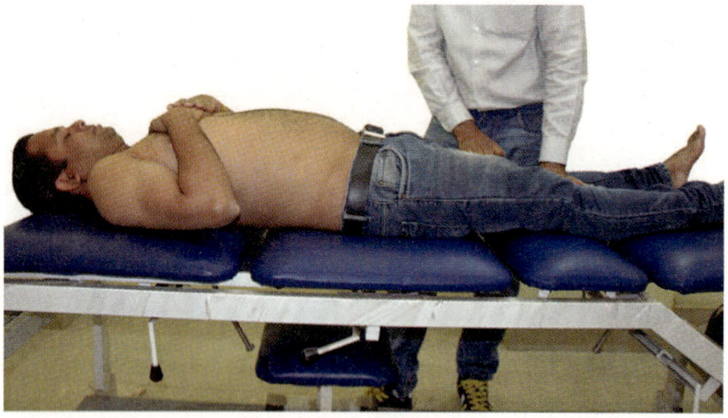

Fig. 6.359a: Testing of obliqus externus and obliqus internus for grade 4

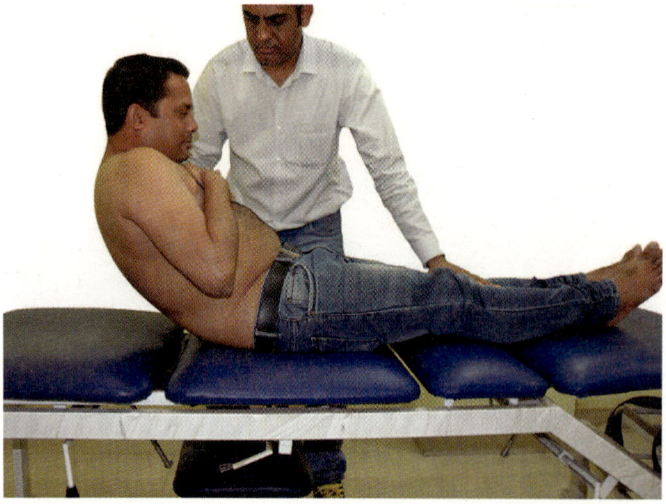

Fig. 6.359b: Testing of obliqus externus and obliqus internus for grade 4

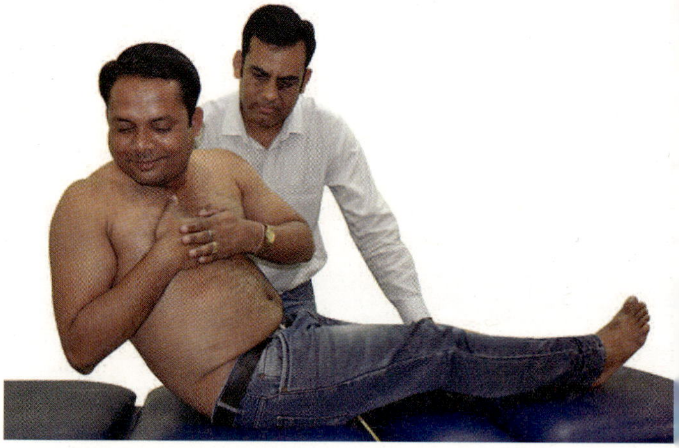

Fig. 6.359c: Testing of obliquus externus and obliqus internus for grade 4

Grade 5

If patient rotates the trunk to the left side with hands clasped behind the head while maintaining the head and shoulders lifted off the table. Examiner assists the patient in lifting the head and shoulders off the table (Figs. 6.360a and b).

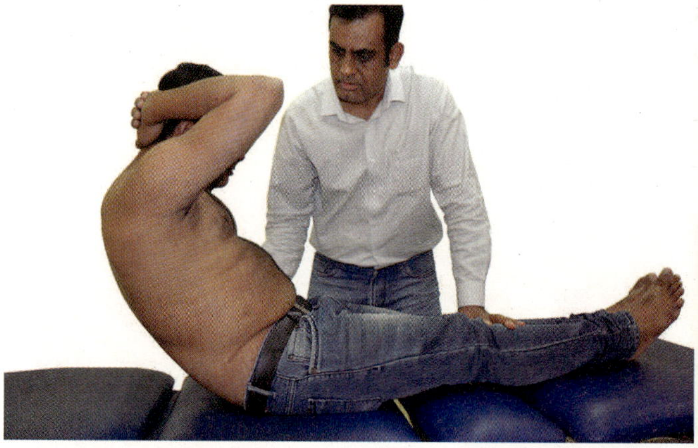

Fig. 6.360a: Testing of obliqus externus and obliqus internus for grade 5

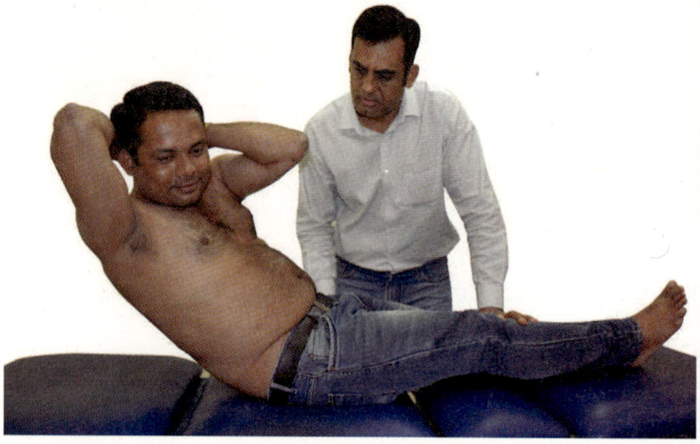

Fig. 6.360b: Testing of right obliqus externus and obliqus internus for grade 5

GONIOMETRY

INTRODUCTION

Goniometry is derived from two Greek words **gonia-angle, meton-measurement**. It means measurement of angles created at the joints by the bones of the human body.

The study of medical science in which the range of motion of the joint of human body is measured by an instrument is known a Goniometry.

INSTRUMENT

To measure the range of motion of the joint several instruments have been provided by **persons of varied professional and academic background** since early Nineteenth century.

In 1995, Salter offered a good survey of the literature but did not include references from the United States in the fields of physical therapy and occupational therapy, each of which have contributed significant studies on joint mobility.

The most widely accepted and recommended instrument is the universal goniometer called an arthrometer (Figs. 6.361a and b).

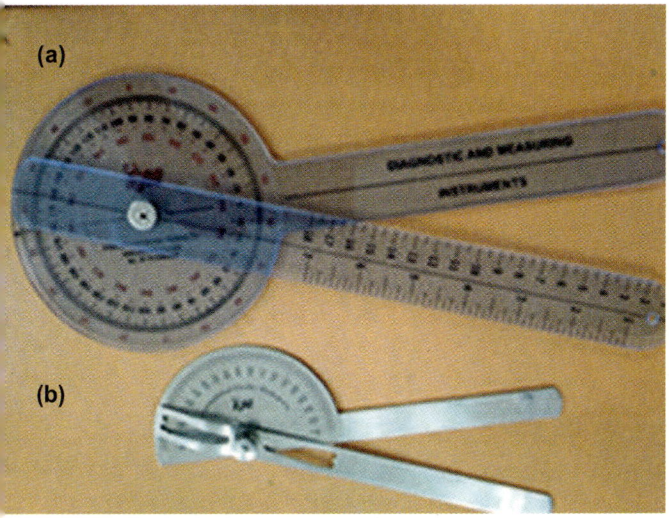

Fig. 6.361: (a) Full circle, (b) Half circle

Many goniometers are recommended to measure the range of motion of the joint but now-a-days the selection of instrument by an examiner depends on the instrument's accuracy, cost and availability.

1. Universal Goniometer

The most widely accepted and recommended instrument to measure the joint range of motion of almost all joints of human body, designed by Moore, is known as universal goniometer. It is a type of protractor with two thin arms made of plastic or metal. The instrument is available in different sizes and shapes but the features (protractor and two arms) remain same in all universal goniometers. There are three parts of universal goniometer.

1. Body or protractor.
2. Two arms.
3. Fulcrum.

Body of Goniometer

It is basically a protractor on which scales are located, if the protractor is full circle then it is called a full circle goniometer in which scales are located on one or both side from 0°-360° and 360°-0° or 0°-180° and from 180°-0°.

If the protractor is half circle, then it is called as half circle goniometer and scales are located on either side from 0°-180° and 180° to 0°.

The graduation should be large enough to be read by naked eyes. The interval on the scale may vary from 1 to 10°.

Fulcrum

The part where moving arm attached with the body is known as fulcrum. It is the type of screw which gives degree of freedom to moving arm. Fulcrum is generally placed over the joint line (Fig. 6.362).

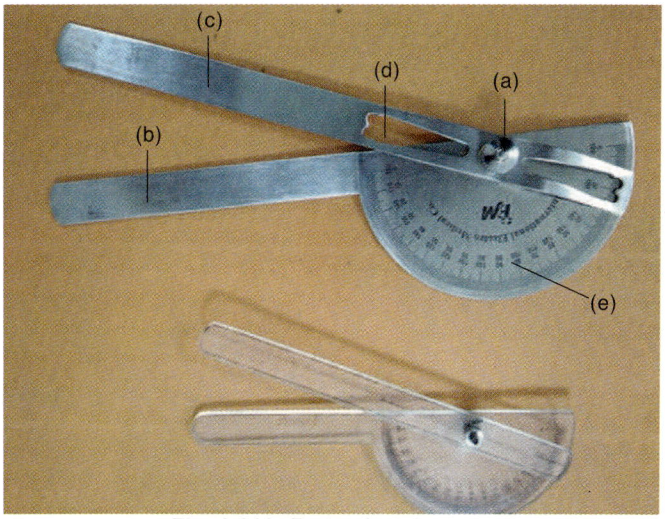

Fig. 6.362: Parts of goniometer
(a) Fulcrum; (b) Stationary arm; (c) Moving arm; (d) Keyhole; (e) Body

Arms

The two arms are **attached on body**, (a) stationary and (b) moving.

a. *Stationary arm:* It is fixed on body and cannot be moved over it, generally stationary arm is placed over the proximal or stabilised part of the limb or extremity.

b. *Moving arm:* It is also attached on body at the centre with screw which allows it to move. Moving arm is placed on the distal part of the limb and moves along with it. Every moving arm should have one of the following character.

   i. *Keyhole indicator or cut out portion*—At the centre of moving arm over the scale a whole is made, which allows the transparency to read out the scale (degree).

   ii. A prominent line should extend from the point to the distal tip of the moving arm.

   iii. A black or white line on middle of the moving arm should extend from screw (fulcrum) to the distal tip of the moving arm.

2. Electrogoniometers

This goniometer was designed by Kar Pavich and Karvich in 1959. It is a type of goniometer, like universal goniometer most of devices have two arms which are connected with potentiometer. The both arms of electrogoniometer placed on the proximal and distal part of the joint and a potentiometer is connected to them. Movement of the arms cause resistance in the potentiometer to vary. The resulting change in voltage can be used to indicate the amount of joint motion. Electrogoniometers are used primarily in research to obtain dynamic joint range measurement (Figs. 6.363a,b and c).

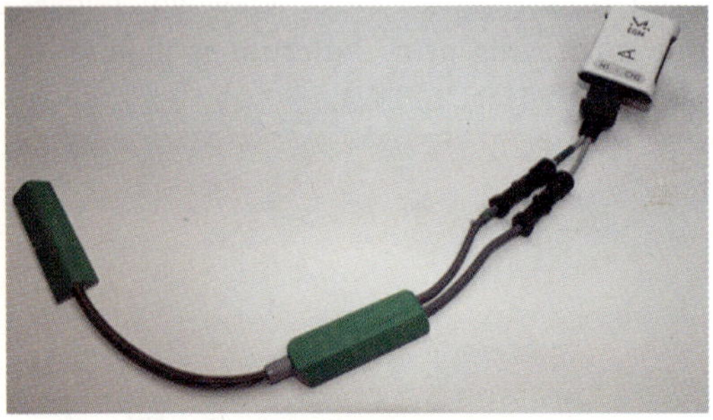

Fig. 6.363a: Electrogoniometer

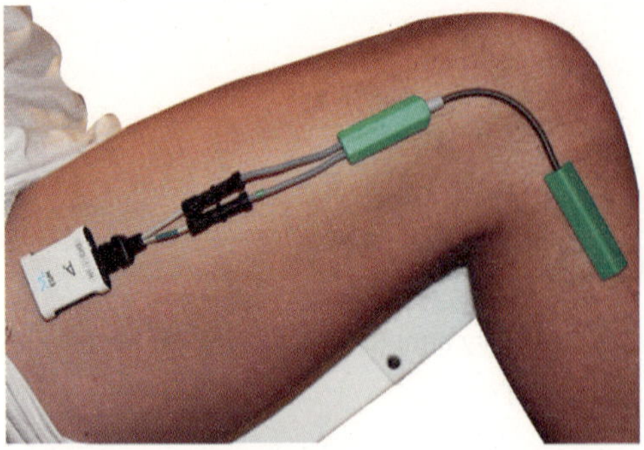

Fig. 6.363b: Placement of electrogoniometer for measurement of knee flexion and extension ROM

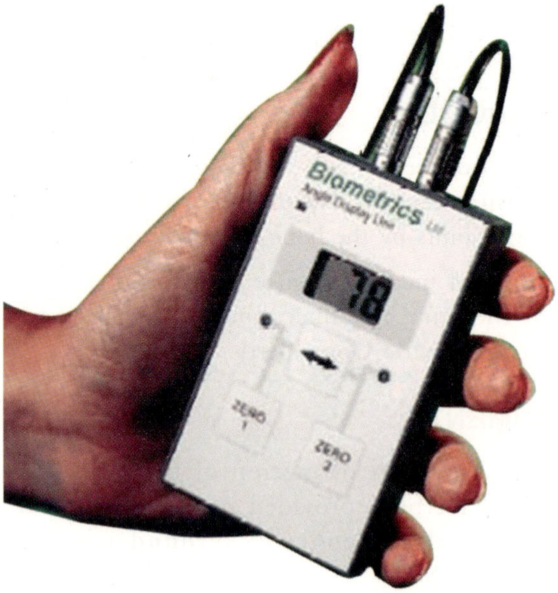

Fig. 6.363c: Potentiometer of the electrogoniometer

3. Gravity Dependent Goniometers

These are sometimes called as inclinometers (Fig. 6.364). To measure the joint range of motion the effect of gravity is used on pointers and fluid levels. These are basically of two types:

1. *Pendulum Goniometer:* It was first devised by Fox and Van Breemen in 1934. It consist a 360° protractor with a weighted pointer hanging from the center of the protractor.

2. *Fluid (Bubble) Goniometer:* It was devised by Schenkar in 1956, has fluid filled circular chamber containing an air bubble.

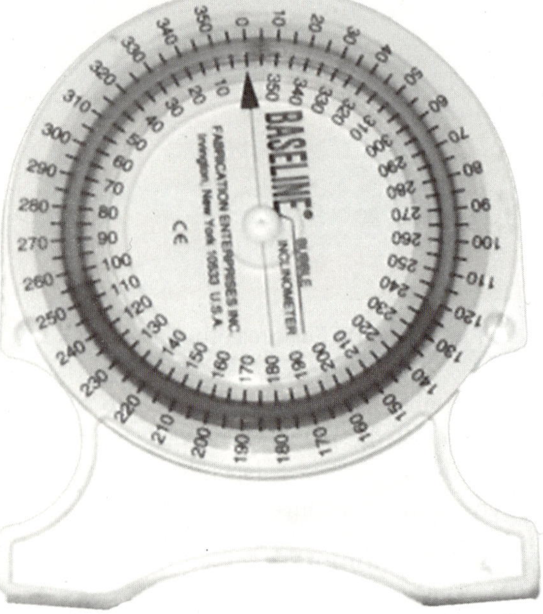

Fig. 6.364: Inclinometer (Gravity dependent goniometer)

END FEEL—NORMAL

The feeling which is experienced by the therapist at the end of passive range of motion. The end range of motion of the normal joint is prevented by the soft tissue structures or bones, for example:

The normal end range of elbow extension is prevented as olecranon process of ulna contacts with the olecranon fossa of humerus, and when joint is extended passively, the hands of the therapist experience hard end feel (bone contacts with the bone). Every joint is having its own unique structures which prevent the motion at end range.

Normally end feels are of three types:

1. **Hard**
   - Bone contacting bone, example–elbow extension.
2. **Firm:** Firm as the name suggests, a firm feeling by the hands of the therapist is because of stretching of soft tissue structures (mainly joint capsule, ligaments and muscles) at the end range of movement.
   i. **Stretching of capsule** example—The anterior joint capsule (MCP) gets stretched and prevents further extension as metacarpophalangeal joints are extended passively.
   ii. **Stretching of muscle** example—When hip joint is flexed with knee extended, the hamstring muscles get stretched and prevents the further hip flexion.
   iii. **Stretching of ligaments** example—Supination of forearm places **extension** in the proximal radioulnar joint, interosseous membrane, oblique cord.
3. **Soft:** Soft tissue approximation mainly because of contact of soft tissues of the proximal and distal segments of the joint (e.g., at end of knee flexion calf muscles contact with the posterior thigh).

END FEELS—PATHOLOGICAL (BY CYRIAX, KALTEN BORN AND PARIS)

Restriction in the range of motion is generally caused by tightness of the soft tissue structures (muscles, ligaments and joint capsule) or pathological changes in the intra-articular structures of the joint. These pathological changes can change the normal end feel of the joint.

Precautions and Contraindications

A. Measurement of joint range of motion is contraindicated in case of following conditions:
   1. Joint dislocation.
   2. Fracture.
   3. Immediate following surgery of soft tissue structures.

B. Extra precautions should be taken in case of following conditions:
   1. Acute joint inflammation.
   2. Osteoporosis.
   3. Haemophilia.
   4. Haematoma.

There are four types of end feels–Soft, firm, hard and empty (Table 6.2).

PROCEDURES

1. To measure the ROM of the joint it is very important to select the comfortable position of patient so that he/she does not move during measurement of range of motion. The joint which is being evaluated should be adequately exposed (remove clothing), to palpate and observe the anatomical landmarks.

Table 6.2: Pathological end feels

	End Feel	*Examples*
Soft	Occurs sooner or later in the range of motion that is usual, or in a joint that normally has a firm or hard end feel.	Soft tissue oedema synovitis
Firm	Occurs sooner or later in the range of motion that is usual, or in a joint that normally has a soft or hard end feel.	Increased muscular tonus capsular, muscular, ligamentous shortening
Hard	Occurs sooner or later in the range of motion than is usual, or in a joint that normally has a soft or end feel a bony grating or bony block is felt.	Chondromalacia Osteoarthritis, loose bodies in joint, myositis ossification, fracture
Empty	No real end feel because pain prevents reaching end of range of motion. No resistance is felt except for patient's protective muscle splinting or muscle spasm.	Acute joint inflammation: – Bursitis – Abscess – Fracture – Psychogenic disorder

2. The therapist stands or sits comfortably according to his convenience and should not change the stance during measurement of ROM, as it may change the alignment/position of goniometer and can cause error in the measurement.
3. *Selection of goniometer:* Different sizes and shapes of universal goniometers are available therefore suitable size and shape of goniometer should be selected depends upon joint being evaluated.
4. The fulcrum of the goniometer is placed over joint line or approximate location of the axis of motion of the joint. Moore suggests that proper alignment of the arms of the goniometer ensure that the fulcrum of goniometer is located at the approximate axis of motion of the joint.
5. **Alignment of arms:**
   i. The *stationary arm* of goniometer is often aligned parallel to the longitudinal axis of the proximal segment or part of the joint (Proximal part of the joint always remains stable during the movement (Fig. 6.365).
   ii. *Moving arm*–is aligned parallel to the longitudinal axis of the distal part of the joint (Fig. 6.365).

   In almost all cases the alignment of arms remain constant but in some circumstances alignment of arms may be vice versa (stationary arm is aligned parallel to the longitudinal axis of the distal segment while moving arm is placed over the proximal segment/part of the joint.

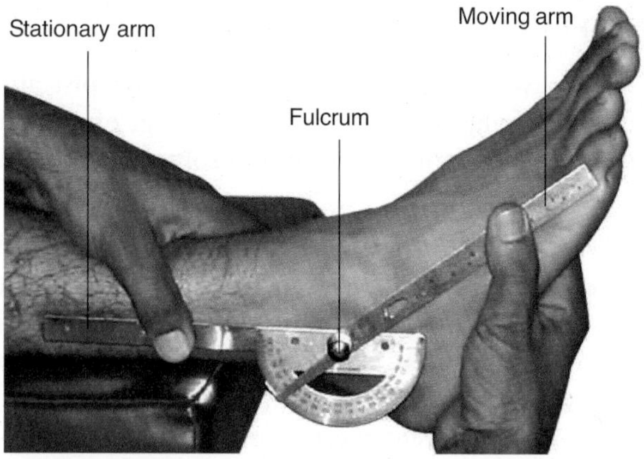

Fig. 6.365: Placement of goniometer for ankle joint (showing fulcrum on lateral malleolus; stationary arm over the proximal part of the joint and moving arm over the distal part of the joint)

6. After placement of fulcrum, stationary arm and moving arm, the examiner stabilizes the stationary arm with the proximal segment of the joint, while moving arm is held with the distal segment of the joint, and patient is asked to move the distal segment of joint in the available range of motion. During motion the arms of the goniometer should be kept with the proximal and distal segment of joint do not allow them to change the position, although slight adjustments are needed to be done. Active and passive ranges are measured.

SHOULDER ROM

FLEXION

The normal flexion range is 0° to 180°, out of which 120° movement occurs at the glenohumeral and 60° movement occurs at the scapulothoracic joint. In addition to this flexion is also accompanied by the motion at the acromioclavicular and sternoclavicular joints. Pain and pathology in any one joints can limit the flexion of the shoulder joint. The normal end feel of the flexion is firm due to tension in the posterior band of the coracohumeral ligament, and in the posterior joint capsule. Tension in the deltoid posterior fibers, teres minor, teres major and infraspinatus is also produced to limit the flexion. Examiner stabilizes the shoulder to prevent excessive posterior tilting and upward rotation of scapula as these movements compensate the flexion range (Figs. 6.366a, b and c).

(a)

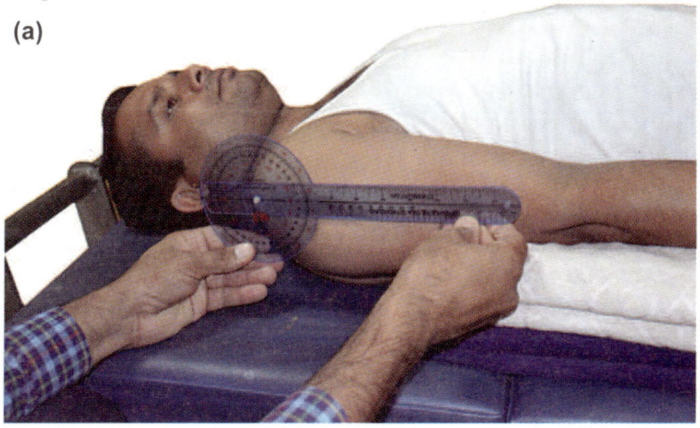

(b)

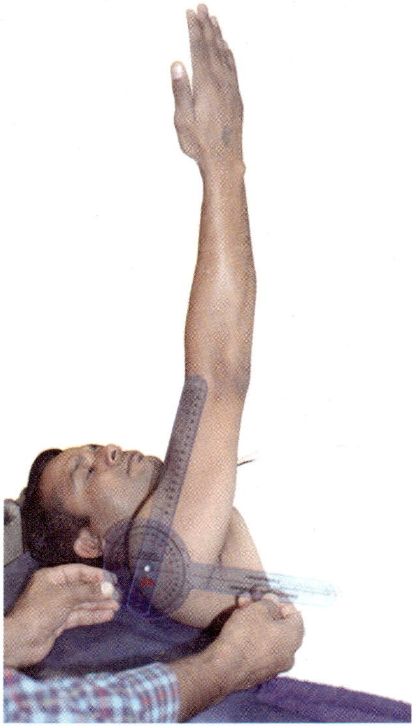

(c)

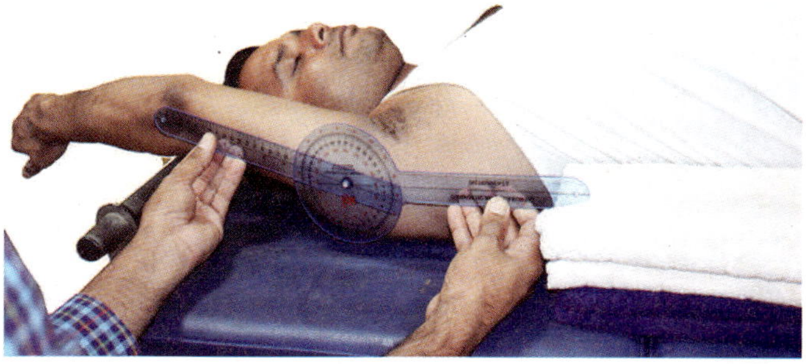

Figs. 6.366 a,b and c: Measurement of shoulder flexion ROM

Measurement of Shoulder Flexion Range of Motion

Plane and Axis: The movement occurs in the sagittal plane around a medial lateral axis.

Position of Patient: Subject is placed in the supine position with shoulder, elbow and wrist in the neutral position. Knees and hip joints are flexed to 90° and 45°, respectively, to flatten the lumbar spine.

Position of Examiner: Examiner stands at side of patient.

Position of Goniometer: Fulcrum of the goniometer is placed over the lateral aspect of the greater tubercle of the humerus. Stationary or proximal arm is placed parallel to the midaxillary line of the thorax. The distal or moving arm is placed with the midline of the humerus. The lateral epicondyle of the humerus is taken reference.

Stabilization: Shoulder girdle is stabilized to prevent excessive posterior tilting of the scapula.

Procedure: After placement of fulcrum, stationary and moving arm, examiner maintains the position of stationary arm along the midaxillary line of the thorax and instructs the subject to flex the shoulder joint. The moving arm moves with the lateral midline of humerus upto the full range of motion or upto available range of motion.

EXTENSION

The normal extension range is 0° to 50° which occurs in the sagittal plane around medial lateral axis. The normal end feel of extension is firm because of tension in the anterior band of coracohumeral ligament, anterior joint capsule. The clavicular fibres of pectoralis major, coracobrachialis and deltoid anterior fibres also limit the end of extension.

Stabilization: The examiner stabilizes the shoulder to prevent elevation and anterior tilting as these movements compensate the extension (Figs. 6.367a and b).

(a)

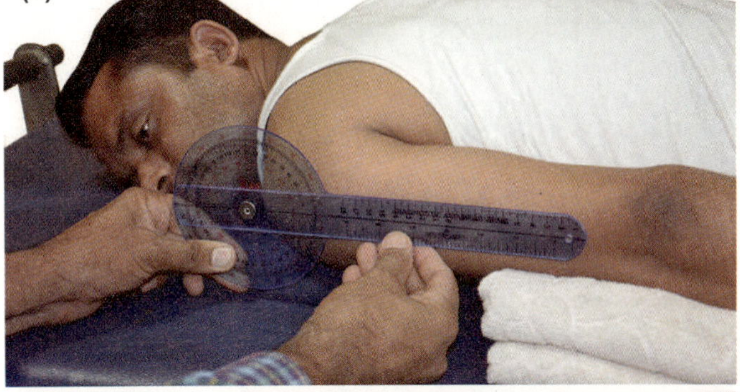

(b)

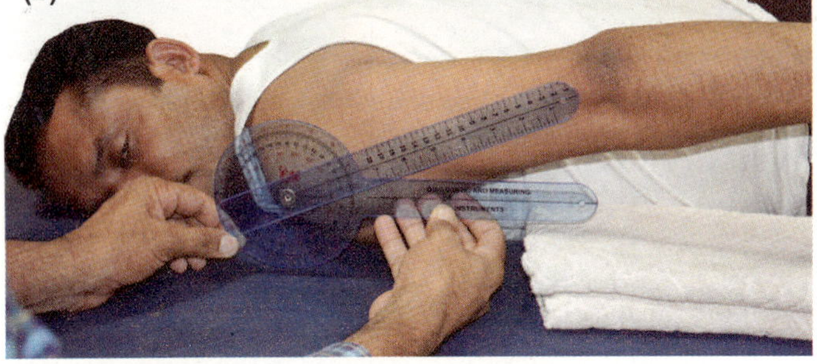

Figs. 6.367a and b: Measurement of shoulder extension range of motion (ROM)

Measurement of Shoulder Extension

Position of Patient: Subject is placed in supine position with shoulder, elbows and wrist joint in the neutral position. A towel roll is placed under the elbow and forearm to bring the arm to the level of mid thorax, this brings the shoulder joint to the neutral position.

Position of Goniometer: Fulcrum of the goniometer is placed over the lateral aspect of greater tubercle of the humerus. Stationary or proximal arm is placed parallel to the midaxillary line of the thorax; and moving or distal arm is placed with the lateral midline of humerus.

Procedure: After placement of goniometer, examiner maintains the position of stationary arm throughout the process. Examiner instructs the patient to flex the shoulder joint upto the full range or available range of motion. Examiner moves the moving arm either with the extremity (arm) or moves it after completing the range.

ABDUCTION

The normal abduction range is 0° to 180° which occurs in the frontal plane around an anterior posterior axis. 120° movement occurs in the glenohumeral and 60° movement occurs in the scapulohumeral joint. In addition to that abduction is accompanied by motion in the acromioclavicular and sternoclavicular joints. The normal end feel of abduction is firm due to tension in the middle and inferior bands of the glenohumeral ligament, and inferior joint capsule. Tension in the teres major and clavicular fibres of pectoralis major is also produced at the end range to limit the motion (Figs. 6.368a and b).

(a)

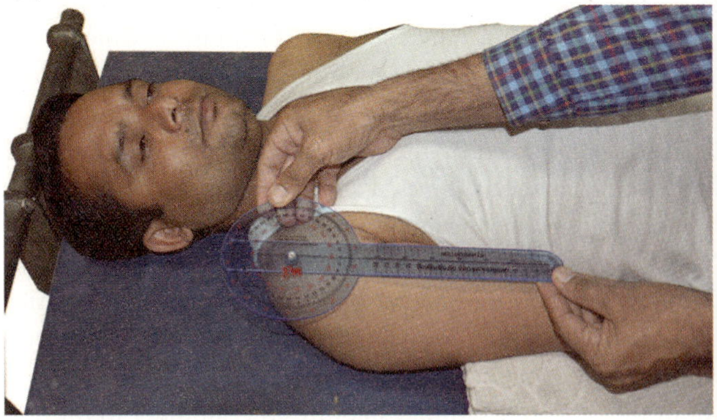

(b)

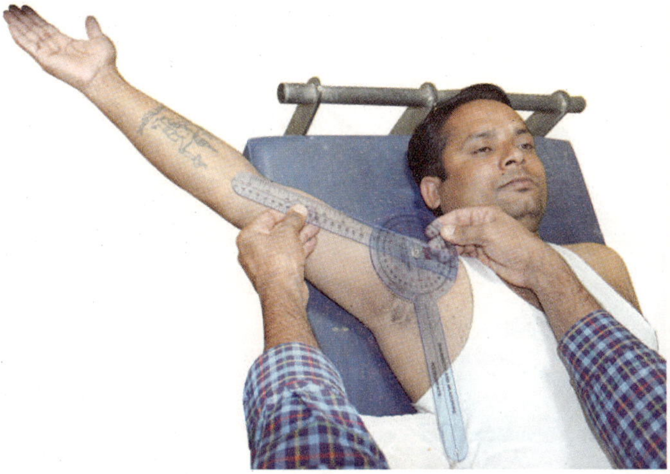

Figs. 6.368a and b: Measurement of shoulder abduction ROM

Position of Patient: Subject is placed in the supine position with shoulder and elbow at the neutral. A towel roll is placed under the elbow and forearm to bring the shoulder joint into the neutral position.

Position of Goniometer: Fulcrum of the goniometer is placed over the anterior aspect of acromian process. Proximal or stationary arm is placed parallel to the midline of the anterior aspect of the sternum. The distal arm or moving arm is placed with anterior midline of the humerus. The medial epicondyle of humerus may be taken as a reference point. After placement of the goniometer, examiner maintains the position of the proximal arm and instructs the subject to elevate the arm (abduction) in the side upto the available range of motion. Examiner moves the moving arm either with the extremity or moves it after completing the range of motion.

ADDUCTION

Adduction is the reverse of abduction. Its normal range is 180° to 0° in the frontal plane around an anteroposterior axis.

MEDIAL AND LATERAL ROTATION

The normal range of medial and lateral rotation is 0° to 80° and 0° to 90° respectively which occur in the transverse plane around a vertical axis. The end feel of medial rotation and lateral rotation is firm. The medial rotation at the end is restricted due to tension in the posterior joint capsule, infraspinatus and teres minor muscles. The lateral rotation at the end is restricted due to tension in the anterior joint capsule, all three bands of glenohumeral ligament, subscapularis, teres major, and the clavicular fibers of the pectoralis major muscles.

Stabilization: The shoulder girdle is stabilized to prevent anterior tilting, posterior tilting, retraction and protraction. The anterior tilting and protraction compensates the medial rotation whereas, posterior tilting and retraction compensates the lateral rotation of the shoulder joint (Figs. 6.369a, b and c).

(a)

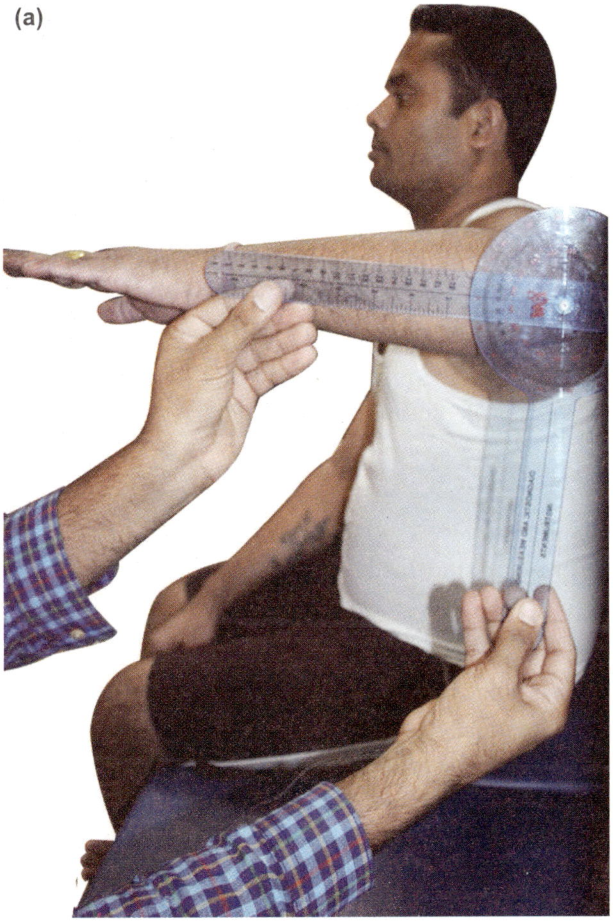

(b)

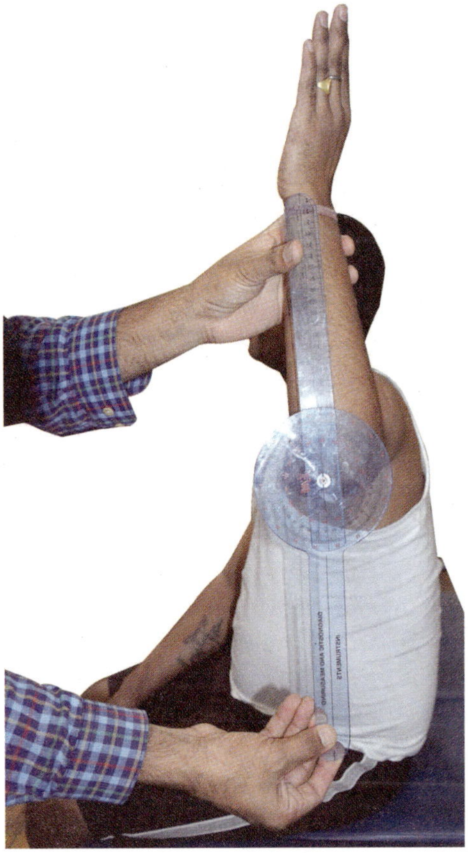

(c)

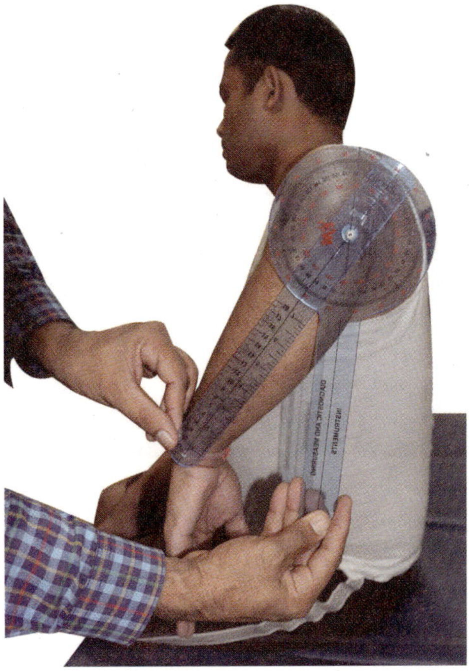

Figs. 6.369a, b and c: Measurement of medial and lateral rotation of the shoulder joint

Position of Patient: Patient is placed in the supine position with the shoulder joint abducted to 90° and elbow joint flexed to 90°. The hand faces the ceiling. A towel roll is placed under the arm to raise it to the shoulder level in order to bring the shoulder into the neutral position.

Position of Goniometer: Fulcrum of the goniometer is placed over the olecranon process of ulna. Proximal or stationary arm hangs freely so that it remains perpendicular to the floor. The proximal arm may also be placed along the mid axillary line so that it remain parallel to the floor. The moving or distal arm of the goniometer is placed along the ulna. The ulnar styloid process is taken as a reference.

Procedure: After placement of the goniometer, the examiner maintains the position of stationary arm and instructs the patient to move the hand and forearm towards the waist for the medial rotation and towards the head for the lateral rotation. Examiner moves the moving arm of the goniometer either with the forearm or after completing the range of motion.

FLEXION

The normal range of elbow flexion is 0° to 140°, which may vary 5°-10° from individual to individual due to hypertrophy or atrophy of the muscles. The movement occurs in the sagittal plane around a medial lateral axis. The normal end feel of the flexion is soft due to approximation of the soft tissues between arm and forearm. However, the end feel may be hard if there is atrophy of the elbow flexors as it allows the contact between coronoid process of ulna and the coronoid fossa of the humerus. Sometimes the end may be firm due to tension in the posterior joint capsule and triceps muscles (Figs. 6.370a, b and c).

(a)

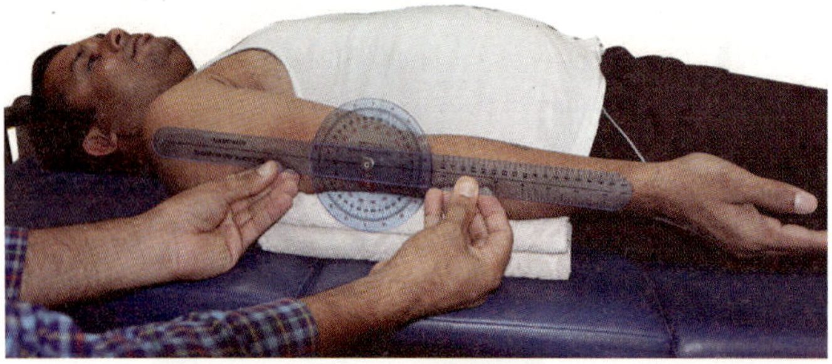

(b)

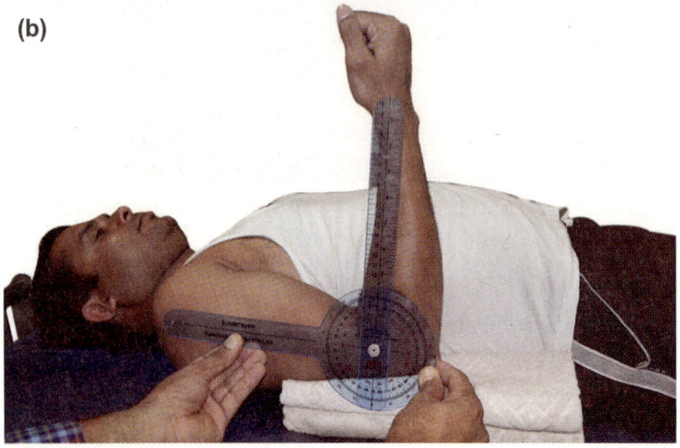

(c)

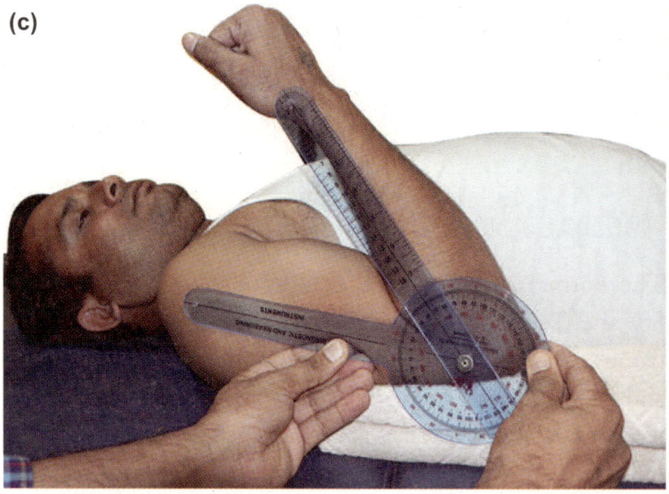

Figs. 6.370a, b and c: Measurement of elbow flexion ROM

Position of Patient: The subject is placed in a supine position with shoulder and elbow joints in the neutral position. A towel roll is placed under arm and forearm to bring the shoulder joint into neutral position. Examiner stands at the side of patient.

Position of Goniometer: Fulcrum of the goniometer over the lateral epicondyle of the humerus. The distal or moving arm is placed over the lateral midline of humerus and proximal or stationary arm is placed over the lateral midline of humerus. The radial styloid and acromion process may be taken the reference points for distal and proximal arms of goniometer respectively.

Procedure: After placement of the goniometer the examiner maintains the position of proximal or stationary arm over the lateral epicondyle of humerus throughout the process with one hand. Examiner instructs the patient to flex the elbow joint upto the full range or available range of motion. Examiner moves the distal arm of the goniometer with the forearm or after completion of range of motion.

Stabilization: Examiner should stabilize the arm to prevent flexion of the shoulder and retraction of scapula.

EXTENSION

Extension is the reverse of flexion from 140° to 0° in the sagittal plane around medial lateral axis.

FOREARM SUPINATION

The normal range of forearm supination is 0° to 80° which occurs in the transverse plane around vertical axis when the forearm is in the anatomical position. The normal end feel of supination is firm due to tension in the palmar radioulnar ligament of the inferior radioulnar joint, interosseous membrane, and pronator teres and pronator quadratus muscles (Figs. 6.371a and b).

(a)

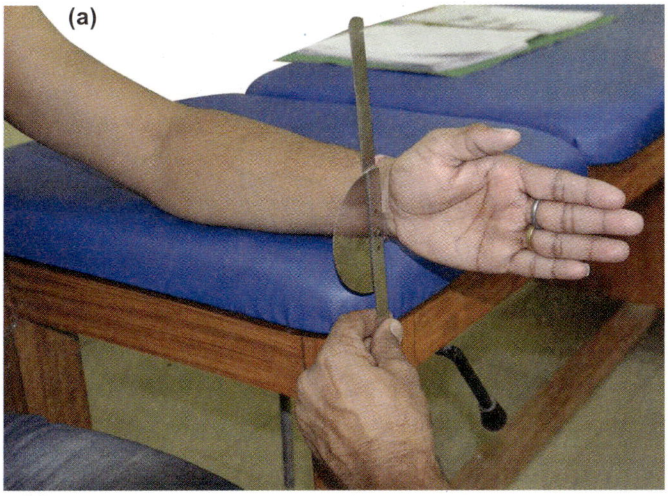

(b)

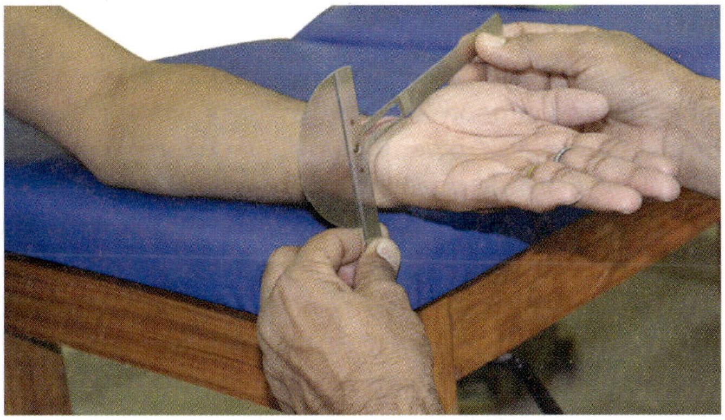

Figs. 6.371a and b: Measurement of forearm supination ROM

Measurement of Forearm Supination

Position of Patient: Subject is placed in the high sitting position with shoulder joint at neutral, elbow joint flexed to 90° and forearm at mid-prone position (thumb points towards ceiling). Examiner sits comfortably on the stool in front of the patient.

Position of Goniometer: Fulcrum of the goniometer is placed medially and proximally to the ulnar styloid process. The proximal or stationary arm is aligned parallel to the anterior midline of humerus and distal arm is aligned across the palmar surface of the distal forearm. So that it remains parallel to the radial and ulnar styloids. Examiner holds the stationary arm firmly and maintains its position throughout the procedure.

Procedure: Examiner instructs the patient to rotate the forearm outwards so that thumb goes out parallel to the floor. Examiner must ensure that the fulcrum of the goniometer remains at the proximal and medial to the ulnar styloid process. It is obvious that there is change of position of the ulnar styloid during supination, hence, fulcrum should also be shifted with the ulnar styloid. The distal or moving arm is moved either with the forearm supination or after completion of range. It is essential to keep the distal arm parallel to the styloid process of radial ulnar styloid.

Stabilization: Distal end of humerus is stabilized to prevent lateral rotation and adduction of the shoulder joint.

FOREARM PRONATION

The normal range of forearm pronation is 0°-75° which occurs in the transverse plane around vertical or longitudinal axis. The normal end feel of pronation is hard because of contact between the ulna and radius, or it may be firm due to tension in the dorsal radioulnar ligament of the inferior radioulnar joint, interosseous membrane, and the supinator muscle (Figs. 6.372a and b).

(a)

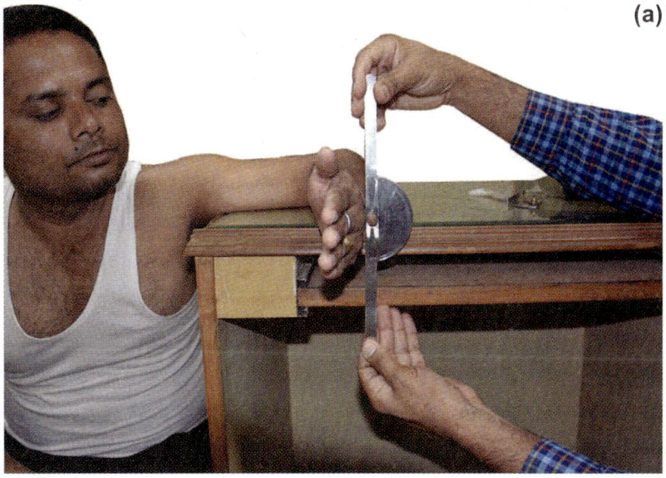

(b)

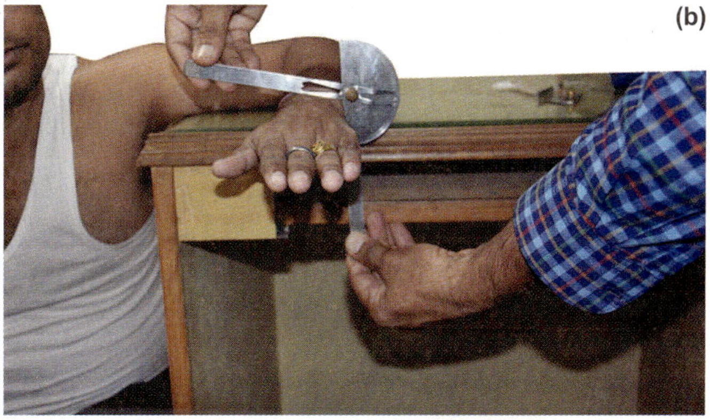

Figs. 6.372a and b: Measurement of forearm pronation ROM

Position of Patient: High sitting with shoulder at neutral, elbow flexed to 90° and forearm in mid-prone position.

Position of Examiner: Examiner sits comfortably on a stool in front of the patient, or at the side of patient.

Position of Goniometer: Fulcrum of the goniometer is positioned lateral and proximal to the ulnar styloid process. Proximal or stationary arm is positioned parallel to the anterior midline of the humerus. Distal or moving arm is positioned across the dorsal aspect of the distal forearm that should be parallel to the styloid process of radius and ulna.

Stabilization: The distal arm is stabilized to prevent medial rotation and abduction of the shoulder joint.

Procedure: After placement of goniometer, examiner maintains the position of goniometer and instructs the patient to rotate the forearm inwards so that thumb faces the body. Examiner may move the moving arm of goniometer along with the distal forearm pronation or move after completion of the pronation. It is obvious that there is change in the position of goniometer to follow the ulnar styloid.

WRIST FLEXION

Normal Range of Motion: 0° – 75°.

Plane and Axis: Sagittal around medial lateral axis.

Normal End Feel: Firm due to tension in the dorsal radiocarpal ligament and the dorsal joint capsule. The muscles which limit the end range are extensor carpi radialis brevis, extensor carpi radialis longus, and extensor carpi ulnaris.

Position of Patient: High sitting with back supported well, shoulder abducted to 90°, elbow flexed to 90°, forearm in midprone position and placed on the supporting surface with the hand and wrist out of the supporting surface. The palm faces downward to the floor.

Position of Examiner: Examiner sits comfortably on chair at the side which is being tested, and tests the end feel of the joint by moving it passively.

Position of Goniometer: Fulcrum of the goniometer is placed on the triquetrum bone to the ulnar side. Proximal arm is positioned on the midline of ulna with reference to the olecranon process and ulnar styloid. Distal or moving arm is placed on the midline of the fifth metacarpal bone with reference to its head. The middle proximal and distal phalanx should not be taken a reference for distal arm of the goniometer (Figs. 6.373a and b).

(a)

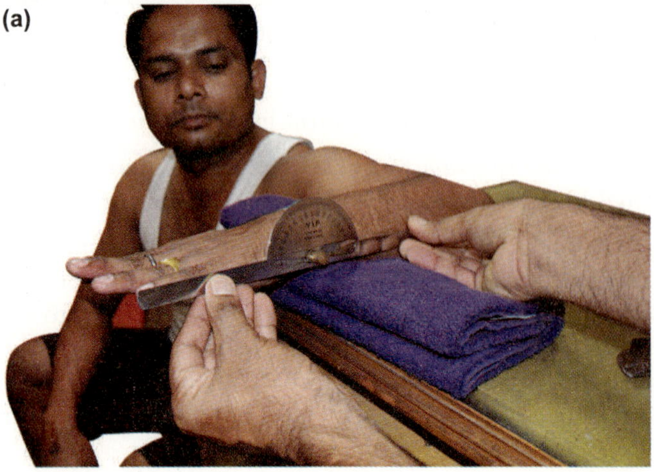

(b)

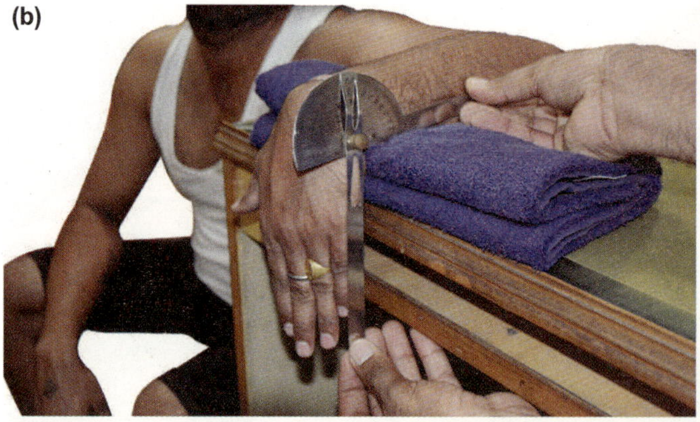

Figs. 6.373a and b: Measurement of wrist flexion ROM

Stabilization: Forearm is stabilized to prevent supination and pronation and elbow joint to prevent flexion and extension.

Procedure: After placement of goniometer, examiner maintains the position of stationary or proximal arm and instructs the subject to flex the wrist joint. Distal or moving arm of the goniometer is moved either along with the fifth metacarpal bone or moved after completion of the wrist flexion.

Alternative Position of the Goniometer: The fulcrum of the goniometer may be placed on the dorsal surface of capitate bone. Proximal arm is positioned over the dorsal midline of the forearm and distal arm is positioned over the dorsal midline of the third metacarpal bone. Forearm is stabilized to prevent supination and pronation, and elbow is stabilized to prevent flexion and extension. Examiner maintains the proximal arm and instructs the subject to take your hand downward as much as possible. The supporting surface should not hinder the wrist flexion. The head of third metacarpal bone is taken as a reference point. The digits should not be taken as a reference point for the distal arm. Distal arm of the goniometer is moved alongwith the third metacarpal bone, or after completion of the motion (Figs. 6.374a and b).

(a)

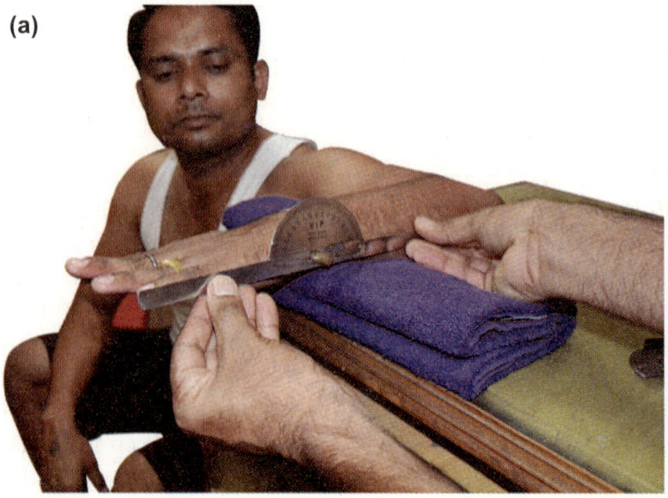

(b)

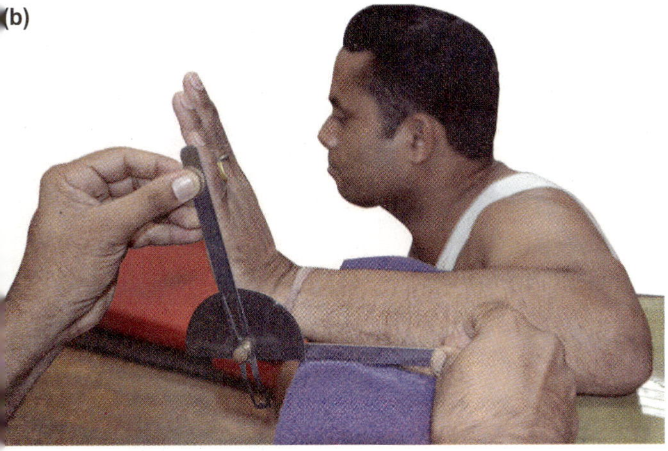

Figs. 6.374a and b: Measurement of wrist extension ROM

WRIST EXTENSION

Normal ROM: 0° to 75°.

Plane and Axis: Sagittal plane around medial lateral axis.

Normal End Feel: Usually it is firm, however, it may also be hard. The firm end feel is due to tension in the palmar radiocarpal ligament, ulnocarpal ligament, and palmar joint capsule. The muscle which limit the wrist extension at the end range are palmaris longus, flexor carpi radialis and flexor carpi ulnaris. The hard end feel is due to the contact between radius and carpal bone.

Position of Patient: Same as for wrist flexion.

Position of Examiner: Same as for wrist flexion.

Position of Goniometer: Same as for wrist flexion.

Stabilization: Forearm is stabilized to prevent supination and pronation, and elbow is stabilized to prevent flexion and extension.

Procedure: After placement of goniometer examiner maintains the position of stationary arm and instructs the patient to move the hand up towards ceiling as much as possible. Distal arm is moved along the third metacarpal bone. The head of third metacarpal bone is taken as a reference point for distal arm.

Alternative Position of Goniometer: Fulcrum of goniometer is positioned on the palmar surface of wrist joint at the level of capitate bone. Proximal arm is placed over the midline of forearm, and distal arm is positioned over the midline of third metacarpal bone (palmar surface). The head of third metacarpal bone is taken a reference point for moving arm. Digits should not be taken as a reference point. Subject is instructed to take the hand up towards ceiling as much as possible the moving arm is moved along the third metacarpal bone (Figs. 6.375a and b).

(a)

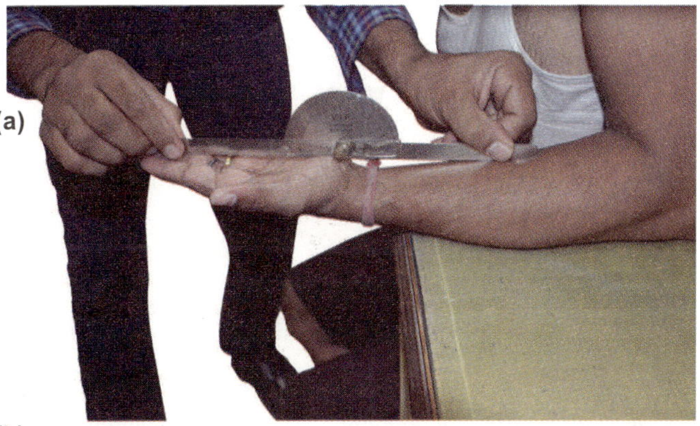

(b)

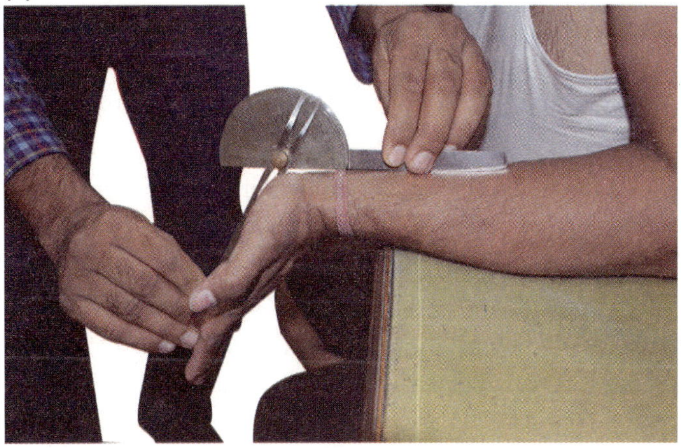

Figs. 6.375a and b: Measurement of wrist extension ROM

WRIST RADIAL DEVIATION

Normal ROM: 0° to 20°.

Plane and Axis: Frontal around anterior posterior axis.

Normal End Feel: Usually end feel is hard, however it may also be firm. Hard end feel is due to contact between the radial styloid process and the scaphoid bone. The firm end feel is because of tension in the ulnar collateral ligament, the ulnocarpal ligament, and the ulnar portion of joint capsule. Tension in the extensor carpi ulnaris and flexion carpi ulnaris may also limit the radial deviation (Figs. 6.376a and b).

(a)

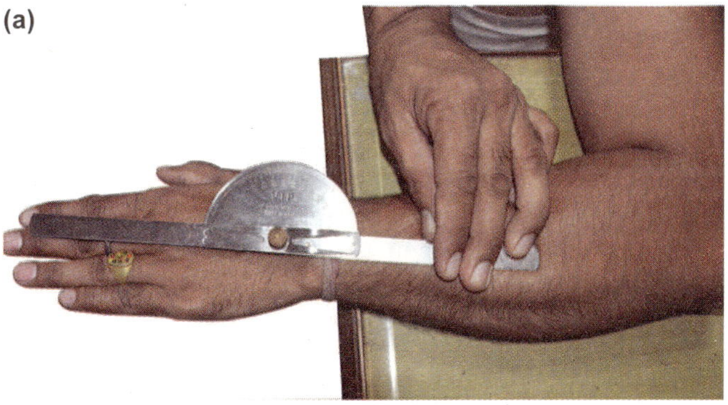

(b)

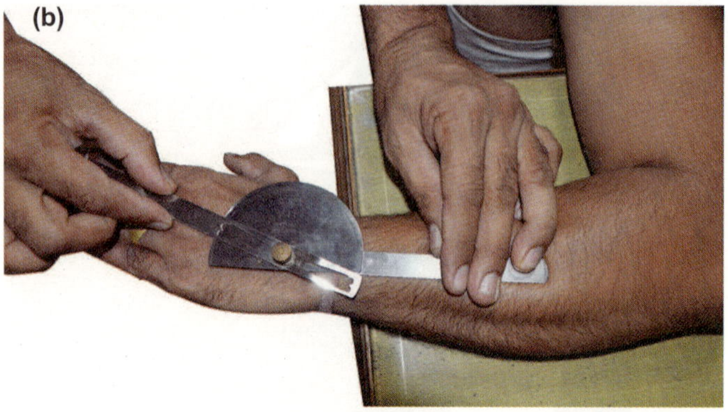

Figs. 6.376a, b: Measurement of wrist radial deviation ROM

Position of Patient: High sitting with back supported well, shoulder abducted to 90°, elbow flexed to 90°, forearm pronated and positioned on the supporting surface with hand out of the supporting surface.

Position of Examiner: Examiner sits comfortably at the side of patient which is being tested.

Position of Goniometer: Fulcrum of the goniometer is placed over the dorsal surface of wrist joint on the capitate bone. Stationary arm is positioned over the dorsal midline of the forearm. Lateral epicondyle of humerus is taken a reference point for the proximal arm. The distal arm is positioned over the dorsal midline of third metacarpal bone, its heal is taken a reference point. The digits should not be taken a reference point for distal arm as abduction or adduction of MCP joints may distort the results.

Stabilization: Forearm is stabilized to prevent supination, promotion, elbow flexion and extension.

Procedure: Examiner maintains the position of proximal arm of the goniometer over the dorsal midline of forearm, and instructs the patient to take the hand towards the chest (radial deviation) without flexion and extension at the wrist joint. The distal arm is moved along with the third metacarpal bone in the available range.

WRIST ULNAR DEVIATION

Normal ROM – 0° to 40°.

Plane and Axis: Frontal plane around anterior posterior axis.

Normal End Feel: Normal end feel is firm due to tension in the radial collateral ligament, and radial portion of the joint capsule. Tension in the extensor pollicis brevis, abductor pollicis longus muscles limit the end range and produce firm end feel (Figs. 6.377a and b).

Position of Patient: Same as for radial deviation.

Position of Examiner: Same as for radial deviation.

(a)

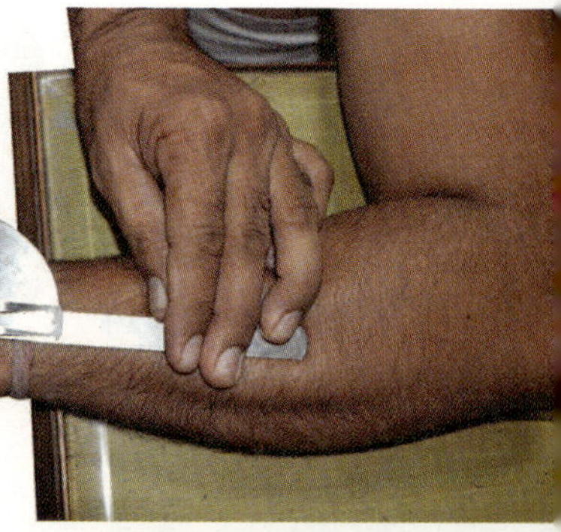

(b)

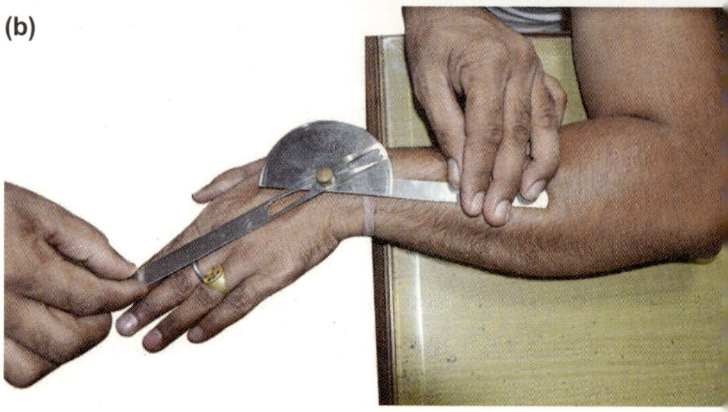

Figs. 6.377a and b: Measurement of wrist ulnar deviation ROM

Position of Goniometer: Same as for radial deviation.

Stabilization: Same as for radial deviation.

Procedure: Examiner maintains the position of stationary arm over the dorsal midline of forearm and instructs the subject to move the hand outwards (away from the midline) without flexion and extension of the wrist joint. The distal/moving arm is moved along the third metacarpal bone.

METACARPOPHALANGEAL FLEXION

Normal ROM: 0° to 90°–100°. Flexion increases slightly from second MCP joint to the fifth MCP joint. Second MCP joint flexion is 90° whereas normal flexion of fifth MCP is 100°.

Plane and Axis: Movement occurs in the sagittal plane around medial-lateral axis.

Normal End Feel: Normal end feel may either be hard or firm. Usually the end feel is hard due to contact between the palmar aspect of the proximal phalanx and the respective metacarpal bone. The end feel may be firm because of tension in the dorsal joint capsule and the collateral ligament (Figs. 6.378a,b,c and d).

Position of Patient: High sitting, with elbow flexion and forearm in midprone position. Hand and forearm rests on the supporting surface. Wrist, PIP, DIP and MCP should be in neutral position.

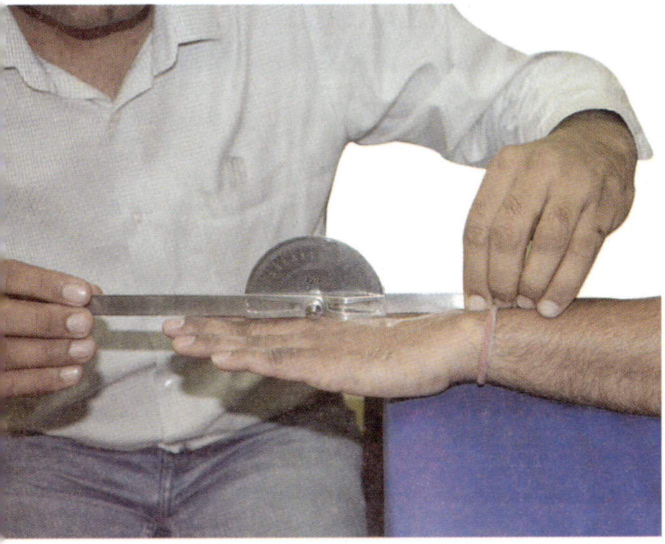

Fig. 6.378a: Measurement of third MCP flexion ROM (Starting)

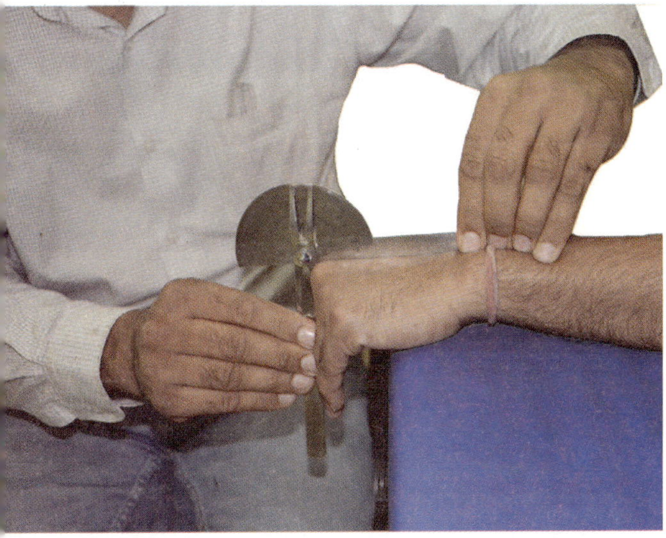

Fig. 6.378b: Measurement of third MCP flexion ROM

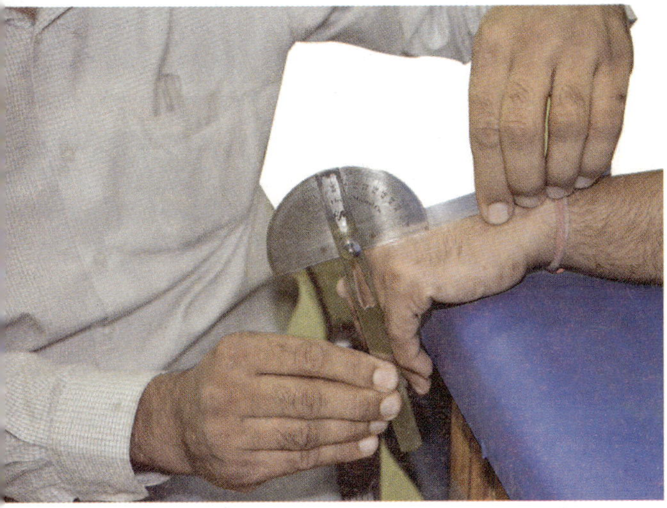

Fig. 6.378c: Measurement of fourth MCP flexion ROM

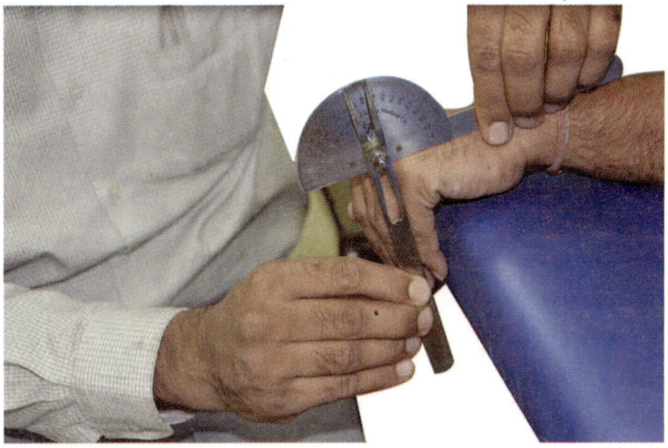

Fig. 6.378d: Measurement of fifth MCP flexion ROM

Position of Examiner: Examiner sits comfortably in chair at the side which is being tested.

Position of Goniometer: Fulcrum of goniometer is positioned over the dorsal aspect of the MCP joint. Proximal arm is aligned over the dorsal midline of the metacarpal bone. The distal arm is aligned over the dorsal midline of the proximal phalanx.

Stabilization: Wrist joint is stabilized to prevent flexion and extension, radial and ulnar deviation of wrist joint. The MCP joints, which are not being tested, should also be stabilized.

Procedure: Examiner stabilizes the stationary arm with the respective metacarpal bone and instructs the patient to take the finger downward. The distal arm is moved along the proximal phalanx which is being tested. Flexion of all the MCP joints from second to fifth can be measured.

METACARPOPHALANGEAL (MCP) EXTENSION

Normal ROM: 0° to 20°.

Plane and Axis: Sagittal around medial lateral axis.

Normal End Feel: Firm because of tension in the palmar joint capsule.

Position of Patient: Same as for MCP flexion.

Position of Examiner: Same as for MCP flexion.

Position of Goniometer: Same as for MCP flexion, however, a half circle plastic goniometer is used especially for this position.

Procedure: Examiner maintains the position of stationary arm along the dorsal midline of respective metacarpal bone and instructs the patient to move the finger upward towards the ceiling as much as possible. The distal arm is moved with the respective phalanx.

Alternative Position for MCP Extension

Fulcrum of goniometer is placed on the palmar surface of MCP joint which is being tested. The proximal arm is placed over the palmar midline of respective metacarpal bone. The distal arm is placed over the proximal phalanx of the respective joint (Figs. 6.379a,b and Fig. 6.380).

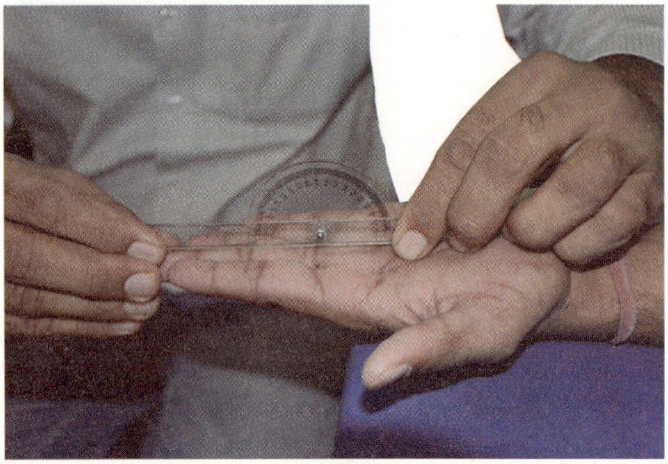

Fig. 6.379a: Measurement of third MCP extension

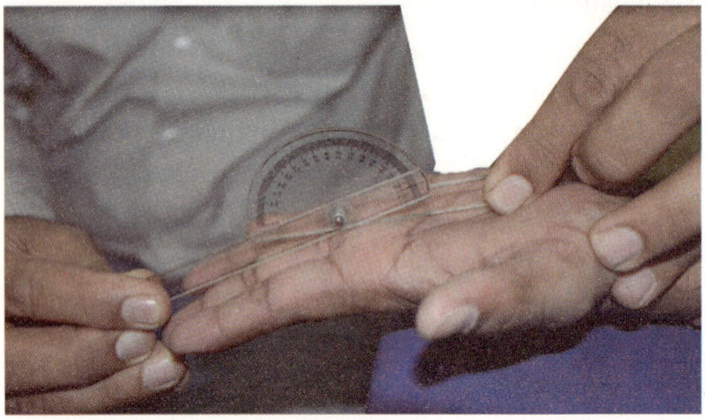

Fig. 6.379b: Measurement of third MCP extension

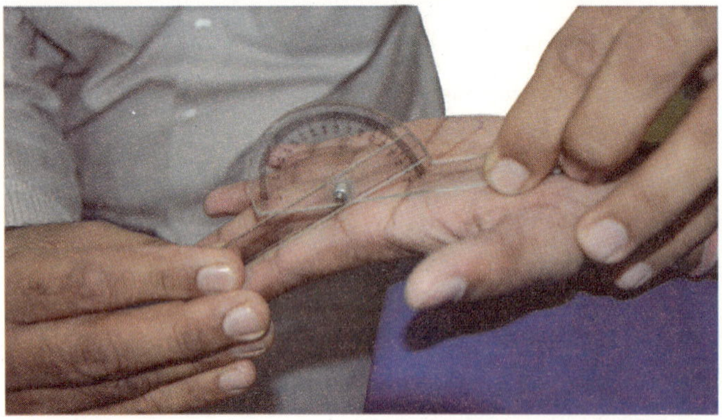

Fig. 6.380: Measurement of second MCP extension

Procedure: Examiner stabilizes the proximal arm with the respective metacarpal bone and instructs the patient to move the finger up towards the ceiling. Distal arm is moved with the phalanx.

METACAROPHALANGEAL (MCP) ABDUCTION

Normal ROM*:* 0° to 30°.

Plane and Axis: Movement occurs in frontal plane around anteroposterior axis.

Normal End Feel: Normal end feel is firm due to tension in the collateral ligament of the MCP joints, fascia of the web space and interossei muscles.

Position of Patient: High sitting with forearm pronated and supported on supporting surface. The MCP joints remain on the supporting surface. PIP, DIP, MCP and wrist joint should be at neutral position.

Position of Examiner: Examiner sits comfortably in a stool in front of patient (Figs. 6.381a to f).

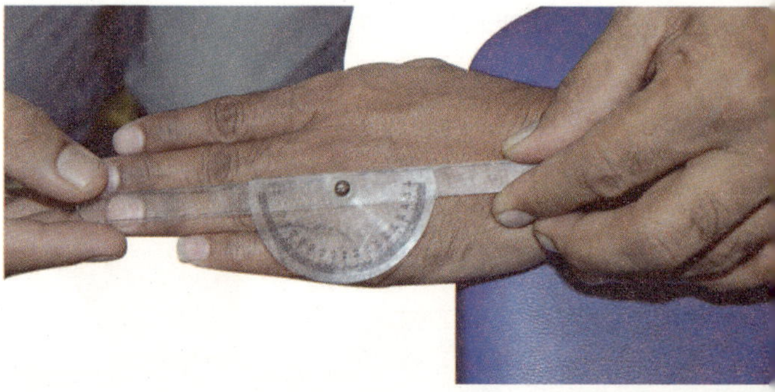

Fig. 6.381a: Measurement of fourth MCP abduction (Starting)

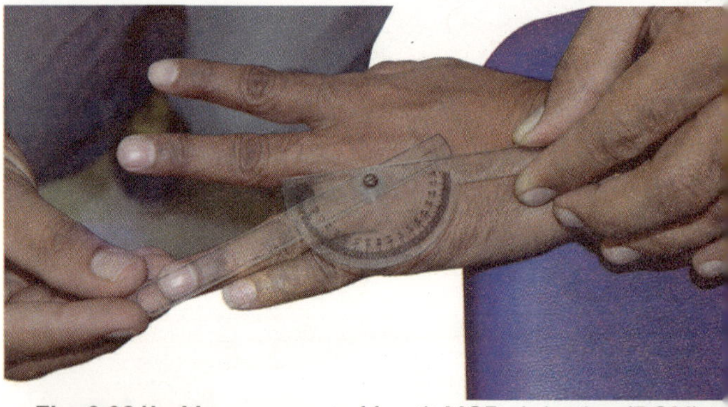

Fig. 6.381b: Measurement of fourth MCP abduction (ROM)

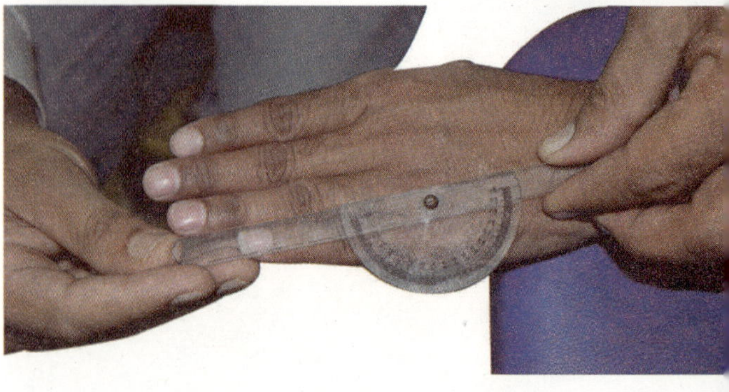

Fig. 6.381c: Measurement of fifth MCP abduction ROM (Starting position)

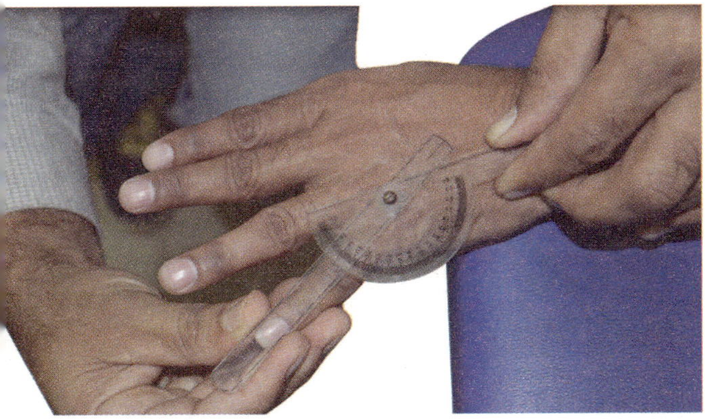

Fig. 6.381d: Measurement of fourth MCP abduction

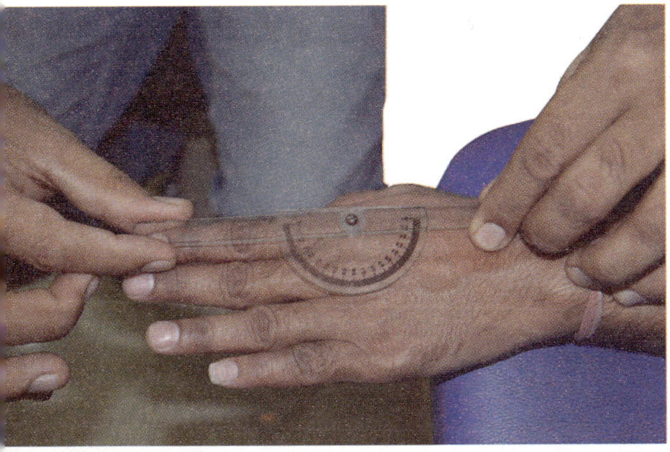

Fig. 6.381e: Measurement of second MCP abduction ROM (Starting position)

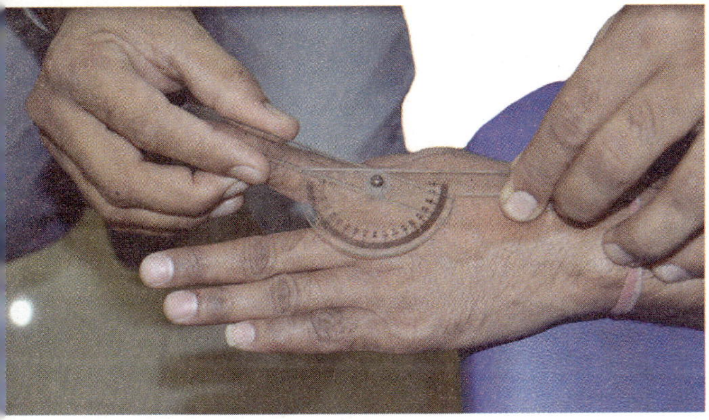

Fig. 6.381f: Measurement of second MCP abduction

Position of Goniometer: Fulcrum is placed on the dorsal aspect of the concerned MCP joint which is being tested. Proximal arm is aligned over the dorsal midline of concerned metacarpal bone and distal arm is aligned over the dorsal midline of concerned phalanx.

Stabilization: Wrist and metacarpal bones are stabilized to prevent flexion and extension.

Procedure: Examiner maintains the position of proximal arm on the concerned metacarpal bone and instructs the patient to take the finger away from the midline of hand (middle finger). The other fingers are stabilized to keep them in the neutral position. The distal arm is moved with the proximal phalanx of the concerned MCP joint.

METACARPOPHALANGEAL ADDUCTION

It is the reverse of MCP abduction.

PROXIMAL INTERPHALANGEAL FLEXION

Normal ROM: 0° to 100°.

Plane and Axis: Sagittal plane around medial lateral axis.

Normal End Feel: The normal end feel of PIP flexion is usually a hard due to contact between the proximal and distal phalanx. The end feel may be soft if there is an approximation of soft tissues of palmar proximal and distal phalanx. Sometimes the end feel may be firm because of tension in the dorsal joint capsule and collateral ligaments (Figs. 6.382a to e).

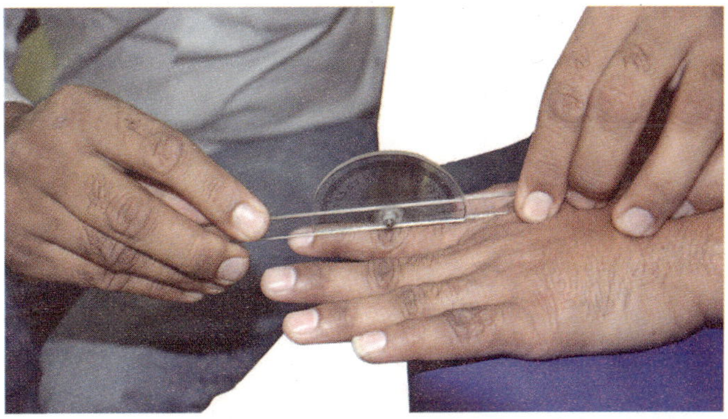

Fig. 6.382a: Measurement of second PIP flexion (Starting position)

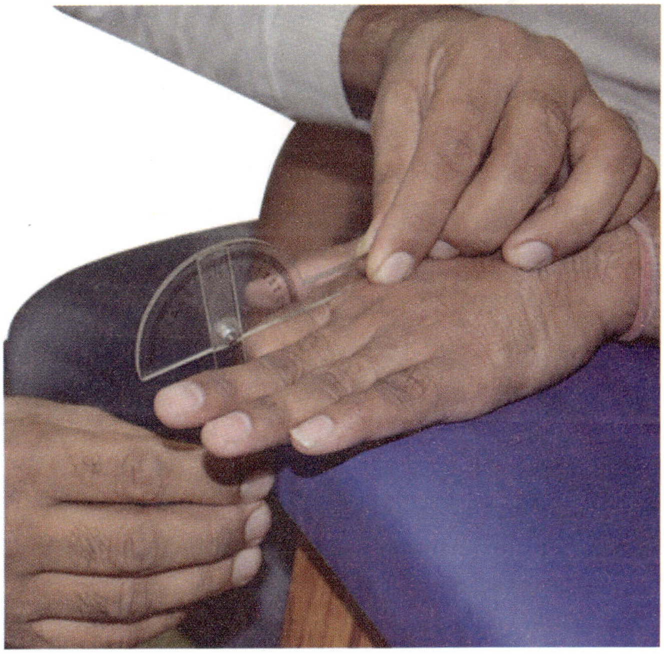

Fig. 6.382b: Measurement of second PIP flexion (Starting position)

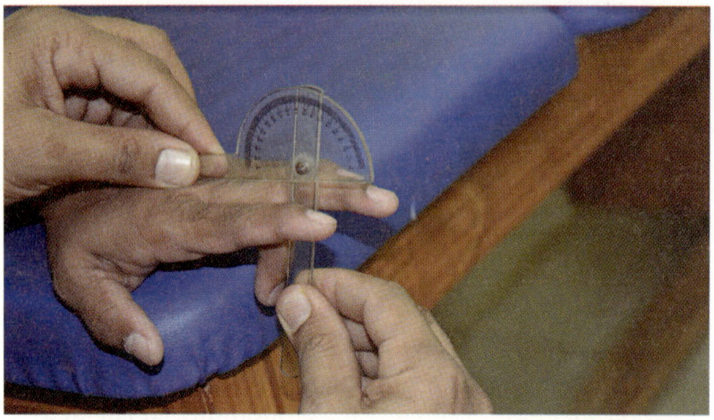

Fig. 6.382c: Measurement of third PIP joint flexion ROM

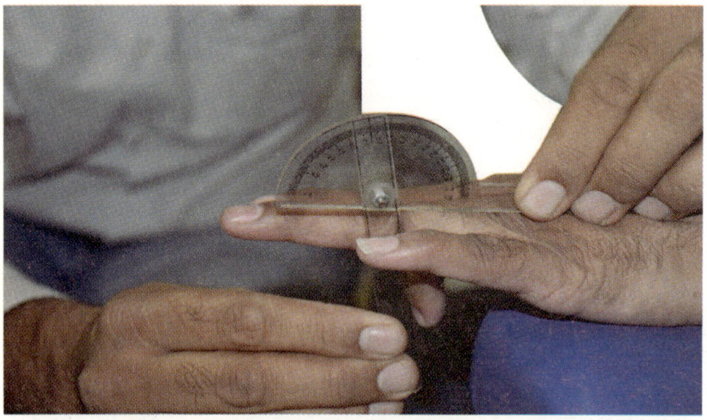

Fig. 6.382d: Measurement of fourth PIP joint flexion ROM

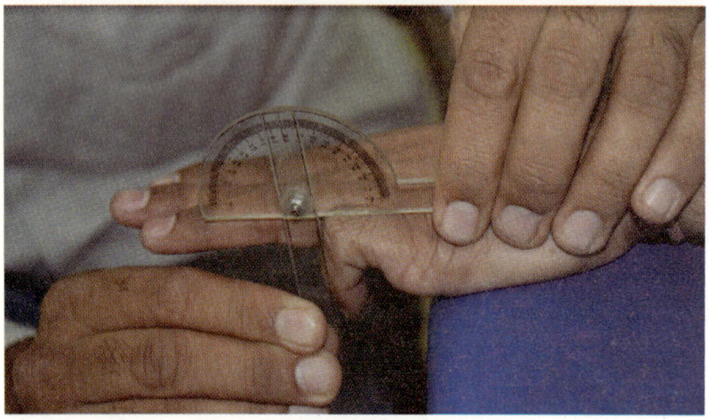

Fig. 6.382e: Measurement of fifth PIP flexion ROM

Position of Patient: High sitting with forearm pronated wrist, MCP, PIP and DIP at neutral position.

Position of Examiner: Examiner sits comfortably in the chair in front of the patient.

Position of Goniometer: Fulcrum of goniometer is positioned over the dorsal aspect of PIP joint which is being tested. Proximal or stationary arm is placed over the dorsal midline of proximal phalanx and distal or moving arm is aligned over the dorsal midline of middle phalanx.

Stabilization: Wrist and MCP joints are stabilized to maintain them at the neutral position.

Procedure: Examiner maintains the proximal stationary arm over the midline of proximal phalanx and instructs the patient to bend the digit down towards the floor as much as possible. The distal arm of the goniometer is moved with the middle phalanx. Flexion of all the PIP joint can be measured with this method.

PROXIMAL INTERPHALANGEAL EXTENSION

Extension is the reverse of flexion.

DISTAL INTERPHALANGEAL FLEXION

Normal ROM: 0° to 80°.

Plane and Axis: Sagittal around medial lateral axis.

Normal End Feel: The normal end feel of DIP flexion is firm because of tension in the dorsal joint capsule, collateral ligaments and oblique retanacular ligament.

Position of Patient: High sitting, forearm fully pronated, wrist, MCP, DIP and PIP at neutral position. The forearm, wrist and hand should be supported on the supporting surface with the DIP out on the edge (Figs. 6.383a to d).

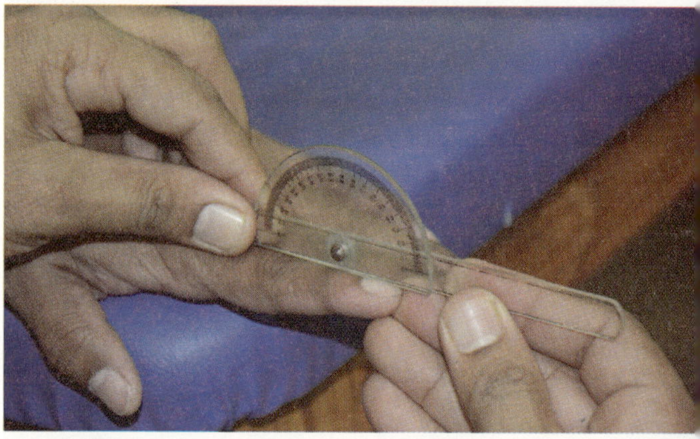

Fig 6.383a: Measurement of second DIP flexion ROM (Starting position)

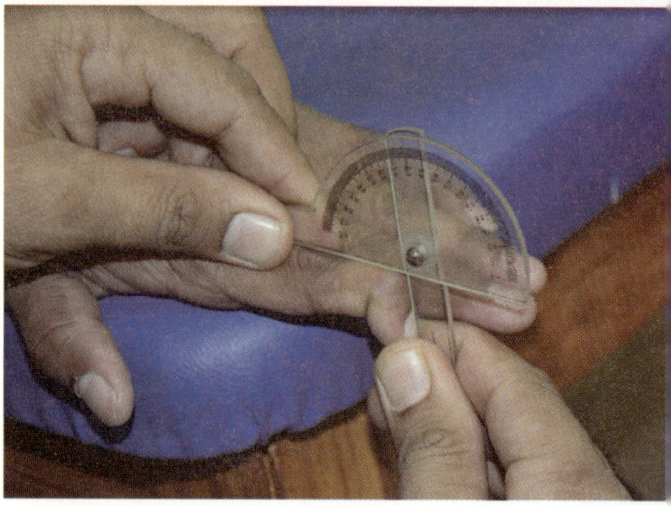

Fig. 6.383b: Measurement of second DIP flexion ROM

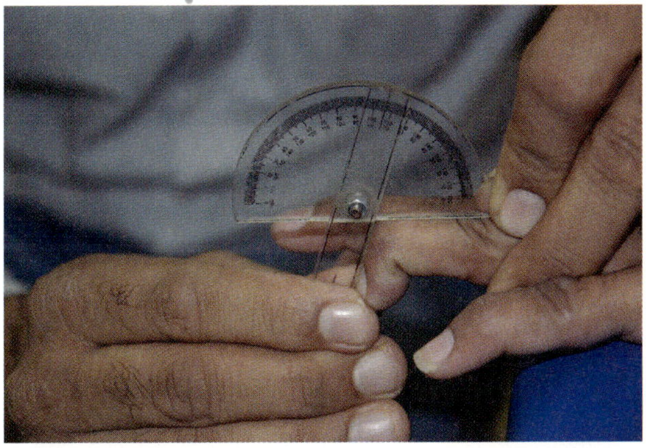

Fig. 6.383c: Measurement of fourth DIP flexion ROM

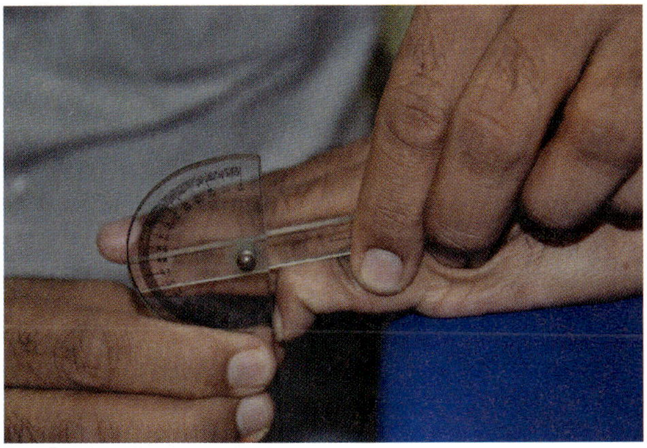

Fig. 6.383d: Measurement of fifth DIP flexion ROM

Position of Examiner: Examiner sits comfortably in the chair at the side which is being tested.

Position of Goniometer: Fulcrum of goniometer is placed on the dorsal surface of DIP joint which is being tested.

The proximal arm of goniometer is aligned over the dorsal midline of middle phalanx and distal or moving arm is aligned over the dorsal midline of distal phalanx.

Stabilization: Wrist, MCP and PIP joints are stabilized to maintain them in the neutral position.

Procedure: Examiner stabilizes the proximal arm over the dorsal midline of middle phalanx and instructs the patient to take the finger down towards the floor as much as possible. The distal arm of goniometer is moved with the distal phalanx. Flexion of all DIP joint can be measured by this method.

FIRST CARPOMETACARPAL FLEXION (THUMB)

Normal ROM: 0° to 15°.

Plane and Axis: Frontal around anterior posterior axis.

Normal End Feel: Normal end feel is usually soft because of contact between the thenar eminence and palm of hand. End feel may be firm due to tension in the dorsal joint capsule and extensor pollicis brevis and abductor pollicis brevis muscles.

Position of Patient: High sitting with back supported, forearm in full supination with wrist and CMC joints at neutral position (Figs. 6.384a and b).

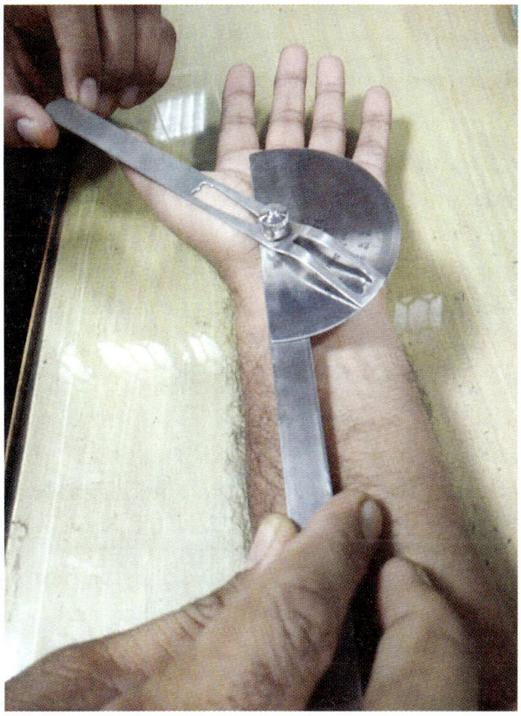

Fig. 6.384a: Measurement of first CMC flexion (Starting)

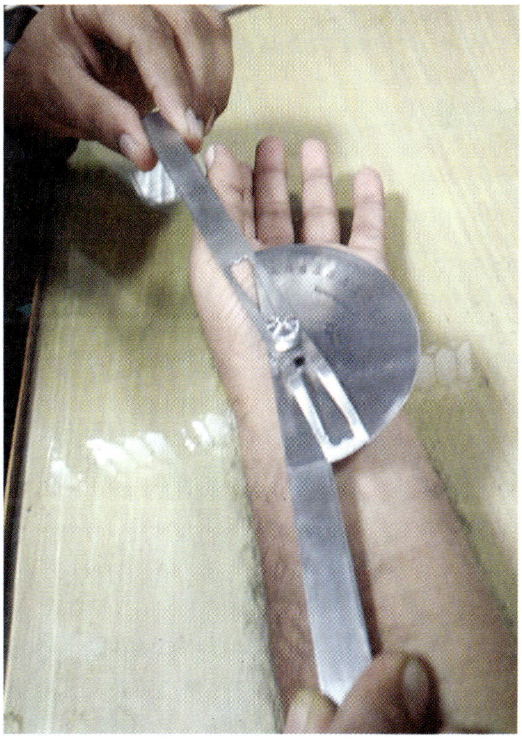

Fig. 6.384b: Measurement of first CMC flexion

Position of Examiner: Sits comfortably in front of the patient.

Position of Goniometer: Fulcrum of the goniometer is placed on the palmar aspect of first CMC joint. Stationary arm is aligned with the palmar midline of the radius. Head of radius in taken a reference for the proximal arm. The distal arm is aligned with the palmar surface of the first metacarpal bone.

Stabilization: Forearm and wrist joint is stabilized to maintain at the neutral position.

Procedure: Examiner maintains the stationary arm over the palmar midline of radius and instructs the patient to draw the thumb (first metacarpal) bone towards little finger across the palm. The distal arm of goniometer is moved along the palmar midline of first metacarpal bone.

FIRST METACARPAL EXTENSION (THUMB)

Normal ROM: 0° to 20°.

Plane and Axis: Frontal around anterior posterior axis.

Normal End Feel: The normal end feel is firm due to tension in the anterior joint capsule and the flexor pollicis brevis, adductor pollicis, opponens pollicis and first dorsal interossei (Figs. 6.385a and b).

Position of Patient: High sitting with back supported. Forearm fully supinated with wrist, MCP joint at neutral position. Thumb should be adducted.

Position of Examiner: Sits comfortably in front of the patient.

Position of Goniometer: Same as for flexion (first CMC).

Stabilization: Forearm and wrist is stabilized to prevent supination, pronation, flexion and extension.

Procedure: Examiner maintains the position of proximal arm along the palmar surface of radius and instructs the patient to extend the thumb (take thumb outwards). Distal arm of the goniometer is moved along the thumb.

FIRST CARPOMETACAPAL ABDUCTION (THUMB)

Normal ROM: 0° to 70°.

Plane and Axis: Sagittal around medial lateral axis.

Normal End Feel: Normal end feel is usually firm because of tension in the fascia and skin of the web between the thumb and index finger. Adductor pollicis and first dorsal

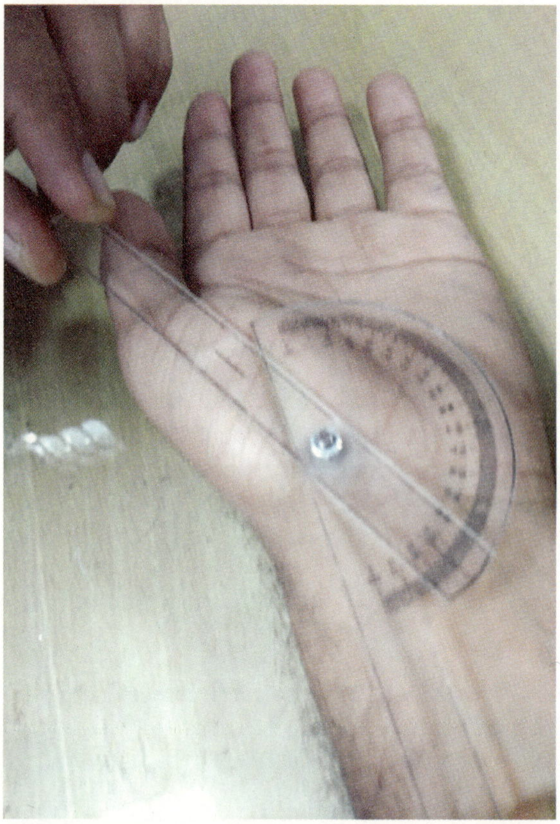

Fig. 6.385a: Measurement of first CMC extension

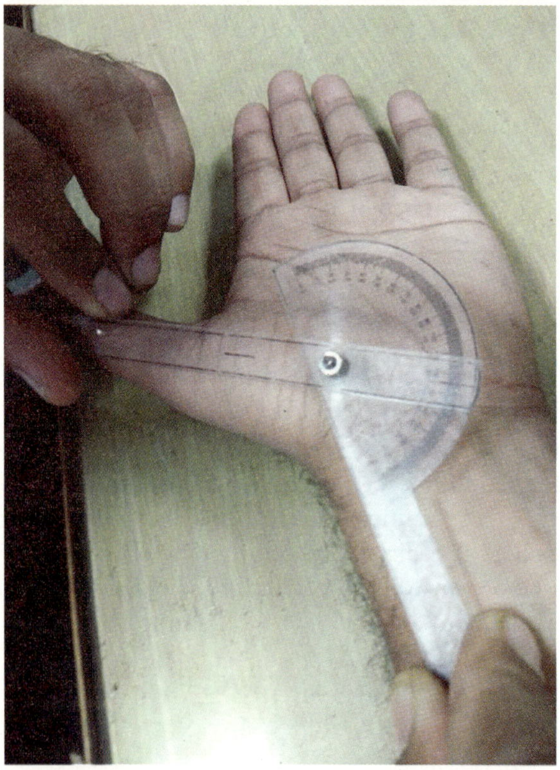

Fig. 6.385b: Measurement of first CMC extension

interossei also limit the end range of abduction (Figs. 6.386a and b).

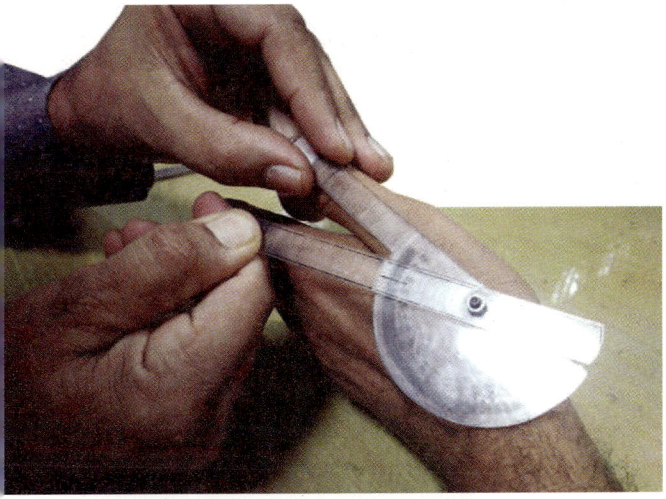

Fig. 6.386a: Measurement of first CMC abduction (Starting)

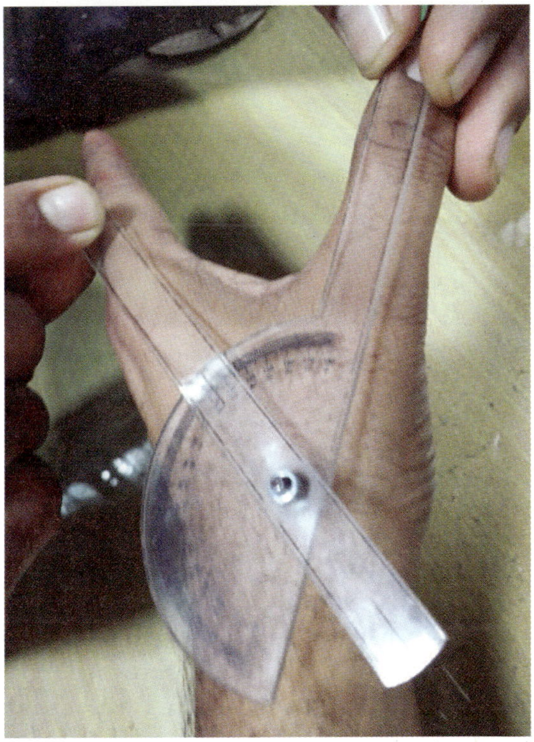

Fig. 6.386b: Measurement of first CMC abduction

Position of Patient: High sitting with back supported. Forearm in midprone, wrist and MCP joint should be at neutral position. The first MCP should be adducted.

Position of Examiner: Examiner sits comfortably in front of the patients.

Position of Goniometer: Fulcrum of goniometer is placed over the lateral aspect of radial styloid process. Proximal arm is aligned with the lateral midline of the second metacarpal bone. Distal arm of goniometer is aligned over the dorsal midline of first metacarpal bone.

Stabilization: Forearm and wrist joint is stabilized to prevent supination, pronation, flexion and extension.

Process: Examiner maintains the proximal and distal arm of the goniometer on the respective surfaces and measures the angle at the starting position. Then after, patient is instructed to take the thumb perpendicular to the palm. The distal arm is moved with the first metacarpal bone. The reading is taken, which is subtracted from starting position reading.

FIRST METACARPOPHALANGEAL FLEXION (THUMB)

Normal ROM: 0° to 60°.

Plane and Axis: Frontal around anterior posterior axis.

Normal End Feel: The end feel is usually hard due to contact between proximal phalanx and first metacarpal bone. End feel may also be firm due to tension in the dorsal joint capsule, the collateral ligaments and the extensor pollicis brevis muscle (Figs. 6.387a and b).

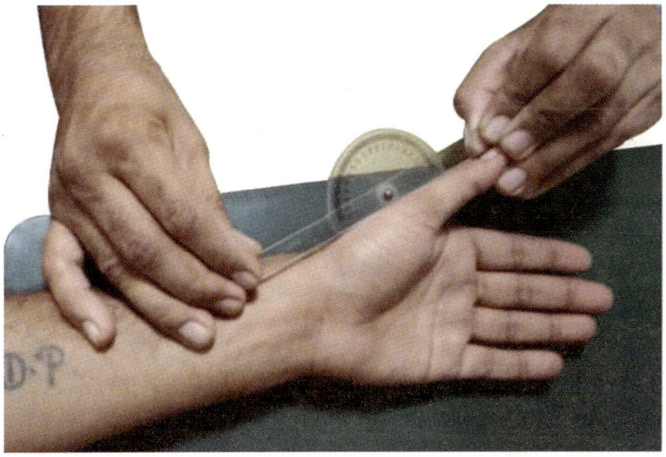

Fig. 6.387a: Measurement of metacarpophalangeal flexion (Starting)

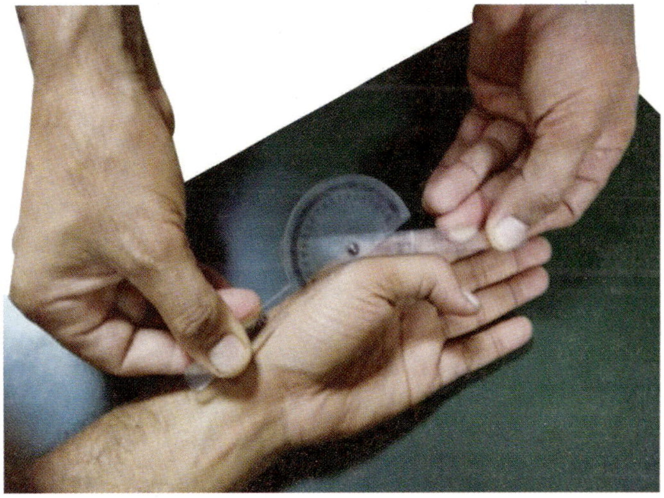

Fig. 6.387b: Measurement of metacarpophalangeal flexion

Position of Patient: High sitting, foreman in midprone, wrist and MCP joints should be at neutral. Forearm and hand should rest on the table on supporting surface.

Position of Examiner: Sitting comfortably in a chair in front of the patient.

Position of Goniometer: Fulcrum of goniometer is placed over the dorsal aspect of first MCP joint. Proximal or stationary arm is placed over the dorsal midline of first metacarpal bone. Distal or moving arm is placed over the dorsal midline of the proximal phalanx.

Stabilization: Forearm, wrist and MCP joints are stabilized to maintain them at neutral position.

Process: Examiner maintains the position of proximal arm over the dorsal midline of first metacarpal and instructs the patient to bring the thumb towards little finger (flexion). The distal arm is moved with the proximal phalanx.

FIRST INTERPHALANGEAL FLEXION (THUMB)

Normal ROM: 0° to 70°.

Plane and Axis: Frontal around anterior posterior axis.

Normal End Feel: The normal end feel is usually firm because of tension in the collateral ligament and dorsal joint capsule. End feel may be hard if there is contact between proximal and distal phalanx.

Position of Patient: Sitting with forearm in midprone position and wrist, MCP at neutral position. The forearm and hand should be supported on supporting surface.

Position of Examiner: Examiner sits comfortably in a chair in front of the patient.

Position of Goniometer: Fulcrum of goniometer is placed on dorsal surface of first interphalangeal joint and proximal arm is aligned over the dorsal midline of proximal phalanx. Distal arm is aligned over the dorsal midline of distal phalanx.

Stabilization: Examiner stabilizes the forearm, wrist and MCP joint to maintain them at neutral position.

Process: Examiner maintains the proximal arm over the dorsal midline of proximal phalanx and notes the reading (angle) of goniometer. The subject or patient is instructed to bend the thumb at the distal as much as possible. Distal arm of goniometer is moved with the distal phalanx. The reading is noted and subtracted from starting position (Figs. 6.388a and b).

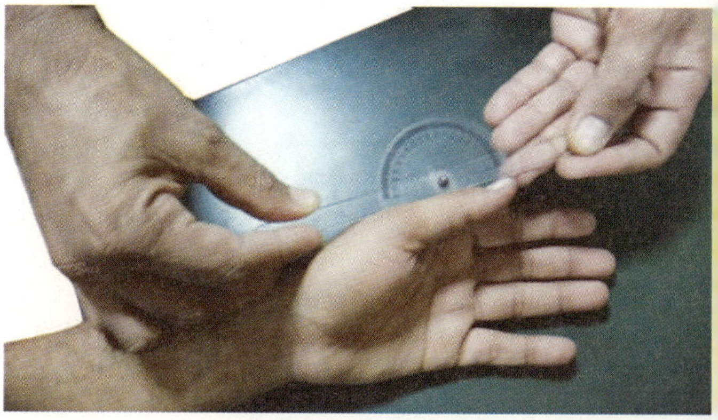

Fig. 6.388a: Measurement of internphalangeal flexion (Starting)

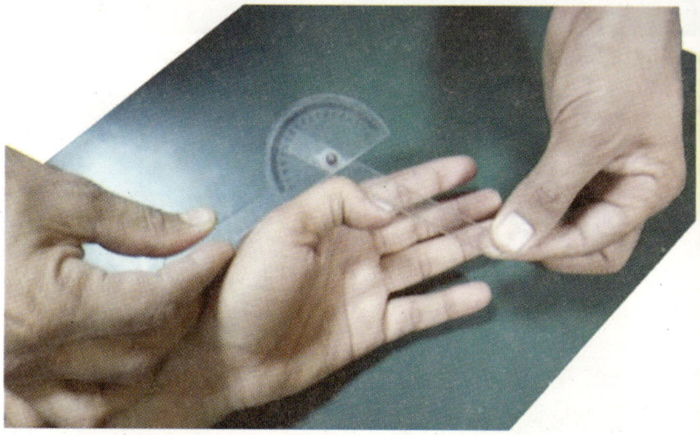

Fig. 6.388b: Measurement of interphalangeal flexion

HIP FLEXION

Normal ROM: 0° to 120° with knee flexion and 0° to 80°-90° with knee joint extended.

Plane and Axis: Sagittal around medial lateral axis.

Normal End Feel: Normal end feel is usually soft because of contact between the soft tissues of anterior thigh and lower abdomen. End feel may also be firm due to posterior joint capsule and gluteus muscles. End feel may be firm due to tension in the hamstrings if the hip joint is flexed with the knee extension.

Position of Patient: Supine with hip joint and knee joint at neutral position (Figs. 6.389a, b and c).

Position of Examiner: Examiner stands at side of patient which is being tested.

Position of Goniometer: Fulcrum of goniometer is placed over the greater trochanter of hip joint. Proximal arm or stationary arm is aligned over the lateral midline of pelvis and moving arm over the lateral midline of femur. Lateral epicondyle of femur may be taken a reference point for distal arm.

Stabilization: Pelvis and trunk is stabilized to prevent posterior tilting and rotation respectively.

(a)

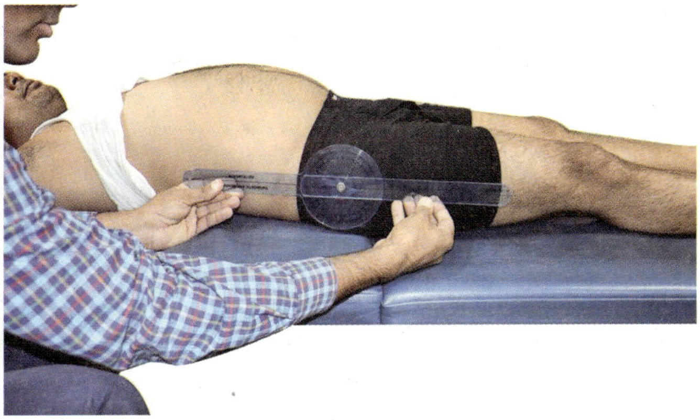

(b)

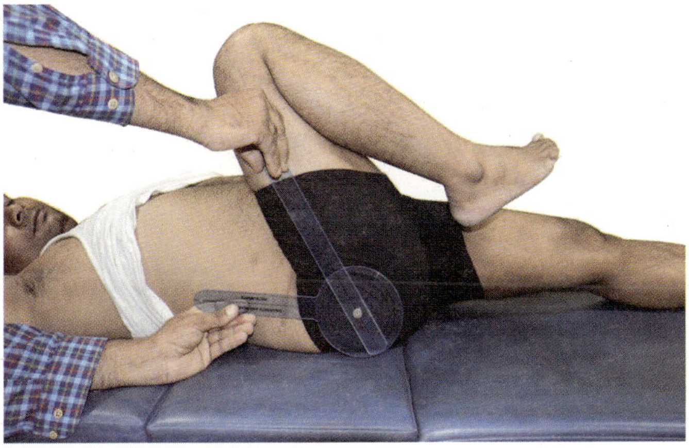

(c)

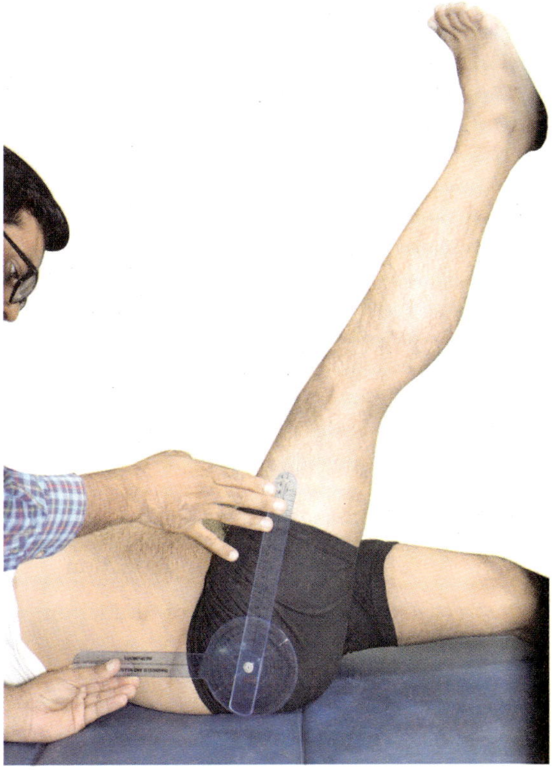

Figs. 6.389a, b and c: Measurement of hip flexion ROM

Process: Examiner maintains the position of proximal arm over the lateral midline of pelvis and thorax and instructs the patient to bring the knee joint towards chest. The distal arm is moved with the thigh.

HIP EXTENSION

Normal ROM: 0° to 30°.

Plane and Axis: Sagittal around medial lateral axis.

Normal End Feel: The normal end feel is usually firm due to tension in anterior joint capsule, ileo-femoral, ischiofemoral and pubofemoral ligaments. Ileopsoas, sartorius, gracilis and TFL also limit the end range of extension.

Position of Patient: Prone with hip and knee joints at neutral position (Figs. 6.390a and b).

(a)

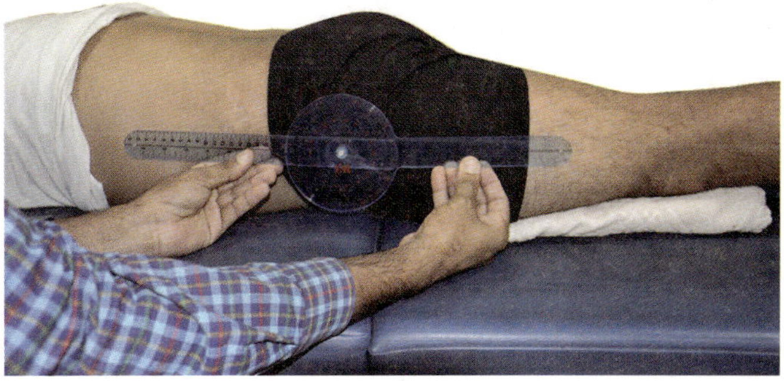

(b)

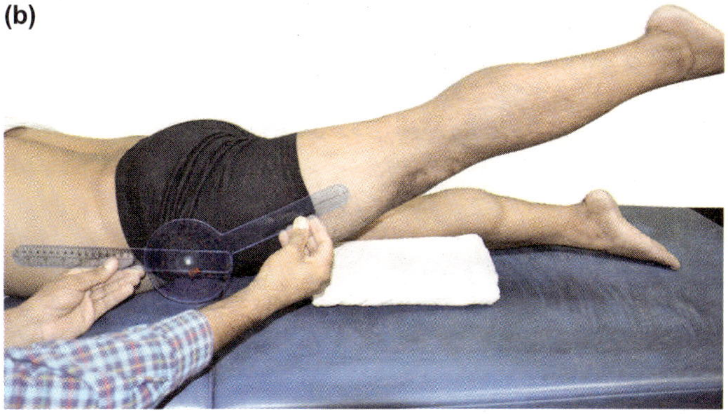

Figs. 6.390a and b: Measurement of hip extension ROM

Position of Patient: Stands at the side which is being tested.

Position of Goniometer: Same as for hip flexion.

Stabilization: Pelvis and trunk is stabilized to prevent pelvic tilting and trunk rotation.

Process: Examiner maintains the stationary arm over the lateral midline of pelvis and trunk, and instructs the patient to extend the hip joint. Distal arm of goniometer is moved with the lateral midline of thigh.

HIP ABDUCTION

Normal ROM: 0° to 45°.

Plane and Axis: Movement occurs in frontal plane around anterior posterior axis.

Normal End Feel: The normal end feel is firm because of tension in the anterior joint capsule, pubofemoral ligament ischiofemoral ligament. The range of abduction is also limited by adductor muscles (magnus, longus and brevis), pectineus and gracilis.

Position of Patient: Supine with hip and knee joints are at the neutral position (Figs. 6.391a and b).

(a)

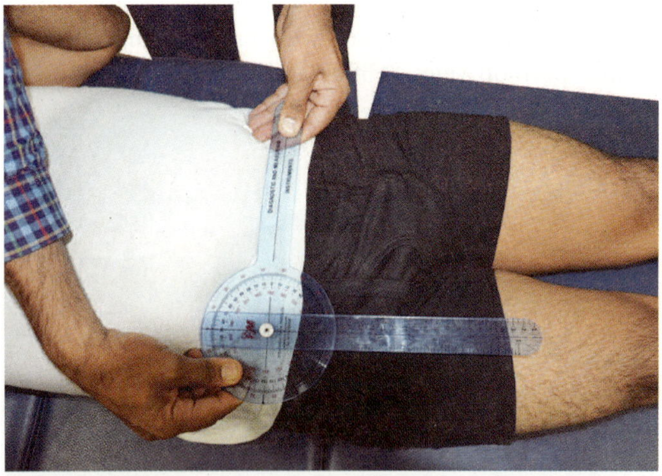

(b)

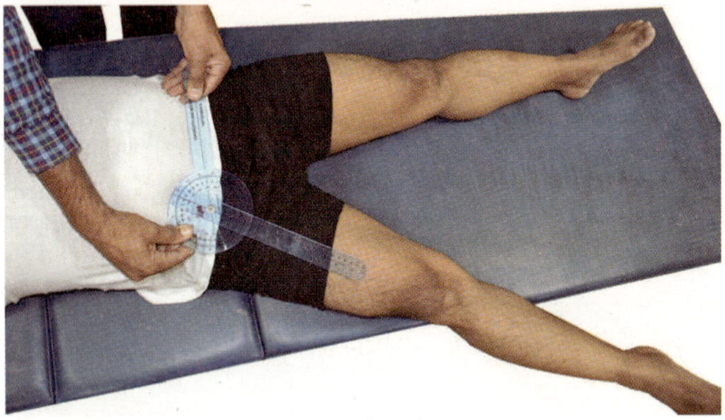

Figs. 6.391a and b: Measurement of hip abduction ROM

Position of Examiner: Examiner stands at the side which is being tested.

Position of Goniometer: Fulcrum of goniometer is placed over the anterior superior iliac spine (ASIS) of the pelvis which is being tested. Proximal arm of goniometer is placed across the pelvis from one ASIS to other ASIS. Distal arm is aligned over the anterior midline of thigh. Midline of patella is taken a reference for the distal arm.

Process: Examiner maintains the position of stationary arm over the pelvis (one ASIS to other) and instructs the patient to move the leg away from the midline (abduction). The distal arm is moved with the anterior midline of thigh.

HIP ADDUCTION

Normal ROM: 0° to 30°.

Plane and Axis: Movement occurs in frontal plane around anterior posterior axis.

Normal End Feel: Normal end feel is firm because of tension in the superior joint capsule and superior band of the iliofermoral ligament. Gluteus medius and gluteus minimus and TFL also limit the adduction at the end range.

Position of Patient: Supine with contralateral hip joint at the abducted position (Figs. 6.392a and b).

(a)

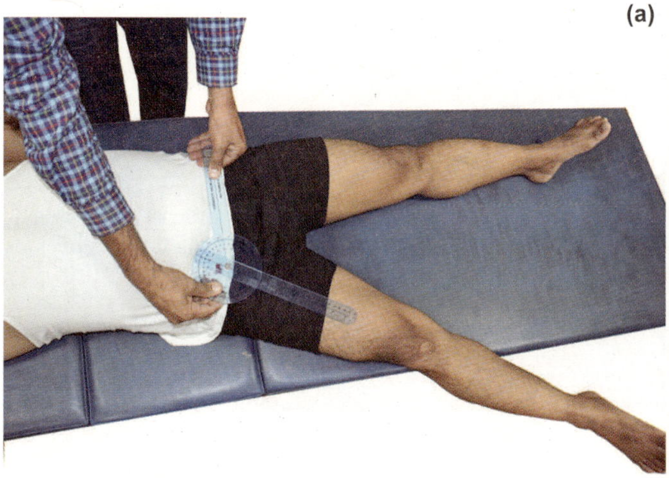

(b)

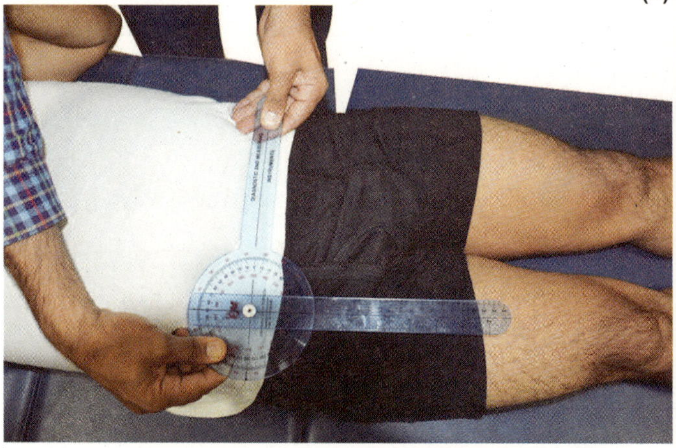

Figs. 6.392a and b: Measurement of hip adduction ROM

Position of Examiner: Same as for abduction.

Position of Goniometer: Same as for abduction.

Stabilization: Same as for abduction.

Process: Examiner maintains the position of proximal arm of goniometer and instructs the patient to move the leg across the midline towards contralateral leg. Distal arm of goniometer is moved with the anterior midline of thigh.

HIP INTERNAL ROTATION

Normal ROM: 0° to 45°.

Plane and Axis: Movement occurs in transverse plane around a vertical axis.

Normal End Feel: Normal end feel is firm due to tension in the anterior joint capsule, iliofermoral ligament, and pubofemoral ligament. End range of external rotation is also limited by the muscles like gluteus medius, gluteus minimus, adductor magnus, adductor longus, pectineus and piriformis.

Position of Patient: High sitting with back supported well, a towel roll is placed under the distal thigh to bring the hip joint into 90° flexion. The contralateral knee is flexed to 100° to allow the testing leg to cross.

Position of Examiner: Examiner stands at the side which is being tested (Figs. 6.393a and b).

Position of Goniometer: Fulcrum of goniometer is placed over the anterior aspect of patella (mid point patella). The proximal arm is aligned perpendicular to the floor and distal (moving) arm is aligned over the anterior midline of leg. A point is marked between the malloli for reference of distal arm of goniometer.

Stabilization: Trunk is stabilized to prevent bending and hip joint is stabilized to prevent abduction.

Process: Examiner maintains the proximal arm perpendicular to the floor and instructs the patient to move the leg across the midline towards contralateral leg. The contralateral knee is flexed to 100° to allow the testing leg to cross. Distal arm of the goniometer is moved with the leg.

HIP EXTERNAL ROTATION

Normal ROM: 0° to 45°.

Plane and Axis: Movement occurs in the transverse plane around vertical axis.

Normal End Feel: Normal end feel of medial rotation is firm due to tension in the posterior joint capsule and ischiofemoral ligament. The muscles such as piriformis,

(a) (b)

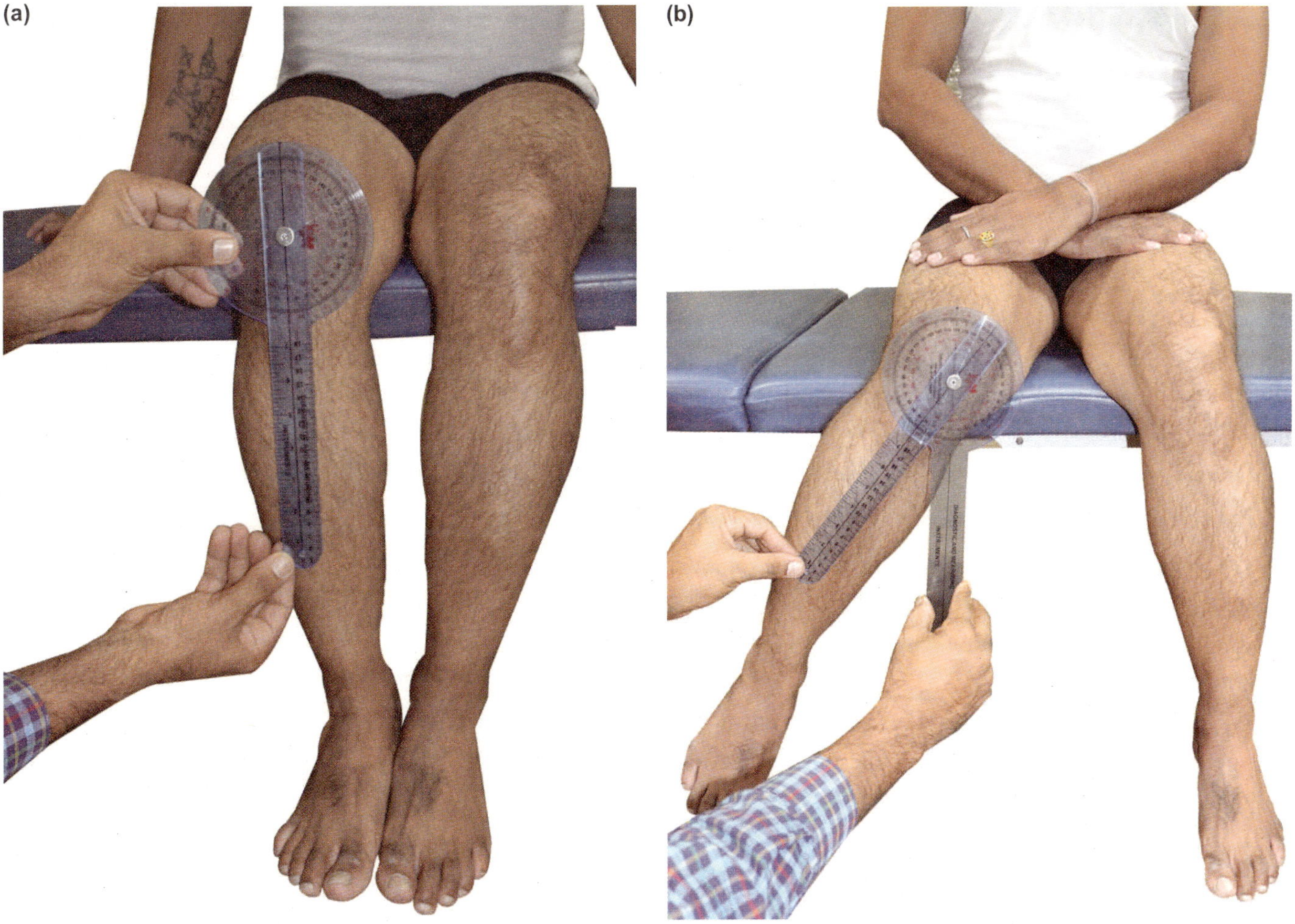

Figs. 6.393a and b: Measurement of hip internal rotation ROM

(a)

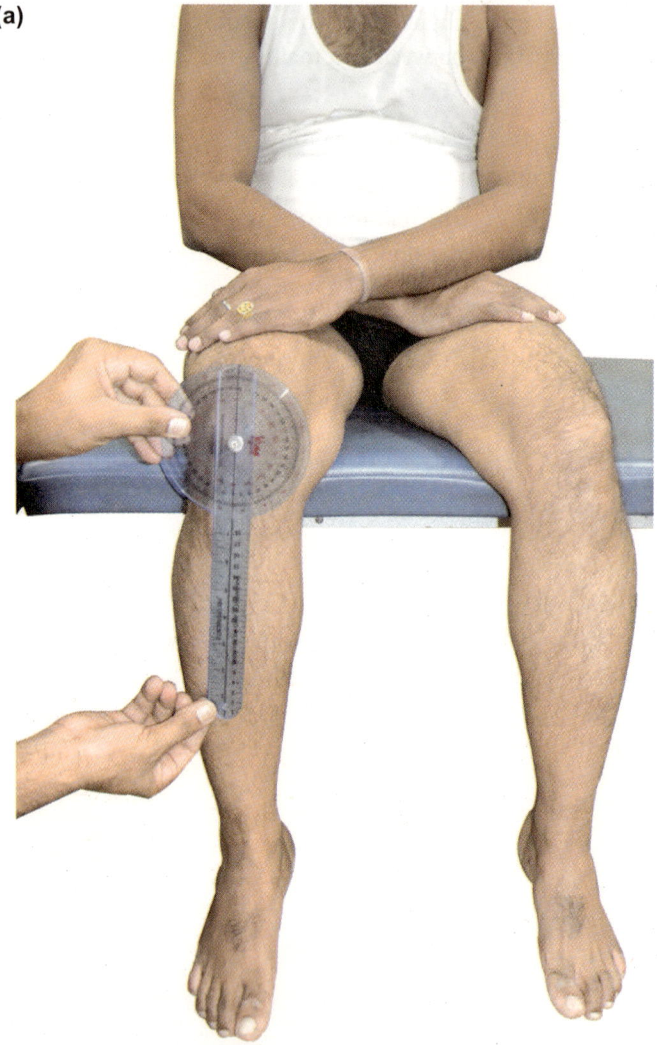

(b)

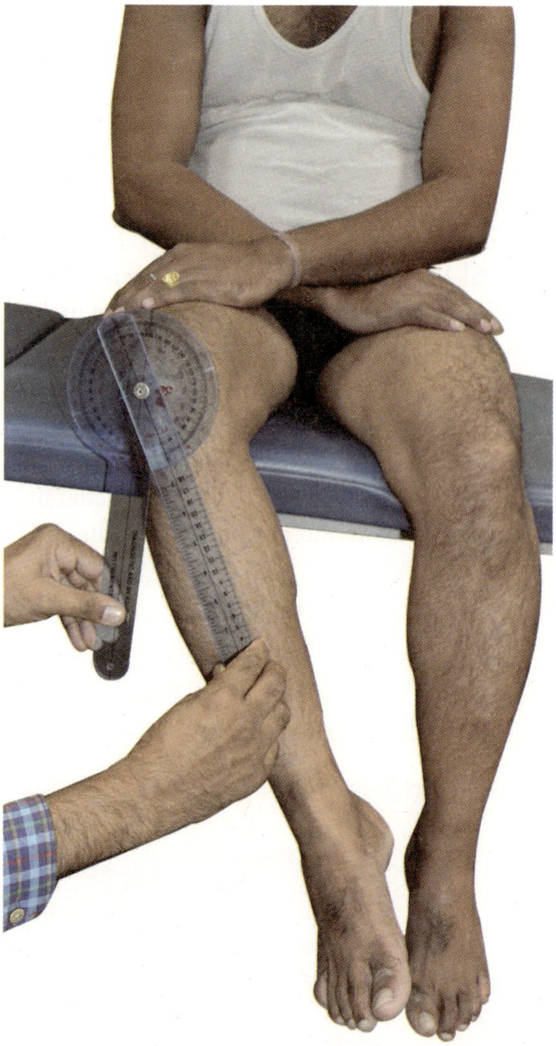

Figs. 6.394a and b: Measurement of hip external rotation ROM

obturato, gemelli, quadratus femoris, gluteus medius and gluteus maximus also limit the end range of medial rotation that results in firm end feel (Figs. 6.394a and b).

Position of Patient: Same as for hip external rotation.

Position of Examiner: Same as for hip external rotation.

Position of Goniometer: Same as for hip external rotation.

Stabilization: Trunk is stabilized to prevent lateral bending and hip is stabilized to prevent adduction and flexion.

Process: Examiner maintains the position of stationary arm perpendicular to the floor and fulcrum on the mid point of patella and instructs the patient to take the leg away from the midline.

KNEE FLEXION

Normal ROM: 0° to 140°.

Plane and Axis: Movement occurs in sagittal plane around medial lateral axis.

Normal End Feel: Normal end feel of knee flexion is usually soft due to approximation of soft tissues of posterior thigh and posterior leg. However, it may be firm if tension in the rectus femoris, vastus medialis, lateralis and intermedialis muscles limit the end range.

Position of Patient: Prone with hip and knee joints at neutral position (Figs. 6.395a and b).

Position of Examiner: Examiner stands at the side which is being tested.

Position of Goniometer: Fulcrum of goniometer is placed over the lateral epicondyle of femur. Proximal arm is placed over the lateral midline of thigh. Greater trochanter is taken a reference point for proximal arm of goniometer. Distal arm of goniometer is placed over the lateral midline of leg. Lateral malleolus is taken as a reference point for distal arm.

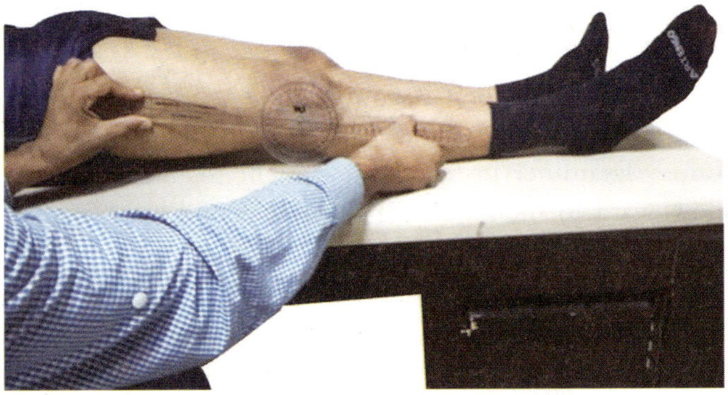

Fig. 6.395a: Knee joint flexion ROM in supine lying (Starting)

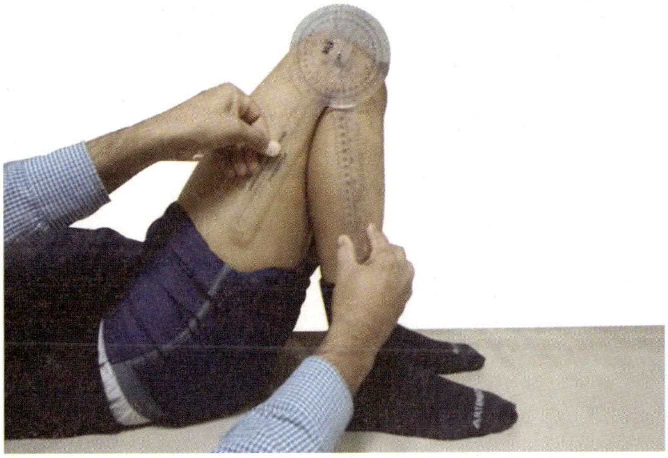

Fig. 6.395b: Knee joint flexion ROM in supine lying

Stabilization: Trunk is stabilized to prevent extension and lateral bending. Hip joint is also stabilized to prevent flexion and rotations.

Process: Examiner maintains the proximal arm over the lateral midline of thigh and instructs the patient to flex the knee joint. Distal arm may be moved either with the leg or after completing the flexion.

KNEE EXTENSION

Normal ROM: 140° to 0° or reverse of flexion.

Plane and Axis: Movement occurs in sagittal plane around medial lateral axis.

Normal End Feel: The normal end feel of knee extension is firm due to stretching of the posterior joint capsule, the oblique and arcuate poplited ligaments, the collateral ligaments, and the anterior and posterior cruciate ligaments.

Position of Patient: Supine with knee full flexion and hip at neutral position (Figs. 6.396a and b).

Position of Examiner: Same as for flexion.

Position of Goniometer: Same as for flexion.

Stabilization: Trunk to prevent flexion and lateral bending and hip to prevent flexion.

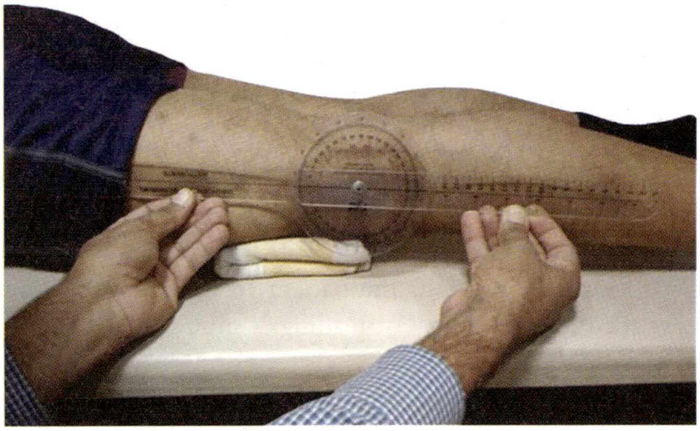

Fig. 6.396a: Knee joint flexion ROM in prone lying (Starting)

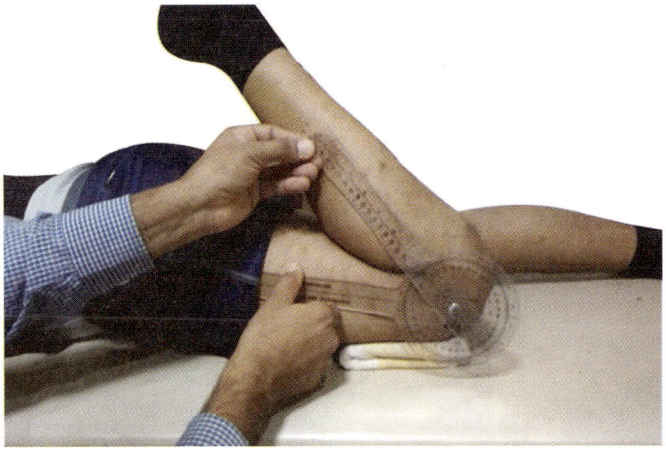

Fig. 6.396b: Knee joint flexion ROM in prone lying

Process: Examiner maintains the proximal arm over the lateral midline of thigh and instructs the patient to extend the knee joint. The distal arm is moved with the leg. If extension is full the goniometer should show the 0° angle. If an extension is limited, goniometer will show less than 0° angle. It is known as extension leg. It is very common in patients with pain in knee joint following injury or trauma. The patients usually walk with slight knee flexion.

ANKLE (TALOCRURAL) JOINT DORSIFLEXION

Normal ROM: 0° to 20°.

Plane and Axis: Movement occurs in sagittal plane around medial lateral axis.

Normal End Feel: Normal end feel is firm due to tension in the posterior joint capsule, gastosoleus muscles, posterior deltoid ligament, posterior talofibular ligament, and the calcaneofibular ligament.

Position of Patient: High sitting.

Position of Examiner: Sitting comfortably in the chair at the side of patient.

Position of Goniometer: Fulcrum of the goniometer is positioned over the lateral malleolus, and proximal arm is aligned over the lateral midline of leg. Head of fibula is taken a reference for proximal arm. The distal arm is aligned over the lateral midline of fifth metacarpal bone.

Process: Examiner maintains the proximal arm over the lateral midline of leg and distal arm over the lateral midline of fifth metacarpal bone. The ankle should be brought into the position so that the reading of the goniometer comes 90°. Examiner instructs the patient to move the foot up towards the body. The last reading is subtracted from 90° (Fig. 6.397).

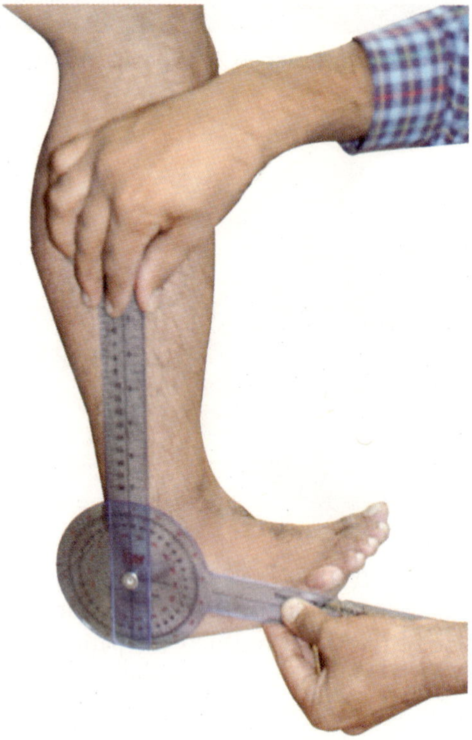

Fig. 6.397: Measurement of dorsiflexion in high sitting

ANKLE (TALOCRURAL) JOINT PLANTAR FLEXION

Normal ROM: 0° to 50°.

Plane and Axis: Movement occurs in the sagittal plane around medial lateral axis.

Normal End Feel: The end feel is usually a firm due to tension in the anterior joint capsule, anterior portion of deltoid ligament, anterior talofibular ligament. The muscles which limit the plantar flexion at the end range are tibialis anterior, extensor hallucis longus and extensor digitorum longus. The end feel may also be hard if there is a contact between talus and tibia.

Position of Patient: Same as for dorsiflexion.

Position of Examiner: Same as for dorsiflexion.

Position of Goniometer: Same as for dorsiflexion.

Stabilization: Knee joint is stabilized to prevent flexion and extension.

Process: Ankle joint is positioned at the neutral so that both the arms of goniometer remain perpendicular to each other. Examiner instructs the patient to move the foot downward to the ground (Figs. 6.398a and b).

(a)

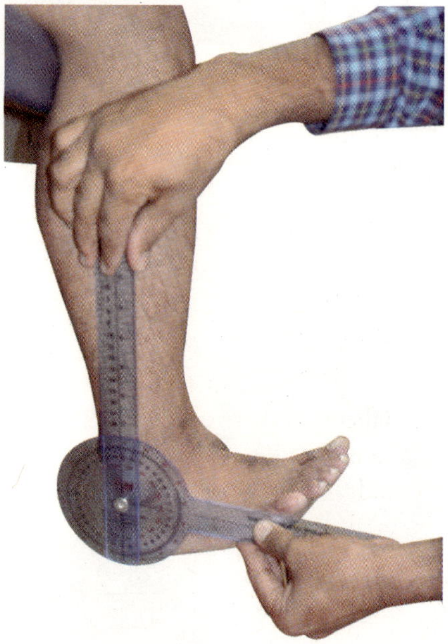

(b)

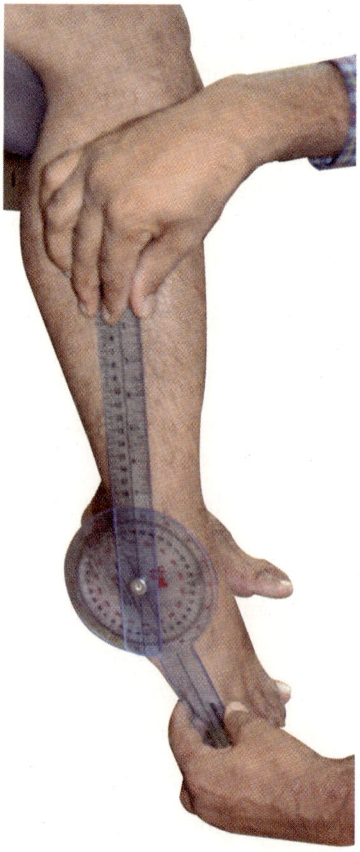

Figs. 6.398a and b: Measurement of plantar flexion ROM

TARSAL JOINTS INVERSION

Normal ROM: 0° to 30°.

Plane and Axis: Movement occurs in frontal plane around anterior posterior axis.

Normal End Feel: End feel is firm due to tension in the joint capsule, anterior and posterior talofibular ligament, calcaneofibular ligament, antero, posterior, lateral and interosseous talocalcaneal ligament, dorsal calcaneal ligament, dorsal calcaneocuboid ligament dorsal talonavicular ligament and transverse metatarsal ligament.

Position of Patient: High sitting with back supported and ankle joint at neutral position.

Position of Examiner: Sitting in a chair comfortably at the side of patient which is being tested.

Position of Goniometer: Fulcrum of goniometer is positioned over the anterior aspect of ankle joint, midway between the malleoli. The proximal arm is placed over the anterior midline of leg. Tibial tuberosity is taken a reference point. The distal arm is aligned over the anterior midline of second metatarsal bone.

Stabilization: Knee joint is stabilized to prevent flexion extension, and tibial rotations. Hip joint may also be kept at neutral position.

Process: Examiner maintains the proximal arm over the anterior tibial shin and instructs the patient to take the foot inwards, towards the midline. Distal arm of goniometer is moved with the second metatarsal bone (Figs. 6.399a and b).

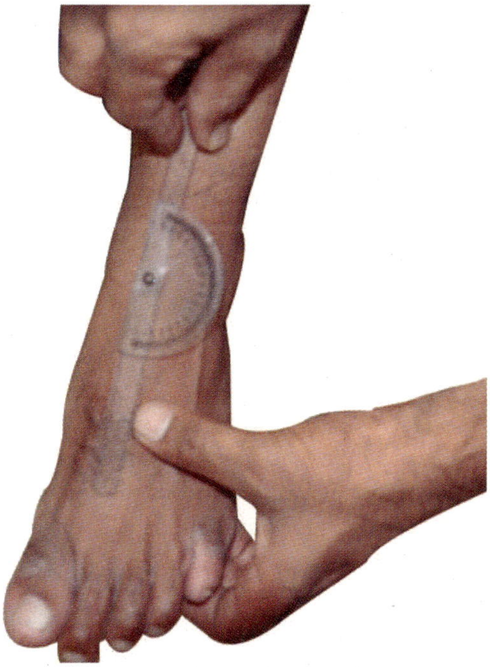

Fig. 6.399a: Measurement of inversion ROM of tarsal joint

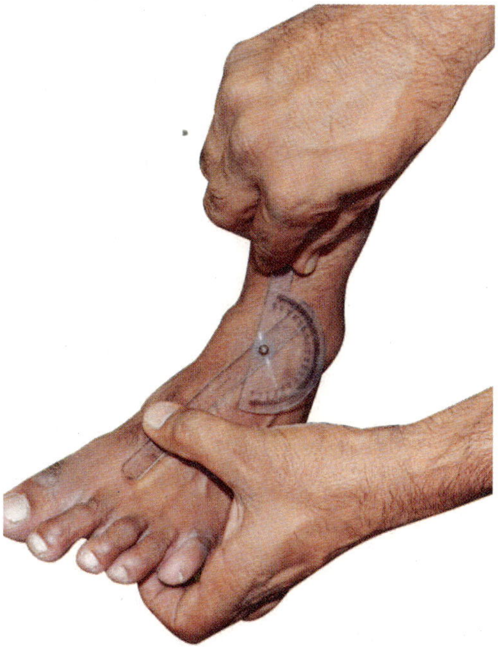

Fig. 6.399b: Measurement of inversion ROM of tarsal joint

TARSAL JOINT EVERSION

Normal ROM: 0° to 80°.

Plane and Axis: Movement occurs in the frontal plane around anterior posterior axis.

Normal End Feel: End feel is usually hard due to contact between calcaneus and the floor of the sinus tarsi. End feel may also be firm due to tension in the joint capsule, deltoid ligament, medial talocalcaneal ligaments, plantar calcaneonavicular and calcaneocuboid ligaments.

Position of Patient: High sitting, ankle at neutral.

Position of Examiner: Sitting in a chair at the side which is being tested.

Position of Goniometer: Same as for tarsal inversion.

Stabilization: Same as for tarsal inversion.

Process: Examiner maintains the position of proximal arm and instructs the patient to take the foot outwards, away from midline. The distal arm is moved with the second metatarsal bone (Figs. 6.400a and b).

SUBTALAR JOINT INVERSION

Normal ROM: 0° to 5°.

Plane and Axis: Movement occurs in the frontal plane around anterior posterior axis.

Normal End Feel: Normal end feel is firm due to tension in the lateral joint capsule, anterior and posterior talofibular ligaments, calcaneofibular ligaments, and the lateral, posterior, anterior and interosseous ligaments.

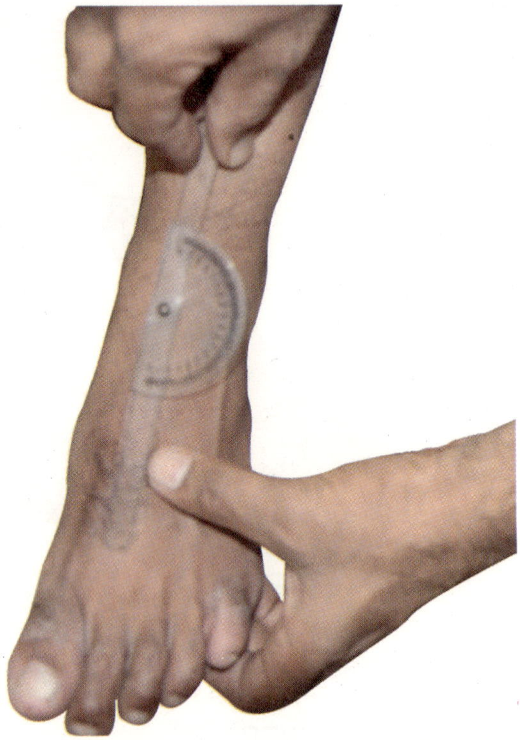

Fig. 6.400a: Measurement of eversion ROM of tarsal joint (Starting)

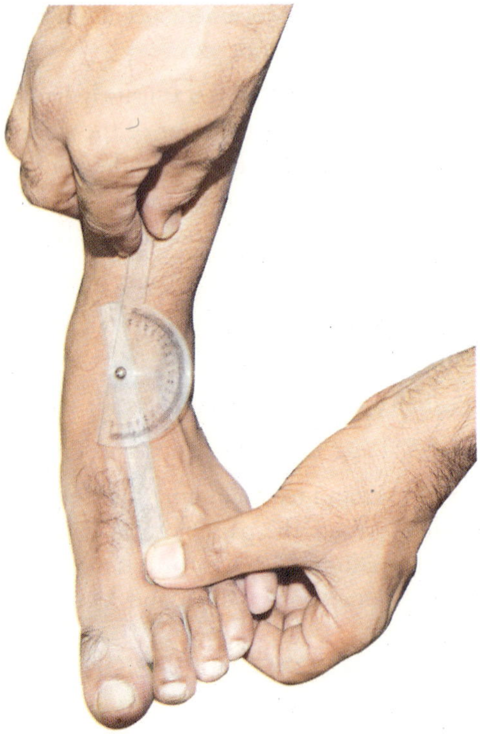

Fig. 6.400b: Measurement of eversion ROM of tarsal joint

Position of Patient: Prone with the ankle joint out of the edge of the table, ankle should be at neutral position.

Position of Examiner: Examiner sits at the side which is being tested.

Position of Goniometer: Fulcrum of goniometer is positioned over the posterior aspect of ankle joint midway between two malleoli. Proximal arm is placed over the posterior midline of leg. Distal arm is aligned over the posterior midline of calcaneum.

Stabilization: Hip and knee joints are stabilized to prevent rotations and flexion respectively.

Process: Examiner maintains the proximal arm over the posterior midline of leg and instructs the patient to bring the heel inwards towards the midline (Figs. 6.401a and b).

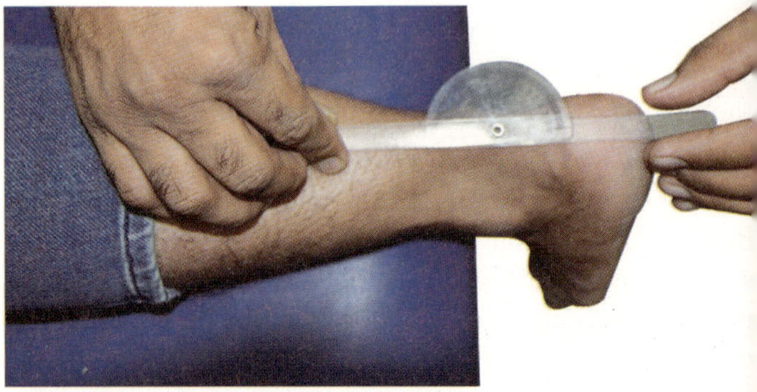

Fig. 6.401a: Measurement of eversion ROM of subtalar joint (Starting)

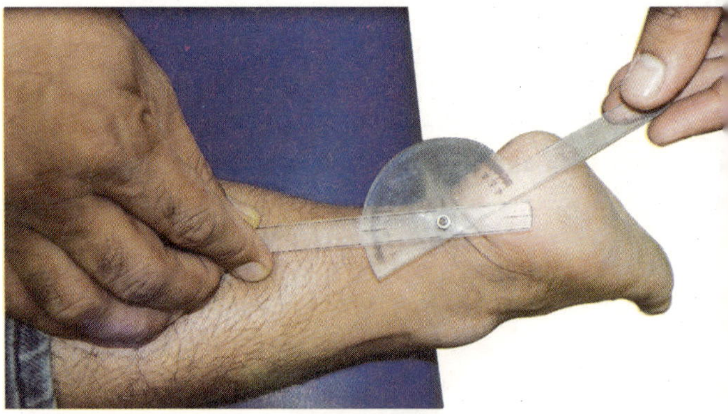

Fig. 6.401b: Measurement of inversion ROM of subtalar joint

SUBTALAR EVERSION

Normal ROM: 0° to 5°.

Plane and Axis: Movement occurs in the frontal plane around anterior posterior axis.

Normal End Feel: End feel is usually hard due to contact between calcaneus and floor of sinus tarsi. End feel may also be firm because of tension in the deltoid ligament, the talocalcaneal ligament, and the tibialis posterior muscles.

Position of Patient: Same as for inversion.

Position of Examiner: Same as for inversion (subtalar).

Position of Goniometer: Same as for inversion (subtalar)

Stabilization: Same as for subtalar inversion.

Process: Examiner maintains the position of proximal arm over the posterior midline of leg and instructs the patient to bring the heel outwards (Figs. 6.402a and b).

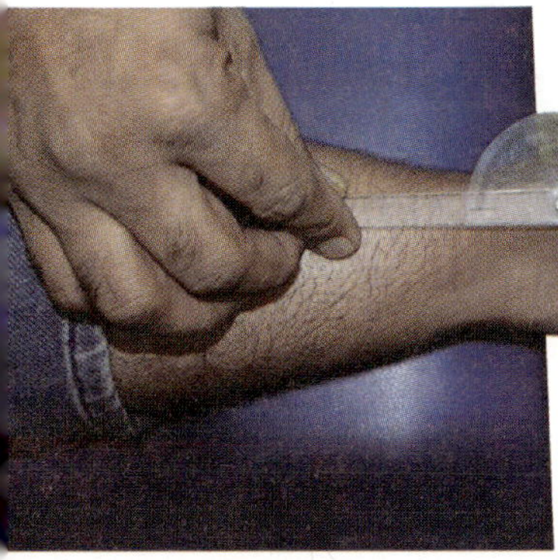

Fig. 6.402a: Measurement of inversion ROM of subtalar joint

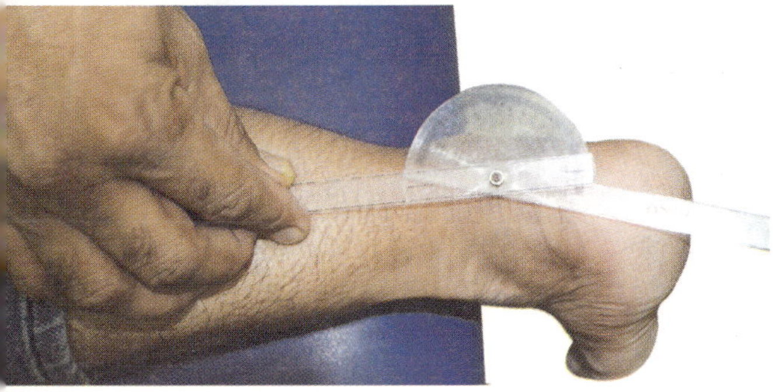

Fig. 6.402b: Measurement of eversion ROM of subtalar joint

TRANSVERSE TARSAL INVERSION

Normal ROM: 0° to 35°.

Plane and Axis: Movement occurs in the frontal plane around anterior posterior axis.

Normal End Feel: End feel is firm due to tension in the joint capsule and ligaments like dorsal calcaneocuboid, dorsal talonavicular, transverse metatarsal and peroneus longus and brevis muscles.

Position of Patient: High sitting with foot hanging freely.

Position of Examiner: Examiner sits comfortably in a chair at the side which is being tested.

Position of Goniometer: Fulcrum of goniometer is positioned over the anterior aspect of the ankle slightly lower to a point midway between the malleoli. The proximal arm is aligned over the anterior midline of leg and distal arm is aligned over the anterior midline of the second metatarsal bone.

Stabilization: Ankle joint is stabilized to prevent dorsiflexion and plantar flexion and subtalar joint is stabilized to prevent inversion.

Process: Examiner maintains the proximal arm over the anterior midline of leg and instructs the patient to move the foot inwards towards the midline (Fig. 6.403).

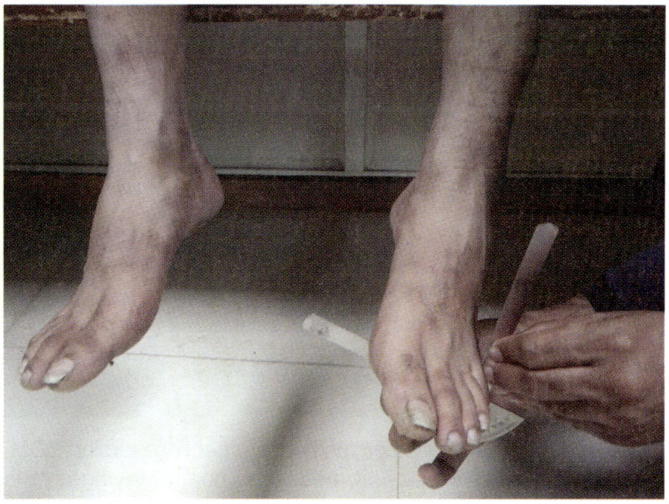

Fig. 6.403: Alternative method for measurement of inversion ROM. Fulcrum is placed at the fifth metatarsal head. Stationary arm remains moving to the plantar surface of metatarsal heads. Stationary arm placed parallel to the tibia

TRANSVERSE TARSAL EVERSION

Normal ROM: 0° to 15°.

Plane and Axis: Movement occurs around frontal plane around anterior posterior axis.

Normal End Feel: The normal end feel is firm due to tension in the joint capsule, and ligaments to line deltoid, plantar calcaneonavicular, the medial band of the bifurcated, transverse metatarsal ligaments and various interosseous ligaments, and tibialis posterior muscles.

Position of Patient: High sitting with the foot hanging.

Position of Examiner: Sitting in a chair comfortably at the side which is being testing.

Position of Goniometer: Fulcrum of goniometer is placed over the anterior aspect of the ankle slightly distal to a point midway between the malleoli. The proximal arm of goniometer is placed on the anterior midline of leg. The tibial tuberosity is taken a reference for proximal arm. The distal arm is aligned over the anterior midline of the second metatarsal bone.

Stabilization: Ankle joint is stabilized to prevent plantar flexion and dorsiflexion and subtalor joint to prevent eversion.

Process: Examiner maintains the position of proximal arm over the anterior midline of leg and instructs the patient to move the foot away from midline outwards (Fig. 6.404).

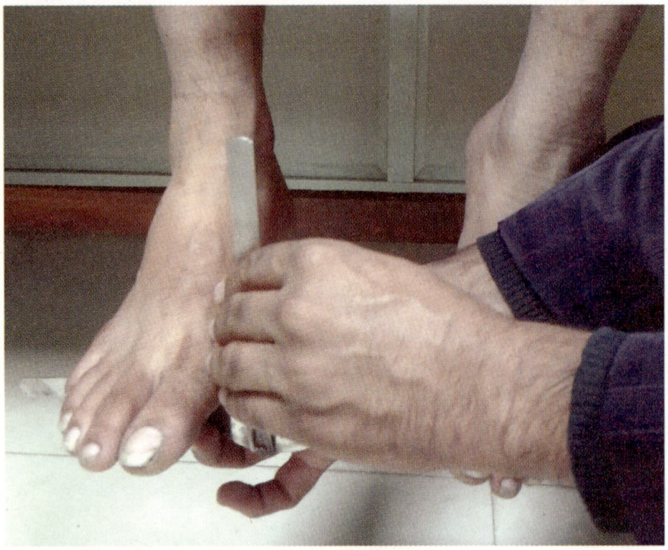

Fig. 6.404: Alternative method for measurement of eversion ROM. Fulcrum is placed at the first metatarsal head. Moving arm is placed along the plantar surface of metatarsal head stationary arm is placed parallel to the tibia

METATARSOPHALANGEAL (MTP) FLEXION

Normal ROM: First MTP: 0° to 45°.

Second to fifth MTP: Between 30° and 45°.

Plane and Axis: Flexion of all the MTP joints occur in the sagittal plane around medial lateral axis.

Normal End Feel: Normal end feel of flexion of all the MTP joints is firm because of tension in the dorsal joint capsule and extensor digitorum, brevis and collateral ligaments.

Position of Patient: Supine or long sitting with the foot out of the edge of the table.

Position of Examiner: Examiner sits comfortably in a chair of the side of the leg which is being tested.

Position of Goniometer: Fulcrum of goniometer is placed over the dorsal aspect of the respective MTP joint. The proximal arm is aligned over the dorsal midline of respective metatarsal bone. The distal arm is aligned over the dorsal midline of respective proximal phalanx. The distal arm is aligned over the dorsal midline of respective metatarsal bone.

Stabilization: Ankle joint is stabilized to prevent plantar flexion, dorsiflexion, inversion and eversion. The metatarsal bones also stabilized to prevent inversion and eversion.

Process: Examiner maintains the position of proximal arm and instructs the patient to bring the respective toe towards the plantar surface (Figs. 6.405a to c).

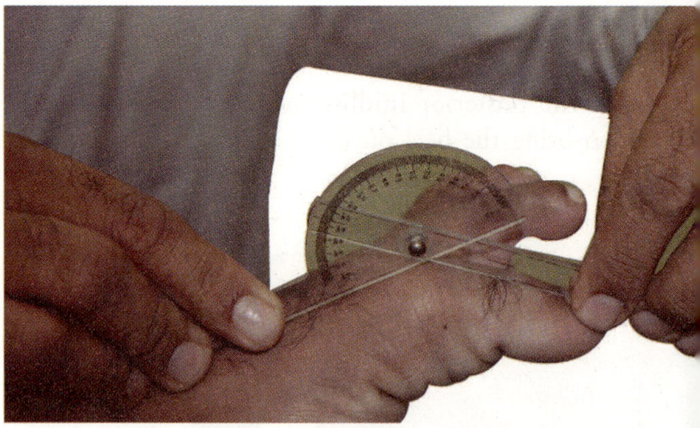

Fig. 6.405a: Measurement of first MTP joint flexion ROM

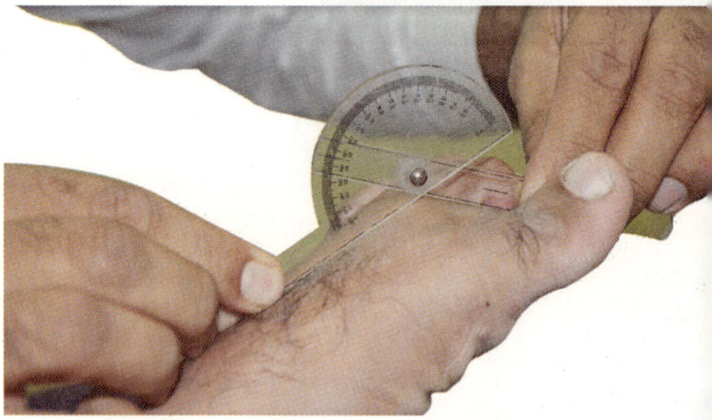

Fig. 6.405b: Measurement of second MTP joint flexion ROM

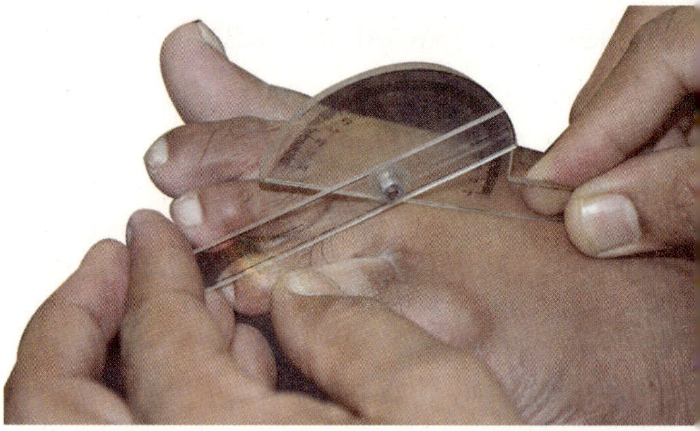

Fig. 6.405c: Measurement of fourth MTP joint flexion ROM

METATARSOPHALANGEAL EXTENSION

Normal ROM: First MTP joint: 0° to 50°.

2nd to 5th MTP joints: 0° to 45°.

Plane and Axis: Movement occurs in the sagittal plane around medial lateral axis.

Normal End Feel: The normal end feel is firm due to tension in the plantar joint capsule, the plantar pad, flexor hallucis, flexor digitorum and flexor digiti minimi muscles.

Position of Patient: Supine or long sitting with the foot out of the edge of table or couch.

Position of Examiner: Examiner sits comfortably in a chair at the side of leg which is being tested.

Position of Goniometer: Same as for MTP flexion.

Stabilization: Same as for MTP flexion.

Process: Examiner maintains the position of proximal arm of the goniometer and instructs the patient to bring the respective toe up towards the dorsum of foot (Figs. 6.406a and b).

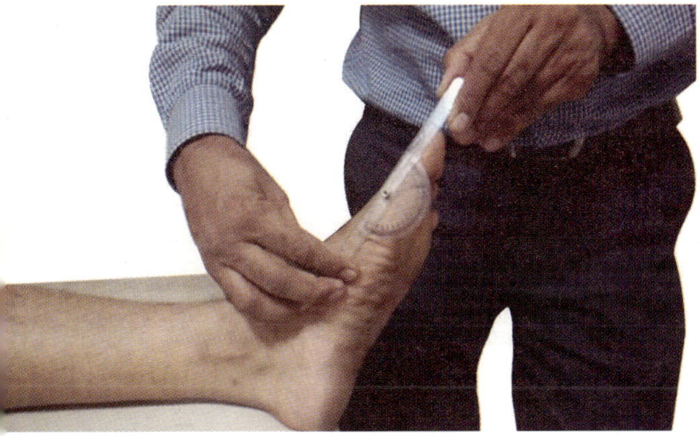

Fig. 6.406a: Measurement of ROM of extension of first MTP joint (starting)

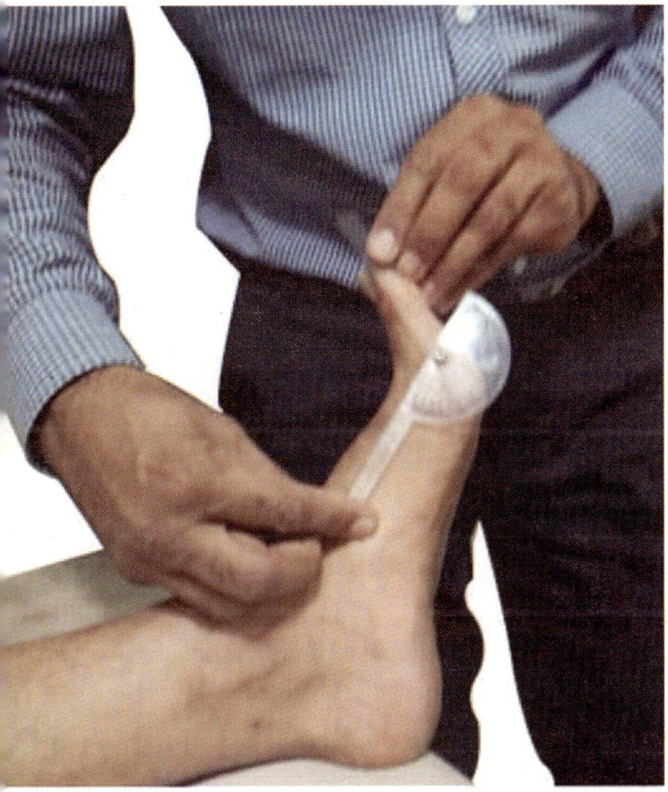

Fig. 6.406b: Measurement of ROM of extension of first MTP joint

METATARSOPHALANGEAL ABDUCTION

Normal ROM: 0° to 25°.

Plane and Axis: Movement occurs in the frontal plane around anterior posterior axis.

Normal End Feel: The normal end feel is firm because of tension in the joint capsule, the fascia of the web space between the toes, collateral ligaments, adductor hallucis, and plantar interossei muscles.

Position of Patient: Supine or long sitting with the foot out of the edge of table.

Position of Examiner: Examiner sits comfortably in a chair at the side of leg which is being tested.

Position of Goniometer: Fulcrum of goniometer is placed over the dorsal aspect of respect MTP joint. The proximal arm is aligned with the dorsal midline of the metatarsal. The distal arm is aligned over the dorsal midline of proximal phalanx of respective MTP joint.

Stabilization: Ankle joint and metatarsal bones are stabilized to prevent inversion and eversion.

Process: Examiner maintains the proximal arm of the goniometer and instructs the patient to take the respective toe away from the midline of foot. Abduction of all the MTP joints can be measured with this procedure (Figs. 6.407a to d).

INTERPHALANGEAL JOINT FLEXION

Normal ROM: First IP joint: 0°-90°.

Second to fifth: 0°-80°(PIP).

Plane and Axis: Movement occurs in sagittal plane around medial lateral axis.

Normal End Feel: The normal end feel is usually soft because of approximation of the soft tissues between the plantar surfaces of phalanges. Sometimes, the end feel is firm due to tension in the dorsal joint capsule and collateral ligaments.

Position of Patient: Supine or long sitting with the foot out of the table or couch.

Position of Examiner: Examiner sits comfortably in the chair at the side of leg which is being tested.

Position of Goniometer: Fulcrum of goniometer is placed on the dorsum surface of respective interphalangeal joint. Proximal arm is aligned over the dorsal midline of respective proximal phalanx and distal arm is aligned over the dorsal midline of respective phalanx.

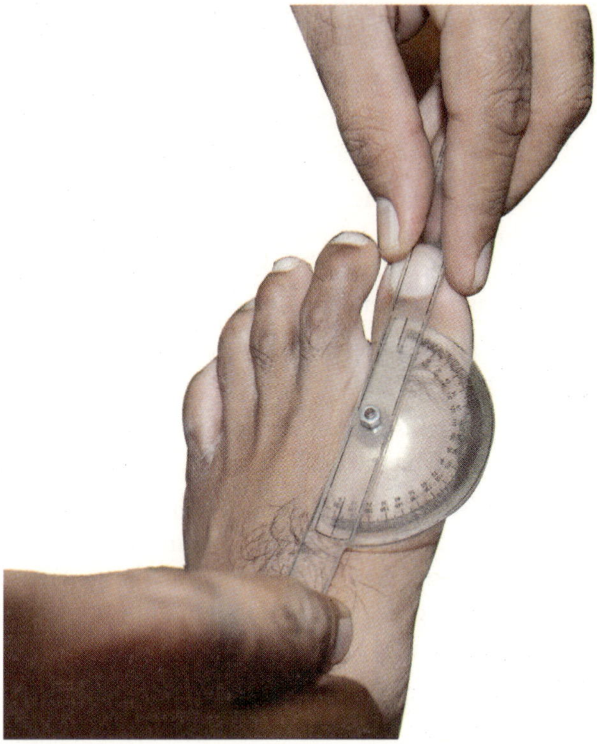

Fig. 6.407a: Measurement of first MTP abduction ROM (Starting position)

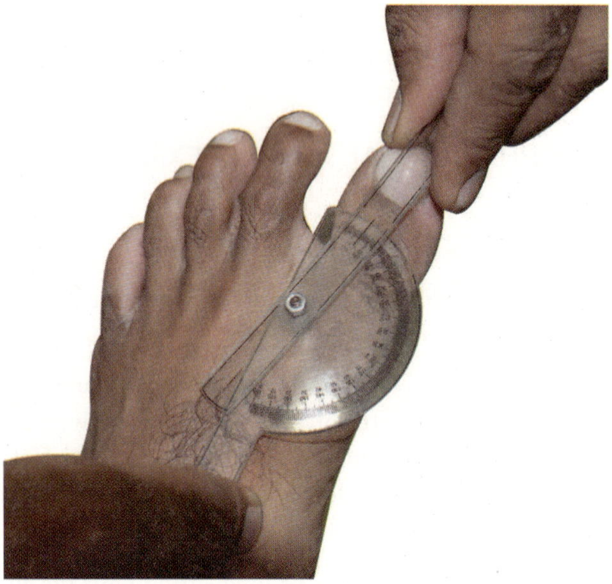

Fig. 6.407b: Measurement of first MTP abduction ROM

Process: Examiner maintains the position of proximal phalanx and instructs the patient to flex the proximal interphalangeal as much as possible.

Stabilization: Ankle and metatarsals are stabilized to maintain MTP joint at the neutral position (Figs. 6.408a to c).

DISTAL INTERPHALANGEAL FLEXION (1 to 4)

Normal ROM: 0° to 30°.

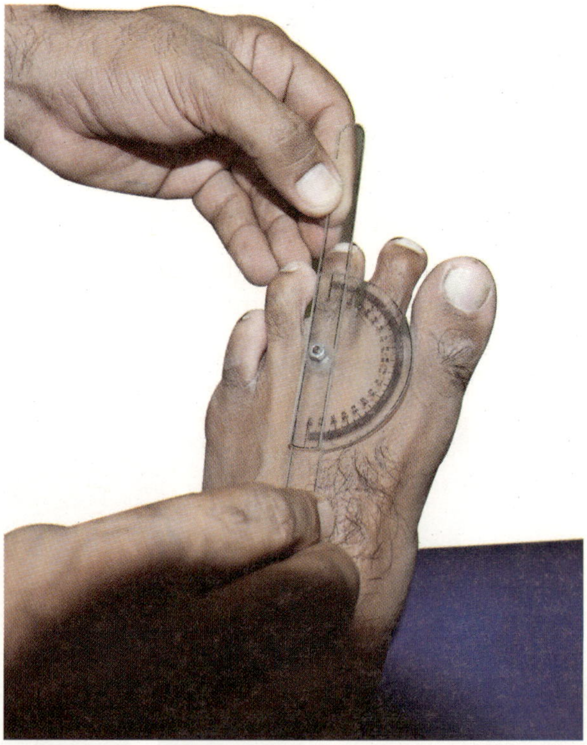

Fig. 6.407c: Measurement of third MTP abduction ROM (Starting position)

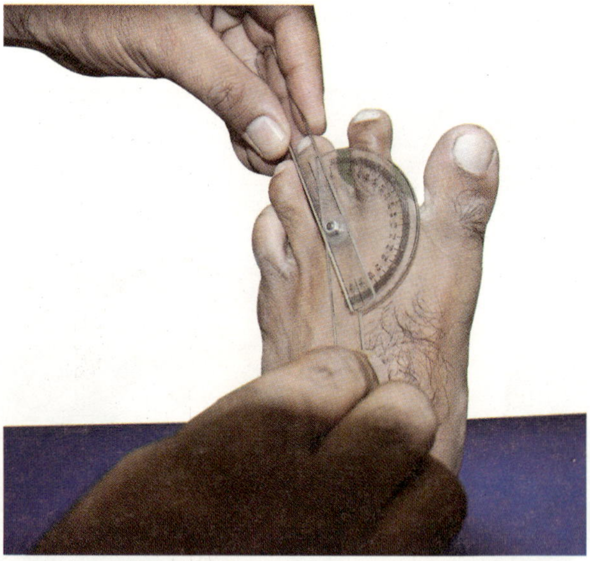

Fig. 6.407d: Measurement of third MTP abduction ROM

Plane and Axis: Sagittal around medial lateral axis.

Normal End Feel: The normal end feel is firm due to tension in the dorsal joint capsule, the collateral ligaments and the oblique retonacular ligaments.

Position of Patient: Supine or long sitting with ankle joint and foot out of the table.

Position of Examiner: Examiner sits comfortably in a chair at the side of leg which is being tested.

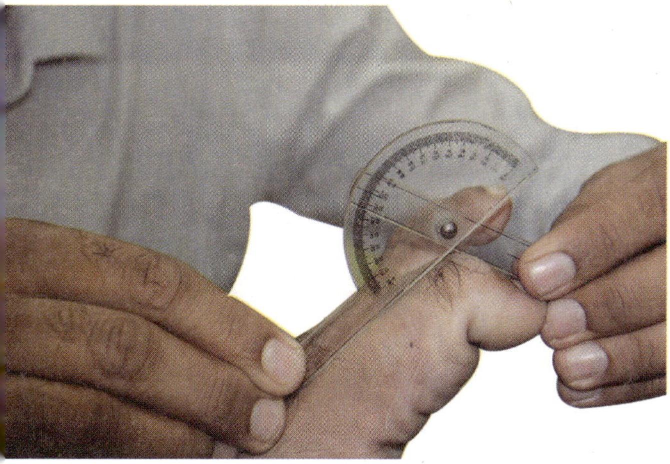

Fig. 6.408a: Measurement of first IP joint flexion ROM

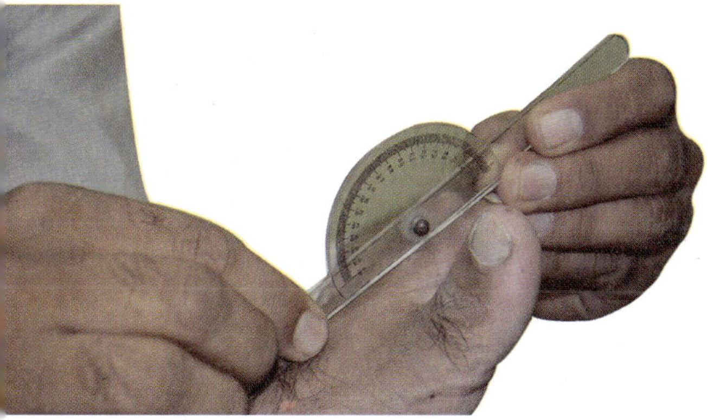

Fig. 6.408b: Measurement of second PIP joint flexion ROM (Starting position)

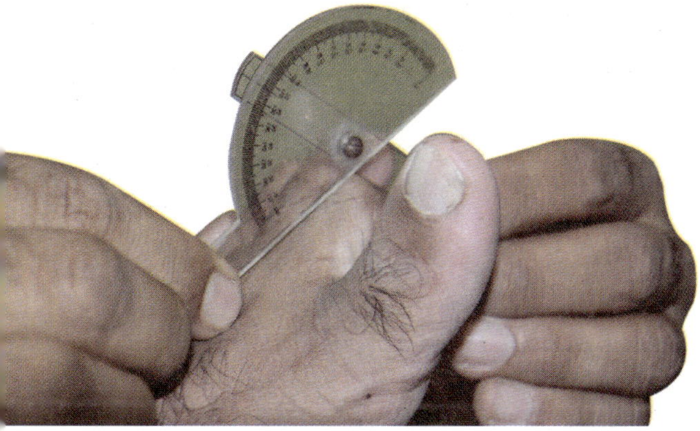

Fig. 6.408c: Measurement of second PIP joint flexion ROM

Stabilization: Metatarsal and proximal phalanx are stabilized to prevent inversion and PIP flexion.

Position of Goniometer: Fulcrum of goniometer is placed on the dorsum aspect of respective DIP joint. Proximal arm is aligned over the dorsal midline of middle phalanx and distal arm is aligned over the dorsal midline of distal phalanx.

Process: Examiner maintains the proximal arm over the middle phalanx and instructs the patient to move the DIP joint into flexion (Figs. 6.409a and d).

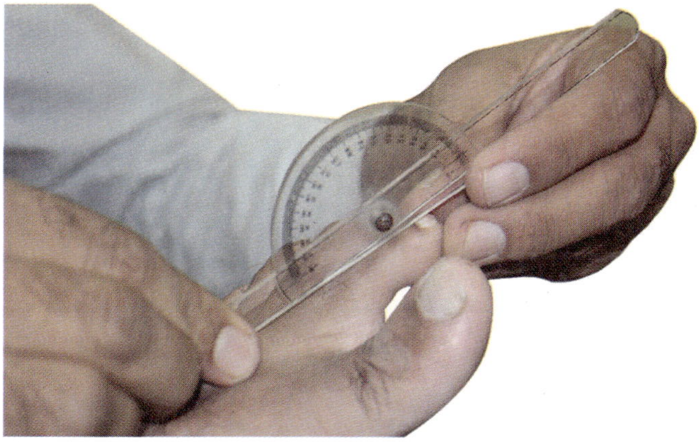

Fig. 6.409a: Measurement of second DIP joint flexion ROM (Starting position)

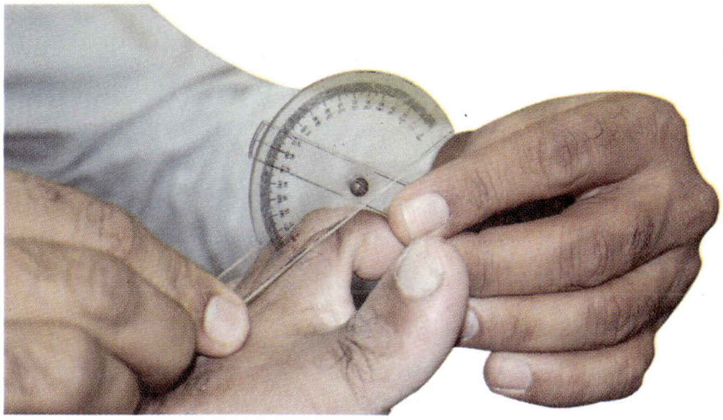

Fig. 6.409b: Measurement of second DIP joint flexion ROM

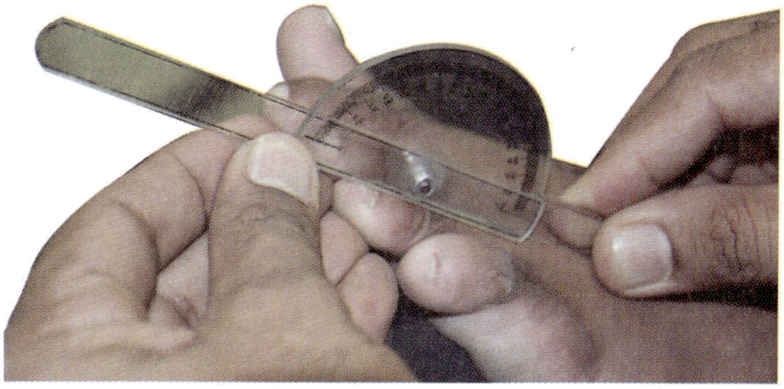

Fig. 6.409c: Measurement of fourth DIP joint flexion ROM (Starting position)

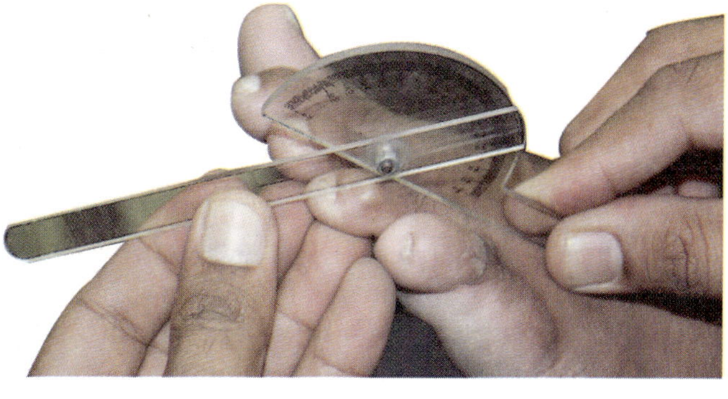

Fig. 6.409d: Measurement of fourth DIP joint flexion ROM

7

MOBILIZATION OF PERIPHERAL JOINT

INTRODUCTION

The technique of mobilization is being used from the time of Hippocrates, a physician in the fourth century, BC. Some time in the past these important techniques of mobilization were lost from practice because earlier, the use of mobilization techniques was based purely on empirical evidence of their effectiveness, there was no scientific basis for their use.

In late 1700s and early 1800s this influence prevailed and joint manipulation remained in the hands of bonesetters. The bonesetters had no basic knowledge of joint structures and manipulation techniques other than their past experience. They tended to guard their knowledge, keeping their secret among family members.

Then rivalry started between physicians and bonesetters. Thomas who was the son and grandson of bonesetters was one of the physician who spoke against the bonesetters and invented the splint, known as Thomas splint.

Hutten was the bonesetter who was famous for his free services to the patients. He suffered from serious illness and was treated by Dr Peter Hood, father of Dr Wharton Hood. In repayment of treatment, Hutten offered Dr Peter to teach all techniques he knew of bonesetting but Dr Peter Hood did not accept the offer. However his son Wharton Hood accepted the offer and learnt the techniques of bonesetting from Hutten. He has written medical book on manipulation which was published in 1870s. In his paper on the subject, published in Lancet in 1871, Hood described Hutten's techniques of spinal and peripheral manipulation. The techniques described by Hutten were always of a high velocity thrust and essentially identical to the manipulations used by manual therapists and even some orthopedists and physiatrist today. Hutten admitted to knowing nothing of anatomy, however, he avoided the techniques on acutely inflammed joints. He employed his techniques primarily on post-immobilization stiffness, displaced cartilage and tendons and ganglionic swellings.

MOBILIZATION AND MANIPULATION

The articular surfaces of a joint move every day in anatomical and physiological ranges as required by normal activities of daily living. Adhesion formation in the region of joint followed by injury or pathological changes restricts the motion of articular surfaces, subsequently the range of motion decreases, and activities of daily living are compromised. Pain becomes the most dominant problem and because of it patient avoids activities. If condition is not treated at the right time, the joint range of motion is severely restricted and gradually the joint space decreases as well, which is called as fibrous ankylosis. Rehabilitation programme which includes mobilization techniques of the joints has significant effect on restricted joints by breaking up the adhesion formation, subsequently increasing range of motion and joint space as well.

Mobilization

- Mobilization is a passive movement directed at the joint without any high velocity thrust and within the range of motion.
- It is a gentle, coaxing, repetitive rhythmic movement of a joint that can be resisted by the patient. Unlike manipulation, it can be performed over a wide range and can thus involve a series of movements, referred to as stages.

Manipulation

- Manipulation is a high velocity thrust of small amplitude.
- It is a very rapid, passive movement at the end of the range of a joint, is far more forceful than mobilization and cannot be controlled by the patient.

EFFECTS OF IMMOBILIZATION ON CONNECTIVE TISSUES

Immobilization and trauma significantly change the histology and normal mechanics of connective tissue.

Macroscopically, fibrofatty infiltrate is evident in the recesses of the immobilized tissues. With prolonged immobilization the infiltrates develop a more fibrotic appearance, creating adhesions in the recesses. These fibrotic changes occur in the absence of trauma. Histologic and histochemical analysis show significant changes primarily in the ground substance, (whose function is to bind the water), with no significant loss of collagen. The changes in the ground substance consist of substantial loss of glycosaminoglycans and water, subsequently the ground substance loses the capacity of hydration. The ground substance also functions to lubricate adjacent collagen fibres and maintain a crucial interfiber distance. *As the ground substance loses this function during immobilization, the collagen fibres approximate too closely, the distance between fibres diminishes, the fibres adhere to one another and form cross links adhesions.* These cross-link create a series of microscopic adhesions that limit the pliability and extensibility of the tissues.

Furthermore because movement affects the orientation of newly synthesized collagen, the collagen in the immobilized joints is laid down in a more haphazard, *"haystack"* arrangement. This orientation restricts tissue mobility, further by adhering to existing collagen fibres.

THE EFFECTS OF MOBILIZATION ON CONNECTIVE TISSUES

Studies suggest that mobility and remobilization prevent the haystack development of collagen fibres and stimulate the production of ground substance. As the movements are employed or connective tissues are mobilized, the ground substance returns to its function (water binding capacity). The rehydration process starts, which diminishes the collagen cross-links, subsequently new collagen is laid down in a more orderly fashion.

The passive and active range of movements also stretch the macroadhesions formed during the immobilization period, subsequently increasing the extensibility of the tissues.

INDICATIONS FOR JOINT MOBILIZATION AND MECHANISM OF ACTION

1. **Pain:** *The international association for the study of pain* has defined pain as an unpleasant sensory or emotional experience associated with actual or potential damage described in terms of such damage.

   Pain is experienced by an individual as the nociceptor fibres myelinated (A delta) and/or unmyelinated (C fibres) situated in the skin reach the conscious brain followed by injury or strong noxious stimuli.

   Both A delta and C fibres project to the spinal cord where they synapse (both directly or via inter-neurons) with neurons in the dorsal horn of the grey matter. These neuron-transmission cells (or T cells) are either involved in local spinal reflex, or project to higher centers of the nervous system via the spinothalamic tracts, it is therefore T cells that receive nociceptors from the peripheral part relay them to the higher centers.

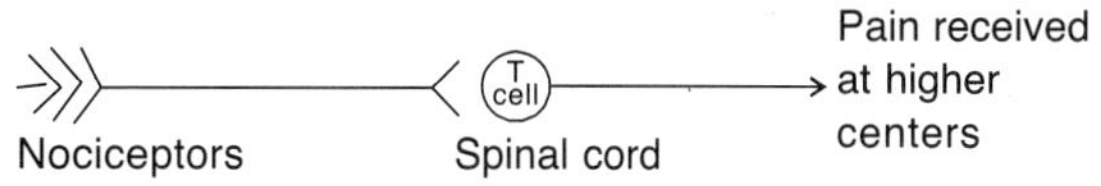

   Large diameter myelinated A beta fibres known as pain inhibitors arise from the peripheral part, terminate on T cells through substantia gelatinosa (S.G.) of the spinal cord dorsal horn grey matter.

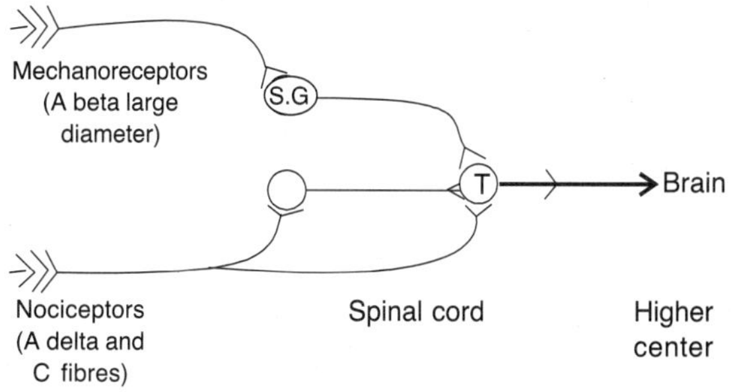

   Now T cells receive excitatory input from the nociceptors and inhibiting input from mechano-receptors through substantia gelatinosa. When nociceptors get excited following an injury, this sensation is relayed from the T cells to the higher centers. If mechanoreceptors also get activated they inhibit the nociceptors at the T cells and prevent the transmission. The inhibitory input caused by activation of the large diameter, mechanosensitive afferents is said to close the gate to nociceptor transmission through the T cells in the spinal cord. This is also known as "Pain Gate Control Theory", which was given by Malzack and Wall in 1965.

   Mobilization techniques such as small amplitude oscillatory, translatory, traction and compression activate large diameter, mechanoreceptors (A beta fibres) which increase the amount of inhibition impinging on the T cells in the spinal cord via the cells of the substantia gelatinosa, and ultimately inhibit nociceptors transmission in the spinal cord by closing the gate. Mobilization of joint in grade 1 and 2 activates the A beta fibres and reduces pain (These grades are discussed later in this chapter).

2. **Muscle Spasm:** Muscles guard the joint by preventing the movements in certain painful conditions. Movements are prevented to such an extent which is not necessary at all. Therefore sustained contraction of the muscles for prolonged period of time causes tightness

of the muscle fibres which is known as protective muscle guarding or muscle spasm. Joint mobilization such as oscillatory techniques in grade-1 and grade-2 in painfree range of motion allows the muscles to lengthen and prevents muscle guarding or spasm.

3. **Joint Stiffness:** Stiffness of the joint is the most common complication following immobilization. Because the collagen fibres approximate too closely, the distance between fibres diminishes, the fibres adhere to one another and form cross link adhesions which prevent the joint to move in full range of motion. The stiffness of the joint depends greatly on the period of immobilization and formation of adhesion between collagen fibres.

   Historically use of mobilization was advocated to improve cartilage nutrition by the synthesis of synovial fluid. The ground substance of synovial fluid which is diminished during immobilization process returns to its function as the mobilization of the joint is started. The rehydration process starts and diminishes the cartilage cross-links, subsequently new collagen is laid down in a more orderly fashion.

The mobilization of the joint also stretches the macroadhesions formed during the immobilization period, subsequently increase the extensibility of the collagen fibres and eventually increase range of motion.

CONTRAINDICATIONS OF JOINT MOBILIZATION

- *Absolute:*
  - Arthrodesis.
  - Bony ankylosis.
  - Any undiagnosed condition.
  - Vertebro bacillary insufficiency (VBI).
  - Rheumatoid arthritic cervical spine.
  - Infective arthritis (an acute osteomyelitis).
  - Acute inflammation.
  - Malignancy involving the vertebral column.
  - Fractures (Acute).
  - Rupture or tear of ligament or tendon.
- *Relative contraindications:*
  - Metabolic bone diseases, such as osteoporosis, Paget's disease and tuberculosis.
  - Joint effusion.
  - Hypermobility.
  - Rheumatoid arthritis.

METHODS OF PERIPHERAL JOINT MOBILIZATION

Range of exercises help in improving range of motion of the joint may be the part of mobilization techniques. However, this chapter will explain only Oscillatory techniques and Sustained translatory techniques as they are the main mobilization techniques.

- *Muscle relaxation techniques:* These are active movements generally not considered mobilization techniques however used to break the muscle spasm and improve range of movement of the joint (explained in Chapter 12).
  - Free exercises.
  - Hold relax.
  - Contract relax.
- *Muscle stretching techniques* (explained in Chapter 13)
  - Forced passive movements.
  - Auto passive stretching or self stretching exercises.
  - Mechanical stretching.
- Oscillatory techniques.
- Sustained translatory joint play techniques.

The Oscillatory Techniques

These techniques are performed in the physiologic range (voluntary movements) or accessory movements (not controlled voluntarily but accompany movements).

Oscillatory techniques are best described by Maitland, who describes oscillations as passive movements to the joint which can be of small or large amplitude and applied anywhere in the range of movement, and can be performed while the joint surfaces are held distracted or compressed.

There are four grades of oscillations:

Grade 1 : is a small–amplitude movement performed at the beginning of range.

Grade 2 : is a large–amplitude movement performed within the range, but not reaching the limit of the range.

Grade 3 : is a large–amplitude movement up to the limit of range.

Grade 4 : is a small–amplitude movement performed at the limit of range.

Grade 1 and Grade 2 are used primarily for neurophysiologic effects and do not engage detectable resistance. Grade 3 and Grade 4 are designed to initiate mechanical changes in the tissue and do engage tissue resistance (Fig. 7.1).

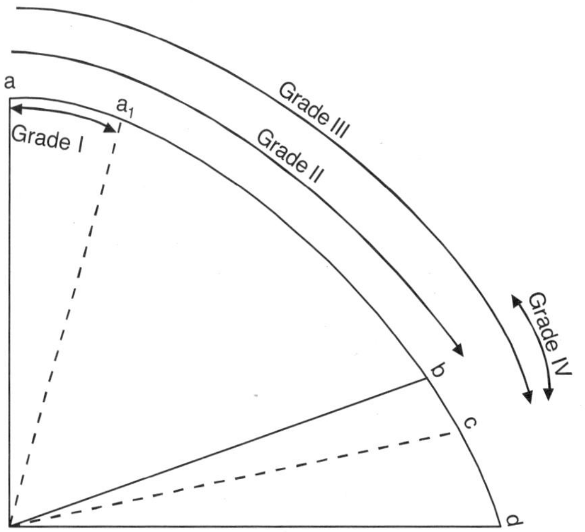

Fig. 7.1: a to d full ROM, a to b available ROM, b to c elastic limit (can be stretched by mobilization), c to d cannot be stretched by mobilization, b to d total limited ROM—a to a_1 = Grade I; a to b = Grade II; a to c = Grade III; b to c = Grade IV

Sustained Translatory Techniques

These are the joint play movements which occur between the joint surfaces and are necessary for joint functioning through the full range of motion. These are demonstrated passively but cannot be performed voluntarily by the patient. The joint play movements include distraction, sliding, compression, rolling and spinning of the joint surfaces. The term arthrokinematics is used to describe the joint play movements. The sustained translatory techniques are graded as:

Grade I

Small amplitude glide or distraction is applied which does not place any stress on joint capsule. Capsule remains loose.

Use–For relief of pain.

Grade II

Sufficient distraction is applied to glide the joint surfaces to stretch the tissues around the joint.

Use–To decrease pain and maintain the joint play movements when physiologic range of motion of the joint is not allowed or contraindicated.

Grade III

A large amplitude glide is applied to place a great or sufficient stretch on the joint capsule and surrounding structures of the joint (periarticular structures).

Use–To increase joint play movements by stretching the joint capsule, subsequently increase physiologic range.

Physiologic movements are the movements that the patient performs and controls voluntarily such as–flexion, extension, abduction, adduction, internal and external rotations. The term osteokinematic is used to describe the physiologic movements.

Accessory movements are the movements that occur between the joint surfaces and surrounding tissues and are necessary for normal joint functioning through the range of motion. These movements cannot be performed or controlled voluntarily but can be performed passively. Accessory movements are categorised into two groups–joint play and component motions.

a. *Joint play*–Occurs between the joint surfaces include distraction or glides, sliding, compression, rolling and spinning of the joint surfaces.

b. *Component motion*–Accompany active movements such as upward rotation of the scapula and clavicle during the shoulder flexion, and rotation of fibula during active movements of the ankle joint.

PRINCIPLES OF PERIPHERAL JOINT MOBILIZATION

Position of Patient

Position of patient should be comfortable. The proximal part of the joint should be stabilized with the weight of body or by the straps, or the hand of therapist.

Position of Therapist

Position of therapist should be convenient to allow the joint to move. Proper body mechanics are essential in application of mobilization techniques. The desired force and direction of movement can be imparted if therapist applies these from wide base of support (position of stability). Therapist should stand close to the area being mobilized and use weight shifting through legs and trunk to assist movement in the vector of mobilization. The therapist's hands and arms should be positioned to act as fulcrums and levers to fine tune mobilization. **The mobilizing hand** should be placed as close as possible to the joint surface and the force applied should be directed at the periarticular tissues. **The stabilizing hand** counter acts the movement of the mobilizing hand by applying an equal but opposite force or by supporting or preventing movement at surrounding joints.

Direction of Movement

Direction of movement during treatment is either parallel or perpendicular to the treatment plane. Treatment plane was described by Kaltenborn as a plane perpendicular to a line running from the axis of rotation to the middle of the concave articular surface. The plane is in the concave partner so its position is determined by the position of the concave bone.

The direction of movement of mobilization should take in account the mechanics of the joint mobilized, the arthrokinematic and osteokinematic impairment of the dysfunction and the current reactivity of the tissue involved.

Glide is applied in the direction in which slide occurs:

a. If the surface of moving bone is convex, slide occurs in the opposite direction of the angular movement of the bone (Fig. 7.2a).

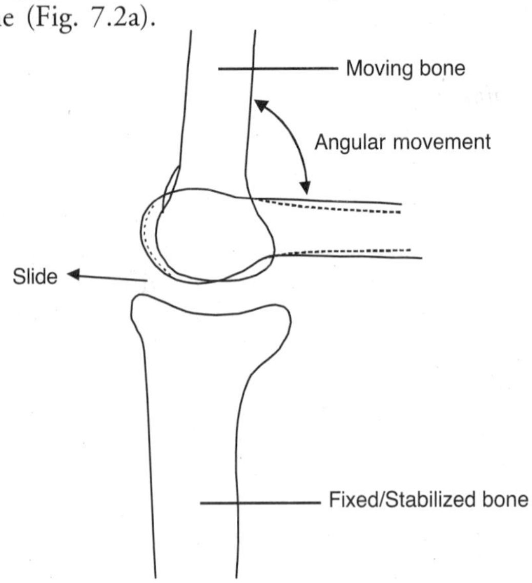

Fig. 7.2a

b. If the surface of the moving bone is concave, sliding occurs in the same direction of angular movement of bone (Fig. 7.2b).

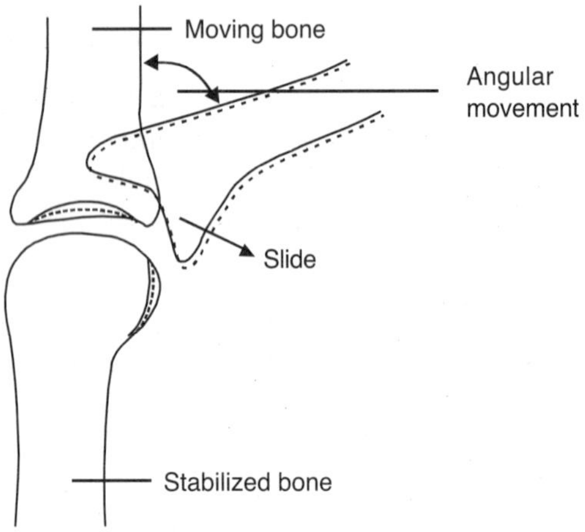

Fig. 7.2b

Intensity and Duration

The several comparative studies (between low load, long duration and heavy load, short duration) have shown that to obtain permanent elongation of collagenous tissues, the long duration with low load mobilization treatment is more effective than short duration with high intensity.

By using sustained translatory techniques the minimum stretch duration should be 6 seconds, however the oscillatory stretch can be applied for 2 to 3 seconds only, every stretch is followed by rest period and several repetitions are performed per treatment session to place effective stretch on joint capsule and surrounding structures of the joint to cause increase extensibility of the collagenous tissues.

Distraction or Traction

It is a separation of the articular surfaces by pulling them apart. Traction places stretch on periarticular structures. This stretching effect on periarticular structures facilitates the movement by lessening resistance between articular surfaces. Therefore, sustained translatory and oscillatory techniques should be performed with the traction. To perform oscillatory mobilization the traction is applied in the form of therapist's hand which can be assisted by belt.

TECHNIQUES OF TRANSLATORY JOINT PLAY MOVEMENTS

Mobilization of Sternoclavicular Joint

1. Superior Glide of the Medial Clavicle

Position of Patient: Supine with arms of the side of body, the hip and knee joints are flexed for flattening the lumbar spine. The sternoclavicular joint is exposed and other area is covered with towel for privacy, especially if the patient is female.

Position of Therapist: At the side of patient. Facing cranially. The palmar surface of the thumb pad is placed over the inferior surface of the medial clavicle. The thumb pushes the proximal end of the clavicle superiorly. If more force is to be delivered, then other thumb may reinforce the mobilizing thumb (Fig. 7.3).

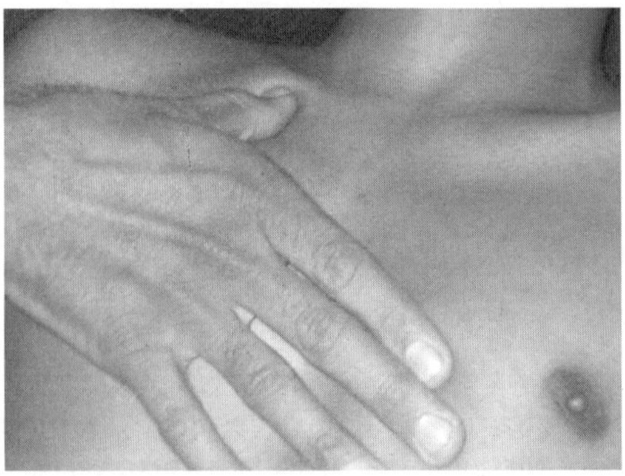

Fig. 7.3: Superior glide of the proximal clavicle

2. Inferior Glide of the Medial Clavicle

Position of Patient and Therapist remain same as superior glide.

Placement of Hand: The palmar aspect of thumb is placed over the superior surface of the medial portion of the clavicle.

The medial clavicle is pushed into caudally, more pressure/ force can be applied by reinforcing the thumb by other thumb (Fig. 7.4).

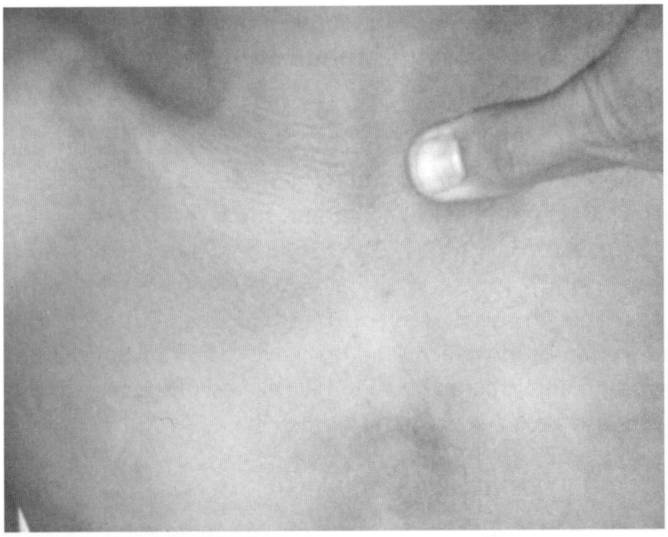

Fig. 7.4: Inferior glide of the proximal clavicle

3. Posterior Glide of the Medial Clavicle

Position of Patient and Therapist remains same as superior glide.

Placement of Hand: The palmar aspect of thumb is placed over the anterior aspect of the medial clavicle. To apply more pressure pisiform aspect of wrist can be placed over the proximal part of clavicle then it is pushed posteriorly (Fig. 7.5).

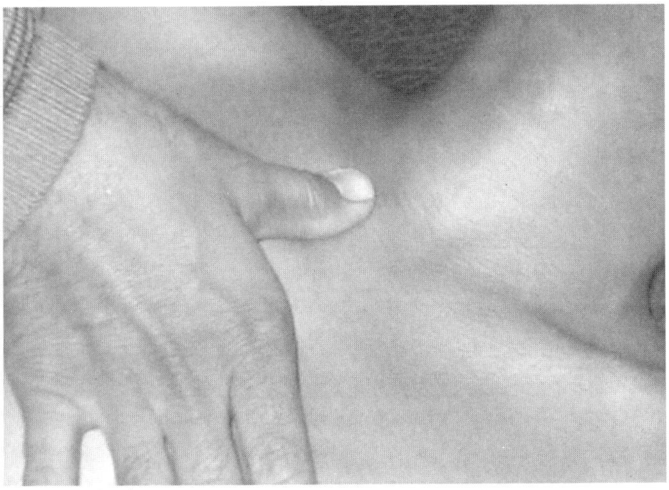

Fig. 7.5: Posterior glide of the proximal clavicle

Mobilization of Acromioclavicular Joint

1. Anterior Glide of the Distal End of Clavicle

Position of Patient: Sitting, back is supported with the back rest of chair. Arms at the side of body and hands are placed on thighs.

Position of Therapist: Stands behind the patient, one hand is used to stabilize the acromion process. The thumb and fingers of other hand grasps the clavicle. While stabilizing the acromion process distal end of the clavicle is glided anteriorly by the thumb and fingers (Fig. 7.6).

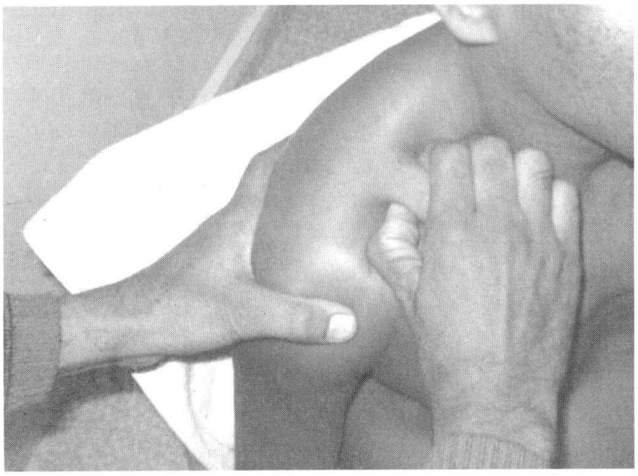

Fig. 7.6: Anterior glide of the distal clavicle

2. Gapping of the Acromioclavicular Joint

Position of Patient: Sitting. Arms at the side of body. Hands on the thighs.

Position of Therapist: Stands behind the patient. One hand is placed over the spine of scapula, other hand over the distal end of clavicle. The force is applied simultaneously by both hands, pushes the bones in opposite direction to each other (Fig. 7.7).

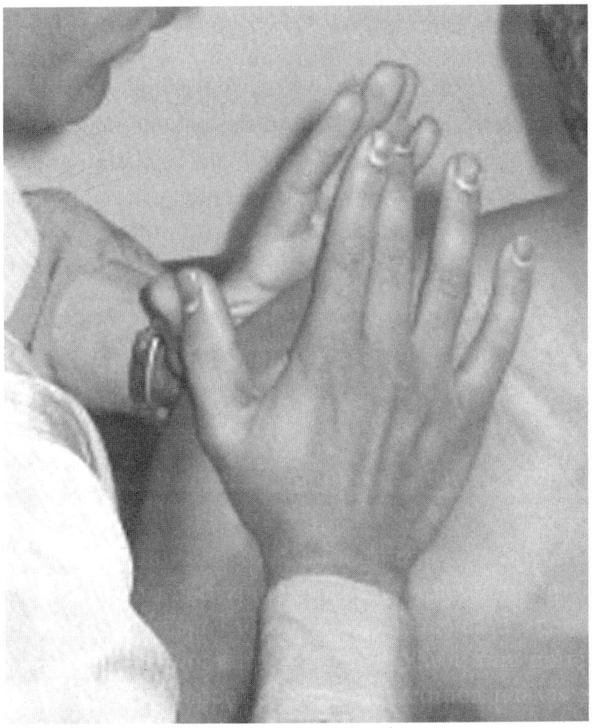

Fig. 7.7: Gapping of the acromioclavicular joint

Scapula Mobilization

1. Scapular Distraction: Technique 1

Position of Patient: Side lying close to the edge of the plinth, the uninvolved hand may be placed under the head, the involved arm rests on the radial side of forearm of therapist with slight abduction.

Position of Therapist: Standing in front of the patient, the anterior aspect of the patient's shoulder rests on the therapist's waist. The one hand holds the inferior angle of the scapula while other hand grasps the vertebral border or medial border of the scapula. The therapist leans forward, distracts the scapula away from the thoracic wall, or both hands pull the scapula toward the body away from the thoracic wall (Fig. 7.8).

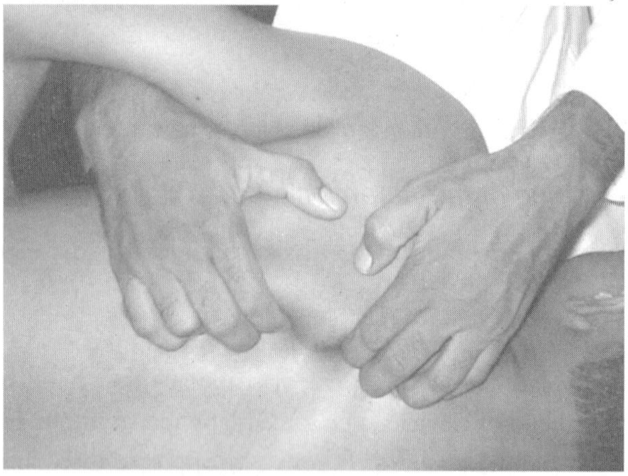

Fig. 7.8: Scapular distraction (Technique 1)

2. Scapular Distraction: Technique 2

Position of Patient: Same as for scapular distraction technique 1.

Position of Therapist: Behind the patient, standing with forward bending of trunk. One hand is placed under the head of humerus and other hand under the inferior angle of the scapula. The force is applied simultaneously which lifts the head of humerus and inferior angle of scapula (Fig. 7.9).

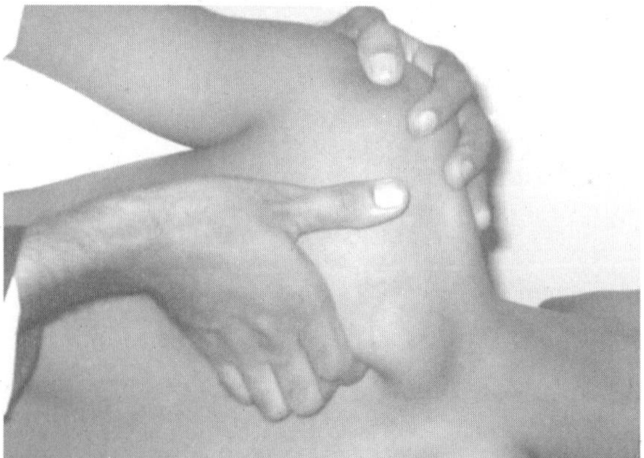

Fig. 7.9: Scapular distraction (Technique 2)

The Shoulder Girdle Complex

The shoulder girdle complex is composed of seven joints, and each joint can be mobilized separately.

Glenohumeral Joint Mobilization

This joint is formed by glenoid fossa of scapula and head of humerus. The head of humerus is glided into the superior, inferior, anterior, lateral and posterior direction with respect to the glenoid fossa. The gliding force must be sufficient enough to place stretch on capsule and periarticular structures. The stretch of the capsule is considered on the resistance to the movement. Improper stabilization, wrong direction of movement and excessive force can cause injury to the joint structures. Glide is applied with traction which can also be achieved by using belt.

1. Longitudinal Distraction

Position of Patient: Supine, the involved side should be as close as possible to the edge of table. The proximal part of the joint (glenoid fossa of scapula) is stabilized with weight of body (straps can also be used to stabilize the proximal part of the joint).

Position of Therapist: At the side of the patient, facing the joint, the mobilizing hand is placed over the shoulder joint and lower hand grasps the distal arm. While maintaining the position the lower hand pulls the arm downward which causes longitudinal traction (Fig. 7.10).

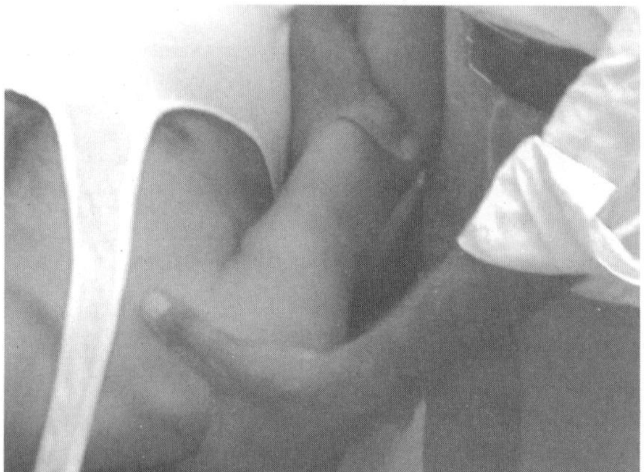

Fig. 7.10: Longitudinal distraction

2. Inferior Glide of Humerus

Position of Patient: Supine, shoulder is abducted at 45°. Strap may be used to stabilize the scapula.

Position of Therapist: At the side of patient, facing the joint by rotating the trunk. The mobilizing hand is placed over the superior aspect of the head of humerus and an assisting hand holds the arm just above the elbow joint. An assisting hand applies traction by pulling the arm toward the body while mobilizing hand pushes the head of humerus into inferior direction with respect to the glenoid fossa (Fig. 7.11).

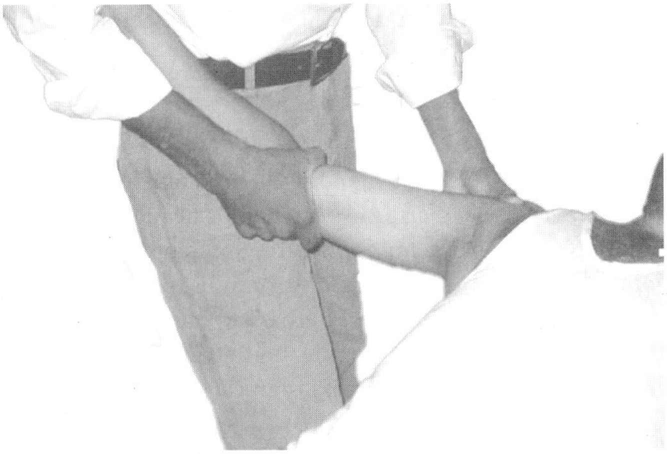

Fig. 7.11: Inferior glide

3. Superior Glide of Humerus

Position of Patient: Supine, arm remains at the side of body or abducted if it is desired to place sufficient stretch on capsule and increase range of motion.

Position of Therapist: Standing at the side of patient, mobilizing hand is placed under the axilla and assisting hand holds the arm just above the elbow. The mobilizing hand pushes the head of humerus up with mild traction to the lateral side. An assisting hand keeps the arm at the side of body (Fig. 7.12). Superior glide in usually not recommended as superior migration of the head of humerus stucks with the acromian arch and impinges the tendon of supraspinatus, long head of biceps and subacromial bursa. This may aggravate the symptoms.

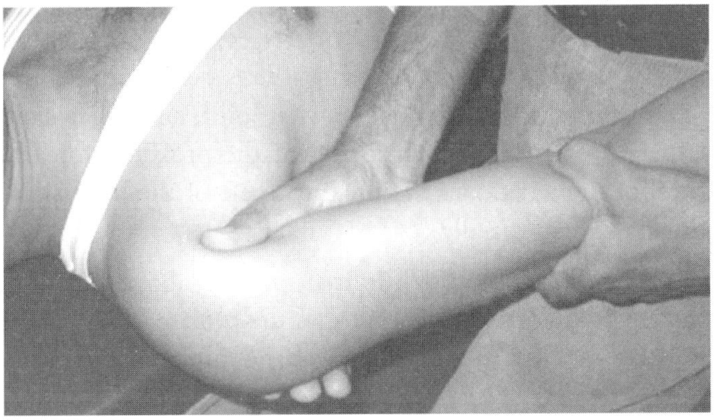

Fig. 7.12: Superior glide

4. Posterior Glide of Humerus (Technique 1)

Position of Patient: Supine, the shoulder is abducted slightly and elbow is flexed at 90° with palm facing the body of therapist. A wedge or pillow is placed under the scapula. The arm rests on therapist's thigh.

Position of Therapist: Sits or stands at the side of patient, facing the joint with slight rotating the trunk. The mobilizing hand (fingers are placed posterolateral aspect of the shoulder and thumb on the head of humerus, during mobilization thumb pushes the head of humerus posteriorly) is placed over the anterior humeral head while assisting hand holds the distal arm and elbow joint of the patient rests on the thigh of therapist. The mobilizing hand pushes the head of humerus downward to the edge of plinth (Fig. 7.13a).

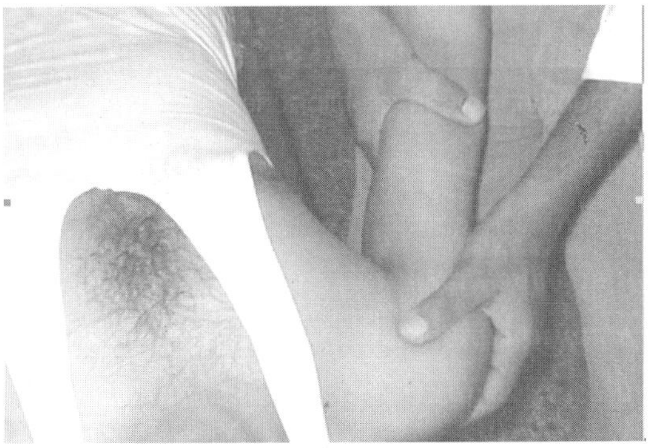

Fig. 7.13a: Posterior glide

5. Posterior Glide (Technique 2)

Position of Patient: Supine, shoulder is flexed to 90°, elbow is flexed at approximately 120°, the hand of patient rests on his or her chest. A wedge or small towel roll may be placed under the scapula which should not prevent the movement of head of humerus.

Position of Therapist: Stands at the side of patient facing the joint. A belt is used to apply traction, which passes from the head of humerus to the therapist's waist/buttocks. Therapist places both hands on the elbow and applies traction through the buttocks by taking them away from the table. The humerus is pushed posteriorly by applying a pressure through hands and body. When buttocks of therapist are taken away, trunk bends automatically which gives a thrust force to the humerus and produces distraction, which facilitates posterior glide of humerus (Fig. 7.13b).

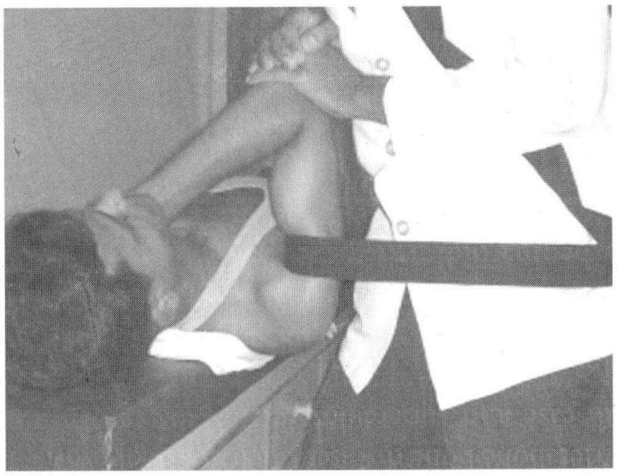

Fig. 7.13b: Posterior glide of head of humerus

6. Anterior Glide

Position of Patient: Prone, with the involved extremity as close as possible to the edge of the table. The shoulder should be off the table.

Position of Therapist: Stands at the side of patient, facing the joint. The mobilizing hand is placed over the posterior **aspect** of the head of humerus, the assisting hand holds the elbow. Arm of patient rests on therapist's thigh. Assisting hand pulls the arm apart from the plinth and mobilizing hand pushes the head of humerus anteriorly causing stretch to the anterior joint capsule (Fig. 7.14).

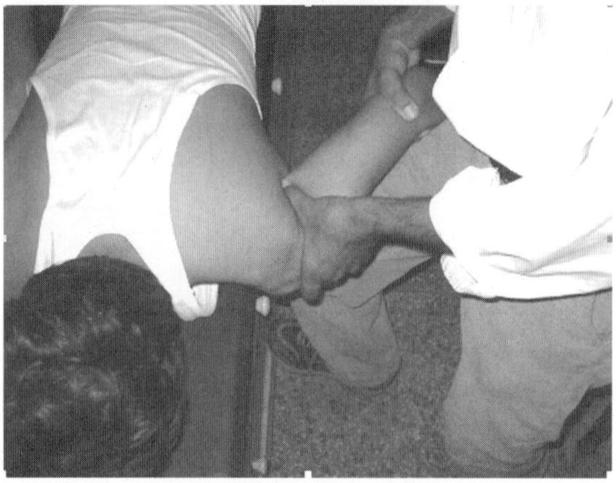

Fig. 7.14: Anterior glide

7. Anterior and Posterior Glide of the Head of Humerus

Position of Patient: Supine, the involved extremity's arm rests on plinth and forearm over the chest.

Position of Therapist: Sits on chair, facing laterally. The thumbs of both hands are placed over the anterior aspect of humerus and fingers are placed over the posterior aspect of humerus head. The head of humerus is glided anteriorly by pushing up by the fingers, the stretched position is held for atleast 6 seconds then released. Now thumbs push the head of humerus posteriorly. These up and down movements of the head of humerus by thumbs and fingers cause anterior and posterior glides alternately (Fig. 7.15).

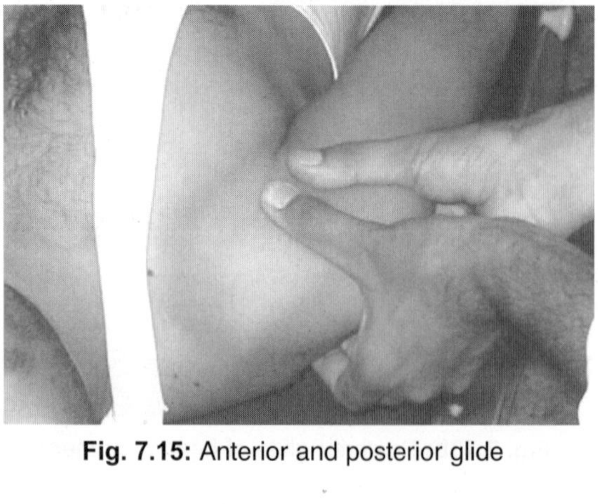

Fig. 7.15: Anterior and posterior glide

8. To Improve External Rotation of the Shoulder

To improve external rotation of the shoulder, the joint is placed into abduction and external rotation (extreme ranges/ stretched ranges) then head of humerus is pushed inferiorly.

Technique

Position of Patient: Supine.

Position of Therapist: Standing. The mobilizing hand is placed over the superior aspect of the head of humerus while assisting hand holds the arm just above the elbow joint. The forearm of patient rests on waist of therapist. An assisting hand abducts and externally rotates the arm with traction, while the mobilizing hand glides the head of humerus anteriorly to place a significant stretch on the anterior joint capsule (Fig. 7.16).

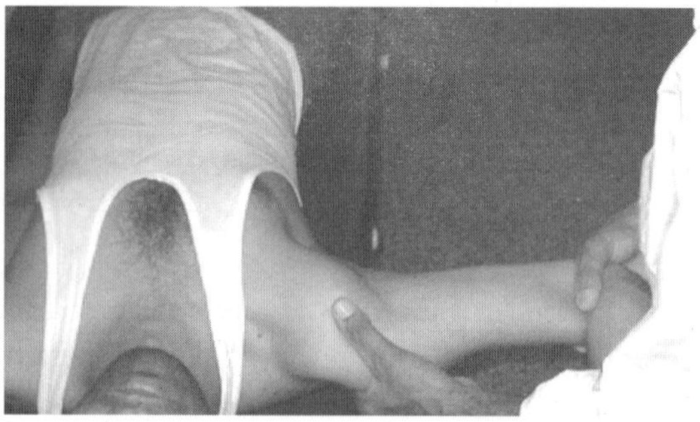

Fig. 7.16: To improve external rotation of the shoulder

Elbow Joint Mobilization

The Humeroulnar Joint

1. Joint Longitudinal Traction

Position of Patient: Supine with elbow flexed at 90° and forearm supinated.

Position of Therapist: Stands at the patient's side. Lower hand grasps the forearm at the wrist joint, and other hand is placed over the palmar aspect of the proximal forearm (heel of the wrist over the proximal part of the joint while fingers spread distally).

Mobilizing Force: While maintaining above position, therapist leans forward and pushes the proximal part of the forearm through the mobilizing hand (upper hand) (Fig. 7.17).

2. Joint Compression

Position of Patient: Supine, elbow is flexed at 90° and shoulder is abducted at 90°.

Position of Therapist: Standing at the side of the patient upper hand stabilizes the distal part of the elbow joint while lower hand grasps the patient's hand.

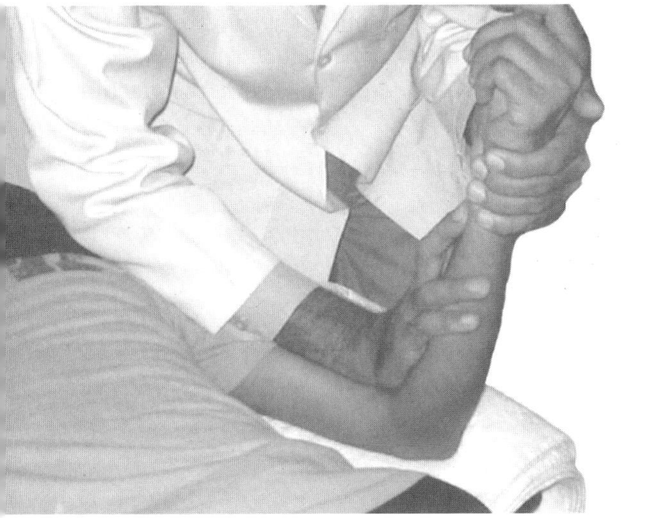

Fig. 7.17: Humeroulnar joint traction

Mobilization Force: While maintaining above position, the mobilizing hand pushes forearm through the hand to the elbow joint (Fig. 7.18).

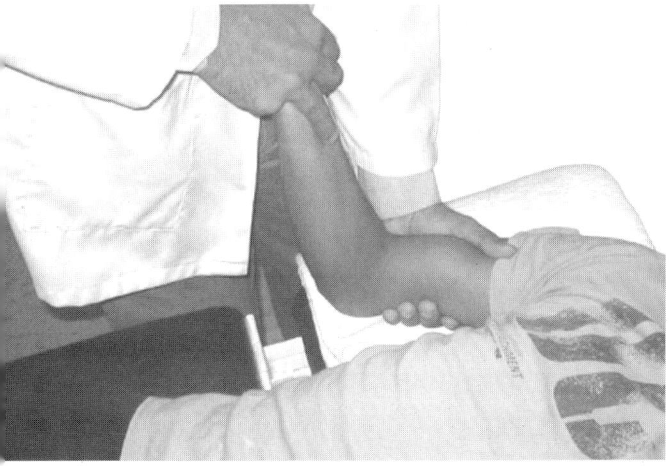

Fig. 7.18: Joint compression (humeroulnar)

3. Dorsal and Volar Glide

Position of Patient: Supine with the elbow extended and forearm supinated.

Position of Therapist: Stands at the side of the patient, one hand grasps the medial distal humerus to stabilize it and other grasps the head of radius (heel on the palmar aspect and fingers on the dorsal aspect).

Mobilization Force: The radial head is pushed dorsally with the heel and volarly with the fingers alternately (Fig. 7.19).

Radioulnar Joint

1. Dorsal and Volar Glide of the Proximal Radioulnar

Position of Patient: Sitting with elbow and forearm in mid range and shoulder slightly abducted.

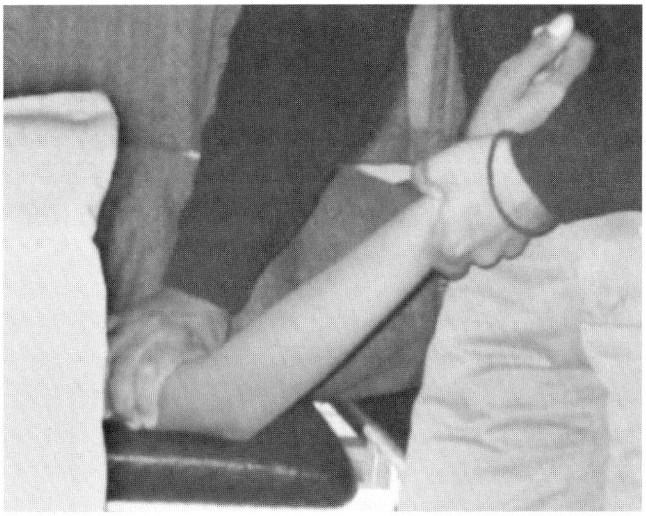

Fig. 7.19: Humeroulnar joint distraction

Position of Therapist: Standing at the side of the patient facing the joint. One hand stabilizes the proximal ulna while other grasps the head of radius (heel on the dorsal aspect and fingers on the palmar).

Mobilization Force: The radial head is pushed with the heel and pulled toward the therapist body with the fingers alternately (Fig. 7.20).

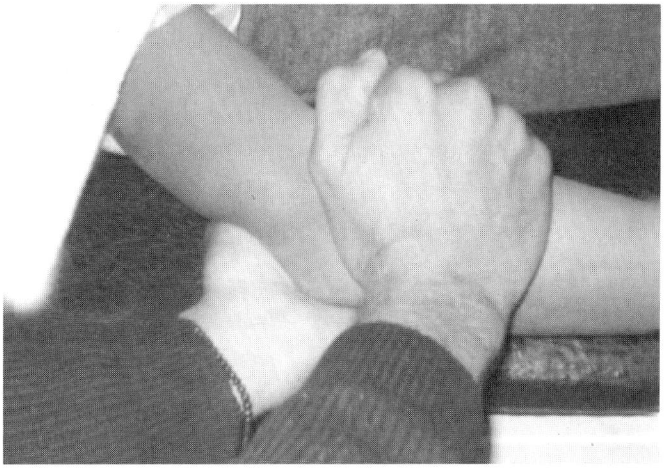

Fig. 7.20: Dorsal and volar glides of the proximal radioulnar joint

2. Dorsal and Volar Glide of the Distal Radioulnar Joint

Position of Patient: Sitting on stool, forearm rests on treatment table in midprone position.

Position of Therapist: Standing at the side of patient one hand grasps the distal ulna to stabilize it and other hand grasps the distal radius (thenar aspect is placed on the dorsal aspect and fingers on the palmar).

Mobilizing Hand: While maintaining above position, the distal radius is glided anteriorly (volar glide) with the thenar aspect and posteriorly (dorsal glide) with the fingers (Fig. 7.21).

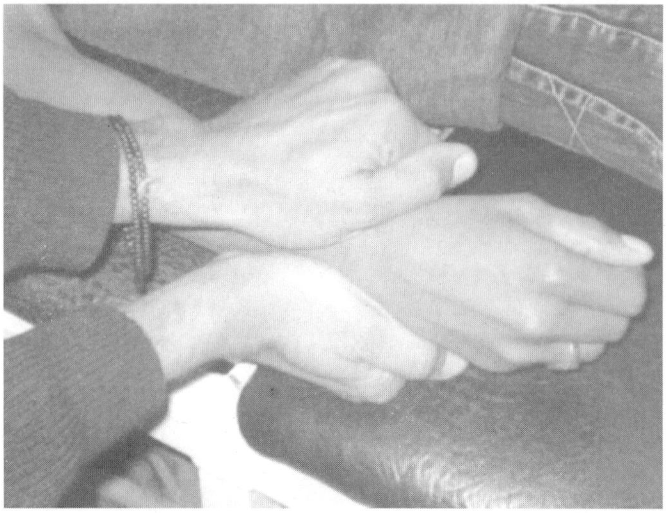

Fig. 7.21: Dorsal and volar glides of the distal radioulnar joint

Wrist Joint

1. Traction

Position of Patient: Sitting on stool, forearm pronated rests on treatment table and wrist over the edge of the table, a towel roll can be placed under the distal forearm.

Position of Therapist: Standing, facing the joint, one hand stabilizes the proximal part while other hand grasps the distal part or hand.

Mobilization Force: While stabilizing the proximal part of the joint the other hand pulls the hand in longitudinal direction (Fig. 7.22).

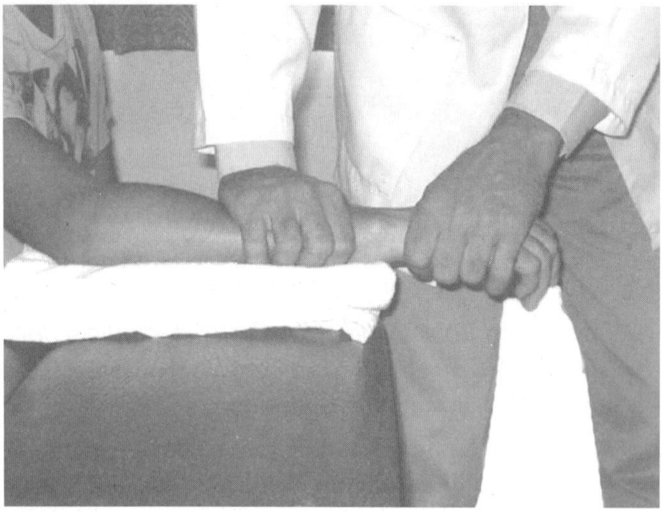

Fig. 7.22: Wrist joint traction

2. Dorsal and Volar Glides

Position of Patient, Therapist and Hands remain same as for traction.

Mobilization Force: While stabilizing the proximal part of the joint, the distal part is glided posteriorly (Dorsal) and anteriorly (volar) alternately with the traction (Figs 7.23a and b).

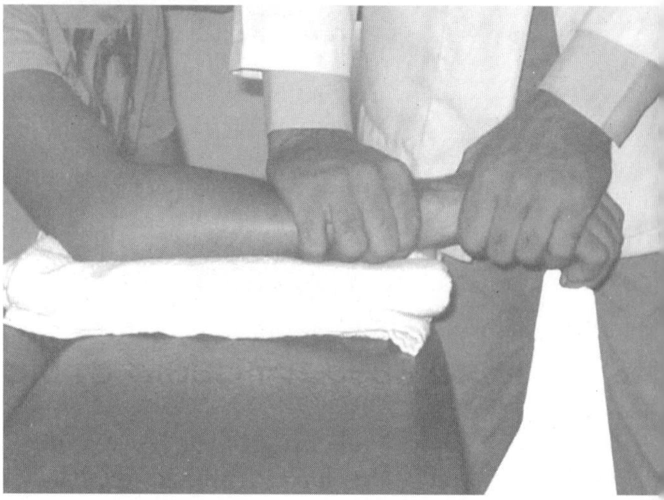

Fig. 7.23a: Wrist joint dorsal glide

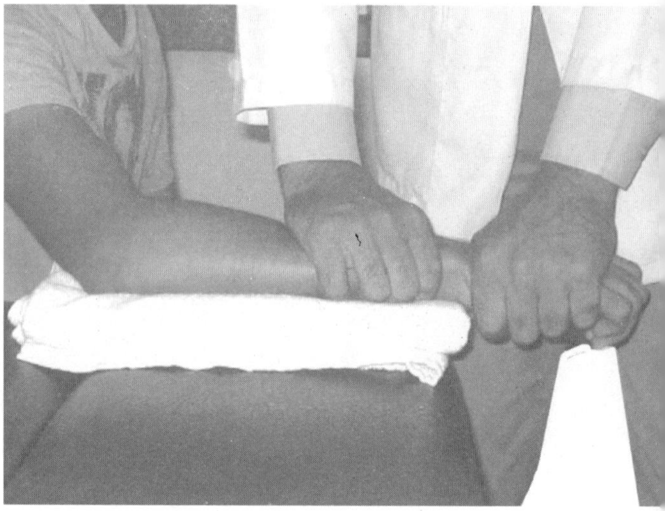

Fig. 7.23b: Wrist joint volar glide

3. Radial Glide and Ulnar Glide

Position of Patient and Therapist remain same as for traction. Therapist stabilizes the proximal part of the joint with one hand the other hand grasps the distal part of the joint.

Mobilization Force: The distal part of the joint is glided alternately toward the radial and ulnar side with the traction (Figs. 7.24a and b).

Intercarpal Joints

1. Volar Glide

Position of Patient: Supine or sitting elbow flexed to 90° and forearm is pronated and rested on treatment table.

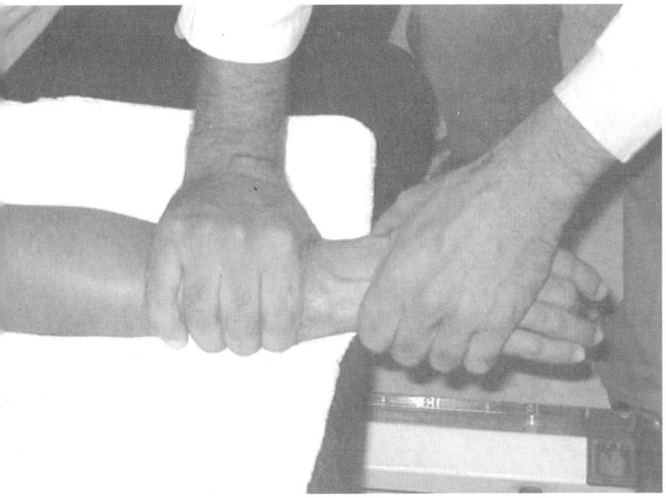

Fig. 7.24a: Wrist joint radial glide

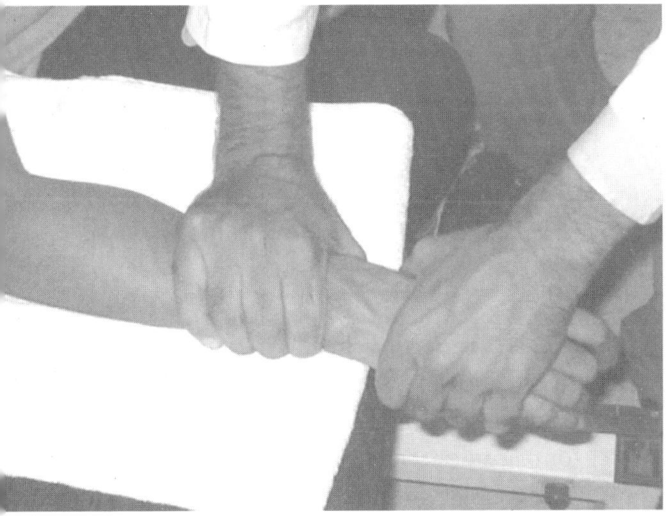

Fig. 7.24b: Wrist joint ulnar glide

Position of Therapist: Standing facing the joint, the thumb of one hand is placed over the dorsal aspect of carpal bone which is not being mobilized (proximal to the mobilizing bone). The thumb of other hand is placed over bone which is to be mobilized. Fingers of both hands rest on palmar surface of the corresponding bones.

Mobilizing Force: While stabilizing the one carpal bone, the other carpal bone is glided anteriorly (volar) (Fig. 7.25).

2. Dorsal Glides

Position of Patient: Supine or sitting elbow is flexed at 90° and forearm is supinated.

Position of Therapist: Standing, facing the joint, thumb of one hand is placed over the palmar aspect of the bone which is not being mobilized (next to the mobilizing bone), and index and middle fingers on the dorsal aspect of the same bone. The thumb of other hand is placed on the

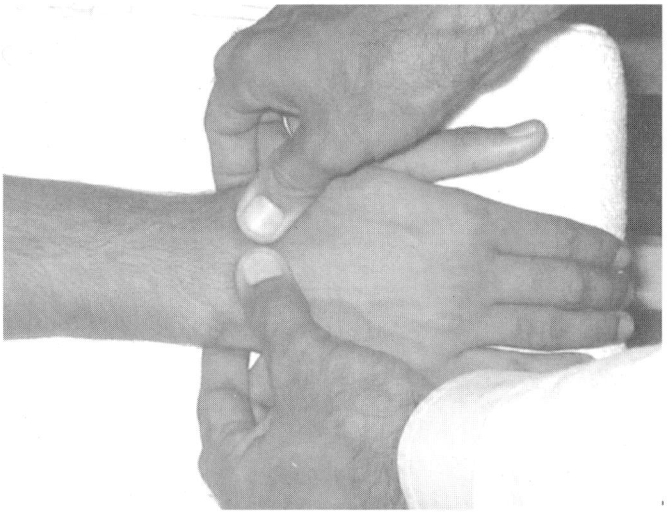

Fig. 7.25: Dorsal glide of intercarpal joint

palmar aspect of the carpal bone which is to be mobilized and fingers on the dorsal aspect of the same bone.

Mobilization Force: The bone which is being mobilized is glided posteriorly (dorsal) (Fig. 7.26).

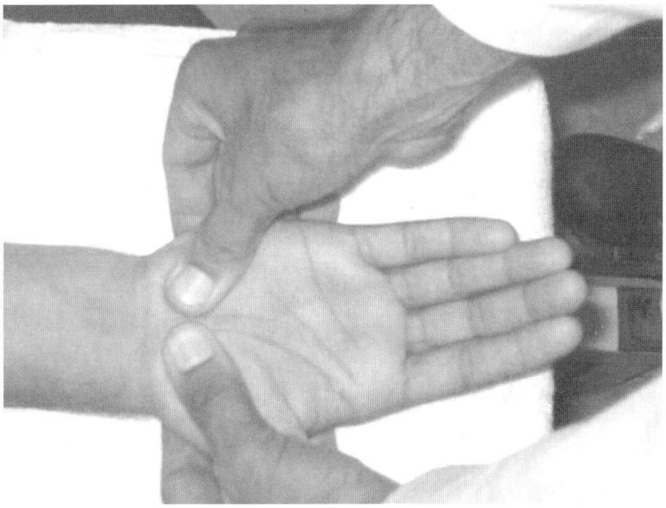

Fig. 7.26: Dorsal glide of intercarpal joint

Carpometacarpal (CMC) Joint

1. Palmar Glide (2nd to 5th Finger)

Position of Patient: Sitting on stool, hand rests on the treatment table with forearm pronated.

Position of Therapist: Standing, facing the joint. The proximal part of the CMC joint which is to be mobilized is stabilized with one hand, and the thumb of other hand is placed over the proximal part of the metacarpal bone, which is to be mobilized.

Mobilization Force: While stabilizing the proximal part of the joint the distal part is glided anteriorly (palmar) (Fig. 7.27).

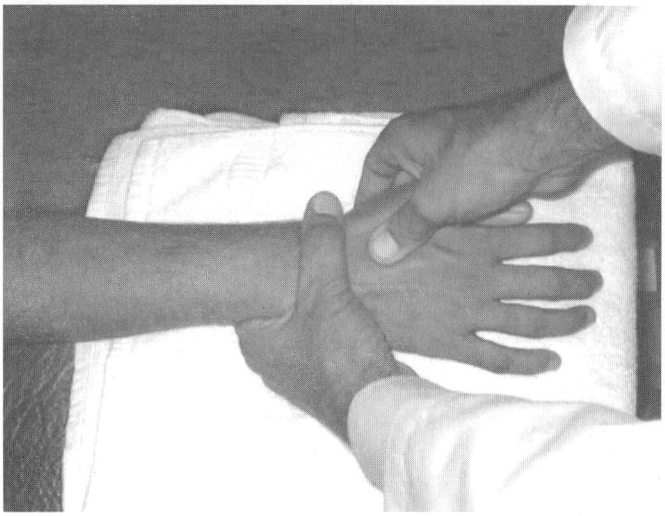

Fig. 7.27: Palmar glide of CMC joint

2. Volar and Dorsal Glide of the 1st CMC Joint

Position of Patient: Sitting, hand rests on treatment table with forearm in midprone position.

Position of Therapist: Standing facing the joint, the trapezium is stabilized with the one hand and other hand grasps the proximal part of 1st metacarpal bone (thumb on palmar aspect and index finger on dorsal).

Mobilization Force: While stabilizing the proximal part of the joint the distal is glided anteriorly (palmar) and posteriorly (dorsal) alternately (Fig. 7.28).

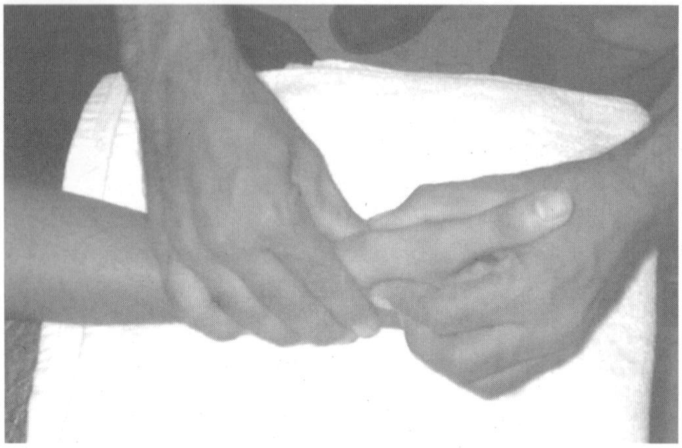

Fig. 7.28: Dorsal and palmar glide of 1st CMC joint

Metacarpophalangeal (MCP) Joint

Volar and Dorsal Glides

Position of Patient: Remains same as above, forearm may be in midprone position.

Position of Therapist: Standing, one hand stabilizes the proximal part of the joint and other grasps the distal part between the thumb and index finger.

Mobilization Force: While stabilizing the proximal par the distal part is glided anteriorly (volar) and posteriorly (dorsal) alternately. Each MCP and IP joint can b mobilized by following this maneuver (Fig. 7.29).

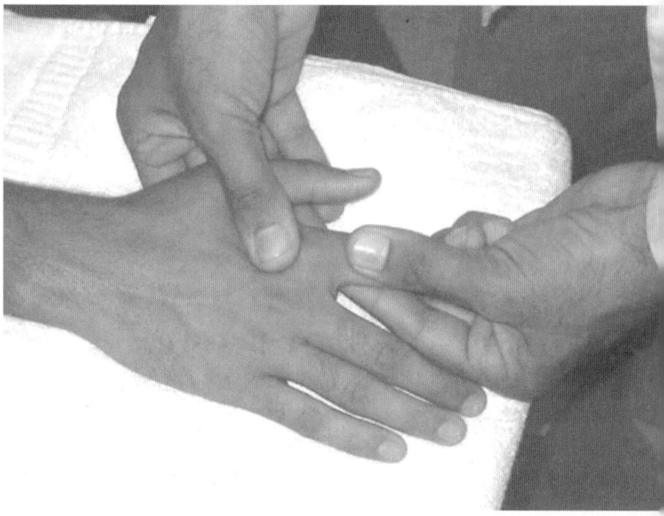

Fig. 7.29: Dorsal and palmar glide of IInd MCP joint

MANUAL MOBILIZATION TECHNIQUES OF LOWER LIMB JOINT

Hip Joint

Hip joint is formed by head of femur (convex) and acetabulum (concave) of the ilium. The joint is surrounded by large and thick muscles, therefore to achieve effective stretch on capsule, the therapist must concentrate on to apply gentle and significant force. To increase range of motion the articular surfaces are brought into the restricted range and then significant force is applied for gliding the joint surface to stretch the joint capsule.

1. Inferior or Caudal Glide

Position of Patient: Supine with hip in resting position with knee extended.

Stabilization: The pelvis is stabilized with the strap or by an assistant.

Position of Therapist: Standing at the end of the treatment table. A belt is used to apply longitudinal pressure force which is wrapped around the waist of the therapist and crosses over just above the ankle joint. The therapist places hands under the belt at the ankle joint as shown in Figures 7.30a and b.

Procedure: While maintaining above position the longitudinal force is applied with hands and the belt as therapist leans backward.

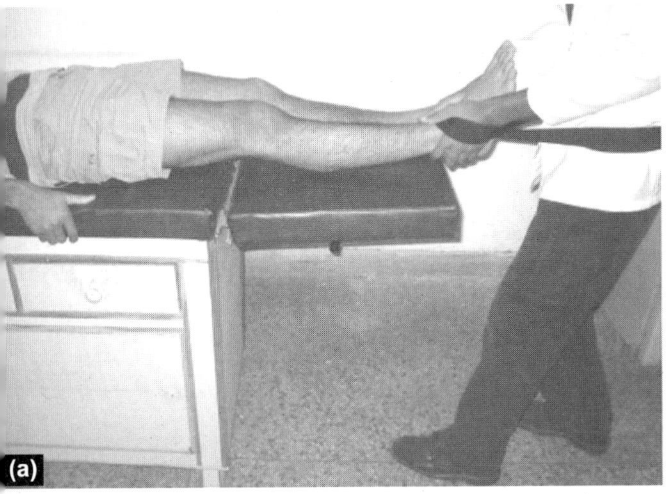

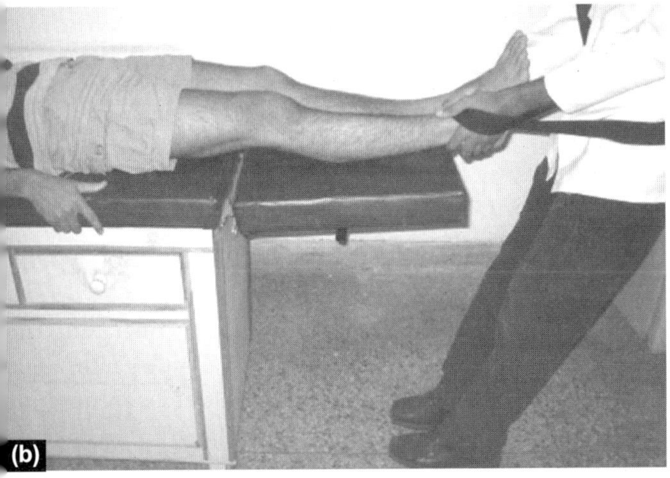

Figs. 7.30a and b: Inferior or caudal glide of the femur

In case of knee joint pain or dysfunction, belt is wrapped around the lower thigh (above patella) and hands are placed under it, the knee is kept flexed. A force is applied through the hands and belt which pulls the femur and causes inferior glide of head of femur.

2. Anterior Glide of the Head of Femur

Position of Patient: Side lying, the lower limb is flexed at hip and knee joints. The upper leg is supported by the pillows.

Position of Therapist: Standing, facing the anterior aspect of joint. A belt is used, which passes around the upper thigh (neck of femur) and wraps around the waist of therapist. Therapist places one hand over the pelvis and other just above the knee joint.

Procedure: While maintaining above position, therapist leans backward, to pull the proximal thigh anteriorly and to apply anterior glide of the head of femur. Both hands stabilize the pelvis and distal thigh (Fig. 7.31).

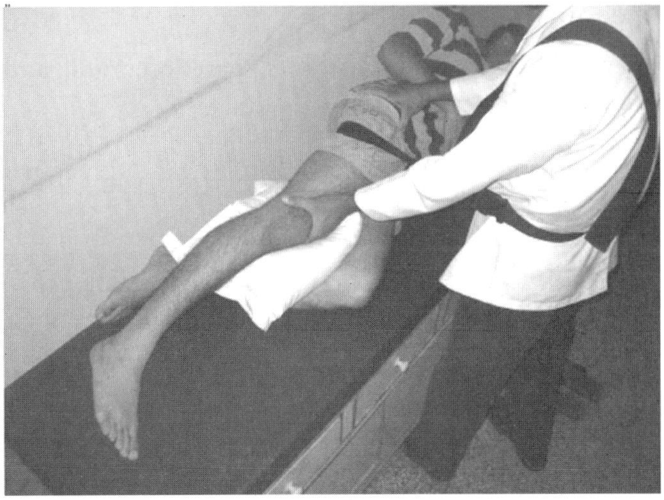

Fig. 7.31: Anterior glide of the head of femur

3. Posterior Glide of the Head of Femur

Position of Patient: Side lying, the lower leg is flexed at hip and knee joints, the upper leg (which is being mobilized may also be flexed slightly at hip and knee joints and supported by the pillows.

Position of Therapist: Standing, behind the patient facing the posterior aspect (gluteal) of the hip joint. A belt is applied around proximal end of the femur of the patient and wrapped around the waist of therapist. Therapist places one hand over the gluteal region and other on the posterior aspect of the distal thigh.

Procedure: While stabilizing the pelvis and distal thigh by the hands, therapist leans backward to pull the proximal thigh (head of femur) posteriorly and to apply posterior glide of the head of femur (Fig. 7.32).

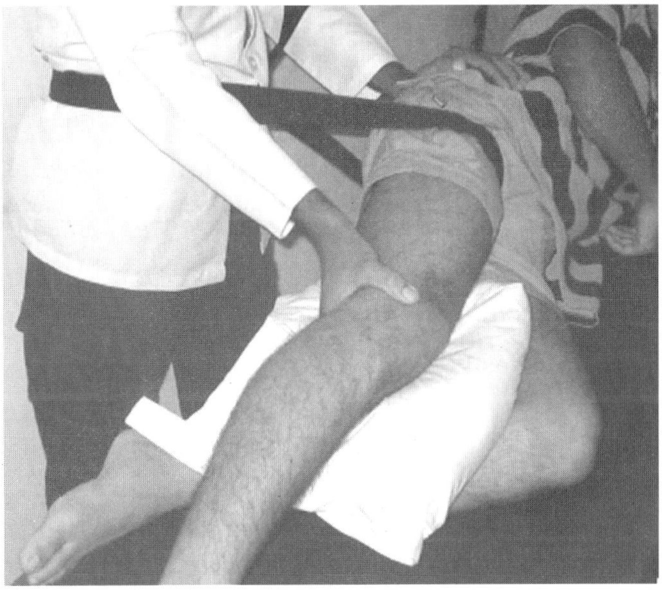

Fig. 7.32: Posterior glide of the head of femur

Knee Joint

The knee comprises two joints, patellofemoral and tibiofemoral:

1. Distraction of Tibiofemoral Joint

Technique No. 1:

Position of Patient: High sitting, knee is flexed slightly (45°).

Position of Therapist: Sitting, facing the anterior aspect of the joint, one hand grasps the leg above the ankle joint, and other is placed over distal thigh.

Procedure: A downward force is applied gently to place significant and effective stretch on capsule (Fig. 7.33).

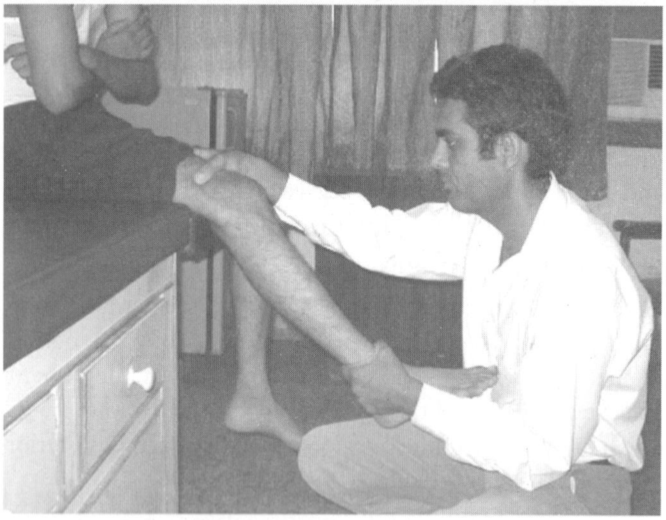

Fig. 7.33: Distraction of tibiofemoral joint

Technique No. 2:

Position of Patient: High sitting, knee is flexed at 45°, a wedge is placed under the knee joint. The proximal part of joint may be stabilized with the strap.

Position of Therapist: Standing at the end of treatment table, facing the joint (antero–inferior part). Both hands grasp the leg just above the ankle joint, then downward force is applied by leaning forward and bending the knees (Fig. 7.34).

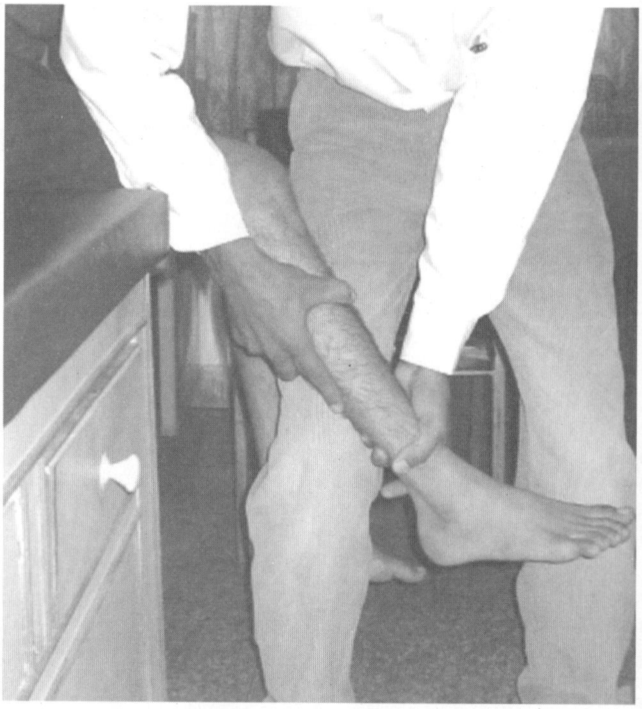

Fig. 7.34: Distraction of tibiofemoral joint

2. Tibiofemoral Joint Anterior Glide

Technique No. 1:

Position of Patient: High sitting, knee flexed to 25°, a wedge is placed under the proximal thigh and it is stabilized with straps.

Position of Therapist: Sitting, facing the anterior aspect of the joint. The ankle joint (involved side) is placed between the knees of therapist. One hand is placed over the knee joint and other grasps the lower leg. A belt is used which passes through posterior aspect of the knee and then around waist of therapist.

Procedure: While maintaining above position, the therapist pulls the proximal part of tibia with gentle force which places significant and effective stretch on anterior joint capsule (Fig. 7.35).

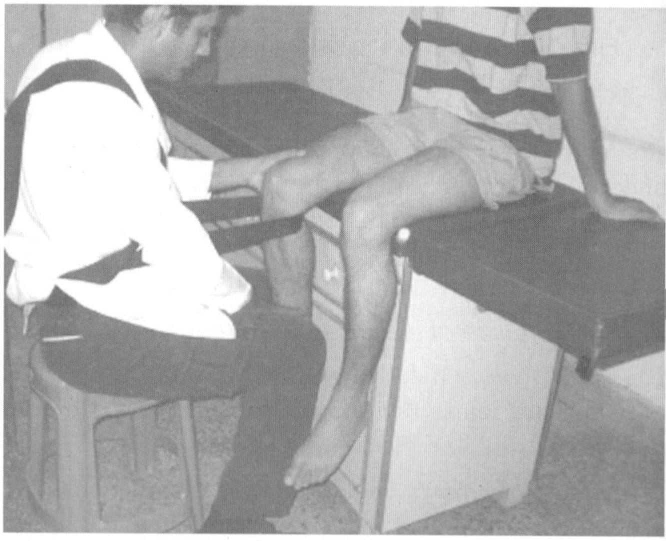

Fig. 7.35: Anterior glide of the proximal tibia

Technique No. 2:

Position of Patient: Supine, knee is flexed to 45°, the foot rests under the therapist's thigh.

Position of Therapist: Sitting on treatment plinth, grasps the proximal tibia (fingers placed on posterior aspect and thumbs on tibial tuberosity).

Procedure: While maintaining above position, a gentle force is applied to pull the upper end of tibia toward the body (Fig. 7.36).

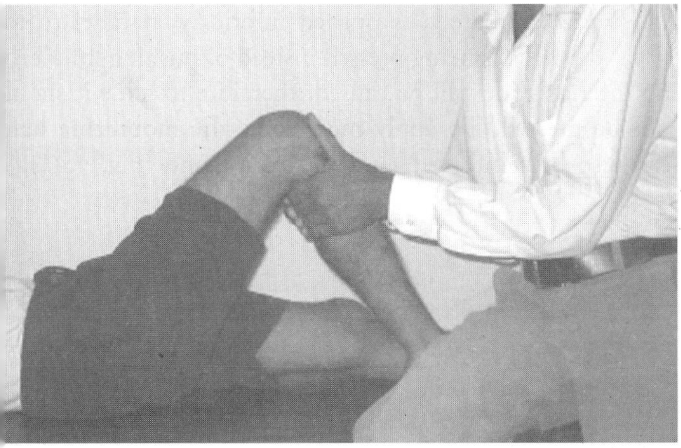

Fig. 7.36: Anterior glide of proximal tibia

Technique No. 3:

Position of Patient: Prone, knee is flexed to 25°. A wedge or small towel may be placed under the knee joint.

Position of Therapist: Standing, facing the joint. The mobilizing hand is placed on the posterior aspect of the tibia and an assisting hand grasps the leg at the ankle joint to maintain the flexion.

Procedure: While maintaining above position, mobilizing hand pushes the tibia with significant force, which glides the tibial condyles anteriorly with respect to the femoral condyles (Fig. 7.37).

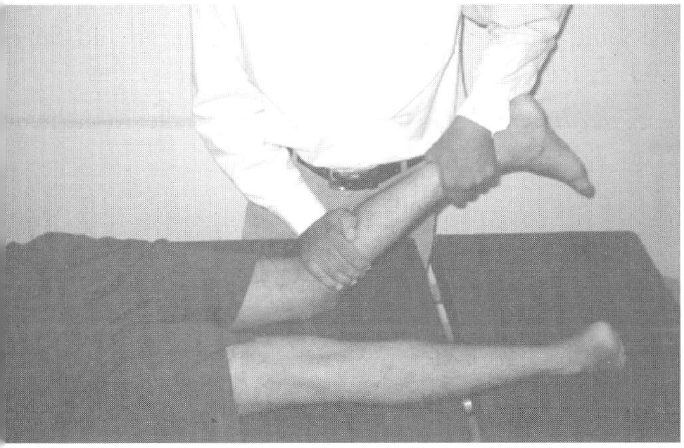

Fig. 7.37: Anterior glide of proximal tibia

3. Tibiofemoral Joint Posterior Glide

Technique No. 1:

Position of Patient: High sitting, knee is flexed to 90°.

Position of Therapist: Sitting, facing the anterior aspect of the joint, the ankle joint (involved side) is placed between the knees of therapist.

Procedure: While maintaining above position, the proximal end of tibia is pushed posteriorly by the thinar aspect of the hand. Force should be sufficient enough to glide the tibia posteriorly. Excessive force can damage the ligament and capsule (Fig. 7.38).

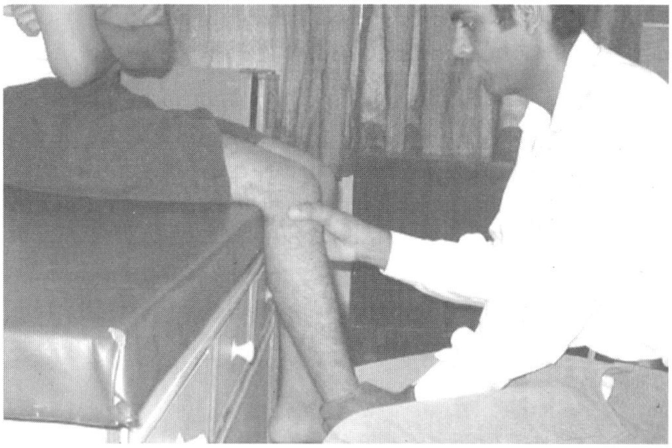

Fig. 7.38: Posterior glide of proximal tibia

Technique No. 2:

Position of Patient: Supine, knee is flexed at 25°, the heel rests on treatment table and toes on therapist's waist (A paper can be placed between toes and therapist's body).

Position of Therapist: Standing at the end of treatment table, leans forward and grasps the upper end of tibia (fingers placed on posterior aspect and thumbs on tibial tuberosity).

Procedure: While maintaining above position, therapist pushes the upper end of tibia with the thumbs and thenar aspect of hands. The force is transmitted through the body by leaning forward. It should be gentle and sufficient enough to cause posterior glide of the tibia (Fig. 7.39).

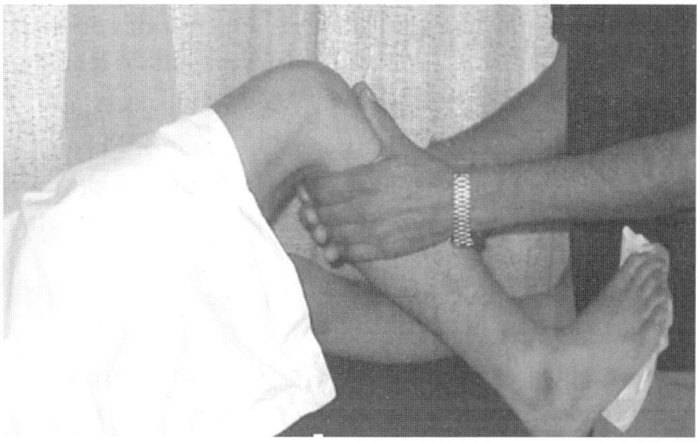

Fig. 7.39: Tibiofemoral joint posterior glide

4. Anteroposterior Glide of the Tibia

Technique 1:

Position of Patient: High sitting, knee is flexed to 25°, a wedge is placed under the popliteal fossa, thigh may be stabilized with straps.

Position of Therapist: Sitting, facing the anterior aspect of the joint. The involved side ankle joint is placed between the knees of therapist. The proximal end of tibia is grasped with both hands (fingers are placed on posterior aspect and thumbs on tibial tuberosity).

Procedure: Therapist pulls the tibia anteriorly then holds it for some time then releases the force gradually and pushes it posteriorly, and again holds it for sometime and releases the force gradually. It includes one cycle (anterior and posterior glides), (every cycle is followed by rest period. Generally to achieve good results and cause sufficient stretch on joint capsule, prolonged stretching of capsule is more effective) (Fig. 7.40).

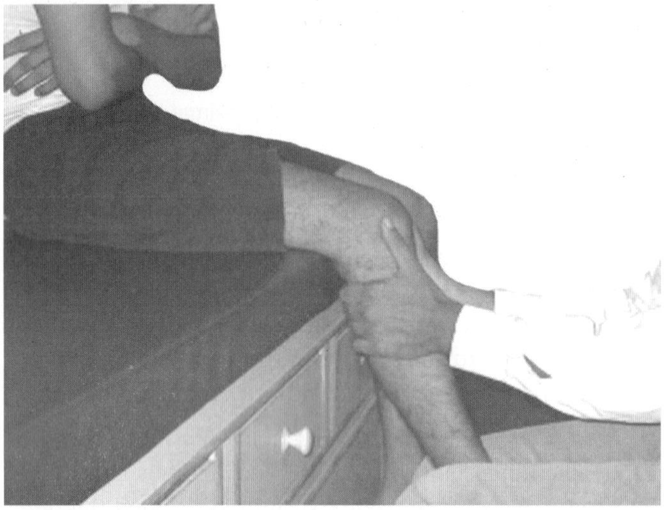

Fig. 7.40: Anterior posterior glide of proximal tibia

Technique No. 2:
The anteroposterior glides can also be performed in same position as in anterior glide of tibiofemoral joint, Technique No. 1.

Note: To increase flexion range of motion, the knee is flexed to its restricted range, then maintain the position and apply anterior and posterior glide of the tibia. After 10–15 repetition with rest period, again flex the knee joint to its next position (progression), maintain the position and apply glides. The procedure can be repeated several times to place sufficient stretch on joint capsule and periarticular structures.

Patellofemoral Joint

1. Inferior Glide of the Patella

Position of Patient: Supine, knee is extended, quadriceps relaxed.

Position of Therapist: Standing, facing the anterior aspec of the joint. A web space (formed by thumb and inde finger) is placed over the superior border of the patella.

Procedure: Patella is pushed inferiorly, parallel to th tibia. If patella is being pressed instead of pushing inferiorl no inferior glide will be caused, therefore to glide it shoul not be pressed. To apply more force the mobilizing han can also be reinforced by an assisting hand (Fig. 7.41).

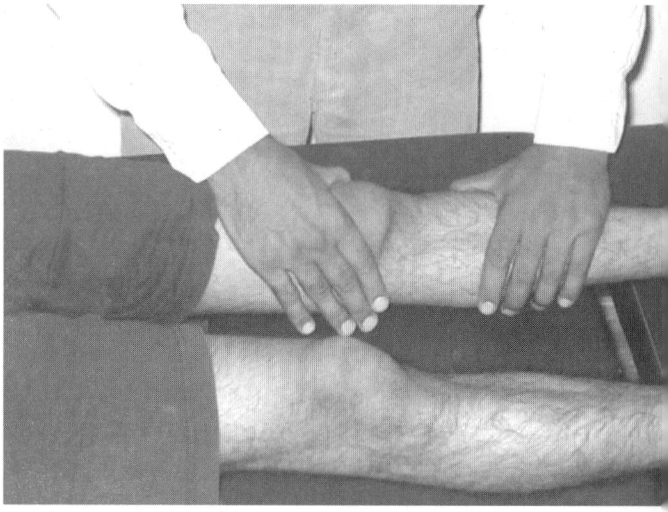

Fig. 7.41: Inferior glide of the patella

2. Superior Glide

Position of Patient: Supine, knee is extended, quadricep relaxed.

Position of Therapist: Standing, facing lateral aspect c the joint, patella is placed between the thumb and finge (web space).

Procedure: The patella is pushed up, parallel to the femu (Fig. 7.42).

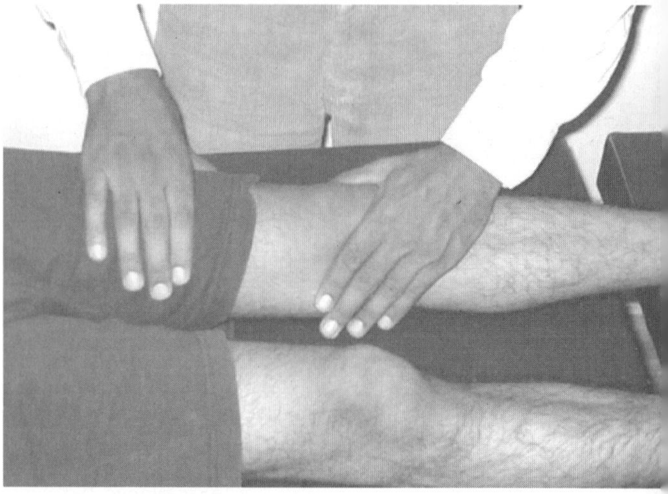

Fig. 7.42: Superior glide of the patella

3. Superoinferior Glide of the Patella

Position of Patient: Supine with knee extended.

Position of Therapist: Standing or sitting, facing anterior aspect of the joint. A web space is made between the thumb and fingers. The superior border of the patella is grasped with the web space of the one hand while other hand is placed over the inferior border of patella.

Procedure: Lower hand pushes the patella up, holds there for some time brings it to the neutral position, then push it down by the upper hand. The superior and inferior glide is followed by a brief rest period.

4. Mediolateral Glide of the Patella

Position of Patient: Supine, knee is extended, quadriceps relaxed.

Position of Therapist: Standing or sitting, facing the joint. The thumbs of both hands are placed over the medial aspect of the patella and fingers are placed over the lateral aspect of the patella.

Procedure: The thumbs push the patella laterally while fingers pull the patella toward the body alternatively (Figs. 7.43a and b).

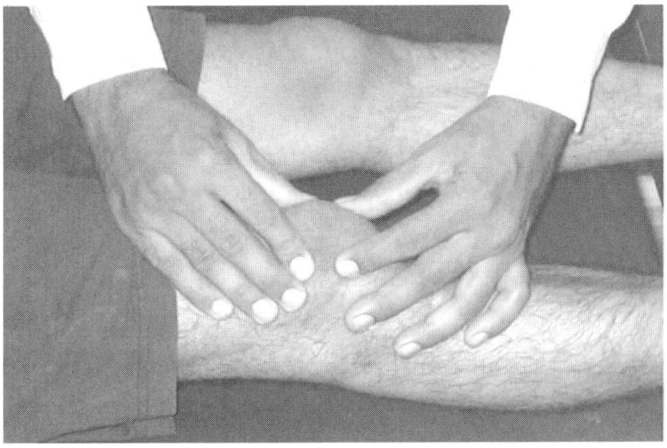

Fig. 7.43a: Medial glide of the patella

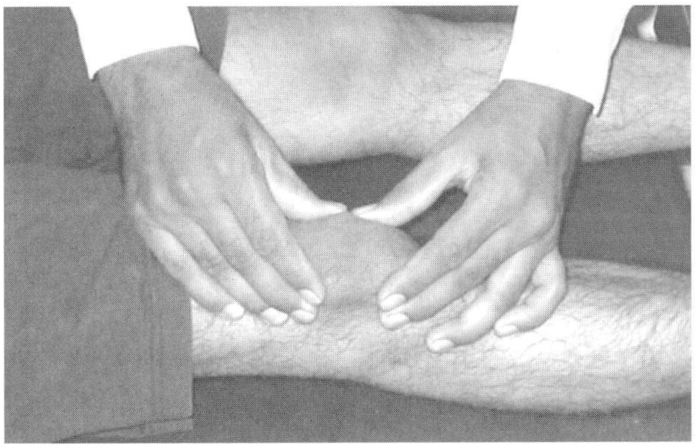

Fig. 7.43b: Lateral glide of the patella

Superior Tibiofibular Joint

1. Posterior Glide

Position of Patient: Side lying, lower limb is flexed at hip and knee joints.

Position of Therapist: Sits in front of the patient, tip of the thumb or pisiform aspect of heel is placed over the fibular head.

Procedure: The posterior directed pressure is exerted against the head of fibula through thumb or heel (Figs. 7.44a and b).

(a)

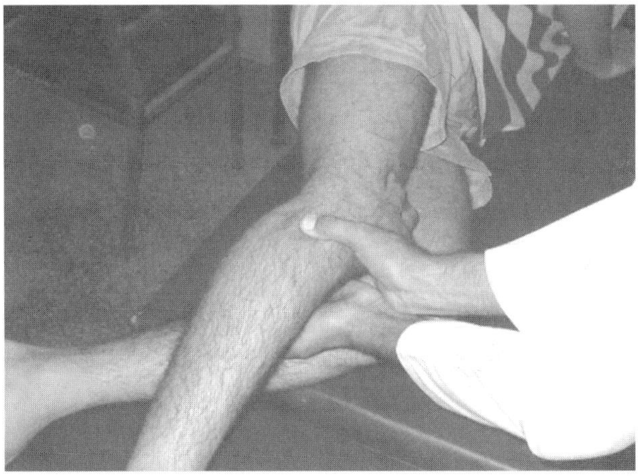

(b)

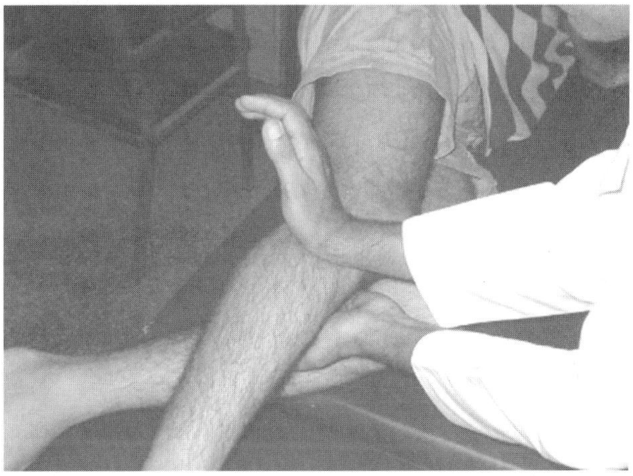

Figs. 7.44a and b: Posterior glide of proximal fibula (superior tibiofibular joint)

2. Anterior Glide

Position of Patient: Side lying, the upper leg is flexed slightly at hip and knee joint, a pillow may be placed under upper knee joint, lower limb rests on the plinth.

Position of Therapist: Stands behind the patient, the thumb or heel of one hand is placed over the posterior aspect of the fibular head, fingers rest on the anterolateral aspect of knee joint. The other hands grasps the tibia from medial side to stabilize it.

Procedure: The anterior directed pressure is exerted against the head of fibula through thumb or heel of mobilizing hand (Fig. 7.45).

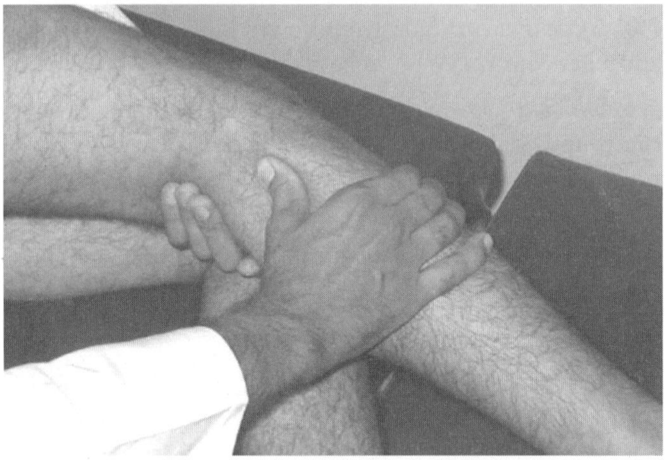

Fig. 7.45: Anterior glide of the proximal fibula

Inferior Tibiofibular Joint

1. Posterior Glide

Position of Patient: Side lying, the ankle rests on pillow and stabilizing hand.

Position of Therapist: Standing at end of treatment table. The heel of one hand is placed over anterior aspect of the lateral malleolus. The other hand grasps tibia at medial malleolus between the heel and fingers to stabilize the tibia.

Procedure: A posterior directed pressure is exerted against the lateral malleolus through the heel of one hand while other hand stabilizes the tibia (Fig. 7.46).

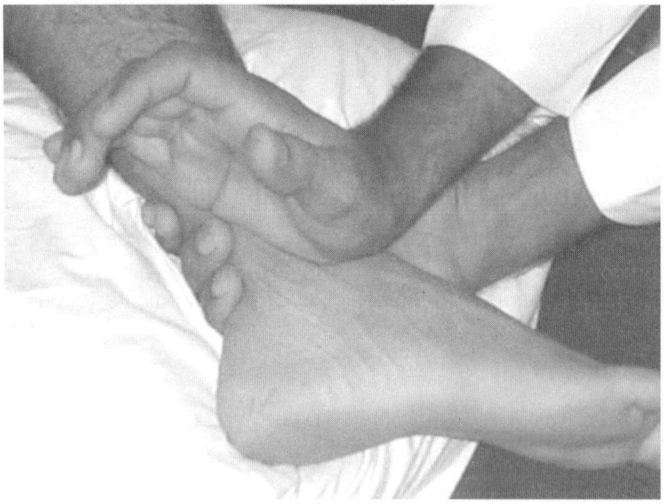

Fig. 7.46: Posterior glide (inferior tibiofibular joint)

2. Anterior Glide

Position of Patient: Side lying, the ankle joint rests on pillow and stabilizing hand.

Position of Therapist: Stands at the side of leg. The heel of upper hand is placed against the posterior border of the lateral malleolus.

Procedure: Anterior directed pressure is exerted against the lateral malleolus through the heel of one hand while other hand stabilizes the tibia (Fig. 7.47).

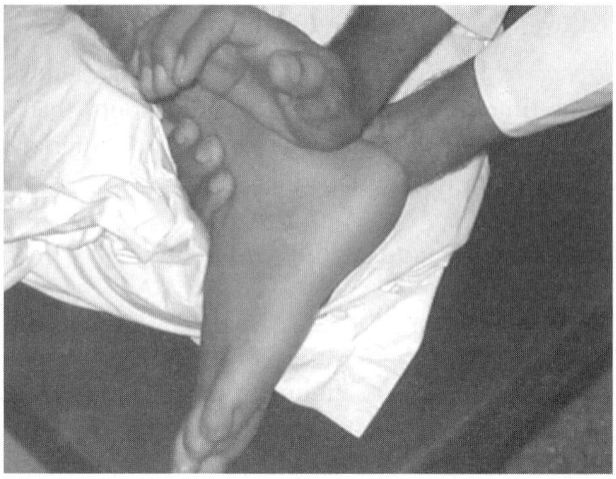

Fig. 7.47: Anterior glide (inferior tibiofibular joint)

Ankle Joint

1. Anterior Glide

Position of Patient: Prone lying with knee flexed to 90°.

Position of Therapist: Stands at the side of the patient. One hand grasps the calcaneum (the heel of hand is placed on posterior aspect of calcaneum and fingers rest on the palmar surface of calcaneum. The other hand is placed against the anterior border of tibia (the heel of hand is over the lower end of tibia while fingers pointing toward proximal part, thumb on the medial aspect of the tibia).

Procedure: The anterior directed pressure is exerted against the calcaneum through the upper hand while lower hand stabilizes the tibia (Fig. 7.48).

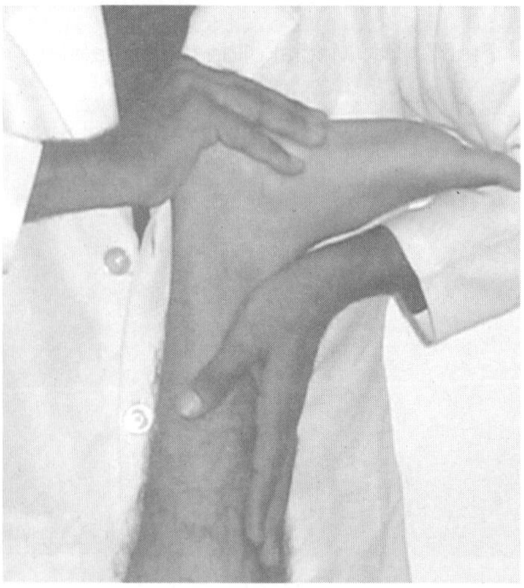

Fig. 7.48: Anterior glide of the ankle joint

2. Posterior Glide

Position of Patient: Prone lying with knee flexed to 90°.

Position of Therapist: Stands at the side of the patient. One hand grasps the distal part of the ankle joint (Index finger rests on the medial malleolus and thumb on the lateral malleolus while web of the 1st interosseous on the neck of the talus. The other hand holds the tibia to stabilize it (thenar and hypothenar aspect on the posterolateral side and fingers on the anteromedial aspect of tibia).

Procedure: The pressure is exerted through the web of upper hand while lower hand stabilizes the tibia (Fig. 7.49).

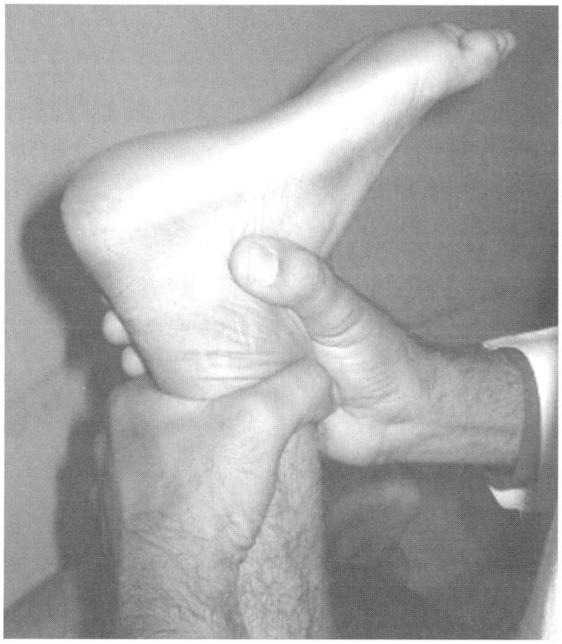

Fig. 7.49: Posterior glide of the ankle joint

3. Ankle Joint Compression

Patient is placed in prone position with knee flexion to 90°. Therapist stands at side of the patient, places both hands on the plantar surface of the heel. Therapist may flex his knee joint and place it on the plinth so that the anterior leg of patient rests on the inner aspect of the therapist's thigh. This is because it stabilizes the leg and controls the force. Therapist applies compression force to the ankle joint through the shoulders by leaning forward (Fig. 7.50).

Ankle Joint Traction: Patient is placed in prone position with the leg flexion. Therapist stands at the side of leg, grasps the distal part of ankle joint with both hands and places his knee joint (proximal part of the leg) over the posterior aspect of the patient's thigh to stabilize the knee joint. While maintaining the position therapist lift the ankle joint towards the ceiling with both arms.

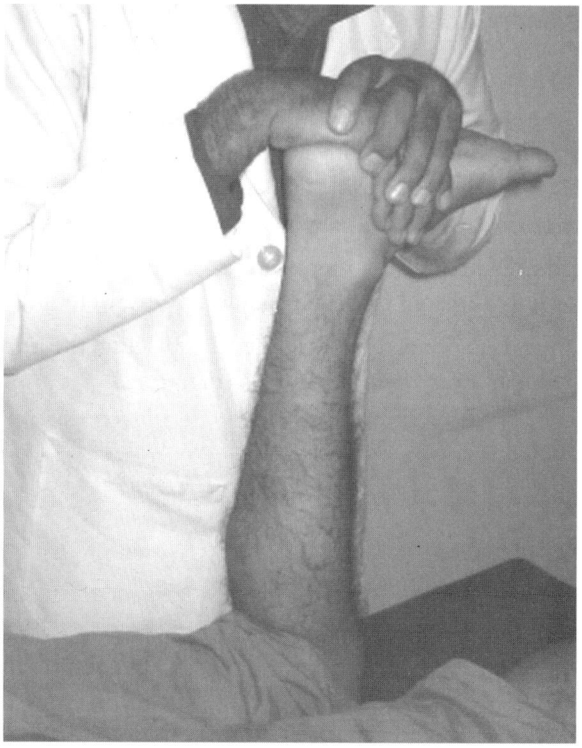

Fig. 7.50: Ankle joint compression

During the traction and compression of the ankle joint, repeated stress comes on the joint, so if patient is having any ailment the techniques should be performed gently or avoided (Fig. 7.51).

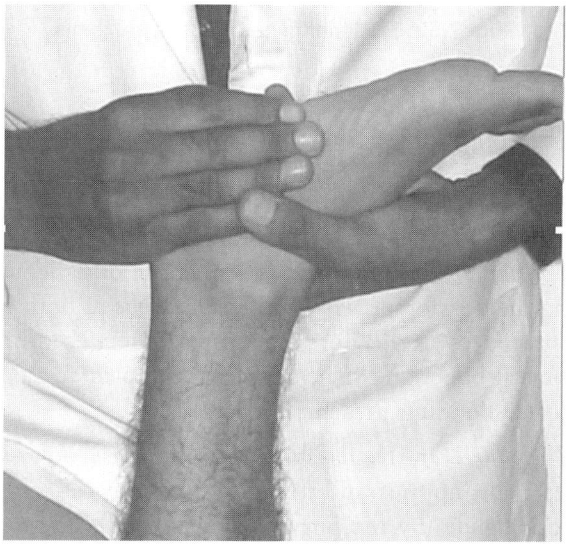

Fig. 7.51: Ankle joint traction

Intertarsal Joints

To perform *anterior and posterior* glides of tarsometatarsal joints the therapist should have knowledge of surface anatomy of the each tarsal bone so that appropriate placement of thumbs and fingers can be achieved satisfactorily.

Posterior Glide

Position of Patient: Supine lying, with hip and knee flexion.

Position of Therapist: At the end of the couch, facing the joint. The thumbs of both hands are placed over the dorsal aspect of tarsal bone which is being mobilized.

Procedure: The posterior directed pressure is exerted by the thumbs to cause posterior glide of tarsal bone. During posteriorly directed force, fingers do not exert any pressure.

All tarsal bones can be glided by placing the thumbs and fingers over them separately (Fig. 7.52).

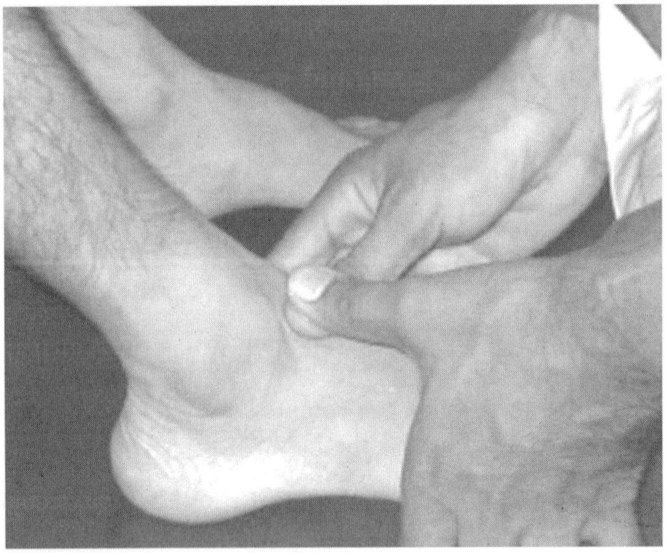

Fig. 7.52: Posterior glide of intertarsal joints

Intermetatarsal

Anteroposterior Glide

Position of Patient: Supine lying, the ankle joint remains out of the edge of treatment table.

Position of Therapist: Stands at the side of patient's leg, facing the dorsal aspect of foot. The thumbs of both hands are placed over the dorsal aspect of the two adjacent metatarsal bones and fingers are over the plantar aspect of the corresponding metatarsal bones.

Procedure: One hand stabilizes the metatarsal bone, while other hand applies anterior glide (by the thumb) and posterior glide (by the fingers of same hand), alternately.

For example, To mobilize the 1st metatarsal bone (anterior and posterior glide) the 2nd metatarsal bone is stabilized by one hand while other hand glides the I metatarsal bone in anterior and posterior direction (Fig. 7.53).

1st MTP Joint: The proximal segment of the joint is stabilized with one hand while other hand grasps the distal and glides it anteriorly and posteriorly (Fig. 7.54).

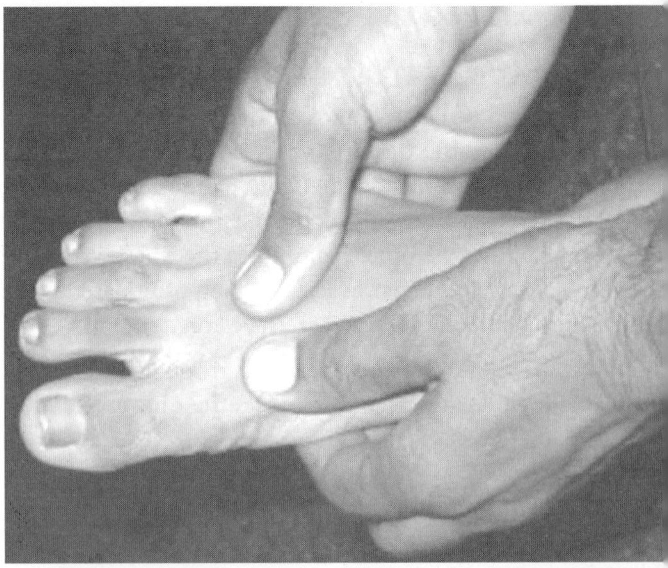

Fig. 7.53: Anterior posterior glides of intermetatarsal joints

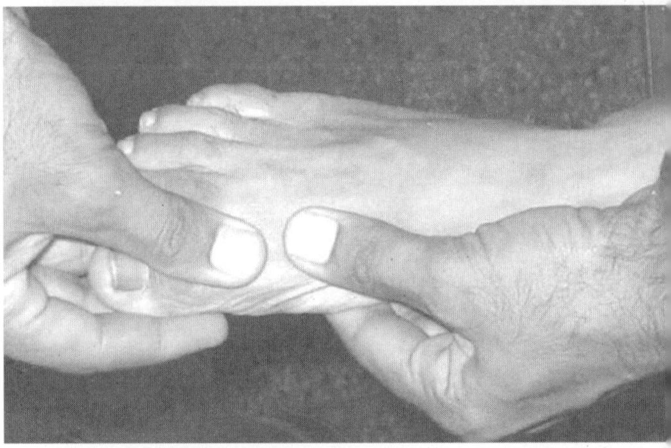

Fig. 7.54: Dorsal and palmar glide of 1st MTP joint

2nd MTP Joint: The proximal segment of the joint is stabilized with one hand while other hand grasps the dista segment and glides it anteriorly and posteriorly (Fig. 7.55)

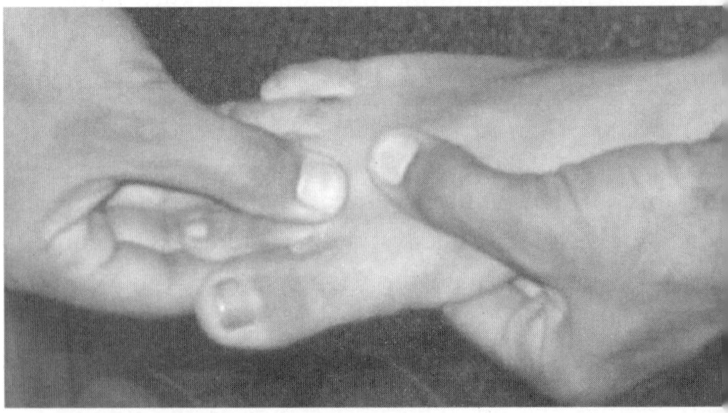

Fig. 7.55: Dorsal and palmar glide of 2nd MTP joint

Interphalangeal Joints

The proximal part of the joint is stabilized with the assisting hand and distal segment is moved anteriorly and posteriorly by the mobilizing hand.

8

BREATHING EXERCISES

INTRODUCTION

Exercises which are given to strengthen the respiratory muscles (Diaphragm, accessory costal and apical muscles) to maintain or increase the range of expiration and inspiration.

INDICATIONS OF BREATHING EXERCISES

1. Acute respiratory distress.
2. Chronic obstructive pulmonary disease (COPD), Asthma, Bronchiectasis.
3. Pneumonia.
4. Nervous system deficits or trauma which cause weakness of respiratory muscles:
   - High level spinal cord injury.
   - Acute, chronic or progressive myopathic or neuropathic diseases.
5. Ankylosing spondylitis.
6. Scoliosis, kyphosis which affect the respiratory function.
7 Stress.

Goals of Breathing Exercises

1. Improve ventilation.
2. Increase the effectiveness of the cough mechanism.
3. Improve the strength and endurance of respiratory muscles.
4. Maintain or improve chest and thoracic mobility.
5. Prevent pulmonary impairments.
6. Promote relaxation.
7. Maintain or improve the lung volumes and capacities.
8. To prevent atlectasis.

Classification of Breathing Exercises

Breathing exercises are classified on the basis of their locations:

1. Costal breathing
   a. Apical.
   b. Upper costal.
   c. Lower costal.
2. Diaphragmatic breathing exercise.
3. Glossopharyngeal breathing.
4. Pursed lip.
5. Pacebreathing.

It is very essential to understand that exercises can be given to patient at clinic or taught to patient so that he or she can learn and perform at home as prescribed by therapist. Whenever breathing exercises are taught following points should be kept in mind:

1. Position of patient.
2. Position of therapist's/patient's hands (placement of hands).
3. Resistance during expiration/inspiration.
4. Assistance during expiration or inspiration.

The best starting positions for these exercises are crook half-lying, crook lying and half lying.

1. Apical Breathing Exercise

Position of Patient: Crook lying, crook half lying, or half lying, adequate pillows can be placed under the knees, back and neck. Patient should be instructed to relax other muscles (shoulder girdle, lower limb and abdominal muscles).

Position of Patient's Hand: The fingers or the palm of patient rests over the clavicle with adduction of the fingers (Fig. 8.1).

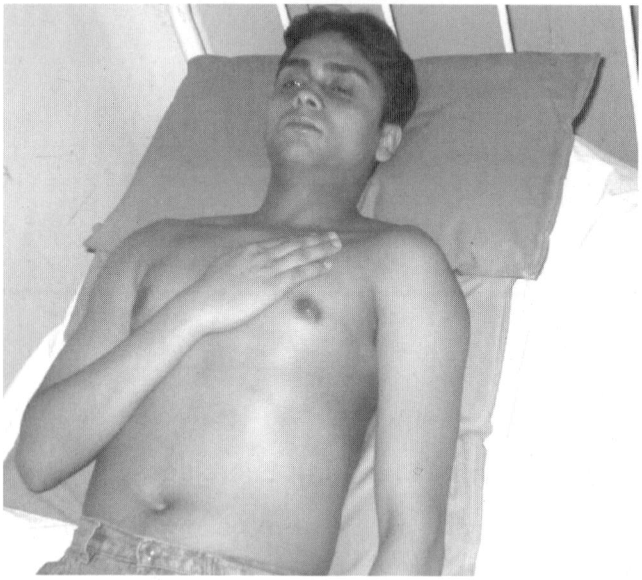

Fig. 8.1: Apical breathing—self resistance with the fingers

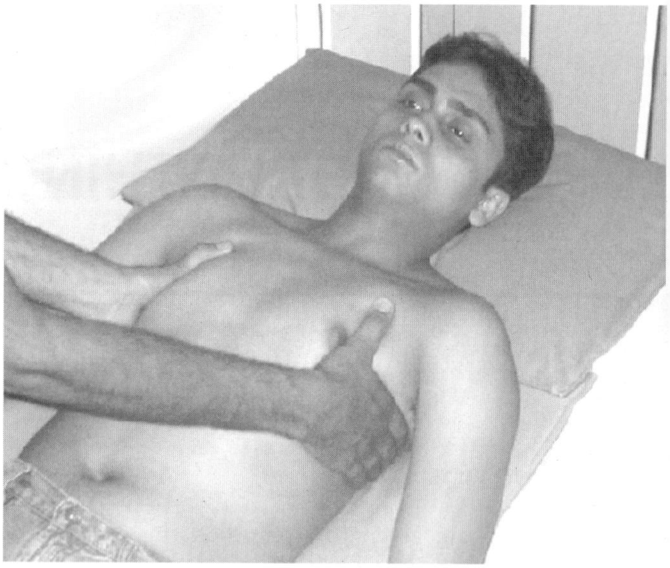

Fig. 8.2a: Upper lateral costal breathing

Resistance

The patient is instructed to 'blow' as he breathes out the therapist applies pressure against the chest. At the end of expiration therapist maintains pressure and asks the patient to breathe in under my hand and allow the chest to expand against the hands. Therapist decrease resistance as the limit of chest expansion is reached which allows maximum expansion to occur. The procedure is repeated for several repetitions. The exercise can be performed by patient himself or herself at home by placing the hand(s) over the apical part (clavicle) and applying resistance during inspiration and expiration as advised by therapist.

2. Costal Breathing

I. Upper Lateral and Lower Costal

Position of Patient: Crook lying, crook half lying, or half lying, adequate pillows can be placed under the knees, and upper back. Patient should be instructed to relax abdominals, shoulder girdle and lower limb muscles (Figs. 8.2a and b).

Position of Therapist: Patient turns his or her neck to the opposite of therapist. Therapist uses both hands and places over the upper lateral costal and lower lateral costal.

Resistance

The therapist instructs the patient to blow. As patient breathes out therapist applies pressure and at the end of expiration therapist maintains it and asks patient to breathe in against my hands. The resistance is decreased as the limit of expansion is reached, which allows maximum expansion to occur. The procedure is repeated several times and therapist changes hands from upper lateral costal to the lower lateral costal, and repeats same procedure. The exercise can also be performed by patient himself or herself by placing hands over lateral costal (upper and lower) (Figs. 8.2c and d).

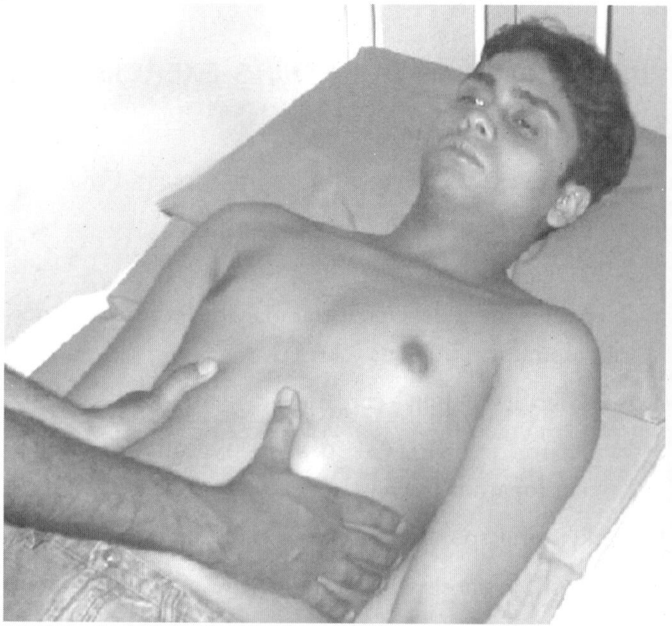

Fig. 8.2b: Lower lateral costal breathing

II. Posterior Basal Costal Breathing

Position of Patient: Arm lean forward crook sitting.

Position of Therapist's Hand: Heels of hands rest on lateral to the rib angles (Fig. 8.3) fingers lie along the line of the eighth, ninth and tenth ribs, and thumb is just below the scapula. Therapist asks patient to breathe out and applies pressure and at the end of expiration therapist maintains

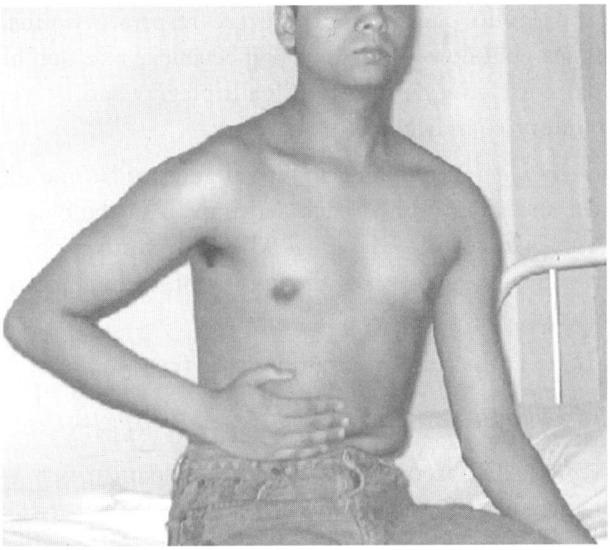

Fig. 8.2c: Self resistance unilateral lower costal breathing with whole hand

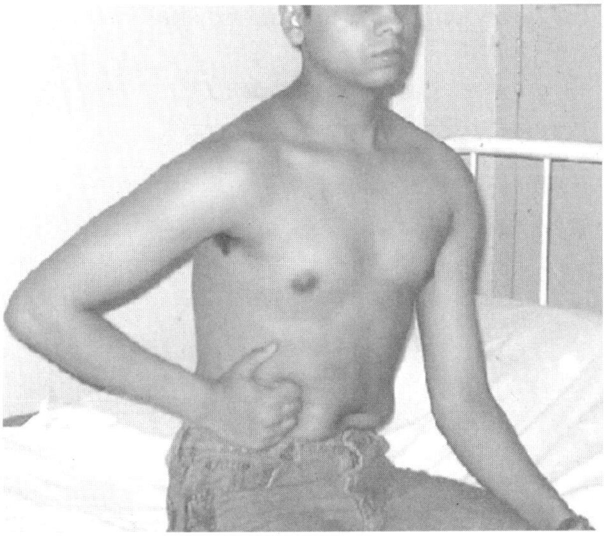

Fig. 8.2d: Self resistance unilateral lower costal breathing with the back of the fingers

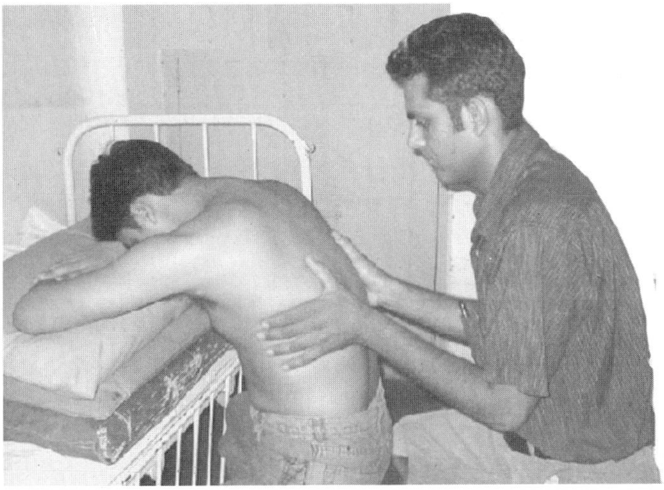

Fig. 8.3: Arm lean forward crook sitting posterior basal breathing–therapist resisting

pressure and asks patient to breathe in and applies resistance against inspiration. The resistance decreases as the limit of expansion is reached, which allows maximum expansion to occur.

3. Diaphragmatic Breathing

Diaphragmatic breathing is the most common form of breathing which has to be caught to a patient to improve the efficiency of ventilation, decrease the work of breathing and improve gas exchange and oxygenation. This exercise helps to strengthen the diaphragm muscle (Figs. 8.4a and b).

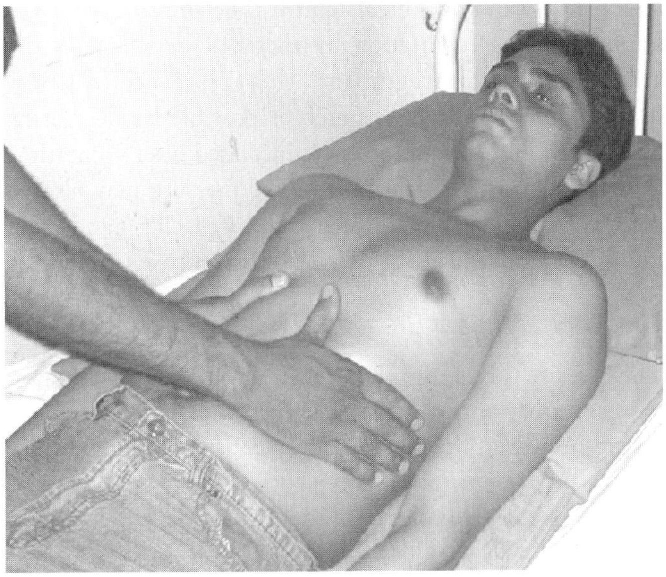

Fig. 8.4a: Diaphragmatic breathing

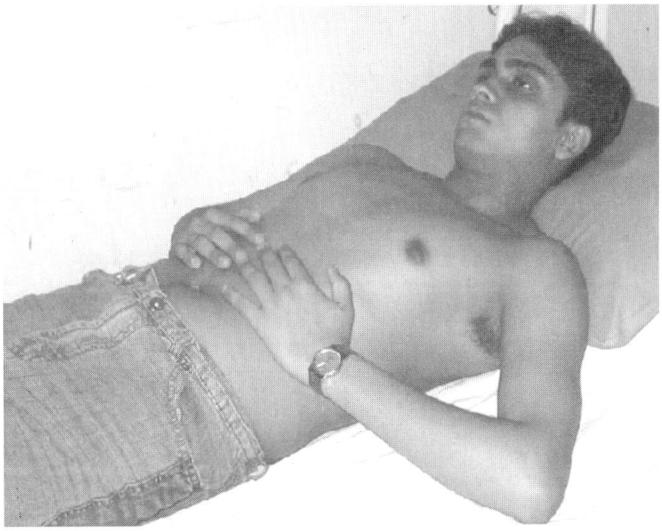

Fig. 8.4b: Half lying practising diaphragmatic breathing

Position of Patient: Crook half lying, adequate pillows are placed under the knees and upper back. The patient is instructed to relax the shoulder girdle and upper chest muscles.

Position of Therapist's Hands: Over the rectus abdominals just below the anterior costal margin. The patient is then instructed to breathe out by asking him to blow gently. This will ensure an expiratory action and he is made aware of the inward movement of the costal margins. The therapist applies gentle pressure at the end of expiration and asks patient to breathe in against my hands. The therapist decreases the pressure as the limit of abdominal expansion is reached to its limit. If the diaphragm is being used in its middle inner range the costal margin will separate whereas the intercostal (central epigastric) area will swell slightly. But if the diaphragm is contracting in its outer range the abdominal wall will bulge slightly. The pressure which is applied during inspiration by therapist depends on the strength of diaphragm and therapist should allow diaphragm to contract as much as possible by decreasing resistance. The pressure may be increased after some time as diaphragm gets strengthened. The pressure may also be applied by patient himself or herself by placing hands over the rectus abdominals below the anterior costal margin.

Glossopharyngeal Breathing

The exercise is basically given when there is severe weakness of respiratory muscles and patients who have difficulty taking in a deep breath. Initially exercise was designed for the postpolio patients with severe respiratory muscle weakness, but now-a-days is having beneficial effect on high spinal cord injury patients (Quadriplegia) and prevents respiratory complications to develop.

Technique: After taking in several gulps of air, mouth is closed and air is pushed back and traps it in the pharynx. The air is forced into the lungs when the glottis is opened. This increases the depth of the inspiration and the patients' vital capacity.

Uses: To increase inspiratory capacity.

Pursed-lip Breathing

Procedure: The procedure is explained to patient very well that forceful expiration should be avoided.

The patient is placed on suitable position, then instructed to breathe in slowly and deeply then have the patient slowly purses the lips and exhale.

Uses:

- COPD.
- Dyspnea.
- Atelectasis
- Bronchiectasis.

9

THERAPEUTIC MASSAGE (SOFT TISSUE MANIPULATION)

INTRODUCTION

Therapeutic massage helps to smooth away stress, unknotting tense and aching muscle, relieving headache and helping sleep problems.

The word massage comes from the Greek *masso* meaning to kneed. In classical Greek culture, massage flourished. The physician, Aesculapius was known as the God of healing in Greek mythology because of his use of massage in healing. Hippocrates (460-377 BC), known as the father of medicine, described the benefits of using oils and massage on joints.

In the Greek countryside, the ruins of healing centres such as Epidourous can be seen today.

In the ancient Roman massage was the part of daily life.

The Traditional Chinese Medicine (TCM) includes various components of massage (Chi Gong exercises, herbals, acupuncture and massage).

Sanskrit word *makeh* means to press softly. In India, rubbing was used in connection with religious ceremonies, cleaning rituals developed into a form of medicine known as Ayurvedic Medicine.

Development

History shows that although the early Egyptians made reference to the benefit of massage but the Chinese were among the first to recognize its healing value at around 3000 BC. Roman and Greek philosophers and physicians prescribed it both for its restorative powers after battle and for general preservation of the body and mind. Although Roman believed in its curative powers.

Ling (Per Hinrik Ling 1776-1839) was a Swede who travelled to China and returned with a detailed insight into their techniques. *From there he developed his own system of massage based on a variety of movements.* The practical knowledge of massage gradually spread all over the world. Today massage is established on the basis of its movements or strokes but in many ways the technique of massage remain same as those early Swedish massage. The benefit of massage is being explored by various medical and non-medical professionals worldwide.

Definitions

The term is used to designate certain manipulations of the soft tissues of the body; these manipulations are most effectively performed with the hands and are administered for the purpose of producing effects on the nervous, muscular, and respiratory systems and the local and general circulation of the blood and lymph (beard).

Maneuvers performed by the hands of a therapist on the skin of a patient and through the skin on the subcutaneous tissues. Massage manipulations may be stationary or progressive; they may be variable in intensity of pressure exerted, surface area treated and frequency of application (Boni and Walthard, 1956).

Massage is the scientific manipulation of the soft tissues of the body, as apart from mere rubbing (Prosser, 1941).

PHYSIOLOGICAL EFFECTS

It is very important for the clinician to understand how the body reacts or responses to the different strokes of soft tissue manipulation (STM) techniques. Any form of STM technique, applied on the tissues causes several physiological changes on the different systems of the body. The body responses to massage in two ways:

1. Mechanical response; and
2. Reflexive response.

Mechanical Response

It refers to the direct effects/influences of STM on the soft tissues being manipulated. Every stroke of soft tissue manipulation technique causes mechanical response. The examples of mechanical response are—increasing blood circulation, reducing swelling and breaking up of scar tissues.

Reflexive Response

It refers to the indirect effects/influences of soft tissue manipulation techniques on tissues. Neural mechanisms are influenced by manual intervention on the tissue. The process is centered on the inter-relationship of the peripheral (cutaneous) and central nervous systems, their reflex patterns and multiple pathways. The reflex effect of massage is perhaps more significant than its mechanical action. The reflexive responses are such as increasing the diameter of blood vessels, reducing blood pressure and general relaxation.

A massage response can be primarily mechanical or reflexive in nature but both responses are closely related and often occur simultaneously. Reflex responses to STM frequently occur due to mechanical stimulation of nerve receptors.

1. *Cardiovascular*

- Increases blood circulation.
- Decreases blood pressure.
- Release of histamine and acetylcholine cause dilatation of the blood vessels.
- Removes metabolic waste products and nutrients.
- Stimulates vasomotor nerves.
- Increases systolic stroke volume.
- Decreases heart rate.
- Increases RBCs, WBCs, Platelets.
- Decreases ischaemia.

2. *Lymph and Lymphatic System*

- Decreases lymphedema (swelling).
- Strengthens immune system.

  Clears away debris, fat and unwanted substances.

3. *Skin*

The sebaceous glands are situated in the skin, these glands get stimulated when the skin is rubbed, and secrets the sebum which improves the skin condition, texture and tone. The superficial effleurage on face causes tone up the face.

The superficial blood vessels (arterioles and capillaries) get dilated as they are massaged and increase the local blood circulation. This effect:

- Keeps the skin healthy.
- Increase insensible perspiration.
- Increases vasomotor activity.
- Decreases formation of superficial keloids and excessive scar formation.

4. *Nervous System*

The sensory receptors situated in the skin, gets stimulated as the skin is pressed, rubbed, squeezed or touched. The information about the type of stimuli is sent to the brain, and makes the brain aware of the stimuli.

The strokes of massage such as superficial effleurage, superficial vibration, superficial friction and shaking soothen the nervous system and causes sedative effect.

The strokes of STM such as deep effleurage, Tapotement, Petrissage (deep), deep transverse friction having stimulating effect on nervous system (These strokes are discussed later in the chapter).

The afferent (sensory) neuron transmits information from the tissues and organs of the body to the central nervous system (CNS). The efferent (motor) neuron transmits information out from the CNS to effector cells (muscle on gland) which receives and reacts to the impulse in following ways:

- Stimulates and soothes the nervous system.
- Releases endorphin, enkephalins, and other pain reducing neurochemicals.
- Stimulates parasympathetic nervous system and promotes relaxation, decreases insomnia and improves sleeping pattern.
- Decreases stress related hormones such as norepinephrine and cortisol.
- Increases in dopamine and serotonin levels.

5. *Muscular System*

1. Increases extensibility of muscle fibres.
2. Decreases stiffness.
3. Breaks adhesion formation between muscle fibres.
4. Decreases muscle spasm.
5. Increases muscular relaxation.
6. Increases blood circulations.

CLASSIFICATION OF MASSAGE (TABLE 9.1)

1. Effleurage.
2. Petrissage.

Table 9.1: Classification of therapeutic massage

Effleurage	1. Superficial	
	2. Deep	
Petrissage	1. Kneeding	: Palmar kneading
		: Finger pad kneading
		: Thumb pad kneading
		: Knucle kneading
		: Reinfinforced kneading
	2. Picking up	
	3. Wringing	
	4. Skin rolling	
Tapotement	1. Clapping	
	2. Beating	
	3. Hacking	
	4. Pouding	
Friction	1. Superficial	
	2. Deep	: Deep Transverse Friction (James Cyriax)
		: Circular Deep Friction
Vibration		
Shaking		

3. Tapotement.
4. Friction.
5. Vibration.
6. Shaking.

PREPARATION OF MATERIALS

Room

The room in which therapeutic massage has to be applied should be free from all sort of noises (telephone, traffic etc). The room should not have bright lights. Curtain should be used to avoid sunlight.

Treatment Plinth

It is an essential tool in the practice of massage. The dimensions of the table should be at least 28 × 72 inches and adjustable for height to accommodate for various needs. It should be solid and firm. Adjustable head support may also be added (Figs. 9.1a to c).

Supports

Towels, pillows of various sizes, bed sheets, wedges; commercially available bolsters etc. can be used to provide support.

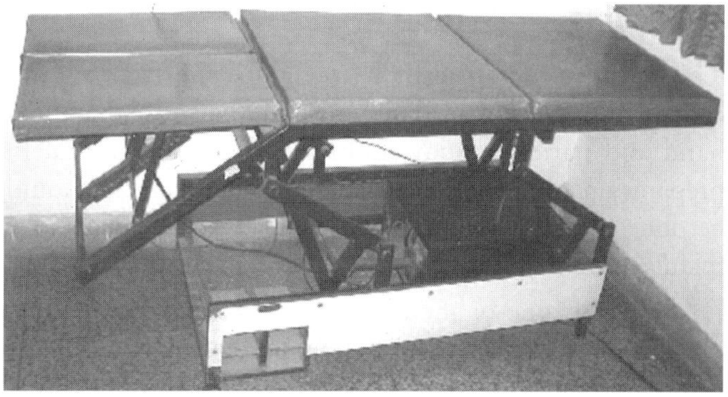

Fig. 9.1a: Treatment plinth

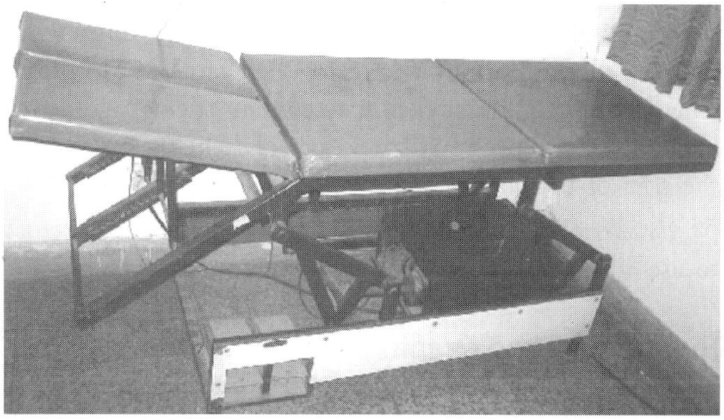

Fig. 9.1b: Inclined treatment plinth (adjustable head support)

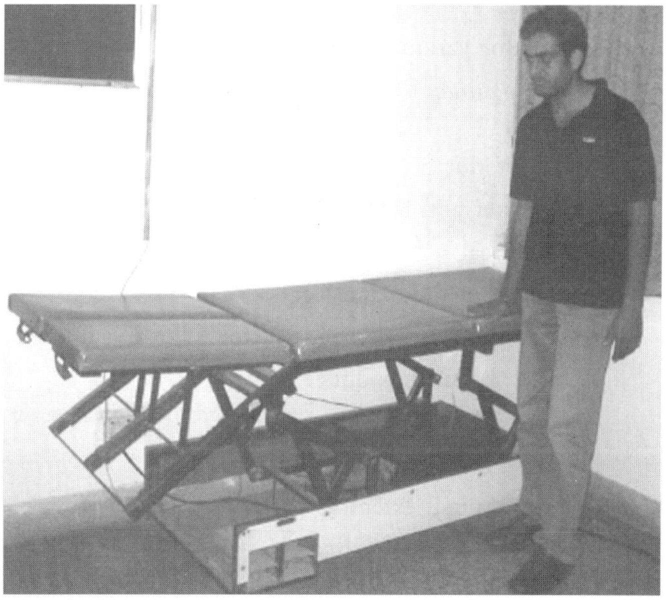

Fig. 9.1c: Measurement of treatment plinth shown by therapist by placing the hand on the plinth with dorsiflexion of wrist (ideal height)

Linen

Cotton material is preferred. All linen should be bleachable. Pillow covers, small and large size towel, bed sheets and blankets are among the common linen supply.

Lubricants

The purpose of lubricant is to reduce the friction and control the amount of drag and glide between therapists hand and patient's body. Lubricants are also helpful in preparation of subcutaneous tissue, but their use should be done as and when need arises. Following lubricants are mainly used in practice:

Oils: It is one of the commonly used lubricants vegetable oil such as olive, coconut, almond etc. are considered to be more nutritious for skin as compared to mineral oil. Unabsorbed oil should be wiped from the client's skin by using tissue paper or small towel.

Creams are thicker suspension. They lie somewhat between oil and lotion in terms of their rate of absorption. They promote glide or they may contain sticky ingredients like lanolin and bee wax that reduce glide helps in dragging the skin of the client.

Powder: Used for gliding and also when patient refuse to use oil. It is also preferred for lymph drainage technique.

Positioning and Draping

Positioning: It depends upon the aim of treatment, the parts to be assessed or treated, client's preference and comfortability. Prone lying, supine, sidelying, seating, seated inclined and long-sitting are commonly used.

Positions for various muscles:

i. *Prone position:* Recommended position for treatment of:
   - Posterior neck muscles.
   - Upper and lower back muscles.
   - Gluteal region.
   - Back of thigh and leg.
   - Position can also be used for following muscles:
     - Latissimus dorsi.
     - Rhomboid.
     - Trapezius.
     - Spinal extensors.
     - Gluteus maximus.
     - Hamstrings.
     - Triceps surae.
     - Foot intrinsics.

ii. *Supine Position:* Recommended for all muscles of head and neck, pectoralis, arm, abdominal, quadriceps and anterior compartment of leg.

iii. *Sidelying*: Scalenes, Rotator cuff, pectoralis minor, serratus anterior, abdominals, quadratus lumborum, intercostals, gluteus medius and minimus, iliotibial tract, peronei, adductors of the hip and triceps surae.

iv. *Seated upright:* Upper trapezius.

v. *Seated inclined:* Muscles of the posterior aspect of the head and neck, Muscles of the upper back, Muscles of posterior aspect of the upper arm.

Draping

Draping should place the client in safe, warm and comfortable position to receive the desired massage. It should maintain the boundary between the patient and therapist in all practice settings including training setup. It sets a symbolic and an actual boundary hence therapist must make draping comfortable, yet precise and secured when exposing the clients body for treatment purposes.

Undraping Rules

- One part should be undraped at a time.
- Undrape only those area which has to be treated.
- Gluteal cleft, perineum, genital and female breast should not be undraped.

  The female breast may be exposed if massage is clinically indicated by taking prior consent from the patient. Similarly pelvis may be undraped by taking prior consent and informing the patient about the importance of massage for that area (such as in labor/delivery).
- Infants under the age of two years may be treated undraped.
- Students must practice the draping technique repeatedly and extend appropriate respect to each other during classroom practice.

Draping Techniques

i. *Undraping the female torso:* A folded towel is placed on top of the sheet over the breasts. The patient holds the edge of the towel while the clinician withdraw the sheet from under the towel. The towel is tucked under the torso or arms then the abdomen is exposed from xiphoid process to the anterior superior iliac spine.

ii. *Undraping the anterior leg:* After exposing and lowering the leg the extra sheet is gathered between the legs. The extra sheet is then pulled underneath the exposed leg back toward the side of the table. Here the sheet is securely anchored by the weight of the leg. The top edge of the drape can be tucked under the gluteal at the level of greater trochanter or the edge can be rolled higher to expose the anterior superior iliac spine and tucked under the lower back.

iii. *To expose the top leg in sidelying:* Fold the posterior portion of the sheet forward, more as much of the extra sheet as possible out of the way in a superior direction.

Edge of the drape is pulled back under the leg. The leg to be exposed is now surrounded by drape. The outer leg is not exposed at any time during the procedure. Again move as much of the extra sheet as possible out of the way in a superior direction. Keep it tight to the leg, gradually pull the drape upto the thigh.

Finally pull the superior edge of the drape toward the groin, toward the gluteral cleft and roll it over the iliac crest. It takes practitioner to get this draping tight and secure. A pillow may be kept under the knee for support.

iv. Undraping the torso in prone:
   - The back is exposed to the level of posterior superior iliac spine.
   - The drape is securely tucked.
   - The arms of client may be kept either on the sides overhead.

Clinician's Posture, Alignment and Body Mechanics

Effectiveness of massage technique is also depend on the therapist's correct use of his feet, leg, pelvis, respiratory apparatus (as in most of shoulder girdle), shoulder, elbow and ofcourse hands. The following general principles of body mechanics should be applied during STM techniques:

i. Posture is aligned as upright as possible except during the controlled transfer of body weight.

ii. Both feet remain in contact with the floor.

iii. Therapist must bend his knee to reduce vertical distance between himself and patient instead of bending trunk.

iv. Similarly therapist must reposition his leg or shift his weight onto his forward leg rather than by bending at the waist or reaching excessively.

v. The therapist orients his navel area toward the body segment of the patient being treated.

vi. Use body weight to increase pressure instead of muscular force.

vii. Therapist's joints are positioned as close to neutral as possible rather than being loaded while they are in a closed-packed position.

viii. Therapist should change his posture frequently by to avoid undue mechanical stress on his body.

ix. Therapist should also avoid unwanted static contraction. Hand muscles must be elongated after few grasps during the massage technique.

x. Therapist should control the amount of his body weight that is being transferred to the patient, precisely and continuously.

STROKING AND EFFLEURAGE

The movement of both stroking and effleurage are so similar that they can be discussed together. Even some authors use the term stroking and effleurage interchangeably.

- *Mennel* has not used the effleurage in his classification, he classified stroking into superficial and deep.
- *Despard:* He used both stroking and effleurage, according to him, the direction of stroking and effleurage remains same (centripetal) but the pressure in stroking is vigorous and in effleurage varies from superficial to deep according to condition.
- *Hoffa* used light pressure at the beginning of the stroke manipulation, increases it over the fleshy part of the muscles and decreases it again at the end of stroke.
- *Ling* said pressure of effleurage varies from the lightest touch to one of considerable force.
- *Murrel* and *Kleen* said that it varies.
- Different authors have different opinions, however, it may be concluded that the stroking and effleurage may be used to produce similar reflex effects, so this book follows the convention used in many texts, and explains that effleurage constitutes pressures from superficial (light) to deep and produces the similar physiological effects such as stroking. In other words the stroking movements are the part of effleurage movements.

EFFLEURAGE

It consists a long, soothing, stroking movements performed by palmar aspect (over the large area) or fingers (over the small area) of one or both hands.

- Effleurage is used to start off any type of massage, soothing the nerve endings and again at the end of massage. It means every soft tissue manipulation technique starts and ends with the effleurage. Effleurage may either be superficial or deep.

Superficial Effleurage

The technique may be performed by single or both hands. The hand(s) should be as relaxed as possible, fingers and thumb may be abducted but not so widely that hand becomes tense. Minimal palmar or radial deviation of wrist is used to enable to conform to local body contours. While maintaining above position, the hands are placed over the patient's body.

Superficial Effleurage (Longitudinal Stroke) for Back Region

Position of Patient: Prone lying, the whole back should be exposed fully. An extra care should be given in case of female patients.

Position of Therapist: Standing at the side of patient, with one foot slightly behind but in line with the other. This position allows therapist to shift the body weight forward and backward.

Lubricants: Talcum, oil.

Procedure: The talcum or oil is poured over the whole back to avoid friction and uneven strokes. Both the hands are placed on the lower back region (one hand on either side of the spine) and are kept relaxed throughout the movement. Both hands move longitudinally from just above the sacrum to the lumbar, thoracic and axilla. As the hands move from sacrum a mild pressure is applied through the hands by shifting the body weight forward on the front leg (slight flexion of the chephalad knee joint). As soon as the hands approach the upper thoracic region, they are slided toward the axilla and pressure is released gradually. After completing stroke at the axilla, hands are returned back to the original position from axilla to the lateral wall of the thorax. When hands return, pressure is not applied but fingers maintain contact with the skin through the return stroke. Again the hands are positioned on the lower back region and prepares for another stroke. Several similar strokes are performed on the back to achieve effective results. Every stroke of effleurage should be in steady rhythm and may take 6 seconds. This technique of effleurage is known as longitudinal effleurage on back (Figs. 9.2a to d).

(a)

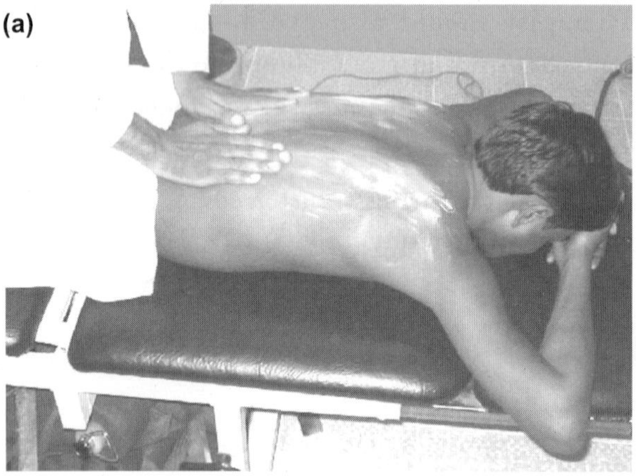

(b)

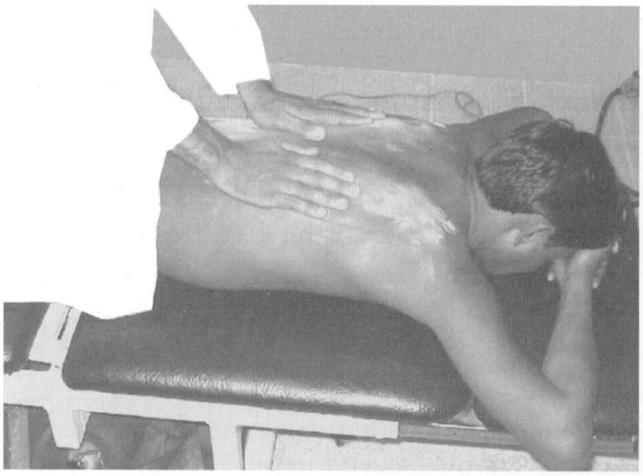

(c)

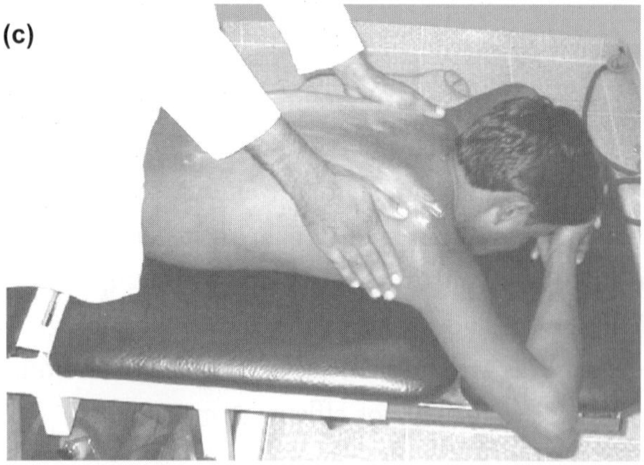

(d)

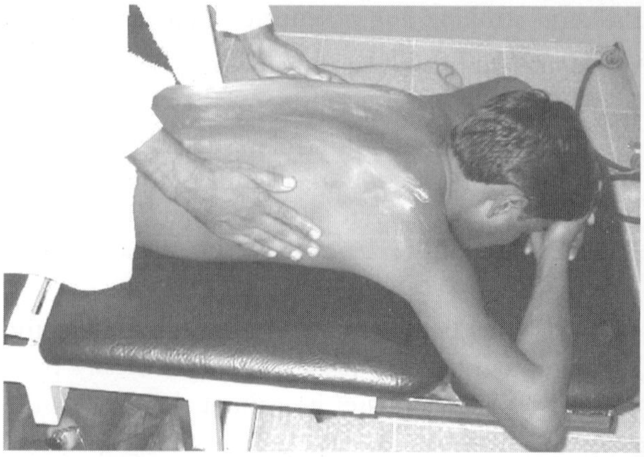

Figs. 9.2a to d: Superficial effleurage (Longitudinal stroke)—(a) Initial, (b) Mid position, (c) End position, and (d) Return stroke

Reverse Longitudinal Stroke of Superficial Effleurage

Position of Patient: Prone lying.

Position of Therapist: Standing at the head, end of the treatment table.

Lubricants: Talcum, oil.

Procedure: Both hands are placed over the upper back (one on either side of the spine). The fingers and thumbs are kept closed. Both the hands are moved with little pressure to the lower back. The pressure is applied through the hands by leaning forward. As soon as hands approach the lower back, they are slided toward the groin (inguinal lymph nodes) and pressure is released gradually. After finishing stroke at groin region, both hands return from groin to the lateral border of the trunk (one hand on either side), shoulders then toward the upper back. During return stroke pressure is not applied but fingers maintain the contact with the skin. When return stroke approaches the upper back from the groin, the direction of fingers remain same (pointing in a caudal direction) but the thumbs opened out away from the fingers. The hands are again placed on upper back and prepare for next stroke (Figs. 9.3a to d).

Five to ten repetitions of strokes are performed. Repetition of strokes may increase if these are performed over large muscles.

When superficial effleurage is performed on extremities (U/L or L/L), the proximal part of the limb is massaged first then the distal part of the limb, and the direction of movement should be from distal to proximal part.

The purpose of effleurage is to drain the fluid, so the strokes of effleurage are performed from distal or proximal part to the lymph nodes, from here the fluid is taken out to the heart, in order to remove swelling effusion or swelling.

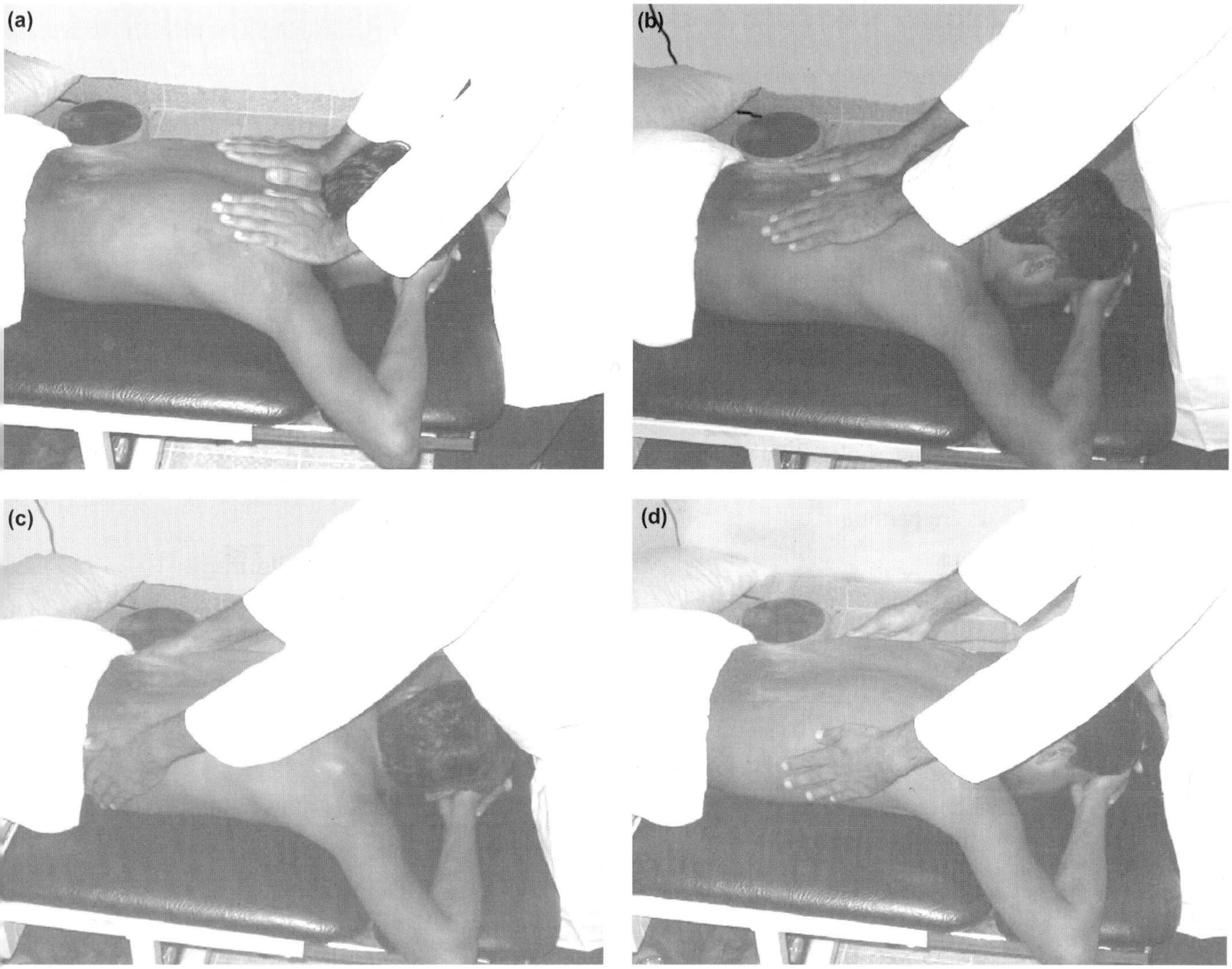

Figs. 9.3a to d: Superficial effleurage (Reverse longitudinal stroke)—(a) Initial stroke, (b) Mid stroke, (c) End stroke and (d) Return stroke

Deep Effleurage

The wrist is maintained in neutral position (no radial or ulnar deviation). If more pressure is required the dorsal surface of hand or wrist is reinforced by the other hand. Mainly its strokes are circular, parallel to the long axis of muscle or muscle group. These strokes may also be performed on whole back region.

Procedure

The pressure and return stroke combine to form circles that are oriented along or across the fibres in the different muscle layers. Most often the long axis of the stroke run parallel to the long axis of the body segment or muscle to which the technique is being applied, especially when significant pressure is requested.

A. ***On whole back region:*** The position of patient and therapist remains same as longitudinal superficial effleurage.

   Lubricants: Talcum or oil.

   Procedure: The procedure also remain same as longitudinal superficial effleurage, but more pressure is applied than the previous technique. To apply more pressure one hand may be reinforced by other hand. One hand is placed over the lower back region and reinforced by the other hand. The pressure is applied as the hand starts moving from lower back to the upper back. As soon as hands approach the upper back they are slided laterally to the axilla and pressure is released gradually. After completing the stroke the hands are returned to the lower back from axilla to the lateral border of trunk. Again hand is placed on lower back, reinforced by other hand and prepares for next stroke. Several similar strokes are performed.

B. ***On neck and upper back:***

   Position of Patient: Prone lying.

   Position of Therapist: Standing at the head, end of the treatment table.

   Procedure: Both hands are placed on the posterolateral aspect of the neck (one hand on either side) and are moved toward the upper back and axilla with the pressure applied through the hands by leaning forward. As the hands approach axilla, pressure is released gradually and hands are return for next stroke with little contact with the skin.

C. ***Deep effleurage with thumbs: (on back)***

   Position of Patient: Prone lying.

   Position of Therapist: Standing at the side of the patient.

   Procedure: Both hands are placed one on each side of the spine over the muscle which is being manipulated. The pressure is applied through the thumbs by leaning slightly forward. The thumbs are moved simultaneously along the long axis of paravertebral muscles in a cephalad direction with slight lateral curve. The hand and fingers may also move with the thumb but pressure is applied only by the thumb. The length of each stroke is 5 cm which may take 2 seconds. Several similar strokes are performed on the same muscle unless satisfactory effect is achieved. An indicator that the tissues are treated sufficiently is a feeling of sinking in with the thumbs. This 'giving' of the tissues however is not quickly accomplished, sometimes not at all. Over treating an area can cause hypersensitivity. If the strokes are performed too quickly and deeply the tension in the muscle tissue may increase.

   After manipulating one area sufficiently and effectively the technique may apply on another adjacent area. Muscles can be manipulated to the thoracic region as far as the lower border of the scapula. The procedure may also be performed with single thumb (Table 9.2).

Therapeutic Effects of Effleurage

1. Increases lymphatics and venous return from the region to which it is applied to the heart.
2. Dilates the superficial arterioles.

Table 9.2: Difference between superficial and deep effleurage

	Superficial effleurage	*Deep effleurage*
Contact	Whole relaxed palmar surface of hand	Whole relaxed palmar surface of hand often reinforce on the wrist or proximal forearm, sometimes thumb
Pressure	Light	Light to heavy
Engages	Skin, superficial fascia	Muscles and associated tissues
Direction	On limbs-centripetal, on torso-towards axillary or inguinal lymph nodes	Circular, parallel to the long axis of muscle or muscles group
Rate	5-50 cm/sec	10-25 cm/sec
Duration	2 min or longer	20-60 sec or more

Therapeutic Uses

- Lymphatic congestion.
- Dependent oedema.
- Oedema or effusion associated with the acute and subacute phase of common musculoskeletal injuries such as bursitis, sprains, strains, dislocation, separation and reflex sympathetic dystrophy (RSD).

Cautions

- Acute cardiac conditions.
- Congestive heart failure.

Contraindication

- Acute orthopaedic injuries.
- Newly forming scars.
- Infected area.
- Hypo and hyperthermia.
- Open wound, burn and ulcers.
- Malignancy.

PETRISSAGE

Petrissage is derived from French word *Petrir* means knead.

It is a technique of soft tissue manipulation which includes various types of strokes in which tissues are compressed, lifted, squeezed and released with varying amount of pressure, drag and glide. Various types of strokes are performed to mobilize skin, subcutaneous tissues and deep structures like muscles. There are four types of petrissage massage:

1. Kneading
2. Picking up
3. Wringing
4. Skin rolling.

Kneading

Kneading is a manipulation in which muscles and subcutaneous tissues are alternately compressed and released. The movement takes place in a circular motion which is divided into two phases pressure and release. During the pressure phase of each stroke, the hand(s) and skin move together on the deeper structure and whereas, in the release phase, the hand glides smoothly over the skin.

Direction of strokes: The basic direction of each stroke is circular.

Techniques

The stroke of kneading are performed in a circulator manner:

The hand or tip of fingers move over the underlying structures with the skin during the one half circle (Ↄ) which is also known as pressure phase, after pressure phase, the pressure is released and the hand(s) glides smoothly over the skin of another half circle (C) which is known as release phase and after performing stroke in full circle the stroke is repeated on adjacent area (Fig. 9.4).

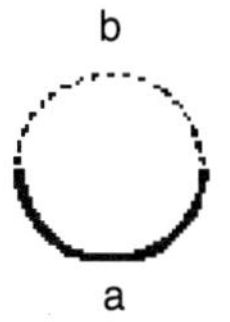

Fig. 9.4: Kneading—a-pressure phase (◡) and b-release phase (⌒)

Rate of Movement

Both pressure phase and release phase should be completed in 3-4 seconds.

Pressure

The pressure is applied during half of the circle but how much pressure will be delivered by the hands or fingers of therapist depends on the parts or structure which is being treated. The delicate structures like face and dorsum of hand require minimal pressure. More pressure can be delivered by using both hands on the back, thighs and calf muscles. The therapist should take an extra precautions while performing the strokes on geriatric patients on osteoporotic bones.

Classification of Kneading

As it is already mentioned that in kneading, tissues are alternately compressed and released by using single or both hands. It is therefore kneading is classified on the basis of the part of hand which is used to deliver the pressure, example—when the whole palm of hands are used to deliver the pressure, this kneading is named as palmar kneading. Following kneadings are clinically used:

- Palmar or compression kneading.

- Finger pad kneading.
- Thumb pad kneading.
- Knuckle kneading.
- Reinforced kneading.
- Squeeze kneading.

Palmar Pad Kneading

Palmar ("compression", "circular", "flat handed" or "whole handed kneading") is performed over large areas, such as, back, thigh, calf, arms and gluteal region. The whole palm is used to direct the pressure upward and inward in a circular motion and the skin moves with hand(s) over the underlying structures. Pressure is applied during half of circle and released during another half of circle and than repeated on the adjacent area.

Finger Pad Kneading

This kneading stroke is used to deliver pressure over the small area. The pads of one or more finger tips are placed over the target structure and movement is performed in a circular manner which includes pressure and release phase. Finger pad may be performed by single or both hands. When it is performed with both hands, the movements of hands take place opposite to each other (Fig. 9.5).

The finger pad kneading is used for tendinitis, fibromyalgia and muscle spasm.

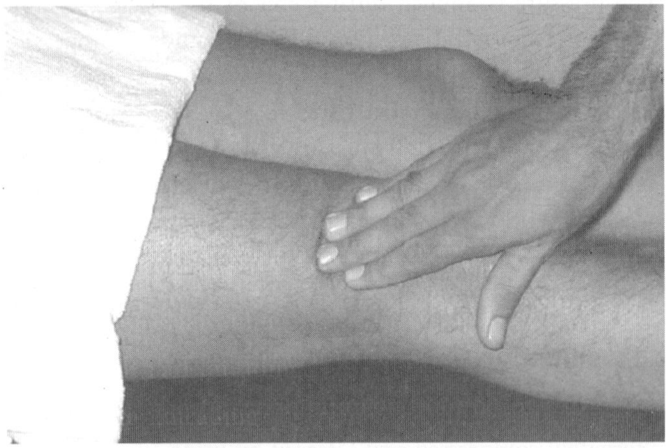

Fig. 9.5: Finger pad kneading

Thumb Pad Kneading

It is performed on small areas (wrist, ankle, elbow joint and face). The pressure over the tissues is applied by the pad of one or both thumbs. The basic direction of movement is circular which includes pressure and release phase. Thumbs of both hands are used to work side by side (Fig. 9.6).

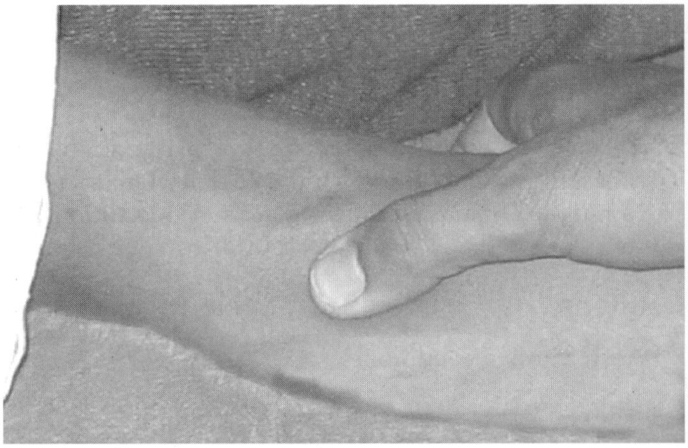

Fig. 9.6: Thumb pad kneading

Knuckle Kneading

It is also performed on small areas. The pressure is applied over the tissues by knuckles (dorsal surface) of the middle or proximal phalanges (Fig. 9.7).

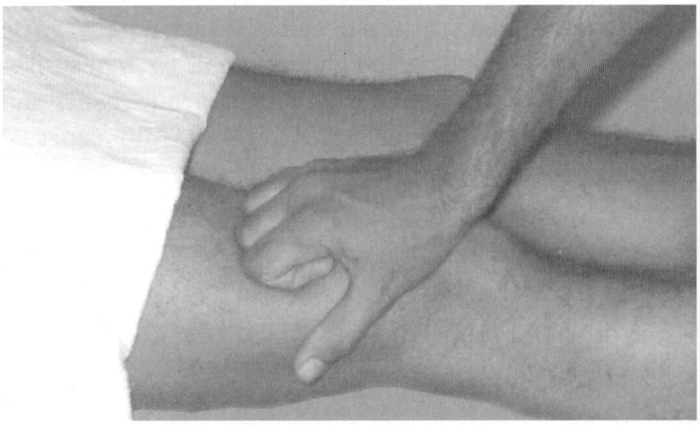

Fig. 9.7: Knuckle kneading

Reinforced Kneading

To deliver more pressure, an extra effort is required for an effective treatment (fat patients) by placing other hand over the hand which is being used to deliver pressure (Fig. 9.8).

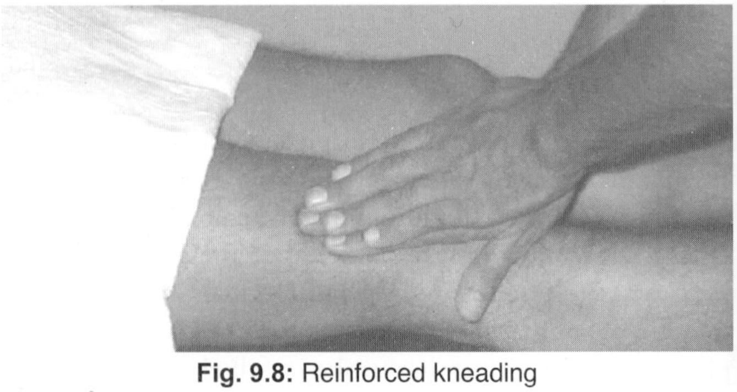

Fig. 9.8: Reinforced kneading

Picking Up

The skin, subcutaneous tissues and muscles are grasped

and lifted away from the underlying structures and then squeezed and released—The sequence of picking up may be followed as:

- Step 1—Compression of tissues–gliding.
- Step 2—Skin, subcutaneous tissues and muscles are grasped, lifted and squeezed.
- Step 3—Compression is released and hand(s) are placed on adjacent area to start the next stroke of picking up.

Technique

Picking up either be single handed or double handed.

One Handed Picking Up: This technique is performed on smaller body segments such as arms, forearms and calf muscles.

Position of Hand: The thumb of the hand is abducted, fingers are adducted, the hand assumes in a C-shaped position (Figs. 9.9a to c).

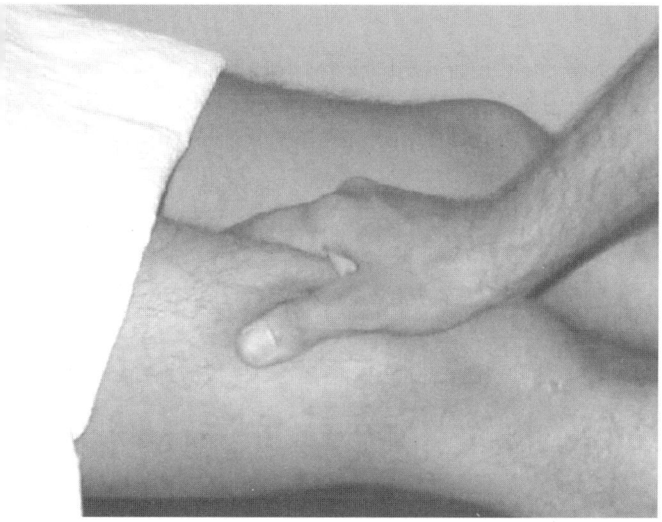

Fig. 9.9a: Picking up of quadriceps muscles

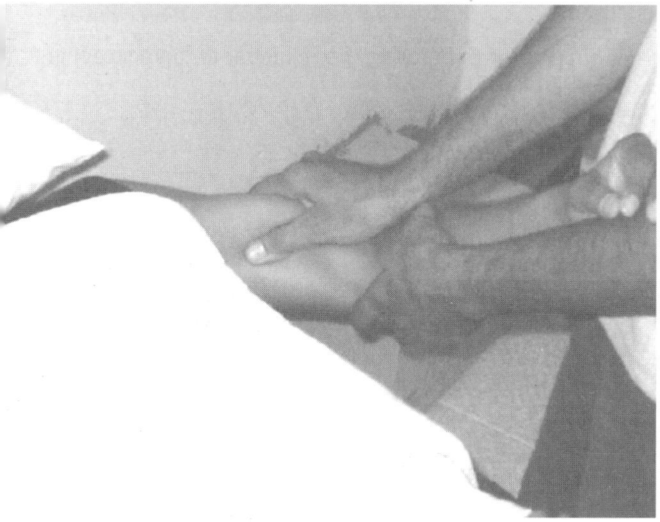

Fig. 9.9b: Picking up of elbow flexors

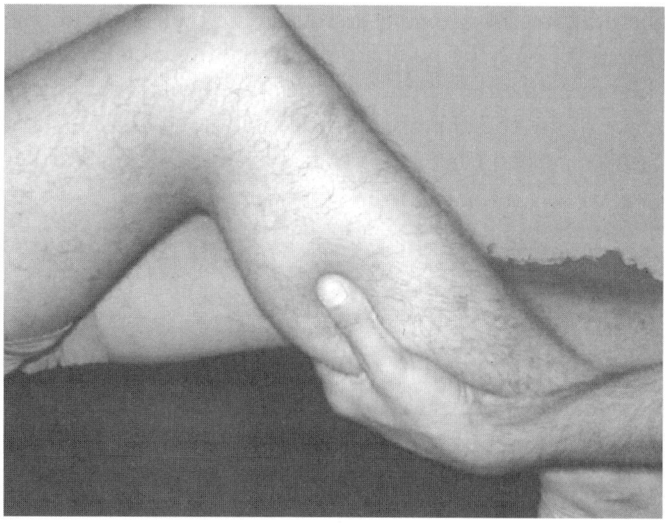

Fig. 9.9c: Picking up of gastrosoleus muscles

While maintaining the C-shape position, hand is placed on the part to be treated and tissues are grasped between the thumb and fingers then lifted away from the underlying structure by using the extension of the wrist. Then tissues are squeezed between thumb and fingers and in the final stage of picking up tissues are released. Hands again assume in a C-shape position for next stroke towards an adjacent part.

Wringing

The skin with muscles is grasped, lifted and squeezed alternately by both hands in opposite direction to each other.

Technique

Position of hands same as in picking up both hands are placed on the skin across the long axis of muscles. The skin with muscles grasped between the thumb and fingers then lifted away from the underlying structures (Fig. 9.10a). In

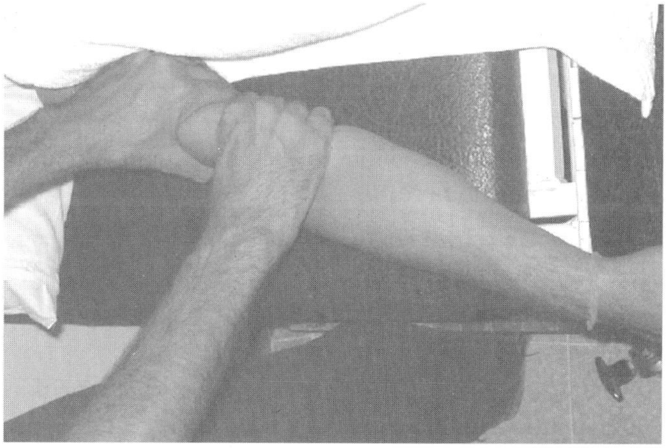

Fig. 9.10a: Wringing of elbow flexors (initial)

the next step of wringing the tissues are pulled toward the therapist's body by pulling the fingers of one hand, and at the same time the thumb of other hand pushes the tissues away from the therapist's body. Tissues assume in a S-shape position between the hands (Fig. 9.10b). Further

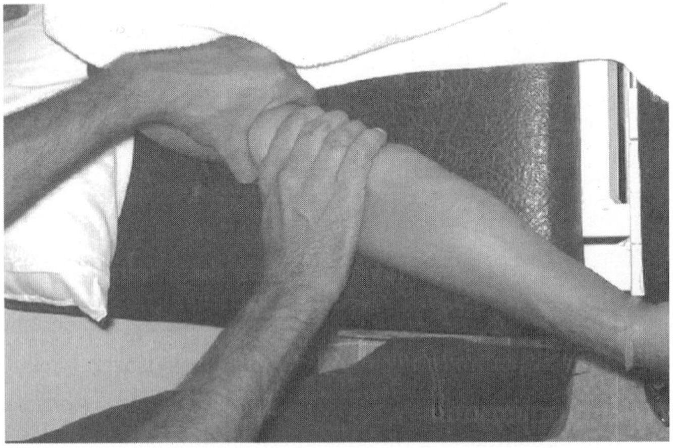

Fig. 9.10b: Wringing of elbow flexors (mid position)

the fingers and thumb move in opposite direction to each other and the tissues assume again in S-shape position (Fig. 9.10c). Therefore, in one cycle of wringing, tissues assume

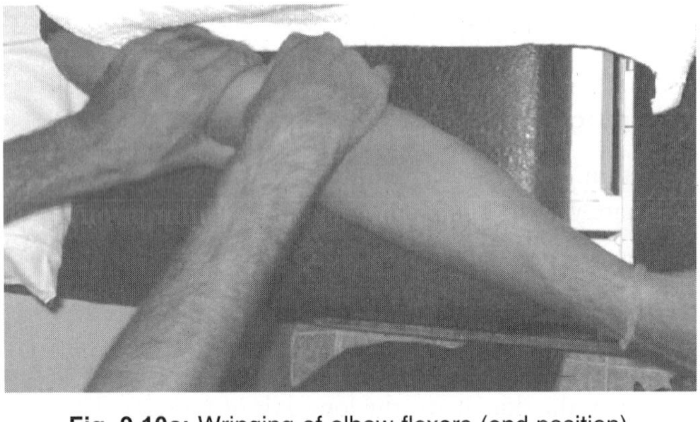

Fig. 9.10c: Wringing of elbow flexors (end position)

in S-shape position for two times. Several repetitions of wringing, may be performed on same tissues if required. In the final step of wringing the tissues are released by both the hands and position of hands is changed for next stroke of wringing towards an adjacent part.

Direction of Movement: Thumb of one hand and fingers of other hand work opposite to each other along the long axis of the muscle fibres.

Rate of Movement: Four to six inch per second, rate may decrease on smaller muscles.

Skin Rolling

It is a soft tissue manipulation technique in which the skin and subcutaneous tissues are rolled over the underlying structures (muscles).

Procedure

Position of Hands: Using the action of lumbricals the metacarpophalangeal joints are flexed at 90° and interphalangeal (IP) joints kept extended and thumb is opposed.

- Wrists are slightly extended.
- Forearms pronated and elbow flexed to 90° shoulder is abducted at 45°.

While maintaining above position both the hands are placed over the skin. The skin is grasped between the thumb and fingers and lifted away from the underlying structures. In the next step of wringing the fingers of right hand move forward and grasp the skin, the thumb of the same hand drags and draws the skin to the fingers. In the next step while maintaining the position of right hand the fingers of left hand move forward and grasp the skin while the thumb of same hand drags and draws the skin to the fingers. It is therefore in this technique the fold of skin between thumb and fingers can be maintained from one part to the other part.

Example: On upper back fold of skin can be maintained between the fingers and thumb from vertebral column to the rib cage and from lumbar to the thoracic spine (Figs. 9.11a and b).

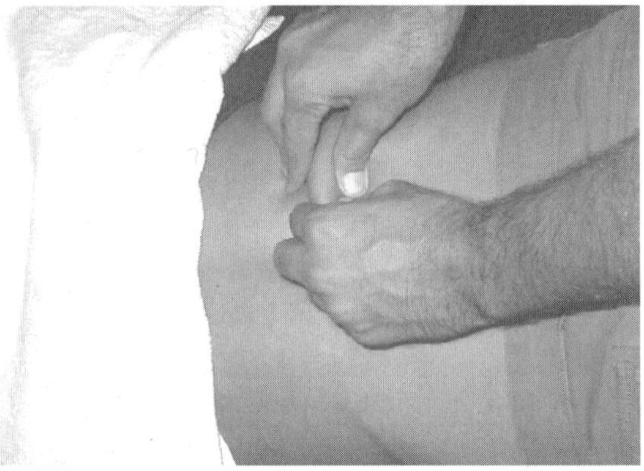

Fig. 9.11a: Skin rolling, from lumbar to thoracic spine

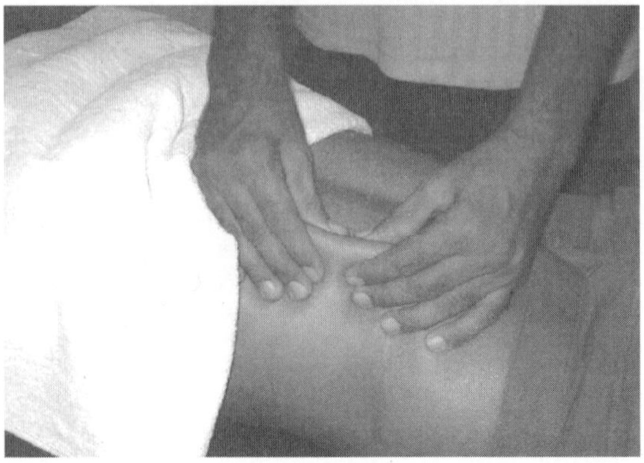

Fig. 9.11b: Skin rolling, from vertebral column to the rib cage

Therapeutic Effects of Petrissage

1. Dilatation of capillaries and arterials increase the blood supply and promote resolution of inflammatory processes of skin and subcutaneous tissues.
2. Increases extensibility and elasticity of skin and subcutaneous tissue.
3. The blood supply of muscles increases, which eliminates the waste metabolic products, thus:
   - Relaxes the muscles.
   - Increases flexibility of muscles.
4. Increase lymphatic blood flow.

Therapeutic uses of Petrissage

1. To increase extensibility and mobility of connective tissues.
2. To reduce anxiety, stress and improve relaxation.
3. To alleviate the behavioural symptoms of depression hyperactivity.
4. To increase joint range of motion (ROM).
5. To mobilize skin and subcutaneous tissues.
6. To decrease chronic oedema.
7. To decrease pain during labour.

The observed positive effect of petrissage on pulmonary conditions such as asthma, chronic obstructive pulmonary disease (COPD) and cystic fibrosis may be as a result of the combined effects of decreased anxiety and increased chest wall mobility, following petrissage manipulations.

Contraindications

- Acute inflammation.
- Infection.
- Confirmed or suspected thrombosis and thrombophlebitis.
- Extra care should be taken if patient is (i) suspected osteoporotic (ii) taking anticoagulants.
- Malignant disease.
- Acute musculoskeletal injuries, fracture, muscle strain, ligaments sprain.

TAPOTEMENT OR PERCUSSION

Tapotement is a technique of soft tissue manipulation in which the part which is being treated strikes repeatedly by the various modified positions of hand(s). In all tapotement movements the fingers, hands and wrists should be as relaxed as possible. Tapotement strokes are fast, precision action, bringing one hand quickly after the other into contact with the patient's body. After few strokes of tapotement the clinician must ask the patient whether the pressure which is being delivered by hands is comfortable or not. There are four types of tapotement techniques:

1. Clapping (cupping).
2. Beating.
3. Hacking.
4. Pounding.

Clapping

Clapping is a soft tissue manipulation technique of tapotement in which the patient's body (skin) is struck alternately by cup shaped hands. To achieve cup shaped position of hands the metacarpophalangeal joints (MCP) are flexed at 45°, interphalangeal joints are kept in neural position (extended) wrist should be as loose as possible (Fig. 9.12). Thumb adducted.

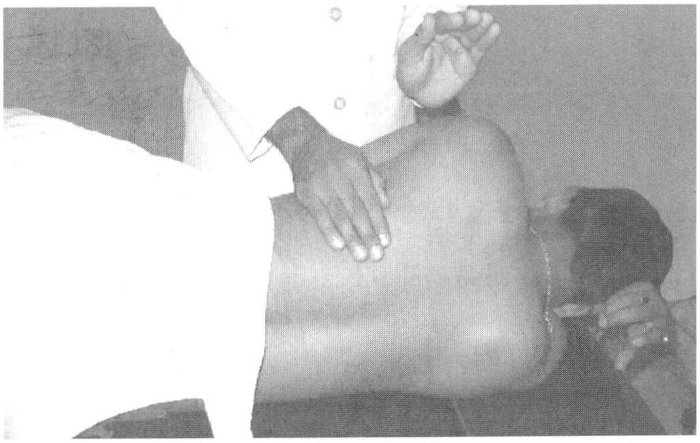

Fig. 9.12: Clapping (cupping)

The cup shaped hands strike alternately over the posterior chest wall and lateral surface of the rib cage by using the alternate flexion and extension of the wrist joints. It is performed rapidly with coordinated hands and pressure should be light. To achieve light pressure the movements (flexion and extension) should be taken place at the wrist joints and elbows remain almost at full extension.

Uses of Clapping

It is performed on posterior chest wall and lateral rib cage to loosen the secretin or drains the fluid from lungs. Therefore, it is important for the clinician to place the patient in appropriate position which helps to drain the fluid while performing clapping. The technique should be followed by postural drainage positions.

- It is also performed on larger muscles group to mobilize and achieve stimulating effect.

Beating

Beating is a soft tissue manipulation technique of tapotement in which the patients skin is struck by the dorsal aspect of the fingers and heel of one or both the hands.

The hands are positioned in a loose fist and tissues are struck by dorsal aspect of the finger's and heel of hand. Beating is a single or double handed technique. When it is performed by both hands, the hands strike the tissues alternately (Fig. 9.13).

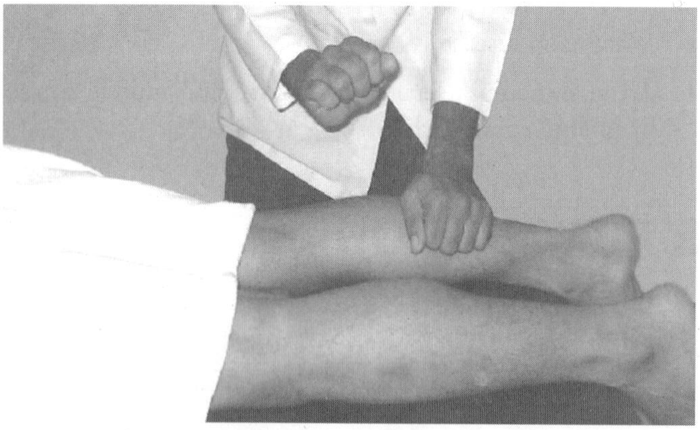

Fig. 9.13: Beating (tapotement)

Pressure: Mild to moderate pressure is applied according to the part of body by the flexion and extension of wrist joints, and the elbow joints remain almost in extension.

Uses of Beating

- To mobilize the muscles.
- To stimulate the skin and subcutaneous tissues.
- To mobilize the joints like lumbosacral junction.

Hacking

Hacking is a soft tissue manipulation technique of tapotement in which the tissues strike alternately by the medial edges and dorsal aspects of the fingers in a rapid succession to create a strong stimulating effect.

The fingers and wrists of clinician should be as relaxed as possible. The repetitive supination and pronation take place at the forearm with slight radial and ulnar deviation at wrist joint. The therapist flexes the elbows and abducts the shoulder joints. The ulnar border of the hand and little finger strike the patient's body, at the same time the medial and dorsal edge of other fingers also strike on skin on each other sequentially which causes an audible sound. The technique is performed on long axis of fleshy muscles with single hand or both hands repeatedly (Figs. 9.14a and b).

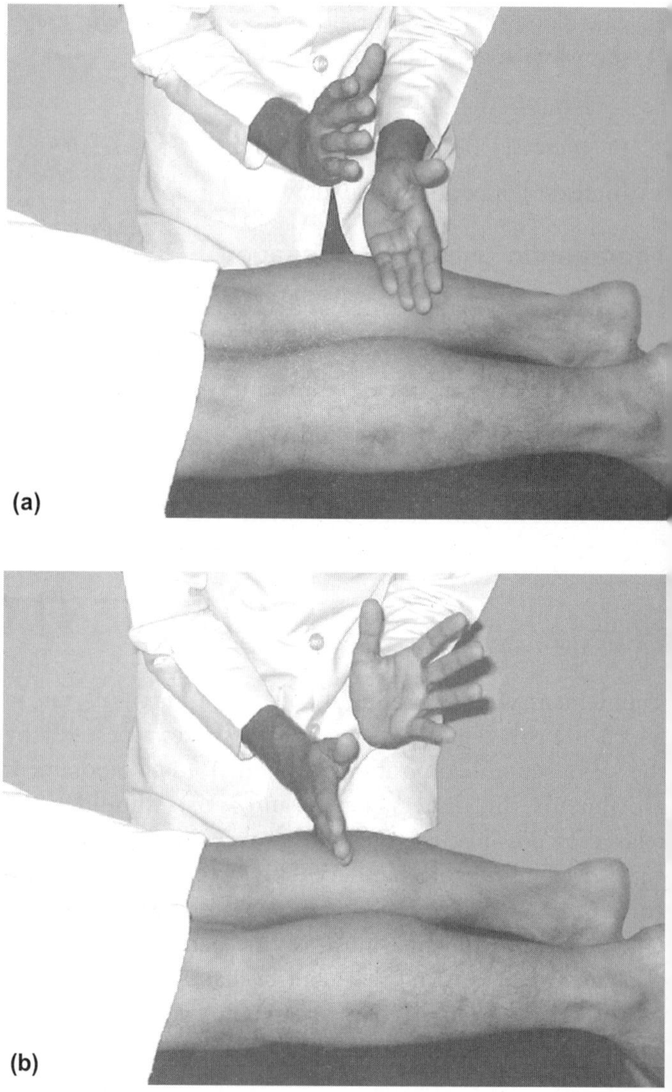

(a)

(b)

Figs. 9.14a and b: Hacking

Rate of Movement

The clinician needs more practice to learn this technique before administrating on the patient's body. The smooth coordinated movements are performed as fast as possible.

Pressure: There is no pressure other than the weight of the relaxed fingers striking the skin surface in rapid succession.

Uses:

- To stimulate the skin and subcutaneous tissues.
- To mobilize the muscles.

Pounding

It is the soft tissue manipulation technique of tapotement in which the tissues are strike or percuss alternately by the ulnar border of the hands.

The clinician loosely clench the fist, but keeps the wrists as relaxed as possible. While maintaining this position the ulnar border of both hands percuss alternately over the long fleshing muscles by flexion and extension of the elbow joints (Figs. 9.15a and b).

(a)

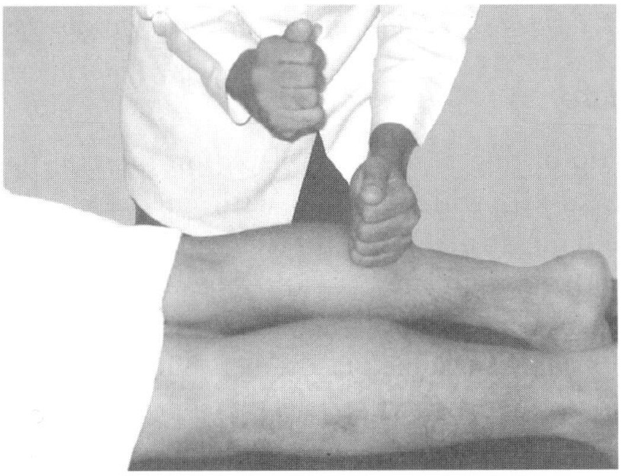

(b)

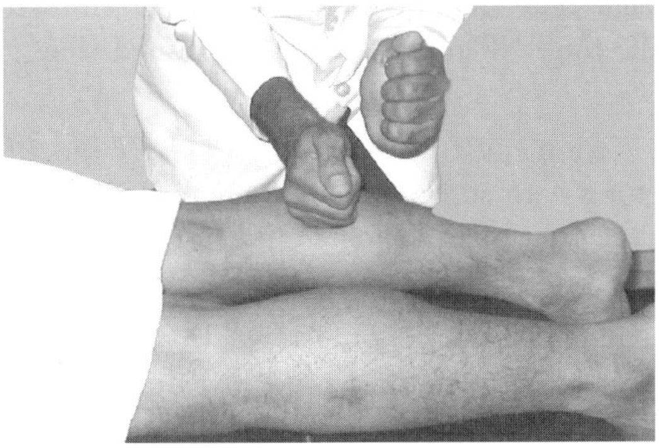

Figs. 9.15a and b: Pounding

Rate of Movements

The movements are rapid but should be controlled and coordinated without thumping the patient's skin/body.

Pressure: The pressure is delivered by the ulnar border of the hand which is deeper than the hacking.

Uses: To mobilize the large fleshy muscles.

- To increase flexibility of skin and subcutaneous tissues.

Therapeutic Effects of Tapotement

Various forms of percussion have different therapeutic effects. Clapping when performed on posterior chest wall and lateral wall it mechanically looses the secretion or mucus from the lungs and facilitates airways clearance while hacking stimulates sensory nerve endings and causes contraction of the muscles.

In cardiopulmonary physiotherapy, percussion is combined with postural drainage and is followed by or alternately with vibration of rib cage.

Contraindications

- Rib fractures.
- Untreated tension pneumothorax.
- Confirmed or possible coronary thrombosis.
- Pulmonary embolism.
- Unstable cardiac condition.
- Spastic muscles.
- Acute traumatic oedema.
- Cancer or tumors.

FRICTION

Friction is derived from Latin word frictio, which means to rub.

It involves brisk, repetitive, specific, compressive strokes which are delivered by hand, tip of fingers, or thumb on the skin. The skin may move with the hand or tip of fingers over the underlying structures (ligamentous, tendons or muscles).

The techniques of friction massage are classified on the basis of direction and amount of force that is applied. There are two types of friction techniques:

1. Superficial friction massage.
2. Deep friction massage.

Superficial Friction Massage

This is a fast rubbing of the body surfaces (Figs. 9.16a and b).

(a)

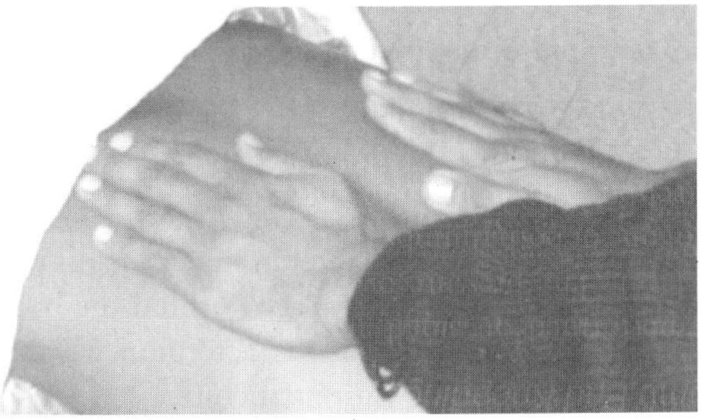

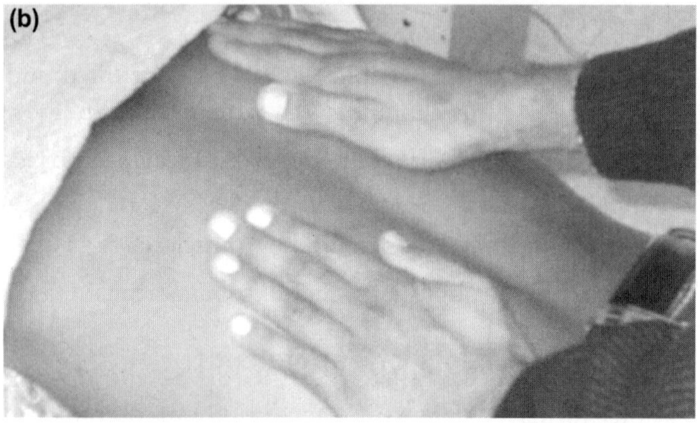
(b)

Figs. 9.16a and b: Superficial friction massage

This requires use of thin lubricant (amount of lubricant depends on hair and speed of movement). Both the hands with fingers and thumb adducted placed over the skin and move simultaneously in opposite directions over the skin. The movements are taken place in the shoulder joint and elbow, while dragging the hands over the skin no movements are taken place at wrist and hand and these should be as relaxed as possible for smooth and rhythmical strokes.

Deep Friction Massage

This is a small, repetitive localised, deep penetrating stroke performed by the tip of fingers, thumb or olecranon process of elbow in a circular or transverse manner on the muscles, ligaments, tendons. The tip of fingers, thumb or olecranon process move with the skin over the underlying structures (muscles, ligamentous and tendon). The strokes of deep friction massage are similar to kneading strokes of petrissage but differ on the basis of length, direction and pressure. Deep friction massage is performed across the connective tissue fibres.

Classification of Deep Friction Massage

A. Transverse friction.

B. Circular friction.

A. Transverse Friction

Also known as cross fibres friction, deep transverse friction and cyriax friction (Figs. 9.17a to e).

Technique: The technique varies slightly from condition to condition ·but the principles remain same.

1. *Treatment part must be brought within reach of the therapist's finger:* For instance, in supraspinatus tendinitis the patients arm must be placed behind the back. This brings the tendon out of the acromion which would otherwise shield the entire structure.
2. *The tissue to receive the massage should be in appropriate tension (except muscle belly):* For intance in lateral epicondylitis if the technique is performed on tendon, then wrist and fingers are flexed, forearm pronated and elbow is extended to put the tendon under tension. If the technique is being performed over the musculotendinous junction or muscle belly then common extensors of wrist should be relaxed (elbow flexed with wrist in neutral), so the massage can penetrate deeply to tease the fibres apart.
3. *The treatment is applied by the therapist's finger tips.*

Procedure

- The tip of finger (index) is placed on the skin (area to be treated), which moves with the skin over the underlying structures. The technique is to move the whole hand with the patient's skin and the therapist's finger moving as one, otherwise a friction burn of the skin may occur. Some practitioners put a piece of tissue paper between fingertips and the skin, this avoids the burn and absorbs sweat which might otherwise cause slippage. The index finger can also be reinforced by middle finger if more pressure is required (Figs. 9.17a to c).
- The friction must be across the fibres of the affected structures with sufficient amplitude of sweep to ensure that the frictional element (and not the pressure) is paramount.
- The strength (pressure) of massage depends on the stage of the lesion. In acute cases it is given extremely gently and in chronic cases with greater rigour.
- *Duration of treatment:* Varies from condition to condition ranging from 5 min to 20 min. The technique is performed at a rate of 2-3 cycles per second for 5-6 minutes in the first treatment session and increases by 2-3 minutes per session with an upper limit of 15-20 minutes.

  Some discomfort may be caused during first few minutes which can be minimised by a gentle start. **If there is continuous discomfort massage should be stopped immediately.**
- The treatment is directed on alternate days for 6 to 12 session although it depends on severity of symptoms.

Deep Transverse Friction Massage on Following Conditions/Structures

1. *Muscular lesions:* The massage breaks down the adhesions formed by the scar tissue between individual muscle fibres.

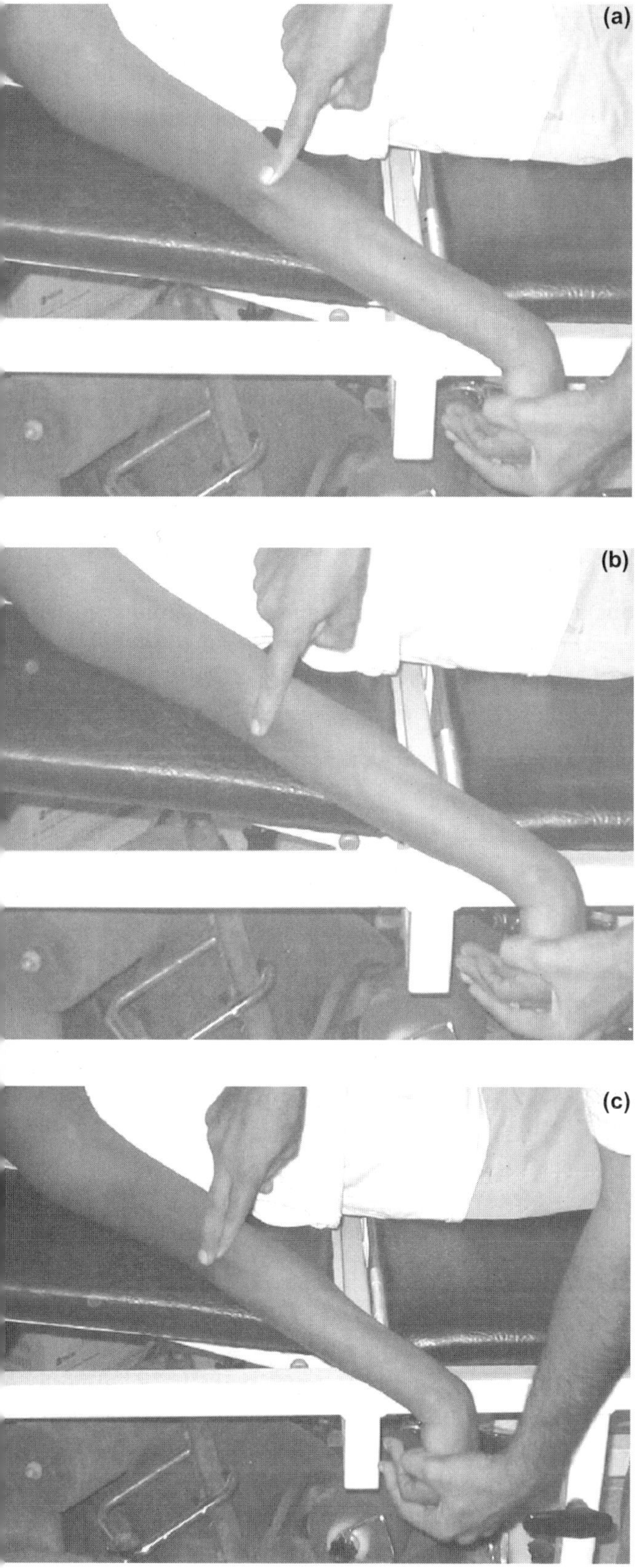

Figs. 9.17a to c: Deep transverse friction massage (a) Initial position—over tendons of extensor communis, (b) End position—over tendons of extensor communis and (c) Reinforcement—over tendons of extensor communis

2. *Muscle tendon:* The scar is eroded by the abrasive action (Fig. 9.17d).
3. *Ligamentous lesions:* The formation of adhesions during the period of healing is prevented by moving the ligament over the bone in limitation of its normal behaviour (Fig. 9.17e).
4. *Tenosynovitis:* It appears that the manual rolling of the tendon sheath to and fro against the tendon serves to smooth off the roughened surfaces.

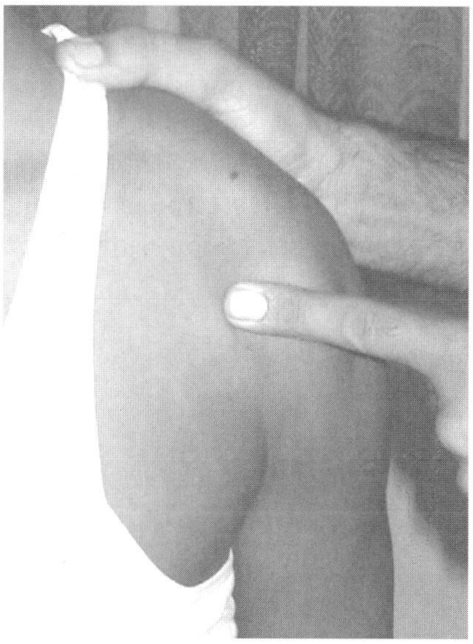

Fig. 9.17d: Deep transverse friction massage over tendon of supraspinatus

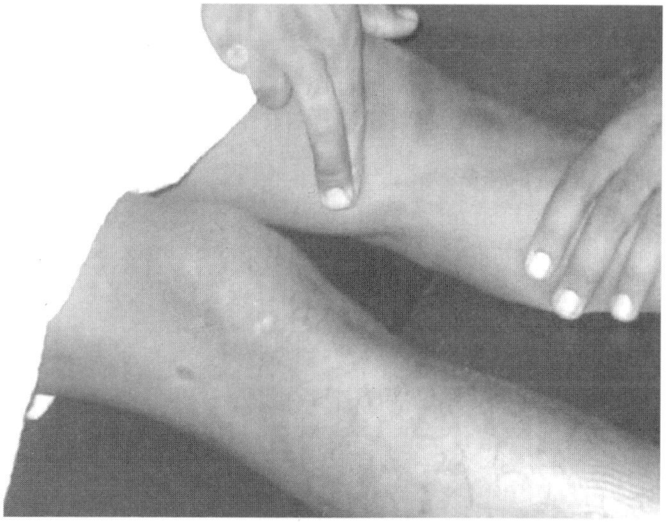

Fig. 9.17e: Deep transverse friction massage over medial collateral ligament of left knee joint

Uses:

- Tendinitis/Tendenosus.
- Joint capsule adhesion.
- Fascia or scar tissue in which the collagen has less regular organisation.

- Trigger points.
- Fibrosis.
- Ligamentous injuries.

B. Circular Friction

Technique: Performed with second, third and fourth digit or thumb. The tip of thumb or fingers are placed over the exact location of the affected structure and moved with the skin over affected structures in a circular direction.

To apply significant pressure the index finger can be reinforced by the middle finger. The technique is performed at a rate of 2 to 3 cycles per second for 5 to 6 minutes in the first treatment session and increases by 2 to 3 minutes per session with an upper limit of 15 to 20 min per session.

Indications

- Tendinitis.
- Fascitis.
- Ligamentous injuries.
- Trigger points.

VIBRATION

Vibration is a soft tissue manipulation technique in which fine shaking strokes are performed over the patients body by single or double hands.

Basic technique: To perform vibration technique single or both hands are placed over the patient's body, then rhythmic, vibrating strokes are delivered from in and out, up and down manner. When technique is performed on the lateral and posterior chest wall to loosen lung secretions, strokes should be delivered during the expiratory phase of the respiration (Fig. 9.18).

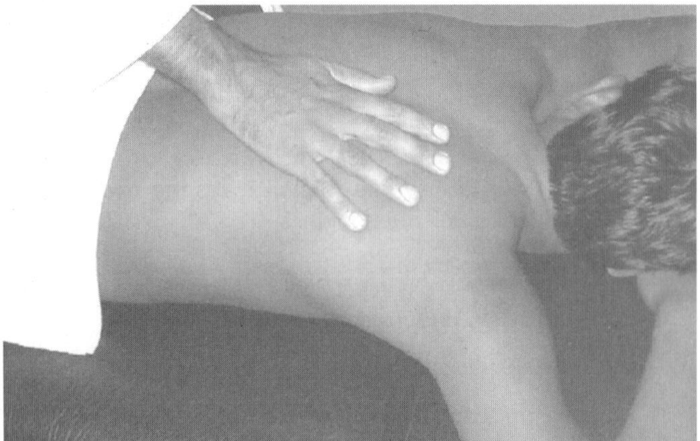

Fig. 9.18: Vibration on posterior chest wall

Indications

1. Chronic obstructive pulmonary disease (COPD).
2. Before and after operation to clear the secretion from lungs.
3. To reduce chronic oedema.

Contraindication

1. Severe rib fractures.
2. Hyperreflexia.
3. Acute pulmonary embolism.
4. Hypertension.
5. Spasticity.

SHAKING

Shaking is a soft tissue manipulation technique in which rhythmic, shaking strokes are delivered over the patient's body, by single or both hands.

Basic technique: Shaking technique can be performed with single or both hands (Fig. 9.19).

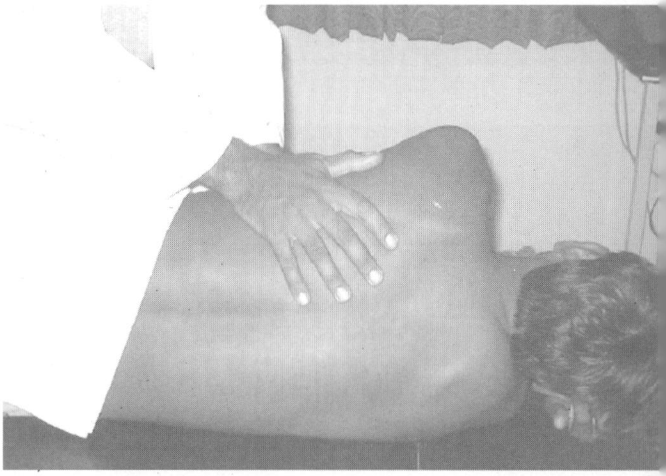

Fig. 9.19: Shaking on lateral costal chest wall with both hands

i. *On lateral or posterior chest wall:* One or both hands are placed over the patient's body (lateral or posterior chest wall), hands should be as relaxed as possible. A relaxed hand that produces minimal tissue compression will result in the freest tissue excursion. A fine rhythmic, shaking strokes are delivered by the hand(s) from side to side or up and down during the expiratory phase of respiration to drain the secretions from lungs.
ii. *On muscles:* One or both hands are placed on the surface. Wrist remains relaxed as the hand moves back and forth rhythmically perpendicular to the

long axis of the limb to produce waves of tissue motion.

Indications

- To loosen the adherent mucus secretion from the lungs.
- To alter the resting muscle tone through stimulating of complex proprioception reflexes.

Contraindication

- Acute muscular injury.
- Muscle spasm.
- Hyperreflexia.
- Spasticity.
- Severe rib fractures.

10

SUSPENSION THERAPY

INTRODUCTION

Suspension therapy is a therapeutic modality of exercise therapy in which the extremity of the body is suspended in the air by ropes and slings attached to fixed point(s) above, so that the effects of gravity upon motion can be used or eliminated. Guthrie Smith frame on which ropes, pulleys and slings are attached to one or two points to suspend the extremity in the air, is most commonly used in the physicial therapy's practice (Fig. 10.1).

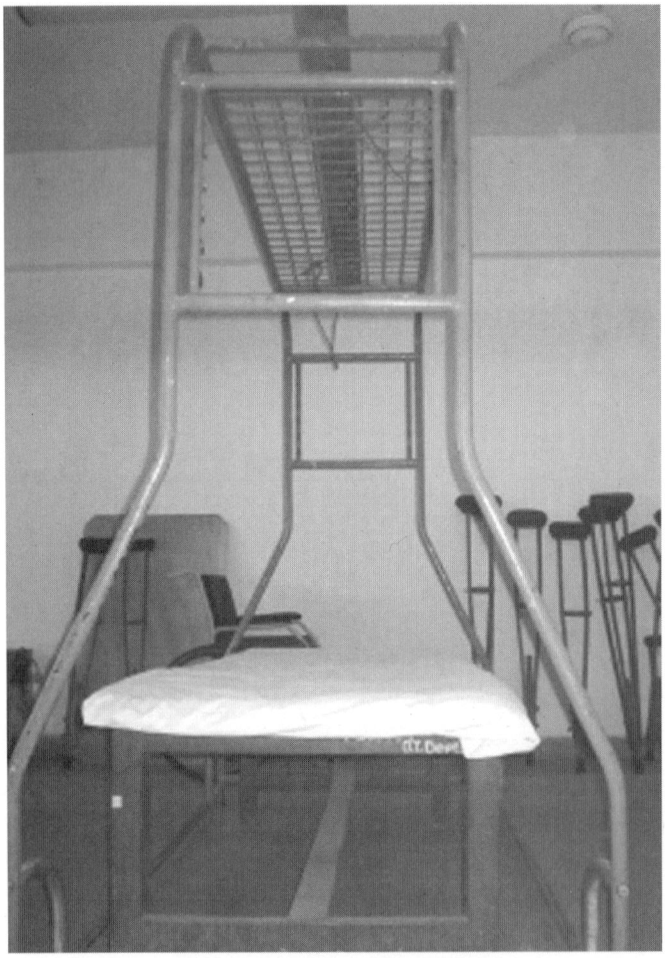

Fig. 10.1: Guthrie Smith frame

The effect of suspension on movement from the resting position is similar to that of an inclined re-education board which supports the limb during movement up the incline but differs from it in that, in suspension friction is virtually eliminated.

Suspension functions as not only to eliminate frictional resistance from the moving body part but also promotes a feeling of weightlessness such as experienced by buoyancy in the hydrotherapy pool.

It is mainly used to allow the muscle to contract actively in the gravity eliminated position or against gravity to improve the muscle strength, joint range of motion and decrease the pain and muscle spasm. There are three types of suspension.

Axial Fixation

The fixation point for all ropes which are attached with the slings to support the moving limb is located immediately above the centre of the moving joint. This type of suspension allows maximum movement of the joint to occur as the limb moves parallel to the floor.

Example: To strengthen the gluteus medius and minimum (hip abductors) the point of fixation is positioned or placed immediately above the anterior marking of the centre of the hip joint. The ropes positioned at the fixation point are attached with the slings at the knee and ankle joints (Fig. 10.2). Patient abducts and adducts the hip joint to move the extremity in parallel to the floor.

Vertical Fixation

The fixation point for all ropes is located over the center of gravity of the moving segment. The vertical suspension is used primarily for support to move the extremity in a small range. To achieve the required outcomes (range of motion and strength) it is often combined with axial fixation.

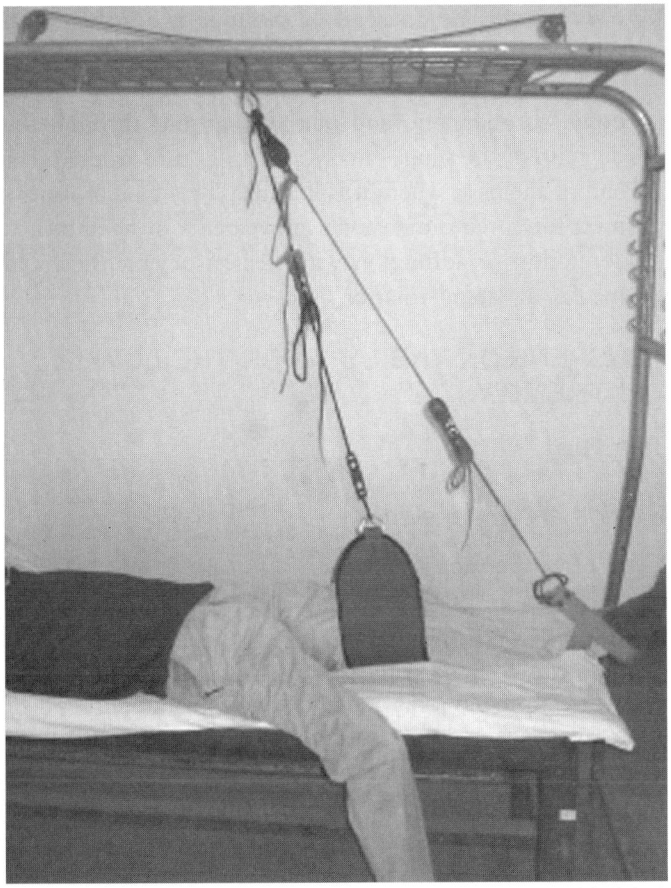

Fig. 10.2: Axial fixation (axial line from fixation point to hip joint)

Pendular Suspension

It is a type of suspension in which the axis of axial suspension is changed to apply resistance to the moving limb. The axis is shifted away from the axial fixation of the hip joint (e.g., patient lies in side lying the axis of the suspension is shifted posterior to the hip joint to strengthen the flexors of the hip joint).

DEVICES USED WITH SUSPENSION THERAPY (Figs. 10.3a to d)

Clips and Hooks

The clips are used to attach the ropes with the slings while hooks are suspended on the suspension unit (fixed point) with one end and other end attached with pulley or rope, generally an 'S' shaped hook is used. The either end of 'S' hook is used according to the fixed point. Common clips and hooks are:

- Carabine clip.
- Dog clip.
- 'S' hook.

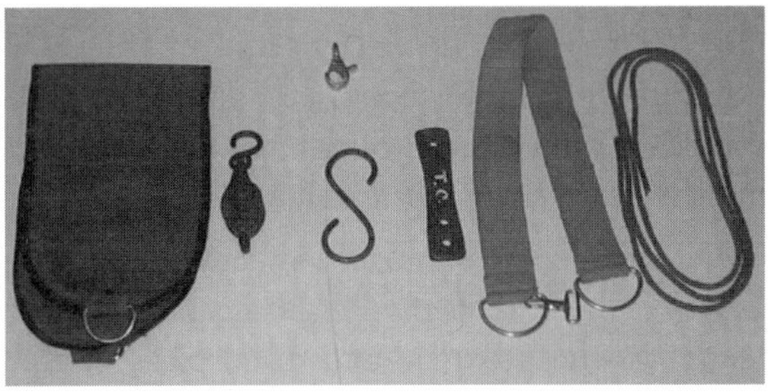

Fig. 10.3a: Devices used in suspension therapy

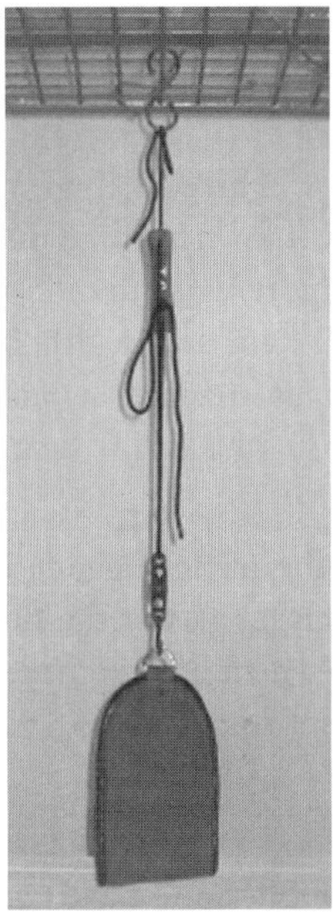

Fig. 10.3b: Pulley rope with single sling

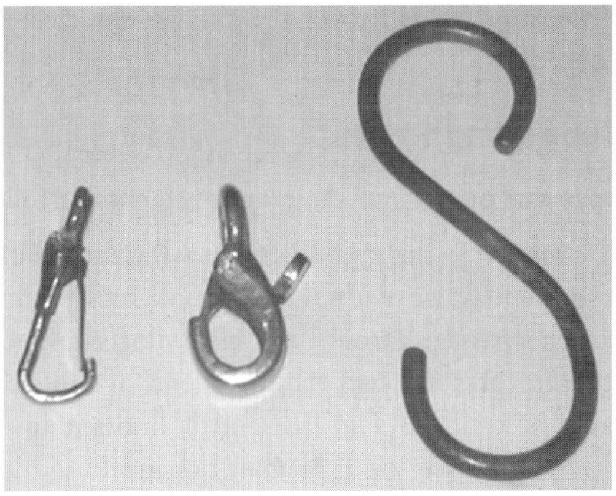

Fig. 10.3c: Carabine clip (left), Dog clip (middle), S-hook (right)

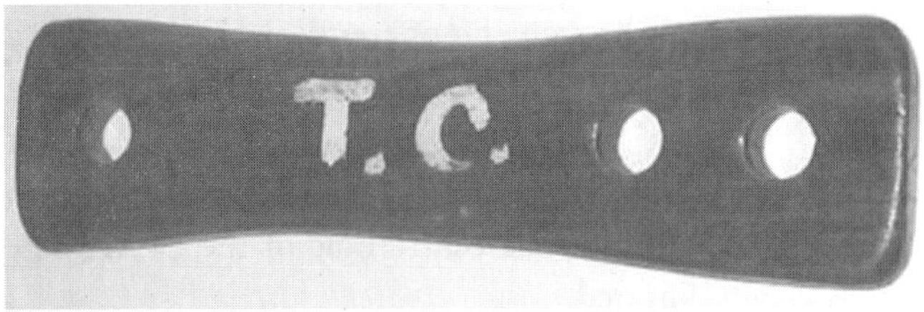

Fig. 10.3d: Cleat

Slings

These are used mainly to support the limbs, and the each end is attached with D ring. Slings are made up of canvas. Common types of slings are as follows:

- *Single Slings:* These are placed usually under the joints to support them. If single sling is used as figure of eight it supports the proximal and distal parts of the joint (for example to support the peripheral joints such as ankle and wrist).
- *Double Slings:* Generally used to support the trunk and pelvis.
- *Three Ring Slings:* Three D rings are attached with the sling so these are known as three ring slings. These slings are used to support wrist, hand, ankle and foot. The length around 71 cm and width 3-4 cm is commonly used. Two D rings attached at both ends to make two loopes and one D ring at the centre is attached to the dog clip.
- *Head Sling:* As the name suggests it is used to support the head. The central part of the sling splits and divided into two halves which are stitched together at an angle to create a central slit.

The Cleat

It is made up of a wooden and have two or three holes. The cleat is used to alter the length of the rope. To alter the length of rope the cleat is held in horizontal position and to hold the rope by its frictional resistance the cleat is held in oblique position.

The Supporting Ropes

The ropes can be used in three arrangements as follows:

- *Single rope:* It is tied at one end at which it is hung up. This end may tie with the 'S' hook or D ring. The other end passage through the cleat, dog clip and takes U turn to pass through the other end of the cleat and then it is knotted. The free end is knotted in such a manner that a tug on it enables quick release.
- *Double rope:* The one end of the rope is attached with the ring or clip same as single rope. The other free end of rope passes through the one end of cleat, rounds a lower pulley wheel (the wheel is attached with the dog clip) then back through the other end of the cleat over the wheel of an upper pulley. The rope then passes down again through the centre hole of the cleat where it is finally knotted.

  Double rope is used to suspend the pelvis, thorax and both thighs.
- *Pulley rope:* The one end of the rope is attached with the dog clip or D ring at the sling. The other free end of the rope passage up over the wheel of a pulley then down through one end of the cleat and through the dog clip of the sling. Finally it takes U turn to the other end of the cleat where it is knotted. This type of rope is used for three dimensional movements of a limb, i.e., abduction or adduction with flexion or extension and medial or lateral rotation.

SUSPENSION THERAPY FOR THE LOWER EXTREMITY

The Hip

Flexion and Extension

Type of Suspension—Axial

The patient is placed in side lying, the lower leg or unaffected leg is flexed at hip and knee joints. For axial fixation, the 'S' hook is fixed to the suspension unit immediately over the hip joint on which two ropes are suspended. The two slings at knee and ankle joint are attached with the D rings and then dog clips and ropes (Figs. 10.4a to c).

The length of ropes is altered by the movements of the cleat until the limb is lifted horizontal. The patient is then allowed to move the joint in flexion or extension.

Abduction and Adduction

Type of Suspension—Axial

The patient is placed in supine lying the unaffected extremity is abducted at hip joint and flexed at knee joint, the foot is placed on stool. The placement of 'S' hook, ropes and slings remain same as flexion and extension (immediately over the hip joint) (Fig. 10.5).

The length of ropes is altered by the movements of the cleat until the limb is lifted horizontal. The patient is then allowed to move the hip joint in abduction and adduction.

Flexion and Extension

Type of Suspension—Vertical

The patient is placed in side lying, the lower unaffected extremity is flexed at hip and knee joints.

The 'S' hook is placed immediately over the center of gravity of the thigh, and is attached with rope than the sling of the knee joint. As vertical fixation is often combined with axial fixation, therefore one 'S' is also placed just above the hip joint and is attached with rope. The three ring sling supports the foot and ankle and its centre ring is attached with the rope. The length of rope is altered by the movement of the cleat until the limb comes in horizontal line. Patient is allowed to move the joint in flexion and extension in available range of motion.

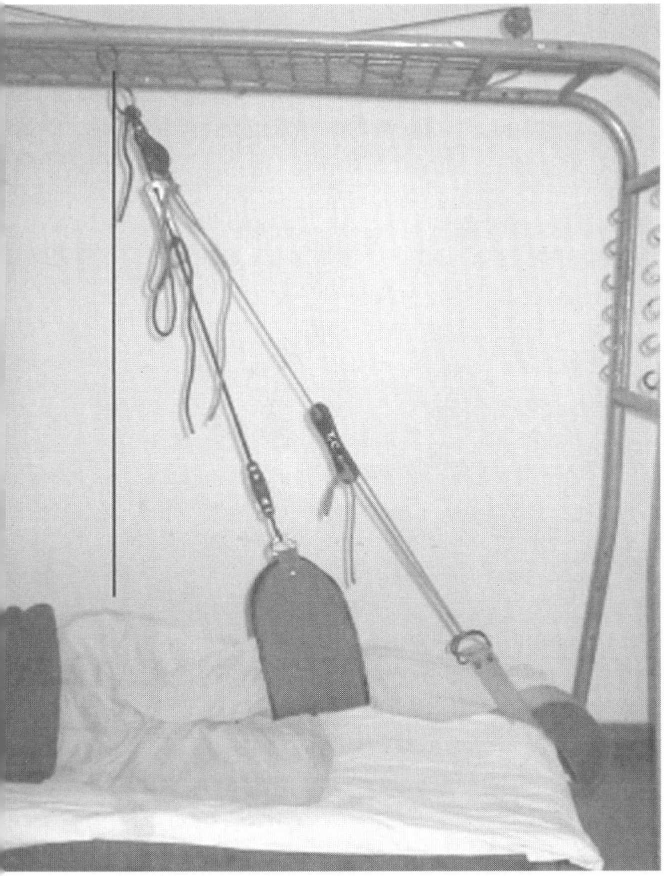

Fig. 10.4a: Hip joint in neutral position

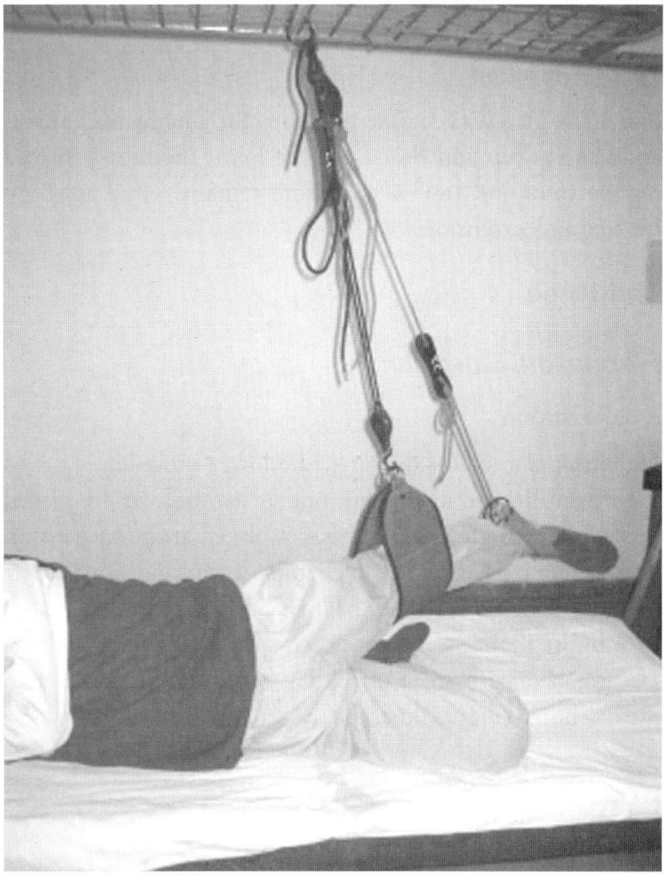

Fig. 10.4c: Hip joint in extension

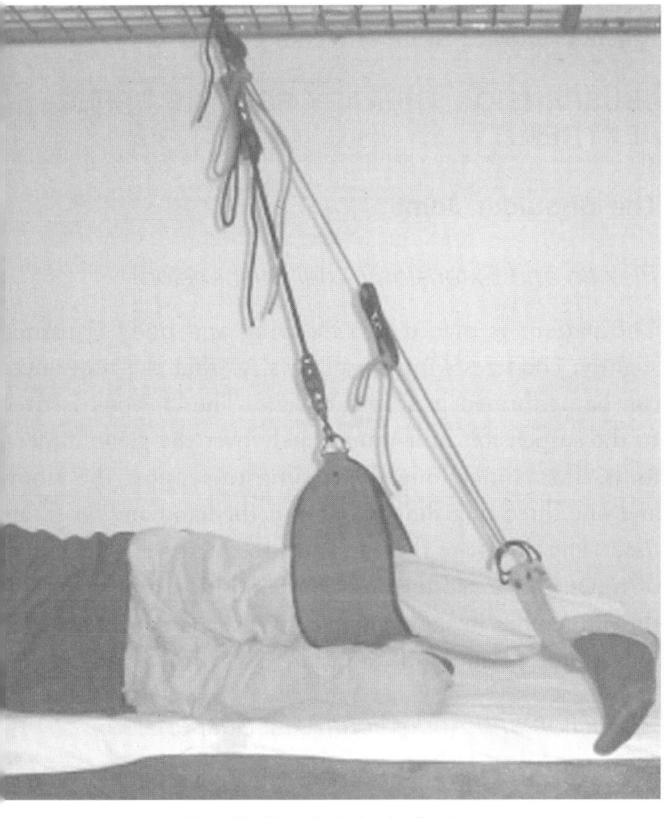

Fig. 10.4b: Hip joint in flexion

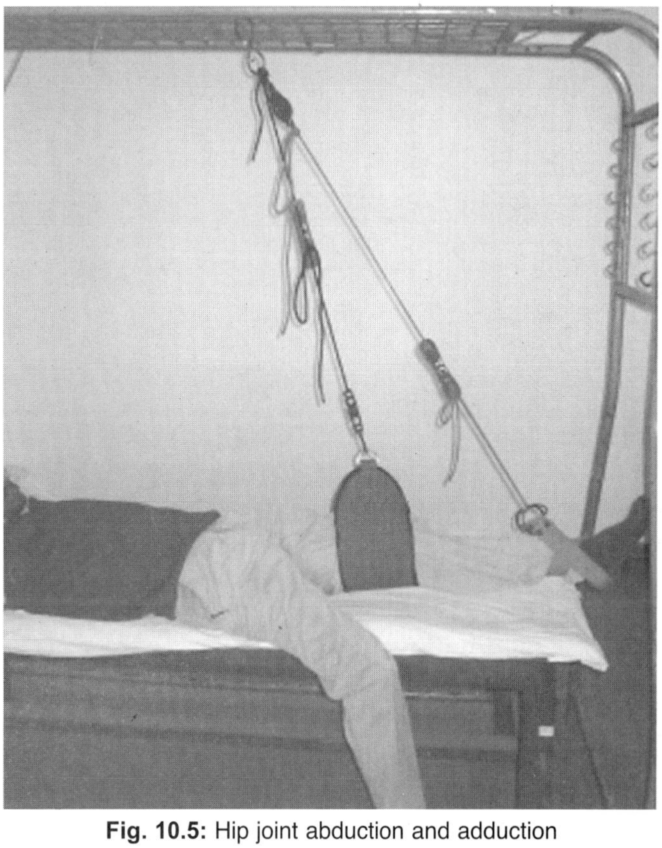

Fig. 10.5: Hip joint abduction and adduction

Abduction and Adduction

Vertical Fixation

Patient is placed in supine position, the unaffected limb is abducted at hip and flexed at knee joint, the foot is placed on the stool and rest of procedure remains same as above flexion and extension.

The Knee

Flexion and Extension

Axial Fixation

Patient is placed in side lying, the lower most leg is flexed slightly at hip and knee joint, one or two pillows are placed between the thighs. The 'S' hook is placed at the suspension unit immediately over the knee joint. Two slings, one single to support the lower thigh or knee and one three ring sling to support the foot and lower leg may be used. The slings are attached with the ropes, then ropes are attached with the 'S' hook (Figs. 10.6a and b).

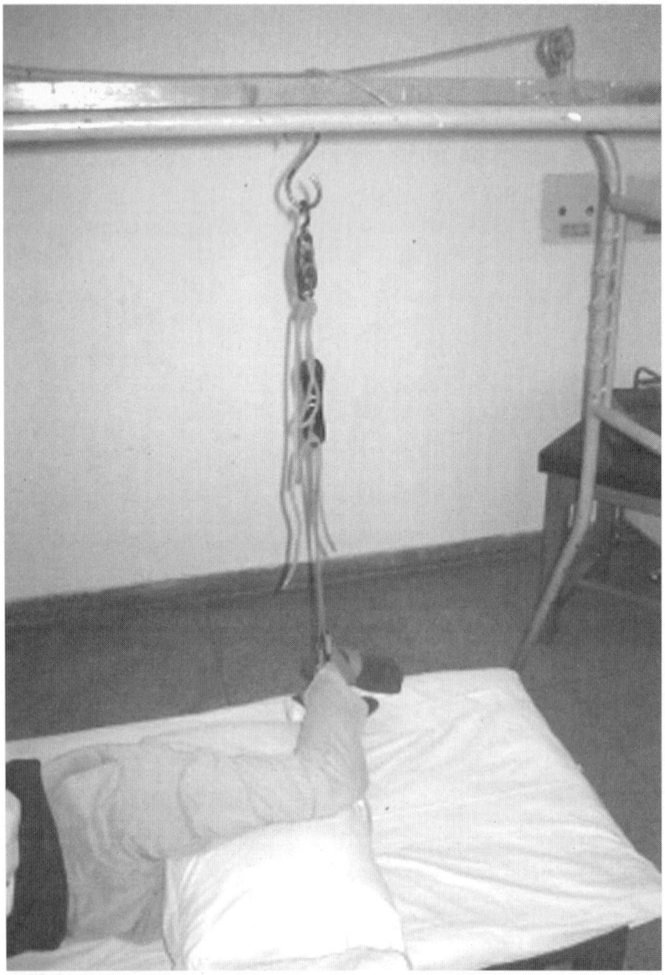

Fig. 10.6a: Knee flexion

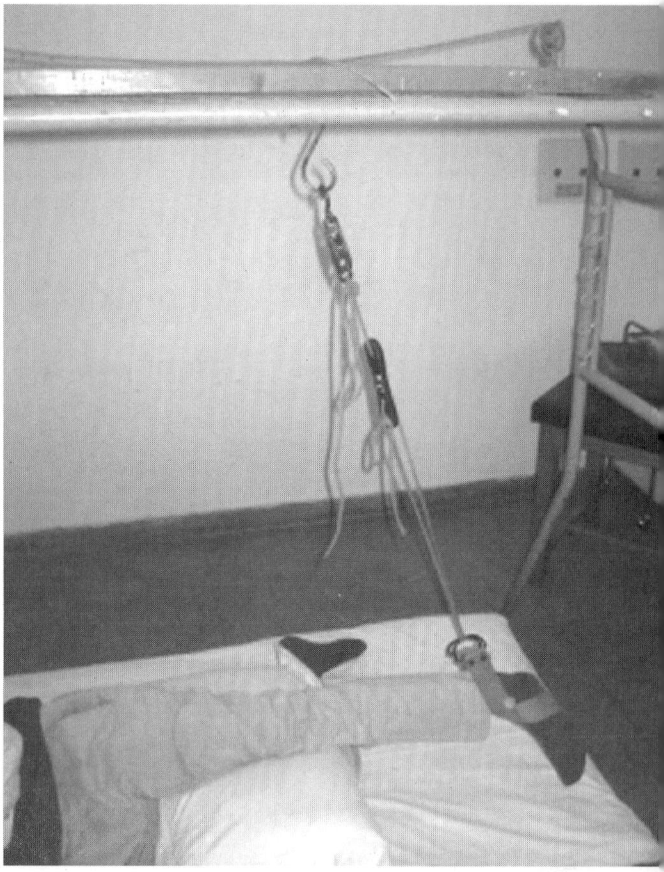

Fig. 10.6b: Knee extension

The limb is lifted up until it comes in horizontal line. Patient is allowed to move the knee joint.

SUSPENSION THERAPY FOR THE UPPER EXTREMITY

The Shoulder Joint

Flexion and Extension (Axial Suspension)

The patient is placed in side lying and body is turned slightly, chest rests on the pillows, so that the movement can be performed in scapular plane. The 'S' hook is fixed to the suspension unit immediately over the glenohumeral joint. Two slings, one single sling to support the elbow and one three ring sling to support the hand and wrist, are used. The slings are then attached to the ropes. The length of ropes is changed by altering the position of cleat and as the arm comes in the plane of scapula, the patient is asked to perform flexion and extension (Figs. 10.7a and b).

Abduction and Adduction (Axial Suspension)

The patient is placed in supine lying, one or two pillows may be placed under the scapula. The 'S' hook is placed

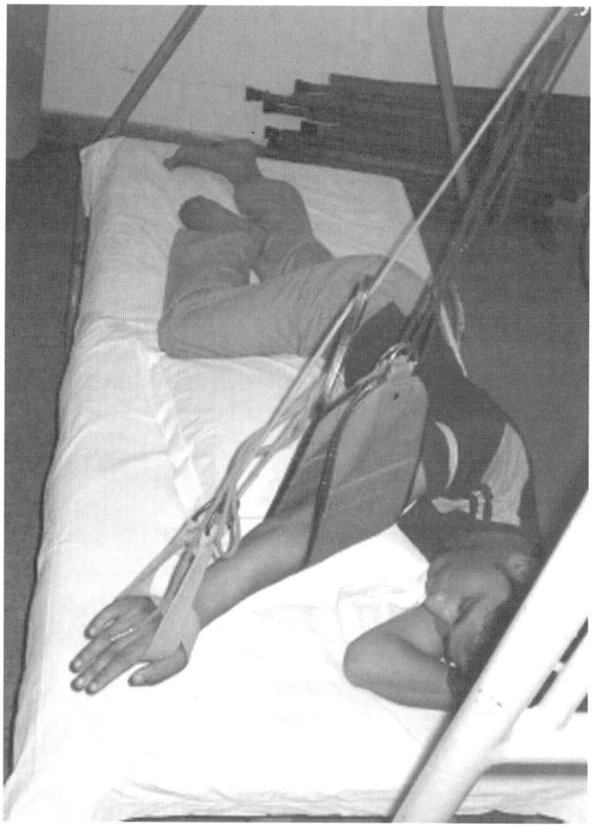

Fig. 10.7a: Shoulder flexion

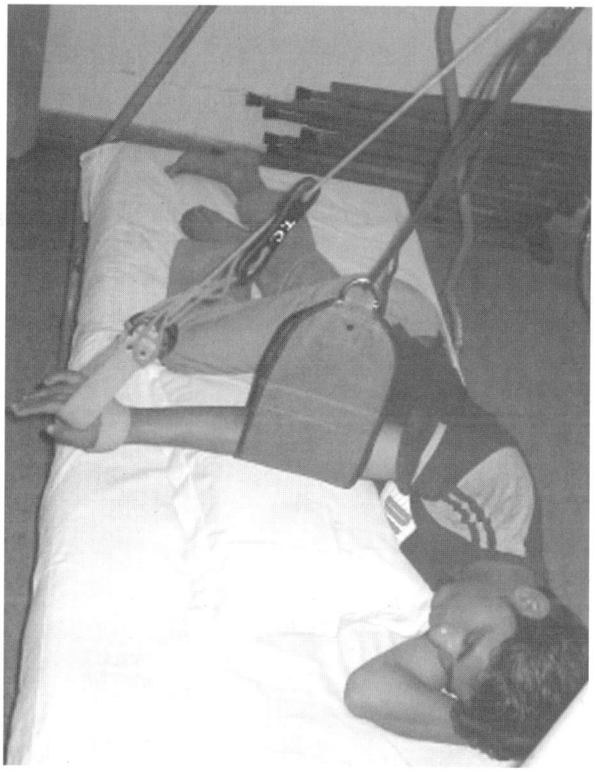

Fig. 10.7b: Shoulder extension

immediately over the glenohumeral joint from which two ropes are suspended. Two slings as in shoulder flexion and extension are used. Rest of procedure remains same as above.

The abduction and adduction may also be performed in prone to see the movement of scapulothoracic joint as well as glenohumeral joint (Fig. 10.8).

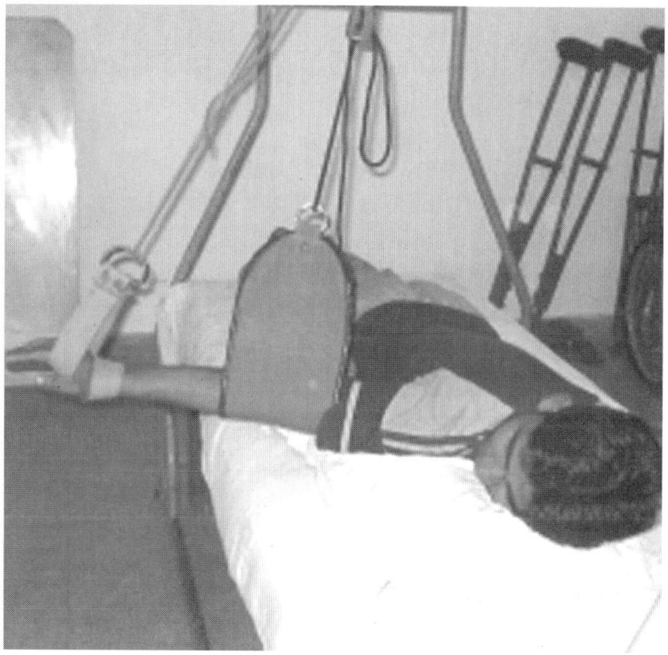

Fig. 10.8: Shoulder abduction and adduction

The Elbow Joint

Flexion and Extension in Lying (Axial Suspension)

The position of patient remains same as in shoulder abduction and adduction. The 'S' hook is fixed just above the elbow joint. Single sling is used to support the distal arm and three ring sling to support the wrist and hand. The flexion and extension is performed as the elbow comes horizontal in the shoulder line.

Flexion and Extension in Sitting

Patient sits on chair and shoulder is abducted to 90°. One 'S' hook is fixed immediately over the elbow joint for axial fixation. Single sling which is attached with axial fixator is used to support the distal arm and three ring sling is attached with 'S' hook to support the wrist and hand (two ring sling may also be used). The arm is lifted up till it comes in horizontal line. Patient is instructed to move the elbow joint (Figs. 10.9a and b) in the available range of motion.

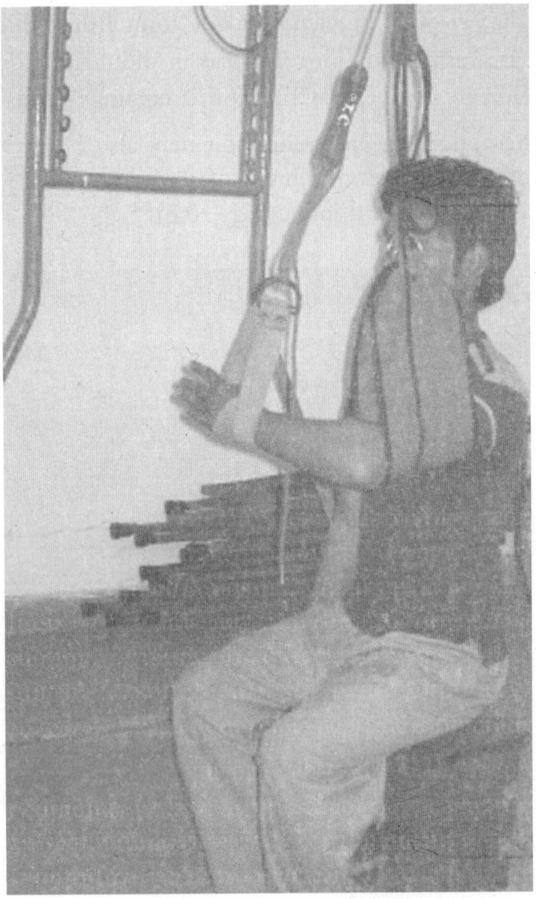

Fig. 10.9a: Elbow flexion

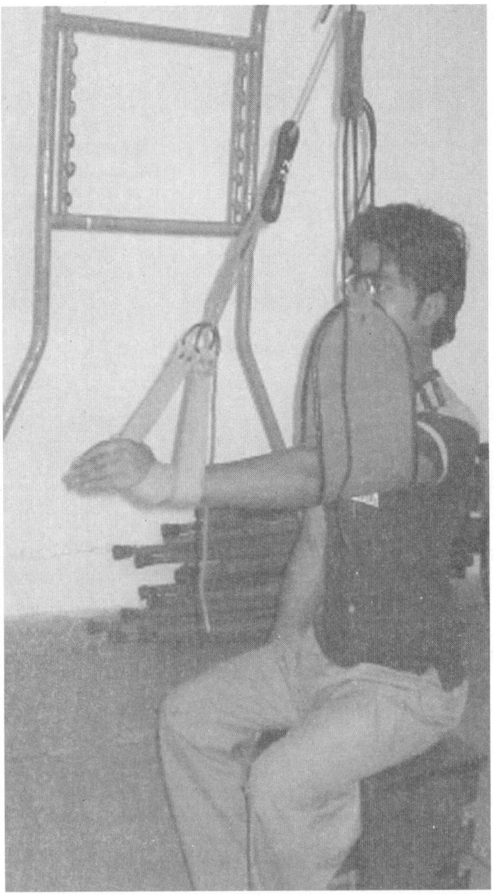

Fig. 10.9b: Elbow extension

Clinical Uses of Suspension Therapy

(i) Muscle relaxation.

(ii) Maintain physical properties of muscles.

(iii) Increase blood circulation.

(iv) Increase various and lymphatic drainage.

(v) Increase, restore and maintain muscle strength and endurance.

(vi) Prevent pressure sores.

(vii) Increase, restore, and maintain range of motion.

11

HYDROTHERAPY

The use of water for various treatments (hydrotherapy) is probably as old as mankind. Hydrotherapy is one of the basic methods of treatment widely used in the system of natural medicine, which is also called as water therapy, aquatic therapy, pool therapy and balneotherapy.[1] Hydrotherapy is the use of water for accelerating healing, repairing and easing various musculoskeletal and neurological ailments. The benefit of 'water healing' or hydrotherapy have been recognized for thousands of years. In Europe, where hydrotherapy is especially popular, there are numerous health spas and health facilities for all types of 'water cures'.

Ancient civilization recognized the healing power of natural hot and cold springs. Back in the 4th century BC the Greek physician Hippocrates prescribed bathing and deinking spring water for its therapeutic effects. The Greek were the first to appreciate the relationship between physical and mental well being. They developed centers near spring and rivers using them for bathing and recreation. The baths were centers where intellectual, recreational activities, and health and hygiene were pursued. Around AD 339 some baths (built by Greek, and extended by Romans) were used solely for healing purposes and treatment was indicated first of all for symptoms of rheumatic disease, paralysis, and the effects of injuries.

RATIONALISM OF USE OF WATER AS A PHYSICAL AGENT

Use of water is one of the oldest, cheapest and safest methods of treating many common ailments. When the body or part of the body is immersed in the water it produces several physiological effects on the body. The buoyancy force generated in the upward direction against the gravity reduces load on the weight bearing joints. The reduction of load on the joints decreases pain and increases the confidence of the patient to exercises in the pool. The hydrostatic pressure exerted by the water on the extremities and body reduces swelling by increasing the venous return.

BIOPHYSICAL CHARACTERISTICS OF WATER

The biophysical characteristics of hydrotherapy rests on the principles and concepts related to the mechanical intrinsic and thermal properties of water.

A. Mechanical Properties

a. **Buoyancy** – There is the upward force in the water which works against the gravity. This fluid force always acts vertically upward. The upward force generated by the water against the gravity is based on Archimedes' Principle, which states that an object or body part, totally or partially immersed in a fluid, experiences an upward, buoyant force equal to the weight of the volume of fluid displaced by that object or body part.[2] The effect of buoyancy reduces the weight and stresses on the weight bearing joints which helps in improving the balance and coordination of patients who find difficulty in standing on ground.

b. **Hydrostatic Pressure** – Hydrostatic pressure is the pressure exerted by the water on the body. According to Pascal's law, when a body part is immersed in the water a pressure is exerted equally at any level in a horizontal direction. This pressure is exerted by the water on all surfaces of the body when it is at rest at a given depth. The hydrostatic pressure increases with the depth and with the density of the fluid (density of the water increases with the depth). Therefore, standing and walking in the water is having greater importance to decrease edema. In standing the distal part of the extremity is the lowest in the water, hence, the pressure gradient between the surface and deeper water favors reduced accumulation of fluid in the distal parts of an extremity. The head out immersion of the body into the water at 35°C facilitates in increasing venous return and shifting of the fluid from the interstitial space to the capillary.

c. **Hydrodynamic Pressure** – It is the pressure caused by movement of either the object or the water. When the person walks in the water resistance is encountered and demand is made on the walking muscles. The faster one walks, the more demands are made on the walking muscles. This pressure offers resistance against the movements of the limbs; therefore, resistance can be used for strengthening of the muscles.

d. **Turbulence** – It is defined as "the velocity at a given point varies erratically in magnitude and direction". The movements of limbs in the water cause circular patterns of the water and create small whirlpools or eddy currents and turbulence. Movement through turbulent water or against the current than through calm water encounters greater resistance which requires more muscular effort. The circular patterns caused by movement of the legs, arms and body of the patient also known as drag force. The drag force is exerted by water on a submerged and moving objects or body segment.[3] The combined effects of buoyancy and hydrostatic is helpful in balancing the body in the water. The pressure supports the body all around to and equal degree in the horizontal direction while buoyancy maintains the vertical position.

B. Intrinsic Properties – Water Exhibits Three Intrinsic Properties such as Density, Specific Gravity and Viscosity

a. **Density** – Different materials usually have different densities, and density may be relevant to buoyancy, purity and packing. The density, or more precisely, the volumetric mass density, of a substance is its mass per unit volume. The symbol most often used for density is P. Mathematically, density is defined as mass divided by volume p = m/V, where p is the density, m is the mass, and V is the volume. the more compactly arranged the molecules, the denser the substance. The density of the material varies with temperature and pressure. Increasing the temperature decreases its density by increasing its volume. Increasing the pressure on an object decreases the volume of the object and thus increases its density.

b. **Specific Gravity** – The specific gravity of the water is unity or 1, because its weight density, as a fluid, equals 9.8 N/L. The object which has the specific gravity greater than 1 would sink in the water. On the other hand the object which has the specific gravity equivalent to the water or less than 1, would float on the water. The specific gravity of human body, which varies depending on the individual's somatotype and residual air volume in the lungs at immersion, is less than 1. Therefore, the human body generally floats on the water when it is totally immersed into the water.

c. **Viscosity** – The viscosity of the water varies from one state to another due to change in the temperature. Viscosity is caused by the chemical binding forces holding the fluid molecules together, such as the forces binding hydrogen to oxygen molecules to form water. The water is more viscous at the lower temperature and its molecules are dispersed at the higher temperatures.

C. Thermal Properties

a. **Specific Heat** – The specific heat value of water is 1 cal/g°C because a heat input of 1 calorie is needed to increase the temperature of 1 g of pure water at 15°C by 1°C. Water has the capacity of holding the heat double of the paraffin wax and four times more than the air at any given temperature. A paraffin wax would contain 50% less heat than water at the same temperature. Hence, the patients can tolerate the paraffin wax bath at the 50°C than the water.

b. **Thermal Conductivity** – Thermal conductivity (often denoted κ, λ, or κ) is the property of a material to conduct heat. It is evaluated primarily in terms of Fourier's Law for heat conduction. The higher the thermal conductivity value of the substance the better the substance performs as a heat conductor. The thermal conductivity value of water at 15°C is 1.42 cal/sec-cm°C. The fat conducts heat 50% slower than the skeletal muscles and 30% slower than the skin. The thermal conductivity of the water is 70 times faster than the air and 2.5 times more rapidly than the paraffin wax.

PHYSIOLOGICAL EFFECTS

Use of water in various forms and in various temperatures can produce different effects on different system of the body. The temperature is the good conductor of the heat. The temperature of water which is slightly higher than the body temperature produces several physiological changes in the body. The normal temperature of the skin and the subcutaneous tissues is 33°C, whereas, the internal temperature of the body is maintained at 37°C. Superficial cold application may cause physiologic reactions such as decrease in local metabolic function, local edema, nerve conduction velocity (NCV), muscle spasm, and increase in local anesthetic effects.[4] The temperature of the skin varies with cold and hot conditions. The living tissues of the body are affected by temperature in two fundamental ways:

A. The direct effects of the temperature on the body includes increase metabolic rate, increase collagen tissue extensibility and decrease viscosity.
   a. **Metabolic Activity** – Metabolic activities are the series of chemical reactions which increase as temperature increases and decrease with fall of temperature. An appropriate rise in temperature increases all cell activities including cell motility and synthesis and release of chemical mediators. Excessive temperature above 45°C of the body causes so much protein, cell and tissue destruction. If the temperature of body rises by 1°C it increases 13% metabolic activities.
   b. **Decrease Viscosity** – The resistance to flow blood in a vessel depends directly on the viscosity of the fluid and inversely on the fourth power of the radius of the vessel. As the temperature rises, the blood vessels get dilated and the viscosity of fluid also decreases. The resistance to flow to the blood decreases.

B. **Systemic Changes** – One hour head-out water immersions (WI) in various temperatures (32°C, 20°C, and 14°C) produced various effects. Immersion at 32°C did not change metabolic rate (MR) and rectal temperature, but it lowered the heart rate (HR) by 15%, systolic blood pressure (SBP) and diastolic blood pressure (DBP) by 11% and 12%, respectively, compared, with controls at ambient air temperature. Along with HR and blood pressure (BP), the plasma renin activity, plasma cortisol, and aldosterone concentrations were also lowered by 46%, 34% and 17%, respectively, while diuresis was increased by 107%.[5]

C. The indirect effects of the temperature on the body are mainly activation of the higher centers to regulate the excess temperature and protect the organs to damage.

INDICATIONS

Hydrotherapy, the use of water as a physical modality for health promotion and treatment of various diseases with different level of temperature has been used widely in ancient culture including India, Egypt and China.[6]

1. **Cerebral Palsy Children** – Hydrotherapy is highly effective form of treatment for cerebral palsy children and adolescents. The buoyancy effect of water relieves load on the lower extremities, whereas, the optimal temperature of the water reduces the spasticity. These effects of water facilitate the voluntary movements. The water offers resistance against the movements during the gait training that further facilitates the voluntary control and balance of the patient. Blohm D[7] conducted the review to evaluate the effectiveness of aquatic interventions for children or adolescents with cerebral palsy. All eight studies reported that aquatic interventions, either as a major component or as a stand alone intervention, were beneficial for children and adolescents with cerebral palsy. Blohm D found improvements in activity for gross motor skills; maintenance of improvement in gross motor function; and increased swimming skills for kindergarten children. The study also reported increases in lower extremity muscle strength[8] and balance; better respiratory function and reduced spasticity in adolescents. Improvements were also reported for range of motion with an increase in passive range of motion of lower extremity joints (one study), and improved active and passive range of motion.
2. **Osteoarthritis** – Exercises in the hydrotherapy pool for knee, ankle and hip osteoarthritic patients with the complaint of pain, lack of confidence, and have high risk of falling may be an excellent alternative to land exercise.[9] Water buoyancy force which is in upward direction against the gravity reduces load or weight of the body on the joints.[10] The warmth water reduces muscle guarding and hydrostatic pressure of water also reduce swelling. These effects promote muscle relaxation and reduces swelling.[11]
3. **Inflammatory Arthritis** – In patients with ankylosing spondylitis (AS), balneotherapy statistically improved pain; physical activity; tiredness and sleep score; on Bath Ankylosing Spondylitis Disease Activity Index (BASDAI). It indicates the effect of balneotherapy in improving disease activity and functional parameters in patients with ankylosing spondylitis.[12] Infrared sauna, a form of total-body hyperthermia was well tolerated; no adverse effects; and no exacerbation of disease were reported in patients with rheumatoid arthritis (RA) and AS in whom pain, stiffness, and fatigue showed clinical improvements during the 4 weeks treatment period.[13] Hydrotherapy is highly valued by RA patients who were treated with hydrotherapy (30-min session/week) reported feeling much better/very much better than those treated with land exercises (similar exercises on land) immediately on completion of the treatment program (6 weeks).[11]
4. **Fibromyalgia** – A systematic review on management of fibromyalgia syndrome (FMS) through hydrotherapy described as "there is strong evidence for the use of hydrotherapy in the management of FMS" and it

showed positive outcomes for pain; tender point count; and health status. Combination of ST (once daily for 3 days/week) and underwater exercise (once daily for 2 days/week) for 12 weeks significantly reduced pain and symptoms (both short- and long-term); and improved QOL in patients with FMS. Pool-based exercise using deep water running three times/week for 8 weeks is safe and effective intervention for FMS because it showed significant improvement in general health and QOL compared with control; and significant improvement in fibromyalgia impact questionnaire score, incorporating pain; fatigue; physical function; stiffness and psychological variables.

5. **Muscle soreness and fatigue** – Leg immersion in warm water (44 ± 1°C) for 45 min before stretch-shortening exercise reduced most of the indirect markers of exercise-induced muscle damage, including muscle soreness, creatine kinase activity in the blood, maximal voluntary contraction force, and jump height. Immersion of extremities of body in the water with the temperature below 15°C lowers ratings of fatigue and potentially improves ratings of physical recovery immediately after immersion with reduction in delayed onset muscle soreness compared with the passive stretching.

CONTRAINDICATIONS

- Pyrexia.
- Active bleeding.
- Acute vomiting or diarrhea.
- Cardiac insufficiency, recent heart attack or resting angina.
- Wound infection.
- Recent neurological event.
- Recent chemotherapy.
- Present history of deep venous thrombosis or pulmonary embolism.
- Stress incontinence.
- AIDS.
- Shortness of breath at rest.
- Uncontrolled epilepsy.

HYDROTHERAPY POOL

Hydrotherapy pool is of different sizes and shapes from a standard pool to large sized to provide therapeutic exercises to treat various musculoskeletal, neurological and sports related injuries. Hydrotherapy is the use of physical properties of water such as temperature and pressure, for therapeutic purposes. The construction and design of the pool depends upon the need of the department.

A **Butterfly Tank** – It is a butterfly shaped hydrotherapy unit designed for arms and legs exercises to be carried out in the unit. It is ideal for the cerebral palsy children. The recessed area at the head and sides of the bath provide good access for the therapist commanding and encouraging the patient for the exercises. The tank is designed for permanent installations with direct connections to hot and cold water supply, overflow and drainage. It is constructed of heavy gauge stainless steel sheet electrically Argon welded tank is shaped to Butterfly (Fig. 11.1).

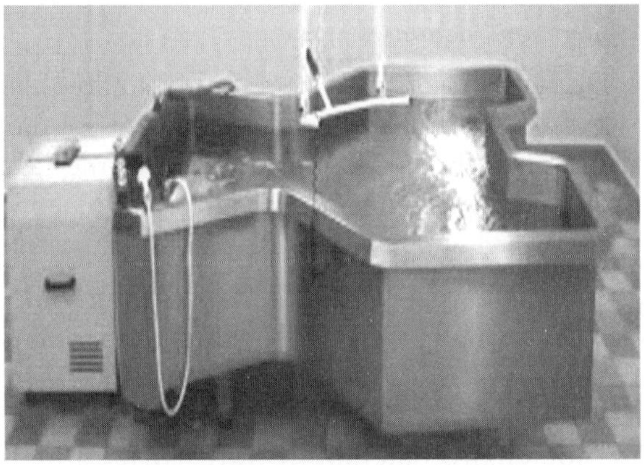

Fig. 11.1: Butterfly unit (Hubbard's tank)

Whirl Pool – Whirl pool bath made of heavy gauge stainless steel is sturdily fabricated with bright finish inside. The unit is fitted with a motorized turbine ejector and aerator on a spring loaded turbine elevator. The jets are strategically directed at the key muscle groups that are vulnerable to stress and soreness. Ten minutes of immersions in whirlpools produce increase in pulse and finger temperature with increased feelings of well-being and decreased state of anxiety.[14] Whirl pool immersion increases metabolic rate, oxygen intake, and removes metabolites and wastages from the body. It accelerates the healing process (Fig. 11.2).

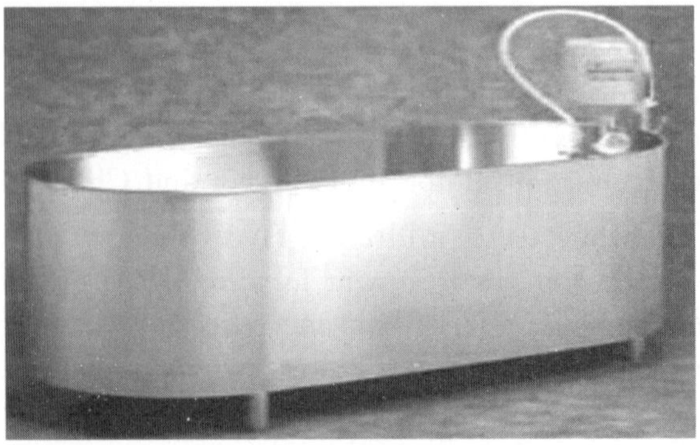

Fig. 11.2: Whirl pool

B. **Hydrotherapy Pool** – Different sizes, shapes, and depths of hydrotherapy pool according to the number of the patients are constructed in the physiotherapy department. Three types of pools are commonly constructed in the department:

a. Below ground.

b. Below ground deck level; and

c. Semi raised or raised.

Below Ground With or Without Deck Pool – Below ground pool with or without deck level is generally advised to construct. The floor of the pool may be of height adjustable with the motorized system. The advantage of the height adjustable pool is that the wheel chair bound patients would enter easily into the pool as the floor is lifted at the ground level and then it is lowered to the desired depth (Fig. 11.3).

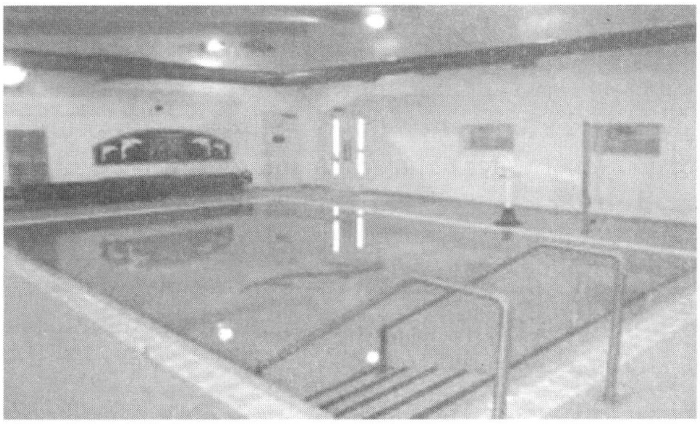

Fig. 11.3: Hydrotherapy pool (Below ground)

Size – In the daily practice the size of the pool should be of 9.24 meter length and 4.57 in the width. This size of pool provides a good working space for approximately eight people at a time and is used for the most of therapeutic activities. However the size may be kept small if the number of patients on pool therapy are not in large size.

Shape – Rectangular shape of pool is strongly recommended.

Depth – The depth of the pool also varies from .84 meter to 1.42 meter.

Floor – The floor may be uniform or stepped. Stepped floor is having advantages of providing several depth. To avoid fear of stepped floor, the edge of each step must be clearly marked. The steps used in the hydrotherapy pool should have height of 150 mm, depth 300 mm and width 600 mm to avoid any inconvenience. Patients may enter into the pool with the help of stairs or they may be shifted into the pool by hoists (a mechanical hydrolytic and electrical). Recently height adjustable floors are introduced to maintain the desired depth and to provide barrier free access to the wheelchair bound patients. However, these pools cost little bit high than the other pools. Parallel bars are installed at appropriate side of the pool with an appropriate height. The handrails at both the side of the stairs are also installed. The assistive devices such as turbulence, underwater jets floats for the activities and to facilitate exercise should be available.

Temperature of Pool – The temperature of pool depends on the condition of the patient. Different authors have suggested different temperature for various conditions. Two main factors affecting oxygen transport during immersion are temperature and hydrostatic pressure. Oxygen transport was improved above neutral temperature, because of increase in cardiac output resulting from the combined actions of hydrostatic counter pressure and body heating. Below neutral temperature, oxygen transport is altered. At any of the temperatures tested, the pulmonary tissue volume and arterial blood gases were not significantly affected.

Exercises in water can be performed in wide range of temperature, but warmer temperature appear to be more favorable for therapeutic activities.[15] Heat is lost from the body much faster in water than when exercising elsewhere, even though the ambient temperature in a gym is likely to be much less than the water temperature. The thin people lose heat more quickly because they do not have such a good layer of subcutaneous fat. On the other hand, obese people have too much insulation, and could theoretically be at risk from overheating. An ideal temperature for exercising with chronic arthritis would be thermoneutral. Some authors believe a pool temperature of 30.5 to 33.3ºC (87 to 92° F) is ideal for therapeutic exercise and general physical programmes providing both sedative and stimulating effects. In the United Kingdom it is not recommended that therapeutic activity takes place if the water is less than 27°C, whereas, in the United States, pool water is generally kept lower than, at about 24°C. In view of the above it can be inferred that the temperature between 32°C (89.6°F) and 35°C (95°F) is suitable for the therapeutic activities. This range of temperature caters all conditions.[16]

Ventilation – The temperature of room should be lower than that of the temperature of water to allow gently cooling. It is maintained at 25°C. A dehumidifier decreases the humidity of the room and maintains humidity at the appropriate level.

Changing Room – There should be a separate room for changing clothes before and after the pool therapy. This should have direct access to the pool. Sometimes it is constructed inside the pool. The privacy of the patient should be the priority of the therapist. The changing room temperature should be maintained 4°C lower than the temperature of the pool.

Preparation of the Patient

- Patient should be examined thoroughly for the contraindication especially for the contaminated diseases.
- Treatment should not be given immediately after meals, nor it is wise to give them too longer after meals.
- The patient should be asked to empty his or her bladder before immersion, since a warm bath often has a diuretic action.
- The patient should be asked to put on shorts or in the case of female patients a proper bathing suit is given.
- Before entering into the pool the patient is asked to take a bath.
- Non ambulatory patients are transferred into the pool with the assistance or electrically or hydraulically operated hoist. The ambulatory patients may walk down the steps if the pool is below ground. If the pool is raised above the ground all the patients can be transferred by the hydraulically or electrically operated hoist.
- Adjustable floor, if available, provide direct access to the pool.
- The temperature of the pool should be as per the condition of the patient.
- The treatment should not exceed the appropriate time.
- After completing session the patient is transferred to the changing room immediately. He or she should be given plenty of water. The patient should leave the room after half an hour of the therapy.

STRENGTHENING EXERCISES IN POOL

Strengthening exercises are carried out in the hydrotherapy pool to strengthen the muscles of lower and upper extremity. The proper assessment of the muscle strength of each muscle needs to be done before starting the exercises. Muscles those are grade 2 are strengthen by using the buoyancy effect. However, grade 3 and grade 4 muscles may be strengthen with resistance offered by the water. The therapist should instruct the patient with an appropriate verbal commands. Free exercises such as mini squat, step up and step down active range of motion against the resistance of water help in improving the strength of the muscles. The progression of exercises in water should be based on the improvement in the strength and balance of the muscle.

OXFORD SCALE FOR MUSCLE POWER GRADING – MODIFIED FOR WATER

This scale is used to grade the strength of the muscle in water but it is limited to the muscles which retain little power but range of movement. The scale of muscle power on land is graded from 0 to 5 where 0 has no contraction and 5 is the normal. In water the scale commences from 1 and continues to 5 but it must be recognized that grade 5 in water is not normal as such function cannot be tested there.

The scale of muscle power modified for water is as under:

1. Contraction with buoyancy assistance.
2. Contraction with buoyancy counter balanced and contraction against buoyancy.
3. Contraction against buoyancy at speed.
4. Contraction against buoyancy and light float.
5. Contraction against buoyancy and heavy float.

GAIT TRAINING IN POOL

Hydrotherapy can reduce weight-bearing to 20%, enabling re-education of gait to commence very early in a patient's recovery. The buoyancy force, hydrostatic pressure and temperature of water reduce pain and swelling. These effects of pool therapy increase the confidence of the patient and encourages for the exercises. The studies found that the patients who find difficulty in standing and walking on the ground have improved the balance, coordination and gait after the pool therapy.

The patient is transferred into the pool manually or by the hoist. To improve standing balance, non-ambulatory patients are made stand in the pool and asked to hold the railings of parallel bar. As the balance improves, patient is asked to raise one hand above the shoulder. Both the hands are raised alternately. In the progression the patient is asked to stand without the support of the railings. Both the hands are raised above the shoulder simultaneously. As the patient gains confidence he or she is asked to throw the ball and catch it. The therapist should throw the ball to the patient little away from the midline.

Once the patient gains confidence in standing he or she is asked to place heel of one leg forward. The same is repeated on the other leg also. An appropriate size of the step is placed before the patient. He or she is instructed to place one foot over the step and then take it down. It is repeatedly performed on both the legs. Three sets of thirty repetitions of mini squat (30 flexion) are done daily. If the patient gains confidence in doing mini squat and step up and down without the support, he or she is asked to ambulate in the pool without the support of the parallel bar. If the patient gains confidence on walking in the pool then he or she should practice gait training on land with the help of parallel bars.

FOOT BATHS

There are two types of foot baths – cold foot bath and warm foot bath. For cold foot bath, a small tub is used with the cold water up to the level of calf muscles. The temperature of the water should not exceed 18°C. Cold foot bath is indicated to the patients with varicose vein, headache, low blood pressure, sweaty foot, contused ankles and circulatory impairment. Both the feet are placed into the water up to the level of calf muscles for at least 15 minutes. Cold bath should be avoided to the patients with cold feet, hypertension, irritable bladder, urinary tract infection and diabetes. The large size of the foot can also be used if the aim of the treatment is exercises in the tub. The warm foot bath is indicated to the patients with cold feet. A small size tub of warm water with the temperature of 97°F is taken. The feet are immersed into the bath and hot water is gradually added till it reaches to the 103°F-104°F. The temperature of the tub is maintained at this level by adding more warm water and procedure should last 10-15 minutes. The procedure can be repeated daily for at least two weeks. The warm foot bath should be avoided to the patients with varicose veins, lymphostasis or edema.

SITZ BATH

The small tub with the warm water with the temperature of 103–104°F is suitable for the sitz bath. The size of the tub should be appropriate so that patient can sit easily on it. Patient sits in the tub and the water covers the glutei. The patient maintains the sitting position for 15–20 minutes. Hot water may be added during the procedure to maintain the temperature of the water at 103°F to 104°F. The sitz bath are indicated to the patient with anal fissures, piles, difficulty in voiding the bladder, and irritable bladder, inflammation or infection of the prostate and preparation for the pregnancy.

BODY WRAPS

Wrap is primarily used as supportive measure for treating fever and local inflammation. For the therapeutic purposes hot wraps and cold wraps are basically used. The treatment period lasts around 45 to 60 minutes sometimes up to three hours. Patient is placed in a comfortable position. A linen cloth is moisturized with cold or hot water. Patient is wrapped with the hot or cold linen for an appropriate time. The cold water wraps are advised for pyrexia and hot packs are for respiratory diseases. They are wrapped properly around the part or body which is being treated. The patient is wrapped in a blanket or another cloth for 45 to 60 minutes. Cold wraps are advised to the rheumatoid arthritis and pyrexia, whereas, hot wraps are advised to the bronchitis, lung diseases, neuralgia, prostatitis, vaginitis, and inflammation in the pelvic cavity.

REFERENCES

1. A Mooventhan and L Nivethitha. Scientific Evidence-Based Effects of Hydrotherapy on Various Systems of the Body, N Am J Med Sci 2014 May; 6(5):199–209.
2. Kreighbaum E, Barthelss KM (1996) Biomechanics: A Qualitative Approach to Studying Human Movement. Allyn and Bacon 98–99.
3. Alain – Yvan Belanger. Therapeutic Electrophysical agents evidence Behind Practice, third edition, Wolters Kluwer 126.
4. Weston M, Taber C, Casagranda L, Cornwall M. Changes in local blood volume during cold gel pack application to traumatized ankles. J Orthop Sports Phys Ther 1994;19:197–99.
5. Srámek P, Simecková M, Janský L, Savlíková J, Vybíral S. Human physiological responses to immersion into water of different temperatures. Eur J Appl Physiol 2000; 81:436–42.
6. Fleming SA, Gutknecht NC. Gutknecht. Naturopathy and the Primary Care Practice. Prim Care 2010;37:119–36.
7. Blohm D effectiveness of aquatic interventions for children with cerebral palsy: Systemic review of the current literature. University of York, Centre of Reviews and Dissemination 24.04.2013.
8. Gorter JW, Currie SJ. Aquatic exercise program for children and adolescents with cerebral palsy: Why do we know and where do we go? University of York, Centre of Reviews and Dissemination 24.07.2014.
9. Arnold CM, Busch AJ, Schachter CL, Harrison EL, Olszynski WP. A Randomized clinical trial of aquatic versus land exercise to improve balance, function, and quality of life in older women with osteoporosis. Physiother Can 2008; 60: 296–306.
10. Biscarini A, Cerulli G. Modeling of the knee joint load in rehabilitative knee extension exercises under water. J Biomech 2006;17:1–11.
11. Eversden L, Maggs F, Nightingale P, Jobanputra P. A pragmatic randomised controlled trial of hydrotherapy and land exercises on overall well being and quality of life in rheumatoid arthritis. BMC Musculoskelet Disord 2007;8:23.
12. Altan L, Bingöl U, Aslan M, Yurtkuran M. The effect of balneotherapy on patients with ankylosing spondylitis. Scand J Rheumatol 2006;35:283–89.
13. Oosterveld FG, Rasker JJ, Floors M, Landkroon R, van Rennes B, Zwijnenberg J, *et al.* Infrared sauna in patients with rheumatoid arthritis and ankylosing spondylitis. A pilot study showing good tolerance, short-term improvement of pain and stiffness, and a trend towards long-term beneficial effects. Clin Rheumatol 2009;28:29–34.
14. Robiner WN. Psychological and physical reactions to whirlpool baths. J Behav Med 1990;13: 157–73.
15. Becker B and Cole A. Comprehensive Aquatic Therapy. Butterworth Heinemann. Woburn MA, 2003.
16. Sova, Ruth. "Exercising in Hot Weather", The AKWA Letter, Vol. 3, #2, July 1989.

12

RELAXATION

INTRODUCTION

Relaxation may be defined as a state in which muscles are free from tension or are in the normal physiological state. This is accompanied by a feeling of diminished consciousness of the external world, drowsiness, passivity, and focussing of the attention on feeling of internal well being *(Rosa 1976)*. Many techniques such as deep breathing, tai chai, yoga, meditation and relaxation exercises are practiced by the people for feeling of internal well being. Healthy diet, regular walk, and enough sleep help in achieving the mental relaxation, necessary for the healthy lifestyle.

Muscle Tension

Normal muscle is never free from tension even when the person is in fully relaxed state. This tension in the muscle is known as physiological muscle tone/tension which is provided or maintained by the intrafusal muscle fibres.

There are two types of muscle fibres, extrafusal and intrafusal. Contraction of extrafusal muscle fibre causes increase in muscle tension or tone, that results in movement at the joint. The tone of extrafusal fibres decreases when they come to the original position or resting state from contracted state. Therefore the tone of extrafusal fibres keeps changing. The tone of intrafusal muscle fibres do not change during the voluntary movement and at the resting state. These are the muscle fibres whose tone remains constant during the activities and at the rest and their fibres provide firmness and maintain the muscle tone/tension during resting state.

There are some abnormal conditions in which the tone of muscle fibres increases as the response of trauma, stress, head injury, stretching of muscle fibres and pathologicals diseases.

Stress

Stress is the "psychological, physiological and behavioural response by an individual when they perceive a lack of equilibrium between the damands placed upon them and their ability to meet those demands, which, over a period of time, leads to ill-health" (Palmer, 1989).

It's believed that stress has remained part of the evolutionary drive because of its usefulness in helping us to survive. Since when it's used at the right time, stress temporarily increases our awareness and improves physical performance (Van Duyne, 2003). Schmidth (1998) states that arousal may be considered as a neutral state that it represents the amount of effort that an individual applies to an action. Stress and motivation represents different type of arousal and are considered to have directional components. Stress is usually considered as negative and motivation as positive component. Mental attitudes such as fear, anger and excitement give rise to general increase in muscular tension which serves a useful purpose by preparing the muscle, for rapid or forceful action (Dina Gardiner).

A small amount of stress can be good, motivating individuals to perform well. But multiple challenges, such as sitting in traffic, meeting deadlines and additional responsibilities to the actual work, can push individuals beyond their ability to cope. Repetitive exposure of the stress response on our body is proven to lead to long-lasting psychological and physical health issues, such as cardiovascular disease, diabetes, anxiety and depression. Stress has been referred to as the "silent killer" as it can silently cause heart disease, high blood pressure, chest pain, and an irregular heartbeat (Chilnick, 2008).

Work-related stress is the response people may have when presented with work demands and pressures that are not matched to their knowledge and abilities and which challenge their ability to cope. Stress occurs in a wide range of work circumstances but is often made worse when employees feel they have little support from seniors and colleagues, as well as little control over work processes. Pressure perceived as acceptable by an individual, may even keep workers alert, motivated, able to work and learn, depending on the available resources and personal characteristics. However, when that pressure becomes excessive or otherwise unmanageable it leads to stress.

Pathological Tension in the Muscles

Every muscle of the body is supplied by the nerve via spinal reflex arc, spinal cord to higher motor centres (brain). Lesion in the pathway above the nucleus of anterior horn cell of spinal cord causes sustained contraction of muscle fibres (spasticity or rigidity). Inflammatory, degenerative conditions of the joint, local trauma or injury to the muscles can cause protective muscle guarding (increase tension in the muscles).

Cortisol is a thyroid hormone produced by the adrenal gland that gets released when the individual is stressed. When cortisol is released for a long period of time, it has adverse effects on body. Cortisol causes glucose to be released into the blood so that it can send a lot of energy to the muscles. When situation lasts for a long period, adverse symptoms such as behavioral changes (irritability, anger, bad mood), hypertension, headache, lack of appetite or excessive hunger and memory loss may occur. According to Texas Heart Institute, stress is one of the factors that most increase the probability of suffering from cardio-vascular illness. The stress increases heart rate and blood pressure, which increases the heart's need for orygen. Tian Xu conducted experiment and revealed that 'stressed' cells can emit signals that induce the generation of tumor, affecting nearby healthy cells. A group of Argentinian researchers identified stress as a trigger for the onset of dementia in their study. They found that stress can trigger a degenerative process in the brain and transfer it to the neuroendocrine and immune systems.

Physiological Manifestation of Relaxation

1. Decrease heart rate.
2. Decrease blood pressure.
3. Decrease O_2 consumption.
4. Decrease CO_2 production and excretion.
5. Decrease blood cholesterol and lactate.
6. Decrease tension in muscle.
7. Decrease metabolic rate.
8. Peripheral vasodilatation.
9. Increased peripheral temperature.
10. Pupil constriction.
11. Increase saliva output.
12. Increase digestive activity.
13. Increase urine output.

Indications of Relaxation

1. Acute neuromuscular hypertension.
2. Chronic neuromuscular hypertension.
3. States of fatigue and exhaustion.
4. States of debility.
5. Various pre-operative and post-operative conditions.
6. Sleep disturbance.
7. Spasticity.
8. Arthritis and related conditions.
9. Bell's palsy.
10. Burns (Post burn contractures).
11. High blood pressure.

RELAXATION TECHNIQUES

- **Local relaxation**
  - Therapeutic massage *(Discussed in Ch-9).*
  - Passive movements *(Discussed in Ch-3).*
  - Muscle energy techniques *(Discussed in Ch-20).*
  - Hold relax.
  - Contract relax.
- **General relaxation**
  - Contrast method.
  - Reciprocal inhibition.
- **Other relaxation techniques.**

Local Relaxation

Therapeutic Massage

It is the technique which is used to improve the blood circulation and remove waste products from the target area. After performing few strokes of massage, the extensibility of the scar tissue/spasmodic muscle increase and patient feels relaxed.

Passive Movements

More beneficial to stretch the muscles, when it is performed on particular muscle or group of muscles followed by *hold relax* or *contract relax.*

Hold Relax

Hold relax is an isometric contraction of the spasmodic muscles at different angles to reduce the spasm, improve range of motion and pain. It is advised, when acute muscle spasm limiting the range severely.

The muscle or group of muscles which are said to be antagonistic to the movement do not allow the joint to move because of spasm. To overcome this problem the resistance against isometric contraction is applied to a muscle or group of muscles which are in tension. The patient is asked to hold the position unless therapist responses 'Relax' or 'let go'. The position (isometric contraction) is maintained for 6 sec or when the therapist feels that the patient has reached the limit of his potential contraction, he grasps the limb firmly, but comfortably and at the same time tells the patient to 'relax' or 'let go' and allow a period of time at least as long as or perhaps longer than the time to build up the maximum contraction.

For example: Spasm in the shoulder adductors can prevent the shoulder abduction. Resistance is applied to adductors of the shoulder joint. Spasm in the shoulder adductors prevent the abduction of the shoulder joint, because when patient attempts to abduct the shoulder joint stretching in the spasmed muscles (adductors) causes pain and thus limits to further abduction.

The procedure is followed as under:

1. The shoulder is abducted slightly by the therapist passively, till the patient complains no pain.
2. Therapist grasps the elbow joint firmly but comfortably (Fig. 12.1a) and instructs the patient to contract the adductors isometrically.
3. Patient adducts the shoulder joint (try to take it to the chest) against the resistance.
4. Therapist maintains the position (isometric contraction) while patient is engaged with contraction of adductors for six seconds and then instructs the patient to relax the adductors (relaxation period should be more than six seconds) (Fig. 12.1b).

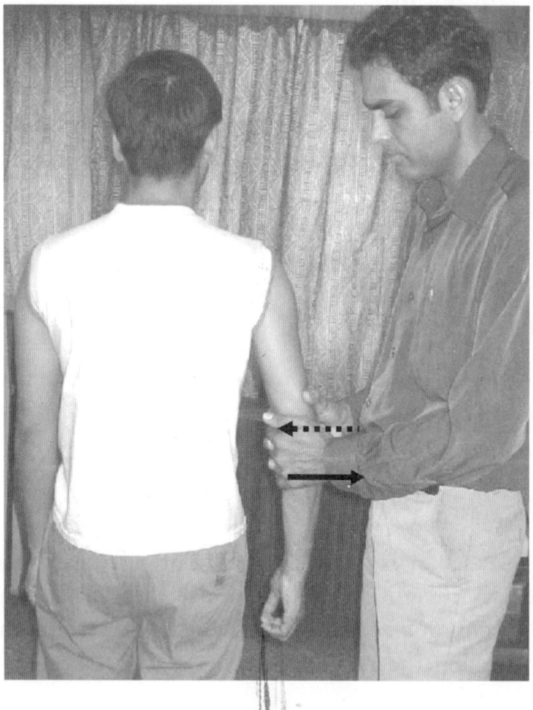

a

- Therapist again abducts the shoulder joint and finds increase in the range of motion and abducts the shoulder joint till the patient complains no pain. The position where patient complains pain, is held firmly but comfortably. Patient is instructed to contract the adductors isometrically against the resistance for six seconds and then let go. The several isometric contractions can be held at different positions as the range increases (Fig. 12.1c).

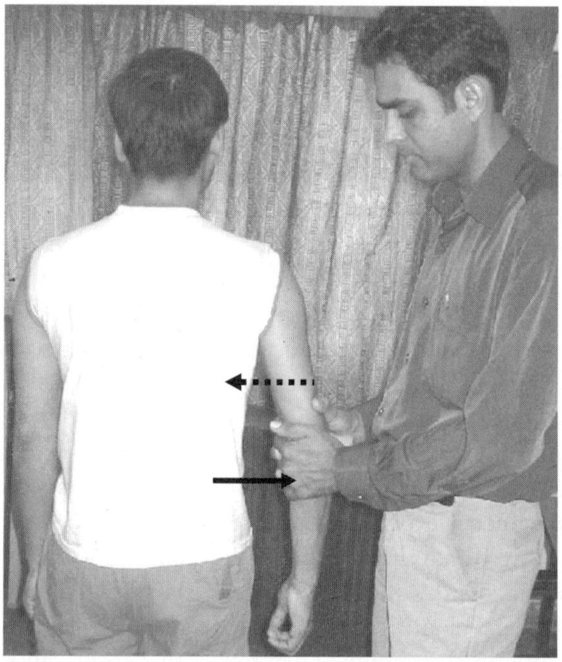

b

Figs. 12.1a and b: Hold relax—(a) Initial position and (b) Dotted arrow shows contraction of shoulder adductors and black arrow shows resistance by therapist

c

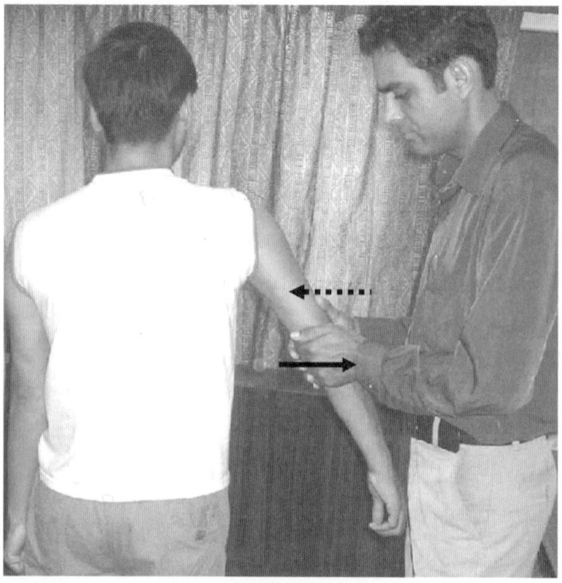

Fig. 12.1c: Hold relax (next angle for hold relax) dotted arrow shows contraction of shoulder adductors and black arrow shows resistance by therapist

- The main purpose of this exercise is to relax the muscles and increase the range of motion.

Contract Relax

Contract relax is an isotonic contraction of the spasmodic muscles at different angles to reduce spasm, and improve range of motion and pain. This technique may be used when a patient has a range of motion but it is prevented from moving further by the spasm of the muscles which are antagonist to the movement.

Technique: The patient is asked to move the joint in painfree range. The range may also be achieved by passive movement. The therapist grasps the limb and patient is asked to make a strong isotonic contraction against resistance back to the original position. At the end of the movement the part is grasped firmly, but comfortably and the patient is told to relax. The period of relaxation should be of adequate time (Figs. 12.2a and b).

The next painfree range should again be attempted with passively or actively. Gain in ROM may be found. Therapist holds the arm at the restricted range firmly but comfortably and instructs the patient to contract the adductors (take the arm towards chest) isotonically against the resistance. Several small arc isotonic contractions can be performed to improve range and spasm.

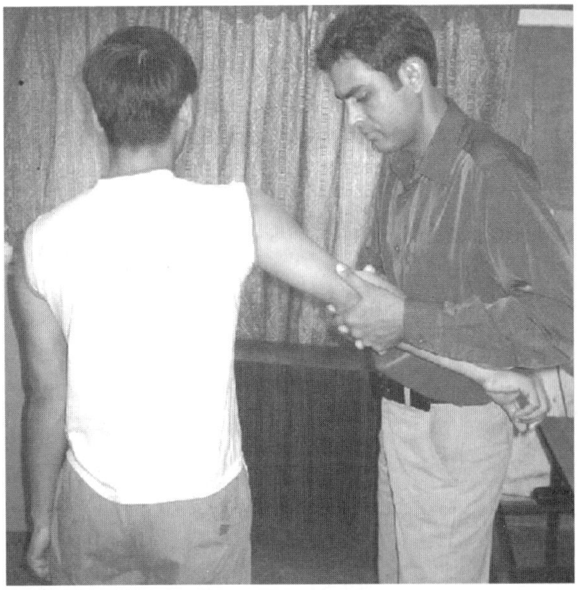

Fig. 12.2a: Contract relax (initial position)

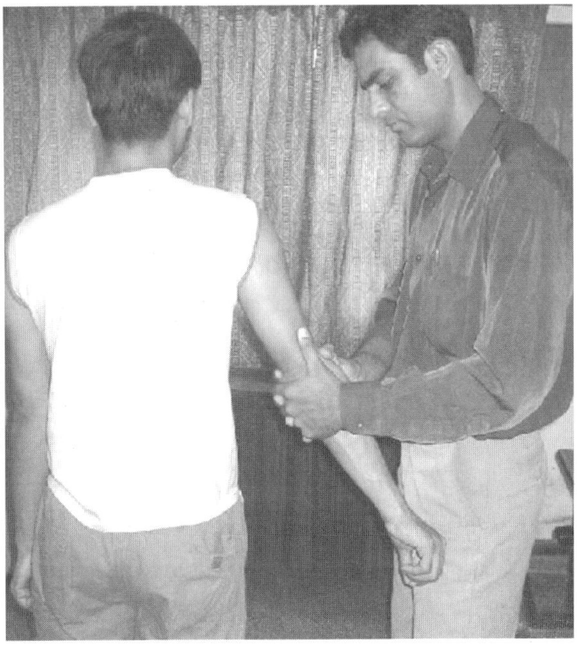

Fig. 12.2b: Contract relax (end position)

General Relaxation

Contrast Method (Progressive Muscular Relaxation)

The physiology of this method is that a strong contraction of a muscle is followed by an equal relaxation of the same muscle (Excitation = Inhibition). Progressive muscular relaxation technique was developed by American Physician Edmund Jacobson in the early 1920s. Jacobson argued that since muscle tension accompanies anxiety, one can reduce anxiety by learning how to relax the muscular tension. PMR entails physical and mental component. The physical component involves the tensing and relaxing of muscle groups over the legs, abdomen, chest and arms with eyes closed. The mental component requires that the individual focuses on the distinction between the feeling of tension an relaxation.

Technique

1. The relaxation technique commences from the distal part of the limb and proceeds to proximal part of the limb in a sequence of contraction of muscles. The therapist commands the patient to contract and relax.
2. Then the muscles of whole limb are allowed to contract from distal to proximal and go for relaxation phase from proximal to distal.
3. The same procedure is repeated on the other limb.
4. The muscles of both limbs contract together from distal to proximal and allowed to relax from proximal to distal.
5. Procedure is repeated in the same manner on upper extremity.
6. Both upper and lower extremity muscles are allowed to contract from distal to proximal and asked for relaxation from proximal to distal.

For Upper Extremity

Command the Patient to:

i. Make a fist and relax.
ii. Contract wrist flexors or extensors and relax.

iii. Contract elbow flexors or extensors and relax.

iv. Contract shoulder adductors and relax.

The muscles of whole upper extremity are contracted simultaneously from distal to proximal and allowed to relax from proximal to distal.

Command is Given as Follows:

i. Make a fist, contract wrist flexors or extensors, elbow flexors and shoulder adductors.

ii. Relax the shoulder muscles, elbow flexors, wrist extensors or flexors and hand muscles.

The same procedure is repeated on the other upper extremity.

For Lower Extremity

Command the Patient to:

i. Contract dorsiflexors or plantar flexors and relax.

ii. Contract the quadriceps or hamstrings and relax.

iii. Contract the gluteus maximus and relax.

The muscles of the extremity are contracted simultaneously from distal to proximal and relaxed from proximal to distal.

Command the Patient as Follows:

1. Contract the plantar flexors or extensors.
2. Contract the knee extensors.
3. Contract the hip extensors.
4. Relax the hip extensors.
5. Relax the knee extensors.
6. Relax the plantar flexors or extensors.

The same procedure is repeated on the other lower extremity.

The technique is then performed on both L/L and U/L muscles simultaneously.

Command the Patient as Follows:

1. Contract the dorsiflexors or plantar flexors, hand and wrists muscle.
2. Contract the knee extensor and elbow flexors.
3. Contract the hip extensor and shoulder adductors.
4. Relax the hip extensor and shoulder adductors.
5. Relax the knee extensor and elbow flexors.
6. Relax the dorsi or plantar flexors, hand and wrist muscles.

Reciprocal Inhibition Method

The physiology of this method is when agonist muscles are contracted, their antagonistic muscles get relaxed reciprocally and equally to the contraction of the agonist muscles.

Contraction of agonist muscles = Reciprocal inhibition or a relaxation of antagonistic muscles

In some circumstances it would be difficult to allow the contraction of the tensed or spasmed muscles because of pain. It is therefore in order to decrease the muscle spasm the agonistic muscles are allowed to contract isometrically to cause relaxation of the tensed muscles.

Agonistic muscle(s) = opposite to tensed muscles

For example: To relieve the tension in elbow flexors, the extensors of elbow are allowed to contract. The contraction of elbow extensors causes relaxation of the elbow flexors reciprocally and equally to the contraction of the agonist muscles (extensors).

Other Relaxation Techniques

1. *Mental Imagery:* It is a relaxation method in which the patient is instructed to imagine himself in a place associated with pleasant memories. *For example*—Sitting at beach, greenery, lake etc. Such images allow the patient to enter a relaxed state. This type of relaxation is useful in reducing stress or anxiety related tensions.
2. *Autogenic Training:* In this technique patient learns to monitor level of body functions such as blood pressure, muscle tension etc. (usually by using biofeedback equipment) and then try to relax himself by do not letting bodily functions crossing the limits.
3. *Yoga and Meditation:* These are two very commonly used techniques in Indian system. In India these techniques have been used since centuries. Now scientific proof has also been made that these two techniques are also very useful in making mental as well as physical relaxation.
4. *Music Therapy:* Research studies have shown that appropriate music causes calming and relaxing effect. Soft, low noise, instrumental music can be used for relaxation.
5. *Pet Therapy:* It has been seen people who have pets are less suffered from hypertension and other cardiac problems. Having pet is a good option to reduce day-to-day stress.
6. *Creational Activities:* Such as dance, swimming etc. can also be utilized as mode of relaxation.
7. *Social Modality:* Family and friends should be valued as they are like shock absorber of once daily life event which helps to maintain mental relaxation.

13

STRETCHING TECHNIQUES OF SOFT TISSUE STRUCTURES

Stretching is a form of physical exercise in which a specific muscle or group of muscles are purposefully stretched to improve their flexibility. The activities of daily living (ADL) such as combing, dressing, putting on shoes, taking bath and fastening bras require optimal flexibility of the muscles and tendons.

Stretching, in its most basic form, is a natural and instinctive activity. It often occurs instinctively after walking from sleep, after long period of inactiviy, or after exiting confined spaces and areas. All the healthy individuals maintain the flexibility of the muscle because of instinctive stretching.

Shortening of the length of muscles (decrease flexibility) usually occurs in response to injury, pathology and muscle guarding. There is limitation in the functions and activities of daily living. Therapeutic stretching performed by the physical therapist deliberately and purposefully elongates and enhances flexibility of the muscles and tendons to improve functional limitations (Flowchart 13.1).

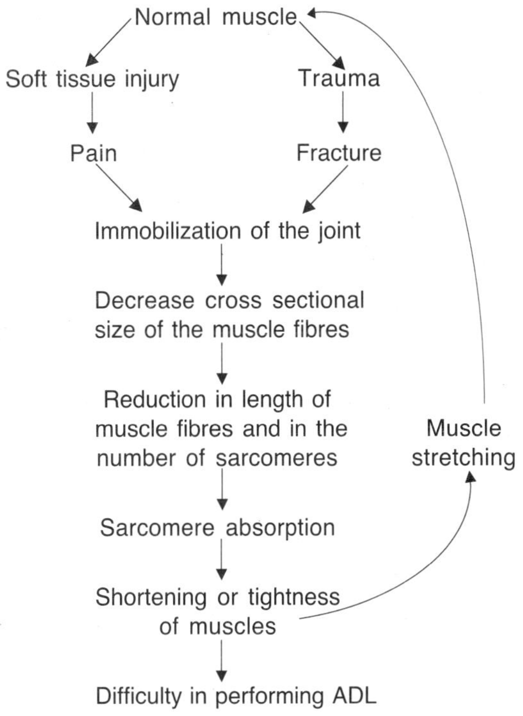

Flowchart 13.1

Some professionals like gymnasts, dancers move their joint beyond the normal range of motion as their soft tissue structures allow the joint to move beyond the range of motion. This is because these professionals start stretching of the soft tissue structures from childhood which is required for their profession.

Effects of Prolonged Immobilization on Muscles

Immobilization of a muscle for a prolong period of time deteriorates the contractile properties and decreases the number of myofibril, resulting in atrophy of muscle. The atrophy of the muscle depends on the duration of immobilization which ranges from as little as few days to a week. The longer the duration of immobilization, the greater the atrophy of muscle fibres.

Lieber suggests the most important factors in atrophy from decreased use to be the degree of immobilization (i.e., number of joints crossed), followed by the degree of change to normal function. For example when knee and ankle joints are immobilized the calf muscles atrophy occurs greatly. The atrophy of the soleus (static postural muscle) is greater than the gastrocnemius (relatively lower use muscle). Atrophy occurs quickly and more extensively in tonic (slow–twitch) postural muscle fibres than in phasic (fast–twitch) fibres. The atrophy of muscles also greatly depends on the positions of muscles during immobilization. The muscle which is immobilized in a lengthened position shows less atrophy than when immobilized in the shortened position.

The profound effects of immobilization on muscles are—decreased cross sectional size of muscle fibres, deterioration in the motor unit recruitment and absorption of sarcomeres. All these above changes lead to decrease in the overall length of the muscle fibres which is the most important cause of the hypomobility of the joint.

Effects of Prestretching

It has been demonstrated in amphibians and in humans that a muscle performs most work when it shortens immediately after being stretched in the concentrically contracted state than when it shortens from a state of isometric contraction (Cuillo and Zarins, 1983). This phenomenon entirely depends on the elastic energy stored in the series elastic component during stretching and energy stored in the contractile component.

Neurological Changes in the Muscle to Stretch

As the muscle is stretched the sensory receptors (composed of intrafusal muscle fibres) located in the central portions of muscle spindle called the nuclear bag and nuclear chain, get stimulated and send information about the intensity, velocity and duration of stretch to the CNS via primary (type Ia) and secondary (type II) afferent fibres. These fibres facilitate the contraction of intrafusal and extrafusal fibres respectively and inhibit the contraction of antagonistic muscle fibres. Excessive tension caused by active contraction or passive stretching is controlled by Golgi Tendon Organ (GTO), situated near the musculotendinous junctions which wraps around the ends of the extrafusal fibres of a muscle, and transmits afferent stimuli via type IIb fibres. Therefore, golgi tendon organ is a protective mechanism that inhibits tension in the muscle, and the effect is known as autogenic inhibition.

Physiological Changes

When a muscle is stretched, some of its fibres lengthen, but other fibres may remain at rest. The length of the entire muscle depends upon the number of stretched fibres. The stretching of muscle fibres begin with the sarcomere, the basic unit of contraction in the muscle fibre. As the sarcomere contracts, the area of overlap between the thick and thin myofilaments increases. When the sarcomeres are stretched, the area of overlap decreases and muscle elongates. As soon as all the sarcomeres reached into full stretched position, additional strecthing places force on the surrounding connective tissues. Hence, in stretching, the muscle fibre is pulled out to its full length sarcomere by sarcomere, and then the connective tissue takes up the remaining slack. This helps in realigning and disorganizing fibres in the direction of the tension.

Indications of Stretching

- Muscle spasm/guarding.
- Muscle tightness.
- Muscle spasticity.
- Muscle rigidity.
- Skin and fascia tightness/post burn stiffness.
- Joint capsule tightness/stiffness.
- Fibrous ankylosis of a joint.

Contraindications of Stretching

- Acute inflammation.
- Muscle strain.
- Ligament sprain.
- Muscle rupture.
- Muscle tear.
- Fracture.
- Subluxation or dislocation of the joint.
- Ligament injuries (acute).
- Myositis ossificans (common in elbow joint).
- Within three weeks of tendon transfer.
- Following the surgical reconstruction of ligaments or tendons (wait for at least three weeks or green signal from surgeon).
- Severe osteoporotic changes (osteomyelitis, tuberculosis) stretching may be done with extra precaution.

Parameters of Soft Tissue Stretching

1. Intensity of stretch.
2. Speed of stretch.
3. Frequency of stretch.
4. Duration of stretch.

1. Intensity of Stretch:

The force which is applied to stretch the soft tissue structures is termed as the intensity of stretch. The intensity of stretch depends on the soft tissue structure which is being stretched. For example—to stretch the trapezius muscles, less intensity of stretch is required than the gastrocnemius. The general rule of intensity to stretch the soft tissues is to be low, though an experienced therapist can only stretch the structure with an optimal intensity.

2. Speed of Stretch:

For the purpose of treatment the exercise should be performed in a smooth, slow and rhythmical manner. High speed of exercise can cause increase in stretch reflex and further tension in the muscles that may prevent stretching of muscles. A slow speed stretch is also easier

Table 13.1: Difference between muscle tightness and muscle contracture

Muscle tightness	*Muscle contracture*
Muscle tightness includes decrease in the length of the muscle and its fibres and in the number of sarcomeres in series within myofibrils as the result of sarcomere absorption. If this state of muscle can be lengthened or elongated by passive stretching is termed the muscle tightness.	Muscle contracture also includes the same physiological changes like muscle tightness but these changes occur severely and decreases the length of muscle permanently which causes deformity at the joint and cannot be stretched by passive stretching and require surgical intervention to elongate the muscle.

for the therapist as well as patient to control and prevent injury to the stretched structures. In addition to that, a slow speed stretch affects the viscoelastic properties of connective tissues making them more compliant.

3. *Frequency of Stretch:*

   It refers to the number of sessions per day or week. The frequency of stretch depends on the severity and underlying cause of tightness of the soft tissue structures. Structures immobilized for long period of time, often require more frequent treatment twice or thrice daily while those structures immobilized for short period of time require only twice or thrice a week.

4. *Duration of Stretch:*

   The structures are held at the stretched position for a sufficient period of time with an optimal intensity to lengthen the soft tissue structures, so that they do not go back to the original position. The length of time a stretch must be held to facilitate muscle flexibility remains a point of disagreement among clinicians. Lantell G *et al.* state that a low load prolonged stretch (15-30 sec) is more effective and that there does not appear to be any advantage to hold the stretch longer than 15-30 seconds.

STRETCHING TECHNIQUES

It has already been mentioned that stretching means elongation of soft tissue structures (especially muscles). To achieve good results it is very essential to apply superficial heat *modalities* or *active contraction* (hold relax, contract relax exercise) to warm up the muscle prior to stretching. The studies show that if hold relax or contract relax is followed by stretching it provides very good results, though the selection of stretching exercise entirely depends on the tightened structure which is being treated. There are some common stretching techniques which are frequently used to stretch the soft tissue structures.

1. Passive stretching—static and intermittent.
2. Active stretching (Self or auto stretching).
3. Isometric stretching.
4. Dynamic stretching.
5. PNF stretching.
6. Ballistic stretching.

1. Passive Stretching

It is the manual technique which is performed by the hands of therapist. The shortened structure are stretched beyond the available range of motion but within anatomical range in a smooth, rhythmic manner. The stretched structures are held at the end of range for some time and released gradually to the normal position, which *consists one cycle of stretching*. Several cyclic stretchings are performed per treatment session. This whole procedure is known as intermittent passive stetching of soft tissue structures.

Generally at the end of range the skeletal structures are held for 5-10 seconds in intermittent passive stretching. But if the tightened structure is held for more than 15 seconds to minutes then it is called as *static passive stretching.* The stretched structure can also be held from almost an hour to several days or weeks by using the mechanical device.

Agonist Contraction with Passive Stretching

It is a type of passive stretching where patient is asked to contract the agonist muscle during stretching, the tightened muscle will reflexively relax and make muscle elongation easier. Some clinician refers to it as a term of neuromuscular inhibition. While patient contracts the muscle, the therapist passively stretches the antagonistic muscles.

2. Active Stretching (Self or Auto Stretching)

It is a type of stretching in which a person/patient is taught the stretching exercise to perform by himself or herself without assistance.

Technique: Patient should choose a comfortable position as therapist advises. During the stretching the patient is taught to relax the antagonistic muscles and allow the tightened muscle to stretch fully.

For example: To stretch the hamstrings and extensors of lower back the patient is advised long sitting position and allowed to touch the toes with the fingers without flexing the knees.

3. Isometric Stretching

It is a type of static stretching of muscles which does not allow the joint to move during the contraction. Resistance is applied against active contraction of the muscle or group of the muscles in the isometric manner. The use of isometric stretching is one of the fastest ways to increase flexibility and is much more effective than either passive stretching or active stretching alone. Isometric stretching also helps to develop strength in the "tensed" muscles (which helps to develop static-active flexibility), and seems to decrease amount of pain usually associated with stretching.

4. Dynamic Stretching

It involves moving parts of body and gradually increasing reach, speed of movement, or both. Dynamic stretching consists of controlled leg and arm movements performed within the limit of range of motion. It improves dynamic flexibility and is quite useful as part of warm up for active or aerobic workout.

The dynamic stretching differs from ballistic as ballistic stretching forces a part of the body beyond its range of motion in a bouncy or jerky manner.

5. PNF Stretching

It is not really a type of stretching but is a technique of combining passive stretching and isometric stretching in order to achieve maximum static flexibility.

In PNF stretching, first muscle(s) is allowed to contract isometrically against the resistance then is stretched passively.

Hold relax—The most common PNF stretching technique is the hold relax. In the first step of this technique muscle is taken passively in extreme stretched position and then patient is allowed to contract the stretched muscle isometrically for 6-10 seconds. In the next step patient is instructed to relax the muscle gradually, and as the patient relaxes the muscle, therapist stretches the muscle passively into extreme range in the smooth and controlled manner. Several repetitions may be performed.

Isometric contraction followed by Passive stretching
= Hold relax stretching

Hold-relax-contract—It is the type of PNF stretching which involves isometric contraction of the both agonist and antagonistic muscles. In the first step of this technique an agonist muscles are allowed to contract isometrically against resistance for 6-10 seconds, then patient is asked to relax the agonist muscle. In the next step of the repetition as the patient relaxes the agonist muscle, the therapist commands the patient to contract antagonistic muscles against the resistance. The position of hand should be in such a manner that it applies resistance to agonist and antagonistic muscles without changing its position.

Isometric contraction of agonist followed by
Isometric contraction of antagonistic =
Hold-relax-contract stretching

Hold-relax-swing—This technique actually involves the use of dynamic or ballistic stretching in conjunction with isometric stretches. The technique is very risky and is successfully used only by the most advanced athletes and dancers that have managed to achieve a high level of control over their muscle stretch reflex.

The hold-relax-swing constitutes, initially isometric contraction for 6-10 seconds which is immediately followed by ballistic stretching.

Isometric contraction followed by Ballistic stretching
= Hold-relax-swing

Hold-relax-bounce—This is the PNF stretching technique which is very similar to hold-relax-swing and involves the use of dynamic or ballistic stretching in conjunction with static and isometric stretching.

Both hold-relax-swing and hold-relax-bounce stretching techniques should be performed by individual or even professional athlete under guidance of therapist as the techniques involve quick stretching. Both techniques have the greatest potential for rapid flexibility gains, but only performed by people who have sufficiently high level of control of the stretch reflex of the muscles which are being stretched.

6. Ballistic Stretching

Ballistic stretching imposes repetitive bouncing or jerking movements on the muscles to be stretched. The athlete uses the momentum of a moving body or limb in an attempt to force it beyond its normal range of motion. This is stretching or "warming up", by bouncing into a stretched position, using the stretched muscle as a spring which pulls out of the stretched position (e.g., bouncing down repeatedly to touch the toes).

It is a type of passive stretching which involves quick forceful, intermittent stretch with high speed and high intensity stretching of muscles and tissues through bobbing or bouncing movements involving active antagonist muscle contractions. This type of stretch can elongate muscles and subsequently increase range of motion in young, healthy patients but is associated with high rates of microtrauma and injury. Ballistic stretching is generally viewed as inappropriate for the sedentary or elderly patients with musculoskeletal pathology or chronic condition (Fig. 13.1)

Technique of Passive Stretching

Every stretching exercise requires suitable and comfortable position of the patient. Though the position varies from

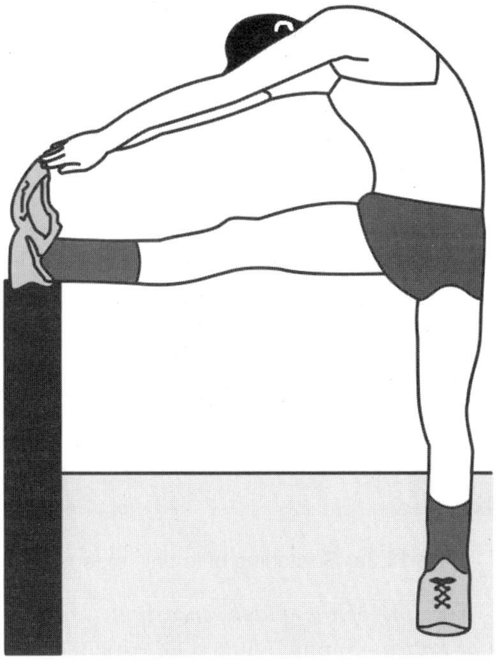

Fig. 13.1: Ballistic stretching. The individual stands on the ground with one leg straight out on the table. He reaches the hands forward as far as the toes possible. Leaning forward by contracting the abdominal muscles, the individual quickly reaches towards the toes or possibly past the toes, and immediately returns to the original position. The stretching is repeated 10 to15 times, with each bounce extending the arms a bit farther

athletes to the persons with health related problems. Athletes do not require specific position to stretch the muscle because of flexibility.

For example: A 65-year-old patient with lower back pain requires long sitting position to stretch the hamstrings as well as back extensors to avoid further strain of the lower back region which already has pathological changes. On the other hand, a 25-year-old athlete can stretch the muscle in standing by touching the toes with fingers.

The proximal part of the joint should be stabilised but the muscle which is being stretched should not be stabilised or compressed by straps. The patient is asked to relax the muscle and not allow the tightened muscle to contract. The therapist holds the distal part of the limb and moves the limb slowly, smoothly in a controlled manner through the available range of motion.

After a repetition of intermittent passive stretching the structure may retain the original position *(tightened position)*, hence, number of repetitions are performed, so that the structure should not go back to the tightened position and remain stretched even after releasing the intensity of stretch.

In mechanical static stretching where tightened muscles are held in elongated position for an hour to days, they do not return to the shortened position after releasing the intensity, the structures remain stretched.

- Stabilisation of the proximal part of the joint can be achieved by body weight.
- The intensity, speed, duration and frequency of stretching exercise should be optimal and should not cause any injury to the other structures as well.
- *Emphasis* should be given on warming up the tissues with mild heat or gentle rhythm activities, such as cycling, push ups, jogging etc.
- The movement should be carried out in the anatomical range of motion to avoid any injury to other structures.

LOWER EXTREMITY MUSCLES STRETCHING

Iliacus and Psoas Major

Position of Patient: Prone.

A. *In prone lying*—Therapist places one hand on the gluteal region to stabilise the pelvis, other hand grasps the knee joint. The leg of the patient rests on the therapist's chest and shoulder. The therapist extends the hip joint by pulling the knee joint upward. The joint is kept in stretched position for brief time of period then the stretched muscles released to the starting position, several repetitions are performed to bring the effect of plasticity (Fig. 13.2a).

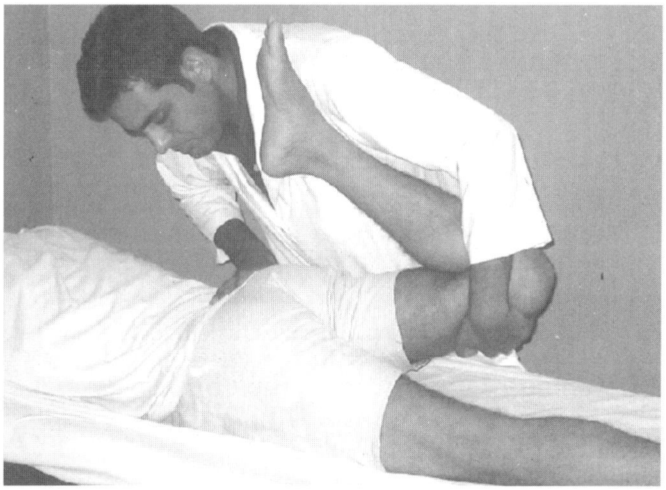

Fig. 13.2a: Stretching of hip flexors (right side)—Prone (Complete flexion of knee joint should be avoided as it causes tension in the quadriceps and restricts hip extension)

The tightness of iliopsoas is very common in patient with below and above knee amputations where limb is kept in flexed (elevated) position to avoid oedema.

B. *In supine lying*—Therapist stands at side of patient, places upper hand on the flexed knee and lower hand on the right knee. While stabilizing the right knee joint, therapist flexes the left hip and knee joints (Fig. 13.2b).

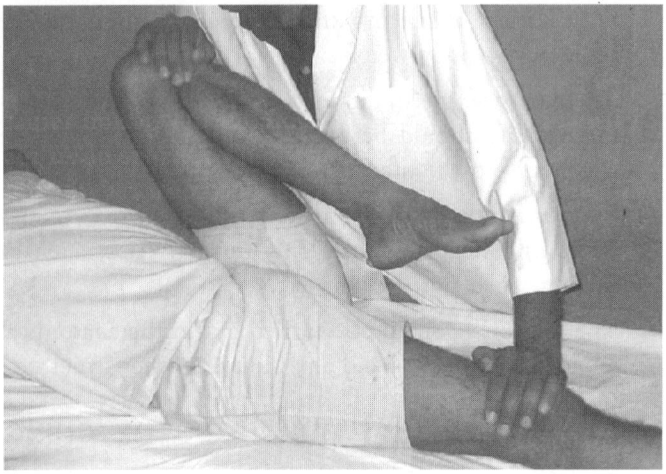

Fig. 13.2b: Stretching of hip flexors (right side)–Supine

C. *In side lying*—Therapist stands behind the patient, places one hand on the pelvis to stabilize the trunk and grasps the knee joint with other hand. The leg of patient rests on the therapist's forearm. While stabilizing the pelvis and trunk therapist extends the hip joint. Stabilize trunk to avoid excessive lumbar lordosis during stretching (Fig. 13.2c).

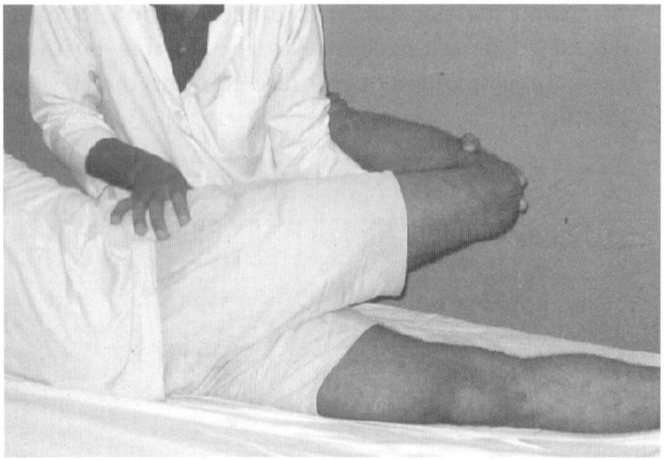

Fig. 13.2c: Stretching of hip flexors (left)–Side lying

Stretching of Extensors of Hip Joint

Tightness of extensors is very rare, however, it is easy to stretch.

Position of Patient: Supine—The therapist stands at the same side of the affected muscle. The knee is grasped with the hand and hip is flexed at the point where restriction starts. Therapist stretches the muscle by bringing the knee joint to the chest. The therapist can place his other hand on the contralateral knee to stabilize the hip (Fig. 13.3a). To stretch the bilateral gluteus maximus muscles the therapist grasps both the knees and brings to the chest, as the knees approaches chest overpressure is applied at the end range.

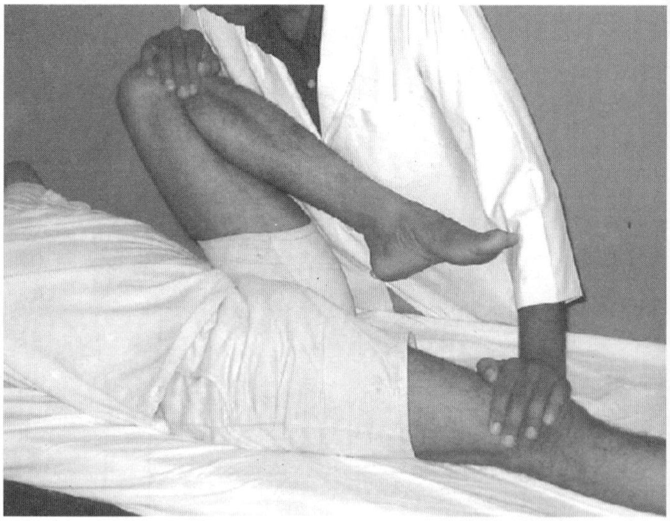

Fig. 13.3a: Stretching of left hip extensors

Self stretching of the gluteus maximus (knee to chest)—Position of Patient–Supine lying. The patient flexes the hip and knee joint gradually toward the chest where it is held for 10-15 seconds and then released (Fig. 13.3b).

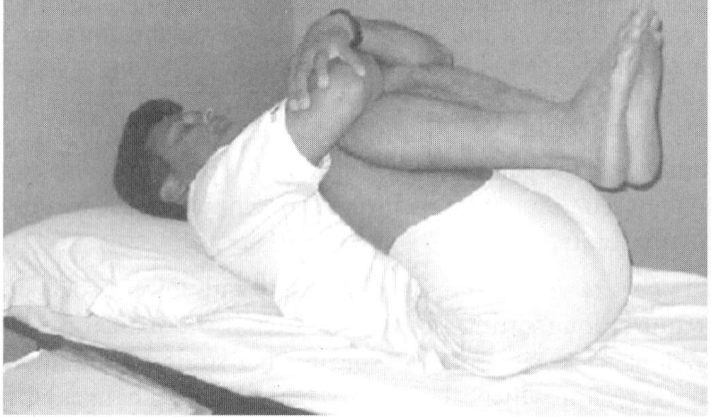

Fig. 13.3b: Self stretching of hip extensors

Adductors of Hip Joint

Position of Patient: Supine—The unaffected leg may be stabilised with the straps or hand of therapist stabilizes the pelvis. The therapist grasps the knee joint of affected side (the calf muscles rest on the forearm of the therapist) while maintaining the above position he abducts or pulls the leg toward his body (Fig. 13.4a).

Self stretching of adductors of hip joint—Position of Patient: Standing in front of wall. The patient holds the grill or wall with both hands and gradually slides both the feet apart (abduction) (Fig. 13.4b).

Alternative technique of adductors—The patient is placed in supine position with flexion of both the knees. Therapist stands at the feet of the patient, and grasps both the knees. Patient is instructed to relax the muscles and then knees

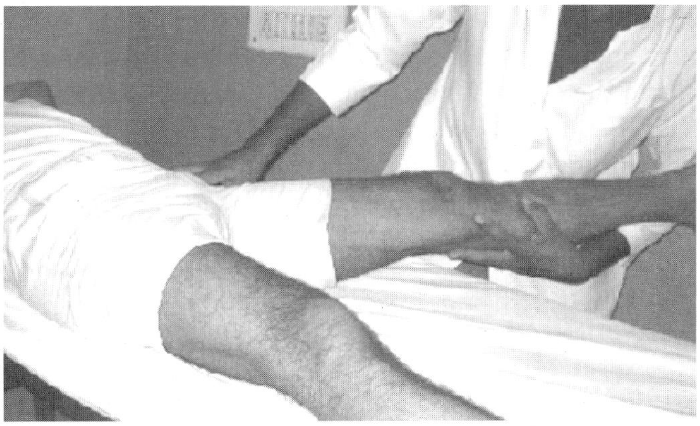

Fig. 13.4a: Stretching of hip adductors (left side)

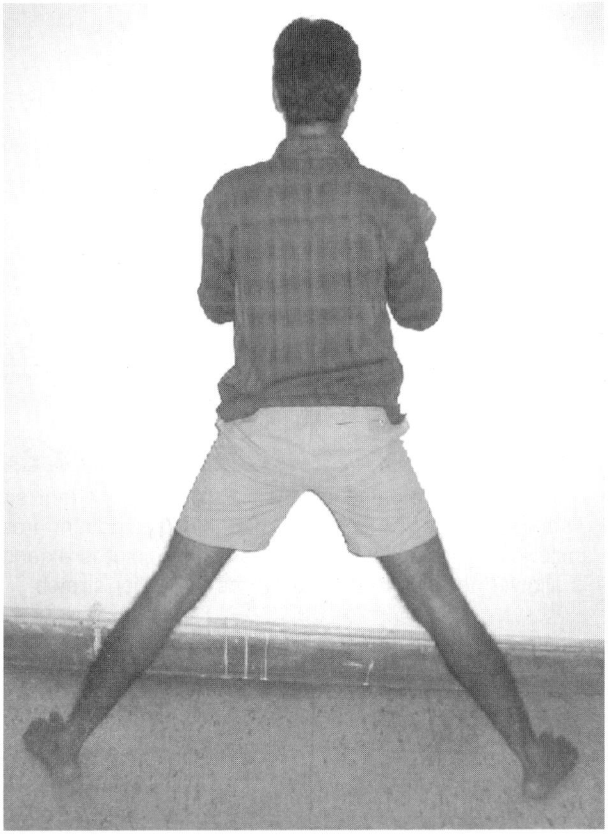

Fig. 13.4b: Adductors self stretching—Legs slide apart from each other while holding the grill or wall

are taken apart, this position is used to stretch the adductors of cerebral palsy children.

Hamstring Muscles

Position of Patient: Supine—The contralateral leg is stabilised with the straps to avoid lifting or therapist can place one hand on the thigh of patient to stabilise the limb. The posterior aspect of the lower leg of the affected side is placed over the shoulder of therapist. While keeping the knee joint straight, the therapist flexes the hip joint by raising the straight leg (Fig. 13.5a).

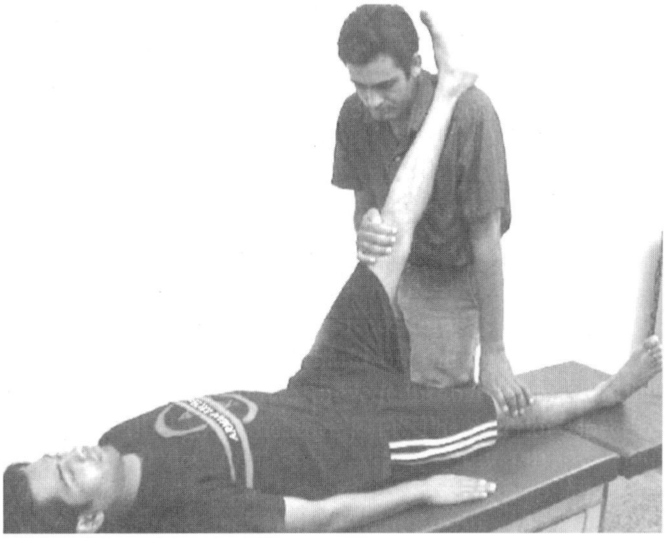

Fig. 13.5a: Stretching of left hamstrings

An Autostretching or Self Stretching of Hamstring Muscles

Position of Patient: Long sitting on plinth or couch. The patient flexes the trunk and hip joints to touch the toes with hands. The hands are further slide down the leg with the flexion of hip joint. During sliding of hands down the leg patient should emphasise more on hip flexion rather than trunk flexion (Fig. 13.5b).

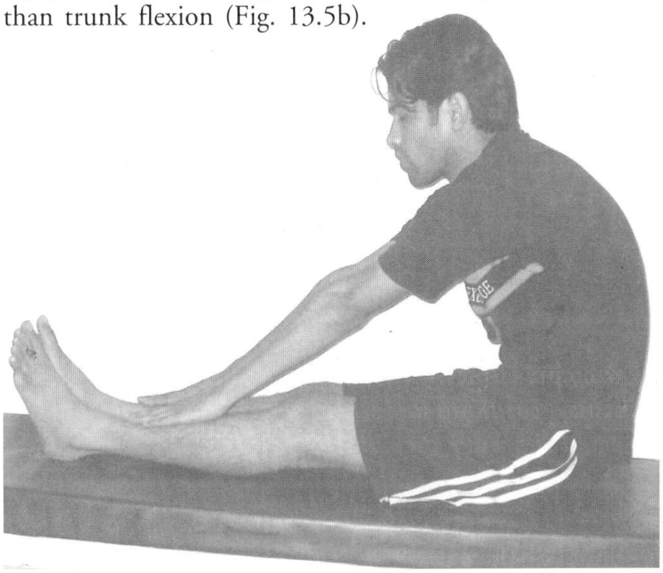

Fig. 13.5b: Self stretching of hamstrings (bilateral)

Rectus Femoris

It is a prime mover of the knee extension which gets tightened when there is immobilization of knee joint due to pain, injury or facture (Fig. 13.6a).

Position of Patient: Prone–Knee joint is flexed beyond 90°. Therapist places one hand on the gluteal region to stabilize the pelvis and to prevent lumbar lordosis, other hand is used to grasp the knee joint. The anterior aspect of

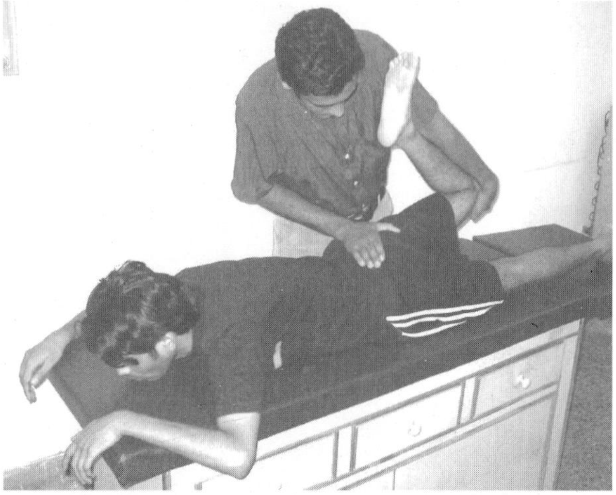

Fig. 13.6a: Stretching of right rectus femoris

leg rests on the forearm of the therapist, which helps to keep the knee joint flexed. While maintaining the above position the therapist extends the hip joint. Discomfort in the anterior thigh indicates stretching of rectus femoris.

Self Stretching of Quadriceps Muscles (Rectus Femoris)

Position of Patient: Standing—Patient stands in front of table and holds the table with one hand. The knee (stretching side) is flexed and the ankle joint is grasped with the same side of hand. The hip joint is brought into the neutral or slightly in extension position. A mild pain in the anterior of the thigh indicates stretching of the quadriceps muscles or rectus femoris (Fig. 13.6b).

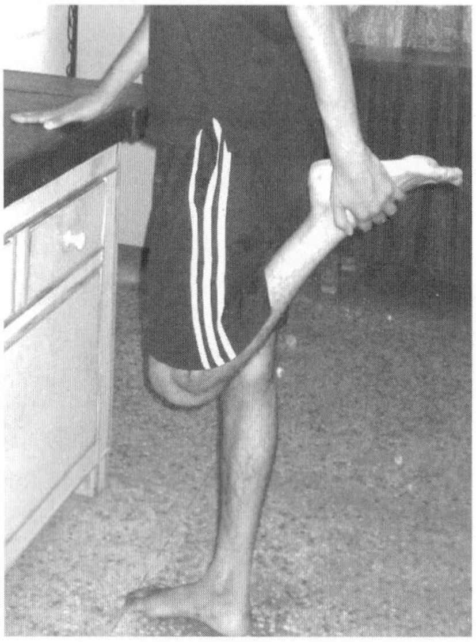

Fig. 13.6b: Self stretching of left rectus femoris

Tensor Fascia Latae (TFL)

Position of Patient: Side lying—The affected leg remains upper most and unaffected leg is flexed at hip and knee joints to widen the base of support. Therapist places one hand over the iliac crest to stabilise the pelvis and other hand grasps the knee joint. Patient's leg rests on the forearm of the therapist. While maintaining above position the therapist adducts, extends and rotates the limb laterally to stretch the TFL holds. Several repetitions are performed (Fig. 13.7a). This procedure is known as reverse Ober test.

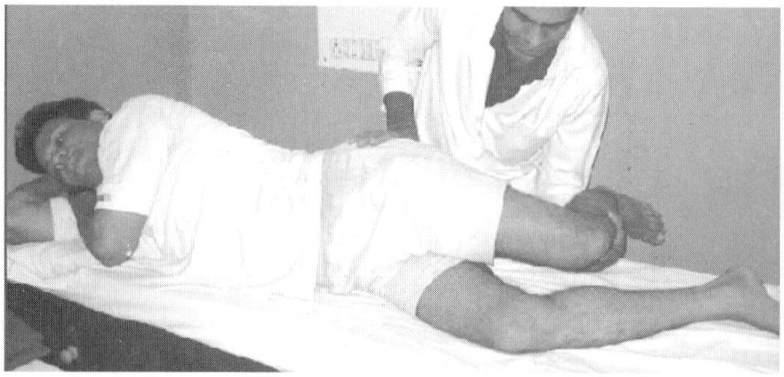

Fig. 13.7a: Stretching of tensor fascia latae

Self Stretching of TFL (Figs. 13.7b and 13.7c).

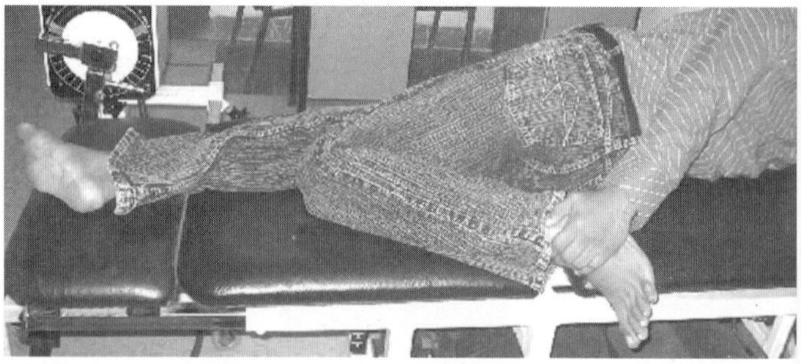

Fig. 13.7b: Self stretching of TFL—Position of patient side-lying, the involved leg is flexed at knee joint and patient grasps the ankle joint. In the next procedure the hip joint is extended and is allowed to adduct. It is known as self-Ober stretch

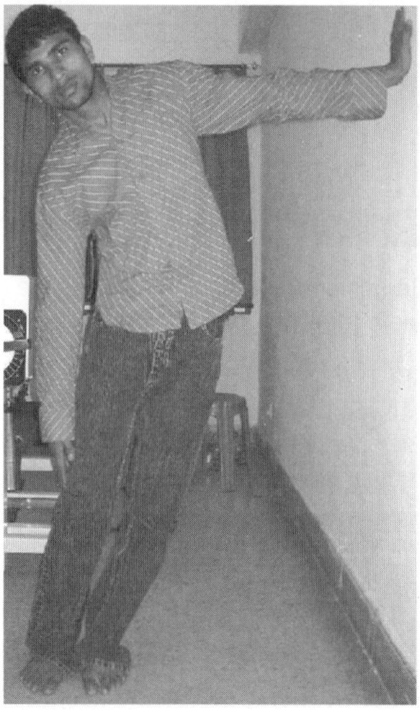

Fig. 13.7c: Self stretching of TFL—Patient stands and places one hand on the wall, the involved leg is closer to the wall. Patient slides the contralateral hand down the leg

Tendo Achilles (Gastrocnemius and Soleus)

Position of Patient: Supine—The ankle joint is placed out of the edge of the treatment table. A towel roll can be placed under the knee joint to flex it slightly. Therapist places one hand over the leg and other hand grasps the heel (calcaneal part), the plantar aspect (sole) of foot rests on the forearm of the therapist. While maintaining the above position therapist pulls the heel into the dorsiflexion, at the same time forearm also transmits the force to the plantar aspect into the dorsiflexion, the force must be able to cause movement at the ankle joint to get effective results. Sometimes movement occurs at the metatarsal joints only and therapist feels that TA is getting stretched. To stretch the TA the heel should be held firmly and pulled into the dorsiflexion which must cause tension in the gastrocnemius muscle (Fig. 13.8a).

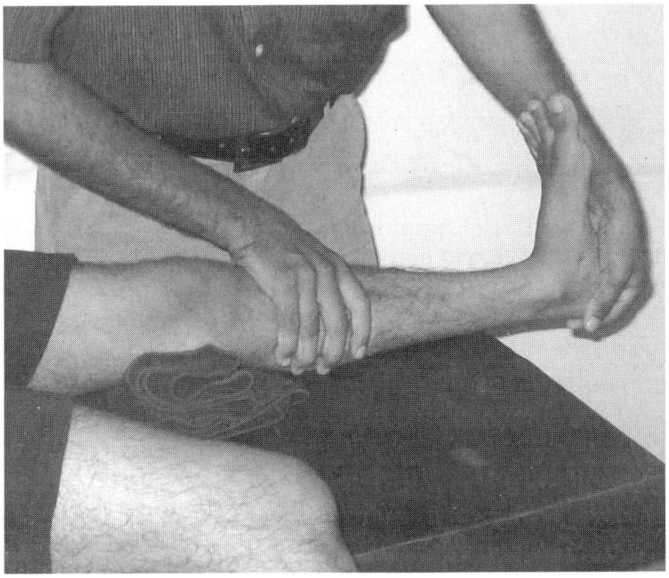

Fig. 13.8a: Stretching of plantar flexors (Gastrosoleus)

Self Stretching of Gastrosoleus Muscle

Patient stands in front of wall. The forefoot of involved leg is placed on the wooden board/stool. A stretch is applied by delivering the weight of body toward the forefoot that results in dorsiflexion. A stretch may be felt in the posterior leg during dorsiflexion of the ankle joint which indicates stretching of gastrocnemius muscle (Fig. 13.8b).

Self Stretching of Soleus Muscle

In standing position with knee flexion the forefoot is placed on the stool (this places the knee joint at 90° flexion). The patient may place both hands on the flexed knee joint. A stretch is applied by shifting the body weight on the flexed knee joint. Patient may feel stretch during extreme dorsiflexion of the ankle joint (Fig. 13.8c).

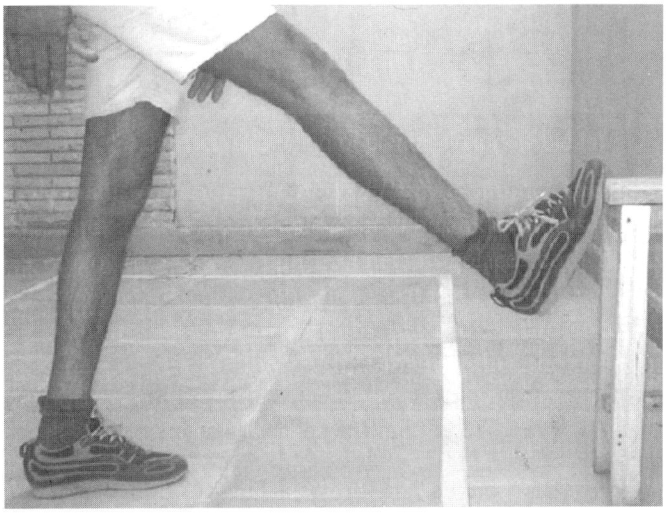

Fig. 13.8b: Self stretching of plantar flexors (Gastrosoleus)

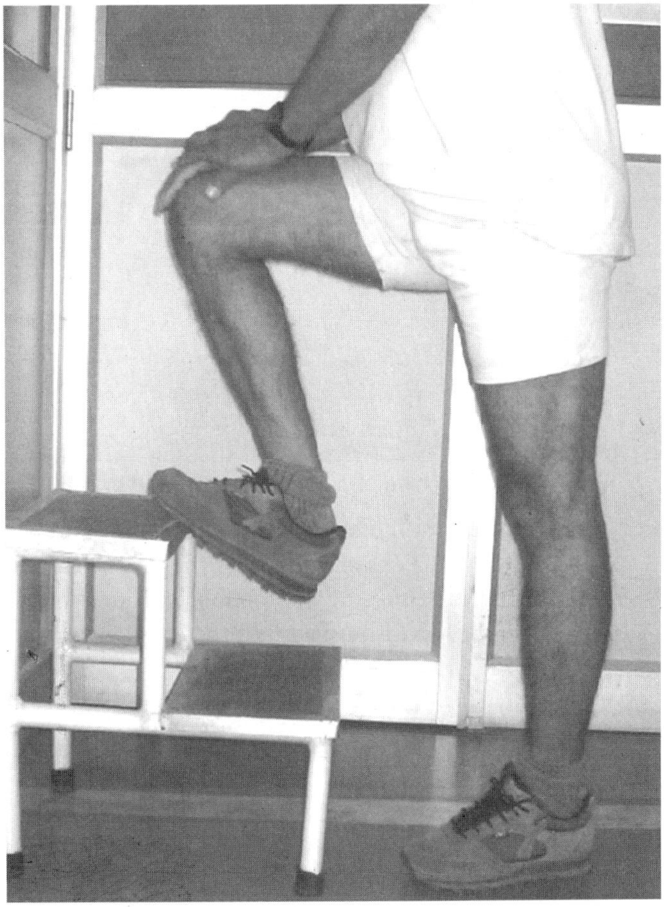

Fig. 13.8c: Self stretching of plantar flexors (Soleus)

- **Tibialis Anterior**—*Position of Patient*–Supine. Therapist stands at the side of ankle joint. The ankle joint is placed out of the edge of plinth. Therapist places both hands over the ankle joint, the fingers of both hands grasp the plantar surface and thumbs place over the anterior aspect of the forefoot. While maintaining the position both thumbs push the dorsum of foot into plantar flexion (Fig. 13.9) and eversion.

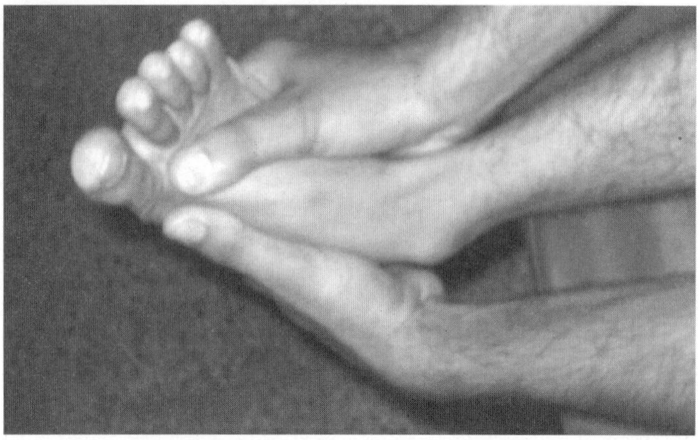

Fig. 13.9: Stretching of tibialis anterior

- **Peroneus Longus and Brevis**—The position of patient and placement of hands remain almost same as for tibialis anterior. Therapist pushes the dorsum of foot into plantar flexion and inversion (Fig. 13.10).

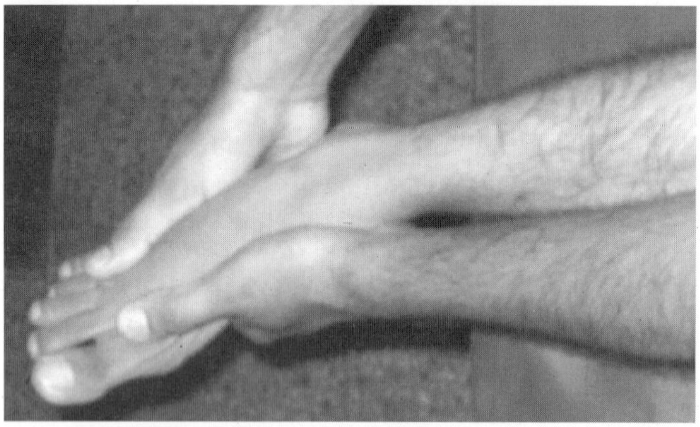

Fig. 13.10: Stretching of peroneus longus and brevis

- **Tibialis Posterior**—Position of patient remain same as for tibialis anterior. Therapist grasps the heel with one hand and lateral aspect of the forefoot by other hand, and then ankle joint is pushed into the dorsiflexion and eversion (Fig. 13.11).

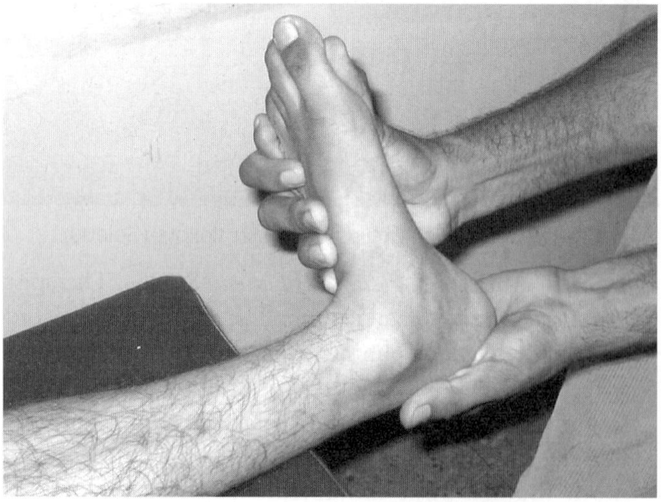

Fig. 13.11: Stretching of tibialis posterior

- **Peroneus Tertius**—Position of patient remain same as for tibialis anterior. Therapist pushes the foot into dorsiflexion and inversion.
- **Extensor Hallusis Longus, Extensor Digitorum Longus and Brevis**—Position of patient remains same, the therapist places fingers over the toes and then pushes the toes into plantar flexion. An individual muscle may be stretched by pushing the individual toe (Fig. 13.12). Plantar flexion of ankle adds more stretching.

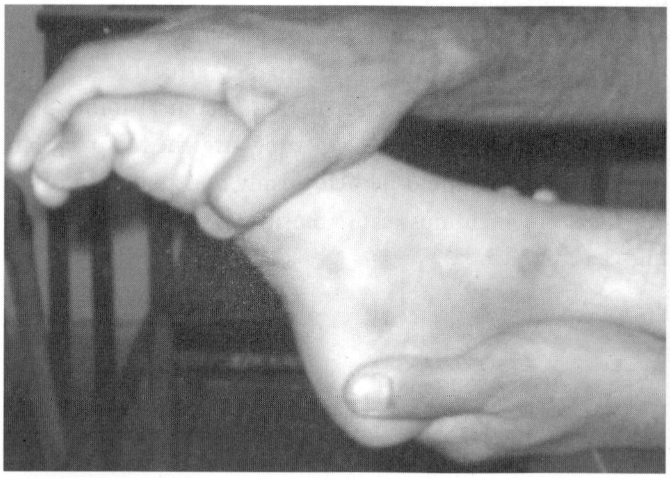

Fig. 13.12: Stretching of extensor hallucis longus, extensor digitorum longus and brevis

- **Flexor Hallucis Longus, Flexor Digitorum Longus and Brevis**—The patient is placed in prone or supine position with the ankle joint out of the treatment plinth. The therapist places fingers over the plantar aspect of the toes. The ankle joint may remain at neutral position or slightly in dorsiflexion. The therapist pushes the toes into extension (Fig. 13.13a). The same procedure is also used to stretch the plantar fascia.

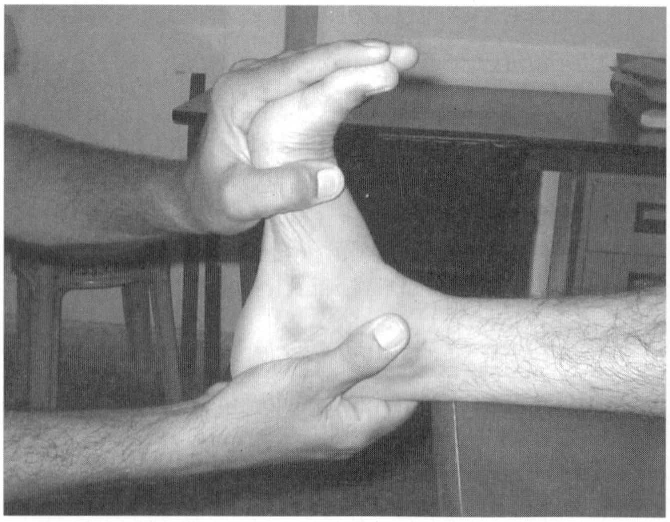

Fig. 13.13a: Stretching of flexor hallucis longus, flexor digitorum longus and brevis

- **Plantar Fascia**—The maneuver is the same as for the flexors of the toes. Patient sits with the knee flexed and heel rests on the plinth. The patient places the fingers over the plantar surface of the toes and gently extends the toes toward the leg (dorsiflexion of the MTP joints (Fig. 13.13b).

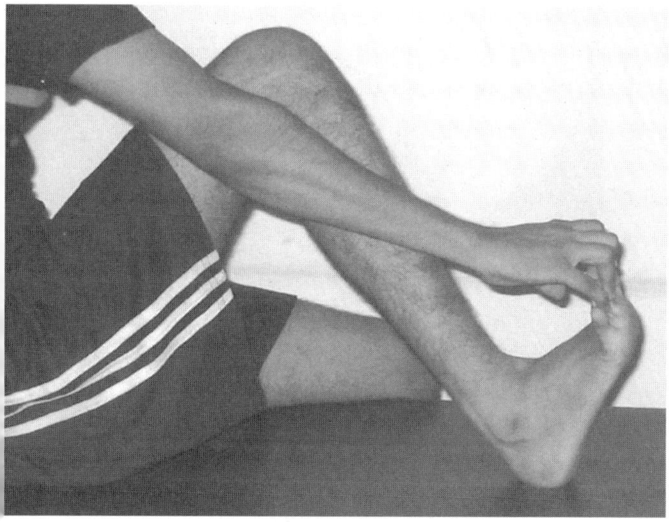

Fig. 13.13b: Stretching of plantar fascia

- **Alternative Plantar Fascia Stretch**—Patient kneels with the toes curled up under the feet (MTP joint extension). The buttocks are gently lowered to the heels until a mild tension is felt in the bottom of the feet. Patient holds the position for 30 seconds and repeats five times per session (Fig. 13.13c).

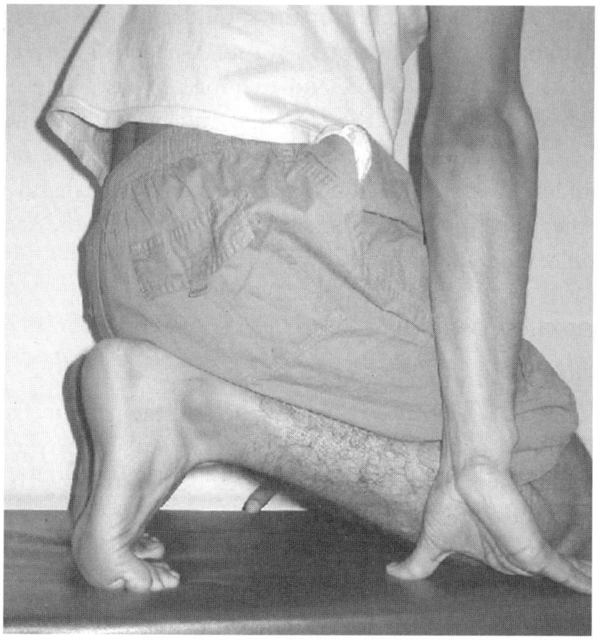

Fig. 13.13c: Plantar fascia stretching—Patient kneels with the toes curled up under the feet

- **Piriformis Muscle**—Patient is positioned in sidelying with the treatment side uppermost. The hip joint is flexed to 90° with adduction and medial rotation. The lower limb may be flexed at hip and knee joints (Fig. 13.14a) for stability.

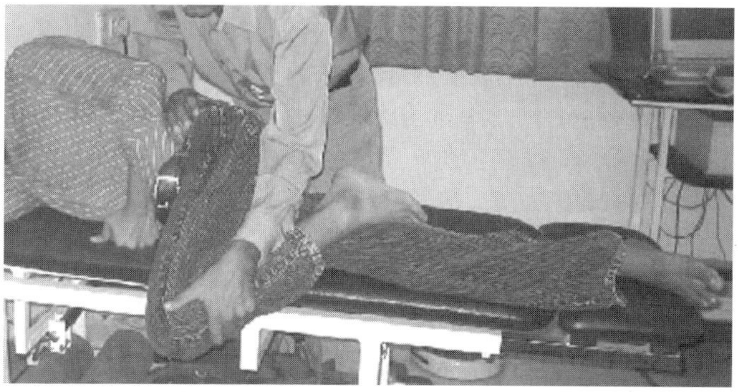

Fig. 13.14a: Stretching of piriformis

- **Alternative Position for Piriformis Muscle**—Patient lies in supine position, therapist stands at the side of the patient and places one hand over the pelvis to stabilize it. The therapist grasps the knee joint and flexes it with the hip joint, as the hip approaches 90° of flexion therapist adducts it with medial rotation (Fig. 13.14b).

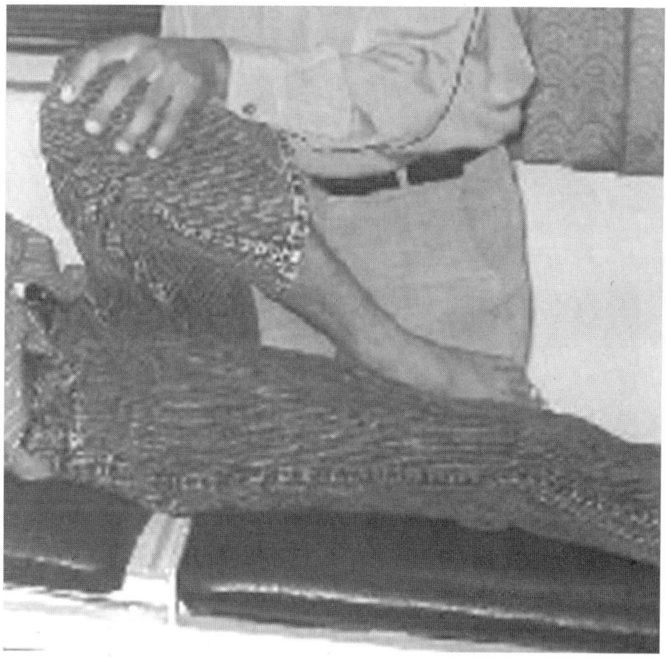

Fig. 13.14b: Stretching of piriformis (alternate)

Self stretching of piriformis muscle: Position of patient is side lying. Patient places the hand on the lateral aspect of the knee joint and then flexes the hip joint to 90° with adduction and medial rotation. The lower limb may be flexed at hip and knee joints (Fig. 13.14c) for stability.

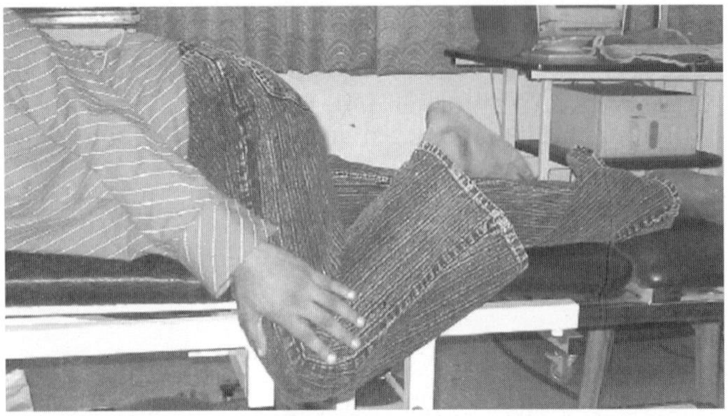

Fig. 13.14c: Self stretching of piriformis

TRUNK AND UPPER EXTREMITY MUSCLE STRETCHING

Lower back extensors: Position of Patient: High sitting—While maintaining the position the patient flexes the lumbar spine by trying to touch the shoulders to the knees. Therapist pushes both shoulders to the knees (Fig. 13.15a).

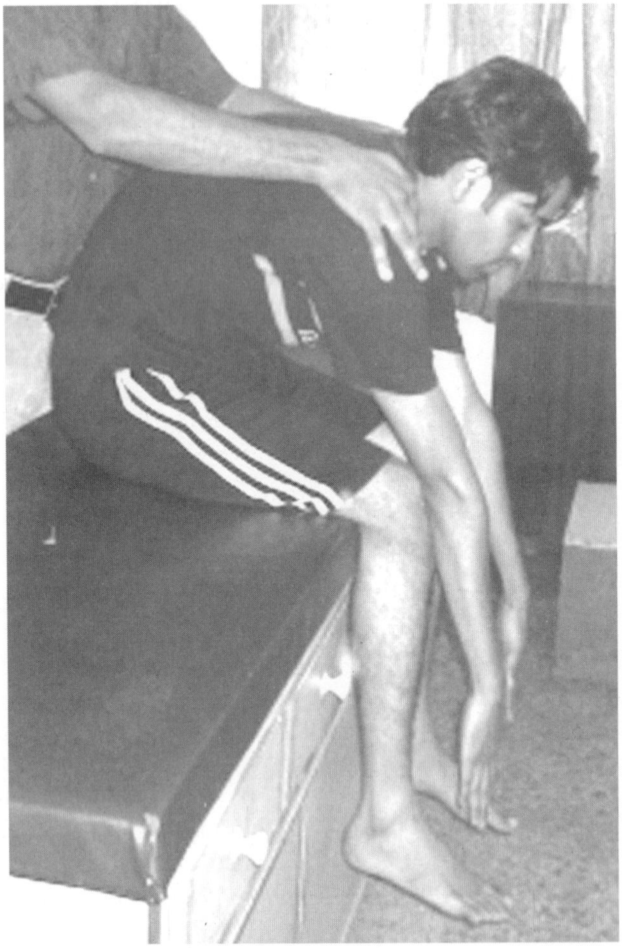

Fig. 13.15a: Stretching of lower back extensors

Self Stretching of Extensors of Back: The procedure remains same as above (the technique is performed without the assistance of therapist) (Fig. 13.15b).

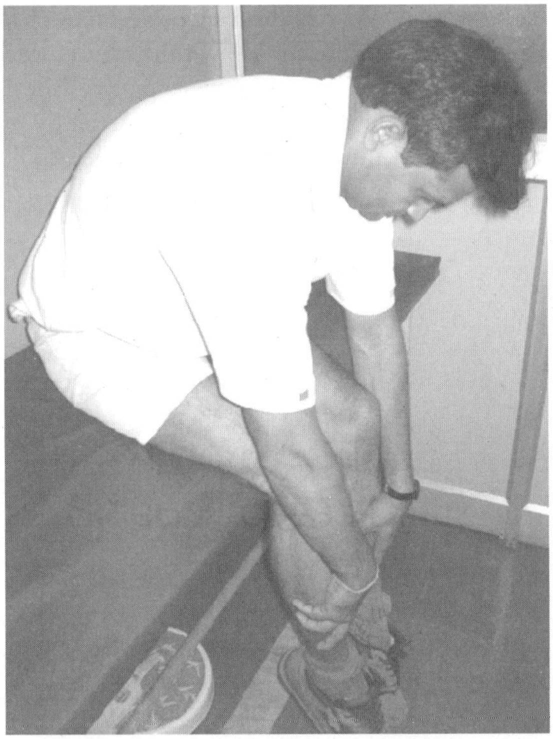

Fig. 13.15b: Self stretching of lower back extensors

Stretching of Levator Scapulae and Trapezius (Upper Fibres)

Position of Patient: Supine lying.

Position of Therapist: Standing at the head of patient or end of treatment table. One hand is placed under the occiput and other hand over the shoulder joint. The vertex of patient rests on therapist's waist. A paper or towel can be placed between vertex and therapist's waist. The hand which is placed over the shoulder, pushes it downward, while other hand flexes the neck to the opposite side of the shoulder. The side flexion is carried out by the hand and the therapist's body together. It brings tension in the levator scapulae and upper fibres of trapezius.

Alternate Position

Position of Patient: Sitting on stool.

Position of Therapist: Standing behind the patient, facing posterior aspect of neck. One hand is placed over the shoulder (same side of the muscles being stretched), the other hand is rest on the head (palmar surface of hand on the vertex and fingers on the temporal aspect of the same side). While maintaining the position of hands, therapist depresses the shoulder by one hand, and simultaneously flexes the neck to the opposite side by the other hand (Figs. 13.16a and b). To put significant pressure on the levator scapulae muscle, neck is rotated to the opposite side with lateral flexion.

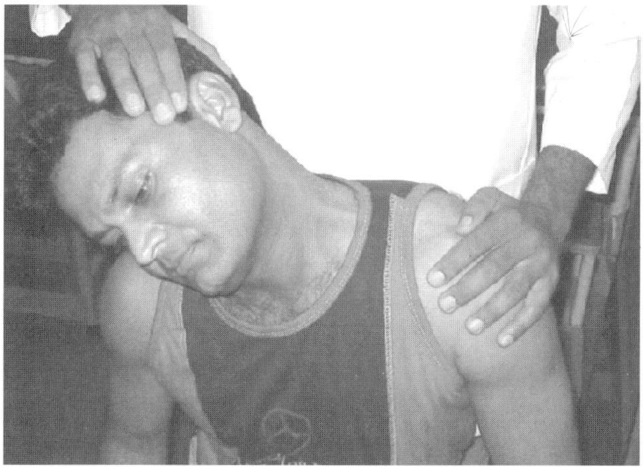

Fig. 13.16a: Stretching of levator scapulae and trapezius upper fibres (opposite side flexion of the neck)

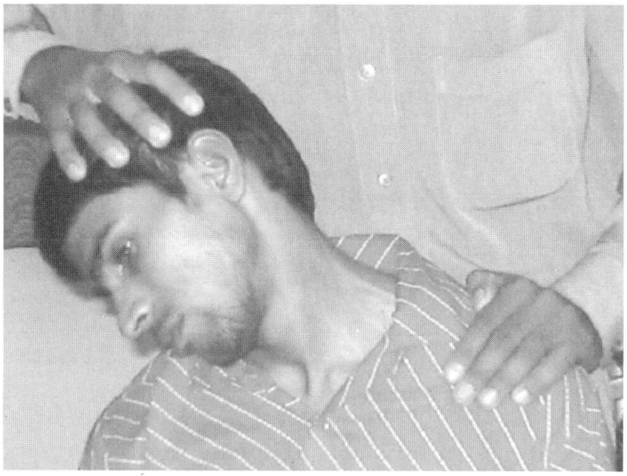

Fig. 13.16b: Stretching of levator scapulae (opposite side flexion and rotation of the neck)

Stretching of Middle Fibres of Trapezius, Rhomboids Major and Minor

Position of Patient: Sitting on stool.

Position of Therapist: Standing behind the patient facing the back of shoulder (Fig. 13.17).

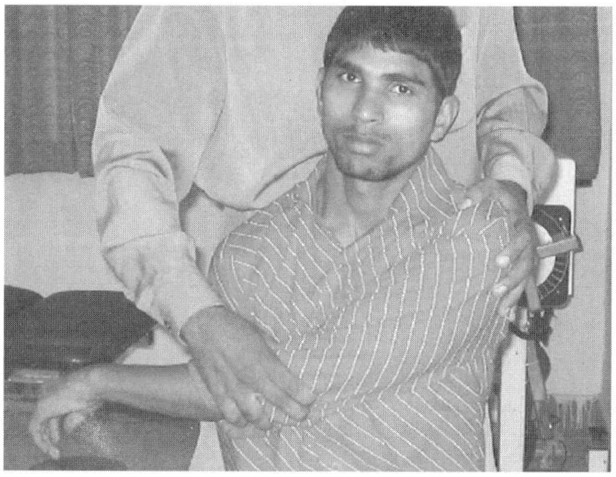

Fig. 13.17: Stretching of middle fibres of trapezius, rhomboids major and minor

One hand is placed over the acromion process and spine of scapula and other hand passes over the shoulder and grasps the arm of the same side of the muscle being stretched.

Stabilization: The trunk of the patient rests on the therapist's thighs which stabilize the trunk to prevent rotation.

Procedure: The arm is pulled diagonally downward by one hand, at the same time other hand pushes the scapula forward in the direction of protraction and slight depression.

For example: To stretch the left side of the muscles— The therapist stands behind the patient places his left hand over the acromian process and spine of left scapula, while other hand passes over the patient's right shoulder and grasps the left arm of the patient. The left arm of the patient is pulled diagonally downward by the right hand. At the same time the left scapula is pushed forward in the direction of protraction and slight depression.

Stretching of Lower Fibres of Trapezius

Position of Patient: Patient sitting on stool.

Position of Therapist: Standing behind the patient.

Placement of Hands: One hand on the opposite shoulder and other hold the arm of same side being stretched.

Procedure: Therapist moves the arm diagonally upward (in the direction of flexion and adduction). The other hand is used to stabilize the opposite shoulders (Fig. 13.18).

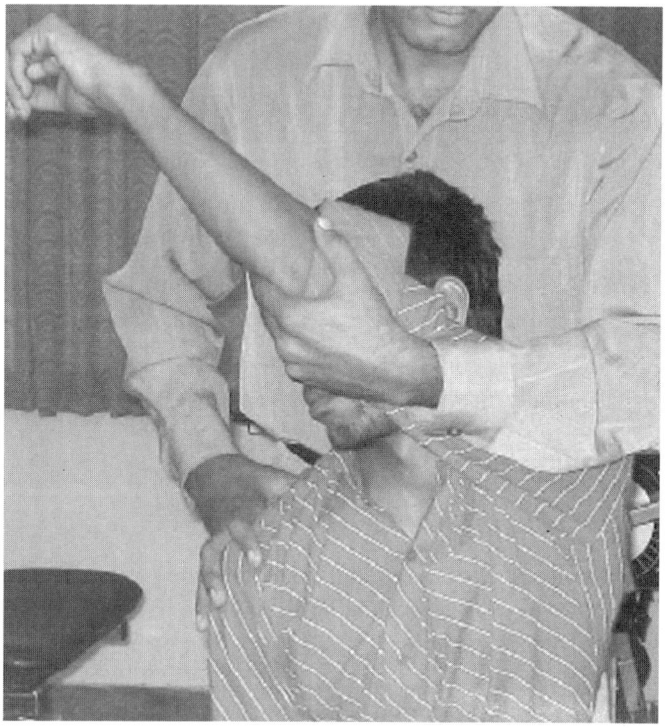

Fig. 13.18: Lower fibres of trapezius

Stretching of Pectoralis Major

Position of Patient: Sitting on stool.

Position of Therapist: Standing behind the patient.

Placement of Hands: Therapist holds the hand of patient with one hand and other hand stabilizes the shoulder (Fig. 13.19a).

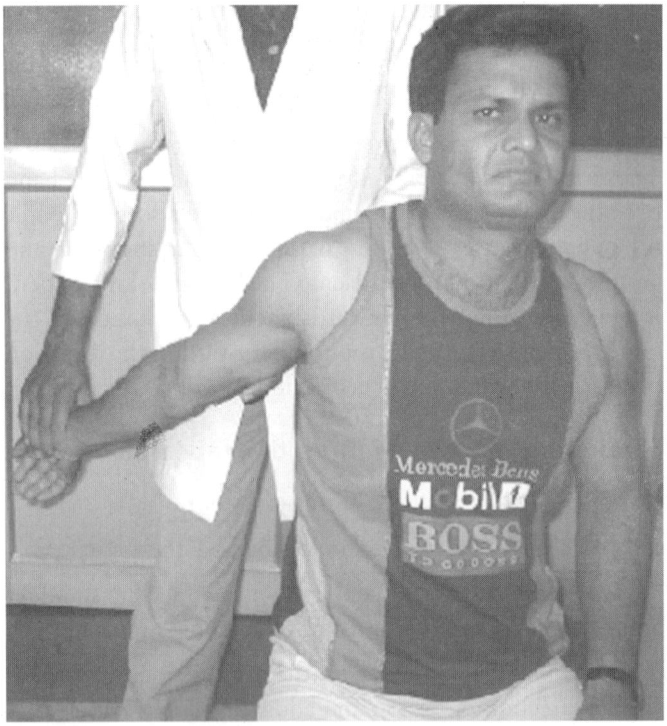

Fig. 13.19a: Stretching of pectoralis major (upper fibres)

Procedure:

i. For upper fibres (clavicular) therapist horizontally abducts the arm as much as possible while stabilizing the opposite shoulder.

   Therapist then comes back to the starting position; extends the shoulder completely by taking the arm in backward direction.

   (The upper 2 methods stretch almost all upper fibres).

ii. For lower fibres (sternal) therapist takes the arm diagonally upward (Fig. 13.19b).

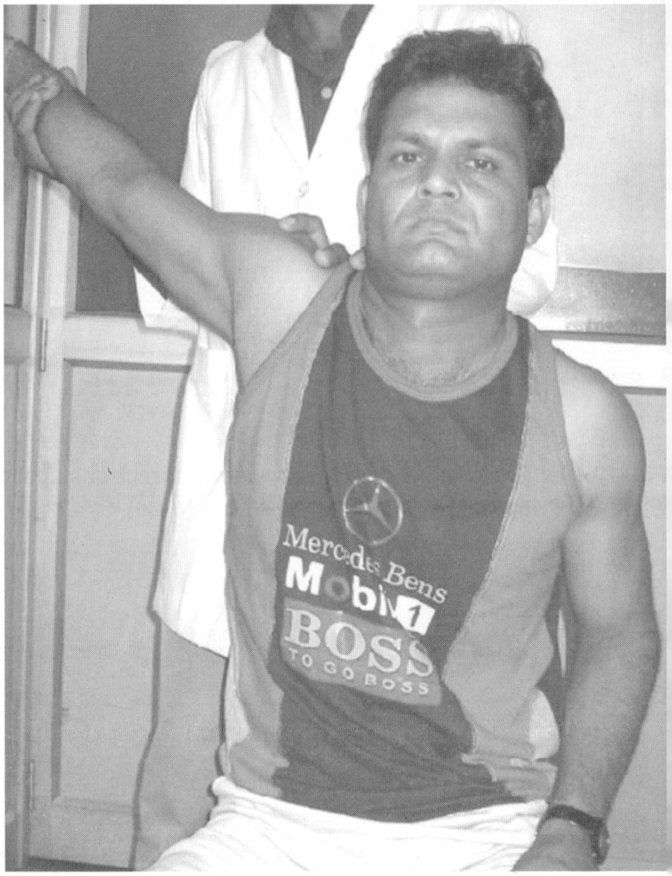

Fig. 13.19b: Stretching of pectoralis major (lower fibre)

Stretching of Supra Spinatus Muscle

Position of Patient: Standing.

Position of Therapist: Standing behind the patient, facing the posterior aspect of shoulder joint. One hand holds the patient's hand, while other hand grasps the patient's elbow.

Procedure: The therapist extends and internally rotates the shoulder joint passively and flexes the elbow joint, so that forearm of patient rests on his back. While maintaining the position the therapist pushes the elbow toward the midline by both the hands. The elbow which rests on patient's back, remains flexed at 80-90°. The procedure may also be repeated on high sitting or supine (Fig. 13.20).

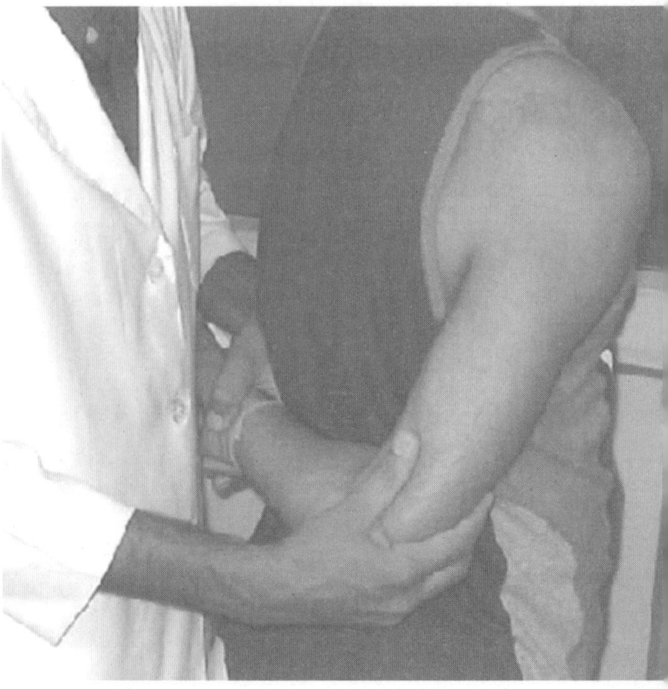

Fig. 13.20: Stretching of supraspinatus in standing position

Stretching of Subscapularis

Position of Patient: Supine.

Position of Therapist: Standing at the side of patient, facing the shoulder joint. One hand grasps the elbow while other grasps the wrist joint.

Procedure: The shoulder is abducted to 90° and elbow is flexed to 90°. While maintaining the position, the shoulder is rotated laterally by taking the hand up (toward the head) (Fig. 13.21). Shoulder is stabilized to prevent retraction of scapula.

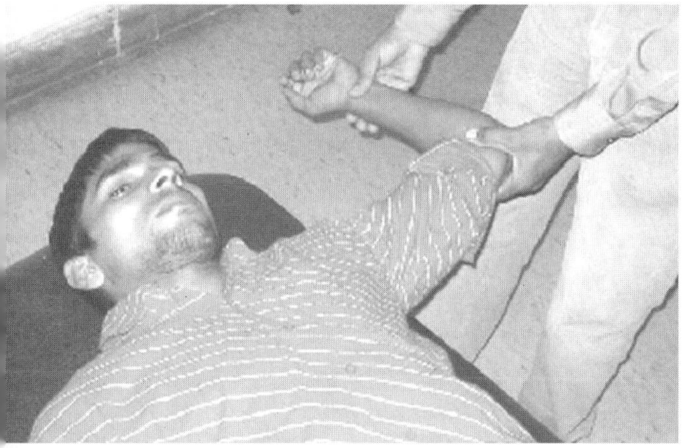

Fig. 13.21: Supine, therapist laterally rotates the shoulder

Stretching of Infraspinatus and Teres Minor

Position of Patient and Therapist: Same as for stretching of subscapularis.

Procedure: The shoulder is abducted to 90° and elbow is kept to 90° flexion. While maintaining the position the shoulder is rotated medially, by taking the hand toward the waist (Fig. 13.22). Shoulder is stabilized to prevent protraction of scapula.

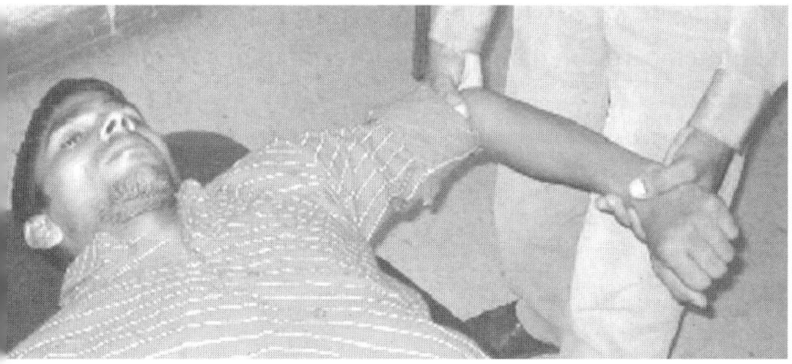

Fig. 13.22: Stretching of infraspinatus

Stretching of Latissimus Dorsi

Position of Patient: Supine lying.

Position of Therapist: Standing at the side of patient, facing the joint. One hand is placed over the lateral border of scapula while other hand grasp the elbow joint.

Procedure: The upper hand abducts the shoulder with external rotation, while lower hand stabilizes the scapula. The lower hand should not press the scapula tightly, as latissimus dorsi might get compressed (Fig. 13.23).

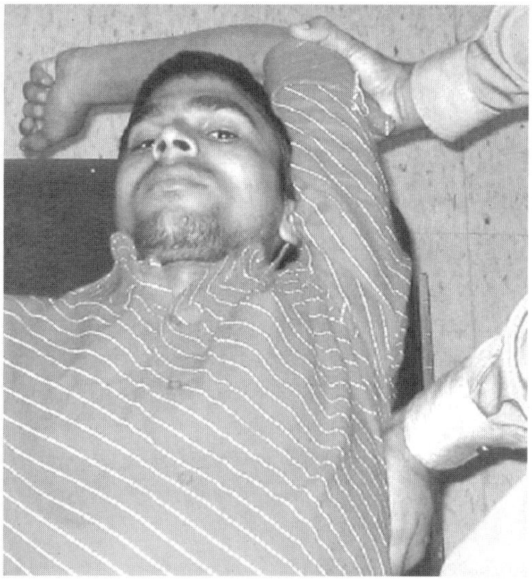

Fig. 13.23: Stretching of latissimus dorsi

Alternate Method of Latissimus Dorsi

Position of Patient: Standing.

Position of Therapist: Standing behind the patient, one hand is placed over the waist opposite to the side of muscle being stretched and the other grasp the arm.

Procedure: The upper hand of therapist abducts the shoulder with elbow to 90° flexion. The trunk is flexed towards opposite side by pushing the arm. At the same time the other hand stabilizes the trunk (or facilitates the trunk bending) by counterbalancing the weight of the body. Further stabilization at the pelvis is given by therapists thigh on the side of stretching (Fig. 13.24).

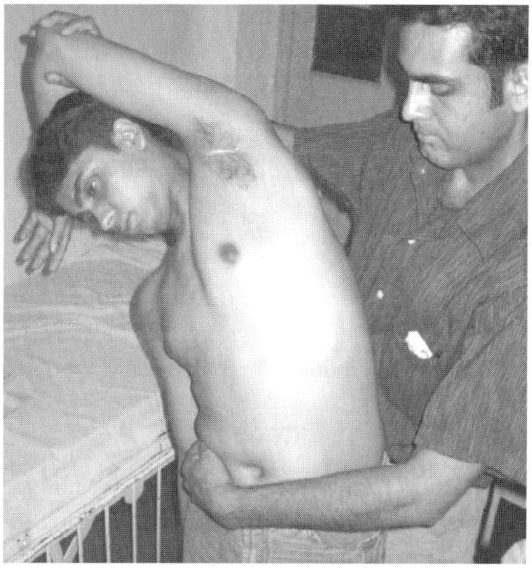

Fig. 13.24: Stretching of latissimus dorsi

For example: To stretch left latissimus dorsi, therapist places his right hand on arm and left hand on the opposite waist. Therapist uses his left thigh to stabilize patient's pelvis from left side (procedure is followed as above). While maintaining the position, therapist grasps the left arm of the patient and bends the trunk to the opposite side with shoulder abduction.

Stretching of Elbow Flexors

Position of Patient: Standing.

Position of Therapist: Standing behind the patient. One hand is placed at the elbow joint and other hand grasp the forearm at the wrist joint. (Forced passive stretching of elbow flexors may cause myositis ossification, therefore extra care should be taken to avoid complication, specially in children) (Fig. 13.25).

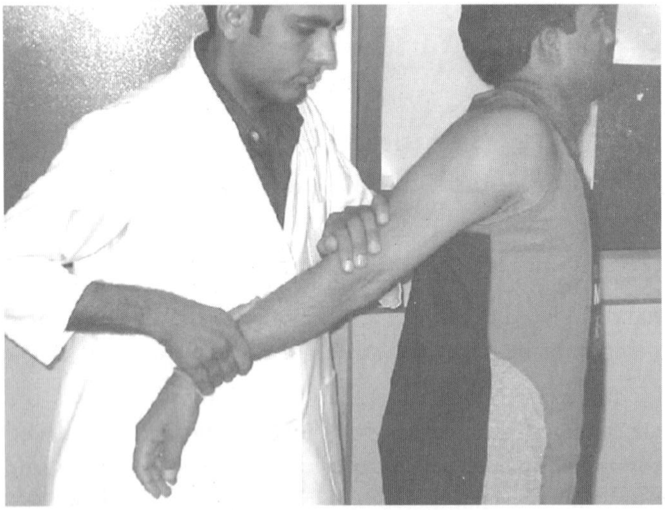

Fig. 13.25: Stretching of biceps

Procedure: The therapist extends the shoulder joint with elbow flexion. In the next step of technique the therapist extends the elbow joint gradually.

Stretching of Elbow Extensors

Position of Patient: Sitting on chair or standing.

Position of Therapist: Standing at the side of patient. One hand grasps the proximal part of elbow while other grasps the wrist joint.

Procedure: The therapist flexes the shoulder joint (full flexion) at 180° with elbow flexion at 90°. In the next step therapist flexes the elbow joint passively (Fig. 13.26).

Stretching of Wrist Extensors

Position of Patient and Therapist: Any comfortable position. The therapist stabilizes the forearm by one hand, while other hand grasps the hand and flexes the wrist joint passively to stretch the extensors (Fig. 13.27).

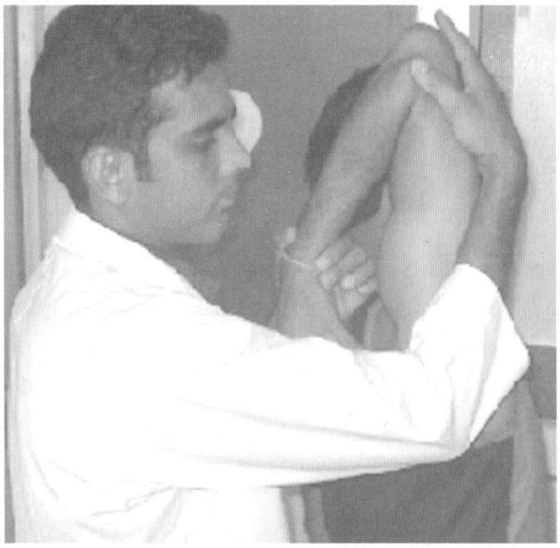

Fig. 13.26: Stretching of triceps

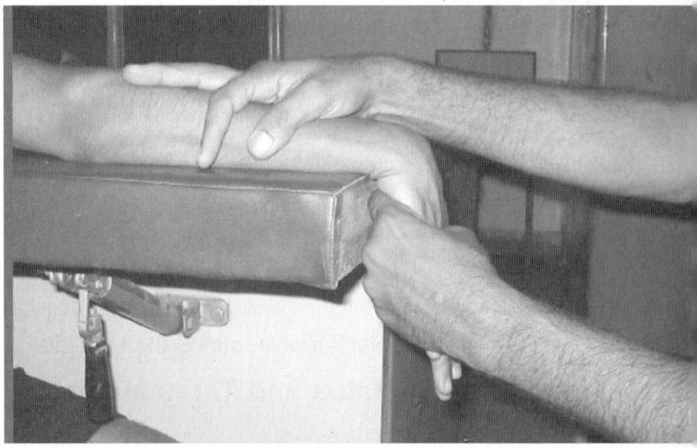

Fig. 13.27: Stretching of wrist extensors

Stretching of Wrist Flexors

Position of Patient and Therapist: Remains same as for wrist extensors stretching. Therapist's one hand stabilizes the forearm and other hand grasps the hand.

Procedure: While stabilizing the forearm by one hand, the other hand passively extends the wrist joint (Fig. 13.28). The metacarpophalangeal and interphalangeal joints remain flexed.

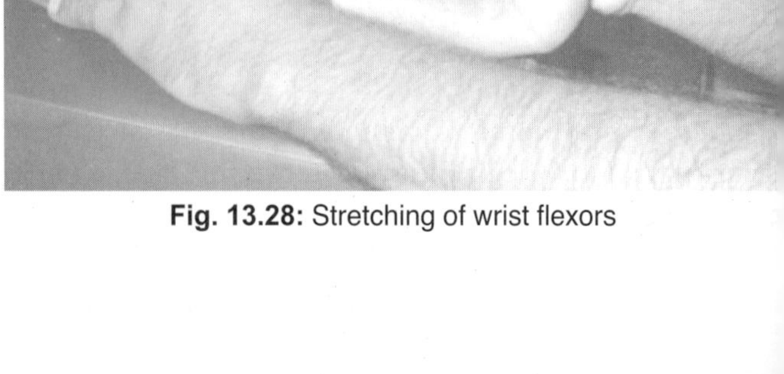

Fig. 13.28: Stretching of wrist flexors

Stretching of Common Extensors (Extensor Carpi Radialis Longus, Extensor Carpi Radialis Brevis, Extensor Carpi Ulnaris, Extensor Digitorum/Communis)

Position of Patient: Sitting on chair, arm rests on table, and wrist out of the edge of the treatment table.

Position of Therapist: Sitting in front of patient (across the table). One hand stabilizes the elbow joint, and other hand grasps the hand of patient.

Procedure: While stabilizing the elbow joint by one hand, the other hand flexes the fingers and wrist joint. In the next step the forearm is pronated and elbow is extended (Fig. 13.29).

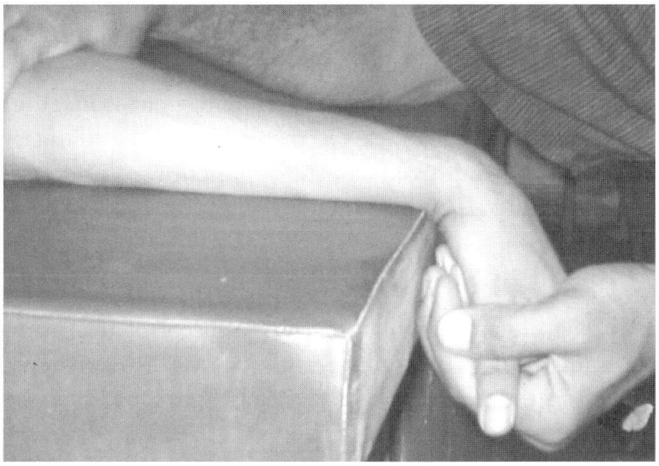

Fig. 13.29: Stretching of wrist common extensors

Stretching of Wrist and Finger Flexors (Flexor Carpi Radialis, Flexor Carpi Ulnaris, Flexor Digitorum Superficialis, Flexor Digitorum Profundus)

Position of Patient: Sitting on chair, arm rests on table.

Position of Therapist: Sitting in front of patient (across the table). One hand grasps the forearm while the fingers of other hand rest on the patient's fingers.

Procedure: Therapist extends the wrist and four fingers (Fig. 13.30).

Stretching of Intrinsic Muscles of Hand (Lumbricals and Interossei)

Position of Patient: Sitting on chair, arm rests on table.

Position of Therapist: Sitting in front of patient (across the table). One hand stabilizes the forearm and wrist joint. The other hand grasps the finger to be stretched.

Procedure: Therapist flexes the PIP joint and hyper extends the MCP joint with one hand while stabilizing wrist and forearm with other hand.

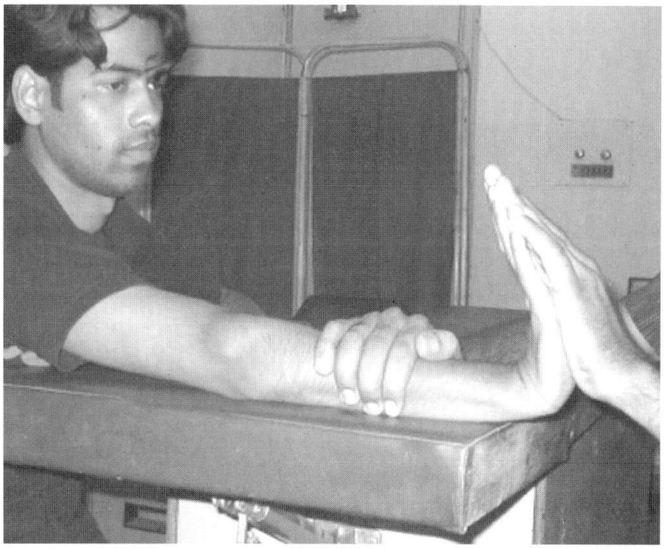

Fig. 13.30: Stretching of wrist and finger flexors

For all fingers together.

Position of Patient: Same.

Position of Therapist: Same.

Therapist flexes proximal interphalangeal (PIP) joints of all fingers and hyperextends the MCP joints with one hand while stabilizing the wrist and wrist with other hand.

Procedure: Therapist flexes all the PIP joints and hyperextends the MCP joints with one hand while stabilizing wrist with other hand.

Alternative Position for Lumbricals and Interossei: The therapist places his/her fingers over the dorsum of the patient's fingers, the tip of the therapist fingers rest on the MCP joints or proximal phalanx. In the first step therapist flexes the PIP and DIP and then hyperextends the MCP joints. The position is maintained for 10-15 seconds (Fig. 13.31).

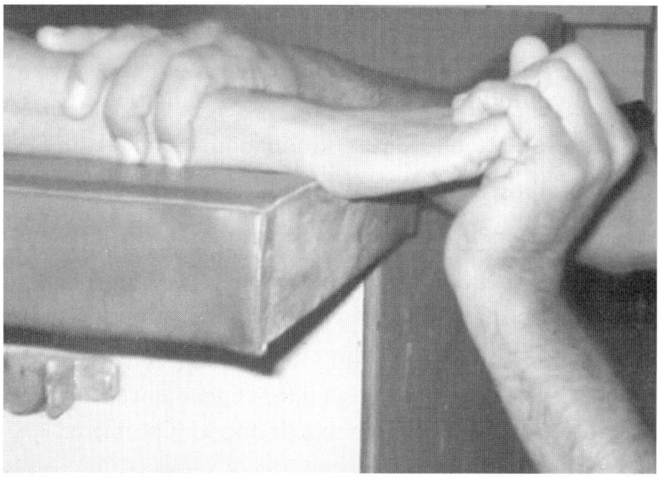

Fig. 13.31: Stretching of lumbricals

14

PROPRIOCEPTIVE NEUROMUSCULAR FACILITATION (PNF)

The nerve endings that relay all the information about the musculoskeletal system to the central nervous system are called proprioceptors. Proprioceptors also called mechanoreceptors, are the source of all proprioception; the perception of one's own body position and movement. The proprioceptors detect any changes in movement or position of limbs and any change in tension, or force, within the body. The proprioceptors are found in the muscle spindles (intrafusal fibers), tendons (Golgi tendon organ), ligaments and joints. A pacinian corpuscle type of proprioceptors located close to the Golgi tendon organ, is responsible for detecting changes in movement and pressure within the body. The Golgi tendon organ (proprioceptor) is sensitive to the change in tension and the rate of change of tension. Proprioceptive neuromuscular facilitation is a therapeutic approach, designed to promote and enhance the response of proprioceptors in order to improve neuromuscular mechanism and functional limitation. The PNF approach includes movements of the joints, contraction and stretching (stimulus) of the muscles to get the proprioceptors (all types) stimulated to facilitated the motor control.

In 1940s, Dr Kabat was the first man who has given the name of proprioceptive facilitation, then after in 1956, Ms Voss (Physiotherapist) added the neuromuscular to Dr Kabat's proprioceptive facilitation, and given the name of PNF (Proprioceptive Neuromuscular Facilitation).

- Proprioception—Means stimulation within tissues.
- Neuromuscular—Pertaining to nerves and muscles.
- Facilitation—Makes response easy.

Therefore PNF may be defined as an approach of promoting or hastening the response of the proprioceptors.

Normal neuromuscular mechanism is capable to produce efficient and purposeful functional movements and activities of daily living without facing any problem.

The response of normal neuromuscular mechanism may be limited as a result of trauma, disease of the nervous system and musculoskeletal system, thus the voluntary effort becomes unable to produce the efficient and purposeful functional movements. Therefore by administering the PNF techniques the response of deficient neuromuscular mechanism can be made easy so that the weakened voluntary effort can be improved for the production of effective, efficient and purposeful functional movement.

PRINCIPLES

PNF is a philosophical approach or concept of treatment. Its underlying philosophy is that all the human being including those with disabilities, have untapped existing potential.

1. The treatment approach is always positive, reinforcing and using that which the patient can do on a physical and psychological level.

   The normal neuromuscular response of an individual is limited to its physical ability, inherent and previously learned neuromuscular responses. However, untapped neuromuscular response may be shown during stressful episodes. Not only that but also the neuromuscular response may be enhanced through environmental influences and voluntary decisions. Based on this philosophy that the individual has untapped neuromuscular potential, the therapist always strives to treat functions, motivates patient to achieve higher levels, and use the patients strength to minimize the weakness.

2. The primary goal of treatment is to help patients achieve their highest level of functions.
3. PNF is an integrated approach; each treatment is directed at a total human being, not at a specific problem or body segment.
4. The PNF patterns are performed according to the normal development process. Development of motion occurs first in the head and neck, then in the trunk and

finally in the extremities. Hence, PNF patterns are strived to the head and neck movements first as they influence the movements of the body. In the next step the patterns are performed on the trunk as it provides foundation of the body. As soon as the patient achieves motor control over the head neck and trunk, the PNF patterns are performed on the extremities to improve their functions.

5. Mass movement patterns performed in spiral and diagonal patterns closely resemble the movements used in sports and in activities of daily living (ADL). The spiral and diagonal character is in keeping the spiral and rotatory characteristic of the skeletal system of bones and muscles and the ligament structures. This type of motion is also in harmony with the topographical alignment of the muscles from origin to insertion and with the structural characteristic of the individual muscles.

PATTERNS OF MOTION

The patterns of PNF are mass motions means during the normal functional activity (to place a specific demand) number of movements occur sequentially from distal part of the limb to the proximal and this activity requires shortening and lengthening of many muscles in varying degrees. There are two main patterns, flexion and extension, performed in the diagonal manner. The patterns of extremities are associated with motion components of the joints.

It is also keeping with Beevor's axiom that the brain knows nothing about the individual muscle action but knows only of movements.

Diagonals

There are two diagonals for each major parts of the body (the head and neck, upper trunk and lower trunk and extremities). It is important to know that the PNF patterns are performed in spiral and diagonal patterns because of the topographical alignment of the muscles from origin to insertion and with the structural characteristic of the individual muscles.

Each diagonal is made up of two patterns which are antagonistic to each other.

- Diagonal$_1$ (D_1) is made up of two patterns–flexion and extension.
- Diagonal$_2$ (D_2) is made up of two patterns–flexion and extension.

Motion Components

It means the movements which take place during the pattern. Each spiral and diagonal pattern is composed of three motion components with respect to all the muscles of action participating in the movement.

These three motion components are as follows:

1. Flexion or Extension.
2. Adduction or Abduction.
3. Internal or External rotation.

BASIC PROCEDURE

Agonists and Antagonists

When muscles contract toward their shortened state the resulting pattern is termed as agonistic pattern. On the contrary when the muscles contract towards their lengthened state, the pattern is called antagonistic pattern.

Traction and Approximation

Traction and approximation is used to *stimulate proprioceptors within* and *around* the joint such as *Ligaments, cartilage,* capsule etc. Approximation is used to facilitate co-contraction around the joint, while traction is used to increase ROM.

Normal Timing

It is the sequence in which the participating muscles in any motor activity contract to carry on coordinated and purposeful movements.

Normally rotation is the movement which is initiated first followed by other components from distal to proximal, if this rotation is blocked other component of motion is not possible.

Stretch Stimulus

The contraction of muscle or group of muscles can be increased if they are stretched before allowing them to contract. Therefore, to achieve more contraction an agonist group of muscles are placed in a lengthened state then a stretch stimulus is given immediately. After stretch stimulus, patient is commanded to contract the muscles (agonist muscles). For example to achieve more contraction of wrist and finger extensors, these group of muscles are placed in a lengthened position and a stretch is given which is followed by contraction of wrist and finger extensors. In PNF all group of motion components are given a stretch stimulus.

The rotation component receives first and last consideration since it is the rotatory component that elongates the muscles in a given pattern. After rotation component the stretch stimulus is given from distal to proximal motion components.

Stretch Reflex

The stretch reflex is given to increase the voluntary contraction of agonist muscles and subsequently the strength. Use of stretch reflex aids the patient with intact innervation to learn and perform the patterns with greater ease.

The difference between stretch stimulus and reflex—In stretch stimulus a gentle stretch is given with low intensity to agonist muscles, while stretch reflex includes a sudden or quick stretch with more intensity which is followed by voluntary contraction of the agonist muscles.

All the motion components (agonist muscles) are placed in an extreme lengthened position then a quick stretch reflex is elicited manually by taking the part past the point of tension. All the components should receive stretch reflex specially proper rotation. To be certain that stretch reflex and contraction of agonist muscles are synchronized, the patient is commanded as "Now push" or pull. This warns the patient to be prepared to attempt the motion.

Manual Contact

The placement of the hands of therapist on the patient's limb or body is termed as manual contact. Appropriate placement of hands facilitates the contraction of agonist muscles. Hands should always be placed over the agonist muscles. When the hand is placed over the patient's skin, it causes tactile stimulation and facilitates the contraction of the underlying muscles or group of muscles.

For example—If finger extensors are the agonist muscles, therapist should place hand over the dorsum of the hand to apply resistance. If the therapist places hand on the palmar aspect of the patient's hand (over the antagonists) the tactile stimulation on palmar surface causes contraction of the finger flexors which decreases the contraction of extensors of the fingers.

When patterns are performed passively, the therapist may place hand on the antagonist muscles as it is difficult to perform without it.

For example—If patient has spasticity in flexor group of muscles of the upper limb and cannot extend the fingers voluntarily then therapist places the tip of fingers on the palmar aspect of patient's finger tips and extends the fingers during the pattern. Here therapist must make efforts to contact the palmar surface of the patient's hand as minimal as possible.

Command and Communication

Patient makes little effort or does not take interest in performing the patterns. Therefore the biggest job of therapist is to make the patient interested and allow him to participate voluntarily in PNF patterns. This can be achieved by giving an adequate command and by appreciating his voluntary efforts during the pattern. There are three types of basic commands: (i) Verbal (ii) Visual (iii) Tactile.

1. *Verbal command:* Tone of voice may influence considerably the quality of response. A tone of voice should be appropriate according to the contraction required. When maximal stimulation of active motion is required a strong, sharp command is given. It simulates a stress situation. A moderate tone of voice should be used when the patient is responding with his best effort. If patient is having musculoskeletal problems such as pain and inflammation the commands should be soft tone of voice. The verbal command is given as "Push", "Pull", "Hold" and "Relax or Let go". The command "Hold" is given during isometric contraction. The "Push" or "Pull" are given during isotonic contraction of muscles while "Relax" or "Let go" used for relaxation.
2. *Visual command:* This type of command is particularly useful in children who do not follow the verbal command. Attractive things or objects are placed in the space/air at different positions (in which the patterns are performed). A child is frequently led to perform by enticing him or her to look at object and his hand tries to follow the direction of object. Several repetitions may be performed in the same manner.

   A visual command is also useful in an adult to make him understand by demonstrating the direction of pattern, if patient finds difficulty to perform the movement in desired direction.
3. *Tactile command:* Therapist places the hand on the agonist muscles and commands the patient by scratching the skin or applying pressure over it. The rubbing and pressing cause tactile stimulation and facilitate the contraction of agonist muscles. Applying pressure or touching the skin also helps to contract the muscle in the desired diagonal.

Line of Movement

The patterns are performed in a diagonal direction from their completely lengthened position to the complete contracting state. The diagonal direction allows the muscles to contract maximum from their fully stretched state.

PNF PATTERNS FOR UPPER EXTREMITIES

The PNF patterns in upper extremities are performed in spiral and diagonal manner (Table 14.1).

Upper extremities consist of two diagonals and each diagonal is made up of two patterns (Flexion and extension). So there are four patterns and two diagonals in upper extremities.

Table 14.1: Upper extremity

Diagonal	*Pattern*	*Motion components*
D_1	Flexion	Shoulder—Flexion, adduction and external rotation. Elbow—May remain flexed or extended. Forearm—Supination. Wrist—Flexion and radial deviation. Fingers—Flexion and adduction. Thumb—Flexion and adduction.
	Extension	Shoulder—Extension, adduction and internal rotation. Elbow—May remain flexed or extended. Forearm—Pronation Wrist—Extension and ulnar deviation. Finger—Extension and abduction. Thumb—Extension and abduction.
D_2	Flexion	Shoulder—Flexion, abduction and external rotation. Elbow—May remain flexed or extended. Forearm—Supination. Wrist—Extension and radial deviation. Finger—Extension and abduction. Thumb—Extension, adduction and external rotation of the first metacarpophalangeal joint.
	Extension	Shoulder—Extension, adduction and internal rotation. Elbow—May remain flexed or extended. Forearm—Pronation. Wrist—Flexion and ulnar deviation. Finger—Flexion and adduction. Thumb—Opposition, adduction and internal rotation of the first metacarpophalangeal joint.

- Diagonal$_1$—D_1 Flexion, D_1 Extension.
- Diagonal$_2$—D_2 Flexion, D_2 Extension.

Common Points for Upper Extremities D_1 and D_2 Patterns

- Shoulder flexion and extension are combined with adduction and abduction.
- External rotation is consistent with flexion.
- Internal rotation is consistent with extension.
- Supination of the forearm and radial deviation of the wrist are combined with flexion and external rotation of the shoulder.
- The pronation of the forearm and ulnar deviation are combined with extension and internal rotation of the shoulder.
- Flexion of wrist with adduction of the finger occurs with flexion of the wrist and adduction of the shoulder.
- Extension of wrist with abduction of the fingers occur with wrist extension and shoulder abduction.
- Adduction of the thumb is consistent with external rotation and flexion of the shoulder.
- Adduction of the thumb is consistent with external rotation and extension.
- Flexion of the thumb is consistent with adduction of the shoulder.
- Extension of thumb is consistent with abduction of the shoulder.
- Distal joints (Hand and Wrist)–The motions are consistent with proximal components.

D_1 Flexion Pattern

Motion Components

Shoulder	–	Flexion, adduction and external rotation
Elbow	–	Flexion or extension
Forearm	–	Supination
Wrist	–	Flexion and radial deviation
Fingers	–	Flexion and adduction
	–	Rotation toward radial side
Thumb	–	Flexion with adduction and external rotation of the first metacarpal joint.

Free Active Motion

Position the patient in standing. This pattern is performed by the patient without the help of therapist. The pattern starts from extreme lengthened position of the agonist to shortened state. Commands may be given as follows:

i. Look at your hand, place it behind your body away from the midline (in extreme lengthened position of agonists) (Fig. 14.1a).

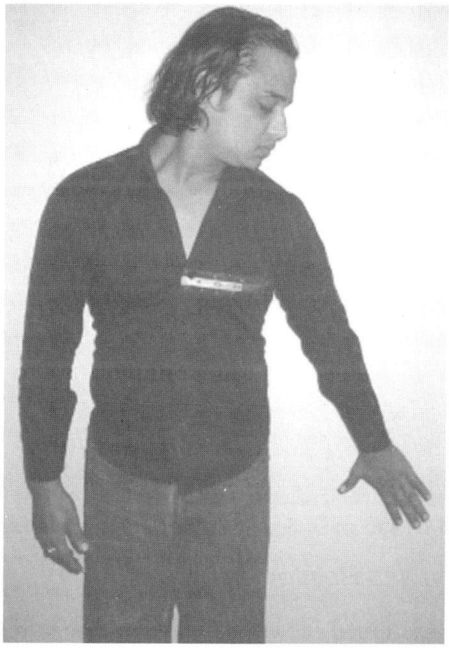

ii. Close the hand and turn it outward (external rotation of the shoulder) (Fig. 14.1b).

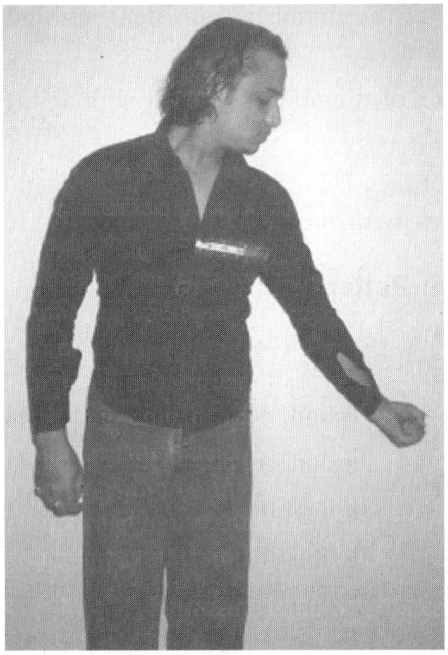

iii. Pull it up across the midline, to the opposite shoulder (Fig. 14.1c).

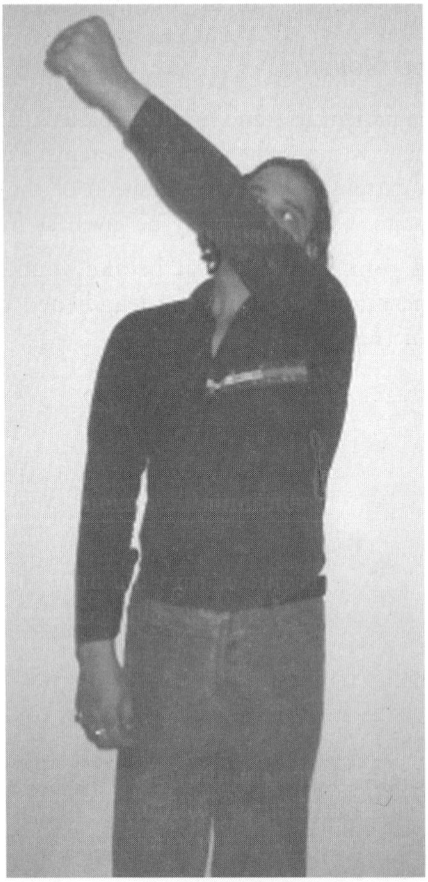

Figs. 14.1a to c: D_1 flexion pattern (free active motion)

Facilitation and Reinforcement

Patient is positioned in supine lying. Therapist places both hands over agonist muscles (one hand over the arm and other over the hand). The extremity is placed in extreme lengthened position. A stretch reflex is given by applying a sudden stretch of the agonists immediately after that patient is commanded to contract the agonists and perform the pattern as demonstrated. As patient starts moving the extremity therapist applies resistance. Therapist must use an appropriate verbal command such as push my both hands in the direction of your opposite shoulder. The proximal joints are given more resistance than distal joints and weaker distal components are guided through their optimal range of motion in accordance with normal timing. This pattern is used to strengthen the muscles if they have fair voluntary control (Figs. 14.2a to c).

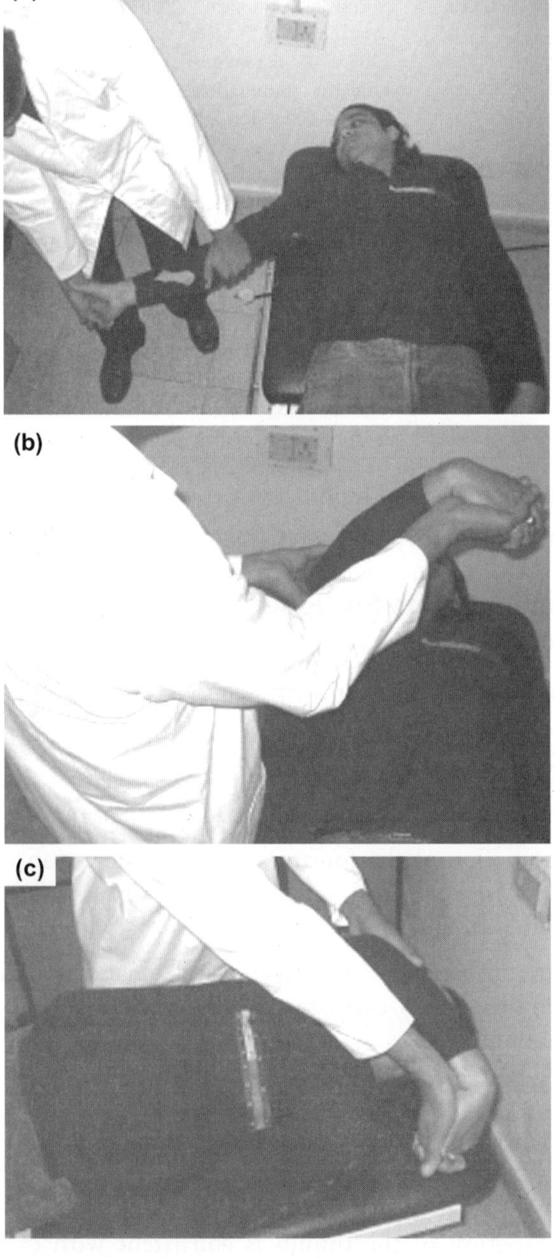

Figs. 14.2a to c: D_1 flexion pattern (facilitation and reinforcement)

D_1 Extension Pattern

Motion Components

Shoulder – Extension, abduction and internal rotation
Elbow – Flexion or extension
Forearm – Pronation
Wrist – Extension, ulnar deviation
Fingers – Extension and abduction
– Rotation toward ulnar side
Thumb – Palmar abduction with abduction and internal rotation of the first metacarpal.

Free Active Motion

The position of patient remains same as D_1 flexion pattern. All agonist muscles are placed in an extreme lengthened position (end of D_1 flexion pattern). The patient is asked to take the hand down to the opposite hip joint (diagonally) and point the fingers downward with palm facing backward. An extremity is taken in an extreme shortened position of the agonist muscles.

Commands may be given as follows:

i. Look at your hand place it up across the midline (in extreme lengthened position of the agonists muscles) (Fig. 14.3a).
ii. Now open your hand (Fig. 14.3b).
iii. Now take it down, away from the midline (Figs. 14.3a to c).

Facilitation and Reinforcement

Patient is positioned in supine lying. Therapist stands at the same side of the extremity and places both hands on the agonist muscles at the elbow and dorsal aspect of the wrist. Agonist muscles are placed in extreme lengthened position then a stretch reflex is given which is synchronized by the contraction of agonist muscles. Patient is instructed to move the limb to the opposite hip joint (diagonally). The resistance is applied by the hands throughout the range of motion (from extreme lengthened state to the extreme shortened state of agonist muscles). The stronger proximal and distal components are resisted but weaker distal components are guided through their optimal range of motion in accordance with normal timing (Figs. 14.4a to c).

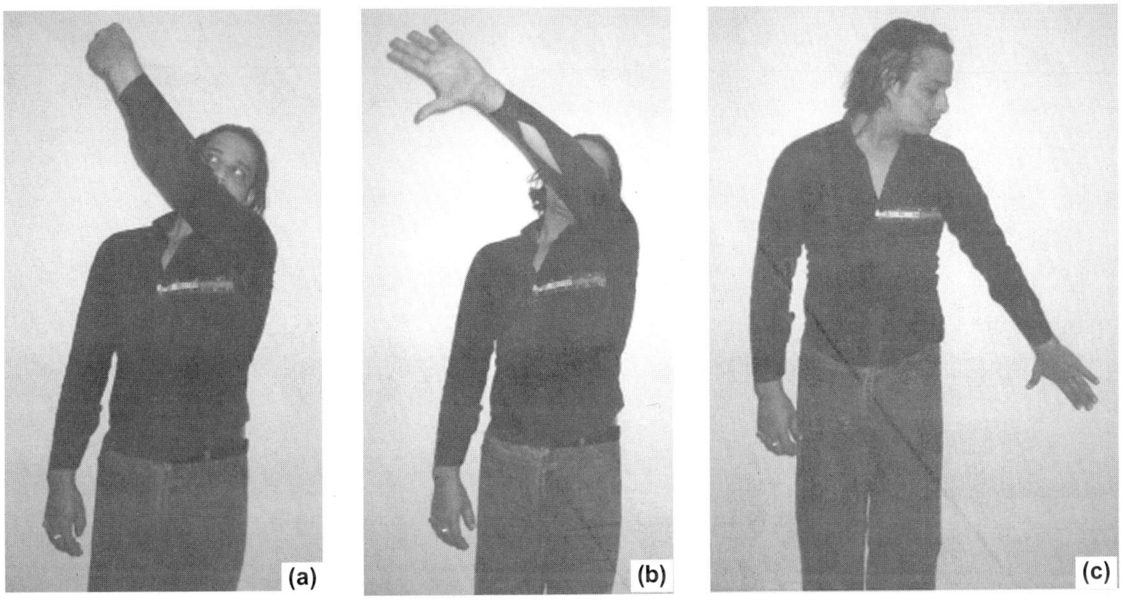

Figs. 14.3a to c: D_1 extension pattern (free active motion)

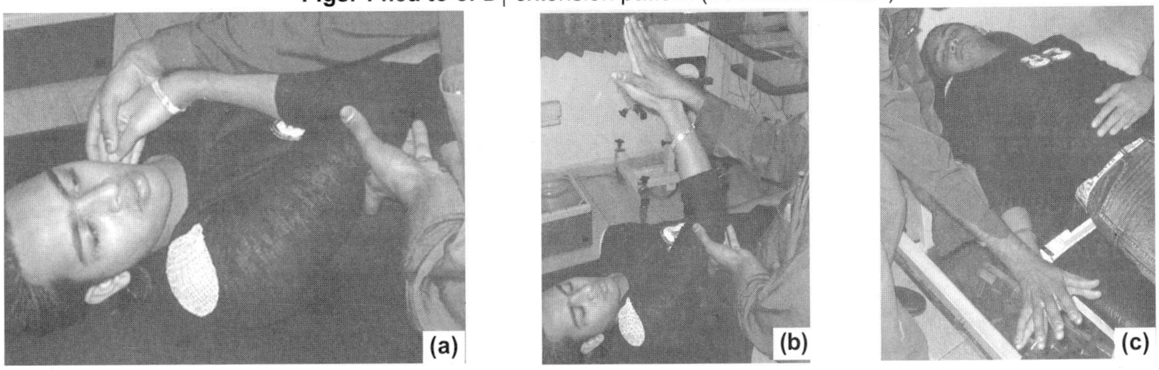

Figs. 14.4a to c: D_1 extension pattern (facilitation and reinforcement)

D_2 Flexion Pattern

Motion Components

Shoulder – Flexion, abduction and external rotation
Elbow – Flexion or extension
Forearm – Supination
Wrist – Extension and radial deviation
Fingers – Extension and abduction
Thumb – Extension, adduction and external rotation of the first metacarpal joint.

Free Active Pattern

Position of the patient is high sitting or standing. All the motion components are flexed in the extreme lengthened position (flexion of finger, wrist, ulnar deviation, thumb flexion, forearm pronation and adduction, flexion and internal rotation of shoulder joints). A stretch reflex is given followed by contraction of agonists.

Commands may be given as follows:

i. Look at your hand place it in front of your body across the midline (in extreme lengthened position of agonist muscles) (Fig. 14.5a).
ii. Open the hand and turn it outward (Fig. 14.5b).
iii. Pull it up away from the midline (Fig. 14.5c).

Facilitation and Reinforcement

The patient is positioned in supine lying. Therapist places both hands on the agonist muscles (one hand over the dorsum of wrist and finger and other over the elbow joint. Agonist muscles are placed in extreme lengthened position then a stretch stimules or reflex is given which is synchronized by an active contraction of agonist muscles.

The stronger proximal and distal components are resisted but weaker distal components are guided through their optimal range of motion in accordance with normal timing (Figs. 14.6a to c).

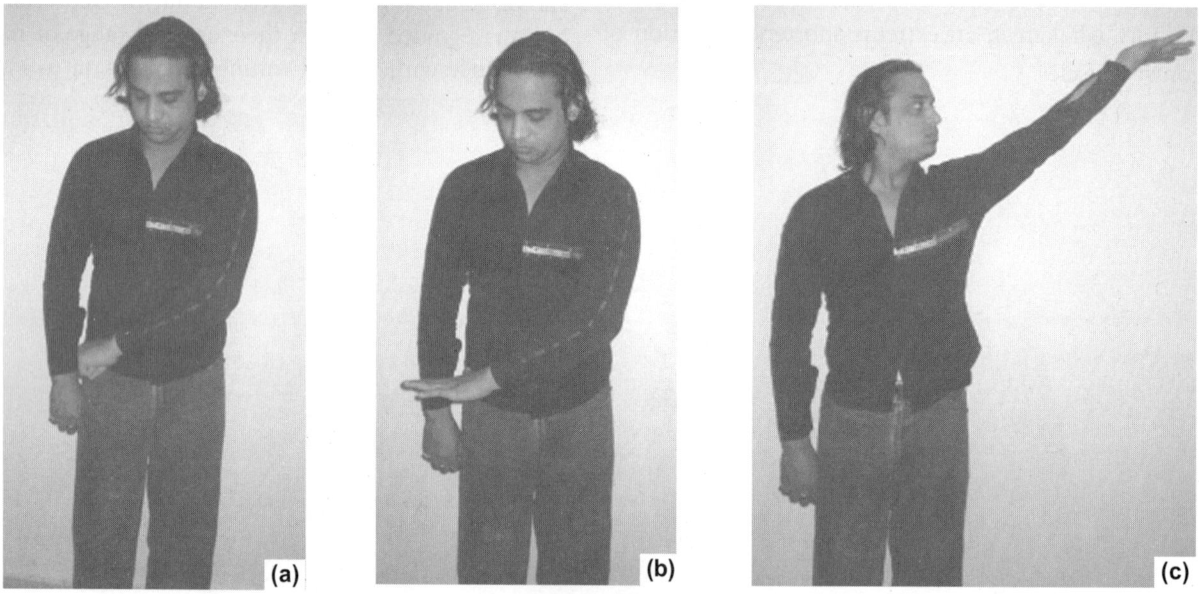

Figs. 14.5a to c: D_2 flexion pattern (free active motion)

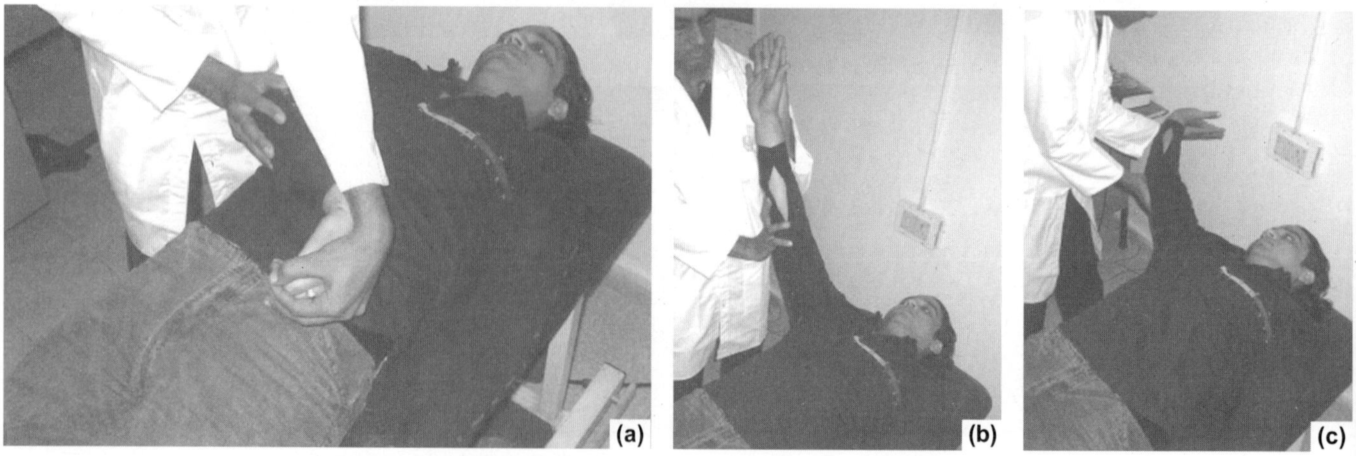

Figs. 14.6a to c: D_2 flexion pattern (facilitation of reinforcement)

D_2 Extension Pattern

Motion Components

Shoulder – Extension, adduction and internal rotation
Elbow – Flexion or extension
Forearm – Supination
Wrist – Flexion and ulnar deviation
Fingers – Flexion and adduction
Thumb – Flexion, abduction and internal rotation of the first metacarpal joint.

Free Active Pattern

This is the reverse of the D_2 flexion pattern. The patient is positioned in high sitting or standing. Agonist muscles are placed in extremely lengthened state and patient is commanded to take the extremity to the opposite buttock (diagonally).

Commands may be given as follows:

i. Look at your hand place it up away from the midline (in an extreme lengthened state of agonist muscles) (Fig. 14.7a).

ii. Now close your hand and turn it inward (Fig. 14.7b).

iii. Pull it down across the midline in front of your body (Fig. 14.7c).

Facilitation and Reinforcement

The patient is positioned in supine lying, therapist stands at the same side of the shoulder joint and places both hands over the agonist muscles (one over the elbow and other over the palmar surface of the hand) the extremity is placed in extreme lengthened position, a stretch reflex is given which is synchronized by an active contraction of agonist muscles. The stronger proximal and distal components are resisted but weaker distal components are guided through their optimal range of motion in accordance with normal timing (Figs. 14.8a to c).

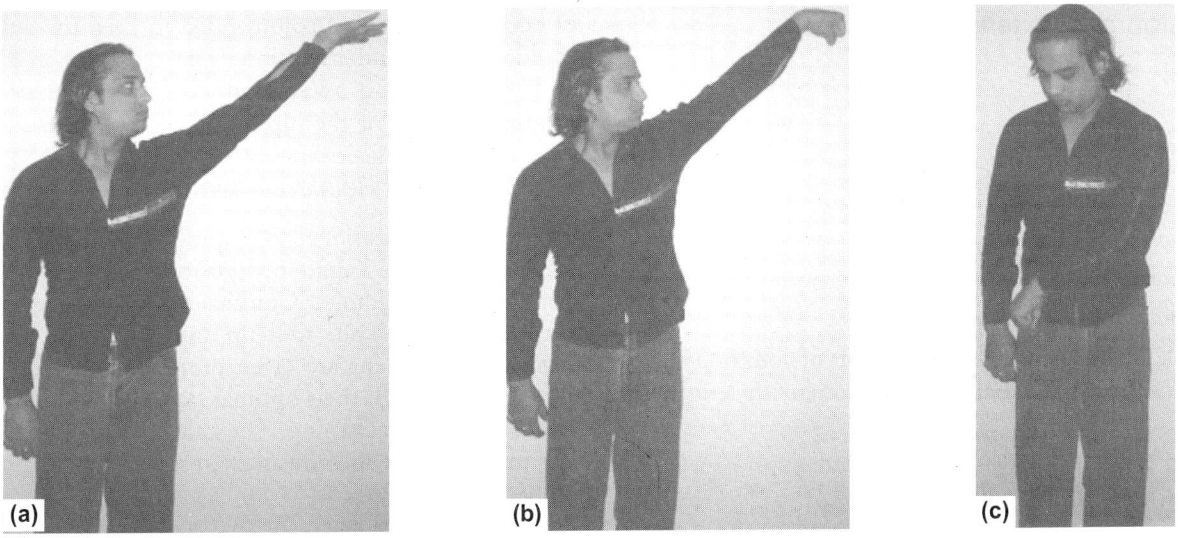

Figs. 14.7a to c: D_2 extension pattern (free active motion)

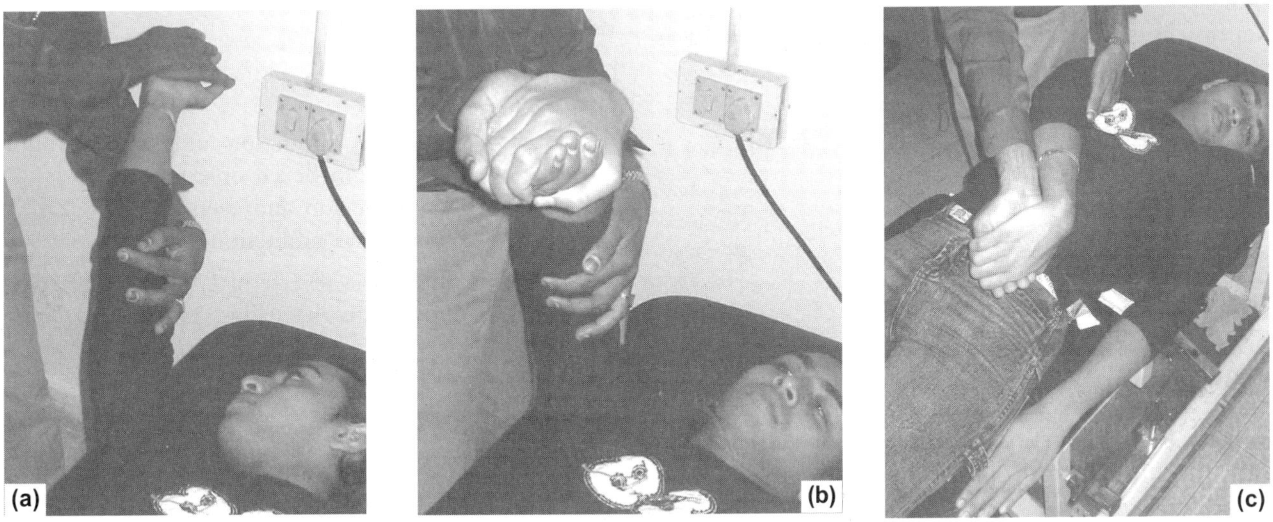

Figs. 14.8a to c: D_2 extension pattern (Facilitation and reinforcement)

D_1 Flexion and Extension Patterns

Diagonal – D_1

Pattern – Flexion and Extension.

Motion Components

Same as D_1 Flexion and Extension.

Position of the Patient: Standing.

Position of the Therapist: Standing in front of patient.

Commands are given as follows:

1. Look at your hand, place it behind your body away from the midline, in extreme lengthened position.
2. "Close the hand! and turn it outward!"
3. Pull it up across the midline.
4. "Now open your hand!"
5. Push it down, back to your body away from the midline.

Repeat the same patterns and speak the command as you perform them.

D_2 Flexion and Extension Patterns

Diagonal – D_1

Pattern – Flexion and Extension.

Motion Components

Same as D_2 Flexion and Extension.

Position of the Patient: Standing.

Position of the Therapist: Standing in front of the patient.

Commands are given as follows:

1. "Look at your hand, place it in front of your body across the midline!" Place all the component in lengthened state.
2. Open the hand and turn it outward.
3. Pull it up! away from the midline.
4. "Now close your hand!" and turn it inward.
5. "Pull it down, across the midline in front of the body!"

Repeat the same patterns and speak the command as you perform the pattern.

PNF PATTERNS FOR LOWER EXTREMITY

D_1 Flexion Pattern

Motion Components

See Table 14.2.

Table 14.2: Lower extremity

Diagonal	*Pattern*	*Motion components*
D_1	Flexion	Hip—Flexion, adduction and external rotation. Knee—May remain flexed or extended. Ankle—Dorsiflexion and inversion. Toes—Extension with abduction, rotation of toes toward tibial side.
	Extension	Hip—Extension, abduction and internal rotation. Knee—May remain flexed or extended. Ankle—Plantar flexion and eversion. Toes—Flexion and adduction, rotation toward fibular side.
D_2	Flexion	Hip—Flexion, abduction and internal rotation. Knee—May remain extended or flexed. Ankle—Dorsiflexion and eversion. Toes—Extension with abduction, rotation toward fibular side.
	Extension	Hip—Extension, adduction and external rotation. Knee—May remain flexed or extended. Ankle—Plantar flexion and inversion. Toes—Flexion with adduction rotation toward tibial side.

Free Active Pattern

The patient is positioned in supine lying. All the components are placed in the lengthened position. A stretch stimulus is given followed by a command to cross the leg over the other leg and touch the wall with the plantar aspect of heel. The patient is commanded to keep the ankle joint at dorsiflexion and inversion. The toes remain extended and abducted and away from the wall to maintain an external rotation of the hip joint.

Facilitation and Reinforcement

The patient is positioned in supine lying, the agonists are placed in extreme lengthened position (lower of the plinth away from the midline). Commands are given as turn your heel in and pull your foot up and across the body. The stronger component are given more resistance but weaker are guided through their optimal range of motion in accordance with normal timing. The ankle is kept at dorsiflexion and inversion, the toes are at extension and abduction (Figs. 14.9a to f).

D_1 Extension Pattern

Motion Components

The motion components are just reverse of the flexion pattern.

Hip – Extension, abduction and internal rotation

Knee – May remain flexed or extended

Ankle – Plantar flexion and eversion

Toes – Flexion and adduction

Procedure: This is the reverse of D_1 flexion pattern and performed as opposite to that (Figs. 14.10a to c).

D_2 Flexion Pattern

Motion Components

Hip – Flexion, abduction and internal rotation

Knee – May remain extended or flexed

Ankle – Dorsiflexion and eversion

Toes – Extension with abduction

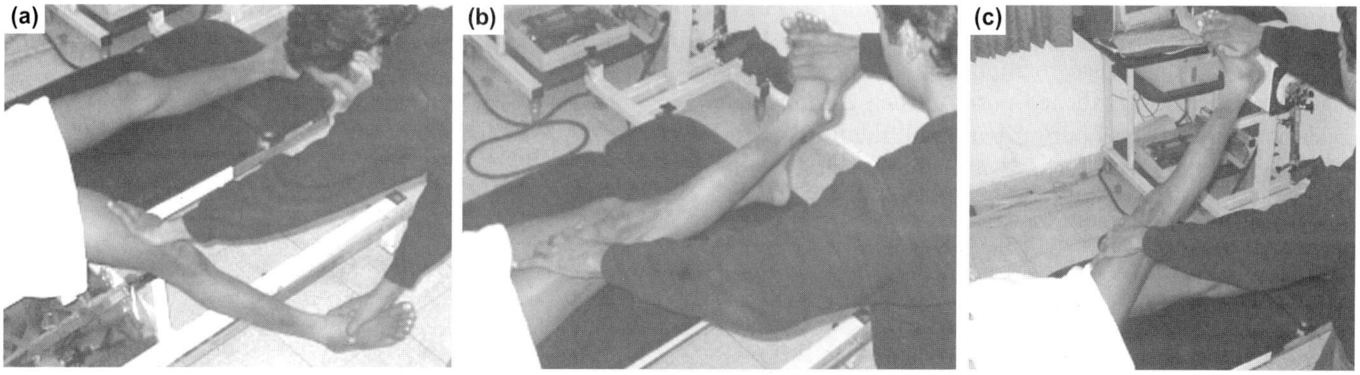

Figs. 14.9a to c: D_1 flexion pattern with knee straight

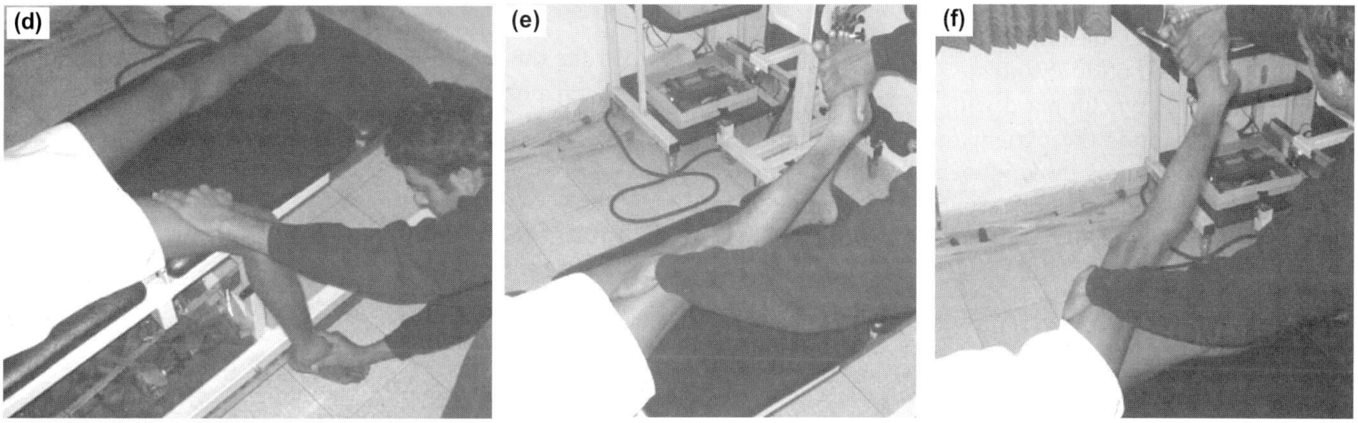

Figs. 14.9d to f: D_1 flexion pattern with knee flexion

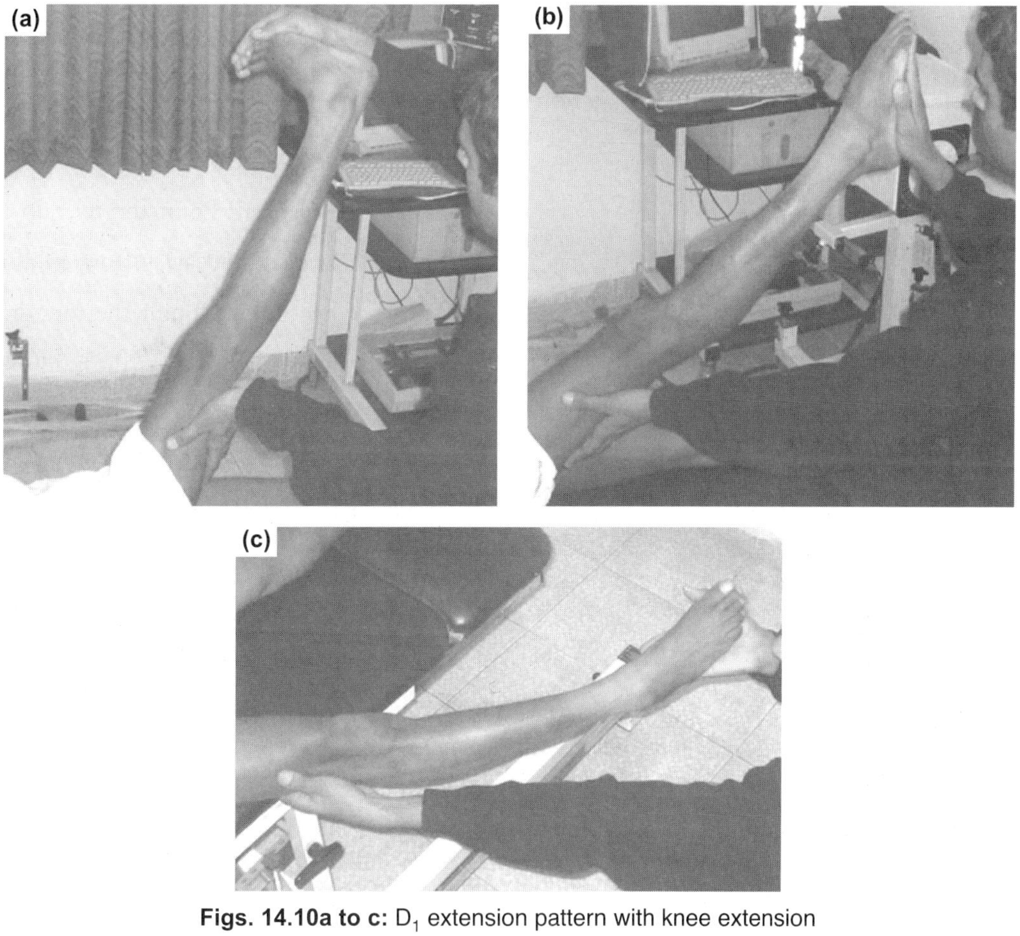

Figs. 14.10a to c: D_1 extension pattern with knee extension

Free Active Pattern

The patient is positioned in supine lying and agonists are placed in extreme lengthened position then commands are given as turn your heel outward and pull the limb up away from the midline as far as possible. The ankle is kept at dorsiflexion and eversion, toes are at extension and abduction.

Facilitation and Reinforcement

The patient is positioned in supine lying, therapist stands at the same side of the extremity and places one hand over the anterolateral aspect of the thigh and other over the dorsum of the foot. All motion components are placed in extreme lengthened position and are given a stretch stimulus or reflex which is synchronized with an active contraction. Therapist commands the patient to push the hands and take the limb up across the midline. All stronger proximal and distal components are resisted but weaker distal components are guided through their optimal range of motion in accordance with their normal timing (Figs. 14.11a to c).

D_2 Extension Pattern

Motion Components

The motion components are just reverse of the flexion pattern of Diagonal D_2.

Hip	–	Extension, adduction and external rotation
Knee	–	May remain extended or flexed
Ankle	–	Plantar flexion with inversion
Toes	–	Flexion with adduction
	–	Rotation toward tibial side.

Diagonal (D_1) Flexion and Extension Pattern with Knee Straight

Motion Components

Same as D_1 Flexion and D_1 Extension.

Position of the Patient: Standing.

Position of the Therapist: Standing in front of the patient.

Commands are given as follows:

1. "Place the limb backward!", "Point your toes down!" (This position places all the flexion components in extreme lengthened state).
2. "Rotate the limb externally, pull the toes up and in! Turn your heel!"
3. "Take the foot up across the midline!"
4. "Now point the toes down, outward and turn the heel in!"
5. "Take the foot down away from the midline toward the initial position!"
6. Now perform the same and speak the commands as you perform.

Diagonal (D_2) Flexion and Extension Pattern with Knee Straight

Motion Components

Same as D_2 Flexion and Extension.

Position of the Patient: Standing.

Position of the Therapist: Standing in front of the patient.

Commands are given as follows:

1. Ready (Place your limb backward across the midline, point the toes down).
2. "Turn the heel out! Point the toes up and out!"
3. Take the foot up and away from midline.
4. Turn the heel in and point the toes down and in.
5. Take the foot down, across the midline.

Repeat the same pattern and speak the commands as you perform.

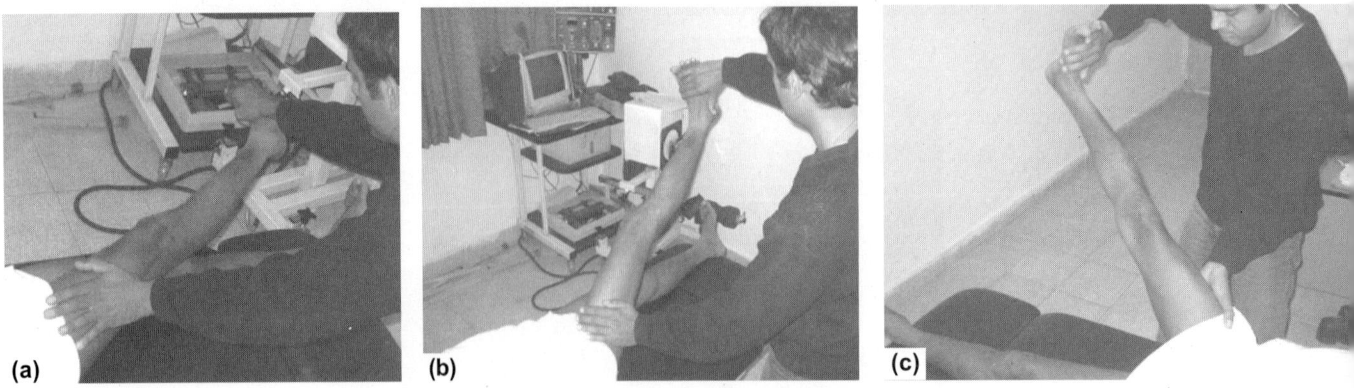

Figs. 14.11a to c: D_2 flexion pattern

HEAD AND NECK

FLEXION WITH ROTATION TO THE RIGHT

Free Active Pattern

Motion Components

- Rotation of head (atlanto-occipital joint) to the right.
- Rotation of cervical spine to right.
- Flexion of the cervical spine to the right.

Position of the Patient: High sitting.

Position of the Therapist: Sitting in front of patient.

Commands are given as under:

- *Preparatory commands* are given to make the patient understand as follows—You are going to turn your head to the right then you have to pull it down to touch the right chest with your chin.
- *Action commands*—"Turn your head!", "Pull your chin down!" and "Pull your head down!"

Repeat the same pattern and speak the commands as you perform.

Facilitation and Reinforcement

Position the patient in supine lying, take the head and neck out of plinth. Therapist stands at the head of patient, grasps the occiput by one hand and chin by other hand. Place all the components in extreme lengthened position.

Commands are given as under:

- *Preparatory command*—You are going to turn your head to the right then you have to pull it down to touch the right chest with your chin.
- *Action commands*—Now "Turn your head!", "Pull your chin down!" and "Pull your head down!"

Therapist resists all the strong components while assists the weak components through their optimal range of motion in accordance with normal timing.

EXTENSION WITH ROTATION TO THE LEFT

Free Active Pattern

Motion Components

- Rotation of the head to the left.
- Rotation of the neck to the left.
- Extension of the neck.

Starting Position: Place all the motion component in extreme lengthened state.

Commands:

- *Preparatory commands*—You are going to turn your head to the left then you have to lift your chin up across the midline.
- *Action commands*—Now "Turn your head to the left!", "Lift your chin up!", "Push your head back".

Repeat the same pattern and speak the commands as you perform.

Facilitation and Reinforcement

Position of patient is supine lying, therapist stands above the head at the edge of treatment table. Therapist grasps the occiput by left hand and chin by the right hand.

Place all the motion components in the extreme lengthened state.

Commands:

- *Preparatory command*—You are going to turn your head to the left then you have to lift your chin up across the midline.
- *Action commands*—Now "Turn your head to the left!", "Lift your chin up!" and "Push your head back!"

Therapist resists the stronger components of neck extension but assists weaker component throughout their optimal range of motion in accordance with normal timing.

UPPER TRUNK

FLEXION WITH ROTATION TO THE RIGHT

Free Active Pattern

Motion Components

- Rotation of the head to the right.
- Flexion with rotation of the cervical spine to the right.
- Flexion with rotation of the thoracic spine to the right.

Position of Patient: Supine lying, the right upper extremity is placed at the initial position of D_1 Extension pattern, while left hand holds the right wrist.

Position of Therapist: Standing at the right side of the patient.

Commands:

- *Preparatory Command*—You are going to turn your head to the right and then you have to pull yourself up and over toward your right hip joint.
- *Action Command*—Now "Pull yourself up!", "Turn toward right!", "Pull your chin down!", "Pull your head down!" and "Pull your arms toward your right hip!"

Repeat the same pattern and speak the commands as you perform.

Facilitation and Reinforcement

Position of Patient and Therapist remains same as free active motion.

Action Command: "Pull yourself up!", "Turn toward right!", "Pull your chin down!", "Pull your head down!" and "Pull your arms toward your right hip joint!"

The therapist resists all the strong component but assists the weak distal components through their optimal range of motion in accordance with normal timing.

EXTENSION WITH ROTATION TO THE LEFT

Facilitation and Reinforcement

Motion Components

- Rotation of head to the left.
- Extension with rotation of cervical spine to the left.
- Extension with rotation of the thoracic spine to the left.

Position of Patient: Supine. The left hand is placed at the right hip joint and right hand grasps it at the wrist joint.

Position of Therapist: Stands at the left side of the patient, places right hand over the occiput while left hand is used to grasp the patient's left hand.

Commands:

- *Preparatory command*—You are going to turn your head up, then pull your arm up away from the midline toward the left shoulder.
- *Action command*—"Push my hands up!", "Turn toward left", "Pull your arm toward left across the away from the midline!" and "Straighten your back!"

The therapist resists all the strong components but assists the weak components through their optimal range of motion accordance with normal timing.

15

MAT ACTIVITIES

INTRODUCTION

A normal individual performs activities such as rolling, getting up from lying position etc. independently day-to-day life usually in the bed or floor. But a person with physical impairment finds difficult to do so. Therapist teaches methods and techniques to carry out such activities independently usually on mat as it provide large base of support (BOS) and low center of gravity (COG), hence known as mat activities. These activities are also prerequisite for independent ambulation.

Exercise mat is a good surface firmer than most beds, making it an easier surface to learn mat activities. At the same time, a mat should be soft enough to allow the inevitable tumbles without injury.

COMMON MAT ACTIVITIES

These activities are:

i. Rolling.

ii. Prone on elbows.

iii. Prone on hands position.

iv. Hook lying.

v. Bridging.

vi. Quadruped position.

vii. Sitting: a. Long.
b. Short.

viii. Kneeling.

ix. Half kneeling.

Rolling

It is roll over from supine to side lying/prone or from prone to side lying/supine.

Rolling generally progresses from log rolling to segmental rolling. Log rolling produces movement of the entire trunk as a unit around the longitudinal axis of the body. Segmental rolling is a progression from log rolling. In segmental rolling either the upper or the lower segment of the trunk moves independently while the other is stabilized.

Techniques to facilitate rolling are:

a. Flexion of the head and neck with rotation may be used to assist movement from supine to prone positions.

b. Extension of the head and neck with rotation may be used to assist movement from prone to supine positions.

c. Both the hands are clasped, elbow fully extended and shoulder flexed upto 100–110°. Patient creates momentum by swinging the extremities from side to side (Fig. 15.1).

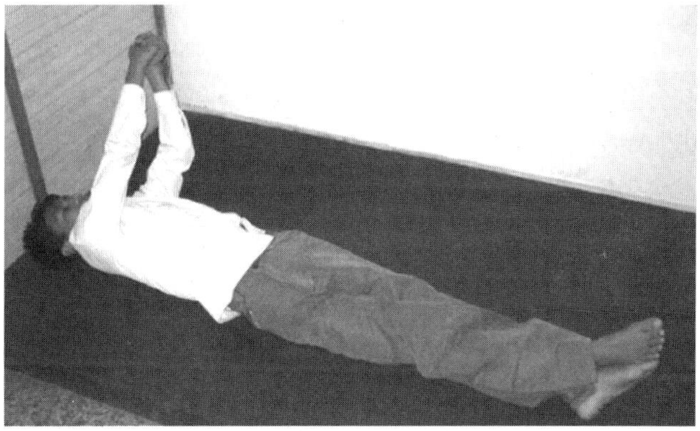

Fig. 15.1: Rolling

d. Crossing the legs one over the other also facilitates in rolling. The upper leg is towards the direction of rolling. For e.g., if a patient wants to roll towards the right side, the left leg should over the right one.

e. PNF patterns such as U/E – D_1 flexion and D_2 extension and L/E – D_1 flexion can also be used to facilitate rolling.

Prone on Elbows

This position provides weight bearing on elbows and

forearm. The posture provides stability of glenohumeral joint co-contraction of scapular musculature, and improving head and neck control (Fig. 15.2).

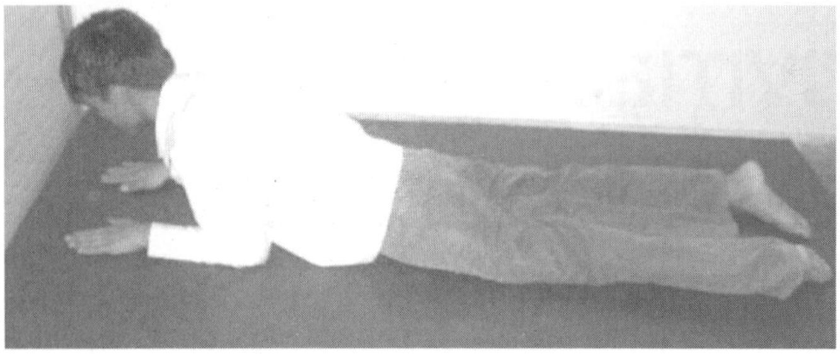

Fig. 15.2: Prone on elbows

Prone on elbows should cautiously be used in patients with:

- Cardiac or respirating problems.
- Shoulder or elbow pathology.
- Marked hip flexor tightness and contracture.
- Excessive lordosis of lumbar spine.

The position should progress in the following manner:

a. Initially patient should try to assume and maintain the position for few to several minutes with or without assistance. During this time activities such as reading, watching TV can be incorporated.
b. Patient should then try to maintain the position independently.
c. Weight shift in lateral directions should then be started which may progress to difficult anterior posterior directions also.
d. Activities such as peg lifting, writing, page turning (during reading), ball squeezing etc. can be used (contact guarding and verbal cues are given wherever necessary).

Prone on Hands

This is the intermediate position between the prone on elbows and quadruped positions. From prone on elbows position, patient fully extends his elbows. In this position BOS reduces and COG becomes more higher. The weight is born on hands, wrists, elbows and shoulders (Fig. 15.3).

Precautions for this position is same as for prone on elbows.

Progression takes place in the following manner:

a. Initially patient should try to assume and maintain the position for few to several minutes with/without assistance.

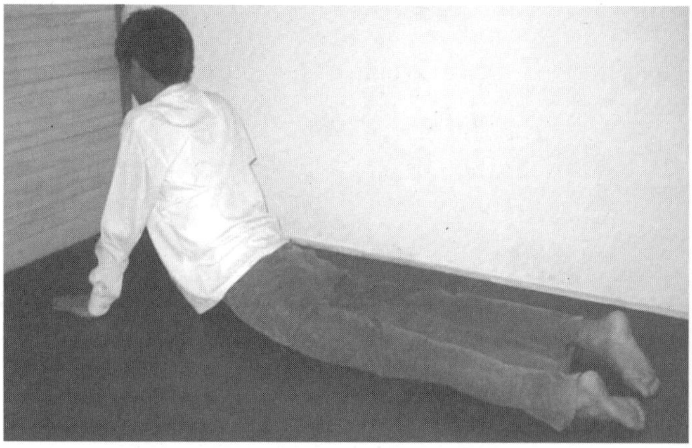

Fig. 15.3: Prone on hands

b. Patient should then try to maintain the position independently.
c. Weight shift in lateral directions should then be incorporated.
d. Final step is performed in the form of push ups in prone position which is also helpful in increasing strength of triceps, brachii and pectoralis major.

Clinical Implications of Prone on Elbows and Prone on Hands Position

Both of these positions are carried over to do floor–to stand transitions by paraplegic patients.

Hook Lying

The patient is in supine position with hips and knees flexed and feet flat on the floor or mat surface. In this position BOS is large and COG is lower than earlier two positions. Patient performs lower trunk rotation by swinging the lower extremity side to side (Fig. 15.4).

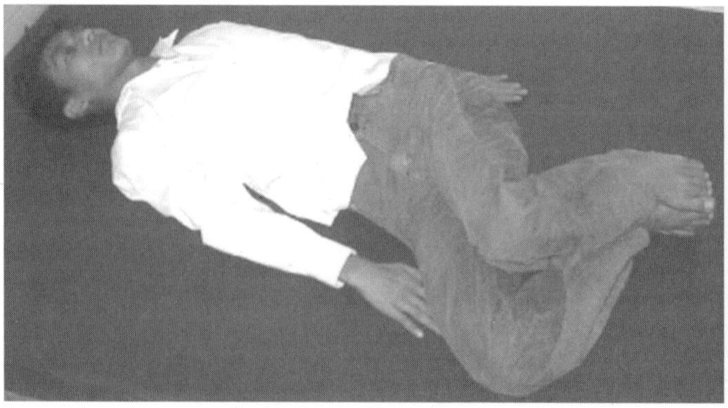

Fig. 15.4: Hook lying

Contanet guarding and verbal cues may be used and gradually weaned off as the progression takes place.

Gradual resistance for lower extremity movement and decrease knee and hip flexion may also be used to increase the level of activity.

Bridging

The patient is in hook lying position, elevates his pelvis off the mat surface. In this position BOS reduces and COG becomes higher (Fig. 15.5).

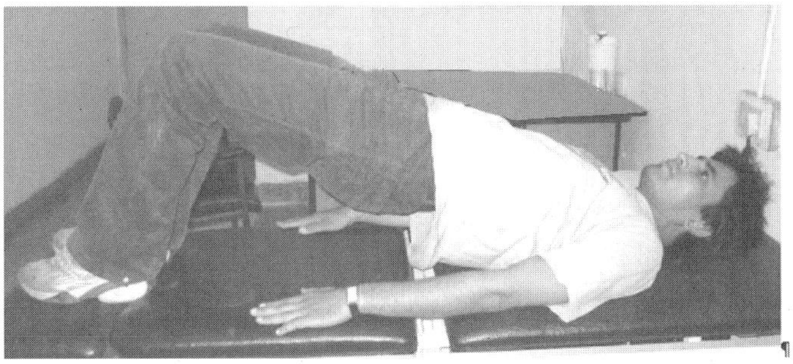

Fig. 15.5: Bridging

Progression of the activity takes place in following sequence:

a. Initially patient assumes and maintains position with or without assistance.
b. Independent maintenance of the position.
c. Elevation of the pelvis off the mat then again depressing it on the mat, is performed several times.
d. Resistance can be given on the anterior superior iliac spine.
e. Decrease the angle of hip and knee flexion.

Clinical Implications of Bridging

- Improves pelvic mobility.
- Strengthens low back and hip extensors.
- Helpful for using bed pan.
- Relieves pressure.
- Lower body dressing (Manual contact and verbal cues are provided as per need).

Quadruped

In this position the patient bears weight on all four limbs (Fig. 15.6).

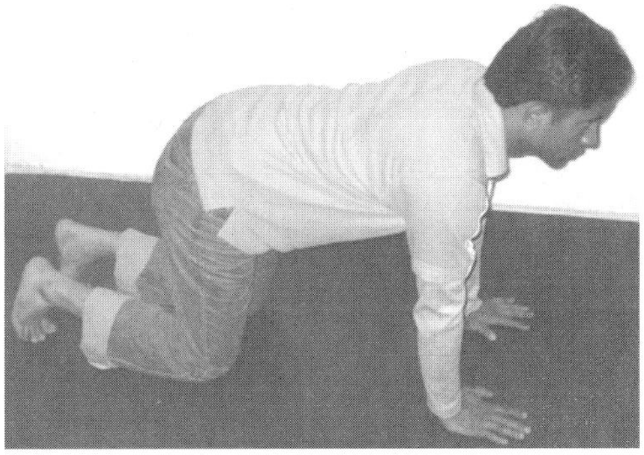

Fig. 15.6: Quadruped

The BOS is smaller the COG is higher than the bridging position.

Patient usually goes in quadruped position from prone on elbows or prone on hands position.

Progression of the activity takes place in the following sequence:

a. Initially patient assumes and maintains the position with assistance for few minutes.
b. Patient should then try to maintain the position independently for several minutes.
c. Weight shifts in forward, backward and side to side direction can be incorporated.
d. Raising of one of upper limb and bearing weight on rest of the 3 limbs.
e. Raising of one of upper limb and contralateral lower limb.

Increase the time gradually for d and e.

Clinical Implications

- Patient weight bearing on lower extremity joints (step towards weight bearing in erect positions).
- Strength and mobility required for so many functional activities by upper extremities.

Functional activities such as cleaning floor, gardening (planting seeds and weeding) can be used to teach static and dynamic stability of quadruped position.

When balance and stability have been achieved in quadruped, crawling may be started. This activity facilitates the co-ordination of the whole body including reciprocal movement of the arms and legs as require in walking.

Sitting

Sitting is the position which requires and facilitates trunk control and balance. It also allows some amount of weight to be borne by upper extremity. There are two forms of sitting needed to be practiced.

a. Long sitting.
b. Short sitting.

Long Sitting

Patient sits with knees fully extended; hips flexed hands may or may not support the upper body weight (hands may be positioned laterally, posteriorly or anteriorly with relation to pelvis) (Fig. 15.7).

Short Sitting

Patient sits on high surface (bed, chair etc) with knees at

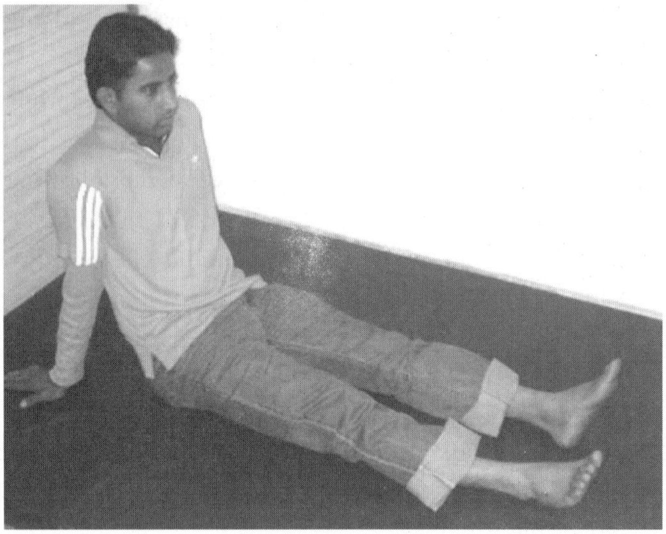

Fig. 15.7: Long sitting

the edge making hip and knees 90° flexed and feet flat on the floor surface. BOS is smaller than long sitting.

Progression of the both positions may take place in following sequence (patient usually progresses from long sitting to short sitting).

a. Initially patient assumes and maintains position with support.
b. Patient raises one hand placing the weight on other one. He repeats the movement with other hand.
c. Patient sits independently without any external or hand support.
d. Patient performs activities such as ball throwing (light to heavy weight), clapping overhead etc.
e. Push ups in both type of sittings should be performed with or without push up blocks. Increase the number of repetitions gradually.

Kneeling

Patient comes into kneeling position (hips extended and knees flexed at 90°) from quadruped position and bears weight on both the joints. This position also improves trunk pelvis control and upright balance. The BOS is smaller and COG is higher as compared to sitting (Fig. 15.8).

Progression may take place in following manner:

a. Initially patient assumes and maintains position with assistance for few seconds.
b. Patient assumes and maintains position independently for few minutes.
c. Patient shifts weight from one to other knee.
d. Ball throwing and other activities should be performed.

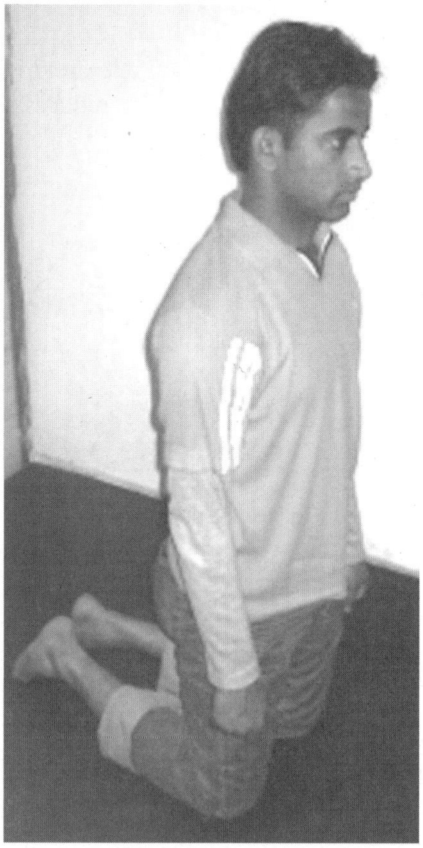

Fig. 15.8: Kneeling

e. Kneel walking would be the final progression for the kneeling position (Fig. 15.9).

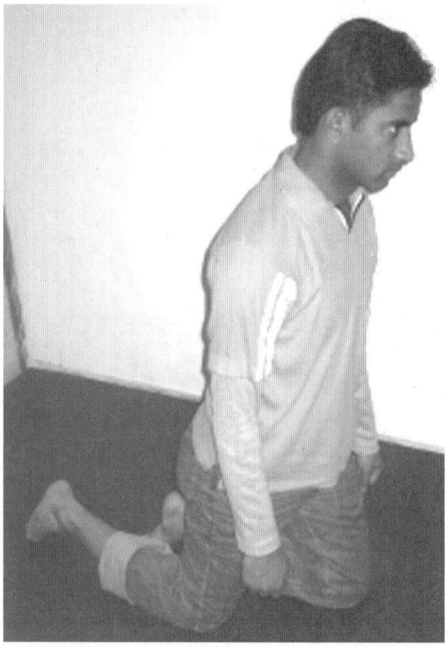

Fig. 15.9: Kneel walking

Half Kneeling

Patient assumes the position as shown in Figure 15.10. The BOS is larger than kneeling while COG is same. The

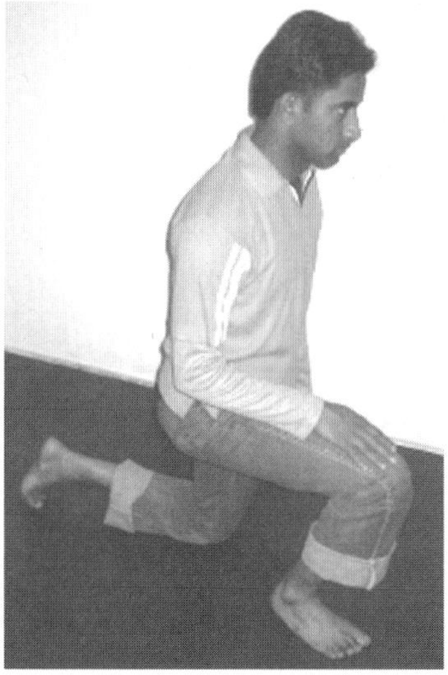

Fig. 15.10: Half kneeling

limb which lies posteriorly bears more weight. This position improves pelvic control (lateral), hip extension and ankle and knee movement.

Progression takes place in the following manner:

a. Initially patient assumes and maintains position with support.
b. Patient then tries to maintain position without support and for longer period of time.
c. Weight shift from one limb to other and even anteriorly and posteriorly.
d. Upper limb activities such as ball throwing (light to heavy weight) peg lifting and clapping etc.

(**Note:** Contact guarding/manual support is given wherever necessary in all the positions or activities).

16

GROUP EXERCISES

INTRODUCTION

Group life has always played an important role in civilization and throughout history, people have considered groups to be essential to survival. We are borne into family group and later expand our social network to include work groups, social groups, recreational groups and the like. Through groups, we avoid isolation and learn about ourselves and other people.

A group is an aggregate of people who shares a common purpose which can be attained by group members interacting and working together. In group exercise the patient gets a measure of individual attention and at the same time learns to take some responsibility for his own effort while working with others. A group for exercise usually comprises 6–8 patients having same type of disability and would benefit from exercises which are similar in character. There is also consideration for modification of exercise in terms of repetition, range, speed etc. to suit the need of every member of the group.

All group members perform the exercises together and get supervised by the therapist for any change and modification in the performance.

Rationale for Doing Exercises in Group

1. The patient gets stimulation from other members of the group to perform the exercise in a more better way.
2. The patient does not feel isolated and depressed which is very common due to disability.
3. The patient tries to compete with other group members and achieves the goal earlier as compared to his performance in isolation.
4. When performed in isolation the patient gets frustrated and stops exercises before prescribed period of time as he observes no or little improvement but in group exercises he observes other's improvement and tries to achieve for himself.
5. The therapist saves time and many patients can be treated simultaneously. It is very practical for the setting where therapist to patient ratio is more.
6. The patient develops in himself a sense of responsibility which further helps in home exercise program.
7. The patient leaves to improve interpersonal relationship which is usually affected after disability.

Disadvantages of Group Exercises

Group exercises might not always be successful due to:

- Improper selection of patients.
- More or uncontrolled number of group members.
- Poor explanation of the instruction etc.

Formation of Group:

- Space and other requirements.
- Selection of patients.
- Number of patients.
- Instruction to patients.
- Group types and levels.
- *Space and other requirements:* Big space is an essential prerequisite for group exercises so that multiple number of patients can perform the exercises together at one place. A big hall with 6–8 plinths or beds and space for mat activities for 6–8 persons is more practical.

  Equipment such as dumbells, sand bags, therabands etc. should also be in multiple numbers.

  Instrumental music or music of other type which suits the rhythm of exercise is always preferred. All the walls of exercise room or hall should be provided with big mirrors to give visual feedback of patient's performance.

- *Selection of patients:* Patients should be selected as per the similarities between their impairments and also the therapeutic needs.

  Clinically patient who has undergone number of individual sessions and expected to do home exercise program, can be selected as a candidate for group exercises.

  If patient does not fit to any of the group its better to continue with the individual treatment.
- *Number of patients:* As already discussed an ideal choice is between 6–8 patients per group, if this number exceeds then it would be difficult for the therapist to explain the instructions properly and to supervise their performance. And if the number of patients are less than 6 then it would not give the effect of group and all the benefits of group may not be obtained.
- *Instructions to the patients:* Therapist should discuss the importance of group exercises. He should give clear instructions to all the group members together in group exercise room or hall. It would be better if therapist demonstrates the exercises to be performed. In some set up video films of the group exercises prior to start the session is also preferred. Written instructions or hand outs can also be used to impart clear understanding of the group exercises.
- *Group types and levels:* Different types of groups are formed on the basis of age, sex, type of impairment, body part involved; patients are assigned to the respective type of group.

  Levels of groups are formed on the basis of intensity and nature of exercises. As the patient progresses, his level may be changed accordingly.

17

BALANCE AND COORDINATION EXERCISE

BALANCE

INTRODUCTION

The most traditional definition of balance is the ability to maintain one's center of gravity over a base of support. But recent researches have changed this definition, emphasizing on various factors affecting balance.

Balance is now defined as the state of physical equilibrium (maintenance of one's center of gravity) achieved when vestibular, visual and somatosensory information which is integrated in the central nervous system.

Constraint in Maintenance of Balance

- Neuromuscular coordination deficits.
- Loss of sensory acuity.
- Musculoskeletal limitations.
- Sensory organization deficits.
- Fine motor control impairment.
- Inability to adapt motor responses.
- Feed forward or predictive deficits.
- Cognitive deficits.

Anatomical Lesions Leading to Balance Dysfunction

- Lesions of the motor cortex.
- Lesions of corticospinal tract.
- Lesions of sensory pathways including cerebellum.
- Lesions of vestibular system.
- Loss of compensatory pathways such as vision.

Diagnostic Conditions Manifested by Balance Dysfunction

- Stroke.
- Guillain-Barré syndrome.
- Multiple scelerosis.
- Peripheral lesions—receptors in the ear, vestibular nerve.
- Ataxia.
- Head injury etc.

Maintaining balance is a complex interaction of the neuromuscular and musculoskeletal systems. Difficulty in maintaining balance may result in apprehension about movement or fear of falling.

Motor or Movement Strategies

These are normal movement patterns used to counteract balance perturbation or disturbances.

i. *Ankle strategy* involves shifting the centre of gravity (CoG) forward and backward by activating muscles in a distal-to-proximal sequence. With forward sway, gastrocnemius is activated first, followed by hamstrings, then paraspinal muscles (Fig. 17.1). With backward sway, the anterior tibialis is activated first, followed by quadriceps, then abdominals.

   This strategy is most commonly used when disturbances are small within the base of support.

ii. *Hip strategy* involves shifts in the CoG by flexing or extending the hips. It has a proximal pattern of muscle activation. With forward sway, abdominals are activated first, followed by quadriceps (Fig. 17.2). With backward sway, paraspinal muscles are activated first followed by hamstrings.

   With sideward sway gluteus medius is primarily activated. This strategy is seen when a greater force challenges balance or when the support surface for the feet is small.

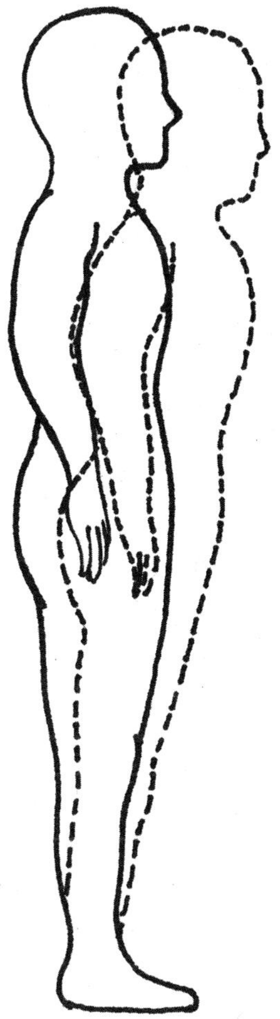

Fig. 17.1: Ankle strategy

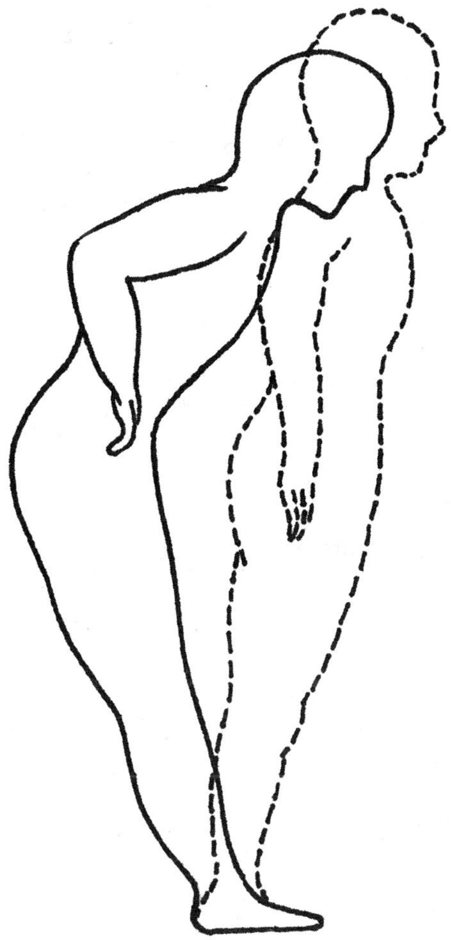

Fig. 17.2: Hip strategy

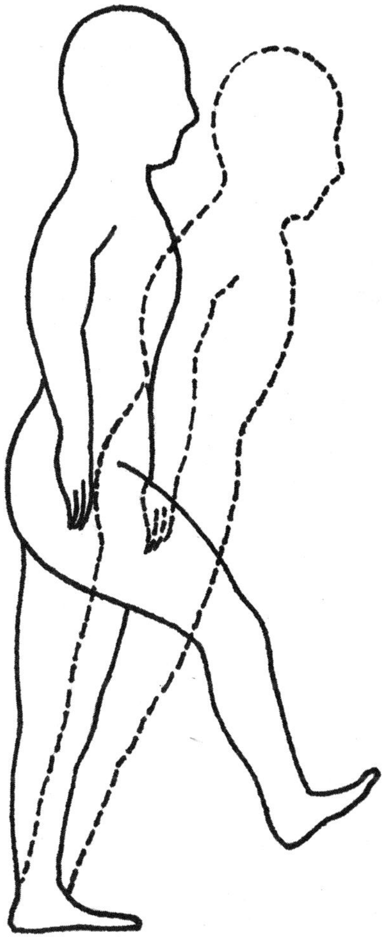

Fig. 17.3: Stepping strategy

iii. *Stepping strategy*—Realigning the base of support with a stepping movement. Stepping can be in forward backward or lateral direction (Fig. 17.3).

This strategy is used in response to fast and large balance disturbances.

iv. *Suspensory strategy*—Lowering the center of gravity towards the base of support, i.e., flexion of the hip, knee and ankle (Fig. 17.4).

This strategy is used during standing or in ambulation to lower the body center of gravity closer to the base of support, which provide more stability. For e.g., Cricketer uses this strategy while catching ball.

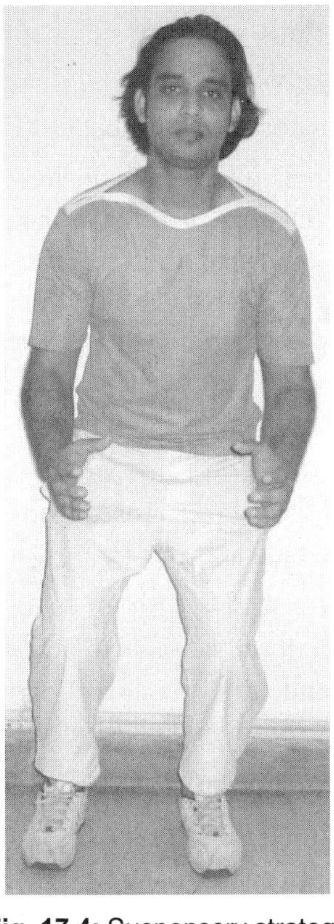

Fig. 17.4: Suspensory strategy

Evaluation for Balance Dysfunction

It is important to determine which component of balance is the cause of dysfunction. Evaluating the cause of balance dysfunction guides the therapist in development of treatment.

Points of Evaluation

- Patient's history.

- Association with head movement.
- Limitation of functional mobility.
- Falling tendency.
- Vertigo/nausea.
- Musculoskeletal system (ROM and Muscle strength).
- Sensory system:
  - Vestibular.
  - Visual and somatosensory (touch, proprioception, kinesthesia etc.).
- Motor/movement strategies
  - Present or normal.
  - Present but limited or delayed.
  - Present but inappropriate for the particular context or situation.
  - Abnormal
  - Absent.
- Function activity/position such as:
  - Rolling.
  - Supine-to-sitting.
  - Stable sitting.
  - Sit-to-stand (Fig. 17.5).
  - Transfers.
  - Ambulation.
  - Climbing stairs.

[*Romberg test (standing balance with eyes closed) suggests a somatosensory problem] (Fig. 17.6).

Hall pike test—The patient is in long sitting position on plinth and instructed to move into supine position. During this movement the therapist guides the head into extended and rotated (45°) off the end of the cervical spine. On reaching supine with the head extended and rotated, the therapist observes for the presence of nystagmus and asks how patient feels (Fig. 17.7).

Repeat the test again with other side of rotation. Complaints of vertigo, nausea and the presence of nystagmus are indication of vestibular dysfunction.

a. *Berg-balance scale*—This ordinal scale (0-4: 0—unable to perform, 4—able to perform the task safely and independently). Evaluates patient performance on 14 tasks commonly performed in day-to-day life.

   Items of the scale are:
   - Sitting to standing.
   - Standing unsupported.

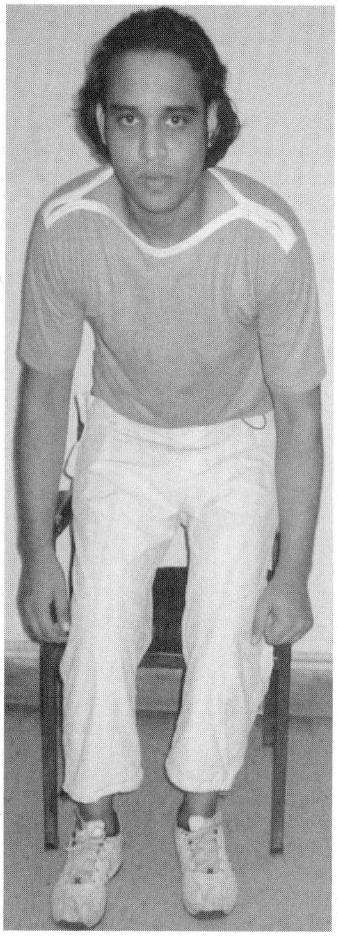

Fig. 17.5: Sit to stand

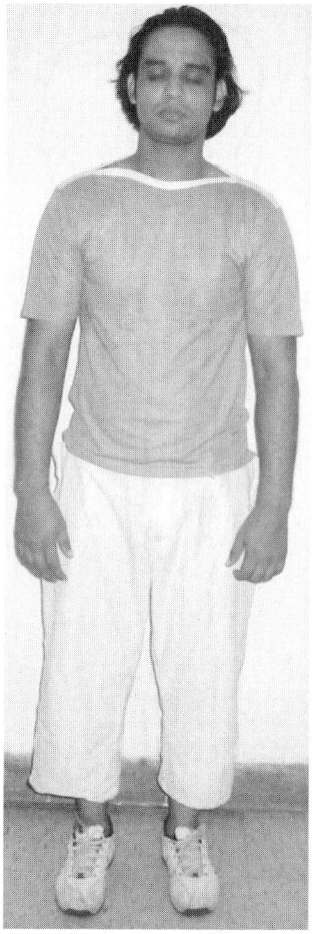

Fig. 17.6: Romberg's test

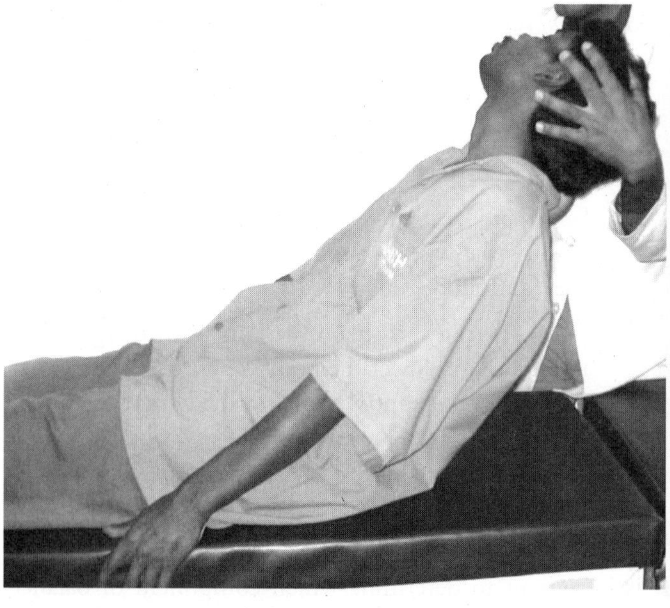

Fig. 17.7: Hall pike test

   - Sitting unsupported.
   - Standing to sitting.
   - Transferring.

- Standing with eyes closed.
- Standing with feet together (Fig. 17.8).
- Reaching forward without stretched arm.
- Retrieving object from floor (Fig. 17.9).
- Turning to look behind (Fig. 17.10).
- Turning 360°.
- Placing alternate foot on stool.
- Standing with one foot in front (Fig. 17.11).
- Standing on one foot (Fig. 17.12).

b. *Functional reach test*—This test uses a yardstick/ marked scale, mounted onto a wall at the height of patient acromion process. The patient stands barefoot in a normal, relaxed stance on footmark, beside the wall (where yardstick is mounted).

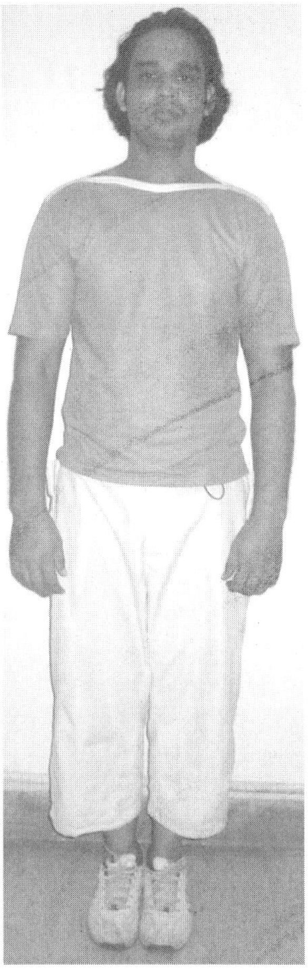

Fig. 17.8: Standing with feet together

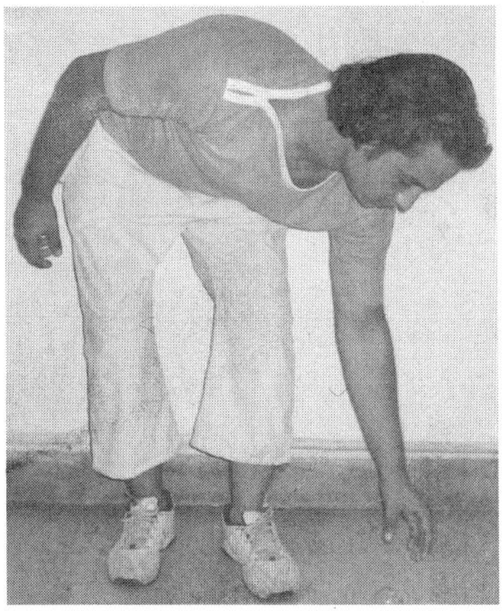

Fig. 17.9: Retrieving object from the floor

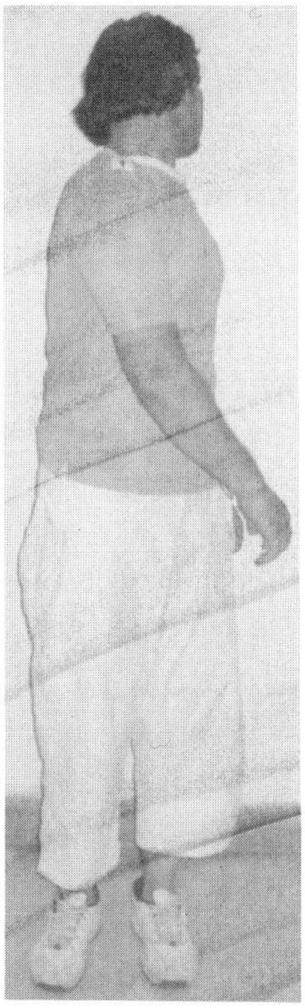

Fig. 17.10: Turning to look behind

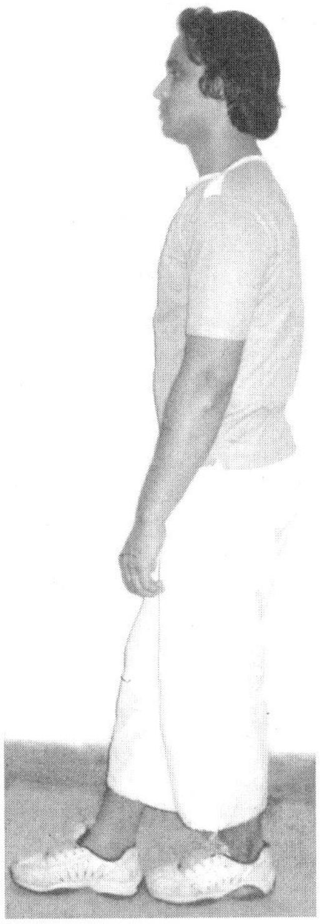

Fig. 17.11: Standing with one foot in front

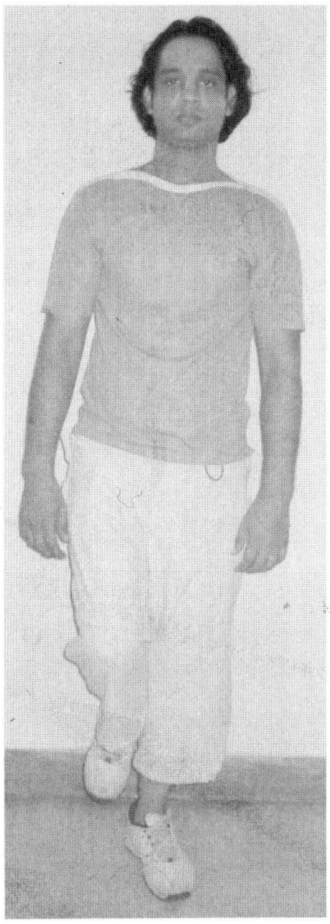

Fig. 17.12: Standing on one foot

The patient then extends one arm, with hand made into fist. Placement of the third metacarpal along the yardstick is recorded. The patient then reaches forward as far as possible without losing balance or take a step forward. Placement of the third metacarpal is again recorded (Figs. 17.13a and b).

(The upper extremity is not allowed to touch the wall during the procedure).

Functional reach = Final measurement – Initial measurement

Duncan *et al.* (1990) reported normal functional reach as per the age:

20-40 years old	:	16.73 inches (men)
		14.64 inches (women)
41-69 years old	:	14.98 inches (men)
		13.81 inches (women)
70-87 years old	:	13.16 inches (men)
		10.47 inches (women).

Balance Exercises

i. *Exercises for weakness*—The muscles which are responsible for postural instability, needs to be strong.

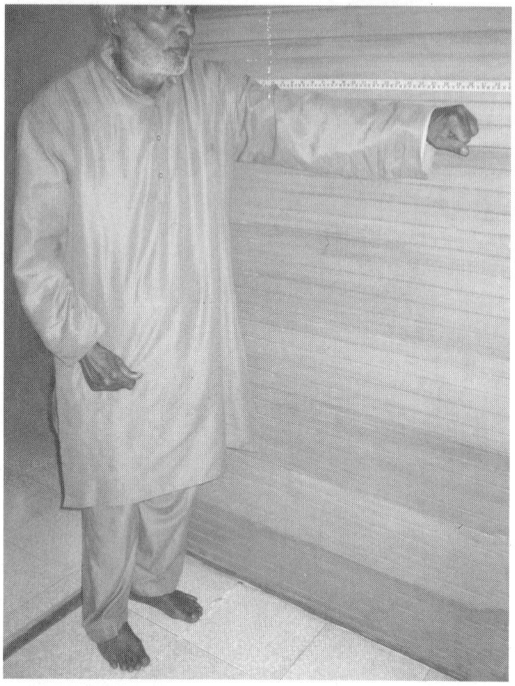

Fig. 17.13a: Functional reach test (initial position)

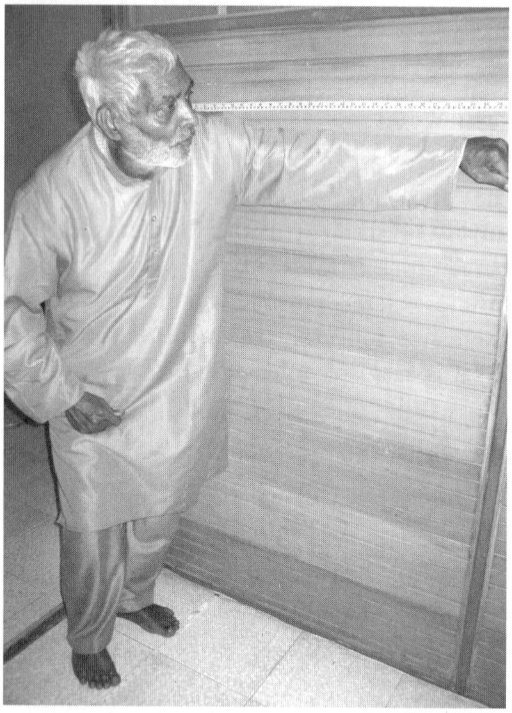

Fig. 17.13b: Functional reach test (final position)

This can be achieved by variety of therapeutic exercises. Such as:

- Active exercises.
- PNF (Proprioceptive neuromuscular facilitation).
- PRE (Progressive resistive exercise).
- Isokinetic etc.

ii. *Exercises for movement strategies*—If patient exhibits weakness or prior control in a particular strategy, he should practice positions which facilitate the activation of muscles require for that strategy.

For e.g., Patient having poor dorsiflexors finds difficulty in using ankle strategy for balance. He should practice following positions to facilitate the dorsiflexors.

a. Sitting on therapeutic ball with feet on the floor, ball is rolled posteriorly by the therapist, dorsiflexors get activated (equilibrium response) (Fig. 17.14).

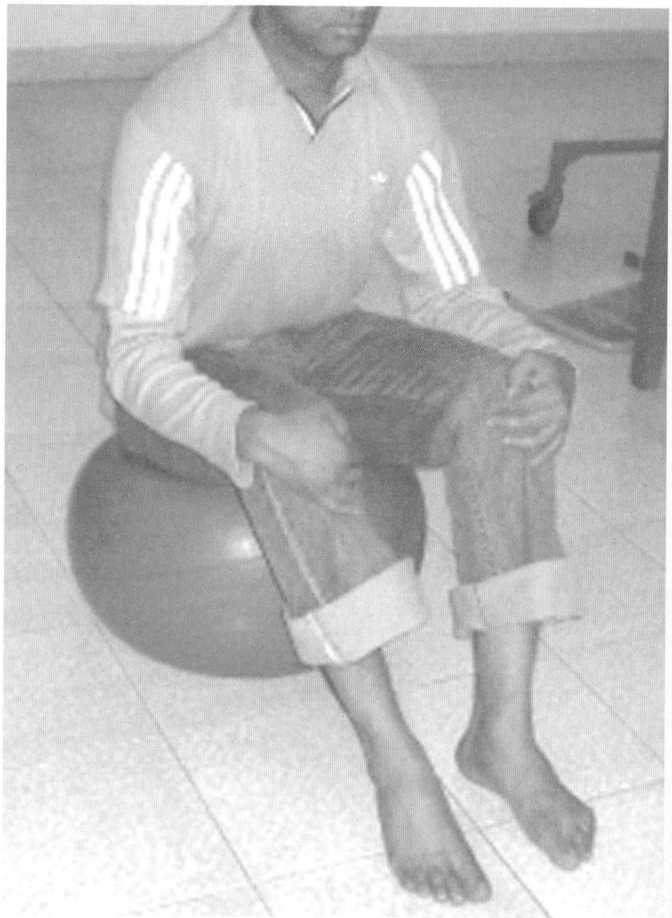

Fig. 17.14: Facilitation of ankle dorsiflexors on therapeutic ball

b. Standing in parallel bar or walker, patient practices leaning posteriorly with small range in starting and then gradually increasing the range. Same facilitation is achieved (Fig. 17.15).

iii. *Static balance exercises*—These are performed to improve control in sitting and standing positions.

Patient follows the following sequence for developing sitting or standing control (he may skip any step in which he has good control).

a. *Sitting:*

- Sitting with two hands support.

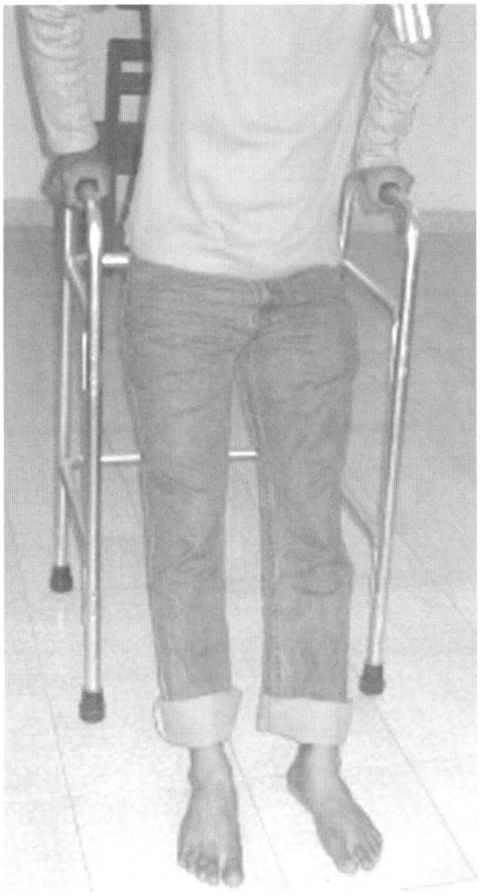

Fig. 17.15: Facilitation of ankle dorsiflexors with walker

- Sitting with one hand support.
- Sitting unsupported.
- Change the sitting surface (hard to soft) (Figs. 17.16a to c).

b. *Standing:*

- Standing in parallel bar with two hands support (Fig. 17.17a).
- Standing with one hand support (Fig. 17.17b).
- Standing unsupported (Fig. 17.17c).
- Change the base of support (wider to narrower).
- Tandem standing (one foot in front of other) (Fig. 17.17d).
- Standing on one leg (Fig. 17.17e).

iv. *Dynamic balance exercises*

- After achieving unsupported sitting, patient is asked to look up and down, and from side to side, which activate the vestibular system.
- Reaching activities on same side and then contralateral side both in sitting and standing position.
- Sitting to standing with both hands support then one hand and then without any support. Equal weight bearing on both lower extremity should be

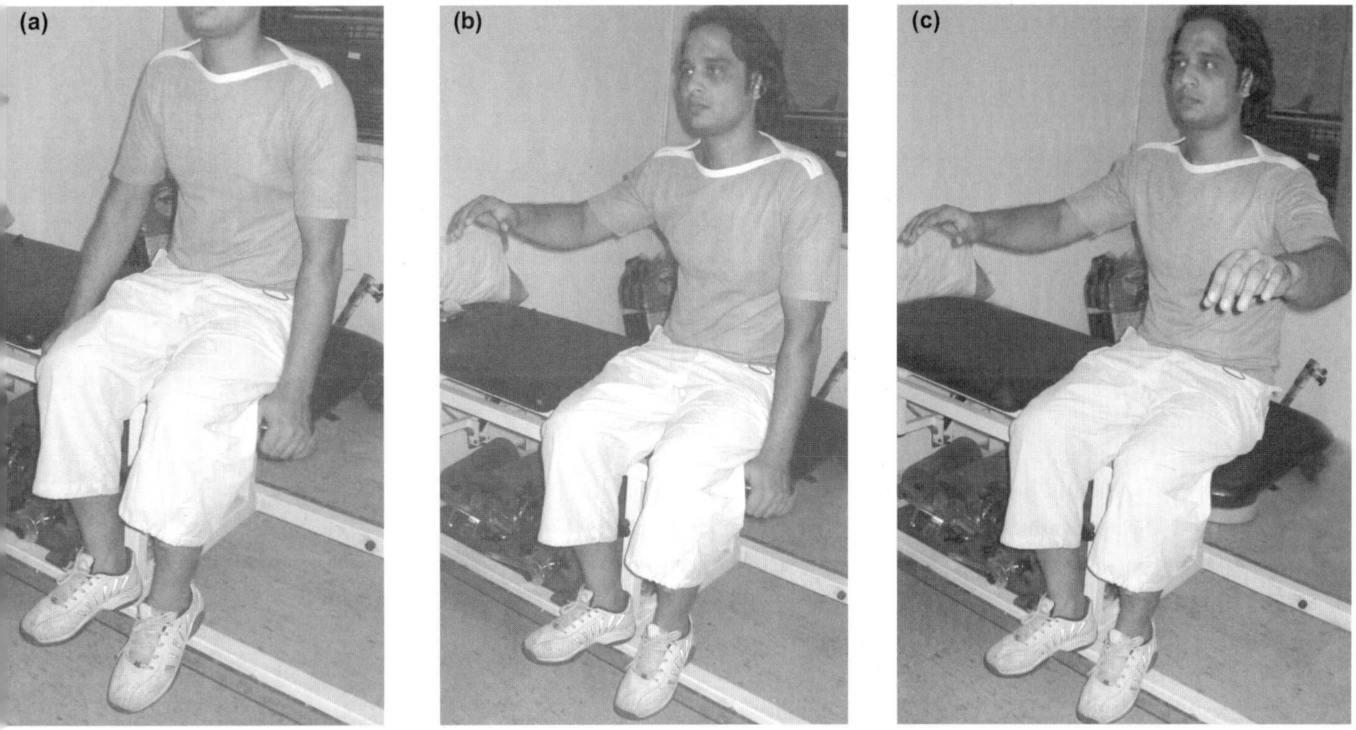

Figs. 17.16a to c: (a) Sitting with both hand support, (b) Sitting with one hand support, and (c) Sitting without hand support

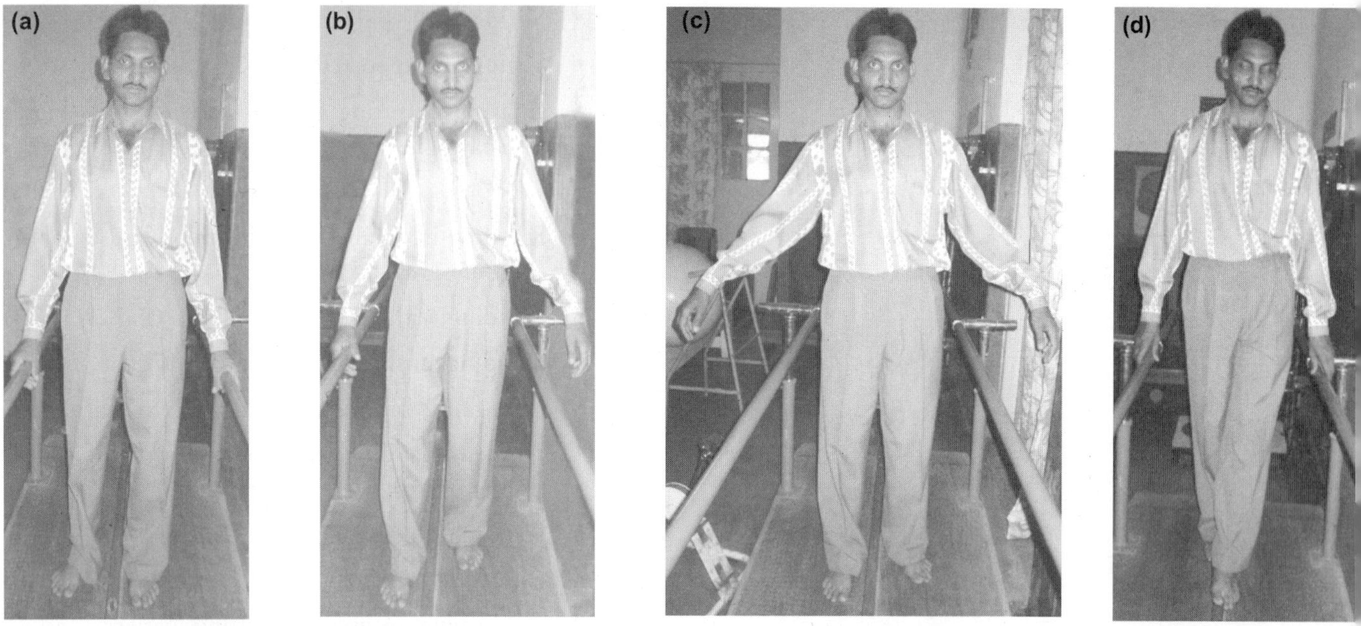

Figs. 17.17a to d: (a) Standing with both hand support, (b) Standing with one hand support, (c) Standing without hand support and (d) Tandem standing

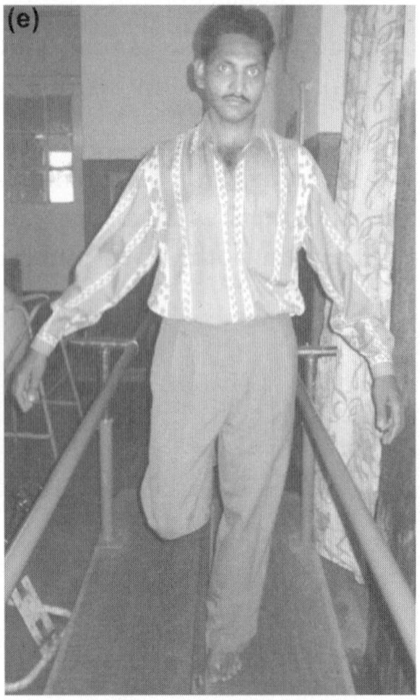

Figs. 17.17e: Standing on one leg

facilitated by visual and verbal feedback (Figs. 17.18a to c).

- Stepping forward and backward can be practised first in parallel bar with one or two hands then without parallel bar.
- Standing to supine on mat and then move back to standing. Same may be practised by going to prone position from standing. Each movement activates the vestibular system in addition to challenging the patient's dynamic balance (Figs. 17.19a to f).
- Trunk dynamic balance and strength can be achieved by throwing and catching (at head level, overhead

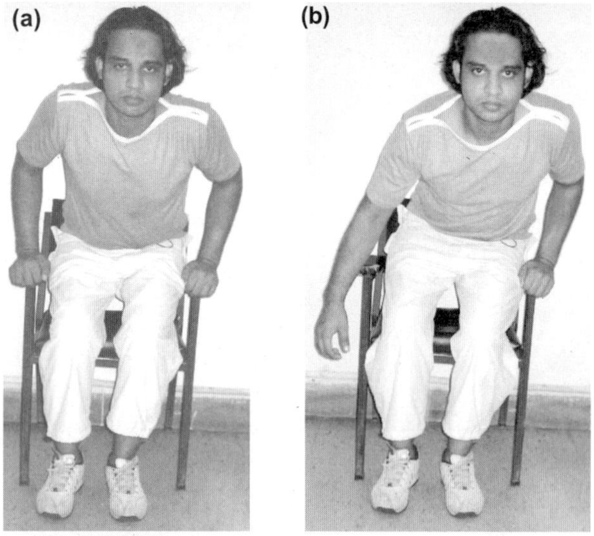

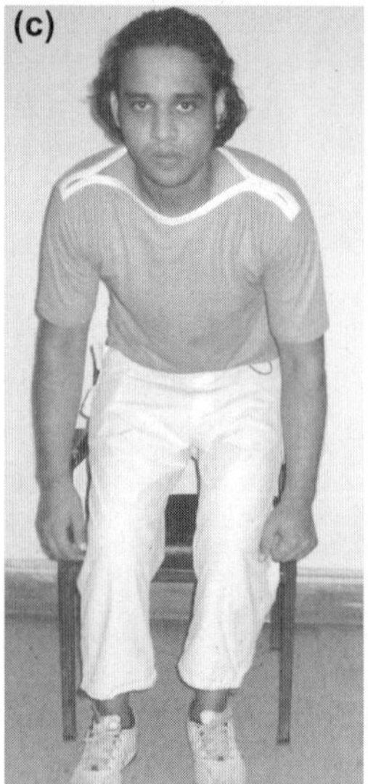

Figs. 17.18a to c: (a) Sit to stand with both hand support, (b) Sit to stand with one hand support and (c) Sit to stand without hand support

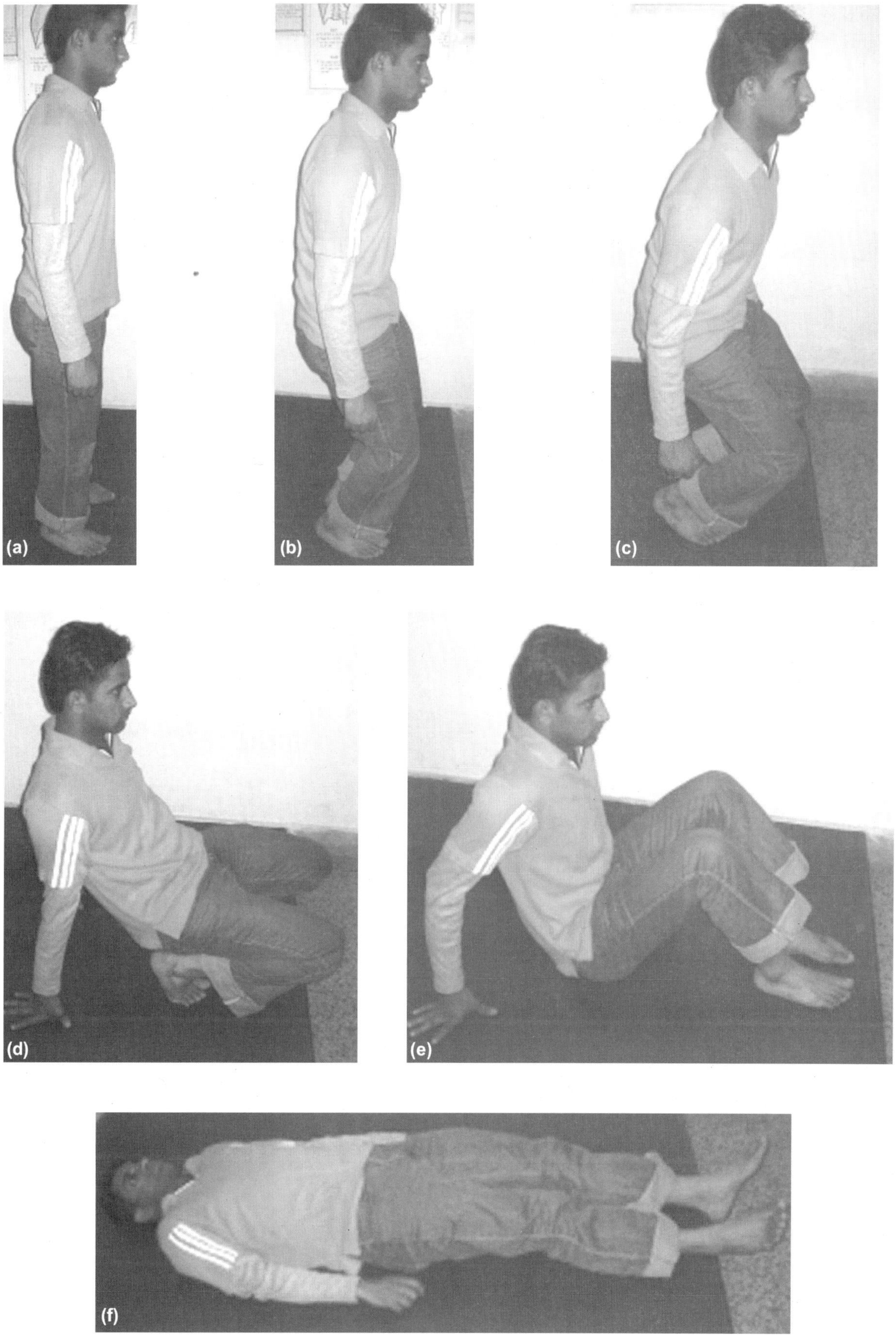

Figs. 17.19a to f: Standing to supine

and either side) by therapy balls of various sizes and weights in a variety of positions such as kneeling, half-kneeling, sitting and standing (Fig. 17.20).

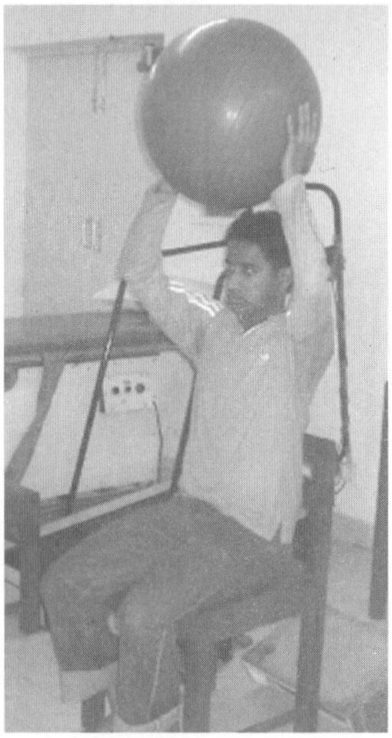

Fig. 17.20: Ball throwing in sitting position

- Gait activities should be practised in parallel bar then with assistive devices (walker → cane) and then without any device (Figs. 17.21a to d).

  Patient should practice:

  - Side stepping (Fig. 17.22a).
  - Walking forward.
  - Crossing legs (Fig. 17.22b).
  - Walking backward (Fig. 17.22c).
  - Walking on heels (Fig. 17.22d).
  - Walking on toes (Fig. 17.22e).

- Balancing on vestibular board or wobble board may be practised to facilitate weight-shift in backward/ forward and side to side direction (Fig. 17.23) (In

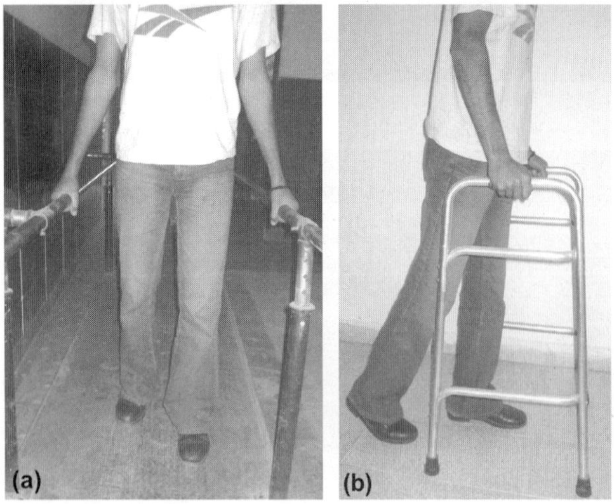

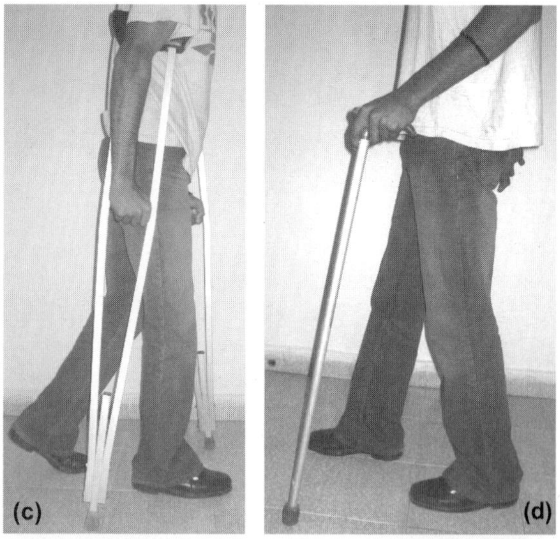

Figs. 17.21a to d: (a) Walking with parallel bar, (b) Walking with walker, (c) Walking with crutches, and (d) Walking with stick

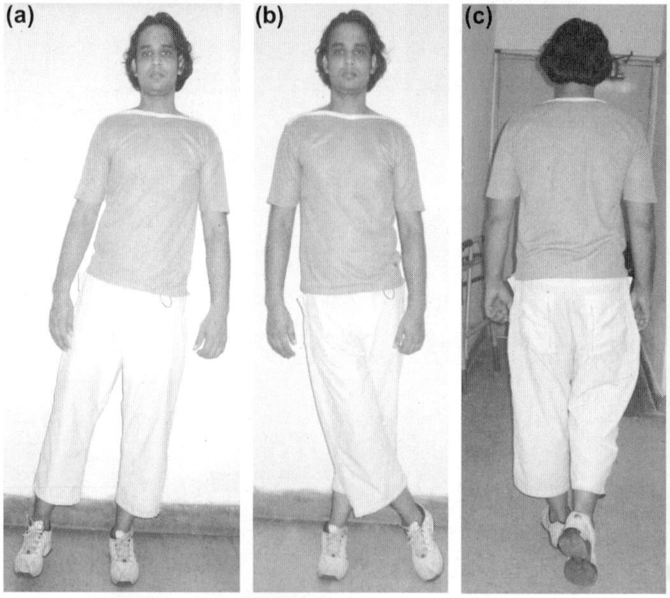

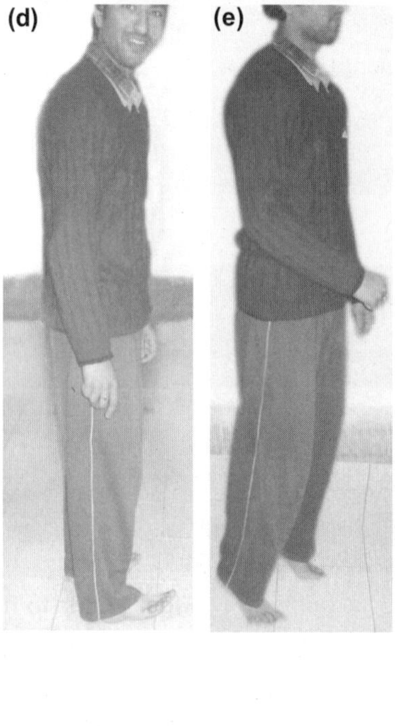

Figs. 17.22a to e: (a) Side stepping, (b) Crossing legs, (c) Backward walking, (d) Walking on heels and (e) Walking on toes

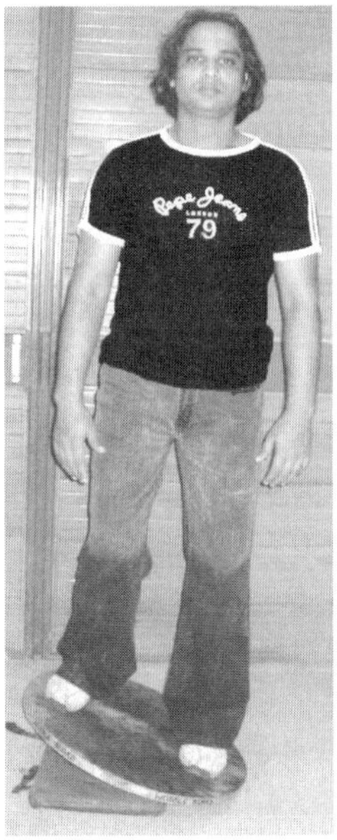

Fig. 17.23: Balancing on wobble board (side to side)

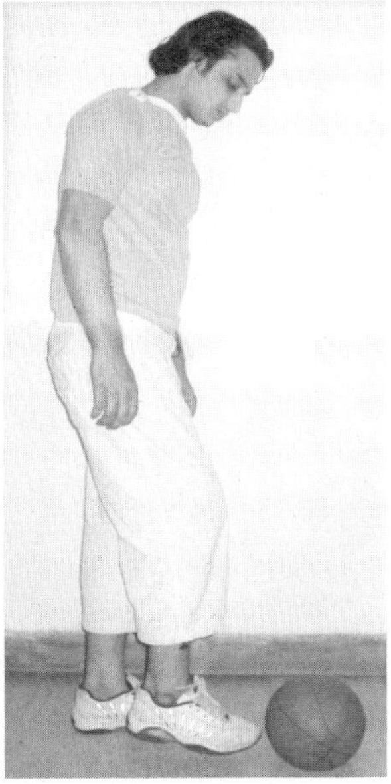

Fig. 17.24: Ball kicking

starting this activity may be performed between the parallel bars).

- Ball kicking activities should be incorporated to improve stability on one leg and dynamic movement with other leg (Fig. 17.24).
- Walking through obstacles (Fig. 17.25).
- Walking on different surfaces (hard to soft) (Fig. 17.26).
- Walking with various speeds (slow to fast).

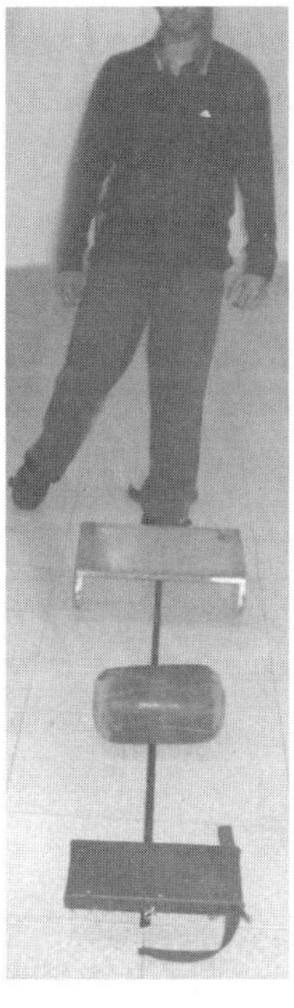

Fig. 17.25: Walking through obstacles

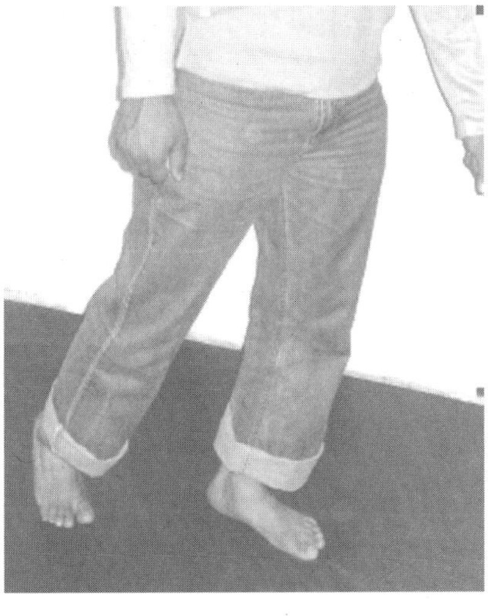

Fig. 17.26: Walking on soft surface

v. *Aerobic exercises*—Patient with balance dysfunction become deconditioned because of self imposed immobility arising from the fear of losing balance.

   Following aerobic exercise can be performed:

   - Static cycling (Fig. 17.27).
   - Upper extremity bicycle ergometer (Fig. 17.28).
   - Walking.
   - Jogging.
   - Rowing (Fig. 17.29).
   - Trampoline etc. (Fig. 17.30).

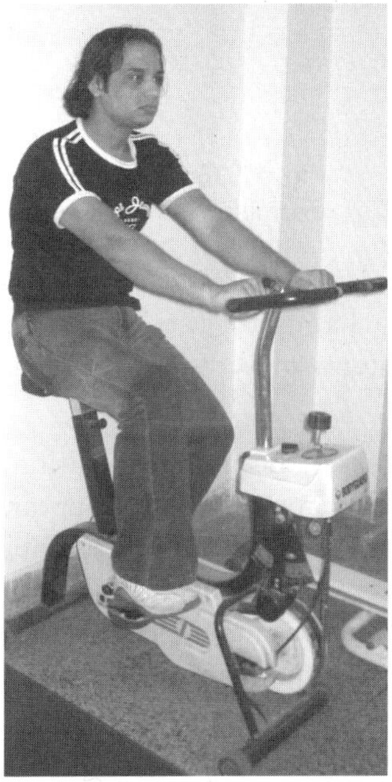

Fig. 17.27: Static cycle

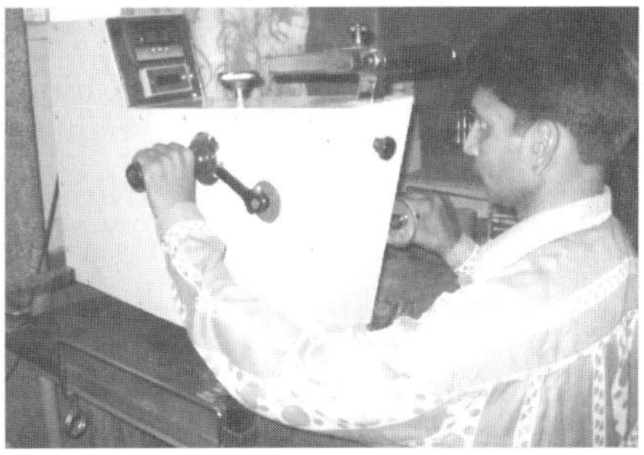

Fig. 17.28: Upper extremity bicycle ergometer

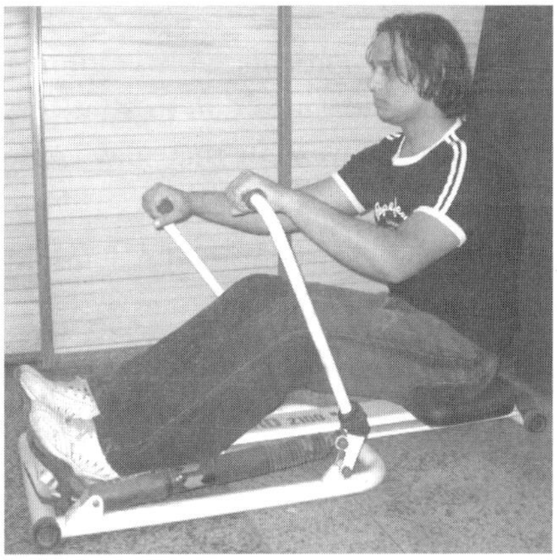

Fig. 17.29: Rowing

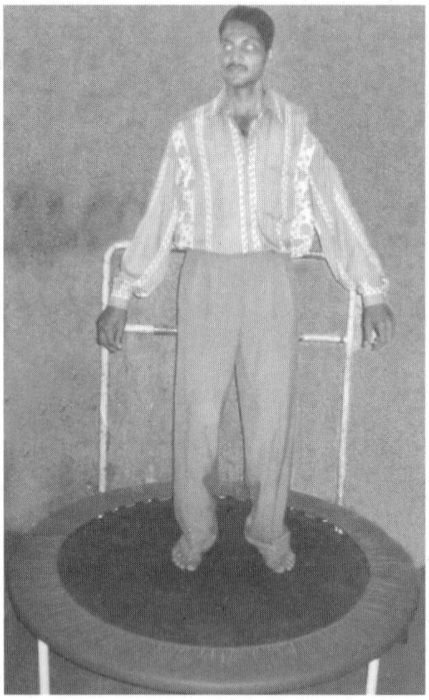

Fig. 17.30: Trampoline exercise

vi. *Balance exercises for vestibular dysfunction habituation exercises*—are those which habituate the patient in positions of eliciting symptoms of vertigo and nystagmus.

Patient is gradually brought to the desired position, with every change in position symptoms might reappear. Positions are maintained at every change until the symptoms disappear. As the symptoms are gone, the change towards the desired position is again made. Moving through the full range without symptoms is the ultimate goal of treatment. Patient may also be moved through the full range if they can tolerate the intensity of treatment.

During the first week, only two movements or positions that elicit symptoms should be addressed. Patient should perform movements and positioning activities 5 to 10 times and repeat them at atleast 3 times a day (Shumway-Cook and Horak 1990). Gradually, other movements and positions that elicit vertigo can be added, until all symptoms diminish and patient is free of vertigo.

Exercises for muscle imbalance—Patients with vestibular dysfunction develop muscle imbalance due to strategies to minimize head and trunk movement that may cause vertigo.

For e.g., Sternocleidomastoid, latissimus dorsi might become tight.

Exercises for vestibular-ocular reflex—The vestibular-ocular reflex may be impaired in patients with vestibular dysfunction. The following exercises may be used to increase vestibular-ocular reflex (Denham, 1996):

a. *Visual tracking exercise:* Instruct the patient to follow tip of pencil/pen moving in various directions with head still. Start with small displacement of the pen/pencil, gradually increase the range. First perform the exercise in sitting then in standing position (Figs. 17.31a and b). Further the exercise may be performed during walking ascending/descending stairs.

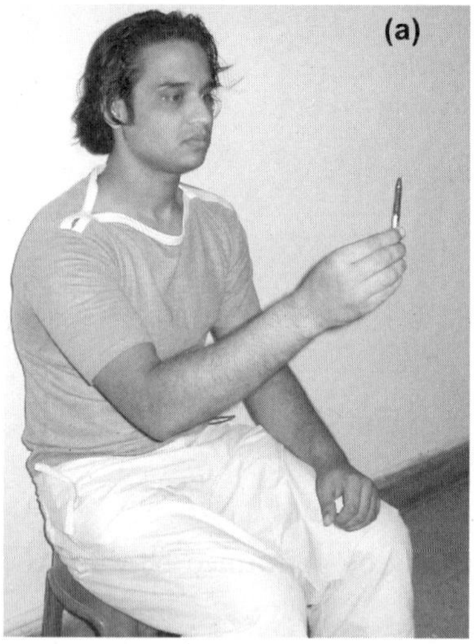

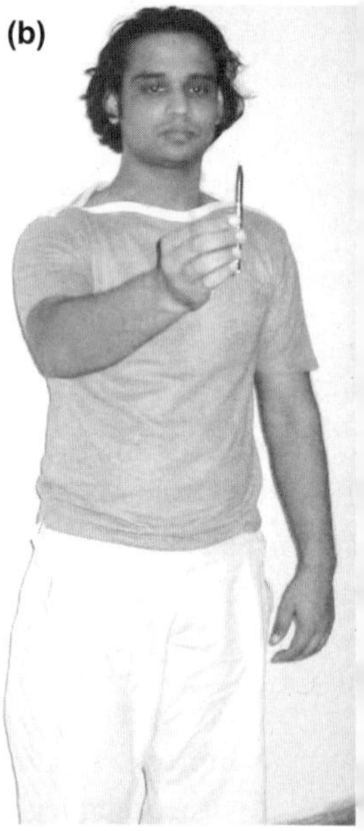

Figs. 17.31a and b: Visual tracking exercise (a) While sitting and (b) While standing

b. *In sitting position:* Eyes are fixed while the head is moved passively by the therapist. First perform slowly, then with increasing speed, progressing to active movement of head.

Once patient can perform actively, exercise may be performed during standing, walking, and walking while reading a magazine (Fig. 17.32).

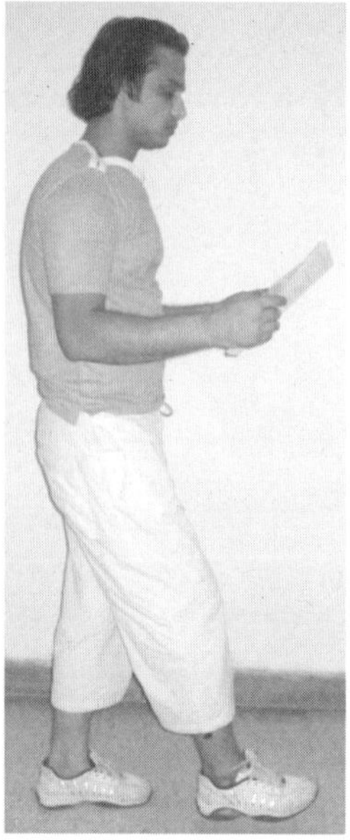

Fig. 17.32: Walking while reading magazine

vii. *Management for somatosensory loss:*

- Modification of external environment.
- Compensation by visual feedback.
- Standing and walking barefoot on different textured surfaces.
- Use of weighted belts, and back support in chairs to improve trunk alignment which is impaired because of somatosensory loss.
- Walking with weight tied on knee and ankle joints (Fig. 17.33).
- Overuse of visual compensation should be discouraged.

Exercises for balance dysfunction may be modified as per the stage of condition, pathology, capability, interest and age of patient.

Precautions must be taken while giving balance exercises. Patient should be provided appropriate support/guidance/supervision as per the need. Environment should be safe enough to prevent any injury from fall during therapy session. Verbal and visual feedback should always be used whenever necessary.

Balance control learnt should be incorporated in real life functional activities.

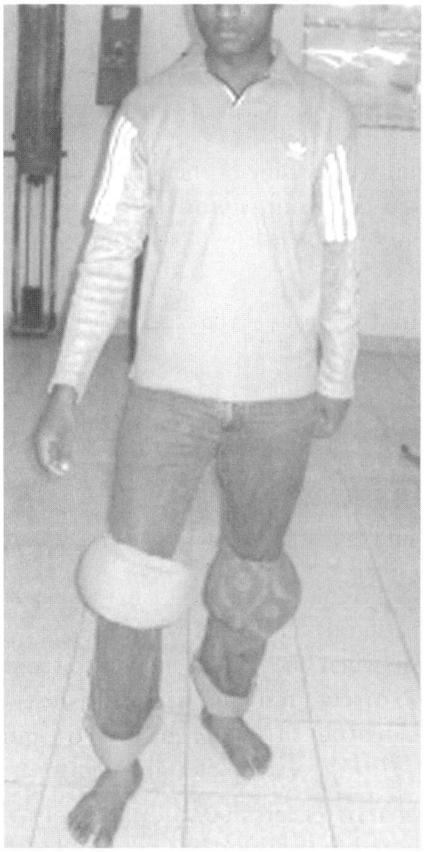

Fig. 17.33: Walking with weight tied on knee

COORDINATION

INTRODUCTION

Coordination is a measure of the quality of movement. It is the ability to carry out smooth, accurate and controlled motor responses which depends on intact neuromuscular system.

Coordinated movements are characterized by appropriate:

- Direction.
- Distance.
- Muscular tension.
- Speed; and
- Timing.

Coordination deficits occur when muscle fails to fire in sequence, or when the central nervous system (CNS) is unable to direct movement activities accurately. Coordinated movement require adequate strength and range of motion (ROM) to complete a particular task.

Incoordination occurs due to CNS lesions—Cerebellar, basal ganglia and dorsal (posterior column) lesion. The most common diagnostic conditions in which incoordination is seen are:

- Parkinsonism.
- Cerebellar ataxia.
- Huntington's disease.
- Sydenham's chorea.
- Vestibular dysfunction.
- Cerebral palsy.

Signs of Incoordination

A. *Due to Cerebellar Dysfunction*

i. *Asthenia*–Generalized muscle weakness.

ii. *Hypotonia*–Decreased in muscle tone. (Decreased in resistance to passive movement and muscle may feel abnormally, soft and flaccid).

iii. *Dysmetria* is an impaired ability to judge the distance or range of a movement (Figs. 17.34a and b):
   - Hypometria–underestimation.
   - Hypermetria–overestimation.

iv. *Dysdiadochokinesia* is an impaired ability to perform rapid alternating movements.

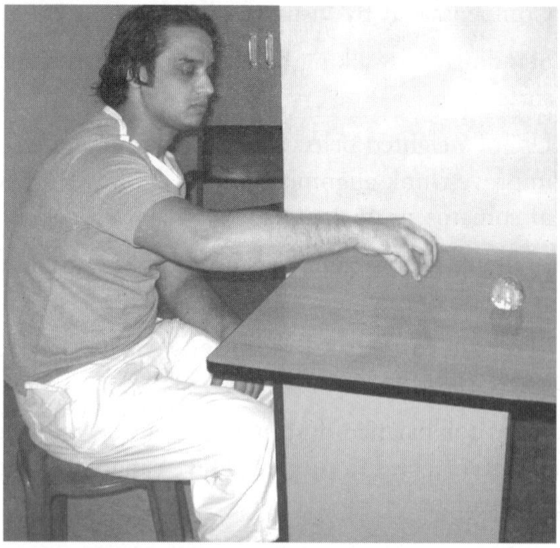

Fig. 17.34a: Dysmetria (hypometria)

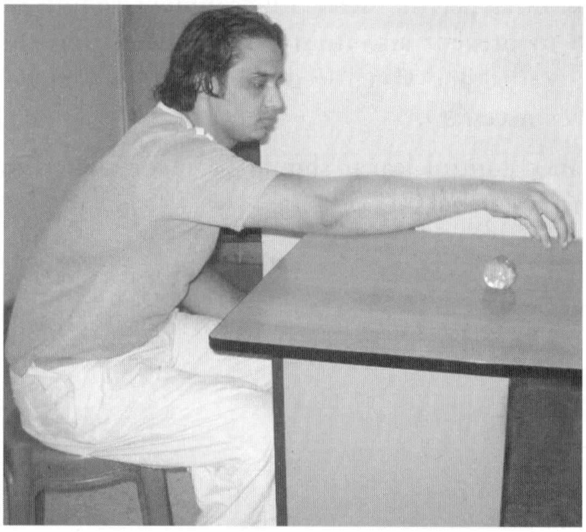

Fig. 17.34b: Dysmetria (hypermetria)

v. *Tremor*–An involuntary oscillatory movement resulting from alternate contractions of opposing muscle groups.

   Kinetic or intentional tremor—occurs during voluntary movement of extremity tends to increase at the end of the desired movement or when the speed increases.

   Postural or static tremor—observed (back-and-forth oscillatory movements) when an individual tries to maintain standing posture.

vi. *Dyssynergia* is the movement decomposition describes a movement performed in a sequence of component part rather than as a single, smooth activity.

vii. *Rebound Phenomenon of Holmes*–Normally, when application of resistance to an isometric contraction is suddenly removed the limb will remain in approximately the same position. This ability gets impaired in patients with cerebellar dysfunction.

viii. *Nystagmus*–Rhythmic oscillatory movements of the eyes.

ix. *Dysarthria*–Disorder of the motor component of speech articulation, characterized by slow, slurred, hesistant, inappropriate pauses and prolonged syllables.

x. *Gait disorder*–Wide base of support.

B. Due to Basal Ganglia Lesion

i. *Bradykinesia*–Slowness of movement manifested by decreased arm swing, slow shuffling gait, lack of facial expressions, difficulty in initiating or changing direction of movement or in stopping a movement once begun.

ii. *Rigidity* is an increase in muscle tone causing greater resistance to passive movement.

Lead pipe rigidity is a uniform constant resistance throughout the range of movement.

Cogwheel rigidity is characterized by 'give' and 'relaxation' and when the extremity is moved passively (combination of lead pipe tremor and tremor).

iii. *Resting tremor*–Tremors observed at rest especially in distal upper extremity in the form a 'pill-rolling' movement. These tremors disappear with movement.

iv. *Chorea*–Involuntary, rapid, irregular and jerky movements.

v. *Athetosis*–Slow, involuntary, writhing, twisting, "worm like" movements usually seen in distal part of upper extremity.

vi. *Dystonia*–Twisting, bizarre movement caused by involuntary contraction of the axial and proximal muscles of the extremities.

vii. *Hemiballismus*–Sudden, jerky, forceful wild, flailing motions of the arm and leg of one side of the body (seen in lesion of contralateral subthalamic nucleus).

C. Due to Dorsal (Posterior) Column Involvement

i. Lack of proprioceptive feedback.

ii. Positive Rhomberg's sign—Inability to stand with eyes closed (as visual compensation for proprioceptive loss is absent).

iii. Dysmetria.

iv. Gait disturbances–Walking with an audible sound by foot (to compensate for proprioceptive loss by auditory feedback).

Tests for Coordination

Presence of incoordination can be tested in standing or during walking (equilibrium) and sitting position (Non-equilibrium). All these tests would make clearly observable one or other signs of incoordination (discussed earlier).

Tests in Standing or During Walking

I. *Standing:*

a. In normal posture.

b. With feet together/narrow base of support (Fig. 17.35).

c. With one foot directly in front of the other (Fig. 17.36).

d. On one foot (Fig. 17.37).

e. Between forward trunk flexion and neutral position (Fig. 17.38).

f. Laterally flex trunk to each side (Fig. 17.39).

g. With eyes closed (Fig. 17.40).

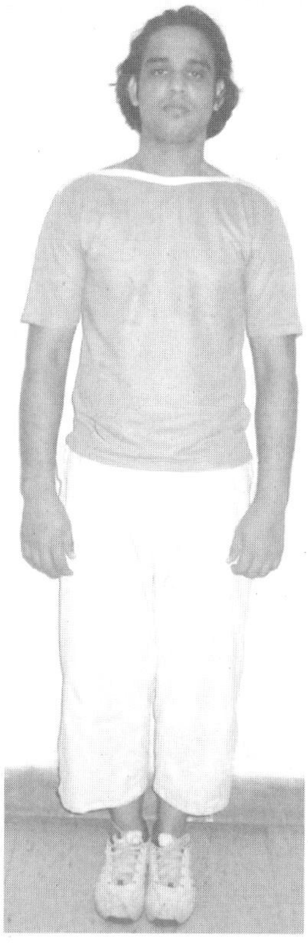

Fig. 17.35: Standing with feet together

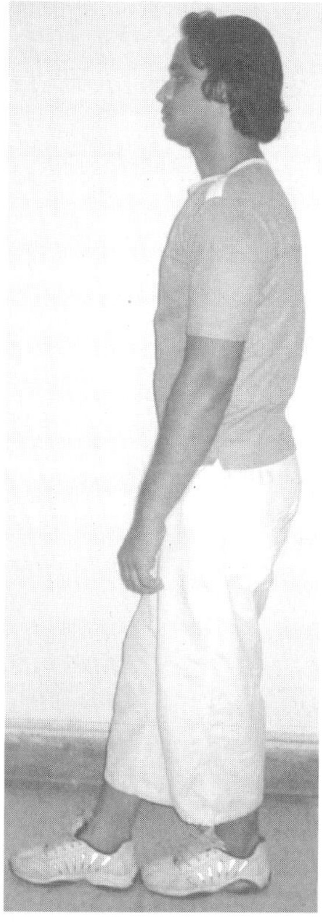

Fig. 17.36: Standing with one foot in front

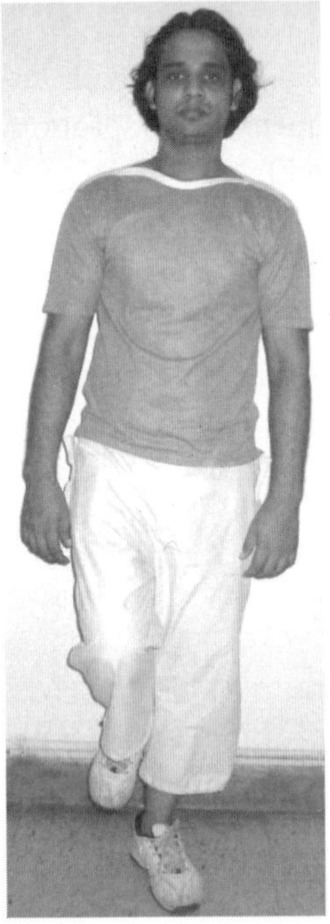

Fig. 17.37: Standing on one foot

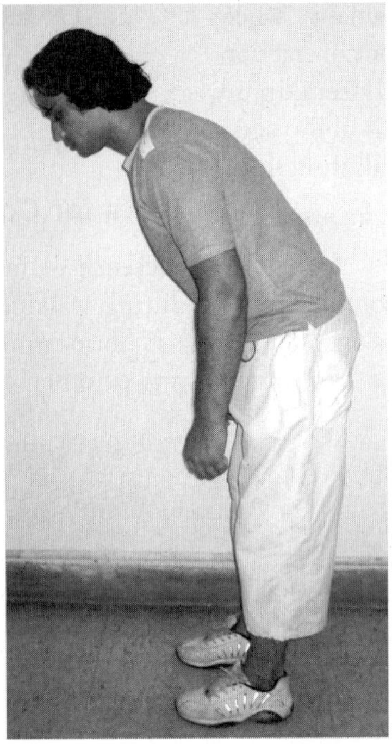

Fig. 17.38: Standing between forward trunk flexion and neutral position

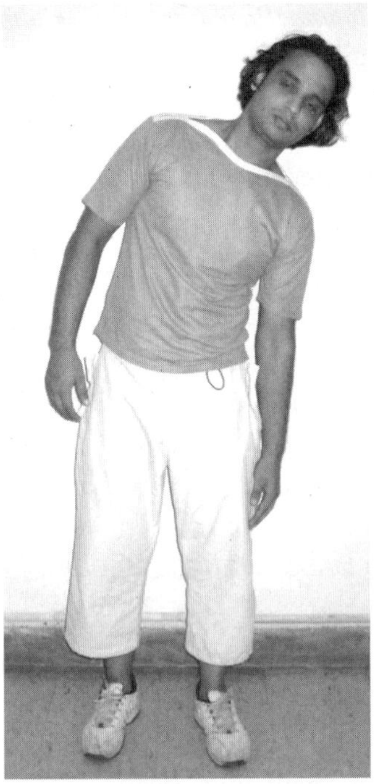

Fig. 17.39: Standing lateral flexion

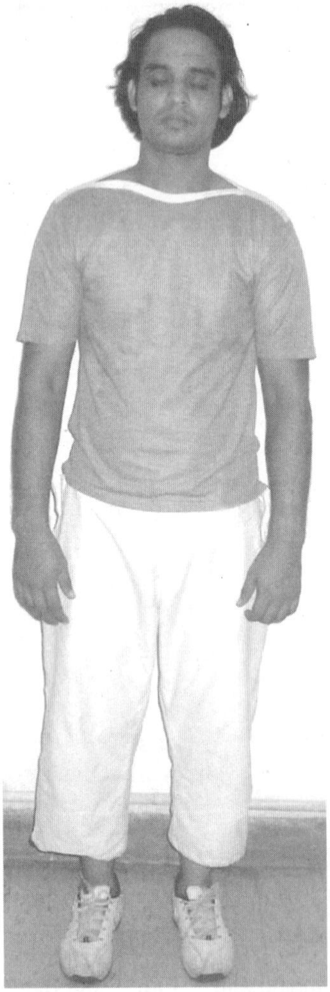

Fig. 17.40: Standing with eyes closed

II. *Walking:*

a. Placing one foot directly in front of the toe of th opposite foot.
b. Along a straight line (Fig. 17.41).
c. On foot prints (Fig. 17.42).
d. Side wards—right and left (Fig. 17.43).
e. Backwards (Fig. 17.44).
f. March in place.
g. Stop and start abruptly.
h. With turning at 90°, 180° and 360°.
i. Around circle (Fig. 17.45).
j. On heels or toes (Figs. 17.46 and 17.47).
k. With step over or around obstacles (Fig. 17.48).
l. With different speeds.

Tests in Sitting or Supine Position (Non-equilibrium)

i. *Finger to Nose*—The patient is asked to bring the tip c the index finger to the tip of the nose. Movement ca be repeated number of times (Fig. 17.49).

ii. *Finger to Therapist Finger*—The patient is asked t touch therapist's finger held in various position (therapist sitting in front of the patient). Movemer can be repeated number of times (Fig. 17.50).

iii. *Finger to Finger*—With shoulders abducted at 90° patient is asked to bring both hands towards th

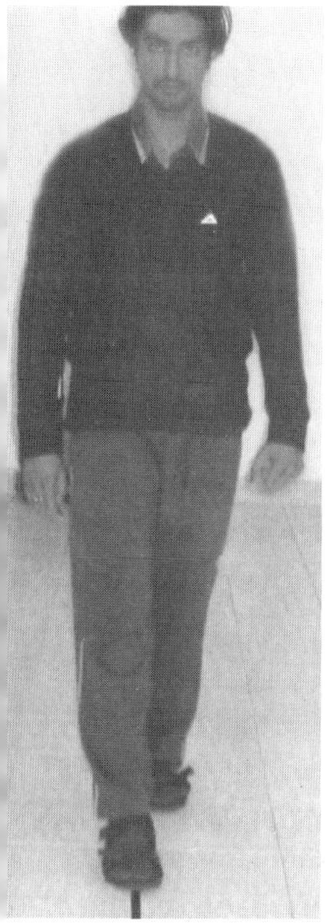

Fig. 17.41: Walking on a straight line

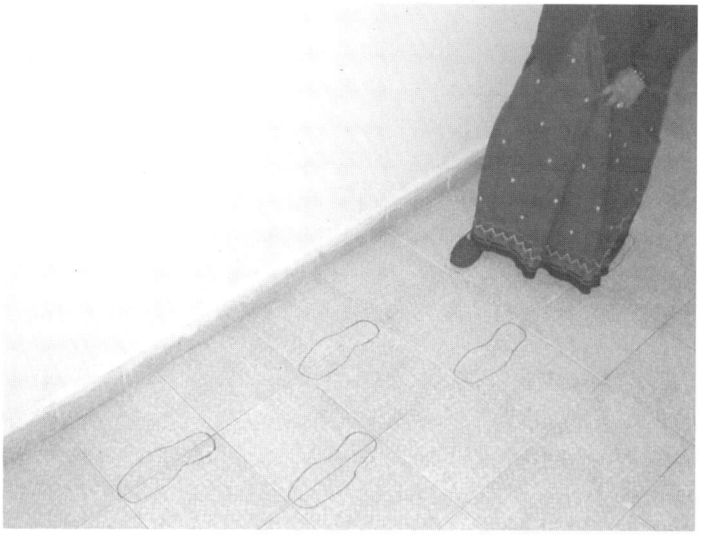

Fig. 17.42: Walking on foot prints

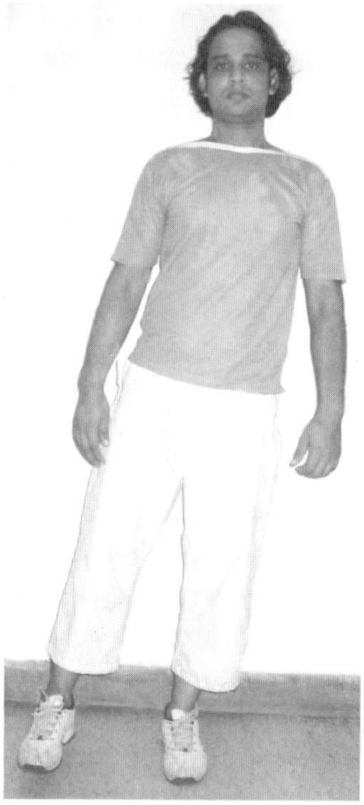

Fig. 17.43: Walking side ward

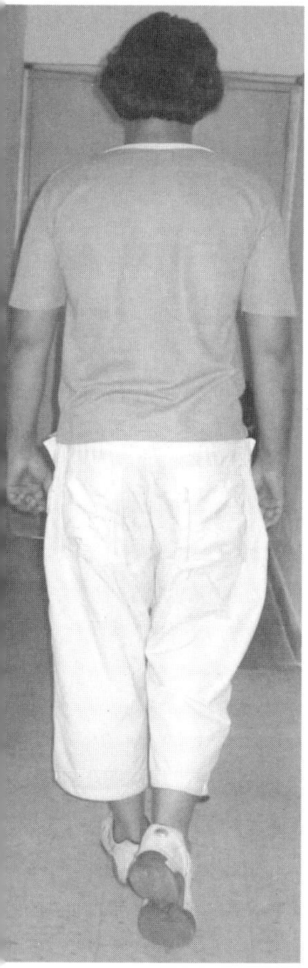

Fig. 17.44: Walking backward

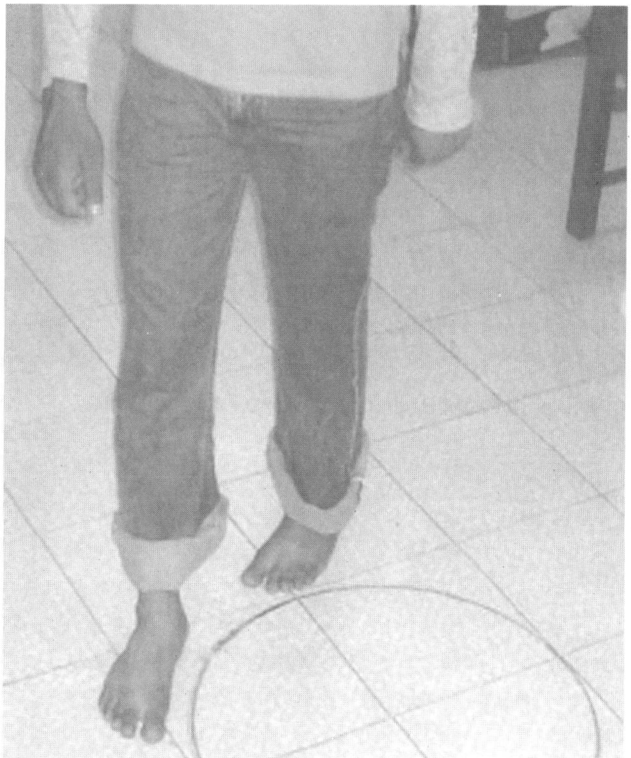

Fig. 17.45: Walking around circle

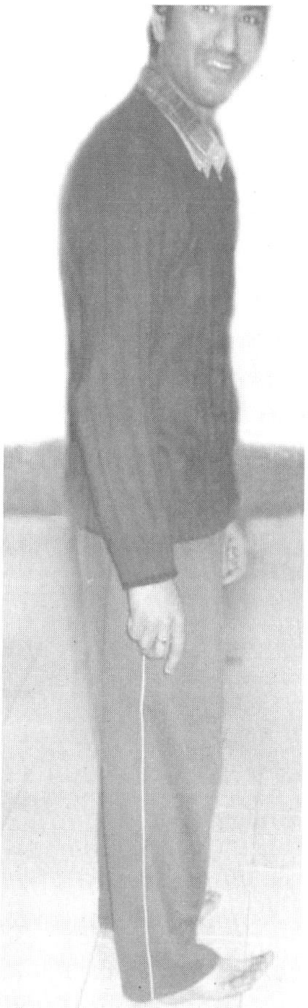

Fig. 17.46: Walking on heels

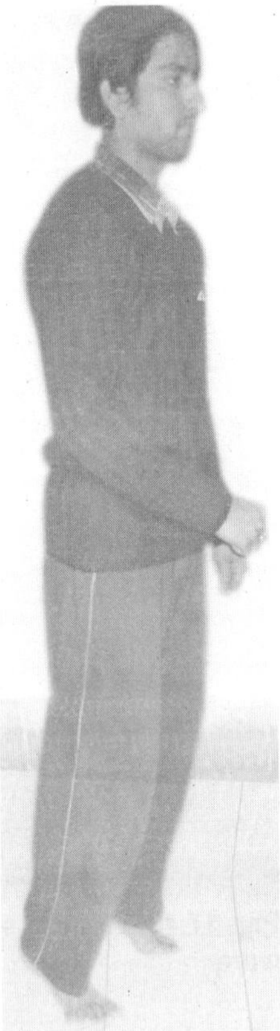

Fig. 17.47: Walking on toes

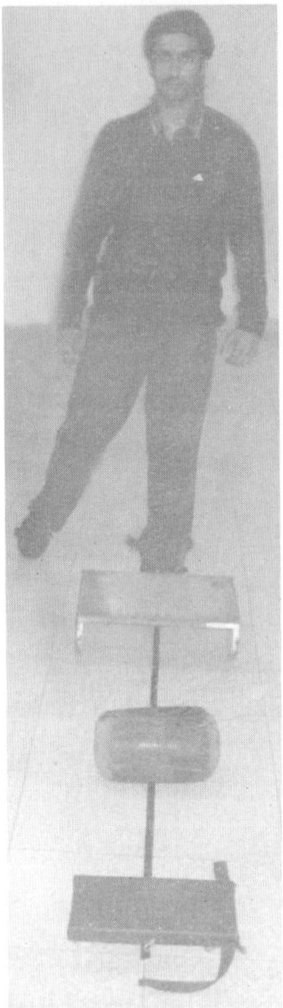

Fig. 17.48: Walking through obstacles

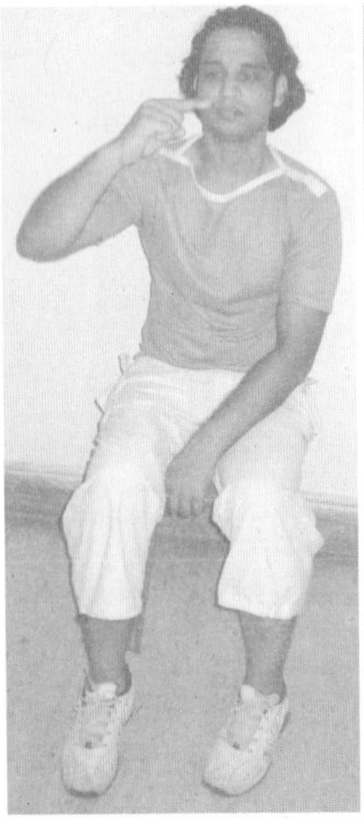

Fig. 17.49: Finger to nose test

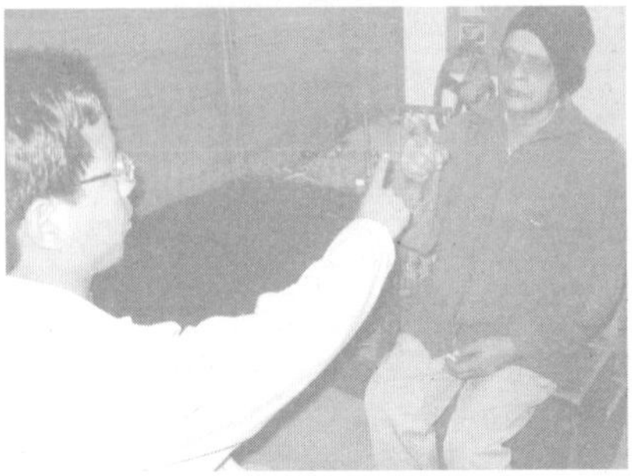

Fig. 17.50: Finger to therapist finger

midline and approximate the index fingers from opposing hand (Fig. 17.51).

iv. *Alternate nose to finger*—The patient alternately touches the tip of his nose and the tip of the therapist's finger (held in various positions) with index finger (Fig. 17.52).

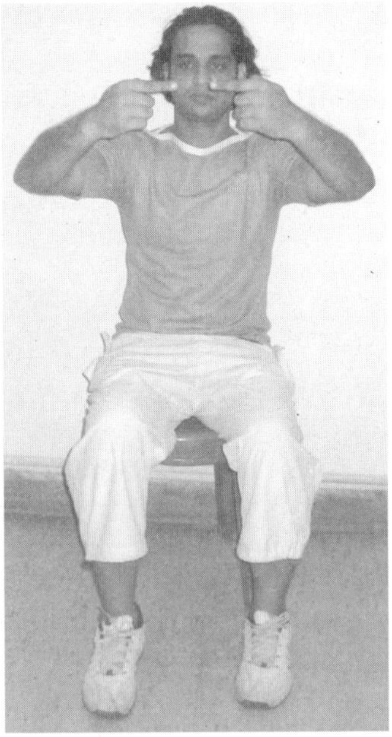

Fig. 17.51: Finger to finger test

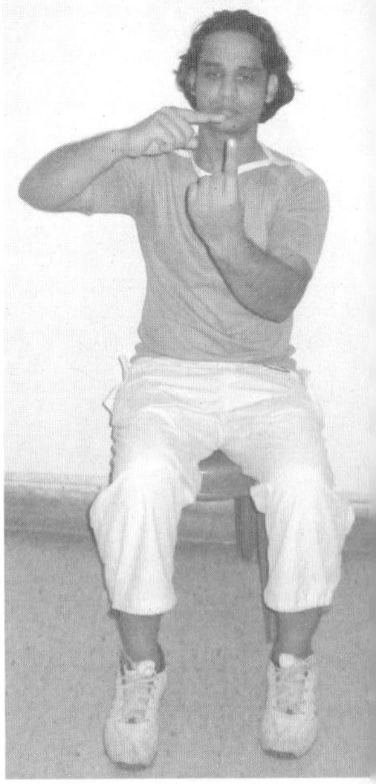

Fig. 17.52: Alternate nose to finger test

v. *Finger opposition*—The patient touches the tip of the thumb to the tip of each finger in sequence.

vi. *Pronation/supination*—The patient is asked to do pronation/supination alternately with elbow flexed at 90°.

vii. *Alternate heel to knee (supine position)*—The patient is asked to touch the knee and big toe alternately with the heel of the opposite extremity (Fig. 17.53).

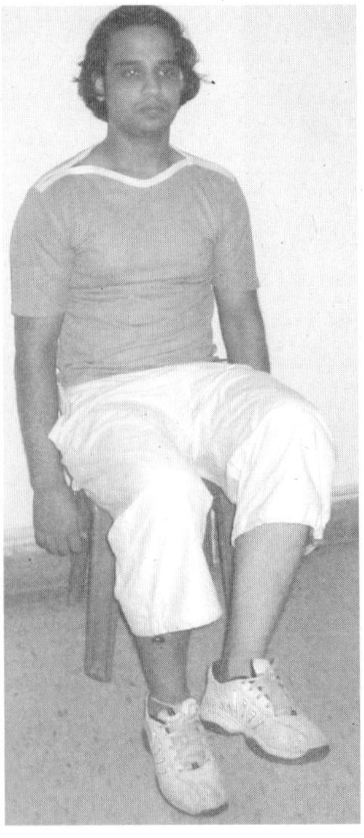

Fig. 17.53: Alternate heel to knee test

viii. *Drawing an imaginary circle in the air with either upper or lower extremity.*

ix. *Position holding*—Patient is asked to hold upper or lower extremity in any position.

x. *Rebound test*—The patient is asked to do elbow extension, the therapist applies resistance to produce an isometric contraction of triceps. Resistance is suddenly released. Normally the opposing muscle group (biceps) will contract and controls the limb. (Other muscle groups such as shoulder abductors and flexors, elbow flexors can also be tested).

COORDINATION EXERCISES

Frenkel's exercises were designed to enable voluntary relearning of movement through repetition and retraining of functional patterns. Frenkel's exercises are performed while patients are supine, sitting or standing. Patients should perform each activity slowly with visual input to help control movement.

The exercises as described by Caliet, cited in Licht (1965) are:

I. *In supine, have the patient perform the following movements:*

i. Flexion and extension of each leg at the knee and hip joints; abduction and adduction with knees flexed; later, abduction and adduction with knees extended (Figs. 17.54a to c).

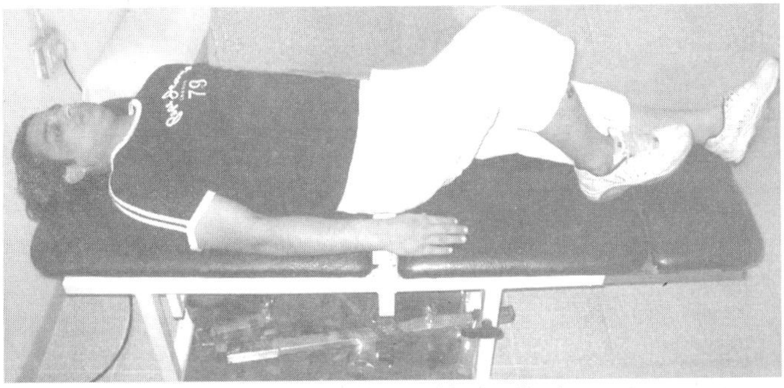

Fig. 17.54a: Hip and knee flexion

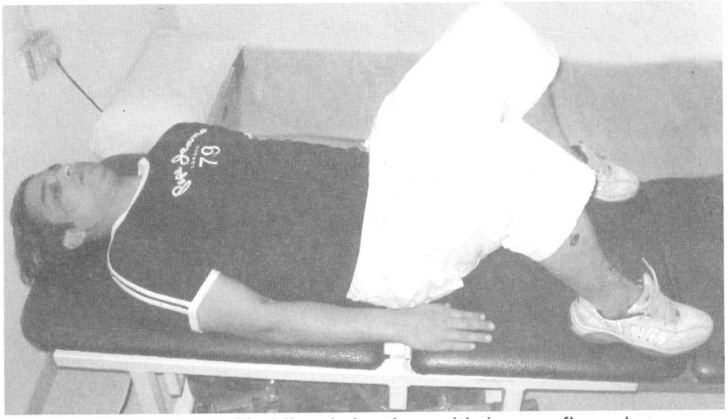

Fig. 17.54b(i): Hip abduction with knees flexed

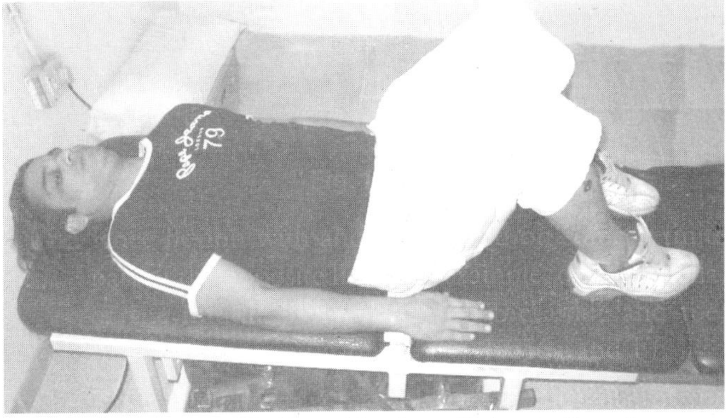

Fig. 17.54b(ii): Hip adduction with knees flexed

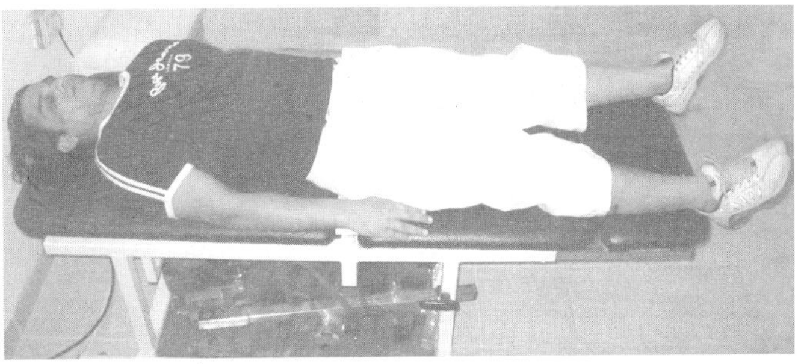

Fig. 17.54c(i): Hip abduction with knees extended

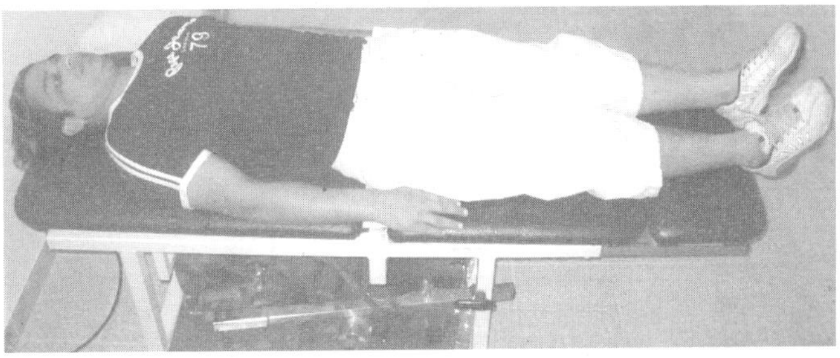

Fig. 17.54c(ii): Hip adduction with knees extended

ii. Flexion and extension of one knee at a time, with heel raised from the bed (Fig. 17.55).

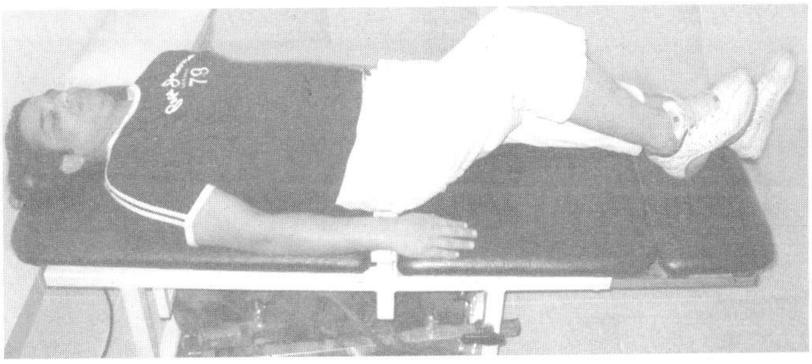

Fig. 17.55

iii. Knee flexion with and heel placed on some definite part of the opposite limb; for example, on the patella, or the middle of the leg, with the ankle and toe, then changing positions (Figs. 17.56a and b).

iv. Knee flexion with, heel placed on the knee of the opposite leg, and is glided down the tibia to the ankle joint and back to the knee (Fig. 17.57).

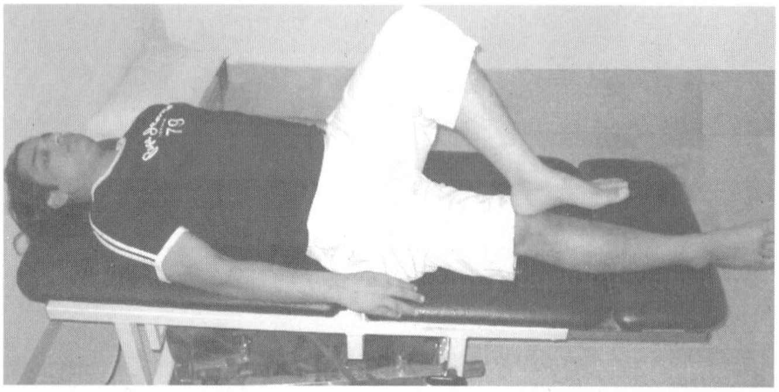

Fig. 17.56a

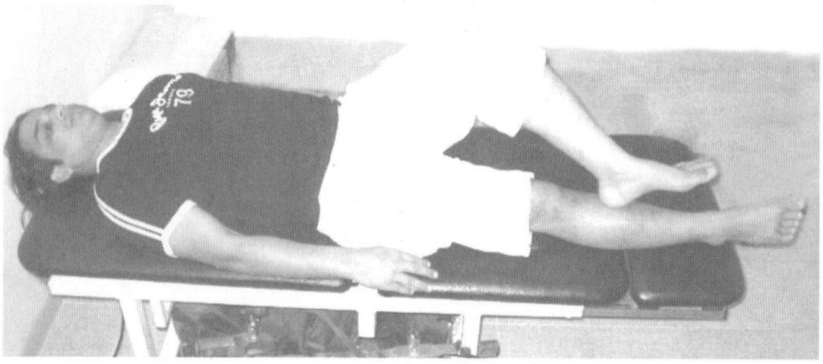

Fig . 17.56b

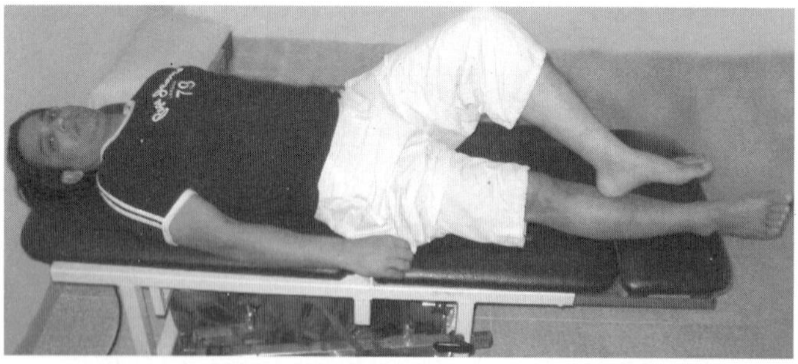

Fig. 17.57

v. Flexion and extension of both legs, together with knees and ankles held close together (Fig. 17.58).

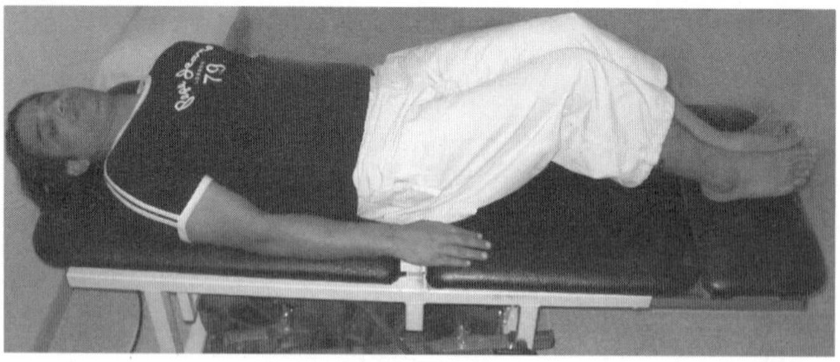

Fig. 17.58

vi. Flexion of one lower extremity during extension of the other (reciprocal) (Fig. 17.59).

vii. Flexion or extension of one leg during adduction or abduction of the other (Fig. 17.60).

II. *When patient can perform exercises (i) to (vii) easily, he should perform them with their eyes closed.*

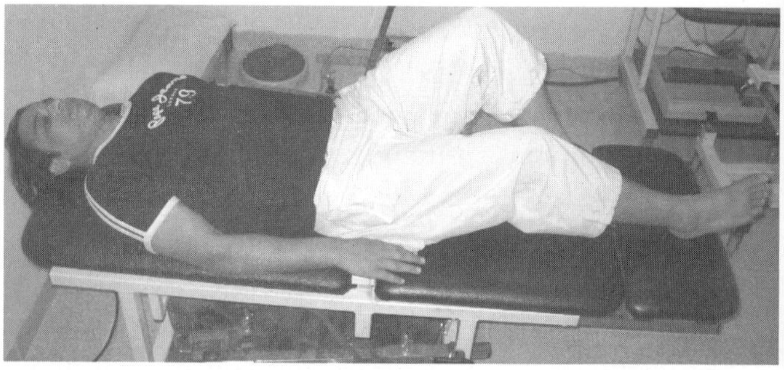

Fig. 17.59

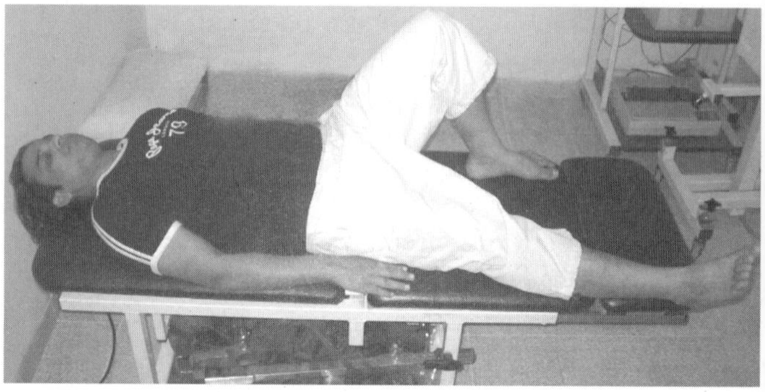

Fig. 17.60

III. *In Sitting:*

i. Try to place the heel of foot into the therapist's hand. The therapist changes the position of his or her hand after each attempt (Fig. 17.61).

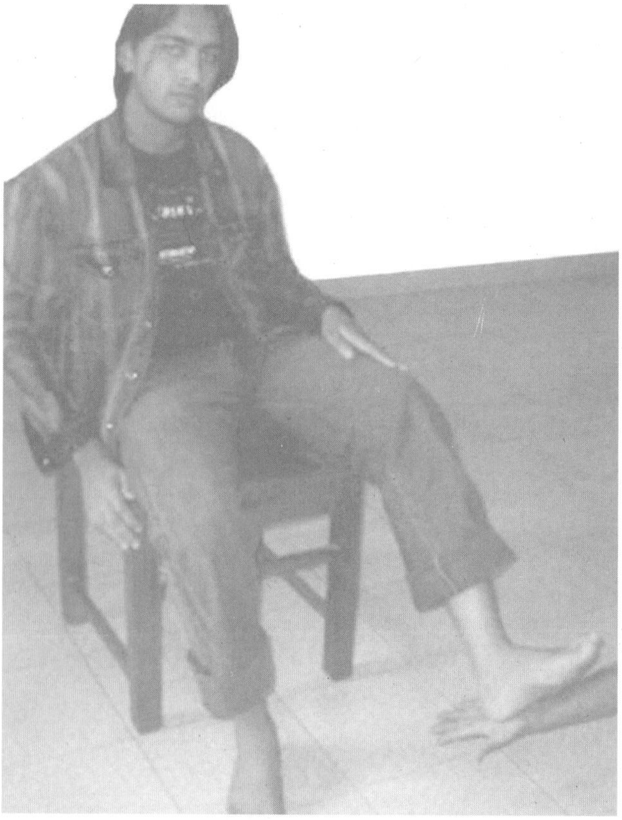

Fig. 17.61: Patient placing heel on therapist's palm

ii. Maintain sitting unsupported for several minutes.

iii. Raise each knee alternately and place each foot firmly on the ground on traced footprint. This task may be performed in sitting or standing position (Fig. 17.62).

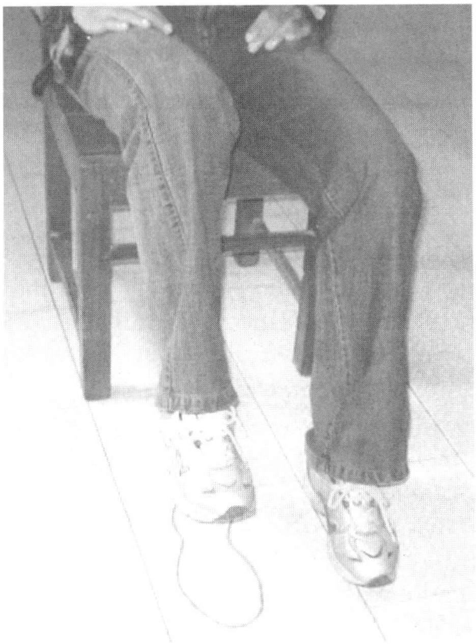

Fig. 17.62: Patient placing foot on marked foot print (in sitting position)

iv. Rise from a chair and then sit again holding knees together (Fig. 17.63).

v. Place feet forward and backward on a straight line, then repeat on a zig-zagged line. These exercises may be performed in both sitting and standing position.

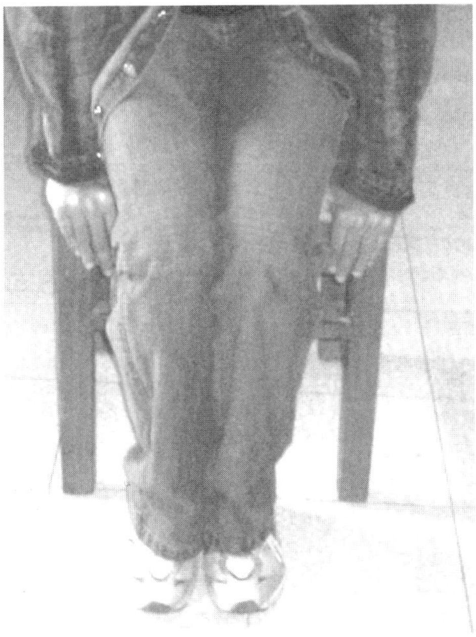

Fig. 17.63: Sit to stand with feet together

IV. *During Walking:*

i. Walk between two parallel lines (Fig. 17.64).

ii. Walk on foot tracings placed on the floor.

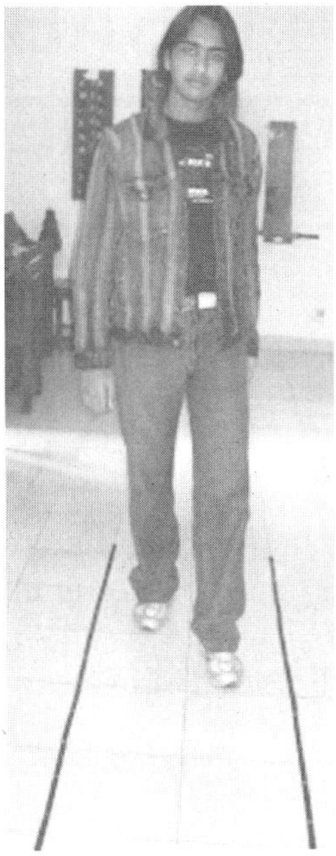

Fig. 17.64: Walking between parallel lines

OTHER ASPECTS OF MANAGEMENT FOR INCOORDINATION

1. *Functional activities*—To improve the coordinated movements of functional task, it is important that the patient repeat those tasks. The key to improving coordination is to vary the distance and speed of the movement to enable successful completion of the task and gradually retrain muscle activity.

   For e.g.:

   a. Draw numbers or alphabet on paper.
   b. Practice writing.
   c. Don and Doff shirts.
   d. Brush teeth.
   e. Comb hair.
   f. Pick up small objects from floor/table.

2. *Proprioceptive neuromuscular facilitation (PNF)* discussed in Chapter 14.

3. *Weight bearing activities through proximal joints* (Standing, kneeling, sitting on mats and weight bearing through involved upper extremity).

4. *Sensory cues*—Use of sensory cues such as visual feedback, manual guidance, verbal cues etc. during exercises or practising functional task enhance the treatment outcome.

18

DISABILITY, FUNCTION AND ACTIVITIES OF DAILY LIVING (ADL)

INTRODUCTION

Before discussing more about function and ADL the concept of disability must be clearly understood.

CONCEPTS OF DISABILITY

As long as human kind has existed there has inevitably been impairment and disability. The life giving processes of gestation and birth themselves can result in physical and mental incapacities that affect individual's activity of daily living. Natural disasters such as earthquakes, tsunami, flood and hurricanes, accidents of all kinds, violent aggression, wars also create disability. Even without all this, the process of life and aging itself guarantees that if we live long enough impairment of some sort will occur.

The definitions of disability describe what the person cannot do. The phrases used are "lack of ability to perform an activity", "reduction of a person's activity", and "inability to engage in any substantial gainful activity". Such definitions are based on the belief that it is the person who cannot do or perform.

"Disability" or "nonability" arise out of an individual's inability to perform a task successfully because of an insufficiency in one or more areas of functional capability: Physical function, mental function, agility, dexterity, coordination, strength, endurance, knowledge, skill, intellectual ability or experience. "Disability" requires a conceptual definition; it is the gap between what a person can do and what the person needs or wants to do. Medically, disability is physical impairment and inability to perform physical functions normally.

Evolution of Models of Disability

Terminology in the field of disablement continues to breed confusion and controversy across and within discipline. Therefore, it is essential to discuss various models of disability (Fig. 18.1).

SAAD NAGI (1969)

Nagi, a sociologist was the first to provide a model of disability process. He suggested four stages in the disability process: active pathology, impairment, functional limitation and disability.

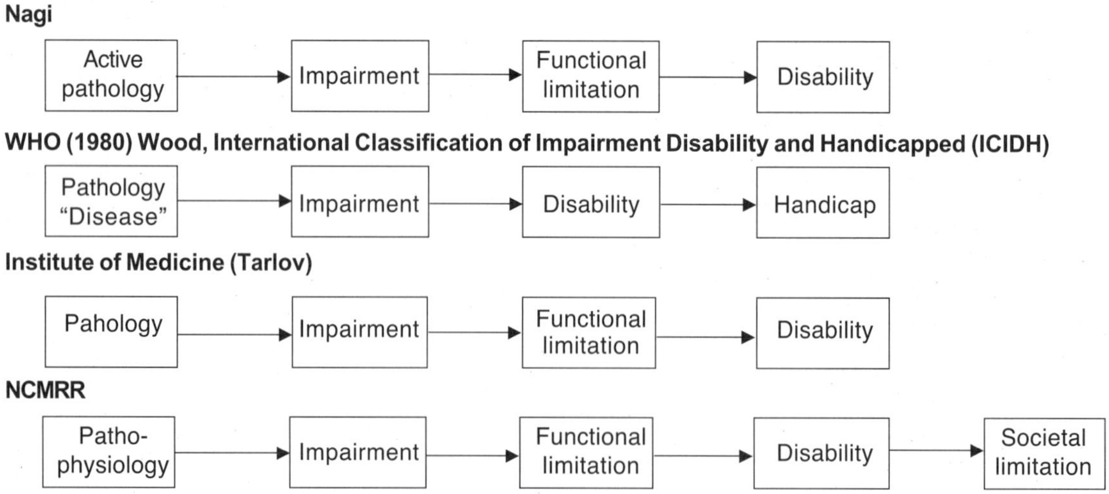

Fig. 18.1: Various models of disability

Active pathology: Interruption or interference with normal processes and efforts of the organism to regain normal state.

Impairment: Anatomical, physiological, mental or emotional abnormalities or loss.

Functional limitation: Limitation in performance at the level of the whole organism or person.

Disability: Limitation in performance of socially defined roles and tasks within a socio-cultural and physical environment.

WORLD HEALTH ORGANIZATION (1980) ICIDH

It is the most commonly used and internationally accepted conceptual model of disablement. It was proposed by Wood, he suggested four levels of disablement.

Pathology: It is a disease or trauma that causes changes in the structure or function of the body or of a specific tissue or organ.

Example: Arthritis.

Impairment: Occurs at the organ level and is defined as "any loss or abnormality of psychological, physiological or anatomical structure or function." Impairment are observable and can be objectively defined and measured in most cases.

Example: Loss of joint motion, amputation.

Disability: Occurs at personal level and is defined as "any restriction or lack (resulting from impairment) of ability to perform an activity in the manner or within the range considered normal for a human being". Disability is most commonly defined in terms of dependent functioning within one's personal sphere.

Example: Dependent activities of daily living.

Handicap: Occurs at societal level is defined as "a disadvantage for a given individual that limits or prevents the fulfillment of a role that is normal (depending upon age, sex, social and cultural factors) for that individual". Handicaps may affect expected roles such as employee, family member, and community member.

Example: Lack of access to a public place because of wheelchair confinement.

The WHO model assumes unidirectional causality (impairments cause disability that cause handicap).

INSTITUTE OF MEDICINE (IOM)

For approximately 10 years, the ICIDH model remained unchallenged. Then two models were published concurrently; IOM and NCMRR. IOM was adapted directly from the Nagi model. The IOM model defines disability as "a function of the interaction of the person with the environment". The IOM model identified a subset of factors that could modify the relationships between impairments, functional limitations and disability. These factors include biology, environment (physical, social and psychological), life style and behavior. These factors are independent variables that can modify all levels of disablement process and affect quality of life.

NCMRR MODEL (1993)

The National Centre for Medical Rehabilitation and Research (NCMRR) changed the structure of model by creating five stages instead of four. The first three are defined similarly to Nagi's model. The term "pathophysiology" is substituted for "active pathology". The difference is in the definition of "disability" and "societal limitation".

Disability is defined as a limitation or inability in performing tasks, activities, and roles to levels expected within physical and social context. Societal limitation is a restriction attributable to social policy or barriers that limit fulfillment of roles.

RECONSIDERATION OF DISABLEMENT MODELS

The multiple models of disability have produced confusion. They limit our ability to define disability. Additionally, there are major criticisms of the existing models. First, they have overemphasized the medical model. A second major criticism is that the models have assumed causal relationships between the different levels. For example in some models disability is directly caused by the observed impairments; whereas in reality, impairments may explain 25% or less of the variance in disability or handicap. A third criticism of the existing models is that a unidirectional relationship exists between the levels. This unidirectional representation does not allow for reverse effects. For example, handicap (role limitation) may cause less mobility (disability), and less mobility causes declines in strength and endurance (impairment). Most importantly, the unidirectional representation implies that disability is not reversible. Lastly, the models are expressed in negative dimensions (handicap) rather than positive (enabling) terms (i.e., residual abilities).

Given these limitations, the two initiatives in 1997 put forth additional models to characterize disability.

MODIFIED IOM MODELS (1997)

The new IOM model clearly defines disability as the interaction of person with the environment and includes a bi-directional dimension (possibility of improvement).

Disability has been moved from being a part of the process to being a product of interaction of the individual with the environment.

NEW WORLD HEALTH ORGANIZATION MODEL (1997-2001)

The WHO has recently modified the 1980 model of the disablement classification with its new name ICF– International Classification of Functioning in 2001.

ICF defines component of health and some health related components of well being (such as education and labour). The ICF domain can, therefore, be seen as health domains and health related domains. These domains are described from body, individual and societal perspectives.

ICF has two parts each with two components (Tables 18.1 and 18.2).

Part I: Functioning and disability

a. Body functions and structures.

b. Activities and participation.

Part II: Contextual factors

a. Environmental factors.

b. Personal factors.

Each component can be expressed in both positive and negative terms.

Table 18.1: Definitions of the component of ICF

1. Functioning: Refers to all body functions, activities and participation as an umbrella term.
2. Disability: Serves as an umbrella term for impairment, activity limitation and participation.
3. Body functions: Are the physiological functions of body systems (including psychological functions).
4. Body structures: Are anatomical parts of the body such as organs, limbs and their components.
5. Impairments: Are problems in body function or structure such as organs, limbs and their components.
6. Activity: Is the execution of a task or action by an individual.
7. Participation: Is involvement in a life situation.
8. Activity limitations: Are difficulties an individual may have in executing activities (activity limitations replaces the term "disability" used in 1980 version of ICIDH).
9. Participation restrictions: Are problems an individual may experience in involvement in life situations (replaces the term "handicap" used in 1980 version of ICIDH).
10. Contextual factors: Are the factors that together constitute the complete context of an individual's life and in particular the background against which the health states are classified in ICF.
11. Environmental factors: Constitute a component of ICF and refers to all aspects of the external or extrinsic world that form the context of an individual's life and as such, have an impact on that person's functioning. Environmental factors include physical world and its features, the human made physical world, other people in different relationships and roles, attitudes and values, social systems and services, and policies; rules and laws.
12. Personal factors: Are contextual factors relate to the individual such as an age, gender, social status, life experiences and so on (which are not currently classified in ICF).

Table. 18.2: An overview of ICF

	Part 1: Functioning and disability		Part 2: Contextual factors	
Components	Body functions and structures	Activities and participation	Environmental factors	Personal factors
Domains	Body functions Body structures	Life areas (tasks, actions)	External influences on functioning and disability	Internal influences on functioning and disability
Constructs	Change in body function (physiological)	Capacity Executing tasks in a standard environment	Facilitating or hindering impact of features of the physical, social and attitudinal world	Impact of attributes of the person
	Change in body structure (anatomical)	Performance Executing task in the current environment		
Positive aspect	Functional and structural integrity	Activities participation	Facilitators	Not applicable
	Functioning			
Negative aspect	Impairment	Activity limitation Participation restriction	Barriers/hindrances	Not applicable
	Disability			

DOMAINS FOR THE ACTIVITIES AND PARTICIPATION

In ICF the domains for the Activities and Participation components are given in a single list that covers the full range of life areas (from basic learning or watching to composite areas such as interpersonal interactions or employment). They are as follows:

1. Learning and applying knowledge.
2. General tasks and demands.
3. Communication.
4. Mobility.
5. Self care.
6. Domestic life.
7. Interpersonal interactions and relationships.
8. Major life areas (education, work and employment and economic life).
9. Community, social and civic life.

INTERACTION BETWEEN THE COMPONENTS OF ICF (Fig. 18.2)

At this time, the new ICIDH-2 (ICF) classification appears to be the best model for conceptualizing impairment and disability. It acknowledges the complex and dynamic interactions between a given health condition, the environment, and personal factors. The relationships between impairment, activity limitations and participation restriction are not assumed to be unidirectional. For example one may have impairment without activity limitations (disability) or limitations in participation (handicap) or one could have activity limitations (disability) without limitations in participation (handicap). On the other hand one could have limitations in activities or participation without documented impairments (e.g., Pain). This model also recognizes that limitations in participation may secondarily produce limitations in activities which may also produce impairments. For example, inability to participate in fitness programs may cause poor performance in daily activities which can produce impairments (decreased cardiovascular endurance and diminished muscle strength).

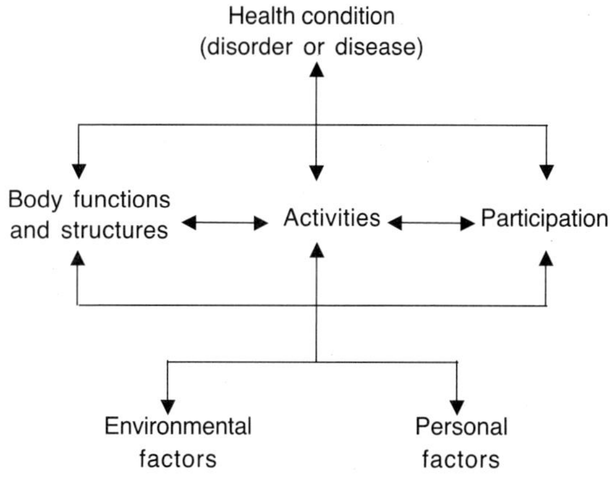

Fig. 18.2: Interaction between the component of ICF

UNIVERSAL APPLICATION OF ICF

There is a widely held misunderstanding that ICF is only about people with disabilities; in fact it about all people. The health and health related states associated with all health conditions can be described using ICF. In other words, ICF has universal application.

FUNCTION

Function, in rehabilitation terms, is what humans do or how humans act. Functional activities encompass all those tasks, activities and roles that makes the individual independent. The ultimate aim of any rehabilitation program is to make the individual independent in all those functions which he used to perform before the trauma/disease.

Human functions can broadly be divided into:

i. Basic or personal activities of daily living (BADLs).
ii. Instrumental activities of daily living (IADLs).
iii. Work activities.
iv. Sports/recreational activities.

Basic ADLs

Basic or personal ADL consists of the following activities:

a. Eating activities (using utensils, cup/glass, taking food/drink to the mouth, breaking bread etc.).
b. Hygiene activities (brushing teeth, bathing, toileting, combing hair, shaving etc.).
c. Bed activities (moving in bed, managing pillows and blankets, reaching for objects etc.).
d. Dressing activities (putting on/taking off shirts, trousers etc.).
e. Transfer activities (bed-to-chair, sit-to-stand from chair and toilet, into a car etc.).
f. Walking activities (walking on level surfaces and uneven surfaces, negotiating curbs, ascending and descending stairs).

Instrumental ADLs

To live independently in a community an individual should be able to perform following functional tasks known as IADLs.

a. Meal preparation (cutting vegetables, stirring etc.).
b. Household work (Dusting, mopping floors, washing dishes etc.).
c. Communication (writing, using telephone etc.).
d. Shopping.
e. Driving.
f. Gardening.
g. Having sex.

Work Activities

These comprises physical demands that a worker may need to perform a job:

a. Lifting
b. Carrying
c. Stooping
d. Pushing
e. Pulling
f. Reaching
g. Manipulating
h. Climbing
i. Sitting
j. Standing
k. Walking.

Sport and Recreational Activities

These skills are required to perform any sport or game:

a. Walking: Forward, retro and side ways.
b. Jogging: Forward, retro, on grass, on a track, on hills in water etc.
c. Jumping: Vertical, forward, retro, side to side, on a level surface, from a height, etc.
d. Throwing: Underhand, overhand, two handed (with different size and weight of ball).
e. Catching: Two handed, one handed (with different size and weight of ball).
f. Batting: Cricket bat, tennis and badminton recquet hockey stick etc.
g. Swimming: Back stroke, crawl stroke, breast stroke etc
h. Sprinting: Forward, retro, on grass, on a track, on a basket ball court etc.

ADL Training is a method to make a particular activity possible for the client to perform with the help of a special device, splint, piece of equipment or specific technique.

Factors Influencing ADL Training

The following factors should be considered before starting ADL training:

i. Physical capability of the client:
   a. Muscle strength.
   b. Joint range of motion.
   c. Coordination.
   d. Sensation.
   e. Balance.
   f. Cognitive and perceptual skills.
   g. Cardiopulmonary endurance.

ii. Culture and values of the client.

iii. Family support.

iv. Environment (in which activity has to be performed).

v. Financial assistance.

Goal of ADL Training

The ultimate aim of any ADL training for the client is to achieve maximal level of independence is different for every client. For e.g., Walking independently may be the maximal level for a person with lower extremity amputation. But self care, feeding and communication with assistance or device may be the maximal level for quadriplegic.

Evaluation of ADL

Consists of evaluation of those activities which the client was performing before the disability or when he is expected to perform as per his socio-cultural context (In case of congenital or early life disability).

Parameters of ADL Evaluation

ADL is evaluated on the basis of three parameters:

1. Level of independence—different levels are:
   - Independent
   - Supervision
   - Minimum assistance
   - Moderate assistance
   - Maximum assistance.
2. Time—Amount of time required to perform an activity.
3. Accuracy—How accurately the client perform the ADL.

Sequence of ADL Training

ADL training has to be given in the following sequence:

- BADL → IADL.

  For self care activities:

  Feeding
  ↓
  Grooming
  ↓
  Continence
  ↓
  Transfer skills
  ↓
  Toileting
  ↓
  Undressing
  ↓
  Dressing
  ↓
  Bathing

Basic Principles of ADL Training

i. Make out which ADLs are possible and which are impossible to achieve.

ii. Explore the alternate methods of performing the activities.

iii. Use any assitive devices that may be helpful.

iv. Determine the amount of assistance required (from no assistance to maximal assistance).

v. Progression of training:

a. Dependent
↓
Maximum assistance
↓
Moderate assistance
↓
Minimum assistance
↓
Supervision
↓
Independent.

b. Few tasks → more tasks
Simple tasks → complex tasks.

vi. Methods of teaching should suit the client's ability.

vii. Each activity should be broken into small tasks and then each task into several small steps. Then step by step teaching should be followed.

viii. Demonstration of each activity/task/step should be done by the therapist.

ix. Method of 'backward' or 'forward' chaining may be used while teaching ADL skills.

- *Backward chaining:* In this method therapist assists the client in all the steps of the task except the last step (which is independently performed by the client).

  When the last step is mastered, the therapist withdraws assistance from the second last step and the client performs the second last independently.

  The process is continued till the client achieves independence over all the steps.

- *Forward chaining:* The client practice and become independent in the first step of the task and rest steps is assisted by the therapist.

  Then therapist withdraws his assistance from the second step and the client performs the second steps.

  The process is continued till the client achieves independence over all the steps.

Guidelines for ADL Training in the Client with Impaired Muscle Strength and/or Limited Range of Motion:

1. **Dressing activities**
   - Use one size larger garments.
   - Use front opening garments.
   - Use larger buttons or zippers.
   - Use velcro if buttons/zippers are difficult to use.
   - Use dressing stick.
   - Use reachers for picking up clothes.
   - Use shoes without laces or with elastic or velcro types fasteners.
   - Use button hooks.
2. **Eating activities**
   - Use adapted or built-up handles of utensils.
   - Use straws if it is difficult to drink with glass.
   - Use universal cuffs.
   - Use high table.
   - Use cups/glass with bilateral handles.
3. **Bathing and grooming**
   - Use hand held shower and flexible hose.
   - Use long-handled bath brush or sponge.
   - Use soap on a rope.
   - Use long or angulated handled comb/toothbrush.
   - Use reacher.
   - Use dressing stick.
   - Use bathing stool with grab bar.
   - Safety issues:
     - Use non skid tiles in bathroom/toilet.
     - Use grab bars.
4. **Communication**
   - Use holder for hand-piece of telephole.
   - Use dialing stick-hand, mouth or head held.
   - Use built up pen and pencils.
   - Use mouth stick or head stick from typewriter or computer.
5. **Mobility and transfers**
   - Use enlarged and padded grips on crutches, canes and walkers.
   - Use walker or crutch, bag or basket to carry objects.
   - Use raised chairs/toilet seats (easy to transfer from).
6. **Home management**

   Use utility cart, reachers, adapted knifes, light weight utensils, etc.

Guidelines ADL Training in the Client with Infcoordination:

1. Weighted devices such as heavy plates or plates with weight attached, etc.
2. Suction bases, non skid mats or plate stabilized can also be used.
3. Weighted wrist cuffs can be used while performing ADLs.
4. Work height should be high enough to prevent bending, leaning or reaching.

Dressing Activities for Hemiplegics

Figures 18.3a to i.

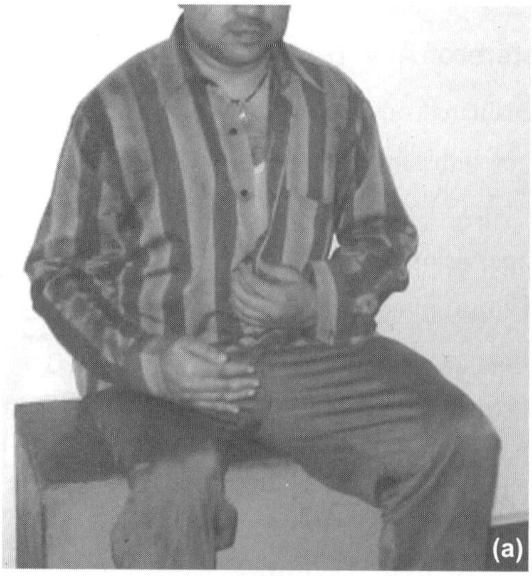

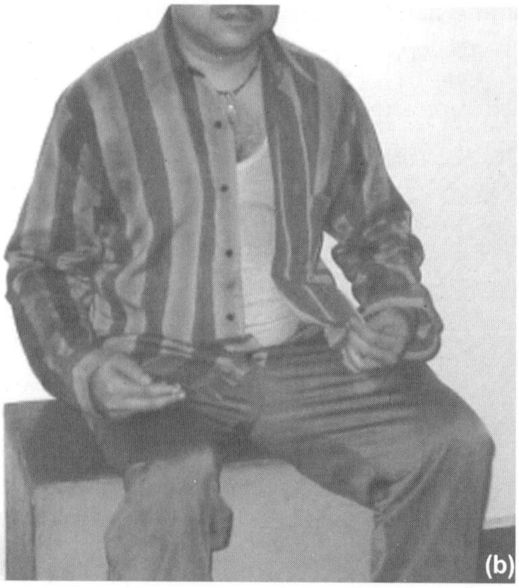

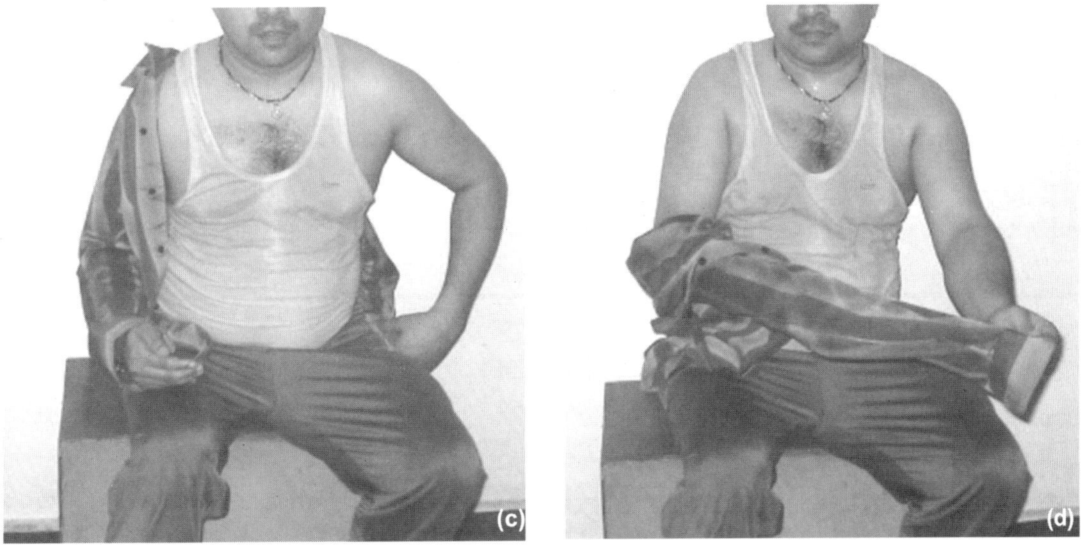

Figs. 18.3a to d: Doffing shirt

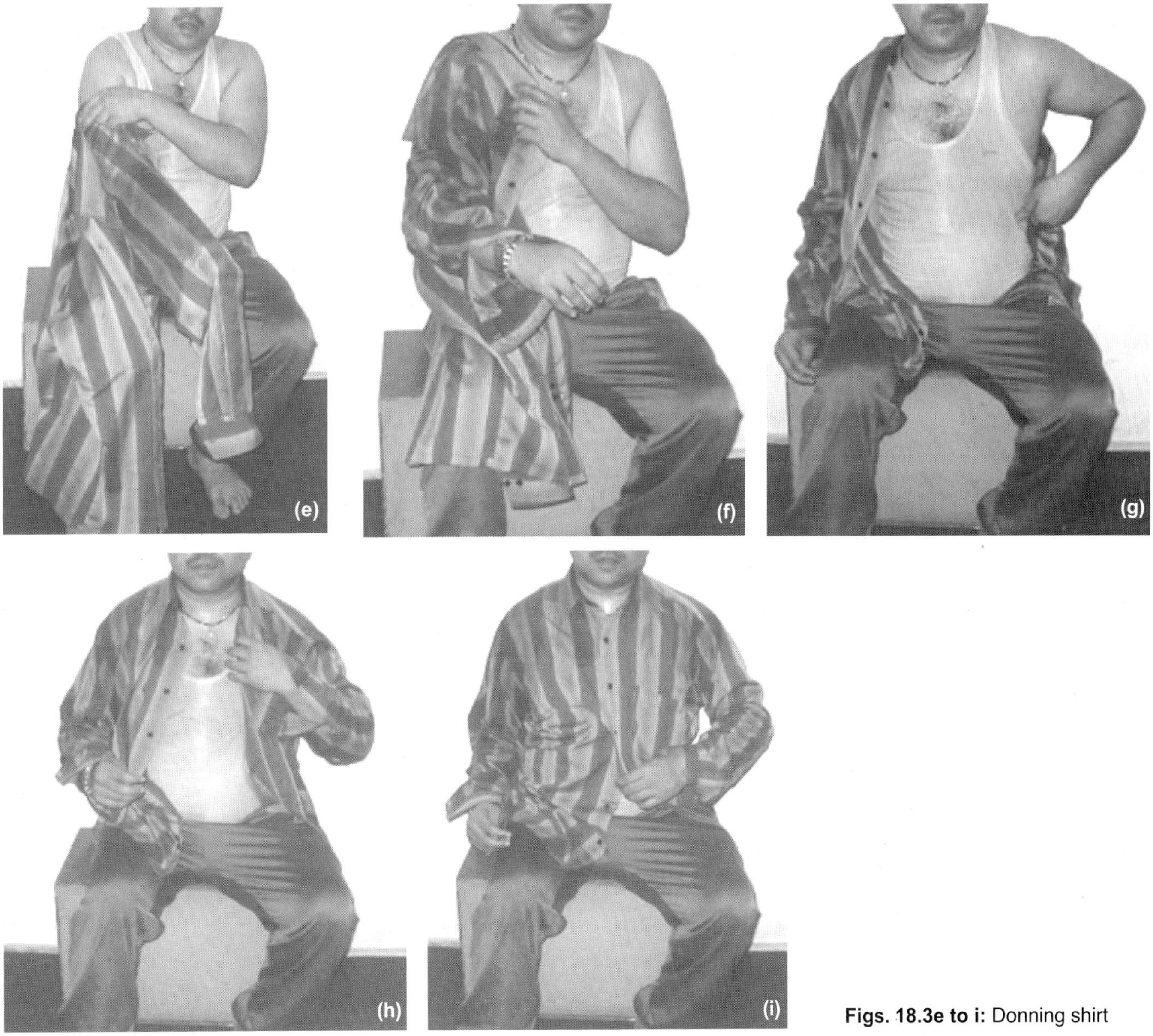

Figs. 18.3e to i: Donning shirt

19

THERAPEUTIC APPROACHES IN NEUROLOGICAL CONDITIONS

ROOD'S APPROACH

INTRODUCTION

Margaret Rood who was both an occupational and a physical therapist designed a treatment originally for cerebral palsy which was also applicable to any patient with motor control problems (Rood, 1976).

Principles

1. Controlled use of sensory stimulation
   - Appropriate sensory stimulus leads to specific motor response.
   - Appropriate sensory stimulus leads to normalization of muscle tone.
2. Use of developmental sequences
   - Sensorimotor development takes place in sequence from lower to higher level.
3. Use of activity to demand a purposeful response.
4. Practice of sensory motor responses is necessary for motor learning.

Levels of Motor Control

1. Supine withdrawal.
2. Roll over.
3. Pivot prone.
4. Neck co-contraction.
5. Prone on elbows.
6. Quadruped.
7. Standing.
8. Walking.

Sensory Inputs

To facilitate/inhibit motor responses:

1. Tactile (cutaneous).
2. Thermal.
3. Olfactory.
4. Gustatory.
5. Auditory.
6. Visual.
7. Proprioceptive (Stretch, resistance).

Method of Treatment

Sensory inputs are applied to facilitate or inhibit motor responses. Patients are made to go in developmental level sequentially starting from the level patient already has sensory inputs can be applied along with the developmental level. Finally use of purpose of activity should be incorporated followed by practice several times.

Rules of Sensory Input

Margaret Rood (1970), described four rules of sensory input:

1. A fast brief stimulus produces a large synchronous motor output. This type of stimulus confirms the reflex are functioning.
2. A fast repetitive sensory input produces a maintained response.
3. A maintained sensory input produces a maintained response.

   For e.g., Gravity—which has a constant effect on the sensory system. In all positions (standing, sitting or lying) the exteroceptors of the skin are in contact with a surface, thus discharging impulses into the nervous system.

4. Slow, rhythmical, repetitive sensory input deactivates body and mind.

   For e.g., Slow rocking or soft music activates the parasympathetic system leads to generalized relaxation.

Sequence of Motor Development

Margaret Rood proposed four sequential phases of motor control:

1. *Reciprocal innervation/inhibition*—A phasic (quick) type of movement that requires contraction of the agonist muscles as the antagonist muscle relaxes. It is an early mobility pattern protective in nature.
2. *Co-contraction*—It is defined as simultaneous contraction of the agonist and antagonist muscles with the antagonist supreme.

   It is a tonic (static) pattern which provides the ability to hold a position or an object for a longer duration.
3. *Heavy work*—It is described by Stock Meyer (1967) as "mobility superimposed on stability." In heavy work the proximal muscles contract and move and the distal segment is fixed.

   For e.g., Creeping, in quadruped position the distal segments—wrist and ankles are in a fixed position. The neck and thorax (proximal joints) are stable whereas the shoulder and hip girdles are free to move.
4. *Skill*—It is the highest level of motor control and combines the effect of mobility and stability. In skilled pattern the proximal segment is stabilized while the distal segment moves freely.

   For e.g., Typing requires stability in proximal joints (shoulder, elbow) while skilled mobility in distal finger joints.

Outogenic Motor Patterns

1. *Supine withdrawal (flexion)*—Is a total flexion response towards the vertebral level of T_{10}. The flexion of the neck and the crossing of the arms and legs protect the anterior surface of the body.

   It is useful in integration of the tonic labyrinthine reflex and for patients who do not have reciprocal flexion pattern and dominated by extensor tone.
2. *Roll over*—Rolling toward side causes:
   - Mobility pattern for the extremities and activates the lateral trunk musculature.
   - Stimulation of the semicircular canals, which in turn activate neck and extra ocular muscles.

   It is useful for patients who are dominated by tonic reflex patterns in the supine position.
3. *Pivot prone*—It is both a mobility pattern and a stability pattern. In this pattern there is full range of extension of the neck, shoulders, trunk and lower extremities. This position is difficult to assume and hold. It prepares the extensor muscles for upright positions and indicates integration of the symmetric tonic neck reflexes and the tonic labyrinthine reflexes.
4. *Neck co-contraction*—It activates both flexors and deep tonic extensors of the neck. It is the first real stability pattern. This pattern elicits the tonic labyrinthine righting reaction when the face is perpendicular to the floor and also promotes neck stability and extraocular control.
5. *Prone on elbows*—Weight bearing on elbows stretches the upper trunk musculature to influence the stability of the scapular and glenohumeral regions. In this position patient has better visibility of the environment and can do weight shift from side to side.

   The symmetric tonic neck reflex gets inhibited in this position.
6. *Quadruped position*—In this pattern lower trunk and lower extremities are in co-contraction. The patient can do weight shifts in forward/backward, side to side and diagonal directions. This provides mobility superimposed on the stability and prepares for equilibrium responses.
7. *Standing*—In this position weight is equally distributed on both legs after that weight shifting begins. The upper extremities are free to perform functions. Also standing brings in integration of righting reactions and equilibrium reacting.
8. *Walking*—Murray (1967) described gait as a normal locomotion that entails the ability to support the body weight, maintains balance and executes the stepping motion. Walking requires coordinated mobility and stability.

FACILITATION TECHNIQUES

1. **Tactile (Cutaneous) Stimulation**—It causes stimulation of exteroceptors (end organs under the skin in subcutaneous tissues). These receptors respond to the external environment causes protective withdrawl responses and produces states of alertness and rapid movements of the limbs.

a. *Light moving touch*—Touch is important for normal growth and development (Montague A, 1978).

It has following effects:

- Increases corticosteroid levels in the blood stream.
- Increases resistance against disease.
- Increases tissue repair.
- Improves fluid and electrolyte balance.

Margaret Rood used a light moving touch or stroking of the skin to activate the superficial mobilizing muscles.

- *Application:* Finger tips, camel hair brush or cotton swab.
- *Frequency:* 3-5 strokes, 30 seconds rest period between strokes.
- *Area:* The first area is the area from the nose to chin, after several stimulation infant may show response of flexion pattern of upper extremity and perhaps lower extremity.
- Light stroking from the corner of the lip to the cheek. It activates neck muscles and the head tilts laterally toward the side of the stimulus.
- Light moving touch to the navel or dermatome T_{10} in a midline to lateral direction-activates unilateral flexion pattern.
- Light moving touch to the dorsal web spaces of the fingers and toes activates a withdrawl pattern of the extremities.
- Light moving touch to the tips of the fingers or soles of feet facilitates a tickle withdrawl response of great magnitude.

b. *Fast brushing*—Fast brushing by battery operated brush (introduced by Margaret Rood in 1964) is applied over the dermatomes of the same segment that supplies the muscle (myotome) to be facilitated.

For e.g., Stimulation of L_{3-4} dermatomes leads to the facilitation of quadriceps, tibialis anterior and detrusor urinae.

The effect of fast brushing lasts for 30 minutes. The stimulus is applied for 3 to 5 seconds and repeated after 30 seconds.

c. *Icing*—Ice is an extreme in thermal facilitation and has been used for facilitation of muscle activity and autonomic nervous system responses (Margaret Rood, 1954). Margaret Rood described three uses of ice:

- Quick icing for patients having hypotonia (3 swipes, blott water after each swipe).
- Pressing ice cubes to the skin of a dermatome corresponding to myotome to be stimulated.
- Ice to stimulate sympathetic nervous system and probably glandular output of the thyroid and adrenal glands.

Ice should be used cautiously especially in patient having cardiac problems.

Note: The exteroceptive stimulation can be unpredictable. In the 1970s M. Rood began to abandon the use of this stimuli and endorse the use of proprioceptive stimuli.

2. **Proprioceptive stimulation**—It refers to the facilitation of:

- Muscle spindles.
- Golgi tendon organs.
- Joint receptors and the vestibular apparatus.

Joint gives more control over the motor response. Proprioceptors adapt more slowly than exteroceptors and can produce sustained postural patterns (Buchwald J, 1967).

a. **Heavy joint compression**—It is defined as joint compression greater than body weight applied through the longitudinal axis of the bone (Ager J, 1974).

It causes co-contraction around joint under compression. This procedure can also be combined with ontogenetic patterns such as prone on elbows, quadruped, sitting and standing positions.

The joint compression can be applied manually or by weighted cuffs or sandbags.

b. **Stretch**—According to Rood stretch is a physiologic stimulus used to activate the proprioceptors in selected muscles of the body.

- *Intrinsic stretch:* According to Rood it is the use of the intrinsic muscles to promote stability of the scapulohumeral rhythm.

  For e.g., In prone on elbows, resistive grasp can enhance shoulder stability. Resistance is a form of stretching as it increases fusimotor activity of the muscle spindle.

- *Resistance:* Rood emphasized the use of heavy resistance to stimulate both primary and secondary endings of the muscle spindle.

When a muscle contracts against resistance it assumes a shortened length that cause the muscle spindles to contract so they readjust to the shorter length.

According to Rood intermittent resistance graded to the desired motion is better than manual stretching for alleviating tight muscles.

- *Stretch pressure:* It affects both the exteroceptors and the Ia afferent of the muscle spindle. The degree of stretch and pressure should be strong enough to cause defomation of skin and underlying superficial muscle:
  - Lubricants can be used.
  - Time of stimulus < 3 seconds.
  - Can be applied directly over muscle or dermatomically.
  - Use thumb, index and middle finger to stretch with pressure.
- *Tapping:* It acts on the muscle spindle (afferent) and increases the tone of the underlying skeletal muscles.
  - It is done by tapping over the belly of muscles with finger tips.
  - 3-5 times over the muscle to be facilitated.
- *Vestibular stimulation:* According to De Quiros JB vestibular stimulation is a powerful proprioceptive input.

  Therapeutic uses:
  - To promote extensor patterns of the neck, trunk and extremities (Static labyrinthine system).
  - To elicit subcortical responses, such as protective extension.
  - To activate antigravity muscles and their antagonist.
  - Fast stimulation such as rocking stimulates while slow rhythmic rocking causes relaxation.
  - Vestibular stimulation affects tone, balance, protective responses, bilateral integration and auditory language development.
- *Vibration:*
  - Frequency—High frequency—100 to 300 cycles/second.

    Low frequency—50 to 60 cycles/second.

    Uses:

    High frequency vibration is used to elicit tonic vibration reflex which stimulates contraction of muscle if applied directly over the belly. It also inhibits contraction of antagonist muscle and suppress stretch reflex.

    Low frequency vibration suppress pain perception, desensitize hypersensitive skin.

    Other factors:

    Vibration should be applied parallel to muscle fibers.

    Do not apply vibration over tendon, it may stimulate surrounding muscle through bone.

    Do not apply vibration with deep pressure as it is inhibitory.

    Duration of application should not be more than 1 to 2 minutes (to avoid heat formation).
- *Osteopressure:* It is defined as pressure on bony prominences to facilitate or inhibit voluntary muscles.

  According to Margaret Rood, osteopressure produces a slower reaction and needs to be preceded by a light moving touch.

  For e.g., If light moving touch is applied to dermatome C_7 of the arm and pressure applied over the lateral epicondyle of the elbow, the arm extends.

  The underlying neurophysiology has not been understood properly.
- *Inhibition Techniques:* According to Rood following techniques may be used for inhibiting abnormal tone.
  - Gentle shaking or rocking.
  - Slow rolling.
  - Light joint compression.
  - Tendinous pressure.
  - Maintained stretch.
  - Rocking in developmental pattern.
- *Use of special senses for inhibition/facilitation:* M. Rood used olfactory and gustatory stimuli to facilitate cranial nerves and to influence.

  Autonomic nervous system: Though she did not provide specific guidelines for their uses: Clinically following can be used:
  - Pleasant orders for calming effect.
  - Unpleasant order to produce primitive protective responses.
  - Noxious substances (such as vinegar) for activating muscles of mastication.

BRUNNSTROM'S APPROACH

INTRODUCTION

Brunnstrom approach or movement was given by sign Brunnstrom, a physical therapist in the year 1970.

This approach is exclusively for the patients with cerebrovascular accidents or stroke.

Principles

1. Reflexes and whole-limb movement patterns are normal stages of development. In stroke, development occurs in reverse pattern.
2. Reflexes and primitive movement patterns should be used to facilitate the recovery of voluntary movement after stroke.
3. Proprioceptive and other somatosensory stimuli can be used to facilitate movement or tonal changes.
4. Recovery in stroke patient takes place in following sequence:

Mass movement
↓
Stereotyped flexor/extensor movement pattern, i.e., SYNERGY
↓
Combination of two pattern
↓
Discrete movements of each joint

5. New correct movements achieved, must be practiced to be learned.
6. Treatment progresses in following sequence.

Reflex movement
↓
Voluntary movement
↓
Functional movement

7. If voluntary effort leads to a response, the following sequence of contraction should be practiced:

Isometric (hold)
↓
Eccentric (controlled lengthening)
↓
Concentric (shortening)

8. Reduce or wean off facilitation as soon as patient shows evidence of voluntary control.
9. Correct elicited movement, repeat to learn it.
10. Practice should include functional activities.

Definition of Terms

Synergy—is a movement pattern in which a group of muscles acting as a bound unit in a primitive and stereotypical manner.

The muscles are neurophysiologically linked and cannot act alone or perform all of their function. If one muscle in the synergy is activated, each muscle in the synergy responds partially or completely.

Associated reactions—are movements seen on the affected side in response to voluntary forceful movements in other parts of the body.

Homolateral limb synkinesis—is a mutual dependency between the synergies of the affected upper and lower limb. Similar type of movement occurs in affected upper and lower limb.

Limitation synkinesis—are associated reactions that facilitate the performance of difficult movement by performing the same movement on the opposite side.

Proximal traction response—is elicited by a stretch to the flexors muscles of one joint of upper limb which evokes contraction of all flexors of that limb including the fingers.

Grasp reflex—When deep pressure is applied to the palm and move distally over the hand and fingers, mostly on the radial side, adduction and flexion of fingers occur.

Instinctive grasp reaction—It is a closure of hand in response to contact of a stationary object with palm of the hand.

Instinctive avoiding reaction—A hyperextension reaction of the fingers and thumb in response to forward-upward elevation of the arm.

Souque's phenomenon—It is the automatic extension of the fingers when the shoulder is flexed.

It can be seen in only few patients though the position is helpful in facilitation of finger extension.

Ramiste's phenomenon—are associated reactions of hip abduction on an adduction. Resistance to hip abduction or adduction of the non involved extremity evokes the same movement of the involved extremity.

Components of Limb Synergies

Upper Extremity Flexor Synergy

It usually develops before the extensor synergy and composed of:

- Scapular retraction and/or elevation.
- Shoulder abduction and external rotation.
- Elbow flexion.
- Forearm supination.
- Wrist and finger—variable position elbow flexion is the strongest component movement to appear or to be facilitated. Shoulder abduction and external rotation are weak components.

Upper Extremity Extensor Synergy

Composed of:

- Scapular protraction.
- Shoulder horizontal adduction and internal rotation.
- Elbow extension.
- Forearm pronation.
- Wrist and finger—variable position.

Shoulder horizontal adduction and internal rotation are the strongest components of this synergy. They are the first movements to appear and to be facilitated. Elbow extension is a weak component.

Lower Extremity Flexor Synergy

Composed of:

- Hip flexion, abduction and external rotation.
- Knee flexion.
- Ankle dorsiflexion and inversion.

Hip flexion is the strongest component whereas hip abduction and external rotation are weak components.

Lower Extremity Extensor Synergy

This synergy usually dominates in the lower extremity and composed of:

- Hip extension adduction and internal rotation.
- Knee extension.
- Ankle plantar flexion and inversion.
- Toes dorsiflexion.

Hip adduction, knee extension, ankle plantar flexion with inversion are all strong component. This synergy is dominant in standing position.

Typical Arm Posture

When both synergies are developing and spasticity is marked, the strongest components of the flexion and extension synergies sometimes combine to produce typical upper limb posture in hemiplegia. The arm is adducted and internally rotated with the elbow flexed, forearm pronated and the wrist and fingers flexed.

Stages of Motor Recovery

Signe Brunnstrom observed that patient progresses through a series of recovery stages in a stereotypical fashion (Table 19.1).

Table 19.1: Stages of motor recovery in hemiplegia

Stage	*Characteristics*		
	Leg	**Arm**	**Hand***
1.	Flaccidity.	Flaccidity; inability to perform any movements.	No hand function.
2.	Spasticity develops; minimal voluntary movements.	Beginning development of spasticity; limb synergies or some of their components begin to appear as associated reactions.	Gross grasp beginning; minimal finger flexion possible.
3.	Spasticity peaks; flexion and extension synergy present; hip-knee-ankle flexion in sitting and standing.	Spasticity increasing; synergy patterns or some of their components can be performed voluntarily.	Gross grasp, hook grasp possible; no release.
4.	Knee flexion past 90° in sitting, with foot sliding backward on floor; dorsiflexion with heel on floor and knee flexed to 90°.	Spasticity declining; movement combinations deviating from synergies are now possible.	Gross grasp present; lateral prehension developing, small amount of finger extension and some thumb movement possible.
5.	Knee flexion with hip extended in standing; ankle dorsiflexion with hip and knee extended.	Synergies no longer dominant; more movement combinations deviating from synergies performed with greater care.	Palmar prehension, spherical and cylindrical grasp and release possible.
6.	Hip abduction in sitting or standing; reciprocal internal and external rotation of hip combined with inversion and eversion of ankle in sitting.	Spasticity absent except when performing rapid movement; isolated joint movements performed with care.	All types of prehension, individual finger motion, and full range of voluntary extension possible.

From Brunnstrom S: Movement therapy in hemiplegia. New York, 1970, Harper and Row.

Evaluation

Evaluation for Brunnstrom's approach includes following:

- Evaluation of sensory status of the patient.
- Level of recovery.
- Voluntary motor control.
- Influence of Reflexes and associated reactions.

S. Brunnstrom gave *Hemiplegia classification and progress record,* but no data exists for its reliability support. Fugl Meyer *et al.* (1975) developed *The Fugl-Meyer Motor Test* whose reliability were determined to be strong and significant.

Goal of Brunnstrom's Approach

The main goal of this approach is to facilitate the patient's progress through the recovery stages that occur after the stroke.

The following techniques can be used to achieve this goal (Table 19.2).

Table 19.2: Techniques
• Postural and attitudinal reflexes (such as tonic neck reflex, equilibrium and protective reactions etc.).
• Associated reaction.
• Homolateral limb synkinesis.
• Limitation synkinesis.
• Proximal traction response.
• Grasp reflex.
• Instinctive grasp reaction.
• Instinctive avoiding reaction.
• Souque's phenomenon.
• Ramiste's phenomenon.
• Resistance.
• Auditory stimuli (e.g., verbal cues).
• Sensory stimulus (e.g., rubbing/stroking skin over the muscle).
• Visual stimuli (e.g., use of mirror).

Treatment

1. *Bed positioning:*
   - Proper positioning begins immediately after the onset of the stroke when the patient is in the flaccid stage.
   - Limbs should be placed in the most favorable position without interference from the hypertonic muscles.
   - In absence of proper bed positioning the lower limb tends to assume a position of hip external rotation, abduction and knee flexion (due to weight of the limb, position is like flexor synergy of lower limb).
   - In case, the extensor synergy dominates in lower limb, the recommended position is:
     - Supine.
     - Slight flexion of hip and knee (use towel or pillow).
     - Later support of leg by towel roll or pillow or sand bag to prevent external rotation and abduction.
     - Ankle supported for neutral position.
   - In case, the flexor synergy dominates in lower limb, the recommended position is:
     - Supine.
     - Knee in extension.
     - Hip external rotation should be prevented as described earlier.
   - The affected upper limb is supported on a pillow in a position that is comfortable for the patient. Abduction of humerus must be avoided. Patient is instructed to use the unaffected hand to support the affected arm when moving in bed.

2. *Bed mobility:*
   - Turning toward the affected side is easier than turning toward the unaffected side.
   - To turn toward the unaffected side, the affected upper limb is grasped by the unaffected hand, both the limbs are elevated upto 80°-90° of shoulder flexion with elbow extended. The affected lower limb is in slight flexion at hip and knee (supported by therapist). Patient turns an unaffected side by swinging the arms and the affected knee across the body towards the unaffected side. The momentum produced by upper limb helps in turning upper body and pelvis.

   As the patient develops control therapist support is withdrawn.

3. *Trunk control:*
   - To improve trunk control, the patient is gently pushed in forward, backward and side to side direction in sitting position.
   - First push towards the affected side to promote contraction on unaffected side then towards the unaffected side to facilitate contraction on affected side.

- Improve control in all directions—trunk flexion, extension and rotation.
- Patient crosses his arms with unaffected hand under the involved elbow and unaffected forearm supports the affected forearm. Therapist sitting in front of patient, supports the patient under the elbow and assists in trunk flexion (avoid any pull on the shoulders). This movement is also helpful in causing some amount of pain free movement of shoulder unconsciously.
- Trunk rotation is facilitated by using tonic neck and tonic lumbar reflexes.

4. *Upper limb training.*
5. *Hand training.*
6. *Lower limb training.*

Guidelines for Treatment

Following are the guidelines given by signe Brunnstrom for treating upper extremity, hand, trunk and lower extremity during various stages.

Upper Extremity

a. *During stages 1 and 2:* The aim of treatment is to elicit muscle tone and the synergy patterns on a reflex basis.
   - To elicit flexor synergy, tap over the upper and middle trapezius, rhomboids and biceps.
   - To elicit extensory synergy tap over the triceps and stretch serratus anterior.
   - Passive movement through each of the synergy pattern.
   - Elicit flexor synergy first which should be followed by facilitation of the weak extension synergy.

b. *Stage 3:* The aim of treatment is to achieve:
   - Voluntary control for the synergy pattern.
   - Repeat alternate performance of synergy patterns.
   - Weight bearing.
   - Use bilateral rowing movements with therapist hold the patient's hands.

c. *Stages 4 and 5:* The aim of treatment is to break away from the synergies by mixing components from antagonistic synergies to perform new and complex patterns of movement:
   - Perform figure of 8 movement on table or board.
   - Following flexion movements can be performed to promote transition between stages 3 and 4.
     - Hand to chin.
     - Hand to ear (first affected then on the unaffected side).
     - Hand to opposite elbow.
     - Hand to opposite shoulder.
     - Hand to forehead.
     - Hand to top of head.
     - Hand to back of head.
   - Other complex movements which represents stage 4, may also be practiced.

     For stage 4:
     - Arm to rear of body.
     - Arm raising forward to horizontal position.
     - Pronation—supination of forearms with elbows flexed.

     For stage 5:
     - Arm raising to side horizontal position.
     - Turning palms up and down, elbows extended.

d. *Stage 6:* Very few patients reached to this stage of upper limb. No specific training method is recommended.

Hand Training

Main objectives of hand training are:

- Achieve mass grasp by using proximal traction response and grasp reflex.
- Achieve wrist fixation for wrist. Facilitate wrist extension by tapping and fist closure simultaneously.
- Achieve active release of grasp:
  - This goal is difficult to achieve due to marked spasticity in finger flexors. Manipulation for active release of grasp—pull the thumb out of the palm, by gripping the thenar eminence while supinating the forearm passively.
  - Roll fingers into flexion to stretch extensors.
  - Pronate forearm while maintaining thumb extension.
  - Use Sougue's phenomenon.
  - Stroke over the interphalangeal joints.
  - Reinforce by individually stretching the finger extensors of each digit.

Trunk

- To elicit balance responses, patient is gently pushed in forward, backward and sideward directions.

- First push toward the affected side (to develop control on non affected side) then toward the non affected side (to develop control on involved side).
- Practice forward flexion of trunk by crossing arms with the non-affected hand under the affected elbow and the non-affected forearm supporting the affected forearm. Therapist may assist by supporting the patient under elbows. This also helps in achieving some pain free movement of shoulder.
- Return from trunk flexion position is actively performed by the patient (without therapist's support).
- Practice forward movement in oblique direction.
- Practice trunk rotation, first with therapist supporting the affected limb then without support.

(Tonic neck and tonic lumbar reflexes can also be used to facilitate the response).

The basic principles for training of lower extremity follows the following sequence:

1. If voluntary control is absent in any movement or position, contraction of muscle is elicited reflexively.
2. Superimpose voluntary effort on the reflex contraction.
3. Use local facilitatory measures to reinforce the patient's voluntary effort.
4. Use the activated muscle in desired situation.

BOBATH APPROACH

INTRODUCTION

Berta Busse (physical therapist) and Karel Bobath (pediatric physician) born in Berlin, Germany, they practiced in London and developed Bobath concepts there.

Bobath has never conducted original research but hypothesized with the popular findings at the time and tried to explain the various theories.

Berta, during her practice, she observed and analyzed the normal movements and methods of relaxation of the muscles. The assessment of the muscle strength, activity of the muscles and their response to special relaxation methods formed the basis of her for abnormal motor coordination patients. She analyzed posture and movements, then practiced them variation until she learned how individuals perfected them. Her hands developed a great sensitivity to a muscle tone, its readiness to move and responsiveness to change.

Neural Development Technique (NDT) focuses on the analysis and treatment of sensorimotor impairments and functional limitations. This is a living concept, a problem solving approach that consists treatment and management of movements dysfunctions in individual with central nervous system pathophysiology.

Concepts

Following a cerebrovascular accident patient typically overuses the uninvolved side due to impaired sensory and motor function on the hemiplegic side. This also adds to posture, balance, strength, tone and coordination disturbances.

In Bobath approach the therapist develops a program to help the patient to avoid abnormal patterns of movement. This approach provides a foundation that promotes the highest level of functional recovery based on relearning normal movement rather than as compensation. One of the central principles of this approach is that alignment and symmetry of the trunk and pelvis are necessary for good alignment and symmetry of the extremities.

Patients with hemiplegia (stroke) exhibit abnormally high or low tone, which has to be inhibited or facilitated respectively.

Theories

Following are the various theories Bobath used for their clinical findings:

1. Reflex/Hierarchical Model.
2. System Theory.
3. Dynamic System Approach.
4. Neuronal Group Selection Theory.

Reflex/Hierarchical Model

It was developed by Jackson. Bobath used this to the maximum at the early stages. This theory states that a lesion in the higher centers would permit expression of normally suppressed patterns of movements which would then dominate the person's posture and movement. Bobath believed and thought that the CNS is organised as a hierarchy and divided into four functional levels of integration.

- Level 1 : Spinal level—Phasic, Primitive reflexes, stretch reflexes.
- Level 2 : Pre pontine/Brainstem—Local, segmental, general tonic reflexes, mass synergies.
- Level 3 : Midbrain—Righting and protective reactions, excitatory and inhibitory control.
- Level 4 : Cortical level—Balance and equilibrium reactions or decrease voluntary control.

These four successive higher levels of neural integrative exert control over the preceding levels. Each level made use of the centrally controlled inhibition so that higher centres have the ability to suppress all but they require part of any intended movement.

The lower centres surrender their autonomy to the higher level during humankind's development. This rigid model is generally being discarded today for in favor of more flexible models.

System Theory in NDT

Nicoli Bernstein a physiologist developed this theory. According to this motor behavior is an end product of a process of self organization of the body system which is not limited to the CNS alone. He has termed a "coordinative structure" because whenever two or more independent parts combine to perform as a functional unit or synergy they act as a unit.

Nicoli states that biological organisms, like other physical systems, are complex, multi-dimensional, cooperative systems in which no one system has a priority for organizing the behavior of the system. In this framework the task and the context of the behaviour becomes equally important parts of the system.

Dynamic System Approach

This is the extension of system theory, incorporating ideas of how complex system work together within physical world. It has emphasized more on the environment and body system as a strategies of intervention. This theory does not seem to support manual guiding and facilitating movement as a strategy for gaining the best movement possible for individual with motor dysfunction.

Neuronal Group Selection Theory

The dynamic theory is extended by Edelman (1987) and Sporns (1994) by offering a balance between maturation and interactive physical systems.

The theory explains that the recovery of the damaged brain can be fasten or achieved:

1. If the individual is engaged in activities that occur in functionally or developmentally appropriate environmental context; and
2. If he or she is allowed to perform the movements which are required for specific tasks.

The Principles of NDT

- The individual should be seen as a whole person with a whole personality.
- A proper evaluation and assessment must be done based on observations and feeling the individual's responses.
- Treatment programmes are tailor made to meet the needs of the individual.
- Reassessment of the individual's responses to treatment is immediate and ongoing. Modifications are made immediately according to that.
- Key points of control are used during treatment to inhibit abnormal movement patterns and facilitate normal movement.
- The Physical Therapist, Occupational Therapist and Speech Therapist must work with the family and teach them how to manage the individual in functional activities, which is essential for effective treatment.
- The normal movements should not be superimposed on abnormal tone.
- All voluntary movements have automatic components.

Normalization of muscle tone may be accomplished by using one or more of the following techniques:

1. Weight-bearing over the affected side.
2. Trunk rotation.
3. Scapular protraction.
4. Anterior pelvic tilt.
5. Facilitation of slow, controlled movements.
6. Proper positioning.

Weight-bearing over the affected side: It is the most effective way of normalizing tone. With patients exhibiting low tone it is facilitative and with patients exhibiting high tone it can be inhibitory. It is helpful in normalization of tone and providing sensory input to the hemiplegic side through proprioception.

Trunk rotation: It is another very effective way of normalization of tone and facilitating normal movement through the upper and lower extremity patients with hemiplegia usually move as a log or block without dissociation. Trunk rotation is helpful in breaking seen non dissociated movement.

Scapular protraction: It is beneficial for patients exhibiting a flexion synergy of the upper extremity.

Anterior pelvic tilt: The posterior pelvic tilt is a position in which patients are usually seen. This position encourages abnormal posture resulting in increased hip extension, kyphosis of upper thoracic region and head and neck extension.

All these can be managed by position the pelvic forward.

Facilitation of slow, controlled movements: It is beneficial for high tone patients. It has been seen that quick movements increase the tone therefore it is recommended to use slower and more controlled movement.

Proper positioning: Abnormal postures promote compensatory movement and should be avoided. Proper positioning is very important during all the stages especially in the acute stage.

In Sitting:

- Feet flat on the floor.
- Hips near 90° of flexion.
- Knees and ankles less than 90° of flexion.
- Trunk extended.
- Head in midline and arm fully supported when working at the table.

In Standing:

- Head should be in midline.
- Trunk symmetric.
- Weight equally distributed on both lower extremity.

MOTOR RELEARNING PROGRAM

INTRODUCTION

The Motor Relearning Program was developed by Australian physical therapists Roberta Carr and Janet Shepherd (1983) from their clinical experience and extensive review of contemporary movement science theory and research.

Characteristics of Motor Relearning Program (MRP)

1. Based on skill acquisition and motor development theories especially cognitive motor learning theory.
2. Considers factors other than central nervous system (CNS) damage that may be affecting performance.
3. Includes remediation of impairment and modification of environment.
4. Stresses on practice that fits the nature of the task.
5. Rejects assumptions of the reflex hierarchical model of motor control and of the traditional developmental theories.

Theoretical Basis of MRP

The Rood, Bobath, Brunnstrom and Proprioceptive neuromuscular facilitation (PNF) approaches are based on a hierarchical model of motor control, which predicts that dysfunction in the motor cortex results in a release from inhibition of the more primitive brainstem and spinal networks. Treatment focuses on decreasing abnormal reflex activity and primitive movement patterns to facilitate normal movement.

Latest theories in movement science emphasize a distributed control, approach rather than a hierarchical model of motor control. According to this new model motor control depends upon number of structures in the central nervous system. Spinal level structures do not completely depend on higher centres for direct movement commands. Other hemispheric structures prepare the motor system to respond most efficiently to changing environment and task demands.

MRP is based on distributed control model and emphasize the interaction between the performer and the environment.

Interaction with environment for motor performance can better be understood by considering an example. Suppose a person wants to reach forward with one arm, reaching forward would depend upon many factors: the person's posture (sitting, standing, kneeling) and postural alignment, the shape and stability of the seat or supporting surface, how far away and in what direction the goal object is located and the presence of any obstacles between the individual and the goal object.

Motor performance skill of any task depends on the ability to perform the task in number of manners. Research has shown that simply practising movements in isolation of a goal or functional task will not lead to skill development. (Higgins and Spaeth 1972, Smyth 1984).

Carr and Shepherd emphasized on following issues which forms the foundation of Motor Relearning Program:

1. ***Postural adjustments:*** It is defined as automatic, anticipatory and ongoing muscle activation that enables an individual to maintain balance against gravity, optimal alignment between body parts and optimal orientation of the head, trunk and limbs in relation to the environment.

   It was advocated that postural adjustments can be learned only in the context of task performance. Furthermore, balance training in one position or for one task cannot be generalized to other position or for other task. That is postural adjustments has to be taught in various positions and number of tasks.
2. ***Compensator strategies:*** These are motor patterns or fixations which develop in response to obstructions to normal movement to enable an individual to achieve short-term success in movement or balance.

   Effects of compensatory strategies may be reduced by:

   a. *Prevention of abnormal muscle shortening:*
      - Postural education.
      - Proper posture in lying, sitting and standing.
      - Practice variety of motor tasks.

      For e.g., Standing up from sitting position with dorsiflexed ankle, several times a day would prevent shortening of gastrocnemius.

   b. *Prevention of fixation patterns:* Normally when we do tasks like skating or cycling for first time we contract maximum number of body muscles (especially flexors and extensors of trunk) to maintain our balance in posturally threatening situations. Similarly patients with neurological deficits use this pattern in normal day-to-day task. Most commonly fixation patterns used by such patients are pelvis-on-lumbar spine and scapula-on-thorax. The consequences of these patterns are difficulty in dissociating pelvis or scapula from their respective adjacent structures and lack of mobility of the limbs girdles limiting normal kinematics of upper and lower extremity.

Motor relearning program stressed on prevention of such patterns by early introduction of training for balance and posture control.

c. *Prevention of muscle weakness:* Motor Relearning Program encourages therapists to "actively search for and detect small amounts of muscle activity as soon as they occur" (Carr and Shepherd 1987). MRP proposes following therapeutic interventions to counteract muscle weakness.
   - Various positions of task performance to improve condition of muscle length and assisstive use of gravity.
   - Educate patient about inefficient compensations and avoiding unnecessary muscle activity.
   - Provide manual guidance to direct patient's performance of task.

3. ***Analysis of normal motor performance of functional tasks:*** One of the important assumption of MRP is that systematic research on how average people perform motor activities can provide a framework from the treatment of physically impaired patients who must relearn what were once habitual, every day tasks. But research on analysis of normal human performance is limited.

   Tools like video cameras, force plate sensors, gait analyser and electromyographic polygraphs can be used to analyse such performance.

4. ***Motor learning:*** Motor learning has been defined as a set of processes associated practice or experience leading to relatively permanent changes in the capability for producing skilled action (Schimd tRA). This definition of motor learning reflects four concepts:
   a. Learning is a process of acquiring the capability for skilled action.
   b. Learning results from experience or practice.
   c. Learning cannot be measured directly.
   d. Learning produces relatively permanent changes in behaviour, thus short-term alterations are not thought of as learning.

   The motor relearning program has a significant different approach to motor learning from the previous approaches designed to improve motor control.

   It was assumed that practice of an exercise will generalize into improved performance of functional activity. But research does not approve this assumption. Therefore MRP proposes use of exercise with functional goal and varied context.

   Approaches like PNF assumes that development takes place in a proper sequence (e.g., rolling → crawling → sitting → standing) as in infants. This forms the foundation for therapy in developing motor control for adult patients. To develop motor control one should follow the proper sequence by developing earlier pattern one would have good control over advanced pattern.

   For e.g., If patient develops good control over sitting it would aid him to develop good control in standing.

   But MRP does not follow a developmental sequence. The MRP also disagree those who suggests that therapeutic intervention should proceed in a proximal to distal sequence.

   For e.g., While working on shoulder girdle, MRP encourages to work on hands, also through functional task.

   In nutshell, previous therapeutic interventions for individuals with neurological deficits have focused on the patient as a recipient of facilitation and inhibition techniques provided by the therapist. In the MRP, the patient is an active participant in learning how to move functionally and to solve problem during performing functional task.

Therapeutic Intervention

The Motor Relearning Program provides guidelines for evaluating and improving motor control in seven functional daily activities:

1. Upper limb function.
2. Orofacial function.
3. Sitting up over the side of the bed.
4. Balanced sitting.
5. Standing up and sitting down.
6. Balanced standing.
7. Walking.

Carr and Shepherd do not propose any specific sequence for intervention among these seven functional categories. A four-step sequence may be followed to improve skill in a selected function:

Step 1 : Analysis of task
(Observation, comparison).

Step 2 : Practice of missing components
(Explanation of goal, visual and verbal feedback, manual guidance).

Step 3 : Practice of functional task

(Explanation of goal, visual and verbal feedback, manual guidance, Re-evaluation).

Step 4 : Transference of training

(Varied context, consistent practice, modification of environment, involvement of family members).

Guidelines for Evaluation

Detailed analysis of patient's performance of tasks within each of the seven categories of daily activities. The therapist observes the patient as he performs each task and then compares his performance with the normal performance associated with the task. Therapist should be keen observer and try to note the following:

1. Any missing components such as a lack of anterior pelvic tilt and hip flexion when rising to stand.
2. The absence of specific muscle activity.
3. The presence of any excessive or inappropriate muscle activity.
4. Compensatory motor behaviour such as hip-hiking during walking.
5. Incorrect timing of components within a movement pattern.

Guidelines for Treatment

The key to therapy is to adapt the task or the environment so that the person can achieve successful performance without compensation.

1. A functional task which is challenging yet attainable without any compensatory strategy, is selected and clearly explained to the patient.
2. Therapist modifies the patient's position and position of goal objects to match the level of motor as per the patient's capabilities.
3. The supporting surface on which the patient sits or stands is also carefully selected as per patient's postural control.
4. The MRP recommends five strategies for teaching the patient what he needs to learn:
   a. Verbal instruction.
   b. Visual demonstration:
      - by therapist.
      - with unaffected side/body parts of the patient.
   c. Manual guidance.
   d. Feedback:
      - About quality of performance of task.
      - Should be timely and accurate.
      - Should inform about movements to be repeated and movements to be avoided.
      - Positive feedback should be genuine.
   e. Consistent practice.
5. Movement component learned should be practised with complete functional task.

   For e.g., Component of bearing weight in elbow extended position should be incorporated in sitting to stand.
6. Once learned a task should be practised in varied context and different environmental and real life situation.

   For e.g., If a patient has learned to reach a glass on table, same task should be practised with cup in different position, at home, with friends etc.

Limitation of MRP

The MRP can't be applicable to patients with severe cognitive deficits which is not uncommon manifestation of stroke and other neurological conditions.

CONCLUSION

In conclusion the MRP is still relatively new and has some inconsistencies between its theoretical basis and actual clinical practice. Carr and Shepherd repeatedly emphasized on functional and goal oriented activities. They state and that they do not consider spasticity to be a significant problem of stroke and they give no recommendations for reducing abnormal tone.

20

THERAPEUTIC APPROACHES IN ORTHOPEDIC CONDITIONS

PROGRESSIVE RESISTIVE EXERCISE (PRE)

Progressive resistance exercise was developed by De Lorme, which is based on 10 repetition maximum (RM). He first executed it on soldiers suffering from muscle weakness following second world war due to musculoskeletal injuries. A set of exercises was repeated 7 to 10 times per treatment session for five days a week. On the last day of the week (Friday) 10 RM was calculated and new exercise programme introduced for the next week. De Lorme called this method "Heavy Resistance Exercises".

The muscles strengthened by him were not disused but had lost strength from disuse. Later he implemented same exercises on poliomyelitis.

In 1948 De Lorme revised his original method and adopted the name progressive resistance exercise (PRE) because he believed the original name bore false implications since even muscles which could not contract against the force of gravity could be strengthened by this method.

Repetition Maximum (RM)

It is used in PRE to measure the strength of the given muscle, so that the muscle can be strengthened onward to its available strength.

For example:

- 1 RM-is the maximum amount of resistance or load that can be lifted only once through available range of motion.
- 2 RM-is the maximum amount of resistance or load that can be lifted twice through available range of motion.
- 10 RM-is the maximum amount of resistance or load that can be lifted ten times through available range of motion.

Assessment of RM (*For example quadriceps muscles*)

Apparatus—Quadriceps table, De Lorme Boot and straps.

Procedure—The patient is asked to sit in quadriceps table with proper back support, thigh is stabilized with straps. Hands should not be allowed to do any trick movements. De Lorme boot is attached with straps at just above ankle joint. Therapist manually assesses the strength of the quadriceps (which gives hypothesis that this patient can lift this much of weight). Then the weight is attached to the De Lorme boot and patient is asked to lift it in full range of motion. If patient lifts it easily then more weight is applied and patient lifts the weight. This involves a series of single repetition with progressively heavier weight until the 1 RM is achieved (Suppose 20 kg weight is lifted by the patient initially, then weight is increased to 20.5 kg and allowed to lift it through available range of motion, if it can also be lifted through full range of motion, weight is increased further to 21 kg and if this time patient is unable to extend it through available range of motion it means the 1 RM of this patient is 20.5 kg or this patient can extend the leg with 20.5 kg of weight once only in the prescribed or available range of motion.

The 10 RM is calculated by using the same method in which weight is applied to the De Lorme Boot and patient is allowed to extend the leg with the weight 10 times through available range of motion. The weight is increased progressively till the 10 RM is achieved (For example leg is extended with 10 kg for 10 times, if it can be lifted, weight is increased and leg is allowed to extend 10 times and is continued till 10 RM is obtained).

RM assessment is done following warm up exercises (cycling, jogging, push ups etc.) to prevent injuries to the muscles.

The following schemes are generally used in daily clinical practice by the therapist and trainers.

1. *De Lorme and Watkins*
   - 10 lifts with 1/2 10 RM
   - 10 lifts with 3/4 10 RM

- 10 lifts with full 10 RM

30 lifts for four times a week, progress 10 RM once weekly. Every 10 repetition.

2. *Mac Queen*
   - 10 lifts with 10 RM
   - 10 lifts with 10 RM
   - 10 lifts with 10 RM
   - 10 lifts with 10 RM

   Progress 10 RM every 1-2 weeks.

3. *Zinovief (Oxford Technique)*
   - 10 lifts with 10 RM
   - 10 lifts with 10 RM minus 1 lb
   - 10 lifts with 10 RM minus 2 lb
   - 10 lifts with 10 RM minus 3 lb
   - 10 lifts with 10 RM minus 4 lb
   - 10 lifts with 10 RM minus 5 lb
   - 10 lifts with 10 RM minus 6 lb
   - 10 lifts with 10 RM minus 7 lb
   - 10 lifts with 10 RM minus 8 lb
   - 10 lifts with 10 RM minus 9 lb

     100 lifts for five times a week, progress 10 RM daily.
   - Every 10 lifts/repetitions are followed by brief period of rest.

HEAVY RESISTANCE EXERCISES

These exercises were first described by De Lorme in 1945 and used to restore the muscular power and volume after injuries. Athletes, sports persons and body builders use these exercises to increase the muscle girth and strength. Metal weights are generally used to apply resistance against the muscular effort after calculating the repetition maximum (RM). The resistance varies from individual to individual, age and the condition from which he or she is suffering.

PLYOMETRIC EXERCISES

It is the quick, powerful movement in which muscle or group of muscles contract eccentrically which is immediately followed by concentric contraction of the same muscle or group of muscles. For example during running or jumping when toes comes in the contact with the ground the gastro-soleus muscles contract first eccentrically than followed by concentric contraction (Figs. 20.1a to c).

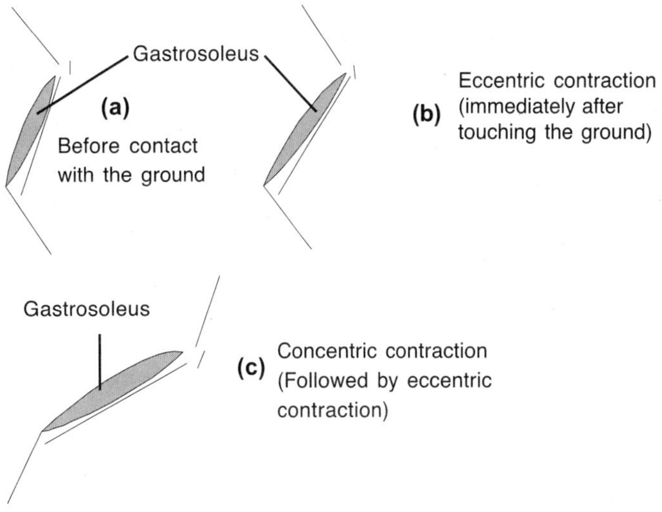

Figs. 20.1a to c: Plyometric exercise

During the eccentric contraction (stretch phase), the work performance is enhanced by storing elastic energy in the muscles and during concentric contraction it is reused as mechanical work. This mechanical work is stored in the sarcomere cross bridges and can be reused during the following positive work if the muscles are contracted immediately after the stretch. The timing of the eccentric and concentric contractions, the velocity, and magnitude of stretch determines the ability of muscle to use the stored energy. A quick transition from eccentric to concentric contraction along with a high-velocity stretch of high magnitude produces the greatest benefits.

Bosco and colleagues found that the amount of elastic energy stored in a muscle during eccentric work determines the recoil of elastic energy during positive work.

Plyometric exercises are used to increase the reactivity of the nervous system and enhance the work performance. Before starting plyometric exercises an individual or athlete should undergo advanced exercise programme to build up muscle power, strength and endurance, because plyometric exercises are high level activities in which the muscle (mostly tendon part) is more susceptible to overuse injury.

Uses: Generally used for athletic training.

CLOSED AND OPEN KINETIC CHAIN EXERCISES OR TRAINING

Closed Kinetic Chain (CKC) Training

It is a method of exercise in which the distal segment is fixed and meets considerable external resistance, which prohibits or restrains its free motion. For example both feet (distal segment of the lower extremity) remain on the ground during partial squat to standing or *vice-versa*. The distal segment remains fixed while multiple proximal joints move in a functional manner with contraction of both agonist and antagonists for stabilization.

Examples of closed kinetic chain in upper extremity are–using the upper extremity to perform a wheel chair to bed transfer and push ups.

Closed kinetic chain exercises are more function-based and used for sport-specific muscle group. For example squating involves series of cocontraction of various muscles such as quadriceps, hamstrings, gastrocnemius, and gluteus maximus, which require in many sports and general activities.

Although most of the scientific literatures concerning CKC activities is focussed on quadriceps rehabilitation after anterior cruciate ligament reconstruction, contrasting research by Hungerford and Barry evaluated patellofemoral contact pressure areas during open kinetic chain exercises and closed kinetic chain exercises.

During closed kinetic chain exercises the cocontraction of the quadriceps and hamstrings decrease the anterior shear force in the knee joint and avoids any stress upon the maturing anterior cruciate ligament (ACL) graft. These exercises (CKC) are safe to start in the first week of the ACL reconstruction because they generate low anterior tibial displacement and put the ACL graft at the lower risk for developing laxity. And this is the only reason why closed kinetic chain exercises favoured over open kinetic chain exercises after ACL reconstruction.

The cocontraction of quadriceps and hamstrings occurs in CKC exercises, with a progressive decrease in the hamstrings activity as the flexion angle of the knee increases, therefore CKC exercises should be limited to mini squat.

In lower extremities closed kinetic chain exercises appear to be more functional than open-kinetic chain exercises (OKC). During squating simultaneous extension occurs at the knee joint and hip joint. As a result of this movement, the rectus femoris muscle contracts concentrically (shortening) at the knee joint while at the same time it contracts eccentrically (lengthening) at the hip joint. Conversely, the hamstrings contract eccentrically (lengthening) at the knee joint and simultaneously contract concentrically across the hip joint. Therefore CKC causes concentric and eccentric contraction of the rectus femoris from half squat to standing and concentric and eccentric contraction of hamstring from standing to half squating. The concentric and same eccentric contractions at opposite ends of the muscle produce a pseudoisometric contraction. This type of contraction is used during functional activities such as walking, stair climbing, running and jumping and cannot be reproduced by isolated open kinetic chain (OKC) knee flexion and extension exercises.

Open Kinetic Chain Training

It is a method of exercise in which the distal segment of the extremity is free to move. *For example,* strengthening of quadriceps muscle on quadriceps table where the end segment of the extremity moves freely. In upper extremity such as throwing, strengthening of elbow flexors with dumbbell are the examples of open kinetic chain exercises. The open kinetic chain exercises are more useful in upper extremity as most of the functions are performed in open kinetic chain form.

Open kinetic chain exercises are recommended, especially in the intermediate phase of "bulking up" a severely atrophied muscle before more functional closed chain work is attempted (or along with low-weight closed chain work that emphasizes proper technique and mechanics).

For the upper extremities, open kinetic chain exercises are essential before return to sport because these exercises are similar to the limb movements used in most sports (e.g., the throwing motion).

MUSCLE ENERGY TECHNIQUES (METs)

The muscle energy techniques are derived from the osteopathy field and now being used most widely by clinician in the field of physiotherapy, orthopedic and osteopathic medicine.

The variety of terms are used to describe the muscle energy techniques—According to:

- Liebenson, 1989 the muscle energy techniques are the "active muscular techniques of relaxation".
- Fred Mitcell Junior, 1958, son of Fred Mitchell Senior M (known for his incredible efforts into osteopathic field)—The patient uses his or her on request, from a precisely controlled position in a specific direction against a distinctly executed counter force.

Thus the muscle energy techniques are the muscle relaxation techniques in which manual resistance is applied against the active contraction of the muscle in the form of isometric or isotonic contraction which may be followed by gentle stretch.

Uses and Indications of METs

1. Severe pain because of severe muscle spasm followed by acute somatic dysfunction such as those with a whiplash injury.

2. Trigger points.
3. Fibrositic changes in the muscle.
4. Restriction of joint range of motion.

Effects of METs

- Muscle relaxation.
- Muscle strengthening.
- Decrease localized oedema/haematoma.
- Relieve passive congestion.
- Increase range of motion of the joint.
- Lengthening of muscles or soft tissues.

PRINCIPLES OF METs

Reciprocal Inhibition

As the name suggests it is the relaxation of antagonistic muscles. In this maneuver the agonist muscles which are shortened or tensed are not allowed to contract, because pain prevents the agonist muscle to contract, therefore opposite group of muscles (antagonist) are allowed to contract isometrically or isotonically against resistance which causes reciprocal inhibition or relaxation of the shortened muscles (antagonist).

Procedure

The shortened muscle is placed between a fully stretched or a fully relaxed state. The limb is held firmly but comfortably. The patient is instructed to contract the muscle (which is opposite to the shortened or tensed muscle), isometrically or isotonically against manual resistance for 6-10 seconds. This technique allows agonist muscles to relax without contracting them (As the reciprocal inhibition is the component of both proprioceptive neuromuscular facilitation and muscle energy techniques, the some degree of rotational or diagonal movement may be incorporated during isotonic contraction).

Postisometric Relaxation (Lewit's PIR)

As the name suggests "The physiological relaxation of muscle after isometric contraction". It is the type of hold relax exercise in which the contracted or tensed muscle is allowed to contract against the manual resistance. In this technique the patient is allowed to use the 10-20 percent of his available strength.

Procedure

The tensed or hypertonic (spasmed) muscle is lengthened into the restricted range of motion. Then the limb is held firmly but comfortably and patient is allowed to use 10-20 percent strength of his muscle against the manual resistance applied by therapist and also allows to take the deep breath during contraction. The contraction is allowed for 6 to 10 seconds.

In the next step of the techniques patient is instructed to relax the muscle and exhale then the muscle is again stretched into the restricted range of motion just short of pain and same step is followed again.

Janda's Postfacilitation Stretch Method

As the name suggest a stretch is given to the muscle just after the contraction. The method is generally used to elongate the muscle length, as well as relax the muscle.

Procedure

The tensed muscle is placed between a fully relaxed and fully stretched state. The limb is held firmly but comfortably and patient is instructed to contract the tensed or shortened muscle with full efforts for 6 to 10 seconds, then allowed to relax the muscle.

In the next step of manuever as the patient relaxes, a rapid stretch is given to the tensed or shortened muscle into restricted range of motion (new position) and held for 10 seconds which is followed by rest of 20 seconds.

The procedure is repeated 3-5 times per session.

Isolytic Technique

This is the type of resisted isotonic eccentric contraction of muscle. The technique is used to elongate the muscle fibres by stretching them.

Suppose a patient has shortened hamstrings. The hip joint is flexed at 30-45° (as it is convenient for therapist) with knee fully extended. The patient is then asked to contract the hamstrings, at the same time therapist maintains the knee extension and flexes the hip joint further which causes eccentric isotonic contraction of the hamstring muscles.

Initially patient offers 20 percent of available strength and the strength increases as the repetitions increase.

WILLIAMS FLEXION EXERCISES

In 1930 William proposed six lumbar flexion exercises. The aim of these exercises were to widen the intervertebral foramen and facet joints to reduce compression on nerve, strengthen the abdominals, stretch the back extensors, hip flexors, and reduce posterior fixation of the lumbosacral junction.

Six exercises are as follows:

1. Patient lies in supine with both knees flexed. While maintaining the position of legs, patient bends the trunk forward with hip flexion and touches the toes.
2. The patient lies in supine with both knees flexed and contracts the abdominals.
3. Patient lies in supine with hip and knee flexion, holds both the knees with the hands and touches the chest with both the knees.
4. In long sitting position repeatedly toes are touched with the hands.
5. In quadruped position one leg remains straightened and other is flexed at hip and knee joint.
6. Patient squats from standing to sitting with slight flexed trunk.

The first three flexion exercises increase the intradiscal pressure and further may increase the bulge of disc therefore should be contraindicated for acute disc herniation. Due to these contraindications William's exercises are rarely used in practice.

SPINAL STABILIZATION

It was first designed by Vollowitz and Morgan for the patients with lower back pain and is also called as functional spinal stabilization.

The stability to the spine is provided by static and dynamic stabilizers. Static stabilizers are—intervertebral disc, vertebral bodies, ligaments and facet joints, these stabilizers do not contract actively but they keep the spinal joints in proper alignment and are known as static stabilizers. Dynamic stabilizers are the structures which contract voluntarily during static and dynamic posture. Both static and dynamic stabilizers act on the spine and maintain the stability of the spinal segments.

Repetitive trauma or strain to the spine can weaken or decrease the ability of static and dynamic stabilizers to stabilize the spine and is the most common cause of pain.

Therapeutic exercises which train the patient to control posturally destabilizing forces during functional activities such as sitting, lifting, squatting and lunging etc. are known as *spinal stabilizing exercises.*

The prime function of these exercises is to increase the endurance and strength of the stabilizers of the spine so that the destabilizing forces can be controlled or eliminated, and this is the only instrument which can prevent chronic and recurrent pain. Learning to stabilize the back and self management skill is the key to prevent recurrence.

These exercises are progressed gradually from non weight bearing position (lying) to the weight bearing positions (sitting, standing) and include isometric contraction, which gradually progresses (as the condition of patient allows) to the functional activities such as—sitting, lifting, squating and lunging.

As the rule of these exercises, the exercise must start in pain free range. The lumbopelvic movement (anterior and posterior tilting) is the range of movement that is both safe and appropriate for the task at hand, and most of spinal stabilizing exercises are started with anterior and posterior tilts of the lumbopelvic joint. Sometimes it may be difficult to find the functional (painfree) range and therefore isometric exercises may only be initiated.

As the painfree range has been determined to be biomechanically safe or stable, it should be used in progressive exercise manner and if the condition of patient improves with the functional range, the exercise may progress form isometric to the isotonic.

In a comprehensive review, compelling evidence was presented that neuromuscular dysfunction is associated with lower back pain with changes in muscular strength and endurance of the trunk muscles and changes in activation amplitudes and synergistic muscle activation pattern reported for a variety of movement patterns.

- The dynamic stability approaches include building muscle strength and endurance and using neuromuscular control strategies required to maintain dynamic trunk stability. These strategies include (1) Selective recruitment of specific muscles and (2) Synergistic coactivation.
- McGill provides an excellent overview of the need for the trunk muscles to act in a synchronous manner to maintain stability, suggesting that even one muscle producing an inappropriate contraction (force) could result in the necessary force disrupt stability.

The present study focused on three exercises commonly prescribed in the management of LBP: the pelvic tilt, abdominal hollowing and trunk stability test level. The latter two emphasize the importance of a neutral spinal position and are claimed to recruit abdominals and trunk muscles in a manner consistent with dynamic stability training, lumbopelvic stability in particular. To date there are no measures other than EMG to substantiate that certain exercises elicit specific muscle activation patterns.

A recent EMG study of healthy subjects performing the three study exercises provided evidence that supported some and refused other previous claims associated with the pelvic tilt and the abdominal hollowing exercises.

Conceptual Model – Flexion

Flexion opens up or distracts the Zygapophyseal joint surfaces. The inferior articular processes of the superior vertebra glide up and forward upon the superior articular surfaces of the vertebra below. Anterior loading of the intervertebral disc occurs with compression of the anterior portion, with relaxation and bulging of the outer anterior annular wall. The posterior annular wall is stretched and pulled taut. The nucleus distorts posteriorly. The vertebral canal lengthens, stretching the cord, dura and root filaments and opening the intervertebral foramina.

Conceptual Model – Extension

Inferior articular processes of the vertebra above glides down and backward on the superior articular surfaces of the vertebra below. Posterior loading of the intervertebral disc occurs with distraction of the anterior portion of the annulus, which is stretched and pulled taut. The posterior annular wall is relaxed and there is posterior bulging of the outer, posterior annular wall. The nucleus distorts anteriorly. The vertebral canal shortens, which relaxes the cord, dura and root filaments, and reduces the size of the intervertebral foramina.

Concepts of Stabilization

1. The movement range (functional range) should be painfree.
2. The segment (Lumbar spine) should be moved in functional painfree range passively.
3. If functional range is not available, initially isometric exercise is recommended.
4. Gradually functional range is improved from isometric to isotonic, squating to sitting, walking and normal course of daily work. Thereafter advanced functional based exercises can be started.

McKENZIE

In 1981, RA McKenzie proposed a different method of treatment to back pain patients which is based on the patient's own normal spinal movements. The symptoms of patient can be reproduced and influenced by the movements and are observed during and after repeated movements or sustained movements.

The diagnosis and management in the McKenzie approach to mechanical disorders are based on the symptoms behaviour observed during and after repeated testing.

The aim of repeated movement testing is to influence the symptoms, and identify the movement which is painless and decrease the symptoms from distal part (peripheral) to the proximal part (central), which is known as centralization phenomenon. The painfree movement is only the treatment tool and is repeatedly performed to centralize the symptoms.

The movement which exacerbates the symptoms from proximal to distal, or during repeated movement testing the movement which exacerbates the symptoms from proximal to distal segment which is known as peri-pheralization, should not be administered as it may further increase the disease process.

The intensity and location of symptoms are identified while at rest, during repeated movements and sustained end range positions and are categorized into Postural, Dysfunction and Derangement syndromes.

Postural Syndrome

Pain is normally not present during repeated movements and end range movements but if the end range movements are sustained then only it can reproduce.

The syndrome can be treated by correction of posture. To achieve this the patient first achieves fully sloughed position (in sitting, shoulders are drooped, trunk flexed, pelvis posterior tilted) and then fully straightened (chest is expanded, shoulder retracted and pelvis tilted anteriorly). The exercise is repeated for twenty times per session.

Dysfunction Syndrome

In this syndrome pain is reproduced at range of repeated movements, stops shortly on release of end range stress, and may radiate slightly. The symptoms remain unchanged after testing (no better or worse).

The symptoms are reproduced at end range of repeated movement as the shortened or tightened structures get stretched.

The dysfunction syndrome can be treated by stretching the shortened structures. Patient generated forces are sufficient in most of cases to stretch the shortened structures. The movement which causes pain at end range is ideally performed in a slow repeated movement fashion in sets of 10-15 every 2 hourly each day. The correction of posture is also the key factor.

Manual stretching procedures may also be introduced if the progress is slow.

Derangement Syndrome

Symptoms are altered during the movement or in the mid range or through the range and painful arc is present.

During repeated movement testing symptoms may centralize or peripheralize.

The treatment is based on evaluation of movements that centralize the symptoms (the movement which reduce the symptoms from peripheral part to the proximal). Once the movement is identified that decreases peripheral symptoms is performed repeatedly in painfree range of motion. The movements which exacerbate or peripheralize the symptoms should be discontinued.

MULLIGAN

Brian R Mulligan is a very familiar name in manipulative physical therapy practice. He has been involved in teaching of manual therapy in New Zealand and an abroad since early 1970s. He alongwith RA McKenzie and JC Cameron established the New Zealand Manipulative Therapists Association in 1968 and was made a life member of this body in 1988.

Mobilization with Movement

He has developed the new term "Mobilization with movement" (MWM), which was first implemented on spine to treat the musculoskeletal disorders of spine with SNAGS (sustained natural apophyseal glides) and then to the extremities. Today movement with mobilization covers all the joints of the body.

Similar to the maitland, Mulligan has also paid attention to the movement plane of the joint (Facet joints), which was described by Freddy M Kaltenborn, as lying across the concave articular surface.

Unlike other mobilization techniques, Mulligan has explained all the spinal mobilization techniques in weight bearing positions of the patient (standing or sitting). He considers this to be extremely important as so often with non weight bearing techniques, improvements gained are lost when the patient resumes in an erect posture (weight bearing position).

With the exception of PRP's (Pain relief phenomenon) all techniques are painless. Which are quite different from the often quoted phases "No pain no gain".

Common techniques described by the Mulligan are as follows:

1. NAGs (Natural Apophyseal Glides).
2. Reverse NAGs.
3. SNAGs (Sustained Natural Apophyseal Glides).
4. Self SNAGs.
5. Spinal mobilization with limb movement.

CYRIAX

The Deep Transverse Friction Massage was given by James Cyriax. A London based orthopedic practitioner. The cyriax massage is recommended to treat most of the musculoskeletal ailments. James Cyriax is also famous for his intraarticular injections.

According to cyriax to treat the musculoskeletal ailments, it is very important for the practitioner to know where exactly is the problem or source or root of the symptoms. Once practitioner finds the location of lesion, the treatment must be directed directly on the lesion. The symptoms cannot be improved if the treatment is being directed elsewhere of the lesion. For example, lateral epicondylitis patient may complaint symptoms over the dorsum of the forearm or down the elbow joint. If treatment is given over the dorsum of forearm, the lateral epicondylitis cannot be treated. It is therefore find out the exact location of lesion (i.e., musculotendinous junction/part of the common extensors) and administer the treatment over the location of lesion.

To find out the location of lesion the practitioner must take proper history of patient and perform following maneuvers.

1. Examine the tender area.
2. Observe active range of movements—Pain during active movement suggests that lesion/problem may be in the contractile structures, such as muscles.
3. Perform active resistive movements—Pain on active resistive movements confirms the lesion may be in the contractile structures.
4. Perform passive movements—If above maneuvers do not reproduce symptoms, it may be said that contractile structures are intact and lesion could be elsewhere. If passive movements reproduce the symptoms of the patient the site of tension may be in the innert or non-contractile structures such as ligaments joint capsule, cartilage, bursae or bones.

Deep Transverse Friction Massage

The technique varies slightly from condition to condition but the principles remain constant.

1. *Lesion must be brought within reach of the therapist's finger.* For instance, in supraspinatus tendinitis the patient's arm must be placed behind the back. This brings the tendon out of the acromion which would otherwise shield the entire structure.

2. *The tissue to receive the massage should be in appropriate tension (except muscle belly):* For instance in lateral epicondylitis if the technique is performed on tendon, the wrist and fingers should be flexed, forearm pronated and elbow is extended to put the tendon under tension. If the technique is being performed on the musculotendinous junction or muscle belly then common extensors of wrist should be relaxed, so the massage can penetrate deeply to tease the fibres apart.
3. *The treatment is applied by the therapist's finger tip.*

Procedure

- The tip of finger (index) is placed on the skin, the finger tip moves with the skin over the underlying structures. The technique is to move the whole hand with the patient's skin and the therapist's finger moving as one, otherwise a friction burn of the skin may occur. Some practitioners put a piece of tissue paper between fingertip and the skin: this avoids the burn and absorbs sweat which might otherwise cause slippage. The index finger can also be reinforced by middle finger if more pressure is required.
- The friction must be across the fibres of the affected structures with sufficient amplitude of sweep to ensure that the frictional element (and not the pressure) is paramount.
- *Intensity:* The strength (pressure) of massage depends on the stage of this lesion. In acute cases it is given extremely gently and in chronic cases with greater rigour.
- *Duration of treatment:* Varies from condition to condition ranging from 5 min to 20 min.

  Some discomfort may be caused during first few minutes which can be minimised by a gentle start. **If there is continuous discomfort, massage should be stopped immediately.**
- The treatment is directed on alternate days for 6 to 12 sessions although it depends on severity of symptoms.

Deep transverse friction massage on following:

1. *Muscular lesions*—The massage breaks down the adhesions formed by the scar tissue between individual muscle fibres.
2. *Muscle tendon*—The scar is eroded by the abrasive action.
3. *Ligamentous lesions*—The formation of adhesions during the period of healing is prevented by moving the ligament over bone in limitation of its normal behaviour.
4. *Tenosynovitis*—It appears that the manual rolling of the tendon sheath to and fro against the tendon serve to smooth off the roughened surfaces.

MYOFASCIAL RELEASE TECHNIQUE

Myofascial release (MFR) technique is given to release restrictions that are secondary to tonal dysfunction in children and adults. The lengthening of superficial and deep soft tissue is accomplished by changing the viscosity of the fascia ground substance and by gentle and sustained stretch of the muscular elastic components of fascia.

This technique is usually given in conditions: Such as cerebral palsy, stroke, head injury etc.

Muscle bending: It is also one of the myofascial lengthening technique like MFR which is performed on tendinous part of the muscles such as hamstrings, biceps brachii, hip adductors and pectoralis major.

Procedure: The muscle is placed in a relaxed position, then its tendinous part is grasped between the thumb and fingers of both hands. In the next step the tendinous part is bent by giving pressure with the thumb and fingers of both hands moving away from each other.

The procedure of MFR on superficial and deep soft tissues is as follows:

Pectoralis—Patient is placed in supine position, therapist places three fingertips on the upper sternal end and moves the fingertips along the length of the muscle to the humeral end upto insertion.

Biceps Brachii—Any comfortable position of the patient is choosed. Therapist places three finger tips on the anterior aspect of the upper arm, over the origin of long or short head of biceps and then moves down vertically along the length of muscle to its insertion.

Forearm Muscles (Wrist flexors)—Thumbs of both hands are placed on origin of flexors (below the cubital fossa) then move in a lateral direction upto the wrist.

Palm—Both the thumbs are placed on the palmar aspect of the wrist and move in a lateral direction upto the base of the metacarpophalangeal joints.

Rectus Abdominalis—The patient is placed in supine lying. Therapist places upper hand close to the xiphisternum and the lower hand close to the pubic symphysis. A pressure is applied with the upper hand in cephal direction and with the lower hand in caudal direction.

Posterior Neck Muscles—The patient (child) is placed in prone position on medicinal ball and therapist sits behind the child. Therapist places one hand on the base of occiput and the other is placed between the occiput and shoulder. The upper hand (occipital hand) stabilises the head and neck while lower hand is used to give a pressure in caudal direction towards the pelvis or towards the shoulder girdle in case of an asymmetry.

Lower Extremity

Hip Flexors—The patient is placed in supine lying, therapist stands at the side of patient. One hand is placed one inch lateral below the umblicus and other hand is placed on anterior aspect of the upper thigh (affected side). A pressure is applied in cephal direction with the upper hand and in caudal direction with the lower hand.

Adductors—The patient is placed in supine lying, therapist stands at the affected side of the patient. The knee is kept straight. Three fingertips are placed on the groin or origin of the adductors and run along the muscle belly of adductors (medial aspect of thigh) upto the insertion of the adductors. The pelvis is stabilized during maneuver to avoid hiking or lateral flexion. After every stroke from groin to knee the hip joint is abducted.

Hamstrings—The patient is placed in prone lying and therapist stands at the side of the patient. Three fingertips are placed on the ischial tuberosity and moved along the muscle fibres upto insertion of hamstrings.

Gastrocnemius—Patient is placed in prone lying, therapist stands at the side of the patient. Three fingertips are placed on the origin of the muscle and move down in a vertical direction upto the heel.

Plantar Fascia—The patient is placed in prone lying with knee flexion at 90°. Therapist stands at the side of the patient and grasps the patient's leg at the ankle joint. The thumb of other hand is placed on little below the heel and move in a lateral direction up to the base of toes.

FUNCTIONAL REHABILITATION IN ORTHOPEDICS

On past, functional rehabilitation was the ultimate goal only for the neurologically impaired patients. Although the patient with neurological deficit may have obvious motor control, motor performance, cognitive and perceptual problem. The orthopedic patient may have subtle but similar problems to overcome.

Most of us have experienced that the patient who regained normal strength and motion could not perform his function. Orthopedic injury may result in abnormal sensory feedback and altered neuromuscular control which may lead to decreased or abnormal movements. Functional training maximizes the use of sensory information mediated by the ligaments, capsule and/or musculotendinous unit.

Many studies have been done on this issue and it has been suggested to therapists to work on functional restoration along with strength and range of motion.

There are three approaches which can be used to achieve this goal:

1. A Total Body Approach.
2. An Activity Oriented Approach.
3. A Realistic Approach.

A Total Body Approach

The functional ability of a person depends on the proper interaction of all the body parts and brain. Hence functional restoration requires treatment of the whole body, not just the affected body part. The emphasis of therapy should not only be on strength, ROM, and gait but should also include balance, proprioception, coordination and agility.

An Activity Oriented Approach

The patient should demonstrate the ability to safely perform all the functional tasks necessary to return to his previous life style.

This tasks can be incorporated into standard strengthening and flexibility programs.

A Realistic Approach

Each patient has different needs and functions. The therapist alongwith patient must define the risks and rewards of desired functional goals and should work together to restore important functional activities as safely as possible.

For e.g., In some conditions running, jogging may not be safe for the patient. To walk safely should be the goal.

Functional Exercise Equipment

The following equipments can be used during functional rehabilitation program for orthopedic conditions:

1. Steps.
2. Balls–Basket ball, Football, Beach ball, Tennis ball, Medicinal ball etc.
3. Bicycles (upper and lower body).
4. Games.
5. Hand equipment—such as Baltimore therapeutic equipment (BTE).
6. Stair climbing machine.

7. Surgical tubing.
8. Therabands.
9. Wobble boards.
10. Trampoline.
11. Work hardening equipment.
12. Tread mills.
13. Rowing machine.
14. Gym equipment–Weights, dumbells, barbells etc.
15. Chairs/Stool with different heights.
16. ADL Boards.
17. Self help devices–Reachers, adapted utensils, adapted writing tool, dressing stick etc.
18. Assistive devices–Walker, crutches and sticks.
19. Mobility devices–Wheel chair.

21

YOGA AND ASANAS

INTRODUCTION

Yoga is a very old Indian practice that goes back to over 5000 years. The term 'yoga' comes from a Sanskrit word 'yuj', it means to yoke, to unite. In the most ordinary sense yoga means uniting the body and the mind with the soul. In a dualistic sense it also means uniting the soul with the supreme self. In yoga, through a step by step process we try to dissolve the ego consciousness in the soul consciousness. We practice yoga by withdrawing the mind and the senses from the myriad distractions of the world in order to obliterate the boundaries of identity and form we create for ourselves. This actually means to bring oneself to a disciplined way of life.

It is believed by ancient yogics that for human being to harmonize with the environment and themselves, they have to unite the spirit, mind and body, and for all of it to be united, there must be a balance in the physical, emotional and spiritual aspect of life. The way to maintain and achieve this balance is through meditation, breathing, and yoga postures. Thus, both the body and the mind are used when practising yoga exercises, as it requires perseverance and will power to be able to perform each of the yoga asanas. Yoga in the eastern countries believed to be a spiritual self-mastery meditation skill to keep the mind, body and soul together, whereas, in the western countries yoga is practised as physical exercise or alternative medicine rather than the spiritual self-mastery meditation.

CONCEPTS

In the history of the vast literature on yoga and in the present times, there have been several different conceptions of yoga. In terms of concepts one yoga may differ from another yoga because of the origin of that particular yoga was for a particular function. *For example,* Hatha yoga and Ashtanga yoga (Raja yoga). The ashtanga yoga emphasizes on the ease and spontaneity in one's bodily postures or asanas while meditating, whereas, the hatha yoga employs hatha or violence and force and requires of hatha yogin, for example to stand on one leg, or hold the arms, or inhale smoke with the head inverted when meditating. Similarly, a kind of yogic samadhi or some sort of sidhi or perfection could be achieved by taking drugs or by reciting some mantras. In view of above, it may be learnt that one should not confuse with the other conception and that one should not speak of yoga without specifying the sense in which one is using the word and kind of yoga one is talking about. Now-a-days in the modern world the people have a concept towards yoga as identical with the practice of yogic asanas with the explicit aim not at spiritual upliftment, but better bodily health and reduction of and maximum possible freedom from psychological tension.

Yoga is neither a philosophy nor a religion but it is art which is value neutral such that it can be adopted as necessary part of the conceptual scheme or the training programme of any religion or philosophy.

Therapeutic Effects

The physical aspect of what is called yoga in recent years, the asanas, has been much popularized in the West. Physically, the practice of asanas is considered to:

- Improve flexibility.
- Improve strength.
- Improve balance.
- Reduce stress and anxiety.
- Reduce symptoms of lower back pain.
- Improve symptoms of asthma and chronic obstructive pulmonary disease (COPD).
- Increase energy and decrease fatigue.

- Shorten labor and improve birth outcomes.
- Improve physical health and quality of life measures in the elderly.
- Improve diabetes management.
- Reduce sleep disturbances.
- Reduce hypertension.

Conditions Required Before Yoga

Warm Up: It is important to perform warm up exercises to prepare the muscles for the yoga. Warm up exercises may be a brisk walk or jogging or simply some form of stretching of the muscles like movements of the neck, trunk, shoulder, hip and knee. These warm up exercises not only relaxes the muscles but also prepares the muscles for the extreme stretches require during the yoga asanas.

Empty Stomach: The stomach should be empty. The best suited time to practice the yoga is morning. Yoga may also be performed in the afternoon, but it should be with empty stomach or after 3-4 hours of the meal. Force or pressure should not be used, and body should not tremble.

Environment: The place where yoga is practised should be cleaned, spacious, fully ventilated and free of noises and pollution. Morning yoga in the park is considered to be the suitable conditions for the yoga practitioners.

Clothes: The yoga practitioners should prefer undergarments with loose and comfortable clothes.

TYPES OF YOGA AND ASANAS

A. YOGA

The Yoga Upanishads identify four types of yoga—Mantra yoga, Laya yoga, Raja yoga and Hatha yoga. In the Bhagavadgita we find karma yoga and bhakti yoga. Karma yoga means performing desire less actions as an offering to God.

Mantra Yoga: Involves continuous mental repetition of a mantra or some sacred syllable till the mind become completely absorbed in it.

Laya Yoga: Involves the dissolution of the lower self and the mental activity and the rising of the kundalini (energy from the base of the spine) to the tip of the head. Its more extreme version is Hatha yoga practised by some schools of Saivism such as the Nath yogis and the Kalamukhas. It involves the practice of some extremely difficult bodily postures, breathing practices and use of certain chemicals to gain complete mastery over the body and the mind.

Raja yoga or the king of the yogas is the most standard form of yoga, described by Patanjali in his Yogasutra it involves the practice of eight fold yoga, hence, it is also known as *Ashtanga Yoga.* Ashtanga means eight limbs (steps), which purify the practitioners' mind, reduce stress and anxiety by performing eight steps. Ashtanga is believed to derive its origin from ancient text yoga *Korunta.* It is aimed at channelling hyperactive young minds and restive bodies with the infinite energy of teenage boys. The concepts of each step (limb) is learned and practised carefully before progressing to the next. The following are the eight steps:

1. **Yama (Control):** It is the practice of restraints or precepts. The five restraints suggested by Patanjali are: not to be violent, not to lie, not to steal, not to indulge in sex and not to be greedy.
2. **Niyama (Rules of Conduct):** It is the practice of five observance or discipline. Patanjali suggested five rules or observances: practice of purity, happiness, austerities or asceticism, study of the scriptures, and surrender to God.
3. **Asanas (Poses):** Asanas are the movements, postures of the body to make the body supple and fit.
4. **Pranayama (Breath Control):** It is the practice of regulating of the inspiration and expiration (breathing) for certain period of time to calm the mind and relax the body to experience higher states of consciousness.
5. **Pratyahara (Withdrawal of Sensory Perceptions):** It is the practice of withdrawal of the senses and mind from the sense objects. This is usually done by closing eyes, looking inwards and by focusing the attention on the area between the eyebrows or on the thoughts and feelings that arise in the consciousness.
6. **Dharana (Concentration):** It is the overcome of the sense of duality to which we are usually subject by concentrating the mind on a single point or object such as the image of deity.
7. **Dhyana (Uninterrupted Meditation):** Dhyana is the meditation, which can either be passive or active. Uninterrupted meditation can bring equanimity, tranquillity and inner happiness.
8. **Samadhi (Complete Equilibrium): Samadhi** is a state of self-absorption in which the movements of the senses and the mind cease and all distinctions between the knower and the known disappear. It is a state of unity and subjectivity in which mind comes to a complete rest while the practitioner remains conscious but absorbed in himself.

B. BASIC YOGA–ASANAS

Asanas are the physical movements or posture of the yoga practice and in combination with yoga it constitutes a style of yoga. In the yoga sutra, Patanjali describes asana as a "firm, comfortable posture" that refers specifically to the seating posture, most basic of all the asanas. Asanas are widely known as "yoga postures" or yoga positions. Raja yoga also known as king of all the yoga, has eight limbs (steps), the third step or limb of raja yoga describes the asanas. The Yogasutras is the most authoritative ancient scripture on yoga.

Asana later became a term for various postures useful for restoring and maintaining a practitioner's well-being and improving the body's flexibility and vitality, with the goal of cultivating the ability to remain in seated meditation for extended periods.

There are number of postures and movements in yoga, and although all of them are beneficial, some are more challenging than others. Initially basic yoga are taught to the clients/patients and as soon as the concepts of basic yoga are learned the therapist may progress to the advanced yoga. Progressing to the advanced yoga is one of the crucial steps and the therapist needs to screen the patients/clients as the advanced yoga require more flexibility and movements. The older population should be progressed carefully to the advanced yoga as they have osteoporotic bones, degenerative changes and limited flexibility of the joints. The following yoga asanas are explained as below:

(a) Sun Salutation or Surya Namaskar

Surya Namaskar or the Sun Salutation, which is very commonly practised in most forms of yoga, originally evolved as a type of worship of Surya, the Vedic solar deity. Surya the Hindu solar deity by concentrating on the Sun, for vitalization. It consists of yogasana and Pranayama. It is useful in all the age groups of people. A full round of surya namaskar is considered to be two sets of the twelve poses with the change in the second set where opposite leg is moved first. The twelve poses are mentioned as under (Figs. 21.1(i-xii)); the practitioner:

i. Stands straight with no lordosis in the lumbar and cervical spine, both the feet together and places both hands on the chest to join them. Inhales and recites some mantras (bija mantras).

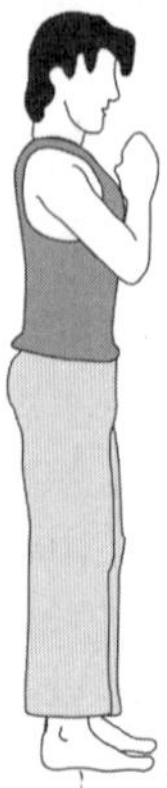

ii. Inhales and raises both the arms overhead, keeping the palms together.

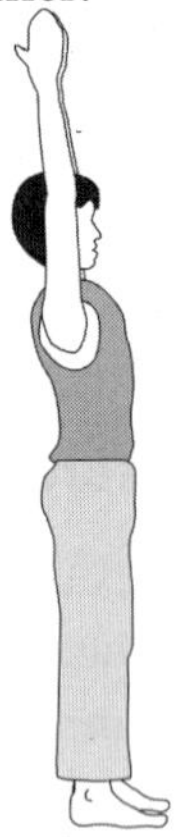

iii. Exhales and bends the trunk forward as much as possible without bending the knees. Patients with PIVD should avoid this asana.

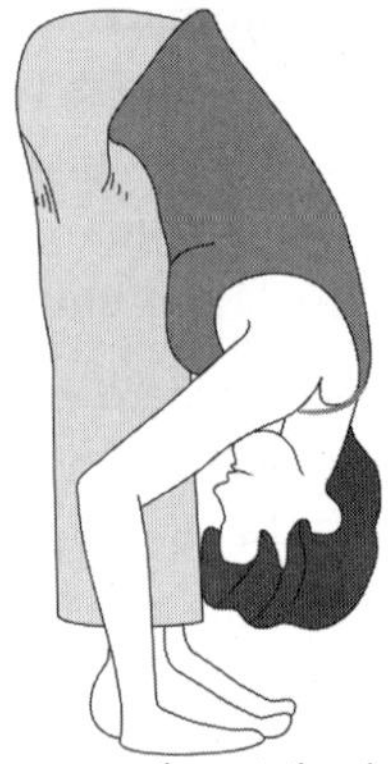

iv. Inhales and steps the right leg backwards, extends the neck, trunk and right hip joint. The left hip and knee is flexed fully.

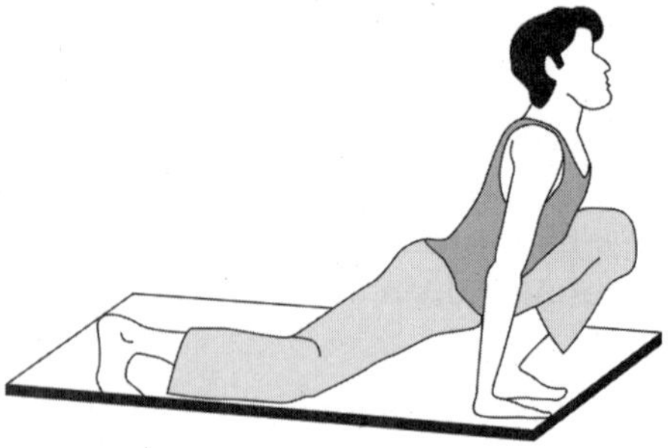

v. Exhales and takes the left leg back into plank position. The body is supported on the hand (palmar aspects). The neck, trunk, hips and ankles remain in the neutral position.

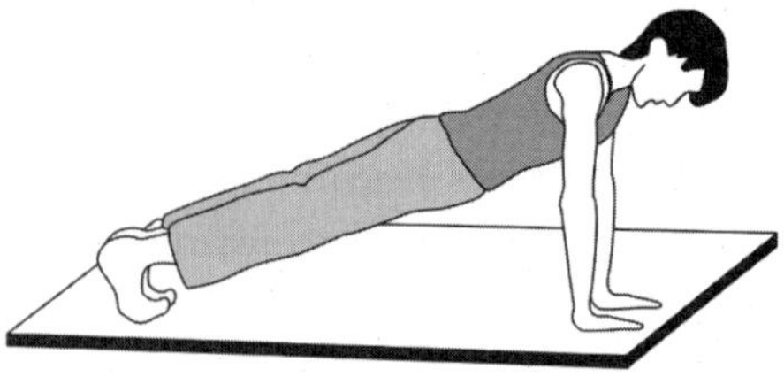

vi. Retaining the breadth, the forehead, chest, and knees are lowered to the floor by extending the shoulders and flexing the elbows. There is strong contraction of the shoulder flexors and elbow extensors, this strengthens the upper corset muscles too.

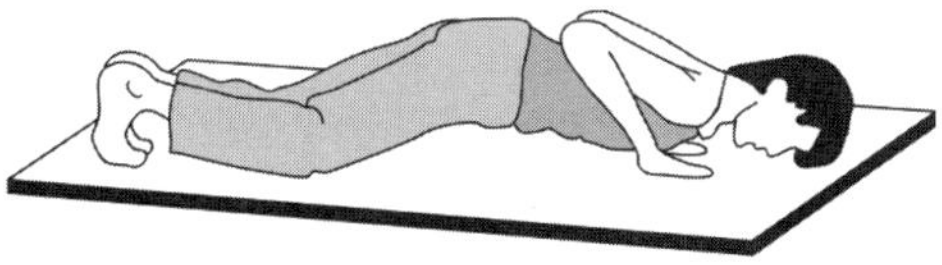

vii. Inhales and extends the spine and hip joints as much as possible. Looks up to the sky.

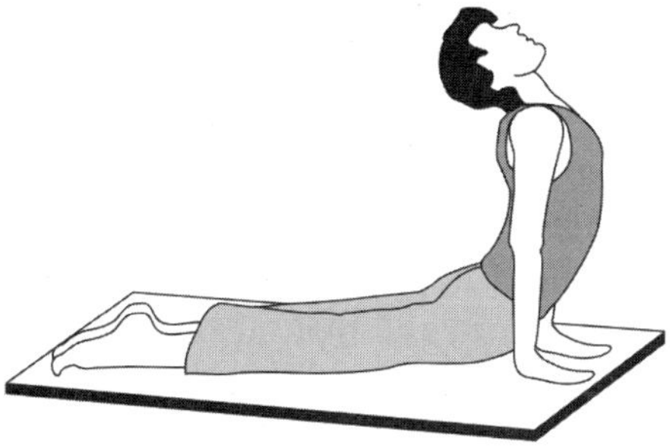

viii. Exhales, curls toes under, flexes the hip joints to 90 degrees the weight of the body is taken on the palmer aspect of the hands with the shoulders fully flexed. The knees are fully extended while the spine remains straight in the line of the arms.

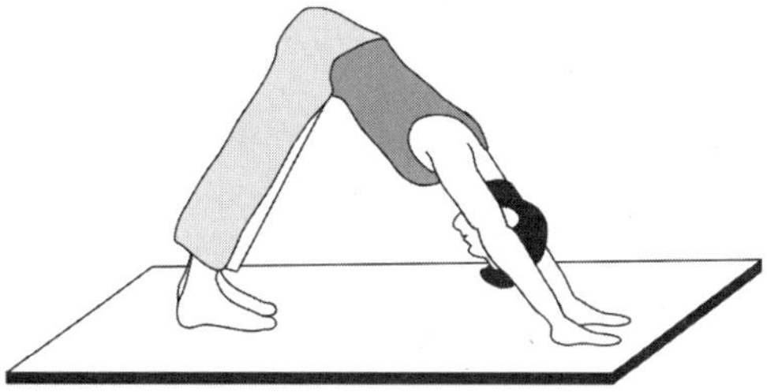

ix. Inhales, brings right leg forward with the hip and knee full flexion. The arms are kept at the side of the body and the spine is extended.

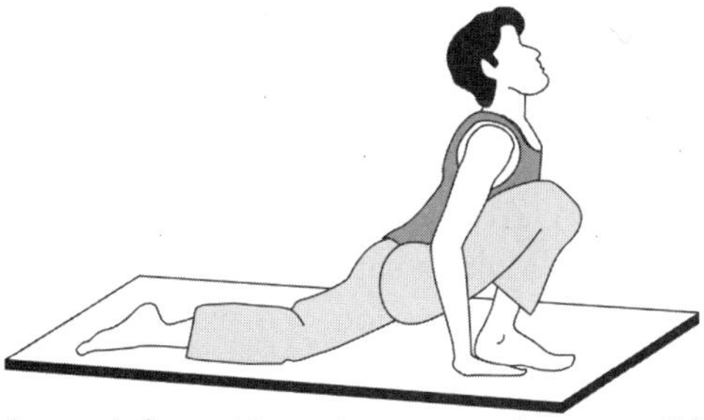

x. Exhales and flexes the spine as much as possible by touching the toes with the hands.

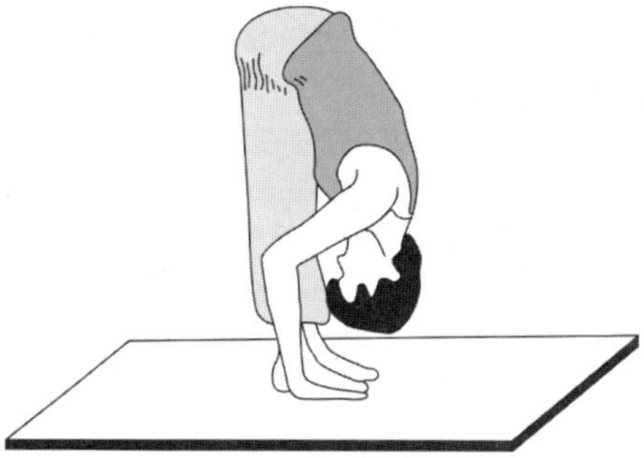

xi. Inhales and extends the knees, hips, spine and shoulders.

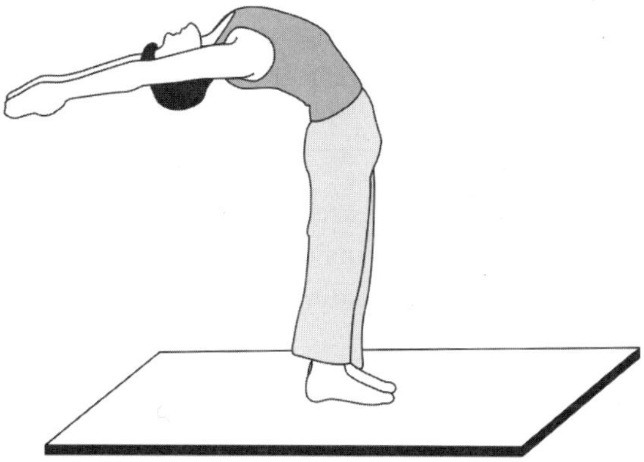

xii. Exhales and comes back to the pose of tadasana.

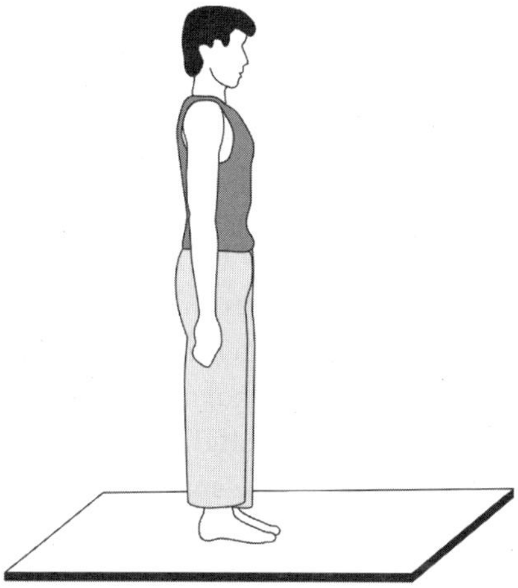

Figs. 21.1 (i-xii)

(b) Pranayama

Pranayama is the fourth limb or step of ashtanga yoga, as set out by Patanjali in the yoga sutra. Pranayama is made up of two words prana means breath or bio energy in the body and yama means control, hence, pranayama is the control of breath or bio (pranic) energy. It is done by regulating the breathing and holding the breath in between for certain periods of time to calm the mind and relax the body to experience higher states of consciousness. The practice is an integral part of both hatha yoga and ashtanga

Pranava Mudra for Pranayama–Body Gesture and Mental Attitudes
It may be performed in six different steps: **Type-1** Keep both the nostrils open and then inhale and exhale with both the nasal passages. This type is nothing but quick breathing with both the nasal cavities. One should inhale and exhale with as much speed as possible and for as much time as feasible. **Type-2** Take up Pranava Mudra and close the right nostril with the help of the thumb of the right hand, and inhale with left nostril and also exhale through the same nasal passage. In brief this type can be described as quick breathing with the left nostril. **Type-3** In this type left nostril is to be closed and the quick breathing is done with the right nostril. **Type-4** In this type close the right nostril and inhale with the left nostril, and then immediately close left nostril and exhale with the right nostril. In this way try quick breathing by changing the nostrils. **Type-5** This type of breathing is just opposite the previous one, that is, the left nostril is closed and inhaling is done with the right nostril, then immediately closing the right nostril, exhaling is done with the left nostril. **Type-6** This type of breathing is designed by combining previous two types, i.e., Type-4 and Type-5. First inhale with left nostril and exhale with right one, then inhale with right nostril and exhale with left nostril. Later continue the same process, i.e., inhaling and exhaling with left and right nostrils alternately. Further switch to fast breathing by increasing the speed of breathing. After sufficient practice the speed of breathing can be increased immensely.

vinayasa yoga in the execution of asanas. Patanjali in yoga sutras mentioned pranayama as means of attaining higher states of awareness, holding of breath is an important practice of reaching samadhi.

Five Types of Prana: Prana, Apana, Vyan, Udana and Samana are responsible for various pranic activities in the body. Out of these Prana and Apana are most important. Prana is upward flowing and Apana is downward flowing. Practice of Pranayama achieves the balance in the activities of these pranas, which results in healthy body and mind.

Pranayama Procedure

The breathing procedure of the pranayama should be taught to the practitioner to avoid any harmful effects. Pranayama involves mainly of two activities inhaling and exhaling. In Yogasutras of Patanjali, inhaling is termed as Puraka and the exhaling is termed as Rechaka. The state when these two activities are made to halt has been termed as Kumbhaka. The breathing rate may be:

i. **Quiet Breathing:** Smooth continuous naturally without any efforts.

ii. **Deep Breathing:** First, the movements concerned with inhaling and exhaling are to be controlled in order to further slow down the breathing, at the same time the need of oxygen for the body is to be lessened, so that the speed of breathing can further, slow down. The constitution of the body is such that if the need or use of oxygen is not reduced, it becomes difficult or rather impossible to control the process of breathing. The easy way to reduce the need of oxygen is to stop the movements of the body and try to relax all the muscles. After some time the practitioner finds it difficult to do the deep breathing further, at this juncture he or she should return to the neutral breathing and rest for a while. After taking rest the deep breathing should start again. After practising deep breathing with equal time and speed successfully, one should start studying it by increasing the time for exhaling. If inhaling (Puraka) is in four seconds, then exhaling (Rechaka) shall take 5 to 6 seconds instead of four. This needs special efforts. When a person succeeds in doing inhaling and exhaling at the ratio of 1: 1 for 10 to 15 minutes, he should double the time for exhalation. The ideal ratio for inhaling-exhaling is 1 : 2.

iii. **Fast Breathing:** When the speed of the inhaling and exhaling is more than the deep breathing is termed as fast breathing. In the fast breathing the practitioner should increase the speed of inhaling and exhaling however short breathing is not practised. The practitioner has to practice continue the cycle of quick breathing with constant practice. This sort of breathing is easy to understand and to practice also. The fast breathing clears the nasal passage and exercises the parts involved in the respiratory system. During fast breathing there is a feeling of whirling sensation in the head which may be considered to be normal, but as soon as it occurs the practitioners should return to the quiet breathing and then after some time comes back to the fast breathing. Making habit of the fast breathing can remove such kind of sensation. To practice the fast breathing the practitioner sits in one of the following asanas

Padmasana, Vajrasana or Swastikasana. The eyes are closed and the practitioner concentrates in the breathing to achieve maximum results.

(c) Dandasana

Dandasana is derived from two words of Sanskrit danda mean stick and asana means posture. The practitioner sits on the floor with both the hip joints flexed to 90 degrees and knees extended fully. The arms should be rested on either side of the body, the whole spine (lumbar, thoracic and cervical) is kept straightened, the whole posture will look like an English alphabet "L". The legs will be parallel, whereas the body will be perpendicular to the floor. The practitioner remains in the dandasana pose for at least 2-3 minutes. The dandasana helps in strengthening core muscles, shoulder girdle and upper back extensors. The pose also helps in hamstrings and neck extensors stretching (Fig. 21.2).

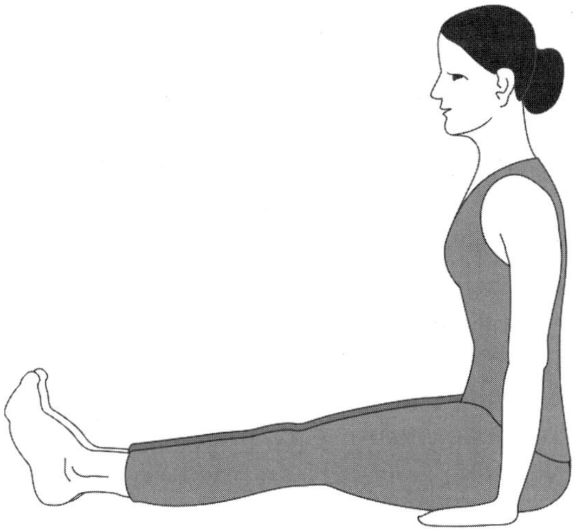

Fig. 21.2

Modifications

(i) The practitioner sits on the floor with the legs extended and spine straight. This pose helps in stretching of the hamstrings and strengthening of the core group muscles.

(ii) Gradually, practitioner expands the chest, drops the shoulder blades down and backward, inhales slowly throughout this entire pose and keeps the chin slightly lowered position. This pose is maintained for a minute or two.

(iii) The neck is flexed forward and then extended backward, this helps in stretching of neck extensors.

(iv) The arms are flexed to 90 degrees with thumb in downward direction. Patient inhales and then flexes the shoulders further to the full range. This helps in improving the chest expansion and pectoralis stretching.

(v) The practitioner presses the thigh with the floor. The hip joints are rotated medially and laterally. The ankle joints are flexed and extended.

(d) Vajrasana

Vajra is derived from Sanskrit mean thunderbolt. Vajrasana makes the body exceptionally strong and healthy. The practitioner sits on the ankle and toes with both the knees flexion. The spine should be extended and both the hands placed on the knees. The practitioner sits on the ankle (dorsum) and toes with both the knees flexion. The spine should be extended and both the hands placed on the knees. The practitioner inhales and exhales slowly. While drawing the abdominal region inward (inhale) and expanding the chest, the practitioner should concentrate on breathing. Vajrasana helps in lowering blood pressure and strengthening of the core stabilizers (Fig. 21.3).

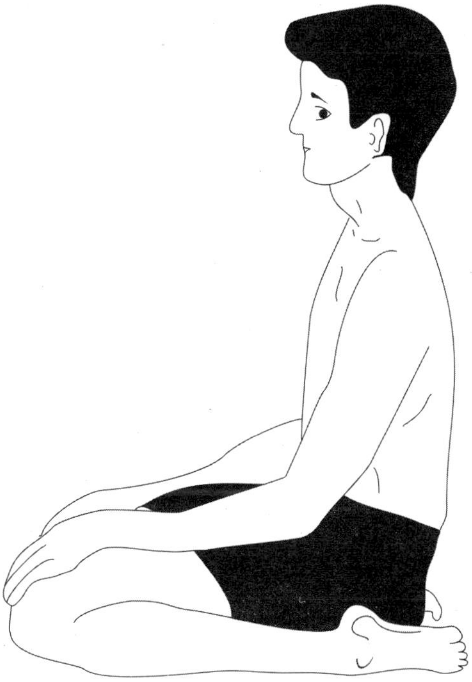

Fig. 21.3

PART II

22

ORTHOPEDIC ASSESSMENT

Assessment is the systematic approach of making a diagnosis to know how to approach treatment and to design an appropriate scheme of management. In order to make a diagnosis, and to design an appropriate scheme of management, it is essential for the examiner to understand each patient as fully as possible, irrespective of their social class and economical or cultural background. Interpretation of the clinical findings obtained during the subjective and objective examination enables the clinician to make a provisional diagnosis and scheme of management. Therefore, assessment is the cornerstone of effective clinical practice. The assessment includes following components:

A. Examination.

B. Evaluation.

C. Diagnosis.

D. Prognosis.

E. Intervention.

A. EXAMINATION

Examination is the process in which clinical data or findings are gathered by obtaining a history, performing a relevant system review, selecting and administrating special tests and measures. Examination has two parts subjective and objective. Moving step by step of the assessment from subjective examination to objective examination the clinician can reproduce the patient's symptoms and determine the level of the dysfunction or injury.

a. Subjective Examination

During subjective examination the examiner gathers information from the patient by asking the questions, such as: "Yes gentleman what is your problem"? When it started? How it started etc? The information collected during the subjective examinations depends on to a large extent on the quality of communication between the examiner and patient. Therefore, the examiner should establish a pleasant relationship with the patient to get an accurate information. Attempts are made to gather accurate information from the patient so that these may give clues in making the diagnosis and designing scheme of management. The examiner should ask the relevant questions. Not every question will need to be asked otherwise patient will get irritated and may distort the information. The subjective examination involves following:

i. ***General Information:*** During the general information the clinician obtains the following information from the patient: Age, Sex, Occupation, Height : Weight ratio, Reaction to stress and pain. *Consideration of Age.* The prevalence of the certain conditions are at the certain ages. The disc degeneration starts at around age of 40 years, while onset of ankylosing spondylitis is before the age of 40 years. The patient over the age of 50 years presents with low back pain may be considered for the malignant disease, while, the patient below the age of 25-30 years with low back pain is considered for the mechanical or traumatic such as dysfunction at the intervertebral disc, appophyseal joints, ligaments, postural problems and malalignment and ruled out for the degenerative disease, hence, examiner must consider the age before progressing to the next element of the assessment. *Sex:* While obtaining general information, clinician should also consider the sex of the patient. The prevalence of some conditions or disease such as ankylosing spondylitis is higher in the males than females, hence, a female patient presents with the low back pain may be ruled out for the AS and may be considered for the mechanical or other conditions of back pain such as dysmenorrhoea, urinary tract and pelvic infection etc. *Occupation:* The people involved in the overhead activities are more prone to the shoulder impingement and anterior instability as overuse of the rotator cuff muscles fail to rotate and depress the head of humerus downward during the elevation. Activities such as lifting and carrying heavy objects with forward flexion of the spine may weaken the annulus fibrosus and end plate, and this may allow nucleus pulposus to bulge towards the annuls fibrosus. Therefore, in order to understand and reach to the exact cause of the problem the examiner should not skip the occupation of the patient taking into account.

ii. Chief Complaint: Why has the patient sought for treatment or referred to the physiotherapy department or clinic? The patient may come to the physiotherapist with following complaints: Stiffeners, giving way, instability, weakness, loss of function, for differential diagnosis, after trauma, surgery, manipulation under anesthesia, plaster removal following dislocation, injury or trauma. The complaint is always written in the patient's language. The therapist should establish a pleasant relationship with the patient and take him into fully confidence and ask the questions such as:

a. **What was the Onset of Symptoms?** The pain and other symptoms may start with gradual or sudden onset. Symptoms start with gradual onset indicate an active pathology such as infection or inflammation if they do not subside with the rest. The mechanical back pain such as disc degeneration and faulty posture has the gradual onset but they respond to the rest and heat modalities. The symptoms start with sudden onset speaks about traumatic lesion, and there is probability of the injury to the ligaments, tendons, joint capsule, menisci, intervertebral disc, appophyseal joints or muscle tear/rupture etc.

b. **What was the Mechanism of Injury?** The patient explains how the injury took place. If patient is able to reveal the exact mechanism of injury, the clinician or examiner can reach to the exact site or structure. For an example below mentioned mechanisms are related to the particular structures. *Forward bending with lifting of heavy weight:* During forward flexion the line of gravity falls anterior to the midline which increases the extension moment arm, and requires more muscle work to stabilize the spine and lift the object. Initially the individual tries but fails to generate that much force in the midway, resulting rupture of the annulus fibrosus, end plate or posterior longitudinal ligaments and strain in the muscles that enables the intervertebral disc (nucleus pulposus) to prolapse posterior, and causes dysfunction at the facet joints and nerve roots. *Patient falls on outstretched hand:* During this mechanism there is excessive load on the distal radius and results in radial styloid fracture. Patient falls on the outstretched shoulder with abduction and external rotation produces large loads on the anterior stabilizers of the shoulder resulting in anterior shoulder subluxation or dislocation. *Twisting of the ankle joint with inversion and plantar flexion:* The anterior wider part of the talus fits snugly in the mortise (space between two malleoli). In plantar flexion and inversion the anterior wider part of the talus comes out of the mortise and leaves the joint unstable, the anterior talofibular ligament fails to control the plantar flexion and inversion, eventually the ligament sprains.

c. **Area of Symptoms:** It is useful to record the area of the pain by using a body chart, because this helps in a quick visual reference. Sometimes the area where symptoms are originated remains silent or less symptomatic, for an example in an acute cervical disc herniation patient complaints more pain in the arm and forearm. Therefore, the examiner should correlate the distal symptoms with the cervical. The examiner should also understand the quality of the pain which helps in determining the area of lesion. The patient may complain on more than one area of symptoms.

d. **Severity or Intensity of Pain:** The patient is asked to indicate the description or number which best describes the intensity of their pain at its least and at its worst.

   i. Mild.

   ii. Moderate.

   iii. Distressing.

   iv. Horrible.

   v. Excruciating.

   Visual Analogue Scale (VAS): It is a ten-point scale starts from 0 to 10. Zero is no pain and ten is the unbearable pain. The patient is asked to indicate the point where his pain falls. This not only helps in understanding the intensity of the pain of the patient but also helps in the prognosis. For example, in the first visit patient marks at five and after five treatment sessions he or she says that the pain is decreased in the intensity and now it is at point 2.

e. **Depth of Pain:** Pain situated deep down may be originated from bone and muscles whereas superficial pain is originated from the joints. The depth of pain may give some indication as to the structure at fault but, like quality, this can also be misleading.

f. **Irritability:** This is the length of time for which the person has to perform the activity to increase the pain, and conversely how long it takes before the pain settles to its former intensity. The purpose of assessing irritability of the disorder is to try to discern just how much movement the patient's disorder can be subjected to without causing an exacerbation. It can be measured as high, moderate or low.

High irritability: The aggravating factor causes the pain to increase very quickly or instantly and then the pain takes a long time to settle back.

Moderate irritability: The aggravating factors take longer to increase the symptoms.

Low irritability: The aggravating factor can be performed for a long time before exacerbating the patient's symptoms and then as stopping the activity the symptoms subside rapidly.

g. **Behavior of Symptoms:** The pain and symptoms of the patient may be constant, intermittent or fluctuating. The examiner should ask when the constant, intermittent or fluctuating symptoms are present? or when they fluctuate? Does the patient has sleep disturbance? If yes, does it because of mechanical or inflammatory reason?

h. **Aggravating and Relieving:** What aggravates and eases the symptoms? The movement or posture that produces or increases the symptoms should be noted carefully. Patients with acute mechanical disorder usually find relief in the symptoms during rest but in chronic stage symptoms may also be present in the rest. These patients respond to the heat therapy treatment. Whereas, patients with inflammatory pain always complaint more pain in the rest and the symptoms decrease in activities probably due to engagement in the activities, however, as the disease progresses symptoms will be present in rest as well as in activities. There is no relief in symptoms with the heat therapy (infection).

i. **Positional Factors:** Most musculoskeletal pain is mechanical in origin and is therefore, made better or worse by adopting particular positions or postures that either stretch or compress the structure that are giving rise to pain.

j. **Time Factors:** Certain pathologies tend to be more painful at characteristic times of the day, for example, chronic changes are characteristically painful and stiff initially and arising from sleep.

k. **Duration of the Symptoms:** How long the symptoms are present? Is there any improvement in the symptoms since they have started? Mechanical pain usually improves with the time whereas, infective or inflammatory pain persists and increases in intensity with the time.

Intermediate: Any relief in the symptoms even for a few minutes is considered intermediate.

Example: Mechanical pain. The patients complaint less severe or no pain while resting in a particular position which releases the stress or load on the faulty structure.

System Review

a. **General Well-being:** Weight, appetites, fever, appearance, sleep mood.
b. **Cardiovascular and Respiratory:** Exercise balance for simple, everyday things laid a flight of stain or moving the lawns. Chest pain, palpitations, swelling, caught and sputters.
c. **Alimentary:** Belly pain, nausea, vomiting bowel habits and nature of stools.
d. **Genitourinary:** Frequency of micturition by day and by night, incontinence, pain, frequency and duration of periods, sexual activity and bladder function.
e. **Nervous System:** Headache, vision and hearing, weakness or disturbed sensation.
f. **Locomotors:** Joint pain, stiffness, range of motion, swelling, crepitus, contracture, tightness and deformity.

iii. History: Previous Treatments: Has the patient received any treatment for this condition in the past, if yes what treatment has been taken? Was it effective or was the improvement partial?

Past Medical History: Has the patient suffered any major operations or illness? This might affect the tissues and be a contraindication to particular treatments.

Examples:

i. Respiratory disease.
ii. Cardiac disease.
iii. Diabetes.
iv. Rheumatoid arthritis.
v. Epilepsy.

Is the patient receiving or received oral steroid medications? Patients having chronic respiratory diseases, inflammatory bowel diseases or R.A., may receive oral steroid therapy. This treatment affects bone and produces tendency towards bruising. Medication used in the past or using for the present condition should also be noted carefully.

iv. Observation: After taking history, the next element of subjective assessment is careful physical observation of the **swelling, redness, muscle atrophy, posture, active movements and gait.** During an observation the patient should be undressed. The posture is reviewed (observed) from anterior, lateral and posterior. The examiner notes down the abnormalities in the posture and restriction in the active range of motion, if any, and the patterns of movements (such as compensatory movements and muscle substitutes to show the maximum results). The best way to find the abnormality in the posture and movements, is compared the clinical findings with the normal subjects (practice to observe the posture and movements on normal subjects). This is known as system review. For an instance the examiner finds the pulse rate of the patient 99 per second and when it is compared with normal it is termed as tachycardia but if the examiner does not know normal value it cannot be said that it is very high.

b. Objective Assessment

On the basis of data received from the patient or caregivers during the history and observation, the therapist establishes a kind of disorder in his mind and progresses to the objective examination for further confirmation of the disorder. It is worth to note before any movement tested, the therapist should have a clear appreciation of the disorder to know whether to limit test movements and so avoid exacerbation. Patients with acute injuries are required to provide history and the mechanism of injury. It is far wiser to delay the objective examination (less important of examination) for such patients over two to three days. Objective examination consists passive movements and some special tests, performed on the patient to produce a degree or kind of pain that is not the normal kind of discomfort that could be considered as an acceptable normal.

i. Palpation: The suspected site of symptoms is palpated for tenderness, temperature, sensation, crepitus and end feel. To elicit the tenderness, a palmar aspect of the thumb is placed directly on the site of symptoms and pressed gently. Pisiform aspect of the wrist may also be used to elicit the pain and symptoms. To feel the temperature, the dorsal aspect of the hand is placed on the suspected area. Increased temperature of the suspect area indicates an active inflammation or infection. To test the sensation, a test tube, cotton or tip of the finger is placed on the suspected area and patient is asked how he or she perceives it. To test the crepitus the examiner places hand on the suspected area of lesion and asks the patient to move the joint actively. Feeling of grinding or jerk during an active movement indicates crepitus. For an example to test the crepitus in the shoulder, the examiner places hand on the shoulder and the patient is asked to elevate the arm actively. The end feel is experienced with passive movements of the joints. The end range may be limited by the pain, swelling, spasm of the muscles, abnormal bony contacts and loose bodies which may give the feeling of empty, soft, firm and hard.

ii. Special Tests: The special tests and measures are performed to generate data by reproducing the symptoms of the patients impairments and functional limitations. These special tests and measures are based on medical safety, patient comfort, emotional, functional, social, vocational needs and financial resources. The following relevant examination may be performed by a therapist: aerobic capacity, joint integrity, and mobility, motor function, range of motion, muscle strength, cardiopulmonary functions (ventilation, respiration and circulation) posture and gait balance.

B. EVALUATION

Interpretation of the examination findings is the evaluation; it is one of the most critical stages in a clinical decision making. Evaluation is the dynamic process in which the therapist makes judgment based on data gathered during the subjective and objective examination. The therapist interprets the subjective and objective examination and clinical findings to understand the source or cause of the patient's impairments, disorder, functional limitations and disabilities. The clinical data may also be analyzed to determine the progression and stage of the sign and symptom, and stability of the condition.

C. DIAGNOSIS

Diagnosis is the dynamic condition of analyzing the clinical data gathered during the subjective and objective examination and evaluation; and organizing them into clusters, syndromes, or categories to help in determining the appropriate intervention and strategy for each patient. American Physical Therapy Association (APTA) has described the diagnosis as a label encompassing a cluster of sign and symptoms commonly associated with a disorder, syndrome or category of impairment, functional limitation or disability. Cluster is set of observations or data that frequently occur as a group for a single patient. Syndrome is an aggregate of sign and symptoms that characterize a given disease or condition.

D. PROGNOSIS

Prognosis is the determination of minimal improvement to maximal improvement expected at various intervals

> **Impairments**
>
> It is the loss or abnormality of physiologic, psychological, or anatomical structure or function.
>
> **Physiologic Impairment:** It can be defined as an alteration in any physiologic function such as reduced force or torque production, reduced endurance, reduced mobility, reduced balance and coordination, and altered posture and movement patterns.
>
> **Anatomic Impairment:** It can be defined as an abnormality or loss of structure, such as hip anteversion, structural genu varum, congenital or traumatic loss of an extremity.
>
> **Psychological Impairment:** It is an abnormality related to the psychological system. It is usual with the physiologic and anatomical patient to have some degree of psychological impairment. Physiotherapy treatment is more effective in improving physiologic impairment in terms of increasing functional strength, range of motion, improving balance and coordination and posture. Physiotherapy treatment has less role in improving the anatomical and psychological impairments.

during the course of physical therapy intervention. The prognosis depends upon the health, underlying condition and age of the patient. A healthy patient shows faster improvement in the sign and symptoms than the patient who is having the history of underlying pathological condition such as diabetes of the same age. For an example a 65-year-old healthy patient with fracture of neck of femur managed with total hip replacement can walk with the toe touch weight bearing with the help of walker in the first week, this is the short term expected improvement of the patient. The long-term expected improvement of this patient is jogging without any pain and gait deviation after three months of the operation. On the other hand an ankylosing patient will be having poor prognosis as the disease is progressive which causes loss of movements of the spine and peripheral joints with the due course of time. The prognosis also depends upon the risk factors and response to previous interventions.

E. INTERVENTION

Intervention is the purposeful and skilled physiotherapeutic treatment of various methods, techniques, modalities and education administered towards the patient in order to improve pain, symptoms and functional impairments. An effective physiotherapeutic treatment requires thorough subjective and objective examination.

Clinical Decision Making

Clinical decision making is the dynamic process which involves vertical thinking and lateral thinking.

Vertical Thinking: It is characterized by logical sequential predictable thinking. It is also known as conventional thinking or process of gathering data or information from the patient. It stays within a problem space.

Lateral Thinking: It is concerned with the generation of new idea, and with looking things in a different way. It tends to restructure the problem space. The lateral thinking focuses not only on the problem space but also on the proximal and distal parts of the problem space. The therapist's assessment is more inclined to the clinical decision making.

Examination

Subjective	*Objective*
• General information	• Palpation
• Chief complaint/History	– Tenderness
– Onset of symptoms	– Temperature
– Mechanism of injury	– Sensation
– Duration of symptoms	– Swelling
– Area of symptoms	
– Nature and quality of symptoms	– End feel
– Intensity of symptoms	– Crepitus
– Aggravating factors	• Special Tests
– Behavior of symptoms	– Functional tests
– Irritability	– Isometric tests
• History	– Joint play tests
• Observation of:	– Neural movement tests
– Posture	
– Active movements	• Radiological Examination
– Swelling	
– Joint contour	
– Muscle atrophy and	
– Gait	

Differential Diagnosis of General Conditions

1. **Infective Conditions:** Severe unremitting pain at rest with no history of injury, persistent pain at night, loss of weight, loss of appetite, unusual growth or lumps, no relief with medication or position or heat therapy.
2. **Inflammatory Conditions:** Pain at rest, morning stiffness, swelling (effusion or thickening), warmth, erythema, diffuse type of tenderness, loss of motion.
3. **Vascular:** Throbbing, diffuse type of pain.
4. **Neurological Conditions: Nerve involvement**—sharp, bright, lightning like. **Nerve root**—sharp, shooting. **Sympathetic nerve**—burning, pressure like, stinging, aching etc. **Upper motor neuron lesion**—spasticity, exaggerated tone, exaggerated reflexes, extensor plantar reflex, spastic gait. **Lower motor neuron lesion**—flaccidity, decrease tone, diminish reflexes muscle wasting.
5. **Systemic Diseases.**

Differential diagnosis of orthopedic conditions

Muscle	*Nerve roots*	*Bone*	*Fracture*	*Mechanical*
Cramping, dull, aching. **Tendinitis:** Localized tenderness, ecchymosis, palpable defect in the muscle, weakness, resisted movement painful. Pain may be in the mid range also. **Strain:** Ecchymosis, palpable defect in the muscle, weakness, pain at extreme ranges on passive stretching.	Sharp, shooting, bright, lightning-like.	Deep situated, dull, nagging.	Sharp, severe in intensity, intolerable.	Pain during activities, tenderness, crepitus, aggravates in particular position/posture which put the pressure on the damaged structure, relieves at rest and night. Mechanical pain may be degenerative, disc herniation, muscle strain, ligaments sprain, and may arise from acute or chronic repetitive injuries. Patients with chronic mechanical pain may have morning stiffness and pain at rest but these respond to the heat therapy and stretching exercise.

Assessment Proforma

Subjective Assessment

- **General Information**
  - Name :
  - Age :
  - Sex:
  - Address :
  - E-mail ID/contact no. :
- **Chief Complaint**
  - Pain :
  - Stiffness :
  - Weakness :
  - Instability :
  - Giving way :
  - Post fracture stiffness/swelling :
  - Referred for differential diagnosis :
- **History of Symptoms**
  - Onset of symptoms: Gradual/sudden :
  - Mechanism of injury :
  - Duration of symptoms :
  - Area of symptoms :
  - Nature and quality of symptoms :
  - Intensity of symptoms (VAS) :
  - Aggravating/relieving factors :
  - Behavior of symptoms :
  - Irritability :
- **Medical History**
  - Hormonal disease
    - q Hypo/hyperthyroidism :
    - q Diabetes :
    - q Parkinson's disease :
  - Hypertension/seizures :
  - Medications, NASAIDs/steroids :
  - Previous surgeries/implants :
  - Drugs interaction/allergy :
- **Observation of:**
  - Posture from
    - Anterior view :

- Posterior view :
- Lateral view :

– Active movements
- Flexion/Extension :
- Abduction/Adduction :
- Medial/Lateral rotation :

– Swelling: Effusion/thickening :
– Joint contour :
– Muscle atrophy :
– Gait :

Objective Assessment

- **Palpation**
  – Tenderness :
  – Temperature :
  – Sensation :
  – End feel :
  – Crepitus :
- **Special Tests**
  – Functional tests
  i.
  ii.
  iii.
  – Isometric tests :
  – Joint play tests :
  – Neural movement tests :
- **Radiological Examination**

....
....
....

Evaluation

- ....
- ....
- ....
- ....
- ....

Diagnosis

- Possible
- Classical
- Definite

Intervention

- ....
- ....
- ....
- ....
- ....
- ....
- ....

Re-Examination/Evaluation/Intervention

....
....
....
....
....
....
....
....
....

23

SOFT TISSUE INJURIES

MUSCLE STRAIN

When the muscle is loaded with an external force, the load is resisted primarily by the collagen fibrils. Initially tissues respond to the load by straightening from their resting crimped state, which may be upto 4% elongation in a linear fashion. The muscle fibers return to its normal resting length as the load is removed. If the load is high and causes elongation of the muscle fibers beyond 4% of its normal length, deformation occurs and muscle fibers never return to the normal length. The muscle is said to be strained.

Elastic Range

Due to external force there is elongation of the muscle fibers upto 4% which return to its normal length as soon as the load is removed.

Plastic Range

Due to extreme load there is elongation of the fiber beyond 4% of its length. The muscle fibers do not return to the normal length after removing the load. Elongation of the fibers beyond 4% of their normal length causes deformation and rupture of the muscle fibers, in turn the load on the remaining fibers increases.

Types of Muscle Strain

Muscle strain may either be an acute or chronic.

Acute Strain: Muscle strain occurs along a continuum from an acute micro traumatic injury to chronic micro traumatic overuse injuries. The acute traumatic injuries can cause muscle strain if a muscle is rapidly overloaded or overstretched and the tension generated in the muscle fibers exceeds the tensile capability of the musculotendinous junction unit. These strains occur near the musculotendinous junction and at random areas within the muscle belly.

Chronic Strain: The chronic traumatic injuries produce muscle strain if the muscles are involved in continuous repetitive activities. During the continuous repetitive activities the proximal muscles of the joint get fatigue, resulting in substitution with distal muscles. The distal muscles will be strained. For example when the shoulder muscles get fatigue during continuous repetitive activities or work, substitution with distal musculature occurs. In lower extremity, following fatigue of the gluteus medius and ilio-psoas muscles, the tensor fascia lata dominates over these muscles and is at risk for an overuse strain. [This situation is very similar to the chairperson of any party sitting on desk along with two members on each side, for press conference. In reply of a particular question, the chairperson apprehended and fails to answer as a lack of knowledge, that allows one of members to dominate over the chairperson and seeks attention of the media. The member has done a good job but he has to pay the price of dominating over the chairperson]. Improving the strength and recruitment patterns of the iliopsoas and gluteus medius can reduce the load on the tensor fascia lata and allow it to recover.

A thorough evaluation can determine the source of the overuse strain which may be due to continuous repetitive activities. Work site assessment is necessary to prevent a recurrence of the muscle performance impairment. If left untreated, this impairment can quickly lead to disability. It should be treated with postural or motor program re-education and resistive exercises. The proximal muscles should be strengthened first followed by distal by using the progressive resistive exercise. The progressive resisted exercise should be directed to the proximal muscles, followed by distal muscles. Two to three sets (each set of ten repetitions) per day to form fatigue is generally recommended, but if not fatigue by 30-40 repetitions, then the resistance should be increased to form fatigue. The exercises will increase muscle performance. These may be progressed to a higher speed to challenge stability. In aforesaid example, to strength the hip abductors, the patient stands with one foot. A resistive theraband around each of the ankle is wrapped. The patient may hold the chair with the one hand for support and then the three sets of PRE are done.

Subtle Strain

This type of muscle strain is common when a muscle is continuously placed in a relatively lengthened, tension producing position. It is a gradual process. In upper crossed syndrome, there is a forward head posture. The head shifts anterior to the midline. This places lower trapezius muscles in a lengthened position. The trapezius lower fibers are at greater risk of overstretch strain. Such patients are need to be educated about the work station ergonomics. Correction of working style can improve the posture and reduce the muscles strain.

A. Hamstrings Strain

Hamstrings strain is frequently reported in clinics, and its diagnosis is one of the challenges for the clinicians. Most common cause of hamstrings strain is overuse of the muscles particularly, biceps femoris. Hamstrings participate in force couples around the lumbopelvic hip complex, contributing to posterior pelvic rotation, hip extension and indirectly hip medial and lateral rotation. However the hamstrings are the prime movers of the knee flexion.

During mid swing to initial contact the hamstrings decelerate the hip joint, while at initial contact and loading response, the biceps femoris is thought to decelerate tibial medial rotation that occurs with foot pronation. Weakness of the gluteus maximus and deep hip external rotators may lead to excess demand on the hamstrings to decelerate hip flexion during late mid swing and hip medial rotation at initial contact. The biceps femoris load is exaggerated (over used) because of force couple it contributes. The condition is aggravated if the weakness of gluteus maximus and deep hip lateral rotators are associated with fore foot varus. Underuse of the oblique abdominal muscles increase anterior tilting of the pelvis which may lead to overuse of the hamstrings because they must exert a posterior rotational force on the lumbopelvic region.

Overuse: Hamstrings strains are managed by strengthening of the gluteus maximus, deep hip external rotators and biomechanical correction of the foot. Sometimes clinicians focus on the symptoms and under estimate the cause of strain. This may improve the symptoms, but there are more chances of recurrence of hamstrings strain, which contributes to the poor performance. Hence, to treat the strains therapist must focus on the cause, not on the symptoms.

The exercises such as stomach-lying hip extension may be taught to the patient. This will not only strengthen gluteus maximus but also strengthens deep external rotators of the hip joint. These two commonly underused synergists (gluteus maximus and deep external rotators) of hamstrings contribute to the hamstrings overuse strain. The aim of stomach-lying hip extension exercise is to improve force generating capability and kinesthetic awareness of the muscle to the extent that is adequate to allow it to fully participate in a function of task. (The patient with overuse hamstrings strain usually give inadequate force generating capability to participate in a functional task).

Stomach-lying Hip Extension

The patient lies on the stomach on a firm surface, and an adequate thickness of pillow is placed under torso. The patient is instructed to pull the belly toward the spine (belly tuck in), in the next hip is extended barely off the floor, and is held for at least six seconds. Three sets of 30 repetition may be performed. As the force generating capability and kinesthetic awareness improves sufficiently, stomach-lying hip extension exercise is progressed to the functional activities such as walk stance, step up and step down.

B. Gluteus Medius Muscle Strain

Gluteus medius strain is not very common, but may strain functioning in a chronic gradual, continuous stretching. Patients with leg length discrepancy (functional or structural) often present with stretched gluteus medius of the normal side due to adduction of the normal side hip joint. The gluteus medius strains are treated with leg length correction in case of structural LLD. If LLD is functional then the treatment should be focused on the strengthening of the muscles contributing to the functional leg length discrepancy in conjunction with stretching. The exercise may progress to the functional activities such as walk stance, step up and step down.

C. Lumbo-Pelvic Musculature Strain

Similar to the hamstrings, the lumbo-pelvic muscles may be strained of trauma, overuse and gradual continuous stretch. Traumatic injuries such as road traffic accident may cause strain to the spinal extensors and multifidus muscles. Overuse strains are usually occur in population whose job involves repetitive flexion and rotation of the lumbo-pelvic region. It often involves the oblique abdominal strain on a crew team.

D. Anterior Scalene Muscle Strain

The anterior scalene muscle is usually strained if it is overused. Patient complains pain in the upper thoracic spine and the area of first rib. The function of the muscles is cervical flexion, ipsilateral side flexion and contralateral cervical rotation. Weakness or underuse of the deep neck flexors, contralateral rotators, ipsilateral side flexors of neck and diaphragmatic muscles force anterior scalene muscle to excessive contraction to maintain the posture and movement of the cervical spine. Sustain and overuse of the muscle results in anterior scalene strain.

Treatment of overuse of the anterior scalene muscle should be focused on strengthening of the underused muscles such as deep neck flexors, ipsilateral side flexors, contralateral rotators and diaphragmatic muscles (anterior scalene muscle also acts as an accessory respiratory muscle). The second part of the treatment should be focused on the stretching of the anterior scalene muscle. To stretch the muscle the first rib is stabilized and patient is instructed to bend the neck to the contralateral side and rotate to the same side. While maintaining the side flexion and rotation the neck is extended for further stretching of the muscle.

E. Middle and Lower Trapezius Strain

The patient with forward head posture (protracted shoulders and head) can place the middle and lower trapezius in an overstretched position. Functioning in overstretched position can cause strain to the middle and lower trapezius muscles. Patients often complaint pain in the middle border of the scapula. Treatment is focused on the correction of the forward head posture (correction of the protracted head and shoulders and upper thoracic kyphosis). This includes strengthening of deep neck flexors, rhomboids, middle and lower trapezius; and stretching of pectoralis major, upper cervical extensors, trapezius upper fibers and anterior scalene muscles.

F. Posterior Deltoid Strain

In patients with anterior instability of the shoulder, the head of humerus translates (excessively) anteriorly as the anterior capsule is lax. Therefore, posterior deltoid muscles contract eccentrically to control anterior excessive translation of the head of humerus. The posterior deltoid fibers are strained as they are overused in order to prevent anterior excessive translation of the head of humerus. These patients complaint pain in the posterior aspect of the shoulder girdle (posterior deltoid).

LIGAMENTOUS SPRAIN

The end range of the joint is mostly resisted by the inert structures such as ligaments and joint capsule. For an example, when the joint is moved beyond its normal limit it is resisted by the joint capsule and ligaments, but if the force is high and beyond the capacity of these structures, there is stretching or disruption in the continuity of the ligaments or joint capsule. Sprains may also be associated with muscle strain injuries. Patients with ligament sprain usually present with pain, swelling, ecchymosis and joint instability. However, mild sprain does not cause significant swelling and instability.

The severity of the sprain depends upon the degree of mechanism of injury. Patients usually complaint pain in the extreme ranges when the disrupted or stretched portion of ligament or joint capsule is stretched. Sometimes patients complaint pain in the end range during the functional activities but the passive movements do not produce these symptoms, this is common in mild injuries, whereas in severe injuries the pain may be present throughout the range of motion. Instability and apprehension tests provoke the symptoms.

Classification

The sprains are graded as mild, moderate and severe, which involve microscopic tearing or stretching of the ligament or joint capsule fibers to complete disruption of the ligament.

- **Grade I or Mild Sprain:** It is a microscopic tearing or stretch of the ligament with little swelling and tenderness. There is no functional impairment and instability of the joint.
- **Grade II or Moderate Sprain:** It involves macroscopic partial tear of ligament with moderate swelling and tenderness. There is loss of functional status of the joint. Joint instability or ligamentous laxity is present.
- **Grade III or Severe Sprain:** Complete or nearly complete tear of the ligament with severe swelling, tenderness and ecchymosis. There is gross functional impairment. Mechanical joint instability is present.

Management

The management depends upon the severity of the sprain. PRICE is administered to improve sign and symptoms. Grade I and Grade II sprains are managed with PRICE, controlled activities and exercises, whereas, grade III sprains may require surgical intervention.

i. **Protection (P):** The activities which put load in the sprained ligament should be avoided. The supportive or assistive devices such as sling, splint, cane, crutches and walker should be used in order to avoid the load on the joint and ligament.

ii. **Rest (R):** The ligament which is sprained should not be allowed to stretch, hence end range movements should be avoided.

iii. **Ice** (I): Ice towel or ice pack over the area should be applied for ten minutes to reduce swelling and accelerate healing of the tissues. The application of ice should not be more than ten minutes for the acute injuries as it may cause dilatation of the vessels that can increase the swelling in the joint. However, it can be repeated every hour.

iv. **Compression** (C): Grade I sprains are usually treated with short term immobilization in the form of elastic crepe bandage to prevent swelling and movements. Grade II sprained joints are immobilized in the elastic crepe bandage or brace with limited weight bearing. Grade III sprained ligaments need to be immobilized in the plaster of paris.

v. **Elevation** (E): Swelling is very usual after ligamentous sprain. The leg should be elevated above the level of heart. To do this two or three pillows may be placed under the ankle joint at night. The leg may also be placed on the stool when the patient is sitting at the work station.

ANTERIOR TALOFIBULAR LIGAMENT (ATFL) SPRAIN

It is estimated that one inversion injury of the ankle occurs for every 10000 people each day. Ankle sprain constitutes 7-10 percent of all admission to the hospital emergency departments. Fifty percent of such injuries occur during sport activities.

The stability of the ankle is provided by the ligaments, muscles and bony configuration. The peroneous longus and brevis on the posterolateral side and tibialis posterior, flexor digitorum longus, and flexor halluces longus on the medial side contribute to the dynamic stability. The passive stability is provided by the medial, lateral, posterior ligaments and the syndesmosis. The lateral ligaments complex such as anterior talofibular ligament (ATFL), calcaneofibular ligament (CFL) and the posterior talofibular ligament is most commonly affected in the ankle injuries (Fig. 23.1).

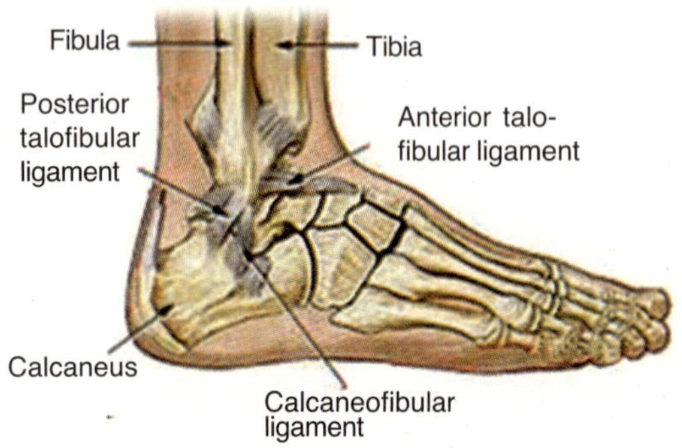

Fig. 23.1: Lateral ligaments complex

The ankle joint remains more stable (closed packed) at the neutral position because the wider anterior portion of the talus fits snugly into the ankle mortise. Plantar flexion of the ankle rotates the posterior narrowed talus into the mortise, resulting in a much loose fit (loose packed), with a particular tendency towards inversion. The anterior talofibular ligament is relaxed at the neutral position and taut in a plantar flexion with inversion. It is the primary restraint against inversion during plantar flexion.

When the ankle is plantar flexed the anterior talofibular ligament becomes taut in order to prevent excessive plantar flexion as the anterior wider portion of the talus is replaced with the narrowed posterior portion of the talus to the mortise and the ankle joint becomes unstable (loose packed). The growth plate in the children is particularly vulnerable to fracture because it is weaker than the surrounding ligaments, bone and the periosteum. Usually anterior talofibular ligament sprain occurs in isolation but if the injury is severe it may be combined with the calcaneofibular ligament sprain. The lateral collateral ligament sprain is classified as grade I, II and III (Fig. 23.2).

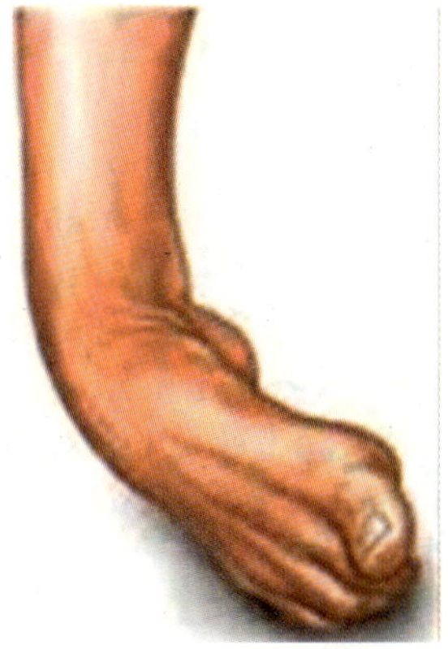

Fig. 23.2: Mechanism of injury, plantar flexion with inversion

- **Grade I or Mild Sprain:** It is a microscopic tearing or stretch of the anterior talofibular ligament with little swelling and tenderness. There is no functional impairment and instability of the joint.
- **Grade II or Moderate Sprain:** It involves macroscopic partial tear of the anterior talofibular ligament with moderate swelling and tenderness. There is loss of functional status of the joint. Joint instability or ligamentous laxity is present.
- **Grade III or Severe Sprain:** Complete or nearly complete tear of the ligament with severe swelling, tenderness and ecchymosis. There is gross functional impairment. Mechanical joint instability is present. Grade III sprains are further classified on the basis of degrees of injury.

First degree sprains: There is complete rupture of the anterior talofibular ligament.

Second degree sprain: There is complete rupture of the anterior talofibular and calcaneofibular ligament.

Third degree sprain: There is a dislocation of the joint with ATFL, CFL and posterior talofibular ligament (PTFL) sprains (Fig. 23.3).

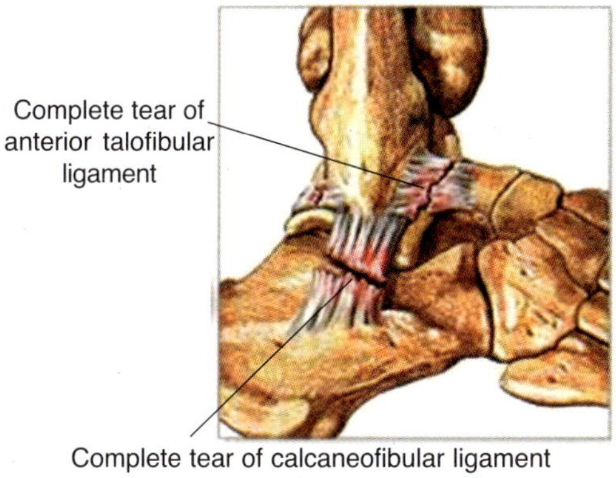

Fig. 23.3: Type III sprain

Clinical Features

The patient usually recalls the mechanism of injury and presents with tenderness on anterior edge and at the tip of the fibula with swelling around the joint, in case of talofibular ligament sprain. Haemorrhage continuous 6 to 12 hours. Patient complaints that pain aggravates when the foot goes into the plantar flexion and inversion, however no or less pain occurs in the dorsiflexion. Ecchymosis may occur, indicating injury to blood vessels in the area (Fig. 23.4).

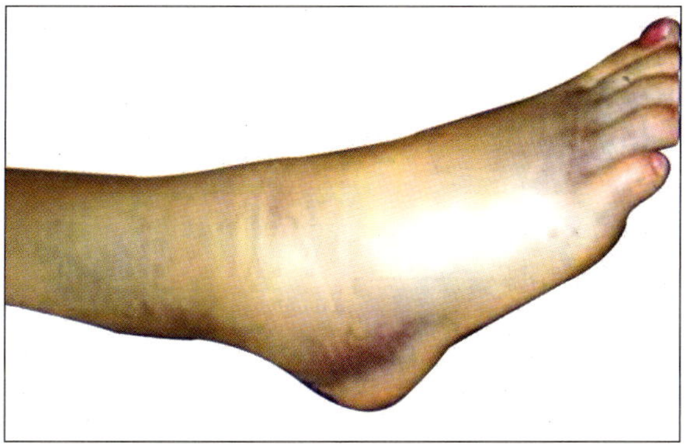

Fig. 23.4: Swelling around the ankle joint

Physical Examination

A comprehensive history and evaluation helps in diagnosing the severity and type of ankle sprain. Radiographic imaging techniques may need to be used to rule out fractures, complete ligament tears, or instability of the ankle mortise. The anterior drawer test and the talar tilt test usually reproduce the symptoms and identify the ligaments sprain.

Anterior Drawer Test: The patient lies supine, ankle joint is taken out of the plinth. The therapist stands at the side of ankle joint, stabilizes distal tibia with one hand and holds the heel in slight plantar flexion with the other hand. While stabilizing the tibia, the heel is drawn anteriorly with respect to the tibia. Translation greater than 5 mm or difference in the anterior translation from the asymptomatic ankle suggests a tear of the ATFL.The test may also be performed in the sitting position (Fig. 23.5).

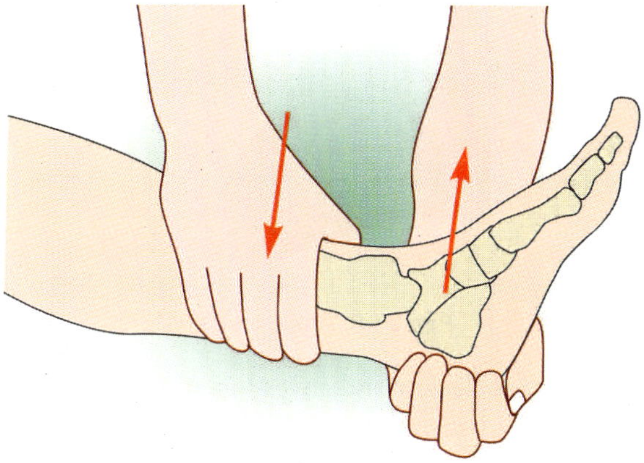

Fig. 23.5: Anterior drawer test

Talar Tilt Test: This tests the integrity of the calcaneofibular ligament. The patient sits comfortably and the therapist stands at the side and stabilizes the distal tibia with one hand. The talus and calcaneus is grasped with other hand by placing the thenar and hypothenar on the dorsum and fingers on the medial aspect of the ankle. While stabilizing the distal tibia the talus and the calcaneus is inverted as a unit with respect to the tibia. A positive finding of more than 5 mm with a soft endpoint indicates a combined injury to the ATFL and CFL.

Management

Based on the diagnosis and an understanding of ligament healing properties, a progressive treatment regimen can be developed. The initial emphasis is made on accelerating healing, controlling inflammation and associated pain and swelling. Healing of a ligament sprain as in most of soft tissue injuries follows a process of inflammation, repair and remodelling. During the reparative and remodelling phase, the goal is to progress the rehabilitation appropriately to facilitate healing and restore the strength and proprioception.The controlled stress helps in promoting healing and results in a stronger repair.

GRADE I AND II SPRAINS MANAGEMENT

Initial Phase

Immediately after injury, PRICE principle is followed to reduce haemorrhage, swelling, inflammation and pain. Most of ankle sprains can be managed successfully with a non-surgical approach.

1. **Protection:** The ankle joint is immobilized (protected) in a functional brace or removable cast boot (for grade II), at the neutral position. Early weight bearing is allowed with the help of axillary crutches (Fig. 23.6).

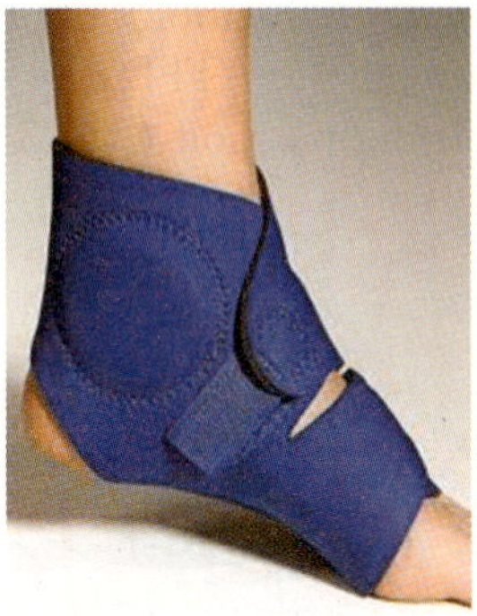

Fig. 23.6: Ankle brace

2. **Rest:** Plantar flexion and inversion must be avoided in order to avoid the stress on ATFL.
3. **Ice:** Ice bag or cryocuff are applied for 10 minutes on the ankle joint to prevent hemorrhage and swelling. During ice application, the vasoconstriction occurs in the first ten minutes which is followed by vasodilatation. The therapist must not allow vasodilatation to occur especially in the acute stage (Fig. 23.7).

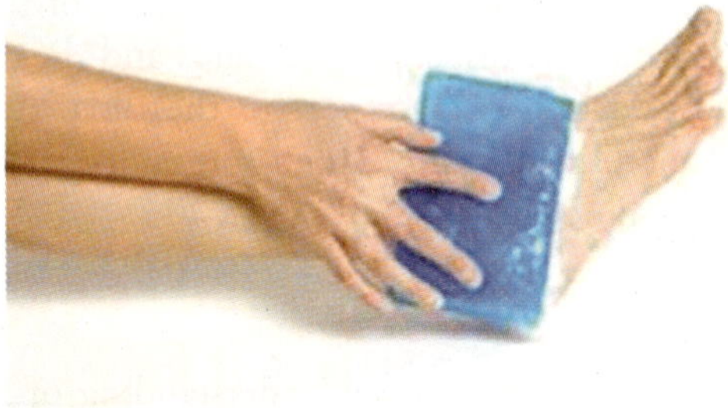

Fig. 23.7: Ice pack over the ATFL

4. **Compression:** Compression with an elastic bandage is beneficial in preventing the swelling especially when the foot is in dependent position such as in sitting and walking. Vasopneumatic compressions are also helpful in controlling pain and swelling (Fig. 23.8).

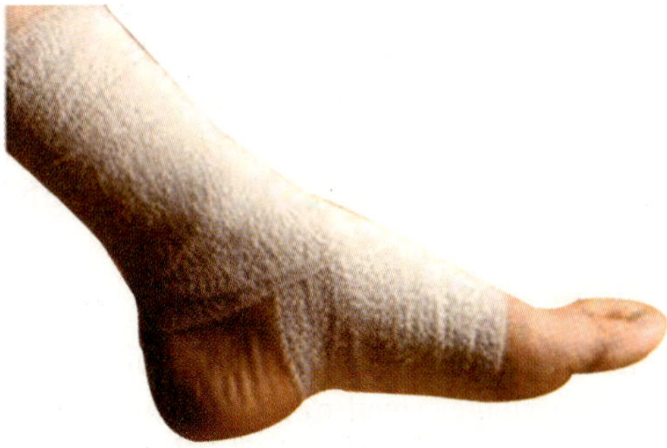

Fig. 23.8: Elastic repe bandage to immobilize the ankle joint

5. **Elevation:** The leg is raised above the heart level in order to increase venous return from distal to the proximal part. The patients are also advised to keep the foot on the stool or chair while sitting instead of hanging in gravity dependent position.

The ankle joint is immobilized (protected) in a functional brace or removable cast boot (for grade II), at the neutral position. Early weight bearing is allowed with the help of axillary crutches. The functional brace or cast boot must be accompanied with the ice, compression and elevation till the end of this phase to achieve optimal results. After 3-4 days of injury, exercises are initiated as the patient shows improvement in the pain and swelling. ***The exercises must not interrupt the repair process***; hence, these should be in a controlled manner. Active dorsiflexion, inversion, foot circles and plantar flexion are initiated in the pain free range. ***Strengthening:*** Submaximal isometric of dorsiflexors, plantar flexors, evertors and invertors in the pain free range are helpful in restoring the strength. ***Stretching***: Calf stretching should be initiated to improve the flexibility. ***Proprioceptive training*** on Seated Biomechanical Ankle Platform System (BAPS) and on the Wobble board are also helpful.

Rehabilitation Phase

This usually starts after one week of the injury when patient reports at least 90% improvement in the sign and symptoms such as pain and swelling. The rehabilitation phase may be delayed if there is no significant improvement in the symptoms. This phase introduces weight bearing exercises such as heel raise, toe raise (initially bilateral followed by unilateral heel raise), stair and mini squatting (30 degrees bilateral knee flexion). The isometric (close kinetic chain) exercises are progressed to the theraband and weight cuff resisted exercises.

Functional Phase

The patient may return to the normal activities. This phase usually starts after second week of the injury. The aim of treatment is to regain full strength, proprioception training, stability of the joint and return to the sport. The theraband and weight cuff resisted exercises remain same but with more resistance. Incorporation of multidirectional agility drills can begin at this stage. Start with controlled exercises that are on both legs.

- Brisk walk followed by figure of eight, zig zag cutting and jogging. Begin jumping forward and backward over a line.
- Progress to jumping laterally over a line.

Syndesmosis Sprains

The syndesmosis sprains are usually occur in combined with other ankle joint sprains. It is the disruption of the distal tibiofibular and interosseous membrane. The distal tibiofibular ligament attaches at the distal end of the tibia and fibula which plays important role in maintaining the mortise space. The anterior wider portion of the talus remains in the mortise at the neutral position.Disruption of tibiofibular ligaments resulting in diastasis, or widening of the mortise at the talocrural joint.

Mechanism of Injury: The tibiofibular ligament disrupts if there is pronation and eversion combined with internal rotation of the leg when the foot is fixed on the ground or extreme dorsiflexion of the ankle joint. The *external rotation* and dorsiflexion forces the talus into the mortise, resulting widening of the talocrural joint which eventually disrupts the tibiofibular ligament and the interosseous membrane. The patients with syndesmosis sprains complaint pain in the anterior and posterior ankle joint particularly when trying to push off of the affected ankle. The patient does not bear the weight on the affected ankle joint.

Physical Evaluation: Pain, swelling and tenderness around the ankle joint with inability to bear the weight on the joint are the common clinical findings of the syndesmosis sprain. The following physical tests may further confirm the sprain. *Squeeze Test:* Patient sits comfortably on the plinth.Therapist stands at the side, stabilizes the knee joint with one hand and grasps the anterior proximal leg with other hand and squeezes gently. If the test elicits pain in the tibiofibular ligament and interosseous membrane or syndesmosis area, it suggests syndesmosis sprain. *External Rotation Stress Test:* The patient sits comfortably on a treatment plinth with knee flexion to 90 degrees. The therapist sits comfortably at the side and stabilizes the distal tibiofibular joint with one hand and grasps the ankle at neutral position with other hand. While stabilizing the joint the foot is rotated externally. In case of positive test, the patient will complaint pain in the syndesmosis area. *Tibiotalar Shuck Test:* The examiner stabilizes the leg with one hand and grasps the talus with other hand. While stabilizing the leg the medial and lateral force is applied to the talus alternatively. Pain in the syndesmosis region or feeling of the looseness may indicate syndesmosis sprain.

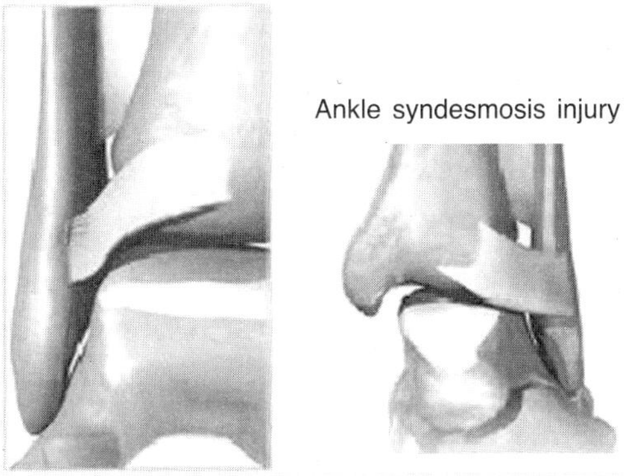

Ankle syndesmosis injury

Management: The syndesmosis sprains are treated conservatively with cast immobilisation for 4-6 weeks followed by rehabilitation program similar to the Grade I and Grade II ATFL sprains. The syndesmosis sprain with unstable and widened mortise is often managed with surgical fixation.

- Progress to box drills: Draw on the floor with tape and number the boxes starting in the upper left corner and progressing clockwise.
- The athlete may return to the sport if he/she gains full confidence, and muscle strength equivalent to the contralateral leg.
- The plyometric and proprioceptive training exercises and running is also started at this phase before return to the sport. On level ground, begin single leg standing exercises incorporating sport specific exercises such as kicking a ball, catching and throwing a ball, or swinging a bat. Progress to standing on an air filled or foam cushion. Begin by keeping the exercise, such as catching a ball, close to the body. Progress to throwing the ball farther from the body to force the athlete to shift his center of gravity.

Prevention of Recurrence of ATFL Sprain

Poor compliance with therapy may predispose to functional instability of the ankle joint, therefore, to prevent reinjury, proprioceptive rehabilitation should continue until the athlete demonstrates improved functional skills particular to the individual's sport. Upon initial return to sport, the athlete should continue to support the ankle with taping or a brace. The patient should be encouraged to continue home exercises program to ensure full restoration. Technique training (on jumping and landing), proprioceptive training, and orthosis have all shown to decrease risk of reinjury.

Grade III Sprain Treatment

The grade III first degree sprains are successfully managed with non-operative conservative treatment. Immediately after injury, PRICE principle is followed to reduce haemorrhage, swelling, inflammation and pain. There has been much debate over the treatment of Grade III sprains whether these should be managed with immobilization or surgical repair. One school of thought recommends surgical repair followed by immobilization and rehabilitation. Others suggest immobilization followed by rehabilitation. It is concluded that the surgery should be recommended if there is involvement of other ligaments sprains such as calcaneofibular and tibiofibular ligament. The rehabilitative management including exercises remain almost same as Grade II and III sprains.

Surgical Management

The surgery should be reserved for the patients with chronic ankle instability. Most surgeons prefer surgical reconstruction of an ATFL especially second and third degree of grade III sprains where other structure such as CFL and syndesmosis sprains are also involved.

A graft is taken from gracillus or semitendinosus tendon. A tunnel is made on the talar neck on the insertion of an ATFL. A transfibular tunnel directed anterior to posterior through the fibula tip to a blind ending tunnel in the calcaneus at the insertion site of the CFL is also made. An ATFL graft is inserted in the tunnel through talus to the fibula. The CFL graft is also inserted in the tunnel through calcaneum to the fibula.

ANTERIOR CRUCIATE LIGAMENT SPRAIN

Anterior cruciate ligament is a primary restraint to the anterior translation of the proximal tibia throughout the range of motion, however, it has more restraining power in the last 30 degrees of the extension. Although functioning independently, an ACL and PCL guide the instant centre of rotation of the knee, thereby controlling the joint arthrokinematics.

An ACL sprains most commonly causes knee joint instability than does sprains to other knee ligaments. In the past, an ACL tear could end the career of the athletes or result in the need for surgery and a year or more of rehabilitation. In the 1970s, ACL reconstruction were done through large arthrotomies, using extraarticular reconstruction followed by immobilization of the knee joint. To get rid of prolong immobilization and arthrotomies new approach of reconstruction "arthroscopy" was introduced in the 1980s. In the 1990s, the concept of "accelerated" rehabilitation evolved in an effort to return to the field quicker than ever.

Anatomy

The anterior cruciate ligament arises from the posteromedial corner of medial aspect of lateral femoral condyle in the intercondylar notch. It inserts in a fossa in front of and lateral to anterior tibial spine. It is made up of multiple collagen fascicles surrounded by an endotendinium and enveloped in a synovial membrane. The anterior cruciate ligament is innervated by the tibial nerve. The blood supply is received from the middle genicular artery. The bony attachments of the ligament at distal and proximal do not receive a significant blood supply from the artery. It is the reason of poor healing of the ligament after the injury (Fig. 23.9).

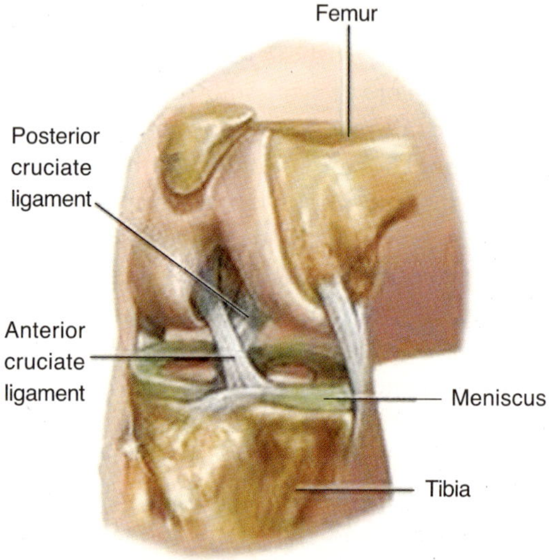

Fig. 23.9: Anterior and posterior cruciate ligaments

The anterior cruciate ligament is composed of two principal parts: small anteromedial band and a larger bulky posterolateral portion. The small anteromedial bundle becomes tight in flexion. The large posterolateral band moves anteriorly and becomes loose in flexion, on the other hand in extension it becomes tight. The posterolateral bulky portion of the ligament limits anterior translation, hyperextension and rotation of the knee joint whereas anteromedial bundle provides more rotational control which is in an axial position.

Epidemiology

Female soccer and basket athletes have the rates of ACL injuries more than the male soccer and basket athletes. Male and female basket athletes have similar rates of contact and non-contact ACL injuries whereas female soccer athletes have more non-contact ACL injuries than male soccer athletes. Women have wider pelvis, shorter femurs, and less developed thigh muscles than males, these differences form a more lateral proximal reference point and increase lateral pull of the quadriceps on the patella and put medial stress on the knee joint.

A notable finding on gender difference in an ACL tears in relationship with physical abilities by researchers (Mountcastle *et al.*) is that women are three times more likely to have an ACL injury than men due to variations of hormone levels and greater ligament strength in men than in women. Most importantly, there is substantial differences in neuromuscular coordination and control in landing. Women also have less hip and knee flexion range of motions. The higher Q angle combined with their weakened hip muscles strength also makes them more prone to an ACL sprain as the greater Q angle increases force on the patella and in turn there is more anterior translation of the proximal tibia on the femur. Some authors have concluded that there is slight difference in gender ACL tear. On the other hand, there were significant gender differences in ACL injury rates when particular specific sports and physical activities were compared.

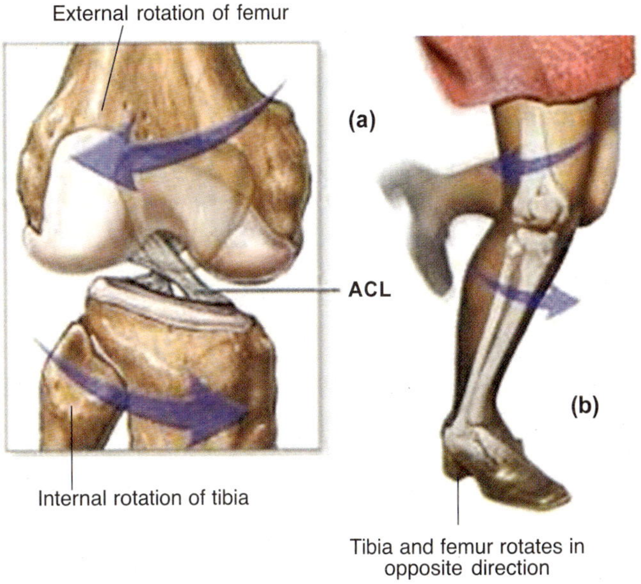

Figs. 23.10a and b: Mechanism of injury

Etiology

The etiology of an ACL injuries has multifactorial theories. Two of them are extrinsic and intrinsic. *Extrinsic:* The athletes who improve their extrinsic elements are not prone to the ACL injuries. The extrinsic elements are improved through attending the different training sessions prior to the play. These training sessions help in improving the body movements in sport, muscle strength and coordination, shoe surface interface, and level of skill and conditioning. *Intrinsic:* The intrinsic elements are the anatomical structures such as joint laxity, limb alignment (valgus or varus), notch dimension, and the size of the ligament. These intrinsic elements also significantly contribute to the ACL injuries.

Mechanism of Injury

An ACL injuries usually occur during soccer and basketball play in young athletes and most often from skiing in the older people. The strong contraction of the quadriceps muscles places a significant stress (anterior tibial shear force on the ACL), especially when the knee is between 0 degree and 30 degrees. An ACL tear often occurs as a result of quick deceleration, hyperextension, or marked internal rotation of the tibia on femur, and does not involve the contact with other individual or athlete. This usually occurs when the athlete lands on the leg and quickly pivots in the opposite direction (valgus twisting injury). In this mechanism the posterolateral large bulky portion of the ACL gets sprained. This possibly disrupts the ACL with minimal injury to other structures such as medial and lateral meniscus and medial collateral ligaments (Figs. 23.10a and b).

The significant stress on an ACL causes plastic deformation (sprain) with loss of collagen cross linkage. Rupture of the ACL usually occurs as a single fibre mass failure rather than sequential fibre failure; this possibly explains why, partial ACL injury is less common than the complete tear (Figs. 23.11a to c).

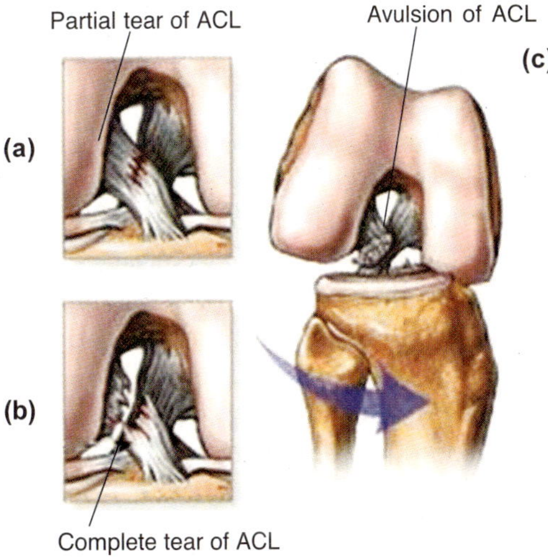

Fig. 23.11a to c: a. Partial tear, b. Complete tear, c. Avulsion of anterior cruciate ligament

Clinical Features

The acute ACL rupture is characterized by hemarthrosis, pain and instability. Athletes may experience a popping sound after impact, swelling and instability usually a "wobbly" feeling. Pain may also be a concerned factor and may range from moderate to severe. However, some patients continue their routine work by neglecting the instability and pain, which can have devastating consequences, resulting in a massive cartilage damage, and increase risk of secondary osteoarthosis.

Physical Examination

The therapist can make a provisional diagnosis of the ACL tear by performing some physical test because some of physical tests have very good sensitivity to the ACL tear. However, the patient needs to get an MRI done to determine the integrity of the ligament especially before arthroscopic treatment.

1. **Anterior Drawer Test:** The patient lies supine with the knee flexion to 90 degrees. Examiner sits on the forefoot of the patient of side which is being examined and holds the proximal tibia with both the hands. The examiner pulls the proximal tibia anteriorly on the femur. A test is positive if there is an excessive displacement of the proximal tibia on the femur without firm end feel compared with normal knee joint (Fig. 23.12a).

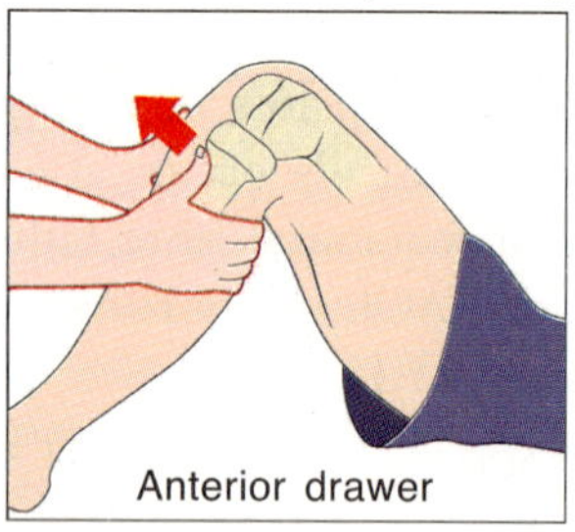

Fig. 23.12a: Anterior drawer

2. **Lachman Test:** This test is named after orthopedic surgeon John Lachman. The test is recognized by most of clinicians as the most reliable and sensitive clinical test for the determination of anterior cruciate ligament integrity, superior to the anterior drawer test commonly used in the past for an ACL evaluation. The patient lies supine with the knee flexion at 20 to 30 degrees with external rotation of the leg (as per Bate's guide to physical examination). The examiner stabilizes the distal femur with one hand and holds the proximal tibia with the other hand. While stabilizing the distal femur the proximal tibia is translated anteriorly on the femur. Anterior translation of tibia more than 12 mm, associated with a soft end-feel indicated a positive test for an ACL sprain or tear (Fig. 23.12b).

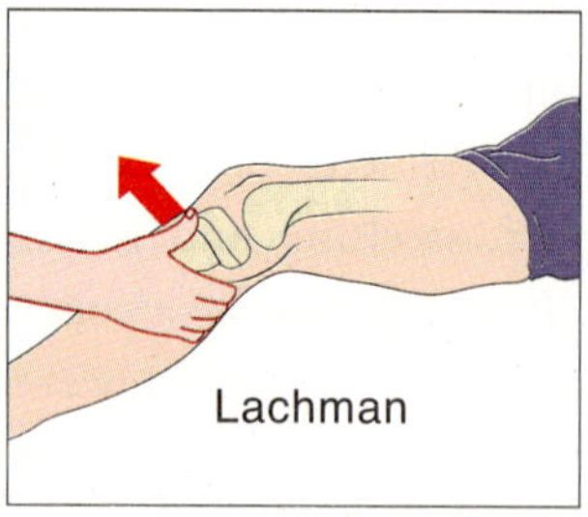

Fig. 23.12b: Lachman test

3. **Pivot Shift Test:** The patient lies supine, therapist stands at the side which is being examined and grasps the heel with the one hand and places other hand on the lateral aspect of the knee to apply valgus stress on it. The leg which is being examined is taken slightly out of the couch edge to flex it upto 30 degrees. At the flexion of 30 degrees a valgus stress is applied to the knee joint and then it is extended gently. A click or pop sound is felt while extending the knee joint with the valgus stress because there is anterior displacement of the lateral tibial plateau on the lateral femoral condyle.This test assess the ACL insufficiency (Fig. 23.13).

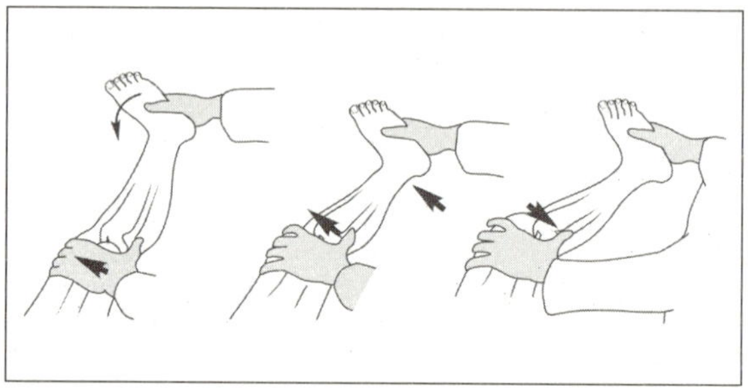

Fig. 23.13: Pivot shift test

Patients who have evaluated for an ACL injury should also be evaluated for other injuries such as meniscus and collateral ligaments, that often occur in combination with an ACL tear.

Management

There is much debate over the management of the ACL sprains, which patient requires reconstruction and which do not is not clear. Athletes with ACL tear, who require high demand sports activities cannot return to the sport without reconstruction of the ligament. However, patients with low demand activities may continue with the torn ACL, but this may lead to secondary osteoarthrosis and meniscal tears especially posterior horn of the medial meniscus.

Partial ACL Tear Management

Partial tears are managed with the conservative treatment especially if the patients are of low demand activities. Immediately after injury, the PRICE principle is followed to reduce haemorrhage, swelling, inflammation and pain. The leg is elevated above the level of the heart and ice is applied for 10 minutes three to four times daily. Elastic crepe bandage is applied over the knee joint to prevent further hemarthrosis. The torn ligament is less likely to restrict the anterior translation of the tibia over the femur, therefore, knee brace or orthosis with the extension lock is advised to prevent the anterior translation of the tibia as it may cause further damage to the torn ligament. The stair climbing and descending is not allowed till the satisfactory improvement in the sign and symptoms is achieved, however, if it is required, the patient should lock the brace in full extension and then do the stairs.

During isometric contraction of the quadriceps, ACL is stressed more at 30 degrees, whereas at 90 degrees ACL remains unstrained. Active knee extension between 50 and 110 degrees does not strain the anterior cruciate ligament. At 90 degrees of flexion, an ACL accounts for approximately 85 percent of resistance to anterior drawer test.

The hyperextension of the knee joint develops much higher forces on ACL than PCL. At 5 degrees of hyperextension, the force on the anterior cruciate ligament is ranged between 50 and 240 newton. In normal ACL, in neutral rotation, application of 100 newtons of anterior force produces: 2-5 mm of anterior translation at full extension, 5-8 mm of anterior translation at 30 degrees of flexion and after 30 degrees as the flexion increases, an anterior translation of the tibia decreases.This biomechanical behaviour of the anterior cruciate ligament has an important clinical significance in administering the exercises especially in the acute stage.

Open Kinetic Chain Exercises

Open kinetic activities generate more isolated muscle contraction and thus allow for more specific muscle strengthening. The stabilizing effect of the muscle may be lost as soon as the fatigue of that particular muscle occurs and can put the ACL at great risk. These exercises place a significant force on the ligament between 0 and 30 degrees, therefore should not be used in the acute phase, particularly between 0 and 30 degrees. The open kinetic strengthening of the quadriceps in the form of isometric can safely be used between 60 and 100 degrees of flexion as the ligament in this range remains unstrained, however the resistance should be mild to moderate. The open kinetic strengthening of the hamstrings muscles is safe and often advised in the treatment of ACL injuries as these exercises do not cause any anterior translation of the tibia.

Closed Kinetic Chain Exercises

Closed kinetic chain exercises cause co-contraction of both the agonist and antagonist group of the muscles with progressive decrease in hamstrings activity as the flexion angle of the knee increases. Closed kinetic chain exercises by allowing agonist muscle activity, may not provide focused strengthening, but may provide a safer environment for an ACL in the setting of fatigue. Closed kinetic chain exercises in the first 30 degrees of the flexion produce less anterior translation of the tibia than the open kinetic chain exercises, this is because contraction of the hamstrings does not allow excessive anterior translation of the tibia. But further increase in flexion angle of the knee decreases the contraction of the hamstrings and increases anterior tibial translation. Therefore, mini squatting (between 0 and 30 degrees) exercise with the brace may be advised to an ACL injury patients.

Arthroscopic Reconstruction of the Anterior Cruciate Ligament

Reconstruction of the ligament is the choice of treatment as an anterior cruciate ligament does not heal independently because of inadequate blood supply to the ligament. Athletes with ACL tear usually require reconstruction in order to perform sharp movements safely with stability. The surgery is advised after swelling and inflammation subsides. This procedure does not repair the ligament, instead, it reconstructs an ACL by using other ligaments or tendons of the body. There are two options for the ACL graft selection; allograft and autograft. Autograft are the patient's own tissues, which may be from hamstrings tendon or patellar tendon. Allografts are cadaveric tissue sourced from a tissue bank. Patella tendon bone autograft and hamstrings tendon autograft are the most common and preferred and tend to produce the best results.

Patellar Tendon Bone Autograft

The central 1/3rd of the patellar tendon is removed along with a piece of bone from patella and tibia. The advantage of this graft is that the patella tendon and ACL are relatively having same length and it uses a bone to bone attachment that helps in accelerating early healing process.The central 1/3rd bone patellar tendon bone graft has an initial failure strength of upto 2977N, which is higher than the intact ACL. The current trend is that the initial strength must exceeds that of the normal ACL to maintain sufficient strength as the strength of graft is decreased during the healing stage. PTB graft has disadvantage of common knee pain due to the removal of the bone from the patella.

Hamstrings Graft: Two tendons are taken from the hamstring muscles, and wrapped together to form a graft (new ACL ligament). This has an advantage of not having pain in the anterior joint and also requires small size incision. The disadvantage of this graft is that it takes longer time to heal because there is no bone to bone healing and tendon to bone connection takes relatively long to become rigid. After implantation, an ACL graft undergoes sequential phases of avascular necrosis, revascularisation, and remodelling. Ultimate load to failure and graft stiffness in a patellar tendon autograft can drop as low as 11% and 13% respectively of the normal ACL.

Femoral and Tibial Tunnel

The appropriate landmarks for femoral and tibial tunnel is one of the key points to be considered before starting the procedure. Most common error is non-isometric tunnel placement within intercondylar notch rather than its normal posterior position. Anterior placement of the graft (femoral) relative to normal anatomical insertion of ACL results in high strain on graft in flexion. Posterior placement of the graft results in excessive tightening of the graft in knee extension. Posterior tibial tunnel placement may be preferred to avoid anterior cruciate ligament graft impingement with the intercondylar roof. More medial starting point for tibial tunnel, may allow for better alignment of femoral tunnel.

Post-Operative Management of the ACL Reconstruction

Post-operative treatment of an ACL reconstruction include: Immobilization in a brace, early motion, strengthening, assisted weight bearing, light sports at 6 months, and competitive at 8 months or later.

- **Bracing:** The knee joint is immobilized in a brace following ACL reconstruction to protect the donor graft. The brace is worn in the first 4-6 weeks all the day and night in a full extension; however, it may be removed or unlocked during the exercises. After six weeks it is replaced with a functional brace, which is advised till the athlete return to the competitive sport. The brace is unlocked while sleeping (after 4-6 weeks). Biomechanical studies of healing ACL graft performed in animals have shown that the graft requires a long time to revascularization and that the biomechanical behaviour of the graft never returns to normal. Functional knee braces provide a protective strain-sheilding effect on the ACL graft when anterior shear loads and internal torque are applied to the knee in the non-weight bearing condition. However, the strain-shielding effect of functional braces decreases as the magnitude of anterior shear and internal torque applied to the knee increase.
- **Weight Bearing:** Toe touch weight bearing with crutches is allowed for 4-6 weeks to prevent anterior translation and any strain on the newly fitted graft. The toe touch weight bearing status of the patient, how long it is recommended, greatly depends upon the surgeon, therefore, further progression of the weight should be done with the consultation of the operating surgeon. Usually after 4-6 weeks weight bearing as tolerance may be initiated with the assistance of crutches followed by full weight bearing.
- **Exercises: Initial Phase: 0-4/6 weeks.** Initially active assisted quadriceps sets, gluteus maximus sets hamstrings sets, ankle pump exercises are started in a brace to prevent the graft. Straight leg raising, and side leg raising initiated with brace in full extension (locking). Assisted active knee flexion and extension in a brace in high sitting position also helps in improving flexion. These exercises are administered for 4-6 weeks. At the end of four weeks patient should achieve full extension and 90 degree flexion and 100 degree flexion by the end of six weeks. Extension lag is one of the complications of the ACL reconstruction, and if not corrected initially, it can cause anterior knee pain quadriceps weakness, and early patella-femoral osteoarthritic changes. Any sign of loss of terminal extension should be observed carefully from the beginning of the exercises, and if, present, it should be managed with locking the brace in full extension especially in the first four to six weeks. Loss of flexion is not a major problem as it does not hamper the functional activities and can be gained easily by using the contract relax exercises, however, anteriorly placed graft may limit the terminal flexion permanently.

  Strengthening Exercises: Isometric resistance exercises of the quadriceps should be started with the angles which do not strain the graft. After four weeks isometric exercises at 80, 90 and 100 degrees can safely be initiated as at these angles the graft remain unstrained. Isometric strengthening of the hamstrings can be started at any angles.

  Closed Kinetic Chain Exercise may also be started after 4-6 weeks. Mini squatting is the choice of close kinetic chain exercise in the first thirty degrees of the flexion as it allows co-contraction of the quadriceps and hamstrings and does not produce much anterior tibial translation, but as the flexion increases the action of the hamstrings decreases on the tibia and anterior tibial translation increases, therefore beyond thirty degree flexion squatting is not advised.

  Eccentric Strengthening Exercises: A muscle force producing capacity is most optimal when an external force exceeds that of the muscle while the muscle lengthens. Hence, the potential to improve muscle strength by overloading the tissue is greater with eccentric strengthening than with concentric strengthening. Recent evidence suggests that the application of progressive, high force eccentric resistance exercises to the involved limb can be used safely to increase muscle volume and strength in ACL reconstructed individual.

TENNIS ELBOW

Lateral elbow tendinopathy, commonly known as tennis elbow, is a condition that can cause significant functional impairment in working-age patients.[1] Tennis elbow, is a common condition thought to be related to overuse injuries to the extensor carpi radialis brevis (ECRB). The natural history of lateral epicondylitis typically involves the resolution of symptoms in 6 to 24 months, with most patients experiencing an improvement in symptoms within 1 year.[2,3] 95% tennis elbow occurs in non tennis players. 10-50% of regular tennis players experience the symptoms of varying degree some time in their life. The use of the term "epicondylitis" was questioned over time, as histological studies failed to show inflammatory cells (macrophages, lymphocytes and neutrophils) in the affected tissue (Fig. 23.14a).

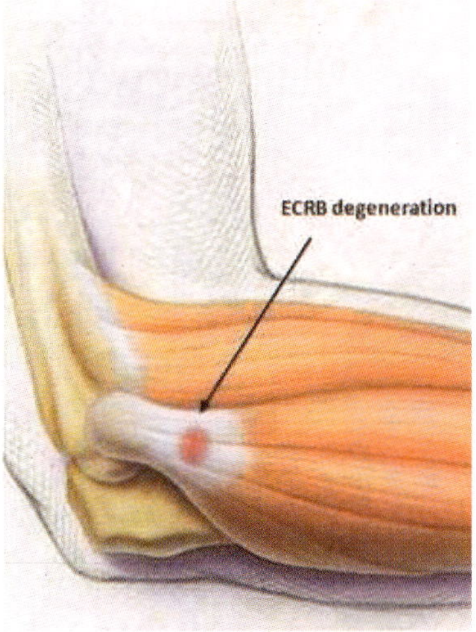

Fig. 23.14a: Lateral epicondylitis

Tennis elbow is a common disorder of the elbow. A recent demographic study described the epidemiology of this condition and investigated its risk factors in a sample of 4783 people aged 30–64 years. The prevalence in this group was 1.3% and did not differ between men and women. The condition was most prevalent in the age group of 45–54 years.

Pathomechanics

The exact cause is unknown but the most common cause in tennis players is a late mechanically poor backhand that places excess force across the extensor wad, that is the elbow leads to the arm (Brotzman). Tennis elbow is thought to result from overuse of the extensor carpi radialis brevis (ECRB) muscle by repetitive microtrauma resulting in a primary tendinosis of the ECRB, with or without involvement of the extensor digitorum communis (EDC).[4] In tennis, the predominant activity of the wrist extensors in all strokes (serve, forehand and one- and two-handed backhand) might be one explanation for predisposition to the condition.[5]

It is generally believed that tennis players using a two-handed backhand rarely develop tennis elbow as the non-dominant arm appears to absorb more energy, which changes the mechanics of the swing. The higher occurrence of tennis elbow amongst recreational tennis players compared to experienced players has been shown to be due to the ability of experienced players to reduce impact transmission from the racquet to the wrist and elbow (Fig. 23.14b).

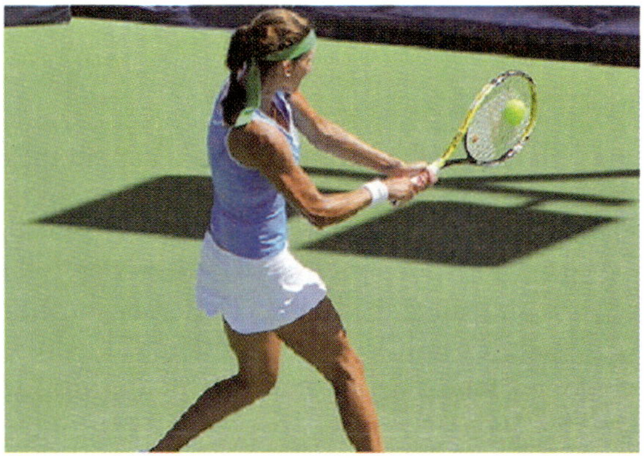

Fig. 23.14b: Back hand stroke

Improper racquet weight and racquet stringing generate high loads on the lateral muscle tendon unit. In addition, harder court services impart a greater momentum to the ball and subsequently increase the force transmitted through the racquet to the extensor mass.[6] Faulty wrist kinematics during the backhand stroke is purposed as another possible explanation for the higher incidence of tennis elbow amongst novice tennis players. The wrist kinematics and EMG data show that novice players eccentrically contract their wrist extensor muscles throughout the stroke, which could contribute to tennis elbow.[7]

The exact molecular profile and processes driving the histopathological changes seen in tendinopathy are yet to be fully understood. It is thought that angiofibroblastic hyperplasia observed after microtrauma is an attempt by the tendon to heal.[8] Resting tenocytes may be activated to multiply and produce collagen by mechanoreceptor stimulation in response to shear stress after an initial insidious injury.[9] The lack of an effective vascular system prevents the influx of any humoral mediators that are necessary for optimal tendon remodeling, leading to progressive degeneration.[10]

Microscopical studies by Nirschl *et al.* showed mainly fibroblastic tissue and vascular invasion that led him to describe the condition in 1999 as "angiofibroblastic tendinosis".[11] It has been postulated that tendinosis or tendinopathy is acquired by overuse of a hypovascular zone, which leads to subsequent neovascularisation.[12] The studies showed sensory fibres containing substance-P and CGRP (calcitonine gene-related peptide)-like immunoreactivity in the origin of the ECRB.[13] The presence of these neuropeptides, which is limited to a subgroup of small vessels, implies the possibility of neurogenic inflammation as a cause of the perceived pain.[7]

There are several other factors contribute to the tennis elbow such as capsular irritation of radiohumeral joint, pain in synovial fold, ligamentous laxity, annular ligament fibrosis, actopic calcification, degenerative condition of radioulnar joint, cervical radiculopathy, and ischaemia of the nerve.

Clinical Feature

Patients with tennis elbow complaint pain around the elbow joint which is aggravated by wrist and forearm movements. Initially pain is confined to the particular point and area, however, it extends into the proximal forearm and sometimes to the wrist joint along the length of extensor muscles. The activities such as holding glass of water and lifting it, kneading, and squeezing become painful and difficult.

Physical Tests

Cozen's Test: Patient sits comfortably on the stool. The examiner stands at the side of the patient which is being examined, stabilizes the patients elbow with one hand and grasps the hand of the patient with other hand. The patient is then instructed to actively make a fist, pronate forearm as well as radially deviate and extend the wrist against a resistance that is being applied by the examiner. A positive test would be the reproduction of pain near the lateral epicondyle (Fig. 23.14c).

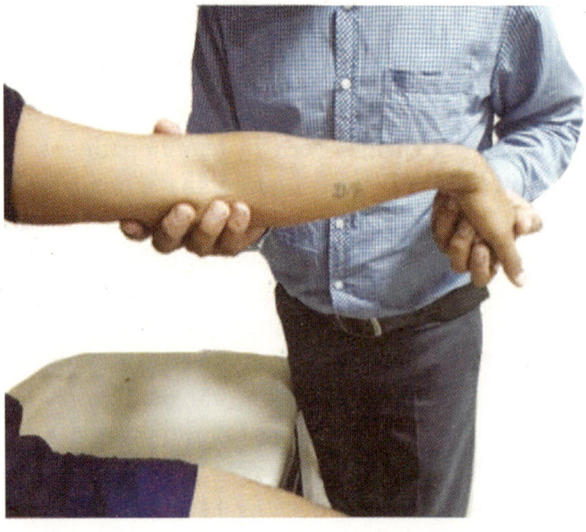

Fig. 23.14c: Cozen's test for lateral epicondylitis

Active Wrist Extension Test: The activity of patient, which involves active extension of the wrist, is observed. Test is considered positive if patient feels pain in the lateral aspect of the forearm.

Thomsen Test: With the shoulder flexed to 60°, elbow extended, forearm pronated and the wrist extended about 30°, pressure was applied to the dorsum of the second and third metacarpal bones in the direction of flexion and ulnar deviation to stress the extensor carpi radialis brevis and longus.

Resisted Middle Finger Extension Test: With the shoulder flexed to 60°, elbow extended, forearm pronated, and the fingers extended, the middle finger is actively extended against resistance.

Mill's Test or Passive Stretching: Stretching the extensor muscles of the wrist by putting the elbow in full extension position and forearm in pronation and then flexing the wrist to get a maximum stretch (Fig. 23.14d).

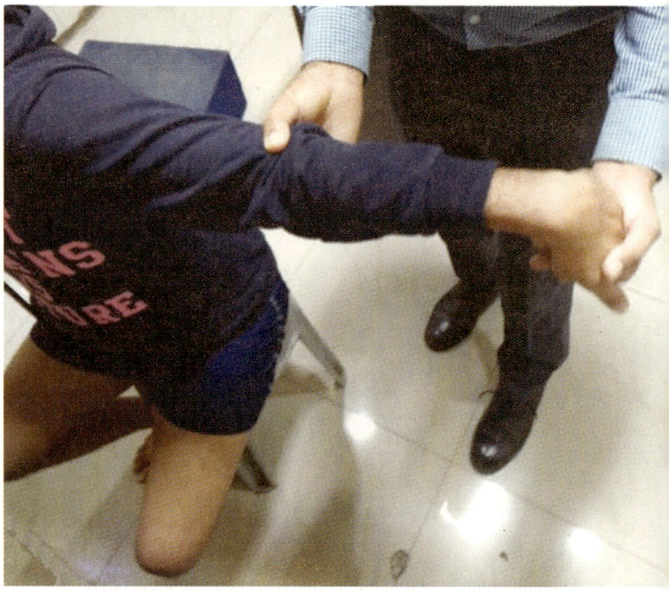

Fig. 23.14d: Mill's test for lateral epicondylitis

Differential Diagnosis

Several conditions can mimic the presentation of lateral epicondylitis and should be considered when tennis elbow is suspected. The differential diagnosis includes radiculopathy (C_6–C_7), entrapment of the posterior interosseus nerve, arthrosis of the radiohumeral joint, osteochondritis dissecans, osteonecrosis (Panner) and plica synovialis.

Management

The aim of treatment is to decrease stress on the tendon, relieve pain, maintain and improve muscle strength, and functional activities of the patient. The clinicians have designed several techniques for treating the tennis elbow effectively, which are explained as under.

Rest

The primary aim of "relative rest" is to halt the injury process by removing mechanical overload, providing the tendon a chance to repair itself through the restriction and modification of provocative daily activities. It has previously been inferred that LET is a self-limiting condition, with pain and symptoms running a "natural course" and resolving spontaneously in up to 89% at 1 year.[26] However, awaiting spontaneous recovery may be associated with the loss of economic productivity and might be an imprudent approach in patients with crippling pain and disability (Fig. 23.14e).[27]

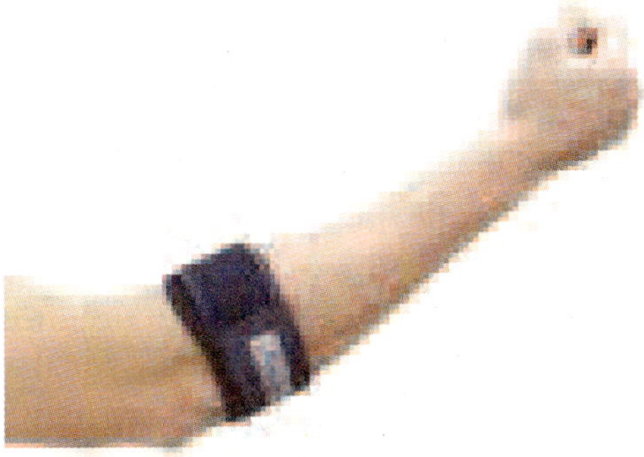

Fig. 23.14e: Tennis elbow support lateral epicondylitis 2

Exercises

Rest may produce adverse effects on the contractability of the connective tissues. There is gross decrease in cross-sectional area of the muscles. Active exercises in pain free range of motion are beneficial in maintaining muscle strength. Exercise, which provoke pain, is the indication of stress on the ECRB tendon, hence, should be avoided. Strengthening of long flexors, supinator, pronator and wrist extensors should be started if patient allows without no pain. Long wrist extensors especially ECRB should be taken care of during the strengthening program.

Mobilization with Movement (MWM)

MWM is a form of manual therapy that includes a sustained lateral glide to the elbow joint with concurrent physiological movement.[14] This mobilization technique is often used to correct the faulty position of the elbow joint. Miller (2000)[15] described in his case report the use of the MWM for lateral epicondylitis as the primary modality for the correction of what Miller diagnosed as a "positional fault of the elbow joint complex mimicking a contractile element pathology of the common extensor bundle". It was found that MWM resulted in reduced pain, improvement of pain-free grip strength (PFGS), and increased ability to tolerate resisted isometric wrist extension, and that, 2 weeks of treatment and 1month follow-up showed full function and absence of pain (Figs. 23.14f, g and h).

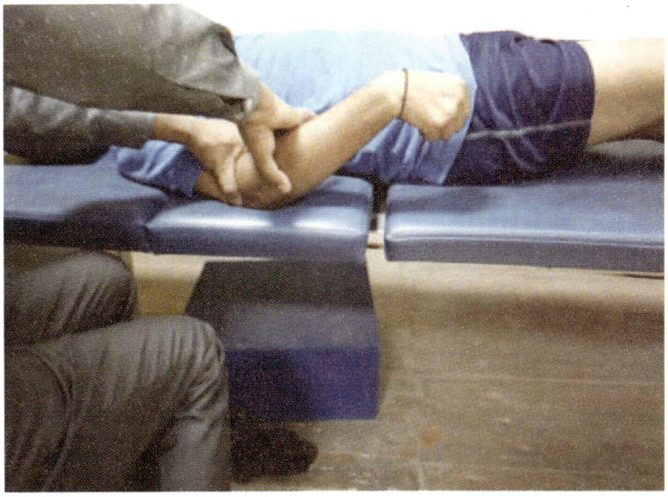

Fig. 23.14f: Mobilization with movement for tennis elbow

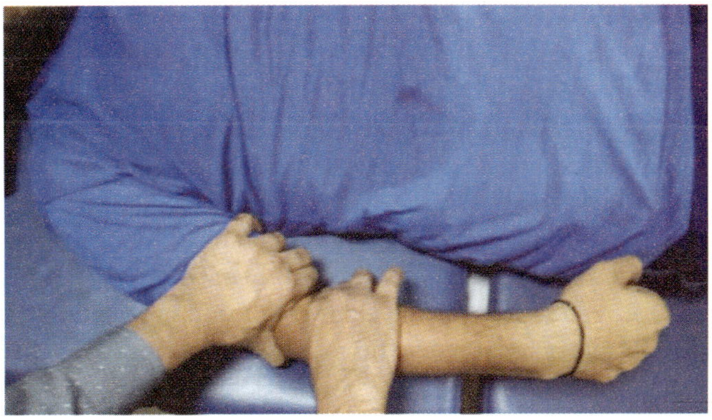

Fig. 23.14g: Mobilization with movement for tennis elbow

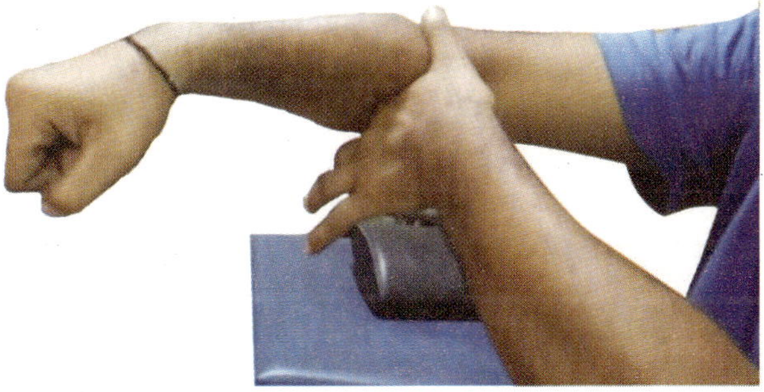

Fig. 23.14h: Mobilization with movement for tennis elbow (self)

The patient is placed in a supine position with the elbow joint in full extension and forearm fully pronated. Therapist stands at the side of the patient, stabilizes the distal arm with one hand, and grasps the proximal forearm medially with the other hand. While stabilizing the distal arm, the proximal forearm is drawn laterally with the other hand and patient is asked to flex the elbow simultaneously with the wrist extension repeatedly for at least ten times to complete one set. A brief period of rest is given between total of three sets. The lateral glide may also be given with the help of belt which is wrapped around the proximal forearm of the patient and then to the west of the therapist. The therapist applies lateral glide by taking the back slightly away from the elbow joint of the patient. Lateral glide of the forearm relative to the humerus produced by a mobilization belt was pain free and now rendered strong resisted isometric wrist extension pain-free. This technique has been described by Mulligan[14] as being effective in the management of "tennis elbow" and supported by early case study research.

Deep Transverse Friction Massage

Deep transverse friction massage is a specific type of connective tissue massage applied precisely to the soft tissue structures such as tendons. It was developed in an empirical way by Cyriax and Cyriax and is currently used extensively in rehabilitation practice.[16-20] The patient is placed in the supine lying with the forearm supination and elbow 90° flexion. Elbow joint is exposed adequately and area of anterolateral elbow is identified. The most common site of pain in the tennis elbow is anterolateral aspect of the joint where the extensor carpi radialis brevis originates. Deep transverse friction must be applied transversely to the specific tissue involved, unlike superficial massage given in the longitudinal direction parallel to the vessels, which enhances circulation and return of fluids. The therapist places lateral border of the thumb or index over the anterolateral aspetct of the elbow joint and applies to and fro pressure across the tendon of ECRB. The thumb of the therapist and the skin of the patient should move together as a unit over the teno osseous junction for ten minutes. The application of deep transverse friction can produce therapeutic movement by breaking down the strong cross links or adhesions that have been formed, softening the scar tissue and mobilizing the cross links between the mutual collagen fibers and the adhesions between repairing connective tissue and surrounding tissues (Fig. 23.14i).

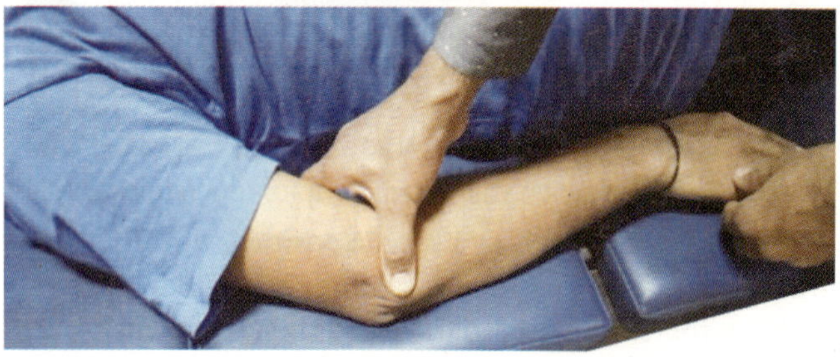

Fig 23.14i: Deep Transverse Friction Massage for Lateral Epicondylitis

Mills Manipulation

Mills manipulation is also one of the therapeutic technique practiced by the physiotherapist for tennis elbow. As per Cyriax and Cyriax it should be performed immediately after ten minutes of deep transverse friction. The patient is positioned on a chair with a backrest and therapist stands behind the patient. Support the patient's arm under the crook of the elbow with the shoulder joint abducted to 90° and medially rotated. The forearm will automatically fall into pronation. Place the thumb of your other hand in the web space between the patient's thumb and index finger and fully flex the patient's wrist and pronate the forearm. Move the hand supporting the crook of the elbow on to the posterior surface of the elbow joint and, while maintaining full wrist flexion and pronation, extend the patient's elbow until you feel that all the slack has been taken up in the tendon. Step sideways to stand behind the patient's head, taking care to prevent the patient from leaning away either forwards or sideways, which would reduce the tension on the tendon. Apply a minimal amplitude, high velocity thrust by simultaneously side flexing the body away from arms and pushing smartly downwards with the hand over the patient's elbow. This manoeuvre is conducted once only at each treatment session because it is not a comfortable procedure for the patient, and the effects of treatment often become fully apparent over the following few days (Figs. 23.14j and k).

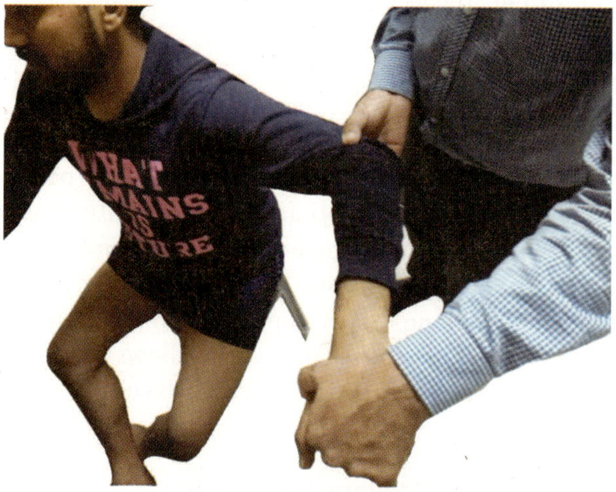

Fig. 23.14j: Mills manipulation

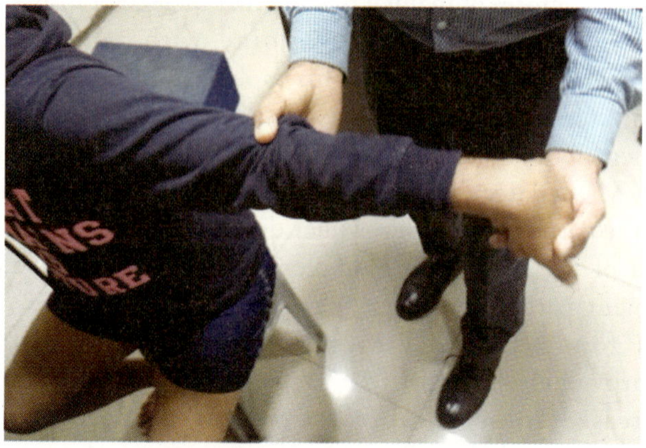

Fig. 23.14k: Mills manipulation

Taping

McConnell has proposed the application of tape as a means of alleviating pain, improving muscle function, and restoring functional movement patterns. Clinically, in musculoskeletal conditions, by minimizing the aggravation of symptoms during the performance of therapeutic exercise, the use of a taping technique may facilitate compliance to exercise rehabilitation programs.[22, 23] Elbow taping technique that was newly used for the treatment of tennis elbow may facilitate the compliance to exercise rehabilitation programs.[24]

The elbow joint is kept slightly flexed, and tape applied around the elbow approximately 2 cm below the lateral epicondyle. Apply the tape firmly to the lateral aspect of the elbow and gently at the middle aspect of the elbow to prevent circulatory problems. 1 – 3 pieces of tape may be used depending on the level of support required. Occasionally this taping technique may be made more effective by rolling up a small section of tape into a small roll and placing it horizontally across the forearm extensors and underneath the tape (Figs. 23.15a and b). The size, shape and exact location of this roll may need to be tailored to the individual to ensure maximal comfort and minimal pain.

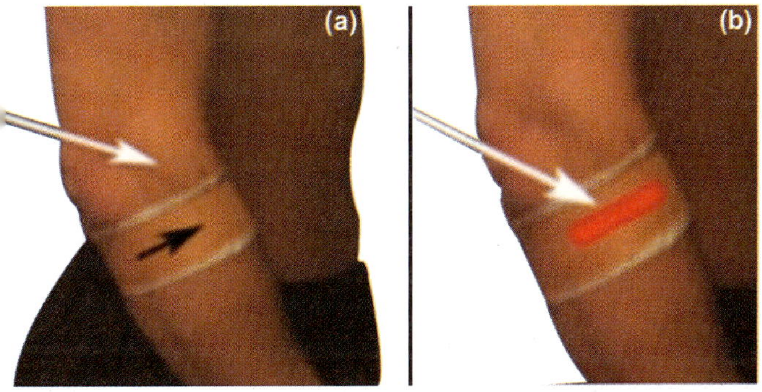

Figs. 23.15a and b: Rolled tape location

Extracorporeal Shockwave Therapy

Extracorporeal shockwave therapy is a safe and effective treatment modality in the management of chronic cases of tennis elbow. ESWT is an increasingly popular therapeutic approach for the treatment of a number of soft tissue complaints including LET. Extracorporeal shock waves are single-pressure pulses of microsecond duration that can be focused on a site using ultrasound guidance.[25] The differences can be attributed to patient selection, the application techniques, the type of devices, and the method of outcome measurements according to Wang (2012). To treat tennis elbow normally moderate to high frequency ranged from 15 Hz for 100-2000 shocks is selected. The pressure bar and energy should be any where from 1.4 bar or 75 mj to 3.0 bar or 120 mj.

GOLFER'S ELBOW

Golfer's elbow also known as medial epicondylitis is characterized by pain at the medial epicondyle of the humerus following overuse and repetitive injury to the common flexor tendon origin. Medial epincondylits is less frequently encountered than lateral epicondylitis with a reported prevalence less than 1% in the general population[28] but as high as 6% in some professions.[29,30] It accounts for 10% to 20% of all epicondylitis cases.[31] The demographics of at-risk patients are very similar to those at risk of lateral epicondylitis and include ages 30 to 50 years, labourers, those performing repetitive tasks demanding wrist flexion, smokers and patients with obesity.[32] In throwing athletes, particularly baseball players, the elbow's medial structures endure the most stress and account for up to 97% of all elbow injuries.[33] The muscles most commonly involved are the flexor-pronator group, including the flexor carpi radialis, palmaris longus, pronator teres, and flexor carpi ulnaris. Histologic studies demonstrate patterns of angiofibroblastic degeneration similar to those seen in lateral epicondylitis.[34]

Clinical Feature

The patients with medial epicondylitis often complaint pain at the origin of common flexors with wrist flexion, supination and pronation. Resisted pronation and/or wrist flexion will reproduce symptoms in most affected patients. Grip strength is decreased in patients with medial epicondylitis compared with normal subjects, although the magnitude of impairment is less than that seen in patients with lateral epicondylitis. Radiological investigation may show calcific or traction osteophytes at the flexor-pronator origin. Similar symptoms may be produced by the medial collateral ligament and ulnar nerve neuritis. To differential from medial collateral ligament insufficiency, the examiner should perform valgus stress test, and tinel sign which should not aggravate the symptoms.

Management

Patients with medial epicondylitis are managed effectively by rest, alleviating stress, activity modification, strengthening of weak and stretching of the short muscles.

Rest and Bracing: Rest and modification in the activities is the mainstay of the conservative treatment. Patient is instructed to reduce the stress on the common wrist flexors by halting that activity for some period of time. There are the activities of daily life which are essential for day-to-day activities and cannot be halted should be performed with an appropriate immobilization. A band or elbow support just 2 cm below the origin of the muscle should be applied during ADLs.

Exercises: Stretching of common wrist flexors and pronator teres is initiated within the comfort zone of the patient. Strengthening exercises of the muscles especially hold relax can be started within the pain free range and these should not provoke the symptoms. Any exercises which aggravate the symptoms should be discarded. However, more vigorous strengthening exercises may be added as the patient shows improvement in the sign and symptoms.

Fascial Spreading: The fascial spreading strokes are performed on the entire anterior forearm over the flexor muscles from proximal to the distal part of the muscles with more pressure in the proximal and lesser towards the distal.

Cyriax Friction: The patient is placed in the supine lying with the forearm supination and elbow 90° flexion. Elbow joint is exposed adequately and area of anteromedial elbow is identified. Therapist places lateral border of the thumb over the tenoperiosteal junction of the origin of common wrist flexors. The thumb and skin moves over the tendons. The technique is performed for 5-10 minutes. The application of deep transverse friction can produce therapeutic movement by breaking down the strong cross links or adhesions that have been formed, softening the scar tissue and mobilizing the cross links between the mutual collagen fibers and the adhesions between repairing connective tissue and surrounding tissues (Figs. 23.16a and b).

If inflammation is present, icing is also an important part of the treatment protocol. Icing can be done before soft tissue manipulation to decrease sensitivity and allow

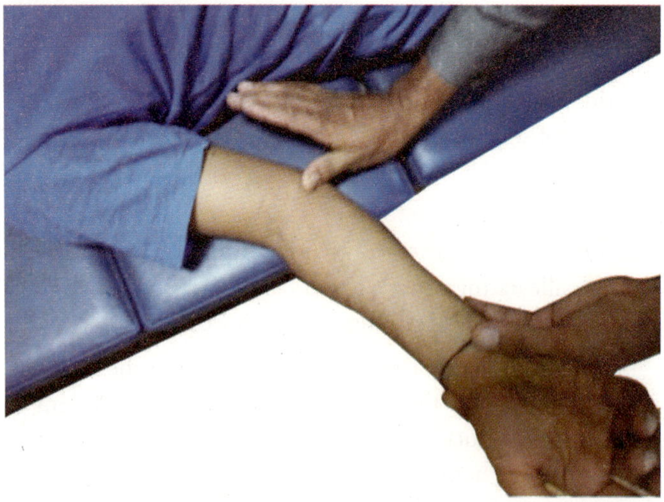

Fig. 23.16a: Deep transverse friction (Cyriax) massage for Golfer's elbow

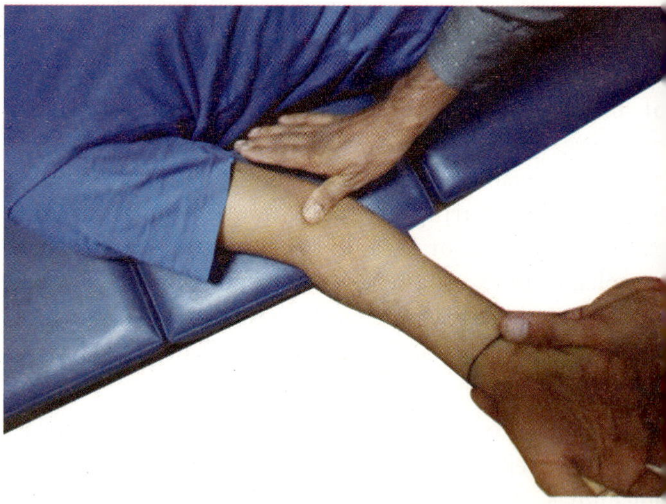

Fig. 23.16b: Deep transverse friction massage (Cyriax) fo[r] Golfer's elbow

for deeper work. It can also be done after soft tissue manipulation to minimize possible swelling as a result of the soft tissue work.

Once direct care to the anterior forearm/wrist/hand region has been done, it is wise to work the entire upper quadrant on that side. Begin at the neck, and work down into the upper back, shoulder region, arm, posterior forearm and hand. Although these regions are not directly responsible for golfer's elbow, they may be involved in dysfunctional postural and movement patterns that may contribute to golfer's elbow.

STUDENTS ELBOW

Olecranon bursitis often refers to the students elbow as repeatedly leaning on the elbows whilst studying can result in pressure on the olecranon process and bursa. Elbow bursitis may occur from one sudden impact such as being hit by a ball, or from repetitive friction. The repeated or constant pressure on the olecranon process causes inflammation in the bursa. The bursa becomes inflamed, swollen, painful and tender. The lining of the bursa becomes inflamed. It then secretes a much greater than normal amount of fluid into the closed cavity of the bursa, from where it has nowhere to go. The bursa therefore inflates, producing a swelling over the proximal end of the ulna, which is usually inflamed and tender (Figs. 23.17a and b).

Swelling, redness, pain on pressure with the history of repeated injury or direct trauma to the elbow joint are the common features of the students elbow. To differentiate from infective bursitis, therapist may refer the patient to the physician especially if there is no history of repeated injury or direct trauma.

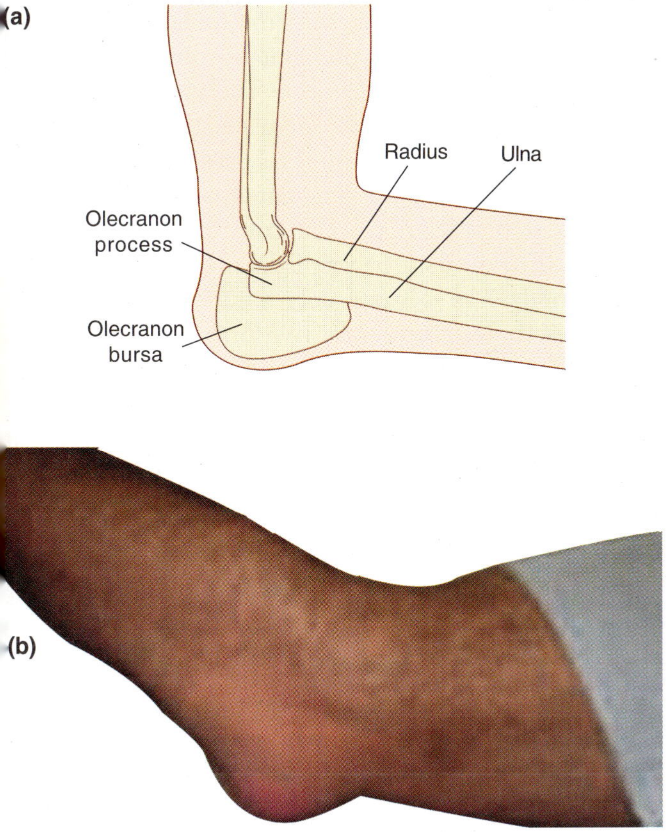

Figs. 23.17a and b: Olecranon bursitis with marked swelling

Management of students elbow includes alleviation of he stress or injury and modification of the activity. The tudents are advised not to place the elbow joint directly over the hard surface while studying. Application of ice for 15 minutes twice is helpful in reducing the inflammation and swelling. Isometric strengthening of the elbow flexors, extensors and forearm supinator and pronator and wrist muscles should be initiated in order to maintain and mprove the strength.

DE QUERVAIN TENOSYNOVITIS

In 1895, a Swiss surgeon, Fritz de Quervain, published five case reports of patients with a tender, thickened first dorsal compartment at the wrist.[35,36] The condition has subsequently borne his name, de Quervain tenosynovitis. The first dorsal compartment at the wrist (dorsolateral) ncludes the tendons of the abductor pollicis longus and extensor pollicis brevis lined by a synovial sheath which eparates it from the five other dorsal wrist compartments. As these tendons pass through an approximately 2 cm long fibrous tunnel passing over the radial styloid and under he transverse fibers of the extensor retinaculum, they are at risk for entrapment, particularly in the setting of acute rauma or repetitive motion (Fig. 23.18).

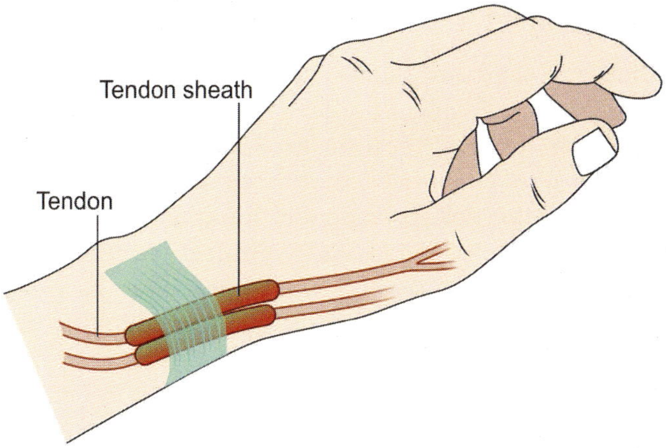

Fig. 23.18: Tendons of APL and EPB passing through fibrous tunnel over the radial styloid

The cause of de Quervain's disease is not established. However, researchers have found personal and work-related factors associated with de Quervain's disease in the working population; wrist bending and movements associated with the twisting or driving of screws were the most significant of the work-related factors. Repetitive strain injury, which holds the thumb in abduction and extension, places greater load on the tendons. Workers who perform rapid repetitive activities involving pinching, grasping, pulling or pushing have been considered at increased risk. Specific activities that have been postulated as potential risk factors include typing, bowling, golf, fly-fishing, piano-playing, sewing, knitting and intensive use of computer mouse and trackball.

The tendons become inflamed and swollen within the compartment. Pain on pressure and tenderness overlying the radial styloid is usually present, and fusiform swelling in this region may also be appreciated. Active and active resisted radial deviation is painful. Finkelstein test reproduces the symptoms. The patient flexes the thumb and holds inside a fist. While maintaining the position of the thumb inside the first examiner deviates the wrist joint into ulnar side. There is a sharp pain along the distal radial and wrist at the first dorsal compartment (Fig. 23.19).

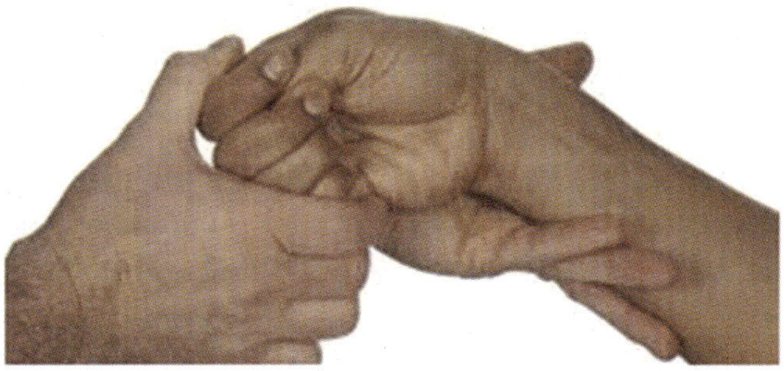

Fig. 23.19: Finkelstein test, examiner deviates the wrist towards ulnar side while maintaining the thumb and fingers in flexed position

Management

Managing hand and thumb injuries is challenging, since most patients frequently use them in their activities of life, thus delaying healing process. There are many recommended conservative treatments, including rest, early immobilization, or corticosteroid injection. Cryotherapy for 15 minutes twice daily reduces swelling and inflammation. Lightweight Thumb Spica splints have been recommended to reduce ulnar deviation and thumb flexion (Fig. 23.20).

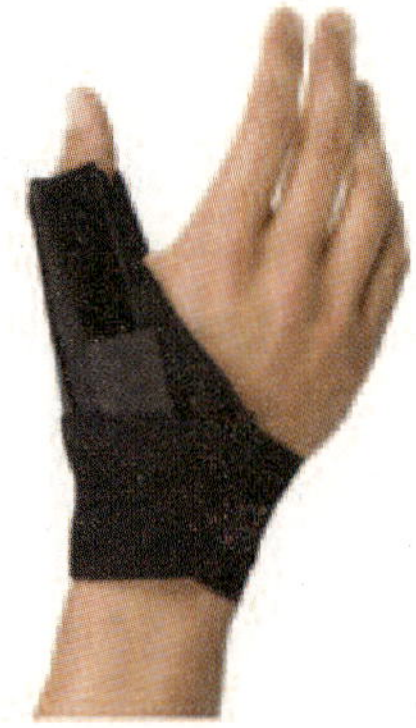

Fig. 23.20: Thumb spica or De Quervain's splint

Kinesiology Tape: To apply kinesio tape for De Quervain's tenosynovitis, the wrist is placed into the radial deviation. This avoids strain on the EPB and APL which helps in reducing inflammation and accelerating healing process (Fig. 23.21).

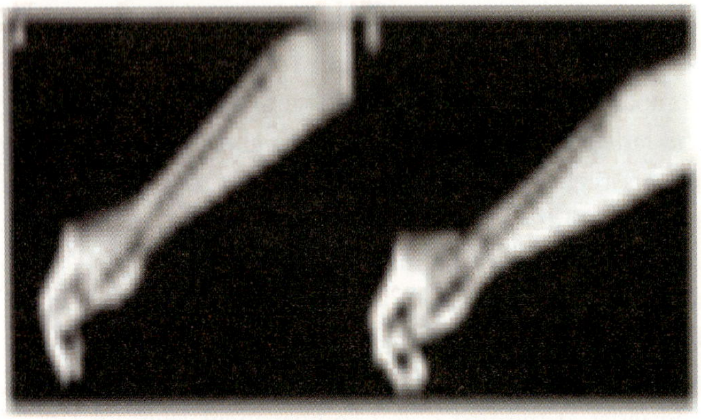

Fig. 23.21: Kinesio tape for De Quervain's disease

Cyriax Deep Transverse Friction Massage: If the condition is chronic which did not respond to the other measure of treatment, there is adhesions of the fibers. The application of deep transverse friction can produce therapeutic movement by breaking down the strong cross links or adhesions that have been formed, softening the scar tissue and mobilizing the cross links between the mutual collagen fibers and the adhesions between repairing connective tissue and surrounding tissues. Friction massage increases scar pliability and facilitates normal collagen fiber orientation as they are produced. The patient is placed in the supine lying or sitting with the forearm supination and elbow 90° flexion. Wrist joint is exposed adequately and area of dorsolateral is identified. Therapist places palmar surface of the index over the anterolateral aspect of styloid process. The thumb and skin moves over the tendons. The technique is performed for 5-10 minutes. In the early stage of fibroblast proliferation when cross links are absent or still weak, friction must be very light and given only over a short period so as to cause only minimal discomfort, in later stages, if strong cross links have formed, intense friction is needed to break these down. Initially the treatment time should not exceed 5 minutes as it produces erythema and pain. The treatment time is increased in the subsequent visits up to ten minutes.

Tendon Gliding Exercises: Tendon thickening and adhesions may result after repeated chronic injury. The formation of adhesions can be prevented by administrating tendon gliding exercises. The exercises allow each tendon to reach its greatest amount of movement; and also help in reducing hand swelling.

- *Tendon gliding for thumb:* The patient is asked to flex the thumb towards palm as far as possible and then stretch it out as far as possible.
- *Tendon gliding for fingers:* Finger tendon gliding exercises: Keep the fingers extended, make a tabletop by keeping the fingers straight, and then bending at the knuckles. Make a straight fist. Make a hook fist. Make a full fist (Figs. 23.22a to e).

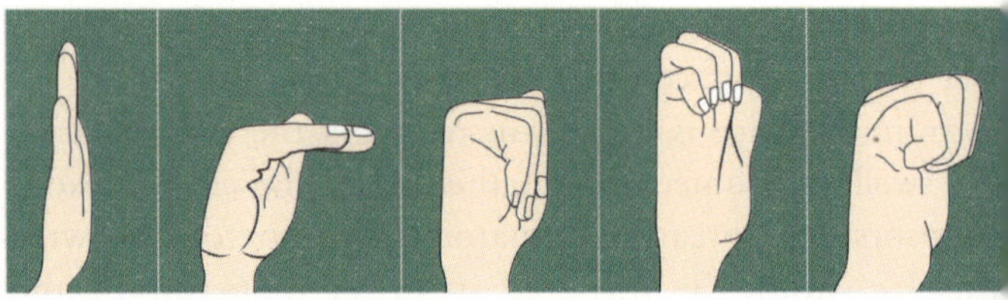

a
Keep all the PIP, DIP, MCP joints and wrist joint at neutral (Starting)

b
Make a tabletop by keeping fingers straight, then bending at the MCP

c
Make a straight fist

d
Make a hook fist

e
Make a full fist

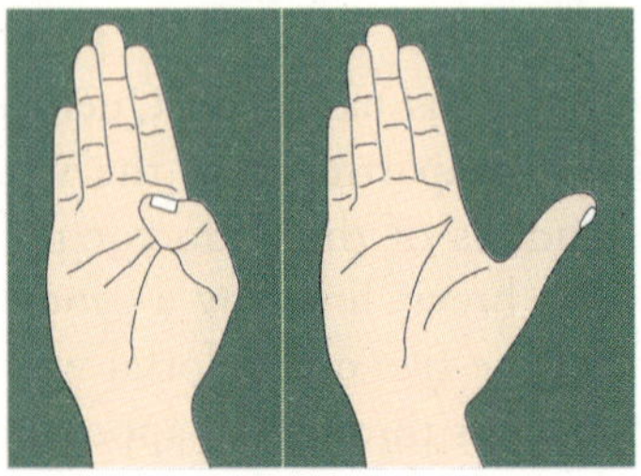

f g

Curl thumb into palm as far as possible and then extend it

Figs. 23.22a-e: Finger tendon gliding exercises, f and g thumb gliding

Stretching and Strengthening Exercises: Stretching of EPB and APL is initiated in the pain free range to maintain the flexibility of the connective tissues. Strengthening exercises may produce pain in the initial stage, however sub isometric exercises in the pain free range are performed to maintain the strength and avoid formation of adhesions. Any active exercise, which aggravates the symptoms, should be discarded immediately. The vigorous strengthening exercises are started as the symptoms such as pain and swelling improves.

CARPAL TUNNEL SYNDROME

Carpal tunnel syndrome has been described as the most common peripheral mononeuropathy characterized by pain, numbness, tingling sensation in the thumb, index, middle and radial side of the ring finger. Carpal tunnel syndrome constitutes a major part of the occupational upper extremity disorder and is associated with considerable health care and indemnity costs.

The carpal tunnel is a narrow passageway on the palm aspect of the wrist made up of carpal bones and ligaments. The median nerve, along with nine flexor tendons runs through this passageway. Normal pressure of the carpal tunnel has been defined as a range of 2–10 mm, and wrist flexion increases this pressure 8-fold, while extension increases it 10-fold.[37] The median nerve can be compressed or impinged in the tunnel if there swelling or inflammation in the tendons the tunnel is narrowed and rigid. The symptoms such as pain, numbness, tingling sensation are produced in the course of median nerve down the wrist joint (Fig. 23.23).

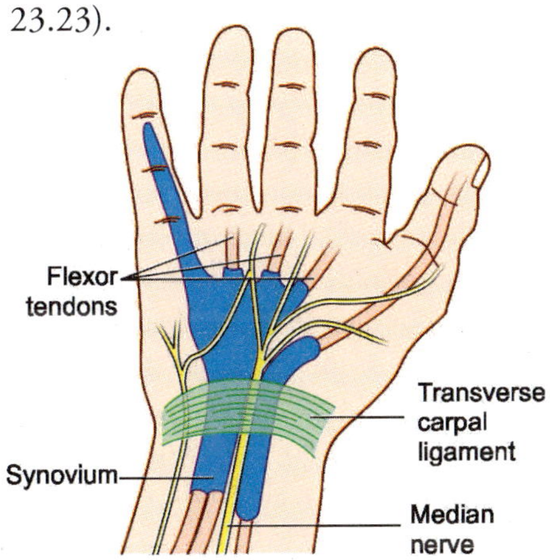

Fig. 23.23: Carpal tunnel with soft tissues

Repetitive flexion and extension in the wrist significantly increase the fluid pressure in the tunnel through thickening of the *synovial* tissue that lines the tendons within the *carpal tunnel*.[38] A review of available scientific data by the *National Institute for Occupational Safety and Health* (*NIOSH*) indicated that job tasks that involve highly repetitive manual acts or specific wrist postures were associated with incidents of CTS, but causation was not established. Women are three times more likely than men to get carpal tunnel syndrome. Some conditions like diabetes, gout, hyperthyroidism, rheumatoid arthritis, and pregnancy can increase the risk of CTS. The *median nerve* can usually move up to 9.6 mm to allow the wrist to flex, and to a lesser extent during extension. Long-term compression of the *median nerve* can inhibit nerve gliding, which may lead to injury and scarring. When scarring occurs, the nerve will adhere to the tissue around it and become locked into a fixed position, so that less movement is apparent.[39]

Symptoms

Carpal tunnel develops slowly. At first, the most likely to notice it at night or when the patient first wakes up in the morning. Patient experiences "pins and needles" sensation when the hand falls asleep. During the day, the patient notices pain or tingling when holding things, like a phone or a book, or when driving. Shaking or moving the fingers often helps. As the condition progresses the patient experiences weakness and muscle wasting on the thenar aspect can be observed. Patient finds difficulty in making a fist, holding a pen, utensils, or buttoning the shirt. Some patients feel like fingers are swollen, even though no swelling is present, or they may have trouble distinguishing between hot and cold.

Management

The initial phases of the conservative treatment methods require corrective splints in the wrist while neutral or in an extension position[40,41,42,43] (Fig. 23.24).

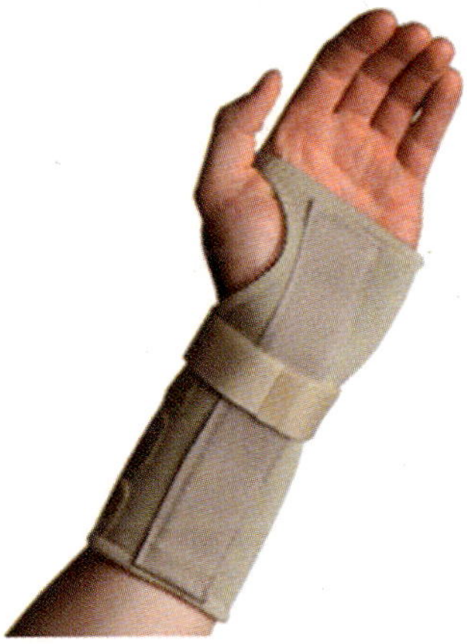

Fig. 23.24: Corrective brace or splint

Recently, several studies reported optimum results with the use of neurodynamic mobilization as a conservative treatment, with neural slipping helping nerve mobilization in relation to musculoskeletal tissues.[44,45] The biomechanical effect of the treatment would restore neural mobilization by decreasing the edema and adhesion in the carpal tunnel.[46,47] Because of the chronicity of CTS, studies also described neuromodulator effects from neural mobilization techniques such as the decrease in nociception of the median nerve; reduction in algogenic and pro-inflammatory substances; and reversibility in the pain pathways.

Neural Mobilization: The patient is placed in a supine position on the couch with the extremity which is being treated rests on the anterior thigh of the therapist. Therapist stands at the side and grasps the hand and elbow of the patient. The shoulder is abducted to 100 degrees with the elbow, wrist and finger flexion. The therapist depresses the shoulder with the thigh. The neck of the patient remains in the neutral position. While maintaining the position of neck, shoulder is rotated externally and elbow joint is extended gradually. In the next step wrist and finger are extended. This whole process produces tension in the median nerve. There are four variations of the neural mobilization. First, the position of the neck is maintained at 45° ipsilateral side flexion by the assistant, and then the extremity is brought into the extreme stretched position. Second, the position of the neck is maintained at 45° contralateral side flexion by the assistant, and then the extremity is brought into the extreme stretched position. Third, the extremity is maintained at its stretched position (shoulder depression, external rotation, elbow extension, wrist (60°) and fingers extension), and then neck is flexed 45° towards the same side. Fourth, the extremity is maintained at its stretched position (shoulder depression, external rotation, elbow extension, wrist (60°) and fingers extension), and then neck is flexed 45° towards the contralateral side. All the movements are performed for three times per treatment session.

Stretching and Strengthening Exercises: Stretching of EPB and APL is initiated in the pain free range to maintain the flexibility of the connective tissues. Strengthening exercises may produce pain in the initial stage, however sub isometric exercises in the pain free range are performed to maintain the strength and avoid formation of adhesions. Any active exercise, which aggravates the symptoms, should be discarded immediately. The vigorous strengthening exercises are started as the symptoms such as pain and swelling improves.

Tendon Gliding Exercises: Tendon thickening and adhesions may result after repeated chronic injury. The formation of adhesions can be prevented by administrating tendon gliding exercises.

- *Tendon gliding for thumb:* The patient is asked to flex the thumb towards palm as far as possible and then stretch it out as far as possible.
- *Tendon gliding for fingers:* Finger tendon gliding exercises: Keep the fingers extended, make a tabletop by keeping the fingers straight, and then bending at the knuckles. Make a straight fist. Make a hook fist. Make a full fist and then extend them.

CONTUSION

Contusion is the disruption of blood vessels below the skin, anywhere in the body. A direct blow to the skin is the main cause of the contusion; however, there is no break in the skin occurs. The blood comes out of the vessels, accumulates in the deeper tissues and forms a clot, known as hematoma. Ecchymosis is seen in the area. It may be absent if the deep tissue hematoma is formed.

Patients complaint pain and swelling in the area with painful movements. If the injury is superficial, ecchymosis is seen on the skin over the contusion. Tenderness is also the dominant feature of the contusion. Patients usually reveal the mechanism of the injury. The severity of this type of injury can be deceptive.

The contusions are managed with PRICE. Contusion of quadriceps and biceps brachii should be treated with caution as these muscles are at risk of ectopic bone formation (myositis ossification).

MUSCLE CRAMP

Muscle cramp is an involuntarily and forcibly contraction of the muscle or group of muscles, that lasts few seconds to minutes or occasionally longer. It is not uncommon for a muscle to recur multiple times until it finally resolves. Typically, cramps cause an abrupt, intense pain in the involved muscle which may be experienced as mild twitches to excruciatingly painful. The cramp may involve few fibers of the muscle or whole muscle or several muscles of same action (agonist or antagonist). Every individual experiences cramp at some time in their life, usually in the third decade of life and become increasingly as the age progresses, however, children may also experience cramps of muscles. Cramp may occur to any skeletal (voluntary) and organ (involuntary) muscles (rarely), however, it is more commoner in the skeletal muscles such as calves ("charley horse"), quadriceps, hamstrings and intrinsic muscles of the foot.

Etiology

The cause of the cramp is unknown, however, it is believed that inadequate stretching before exercises, muscle fatigue, exercising in the heat, and imbalance in the levels of electrolyte such as sodium, potassium, chloride, calcium and phosphate in the blood may contribute to the muscle cramps.

Pathology

The voluntary contraction of the agonistic muscles require relaxation of the antagonistic muscles. Cramps can occur when antagonistic muscles fail to relax properly due to myosin fibers not fully detaching from actin filaments. In skeletal muscle, ATP must attach to the myosin heads for them to disassociate from the actin and allow relaxation. The absence of ATP in sufficient quantities means that the myosin heads remains attached to actin. An attempt to force a muscle cramped in this way to extend (by contracting the opposing muscle) can tear muscle tissue and worsen the pain. The muscle must be allowed to recover (resynthesize ATP), before the myosin fibers can detach and allow the muscle to relax.

Prevention

Adequate conditioning of the muscles and stretching prior to any exercises or sports activities, adequate nutrition and hydration, attention to safety when exercising, and attention to ergonomic factors may help in prevention of the cramps.

Management

Stretching of the muscle may help in relieving the cramps. With exertional heat cramps due to electrolyte abnormalities (primarily sodium loss and not calcium, magnesium and potassium) appropriate fluids and sufficient salt improves symptoms.

BURSITIS

Bursitis is an infection or inflammation of the fluid-filled sac (bursa) that lies between a tendon and skin, or between a tendon and bone. The condition may be acute or chronic. Activities that involve excessive and repetitive forces on the inter-tissue junctions frequently lead to an inflammation to the bursa.

Bursa is a small fluid filled sac lined or water bag similar to synovium; they usually are located at inter-tissue junctions that encounter high friction during movements. The inter-tissue junctions involve skin, tendons, or muscles, ligaments over bony prominence. Bursa may or may not communicate with a joint.

Origin

Bursa is very much similar to tendon sheath and the synovial membrane. Some bursae are simply extension of the synovium membrane, others are formed by external to the capsule. Occasionally the cavity of the bursa communicates with the cavity of the synovial joint (suprapatellar bursa and subscapularis bursa communicates with knee joint and shoulder joint respectively).

There are two types of the bursa:

a. **Anatomical:** Those anatomically or normally present (over the patella and olecranon); and
b. **Adventitious:** Such type of bursa develop over a bunion, an osteochondroma, or on spine due to kyphosis. The adventitious bursa are produced by repeated trauma or constant/prolonged friction or pressure. These bursae have a lack of true endothelial or synovial lining. The adventitious bursa which develops in response to an abnormal and excessive friction (such as subcutaneous bursa) develops over the tendocalcaneous in response to badly fitted shoes should not be confused with anatomic bursa.

Functions

Muscles are the drivers of the joint, their contraction produces movement on the joints (bones move in opposite direction) this encounters high friction in the inter-tissue junctions. The function of the bursae is to reduce friction, protect delicate structure from pressure, help the joint to move with ease, lubricate and cushion pressure points and provide a slippery surface that has no friction.

[*Example:* When a zip lock small water bag is placed between the hands and then hands are rubbed on each other. The movements would be smooth and effortless this is exactly how a bursa functions as a smooth, slippery surface between two moving inter-tissue surfaces].

Causes

Acute or chronic trauma such as overuse, and sustain repetitive stresses can cause excessive load on the bursa. Acute or chronic pyogenic infection, low grade inflammatory conditions such as gout, syphilis, tuberculosis or rheumatoid arthritis may also cause bursitis. Trauma or injury can cause inflammation in the tendon which is termed as tendonitis that may put some degree of stress on the bursa and causes bursitis. However, it is not clear whether tendonitis causes bursitis or bursitis causes tendonitis, but most of time both conditions occur combined (follow each other).

Mechanism

Chronic repeated trauma allows gradual accumulation of synovial fluid in the bursa, in turn the bursa becomes swollen, inflamed and rough. The smooth gliding bursa now acts as gritty and rough within an already confined space that leads to friction in the inter-tissue surfaces. The movements become irritating and painful which further contribute to the bursitis and tendonitis.

Clinical Symptoms

A dull ache, stiffness in the area around the bursa or joint line may be experienced. Symptoms aggravate with movements and pressure. Redness and swelling may be observed occasionally in the area of inflamed bursa in case of superficial (subcutaneous) bursitis. The extreme movements can put the stress/pressure on the bursa and cause pain. The resistance against the contraction at extreme ranges can also aggravate the symptoms.

Hip Joint Bursitis

Bursitis associated with gluteus maximus muscle may be of three types:

- Trochanteric bursitis.
- Subgluteal bursitis.
- Iliopsoas or iliopectineal bursitis.

Trochanteric Bursitis

Trochanteric bursa lies between the insertion of the tendon of the gluteus maximus and the vastus lateralis. Trochanteric bursitis may either be infectious or non-infectious. Infectious trochanteric bursitis may be caused by an acute pyogenic infection or a tuberculosis (Fig. 23.25).

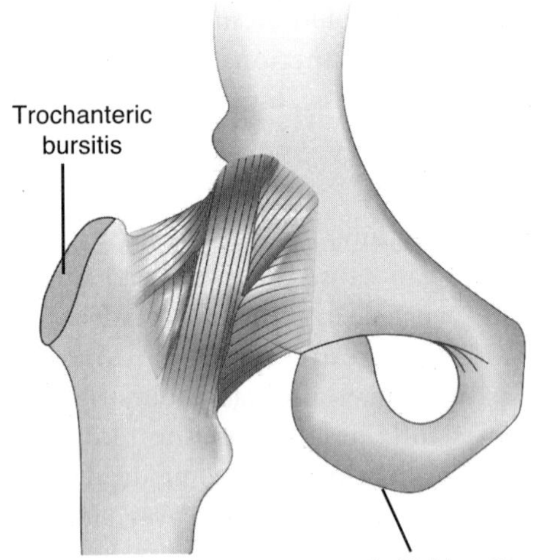

Fig. 23.25: Trochanteric bursitis

a. Tuberculosis is rarely seen now except in some developing countries was fairly common in this bursa in the past. To make a diagnosis, cultures from fluid of bursa should be taken for pyogenic organism and acid fast bacteria. Patients present with localized pain with or without previous history of tuberculosis. Pain aggravates in the night or during rest.
b. Non-infectious or traumatic trochanteric bursitis pain will be around the lateral aspect of the hip. It is common in middle aged older people engaged in sports activities such as running, tennis, gardening etc. Patients typically complain of lateral hip pain over the outer thigh or difficulty in walking. The hip pain is usually aggravated by direct pressure; depending upon the degree of inflammation and swelling, pressure sensitivity ranges from mild morning pain and stiffness to intolerance to sleeping on the affected side. Patients may rub the thigh when describing the pain.

Subgluteal Bursitis

Subgluteal bursa is usually a large and multi locular, separates the deep surface of the gluteus maximus from the greater trochanter and the short rotator of the hip joint. It may be infectious or non-infectious. The pain is experienced in the deep tissues on the posterior aspect of the hip. Extreme hip flexion (with knee flexion) and adduction can elicit the pain in the site of bursa.

Ischiogluteal Bursitis

The ischiogluteal bursa lies between the gluteus maximus and the ischium. It may also be infectious or non-infectious or inflammatory, is more common in individuals who have secondary occupations. The prolonged sitting causes constant irritation in the bursa which becomes swollen and inflamed.

Iliopsoas Bursitis

It is also known as iliopectineal bursitis, the largest bursa around the hip joint, which covers anterior hip joint capsule and extends proximally into the pelvis posterior to the iliopsoas. Iliopsoas bursitis can cause pain in the anterior aspect of hip joint with an ilioinguinal mass. Hip flexion and resistance to the extension of the hip joint may produce pain (Fig. 23.26).

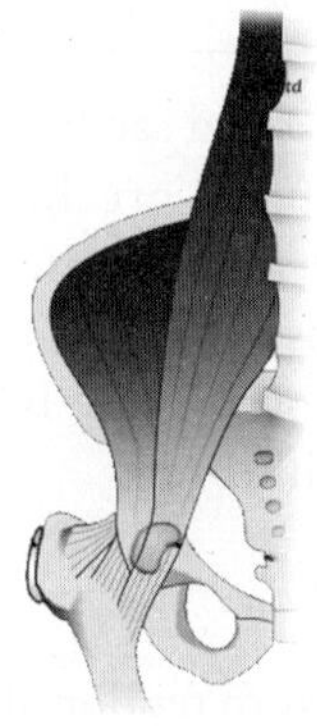

Fig. 23.26: Iliopsoas bursitis

Knee Joint Bursitis

The knee joint has as many as fourteen bursa. They are situated wherever skin, muscle, or tendon rubs against bones. Some important bursae, are discussed as below: (Fig. 23.27).

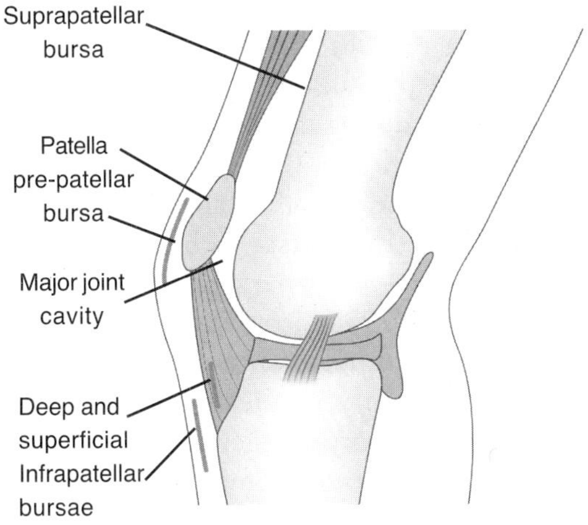

Fig. 23.27: Knee joint bursitis—suprapatellar, infrapatellar and pre-patellar

Suprapatellar Bursitis

In the front of the patellofemoral joint there is no capsule. Quadriceps over the suprapatellar region produce enormous friction during the knee joint movements. To reduce the friction between quadriceps and suprapatellar region an adventitious bursa is formed which is known as suprapatellar bursa. The bursa communicates with the joint. Pain in the superior aspect of the knee joint is usually caused by the suprapatellar bursitis which is more common in runners and jumpers. Suprapatellar bursitis is usually the result of direct trauma to the bursa from either acute injury or repeated microtrauma.

Physical examination may elicit tenderness in the anterior knee just above the patella. Passive flexion as well as active resisted extension of the knee will reproduce the pain. Sudden release of resistance during this maneuver will markedly increase the pain. There may be swelling in the suprapatellar region with boggy feeling on palpation. Occasionally the suprapatellar bursa may become infected which produces systemic symptoms, such as fever and malaise, as well as local symptoms, including rubor, color and dolor.

Infrapatellar Bursitis

Infrapatellar bursa is a small deep situated bursa between the tuberosity of the tibia and the patellar tendon and is separated from the synovium of the knee by a pad of fat. The superficial infrapatellar bursa lies in the subcutaneous tissue between the skin and the front of the lower part of the ligamentum patellae. Patient experiences pain in the site of the bursa, and swelling which may extend on either side of the patellar tendon. Loss of active terminal extension (extension lag), pain on resistance to full flexion and tenderness near the patellar tendon are the common symptoms of the infrapatellar bursitis (Fig. 23.28).

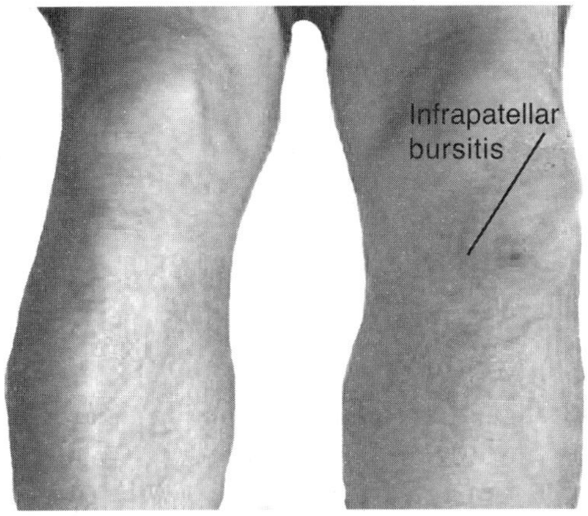

Fig. 23.28: Infrapatellar bursitis with marked swelling

Prepatellar Bursitis

The prepatellar bursa lies in the subcutaneous tissue between the skin and front of the lower half of the patella and the upper part of the ligamentum patellae. The direct trauma such as a fall on the patella, or by recurrent minor injuries (housemaid's and namaaz position) are the common causes of traumatic prepatellar bursitis. Pyogenic prepatellar bursitis especially in children is also common (Figs. 23.29a and b).

(a)

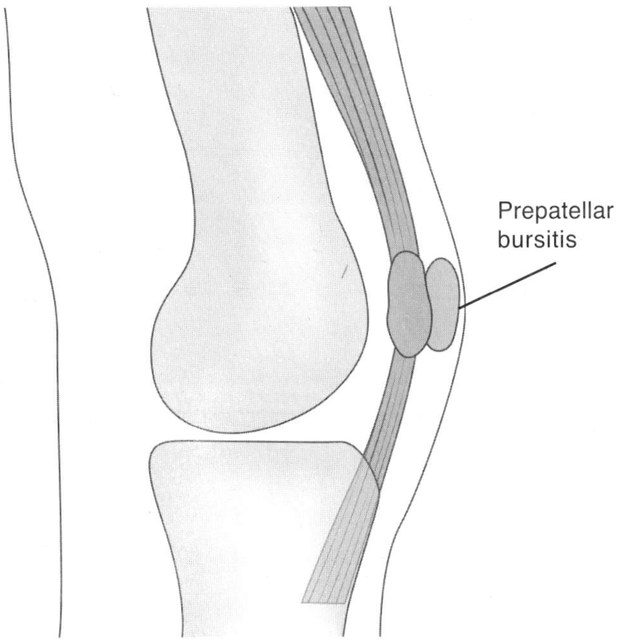

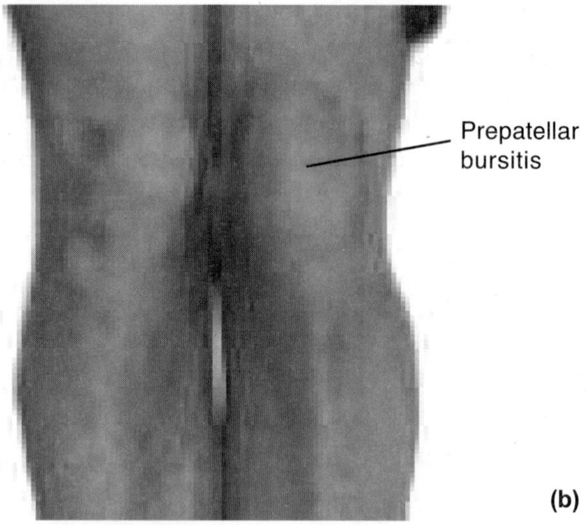

Figs. 23.29a and b: Prepatellar bursitis with redness and swelling

Prepatellar bursitis is very common in those whose occupation demands prolonged kneeling, e.g., carpet layers, housemaid's and namaaz prayers. Indeed, effusion into the bursa sac are popularly known as housemaid's knee because in kneeling, the bursa comes into contact with the ground.

Pes Anserine Bursitis or Voshell's Bursitis

The pes anserine bursa is located between the proximal anteromedial aspect of the tibia and the undersurface of the pes anserinus muscle tendons (gracilis, semitendinosus and sartorius). Pes anserine bursitis also known as Voshell's bursitis is a commonly missed causes of medial knee joint pain (Fig. 23.30).

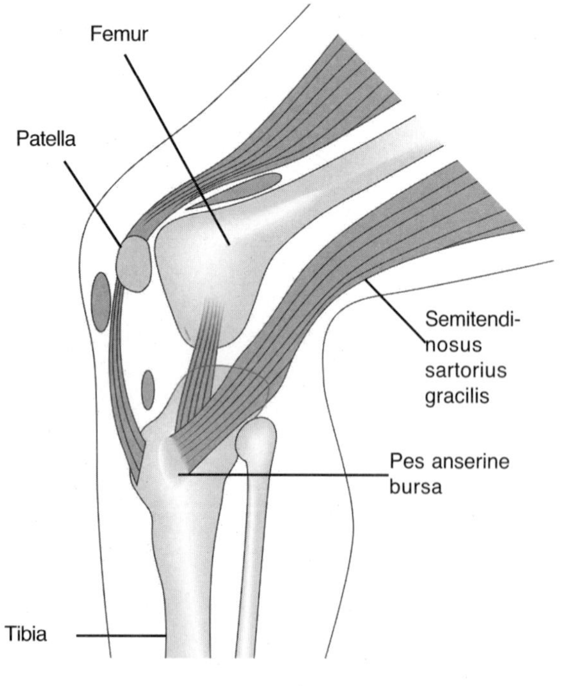

Fig. 23.30: Pes anserinus bursitis

Shoulder Joint Bursitis

Subacromial Bursitis or Sub Deltoid Bursitis

The subacromial bursa lies between the deltoid and supraspinatus muscle. It extends upwards underneath the acromion process and the coracoacromial ligament. The subacromial bursa reduces the friction and permits the greater tuberosity of the humerus to rotate inwards under the acromian process during the abduction and rotation of the shoulder. Although the subacromial bursa becomes inflamed more often than any other bursa, the inflammation is rarely primary in the bursa: rather it results from tendonitis of the rotator cuff of the shoulder with or without calcification. Codman (1934) described bursitis as an entity. The tendon of the supraspinatus lies just below the subacromial bursa. Injury to the supraspinatus tendon produces some inflammatory changes, but it may be painless until the adjacent brusa (subacromial) is involved which, being abundantly supplied with vessels and nerves produces the symptoms of which the patient complains. Pain in the shoulder which may radiate down the lateral arm and aggravates while overhead activities (flexion with internal rotation) is the common symptom of the subacromial bursitis (Figs. 23.31a and b).

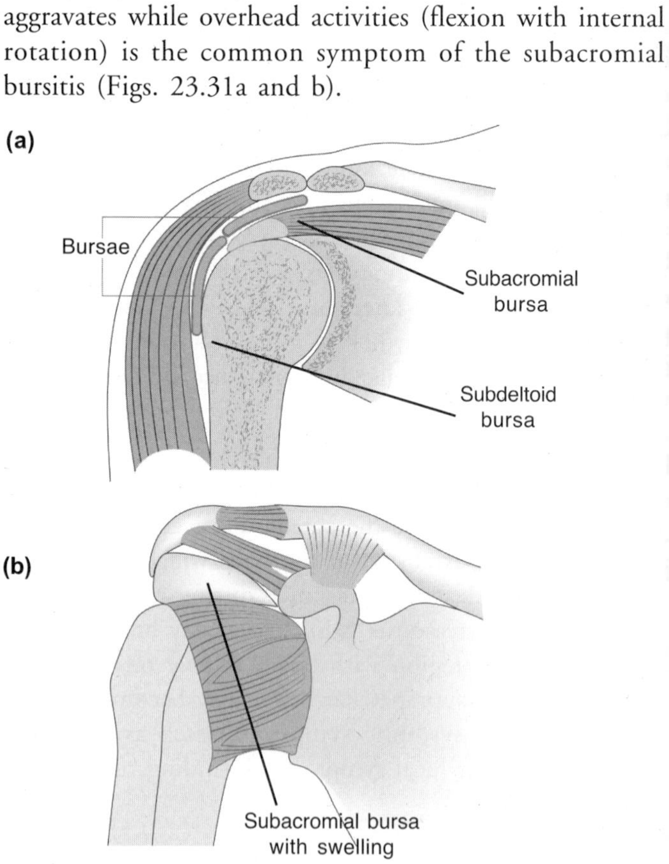

Figs. 23.31a and b: a. Subacromial bursa, b. Subacromial bursa with swelling

Neer has described the maneuver to test the subacromial bursitis as passive shoulder flexion and internal rotation. Patient should complain pain at the end range. The test is not so sensitive to the bursitis as other conditions may also produce the same symptoms. Hawkins and Kennedy described the test which has more sensitivity than Neer. It involves forward flexion at 90° with internal rotation which brings the greater tuberosity under the acromian arch and reduces subacromial space, contributes to further impingement in the bursa.

Subscapularis Bursitis

The subscapularis bursa lies on the anteromedial surface of the humeral head between the tendon of the subscapularis muscle and the capsule of the shoulder and communicates with the joint. Traumatic subscapularis bursitis is not very common.

RETROCALCANEAL BURSITIS

Pain in the posterior aspect of the heel at the insertion of tendo-Achilles may be arisen from retrocalcaneal bursitis. There are two bursae retrocalcaneal and subcutaneous calcaneal bursa. Retrocalcaneal bursa is a deep bursa, situated anterior to the Achilles tendon between calcaneus and Achilles tendon, whereas, subcutaneous calcaneal bursa is a superficial bursa situated posterior to the Achilles tendon between skin and Achilles tendon. Retrocalcaneal bursitis may be caused by bursal impingement between the Achilles tendon and an excessively prominent posterosuperior aspect of the calcaneus (Haglund deformity) during dorsiflexion of the ankle. Retrocalcaneal bursitis may be unilateral or bilateral and may be associated with gout, rheumatoid arthritis, and seronegative spondyloarthropathies. Recent studies suggest that a misaligned subtalar joint axis in relation to the Achilles tendon (measured in terms of joint inclination and deviation) can result in an asymmetrical force load on the tendon disrupting normal biomechanics. Tight or poorly fitted shoes that produce excessive pressure on the posterior heel is also one of the causes of the retrocalcaneal bursitis (Fig. 23.32). This altered joint axis is associated with an increased risk for Achilles pathologies, including bursitis. Swelling and redness with warmth and pain on pressure may clearly be apparent.

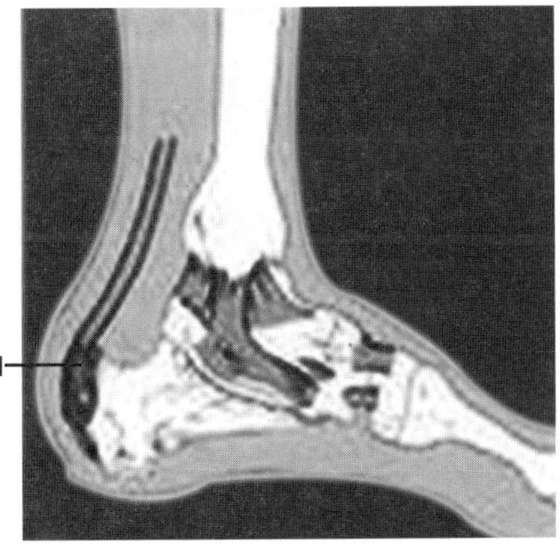

Fig. 23.32: Retrocalcaneal bursitis

Treatment

- Cryotherapy.
- Contrast bath.
- Continuous ultransound with the intensity of .9w/cm^2.
- Gradual progressive stretching of tendo-Achilles.
- Shoe modification.
- Corticosteroid injections–After fair trial of above treatment.

Management

The treatment of bursitis is determined by its cause and secondarily by pathological changes in the bursa. In most of the cases surgery is not needed. Modification in the activities–correction of posture–should be given the priority. Traumatic bursitis often responds favorably to conservative treatment and aspiration and injection of an appropriate steroid preparation, but infectious bursitis may require surgical intervention.

Management of Infectious Bursitis

- Aspiration and injections of an appropriate drugs.
- Incision and drainage when an acute supportive bursitis fails to respond to non-surgical methods.
- Excision of chronically infected and thickened bursa and removal of an underlying bony prominences.

The infected bursa should be examined for organism and also treated with an appropriate antibiotics. Aspiration and injection of antibiotics may be the second step. Dressing should be applied after aspiration, surgical drainage is occasionally needed.

The surgical excision of the bursa is required for repeated bouts of bursitis that interfere with functional activities and for chronically damaged and infected bursa, particularly if calcaneal osteomyelitis is present.

Management of Traumatic Bursitis

Prevention: Any activity which makes the inflammation of the bursa worse, should be avoided.

- Avoid repetitive activities that put excessive load or stress.
- Lose weight if it is needed.
- Modification in the shoe.
- Maintain strength and flexibility of the muscles.

Cryotherapy: Application of ice packs twice or thrice daily with minimum of fifteen minutes can reduce the inflammation. Ice packs are readily available in the market should be recommended at home also.

Pulsed Ultrasound Therapy: 3 MHz ultrasound for subcutaneous bursitis and 1 MHz ultrasound with high intensity and low duty cycle for deep situated bursa can be recommended so that ultrasound energy should reach to the deep situated bursa.

Contrast Bath: Moist heat therapy is effective in relieving the muscle spasm. Contrast bath may also be recommended for retrocalcaneal bursitis.

REFERENCES

1. Gev Bhabra and *et al.* Lateral Elbow Tendinopathy, Development of a Pathophysiology-Based Treatment Algorithm. Orthop J Sports Med. 2016 Nov; 4(11).
2. Binder AI, Hazleman BL. Lateral humeral epicondylitis: A study of natural history and the effect of conservative therapy. Br J Rheumatol 1983;22(2):73–76.
3. Prognostic factors in lateral epicondylitis: A randomized trial with one-year follow-up in 266 new cases treated with minimal occupational intervention or the usual approach in general practice. Haahr JP, Andersen JH. Rheumatology (Oxford) 2003 Oct; 42(10):1216–25.
4. Lateral epicondylitis in tennis: Update on aetiology, biomechanics and treatment. Thomas De Smedt, Andy de Jong, Wim Van Leemput, Dossche Lieven, and Francis Van Glabbeek Br J Sports Med 2007 Nov; 41(11): 816–819. Published online 2007 Jul 6.
5. Electromyographic analysis of elbow function in tennis players. Morris M, Jobe FW, Perry J, Pink M, Healy BS. Am J Sports Med 1989 Mar-Apr; 17(2):241–47.
6. Lateral and Medial Epicondylitis of the Elbow. Jobe FW, Ciccotti MG. J Am Acad Orthop Surg 1994 Jan; 2(1):1–8.
7. Wrist kinematics differ in expert and novice tennis players performing the backhand stroke: Implications for tennis elbow. Blackwell JR, Cole KJ. J Biomech 1994 May; 27(5): 509–16.
8. Fu SC, Rolf C, Cheuk YC, Lui PP, Chan KM. Deciphering the pathogenesis of tendinopathy: A three-stages process. Sports Med Arthrosc Rehabil Ther Technol 2010; 2:30.
9. Kraushaar BS, Nirschl RP. Tendinosis of the elbow (tennis elbow). Clinical features and findings of histological, immunohistochemical, and electron microscopy studies. J Bone Joint Surg Am 1999; 81: 259–78.
10. Maffulli N, Moller HD, Evans CH. Tendon healing: Can it be optimised? Br J Sports Med 2002;36: 315–16.
11. Kraushaar BS, Nirschl RP. Tendinosis of the elbow (tennis elbow). Clinical features and findings of histological, immunohistochemical and electron microscopy studies. J Bone Joint Surg Am 1999; 81: 259–78.
12. Fenwick SA, Hazleman BL, Riley GP. The vasculature and its role in the damaged and healing tendon. Arthritis Res 2002; 4: 252–60.
13. Ljung BO, Forsgren S, Friden J. Substance P and calcitonin gene related peptide expression at the extensor carpi radialis brevis muscle origin: Implications for the etiology of tennis elbow. J Orthop Res 1999; 17: 554–59.
14. B.R. Mulligan. Mobilization with movement. J M Manip Ther 1 (4 1993; 154-56.
15. J Miller. Milligan concept–Management of tennis elbow. Ca Physiother Assoc Ortho Div Rev 2000 May/June, 45–46.
16. Noteboom T, Cruver S, Keller A, *et al.* Tennis elbow: A review. Orthop Sports Phys Ther 1994;19:357–66.
17. Selvier T, Wilson J. Methods utilized in treating lateral epicondylitis Physical Therapy Reviews 2000;5:117–24.
18. Wright A, Sluka K. Nonpharmacological treatments for musculoskeleta pain. Clin J Pain 2001;17:33–46.
19. Chamberlain G. Cyriax's friction massage: A review. J Orthop Sport Phys Ther 1982;4: 16–22.
20. De Bruijn R. Deep transverse friction: Its analgesic effect. Int J Sport Med 1984; 5: 35–36.
21. Gregory M, Deane M, Mars M. Ultrastructural changes in untraumatised rabbit skeletal muscle treated with deep transverse friction. Physiotherapy 2003;89:408–16.
22. A novel approach to pain relief pre-therapeutic exercise. McConnell J J Sci Med Sport 2000 Sep; 3(3):325–34.
23. The initial effects of a cervical spine manipulative physiotherapy treatment on the pain and dysfunction of lateral epicondylalgia Vicenzino B, Collins D, Wright A. Pain 1996 Nov; 68(1): 69–74.
24. Effects of Taping on Pain, Grip Strength and Wrist Extension Force in Patients with Tennis Elbow. Alireza Shamsoddini and Mohammad Taghi Hollisaz. Trauma Mon 2013 Sep; 18(2): 71–74.
25. Lateral Elbow Tendinopathy. Development of a Pathophysiology-Based Treatment Algorithm. Gev Bhabra, MD, FRCS(Orth), Allan Wang, FRACS, PhD, Jay R. Ebert, PhD, Peter Edwards, BSc, Monica Zheng, BPodM and Ming H. Zheng, PhD, MD, FRCPath. Orthop J Sports Med 2016 Nov; 4(11).
26. Smidt N, Lewis M, van der Windt DA, Hay EM, Bouter LM, Croft P. Lateral epicondylitis in general practice: Course and prognostic indicators of outcome. J Rheumatol 2006;33:2053–59.
27. Lateral Elbow Tendinopathy. Development of a Pathophysiology-Based Treatment Algorithm, Gev Bhabra, MD, FRCS(Orth), Allan Wang FRACS, Jay R. Ebert, PhD, First Published November 1, 2016 pubmed.
28. Prevalence and determinants of lateral and medial epicondylitis: A population study. Shiri R, Viikari-Juntura E, Varonen H, Heliövaara M. Am J Epidemiol 2006 Dec 1; 164(11):1065–74.
29. Review Lateral epicondylitis. Whaley AL, Baker CL. Clin Sports Med 2004 Oct; 23(4):677-91.
30. Medial epicondylitis in occupational settings: Prevalence, incidence and associated risk factors. Descatha A, Leclerc A, Chastang JF, Roquelaure Y, Study Group on Repetitive Work. J Occup Environ Med 2003 Sep; 45(9):993–1001.
31. Therapeutic exercises moving towards function, Carrie M, Lori Thein Brody. Lippincott Williams and Wilkins, 648.
32. Evaluation and Management of Elbow Tendinopathy. Samuel A. Taylor, MD and Jo A. Hannafin, MD, PhD Sports Health 2012 Sep; 4(5): 384–93.
33. Review Medial elbow problems in the overhead-throwing athlete. Chen FS, Rokito AS, Jobe FW. J Am Acad Orthop Surg 2001 Mar-Apr; 9(2):99–113.

4. Resection and repair for medial tennis elbow. A prospective analysis. Ollivierre CO, Nirschl RP, Pettrone FA. Am J Sports Med 1995 Mar-Apr; 23(2): 214–21.

5. DeQuervain F. Uebereine Form von chronischer Tendovaginitis. Corresp Blatt Schweizer Arzte 1895; 25: 389–94.

6. DeQuervain F. On a form of chronic tendovaginitis by Dr. Fritz Quervain in la Chaux-de-Fonds. 1895. Am J Orthop 1997, Sep. 26(9):641–44.

7. Ibrahim I, Khan WS; Goddard N; Smitham P (2012). "Suppl 1: Carpal Tunnel Syndrome: A Review of the Recent Literature". The Open Orthopaedics Journal 6: 69–76.

8. Schuind F, Ventura M, Pasteels J. (1990). "Idiopathic carpal tunnel syndrome: Histologic study of flexor tendon synovium". The Journal of Hand Surgery 15 (3): 497–503. doi:10.1016/0363-5023(90) 90070-8.

9. Armstrong T, Chaffin D (1979). "Carpal tunnel syndrome and selected personal attributes". Journal of Occupational Medicine 21 (7).

0. Rozmaryn LM, Dovelle S, Rothman ER, Gorman K, Olvey KM, Bartko JJ. Nerve and tendon gliding exercises and the conservative management of carpal tunnel syndrome J Hand Ther 1998;11(3): 171–79.

1. Verdugo RJ, Salinas RS, Castillo J, Cea JG. Surgical versus non-surgical treatment for carpal tunnel syndrome. Cochrane Database Syst Rev 2003(3):CD001552.

42. Anderson CR, Morris RL, Boeh SD, Panus PC, Sembrowich WL. Effects of iontophoresis current magnitude and duration on dexamethasone deposition and localized drug retention Phys Ther 2003;83(2):161–70.

43. Viera AJ. Management of carpal tunnel syndrome. Am Fam Physician. 2003;68(2): 265–72.

44. Muller M, Tsui D, Schnurr R, Biddulph-Deisroth L, Hard J, MacDermid JC. Effectiveness of hand therapy interventions in primary management of carpal tunnel syndrome: A systematic review. J Hand Ther 2004;17(2):210–28.

45. Duymaz T, Sindel D, Kesiktaþ N, Müslümanoðlu L. Efficacy of some combined conservative methods in the treatment of carpal tunnel syndrome: A randomized controlled clinical and electrophysiological trial. Turk J Rheumatol 2012;27(1): 38–46.

46. Oh J, Zhao C, Zobitz ME, Wold LE, An KN, Amadio PC. Morphological changes of collagen fibrils in the subsynovial connective tissue in carpal tunnel syndrome. J Bone Joint Surg Am 2006;88(4): 824–31.

47. Pinar L, Enhos A, Ada S, Gungor N. Can we use nerve gliding exercises in women with carpal tunnel syndrome? Adv Ther 2005; 22(5): 467–75.

24

ARTHRITIS

Arthritis is derived from two Latin words arth and itis. Arth means joint and itis means inflammation, hence, arthritis is defined as inflammation in the joint. As far as osteoarthritis is concerned, it is an essentially non-inflammatory disease, the disease does not commence with the inflammation, hence, it should not be called as arthritis. Therefore, the latest definition of the arthritis is given as: any process by which a joint is damaged is known as arthritis. There are two processes which involves joint destruction: inflammatory and degenerative.

The Articular Cartilage: The articular cartilage is composed of collagen fibers, proteoglycans and water. These substances contribute to the shape, size and elastic properties of the cartilage which make cartilage more resistant to the repeated mechanical stresses.

- Collagen fibers and proteoglycans (keratin sulphate and condroitin sulphate) contribute upto 20 percent.
- Water contribute upto 80 percent (Figs. 24.1a and b).

In terms of biphasic material, the articular cartilage is composed of a porous permeable collagen proteoglycan solid matrix filled by the freely movable interstitial fluid (approximately 25% by wet weight). In addition to solid and fluid there exists an additional ion phase when considering articular cartilage as a triphasic medium. Therefore biomechanically articular cartilage should be viewed as a triphasic material.

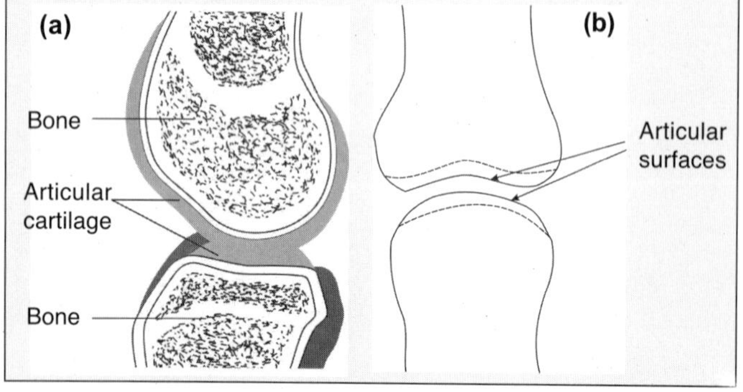

Figs. 24.1a and b: Normal hyaline articular cartilage

OSTEOARTHRITIS

Osteoarthritis is essentially a non-inflammatory degenerative disease of the atricular cartilage which is characterized by thinning and destruction of the joint surface, new bone (osteophyte) formation and capsular fibrosis. As the disease is an essentially non-inflammatory it should be termed as osteoarthrosis instead of osteoarthritis, however, both osteoarthritis and osteoarthrosis terms are used interchageably and has same meaning.

It affects commonly weight bearing joints such as the knee, hip and spine, moreover the individual joints are affected with differing frequency in men and women.

Pathogenesis

It is thought that early failure of the collagen fibers network (loosening of the collagen network) enables the proteoglycans to attract more water molecules. The increased water contents in the cartilage allows abnormal expansion of the proteoglycans and thus tissue swelling. *Associated with this change is a decreased in a cartilage stiffness and increase in cartilage permeability.*

In the next stage of degeneration, the proteoglycans of cartilage contain lower concentration of keratin sulphate than the normal while the concentration of condroitin sulphate increases. *Associated with this change the proteoglycan concentration in the cartilage falls.* At this stage there is decreased in a cartilage stiffness and increased in cartilage permeability. The cartilage losses its elasticity and becomes less resistant to repeated mechanical stresses, and the process of disintegration of cartilage begins. Progressive cartilage destruction contributes further stress to the collagen network. (Some authors claim that proteoglycan synthesis is increased upto the time of cartilage failure and there is an evidence of attempts to the appearance of chondrocytes clusters (cloning) in the matrix-depleted cartilage).

Perpendicularly oriented fissures appear in the superficial ɔne and they gradually extend into the deeper. Due to ıese fissures there is detachment of the small articular ırtilage fragments into the joint space where they are ventually degraded. The progressive loss of thickness of ıe articular cartilage may lead to surface abrasion and ɔmplete exposure of bone in areas of peak overload. ventually there is loss of full thickness of the articular ırtilage, where the articular cartilage is composed of a bony rticular plate polished from the grinding interaction of ɔne articulating with bone. Revascularization of the emaining articular cartilage produces osteophytes which ıay project to the periarticular structures (peripheral nshared areas) (Figs. 24.2a, b and Fig. 24.3).

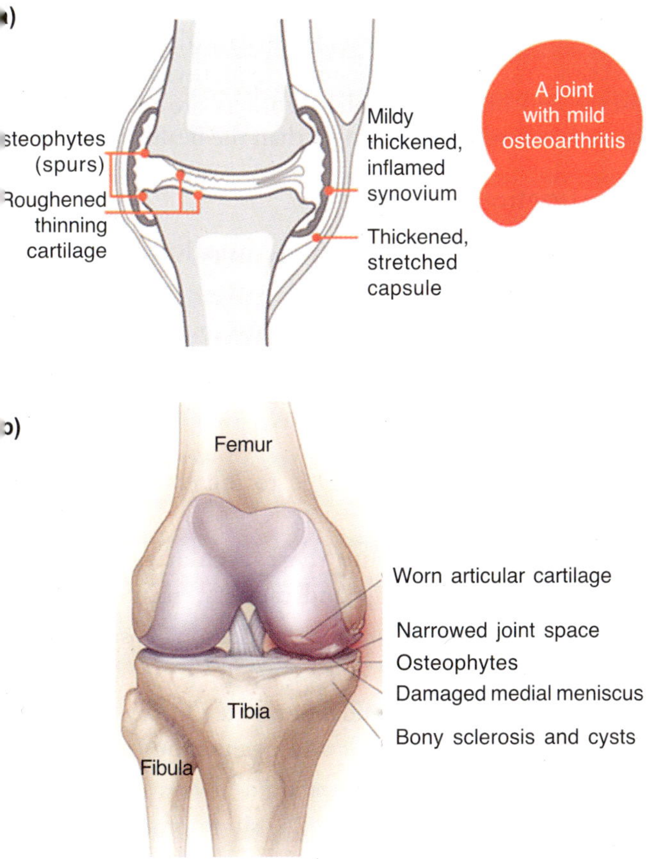

ig. 24.2a and b: Degenerated articular cartilage, loss of joint ɔace and osteophytes

The osteophytes deposit onto the synovium penetrate ɔ the sub synovial layers. The capsule loses its elastic roperties, becomes thickened, and its volume is decreased. inally there is limitation in the range of motion. Loss of ıll thickness of cartilage allows exposure of the ıbchondral bone. 'Cracks' in the subchondral bone plate ermit pressure transmission to the cancellous bone esulting in cyst formation.

The advanced changes include some type of subluxation

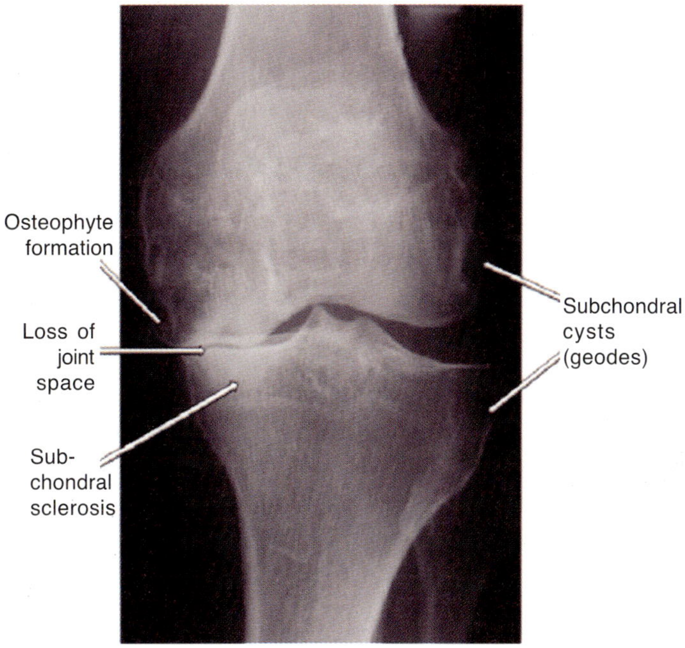

Fig. 24.3: Degenerated articular cartilage with joint space obliteration, osteophytes and subchondral cyst

such as widening of the joint of one side, horizontal translation, angular deviation etc. Small pieces of cartilage may be dislodged and develop loose bodies which can result in locking of the joint and episodic severe pain.

Wear Mechanism of the Cartilage

The wear mechanism of the cartilage begin in three ways:

1. **Interfacial Wear:** There is direct contact of the weight bearing surfaces (articular cartilages) with no lubrication film separating them. This is the common problem in the obese and the individuals whose job is long standing such as nurses, hair dressers. The interaction of the weight bearing joint surfaces causes adhesions:
   - The fragment adhere to each other and abrasion.
   - The tissue is scrapped by harder one.
2. **Fatigue Wear:** The deformation of the underlying weight bearing joint surface may occur if there is repeated micro trauma to the surfaces.
3. **High Impact Wear:** High impact activities such as jumping and running may increase the stress and load on the cartilage with insufficient time for internal fluid distribution.

These wear mechanisms put excessive load and alter the normal load bearing mechanism of the cartilage. This whole phenomenon disrupts the collagen fiber proteoglycan matrix and predisposes cartilage to early degeneration.

Clinical Sign and Symptoms

- Pain.
- Muscles guarding (spasm).
- Stiffness.
- Swelling.
- Tenderness.
- Crepitus.
- Decrease range of motion, flexion contracture, extension lag.
- Angular and rotatory deformities.

Pain is the dominant clinical feature which is aggravated by the activities those put more stress on the affected cartilage. Usually pain is more common in the form of discomfort and stiffness. Initially it is worsen on rising from bed, and again at the end of a day's activities and relieved by the rest. As the disease progresses there is involvement of the synovium and the capsule, which limits the range of motion of the joint and produces swelling (synovial and capsular thickening) and the joint becomes deformed. The muscles guard the joint by preventing the painful movements, resulting in shortening of the muscles which further decreases range of motion. Initially pain is poorly localized and is dull aching nature. It is relieved by rest but when the other structures such as articular, periarticular, and capsule are involved, pain may also be experienced during rest and at night.

Types of Osteoarthrosis

Primary Osteoarthritis

Primary osteoarthritis is a normal phenomenon which commences usually after fifth decade of life. There is no known cause of primary osteoarthritis as it is a part of wear and tear mechanism of the body, however, no cause is barrier for this type of osteoarthritis. All people will show primary osteoarthritic changes in the articular cartilage if they live long life (up to eighty years), however, some of them will have mild changes whereas others may develop severe changes in the joint including deformities. The severity of primary osteoarthritis depends upon the life style, body built and physical activities. The healthy people with an average body weight show osteoarthritic changes on the X-ray but may remain fit and asymptomatic throughout the life.

Secondary Osteoarthritis

Onset of this type of osteoarthritis is associated with some known causes. It may commence after the third decade of life, 10 to 15 years earlier than the primary osteoarthritis. Anything which alters the line of force or put excessive load on the articular cartilage can contribute to the secondary osteoarthritis. The predisposing factors such as injury, trauma or fracture may cause mal-alignment of the joint that results in transfer of load or weight on the particular part of the cartilage. The articular cartilage which transfers excessive weight than the usual due to mal alignment disrupts and disintegrates.

Obesity: According to the Arthritis Foundation, every pound of an extra body weight places three pounds of pressure on the knees and six pounds on the hips. The weight speeds up the wear and tear of joint cartilage.

Inactivity: Inactivity is one of the major causes of the muscle weakness. Muscles are the drivers of the joints. Weakness of the muscles will result in more approximation of the joint surfaces. The nutrition of the articular cartilage depends upon the movements of the joint. Therefore sedentary life style adversely affects the physical properties of articular cartilage. The individuals with history of joint infection, tuberculosis, diabetes, hyperthyroidism, Perthes disease and other metabolic disorders are more prone to the early osteoarthritic changes than the healthy individuals.

Investigations

- Laboratory investigations are usually within normal limits.
- Radiological findings are the most important diagnostic tools. Following changes can be seen on X-rays:
  1. **Loss of Joint Space:** Due to destruction of articular cartilage.
  2. **Subchondral Cyst:** Due to increased cellular and bone deposition.
  3. **Osteophytes:** Due to revascularization of the remaining cartilage and capsular traction.
  4. **Loose Bodies:** Due to fragmentation of osteochondral surface.
  5. **Deformity and Malalignment:** Due to destruction of capsular ligament and ligamentous laxity.

Radiographic evaluation should always be considered in a standing or weight bearing position of anteroposterior view. For patellofemoral joint a lateral view is required as it is a skyline view of the patella. For lateral compartment of the tibiofemoral joint posteroanterior view should be taken in a standing with the knees in 30 degrees of flexion this is because the medial compartment involves degeneration of distal femur and central tibia, and lateral compartment involves degeneration in the posterior femur and posterior tibia.

TIBIOFEMORAL JOINT OSTEOARTHROSIS

The human knee joint, the largest and perhaps most complex joint in the body, is a two joint structure composed of the tibiofemoral and patellofemoral joints. The knee joint transmits loads, participates in motion, aids in conservation of momentum and provides force couple for activities involving the leg.

- 80% of patients develop medial compartment resulting in varus or bow legged deformity.
- 05–10% of patients develop lateral compartment resulting in a valgus or kneed deformity.
- A small percentage of patients develop rotatory deformity of tibia that causes significant patellar maltracking or sublaxation. It is common in an arthritic knee but is surprisingly seldom a source of symptoms.
- **Panarticular Arthritis:** The involvement of both tibiofemoral compartments (medial and lateral) and patellofemoral joint.

Degenerated Articular Cartilage: In the degenerative process the concentration of proteoglycans in the cartilage falls. The proteoglycans organize the collagen fibers in the articular cartilage. As the concentration of the proteoglycans falls the collagen fibers becomes disorganized. At this stage the cartilage looses its elasticity and becomes less resistant to the repeated mechanical stresses and the process of disintegration begins. Perpendicular oriented fissures appear in the superficial zone and gradually extend into deeper zone. These fissures promote detachment of small articular cartilage fragments into the joint space where they are eventually degraded. There is progressive loss of thickness of the articular cartilage. The cartilage looses its full thickness (bone articulating with the bone (Figs. 24.4 a to d).

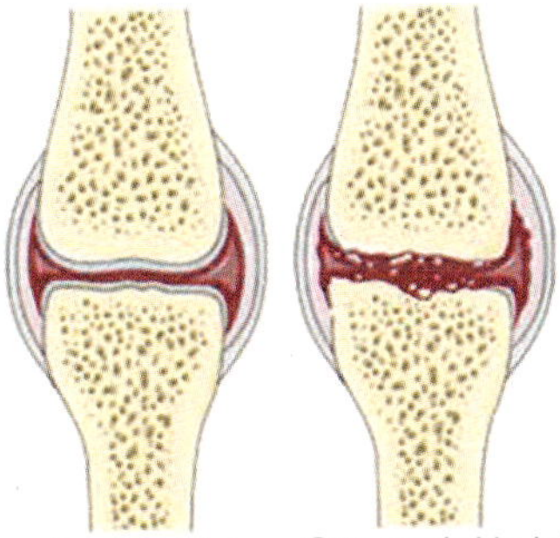

Fig. 24.4a: Knee joint osteoarthritis normal and degenerated cartilage

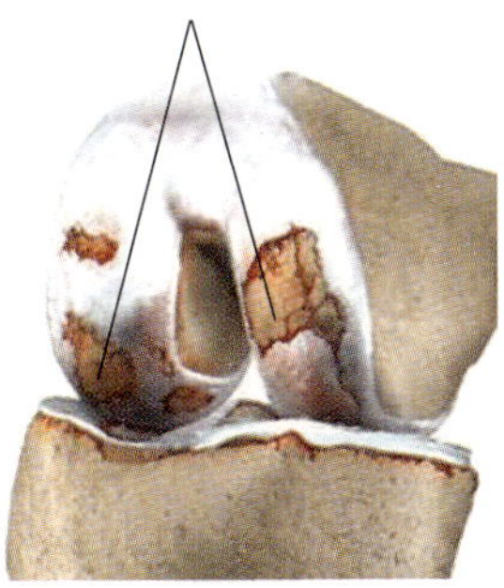

Fig. 24.4b: Knee joint osteoarthritis

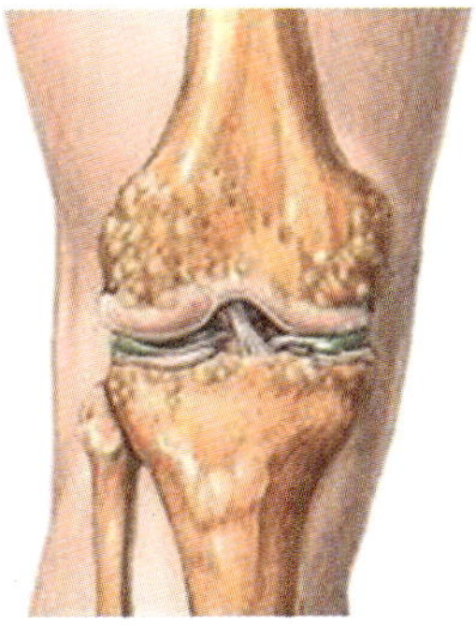

Fig. 24.4c

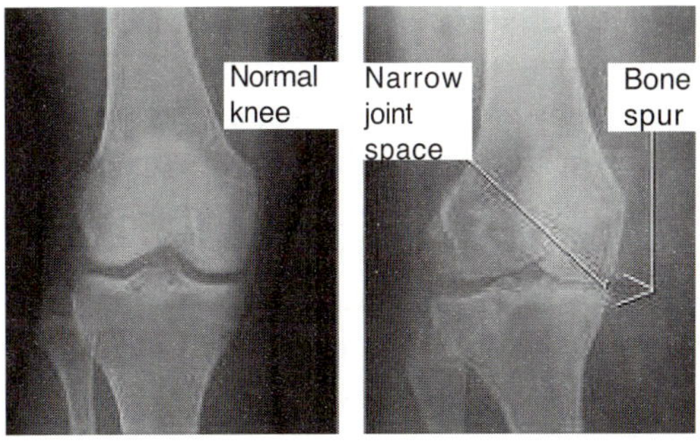

Fig. 24.4d: Knee joint osteoarthritis X-rays

Radiological Grading of the Knee Osteoarthritis

0 – Normal.

1 – Doubtful narrowing of joint space and possible osteophytic lipping.

2 – Definite osteophytes, definite narrowing of joint space.

3 – Moderate multiple osteophytes, definite narrowing of joint space, some sclerosis and possible deformity of bone ends.

4 – Large osteophytes marked narrowing of joint space, severe sclerosis, and definite deformity of bone ends, subchondral cyst may also be present.

Involvement of the Medial Meniscus in Degenerative Disease: The lesion in the meniscus may be of two types: The complete longitudinal tear and horizontal cleavage in the medial meniscus. The fibrocartilage of medial meniscus depends on the synovial fluid for nutrition. Once this portion is damaged in the degenerative process it cannot be healed. *The meniscus then inflicts injury to the articular cartilage of the femoral condyle just as the damaged soft bronze of a bearing inflicts damage to the hard steel of the crankshaft.* The damage to the articular cartilage is mechanical and is *arrested only* by mechanical means, namely, excision of the structure interfering with movement at the limit of extension and in particular with the screw home mechanism (Fig. 24.5).

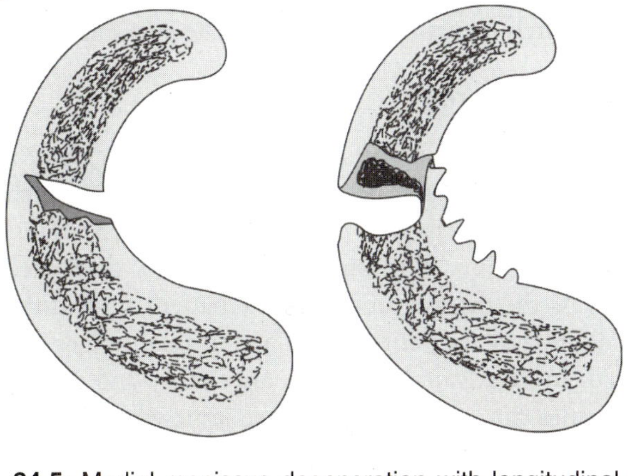

Fig. 24.5: Medial meniscus degeneration with longitudinal tear and horizontal cleavage

Internal Rotation of Tibia: The medial rotation may be associated with varus deformity, however, it is not necessary. The varus deformity and internal rotation of the tibia varies in degrees. If the medial rotation is associated with varus deformity the rotational component takes more responsibility for the degenerative changes. When the tibia a medially rotated in order to produce a gait in which the feet look directly forward instead of crossing over one another in the act of walking the tibia must be rotated laterally by the action of biceps.

In mid stance, tibia rotates laterally on the femur to achieve full extension and closed packed position of the knee joint. This is the most stable position of the tibiofemoral joint. Lateral rotation of the tibia on the femur from flexion to full extension (in mid stance) is termed as "screw home mechanism". The patients with internal tibial torsion or rotation find difficulty in rotating the tibia laterally on the femur. This would compromise the screw home mechanism, and contribute to the further destruction of the medial compartment of the tibiofemoral joint.

Tibial Torsion

The normal lateral tibial rotation is considered as approximately 23 degree. As the osteoarthrosis progresses the lateral tibial torsion decreases. The rate of decrease in lateral tibial torsion in patients with osteoarthrosis is more in the proximal tibia than in the distal. There is a correlation between reduction of lateral torsion with the radiographic stage of osteoarthrosis of the knee and general osteoporosity.

Measurement of Tibial Torsion

A simple clinical method to measure the tibial torsion is to have the patient sit with the legs hanging over the edge of the examination table. The angle formed by the second metatarsal ray and the tibial tuberosity is measured. The tibial torsion is approximately equal to the mean of the two angles. In another similar method of tibial torsion measurement, an angle formed by the transmalleolar axis and the edge of the table is measured. The tibial torsion is approximately equal to the mean of the two angles.

Clinical Features

Pain and stiffness in the knee joint which aggravates in weight bearing are the dominant features of osteoarthritic knee joint. There is pain on pressure (tenderness) on the medial joint line. The knee joint space is decreased on X-rays. As the disease progresses the patient finds difficulty in walking and stair climbing. The terminal ranges may be limited. In an advanced stage an angulatory and translatory deformities can be seen in the knee joint which predispose to the deformities such as bow leg and internal torsion of the tibia.

Baker's Cyst

Baker's cyst or popliteal cyst is an accumulation of the fluid in the gastrocnemius and semi-membranosus bursa, was described first, in 1877, by Baker. He noted communication of the cyst with the joint synovium with fluid that leaks into the bursa but cannot return back to the joint. Sometimes the cyst ruptures and releases the fluid into the semi-membranosus and gastrocnemius tendons which produces immense pain in the posteromedial aspect (medial gastrocnemius and semimembranosus tendons). It is, therefore, sometimes confused with the thrombophlebitis.

The popliteal (Backer) cysts are frequently associated with intra-articular pathology or injury such as meniscal tears, rheumatoid arthritis, osteoarthrosis, conditions causing synovitis, Charcot's joints and tuberculosis.

MANAGEMENT

1. Pain and Stiffness

Pain and spasm in the joint is actually a protective type or muscle guarding. Due to degenerative changes the thickness of the cartilage is decreased and joint space is reduced resulting in laxity of the ligaments. This whole procedure is responsible for instability of the joint. Therefore, during weight bearing or movements there are unwanted movements of articular surfaces. *If patient avoids the movements, pain can be reduced, but limiting the movements can have an adverse effect on the muscles.* The muscles become tight, which further contributes to the pain and stiffness, and limits the range of motion. This whole cycle makes the patient disabled and the activities of the daily living are compromised.

Pain and muscle spasm can be relieved by using some heating modalities such as paraffin wax bath, hot water bag and hot pack. The hot water bag is easily accessible in the market, and can be used by filling the hot water in the bag. The bag covers the painful area. Initially a towel can be placed between the bag and the painful area but it can be removed as the temperature of the water falls. The total time should be at least 15-20 minutes and it can be repeated twice or thrice a day. The hot water bags are preferred over electric pads for their moist heating effects. Short wave diathermy and interferential therapy may also be advised for their deep heating and analgesic effects respectively. Patient may also be advised pocket TENS for its effectiveness in relieving pain and spasm by acting on the pain gait (Fig. 24.6).

2. Strengthening Exercises

Regular exercises may help in strengthening the muscles and potentially stimulating cartilage growth.

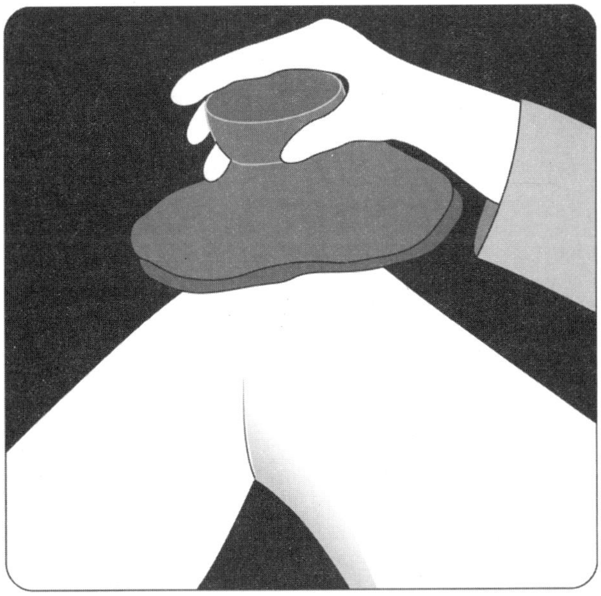

Fig. 24.6: Hot water bag

Restoration of Strength: The muscles are the drivers of the joint and responsible for the movements. Not only that but also they play important role in providing the dynamic stability to the joint. Therefore, restoration of the strength of the muscles is one of the goals of the treatment.

Ten Muscle Strengthening Exercises:

i. **Quadriceps Sets:** In lying with the knee straight a towel roll is placed under the knee joint. While pressing the towel down, knee is extended fully. The position is held for at least 6 seconds. After 6 seconds of contraction muscles is relaxed. 30-40 repetitions may be performed thrice daily (Fig. 24.7).

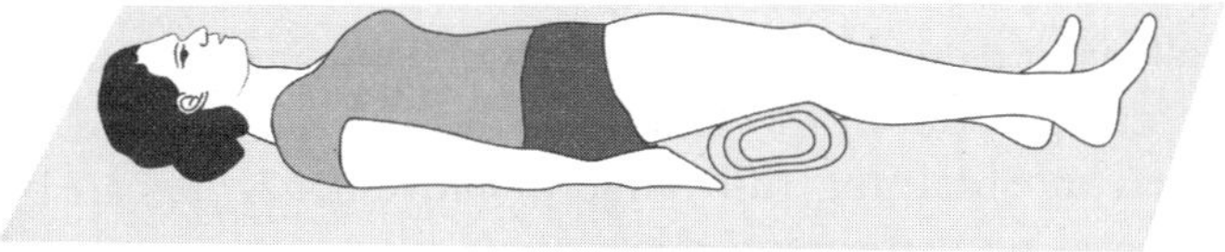

Fig. 24.7: Quadriceps sets

ii. **Gluteus Maximus Set:** In lying with the knee straight a towel roll is placed under the knee joint. The patient is instructed to press the towel down and hold it for at least 6 seconds. 30-40 repetitions may be performed thrice or twice daily (Fig. 24.8).

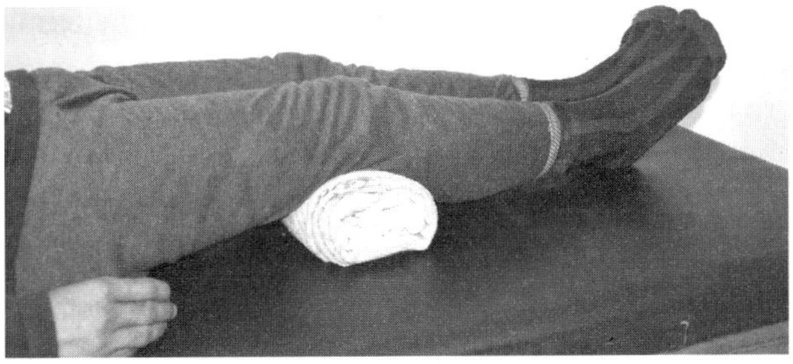

Fig. 24.8: Gluteus maximus set

iii. **Ankle Pump Exercise:** While keeping towel roll under the knee the ankle joint is moved up and down (Figs. 24.9a and b).

(a)

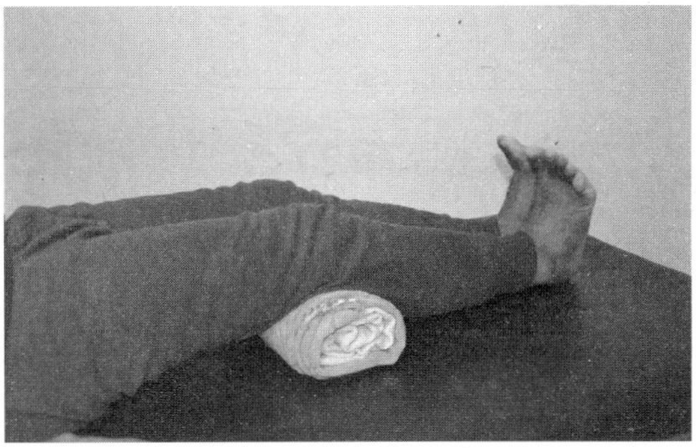

(b)

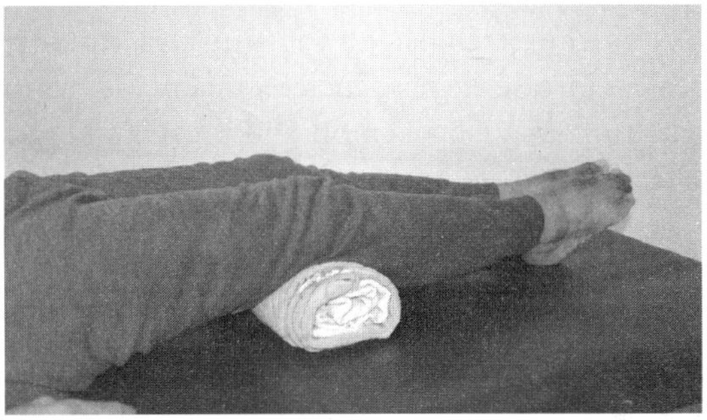

Figs. 24.9a and b: Ankle pump exercise

iv. **Straight Leg Raising:** While keeping the leg straight the patient is asked to raise it above around 60-70 degrees at the hip joint (Fig. 24.10).

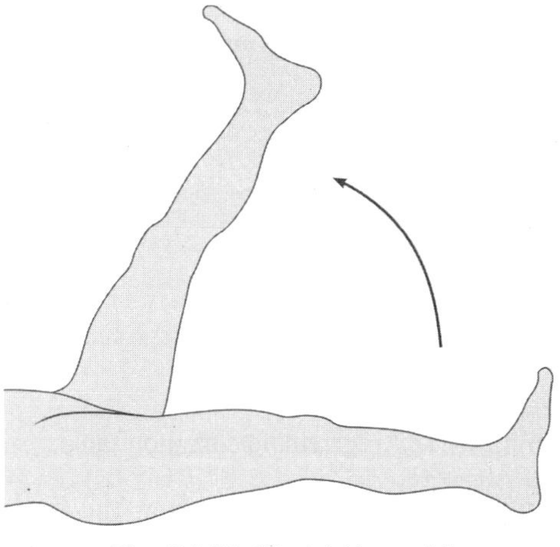

Fig. 24.10: Straight leg raising

v. **Side Leg Raising:** The lower leg is flexed out of the bed at around 20 degrees of the hip and knee joint (supine). In the next the affected leg is raised upto 70 degrees in side lying. 30-40 repetitions, two to thrice daily may be performed (Fig. 24.11).

vi. **High Sitting/Sitting on Table:** The weight cuff of 1/2 kg, 1 kg, or 2 kg, as per tolerance of the patient is tied at the ankle joint. The knee joint is flexed and extended for 10 times. After 10 repetitions patient should take

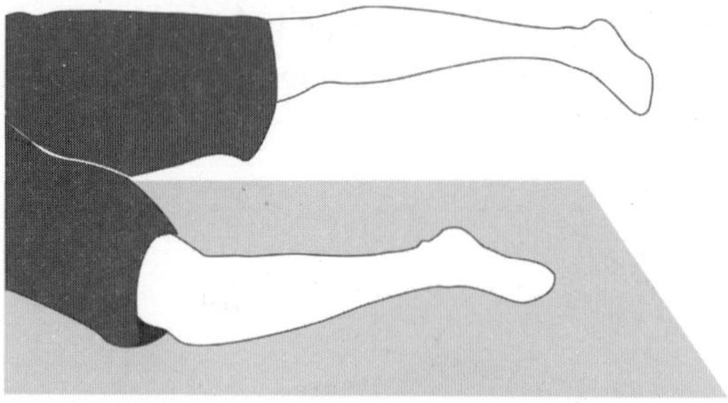

Fig. 24.11: Side straight leg raising

brief period of rest to allow the muscles relaxed. This completes one set (10 repetitions). The total 3 sets may be performed with brief period of relaxation between the sets. The weight can be increased after one or two weeks as the strength of the muscles (quadriceps) increases. In case exercise increases pain and symptoms, weight cuff may be taken off and knee is straighten up and bent down without weight (Fig. 24.12).

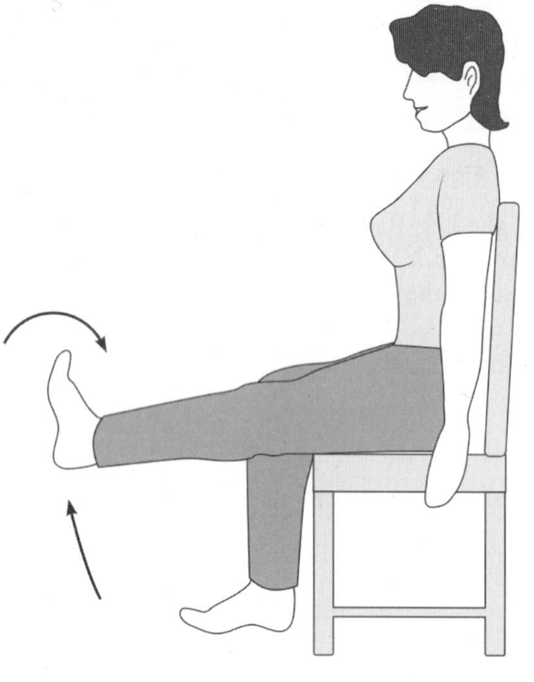

Fig. 24.12: High sitting/sitting on table

vii. **Squatting:** In standing with holding the back rest of chair both the knees are bent for 15-20 degrees. This is also known as mini squat. Squatting produces large loads on the patellofemoral joint, therefore, it should be avoided or limited to the 15-20 degrees (mini squat) (Fig. 24.13).

viii. **Swimming:** Swimming is the best exercise for the patient with osteoarthrosis of the knee and hip joint. The movements are performed against the resistance (water) without placing the excessive load on the joint. The exercise also increases the overall cardiovascular endurance. It reduces weight of the body too.

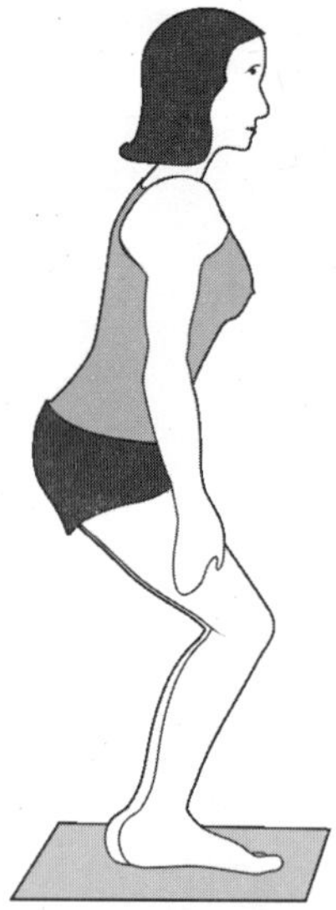

Fig. 24.13: Squatting

ix. **Walking:** If the arthritis changes are chronic, patient should walk with the stick or cane on the opposite hand. Walking is the safe and it produces minimal stresses on the knee joints comparing with the stair climbing and descending. The patient should walk with 90 cadence per minute without bending the trunk excessively for half an hour daily.

x. **Static Cycling:** The static cycling can easily be accessible and patient can do cycling with resistance as per tolerances. Initially the exercise on the bicycle should be started without resistance for a short period of time. After one week as the muscles conditioned, both resistance and the time can be increased as per tolerance.

3. Restoration of Movements

Following reduction of muscle spasm, pain, and restoration of strength the third priority of the therapist should be given in obtaining full range of movements. It can be achieved by performing some exercises.

i. **Exercises to Improve Extension Lag:** Extension lag is an active loss of terminal extension. Once the active and passive extension is lost the joint becomes deformed. Loss of terminal extension is very common in osteoarthrosis. Pain and stiffness are the main factors in preventing the patient to extend the knee to the end (terminal) range. Avoidance of extension in the terminal range causes weakness (disuse) of the quadriceps muscles that further contributes to the extension lag. The posterior capsule of the joint also becomes light.

   a. ***Posterior Capsule Stretching:*** A towel roll is placed under the ankle of the affected leg. Therapist places both the hands on the joint (above and below the patella), and then a posterior directed force is applied and is held for at least 10 seconds. This will increase the flexibility of the posterior capsule. The pressure should be so gentle that it should not aggravate the symptoms. A distraction force may also be applied with one hand to take the joint surfaces apart. A posterior directed force is applied to stretch the posterior joint capsule simultaneously. The exercise must be followed by the active extension. Patient should be taught to do the exercise at home (Figs. 24.14 and 24.15).

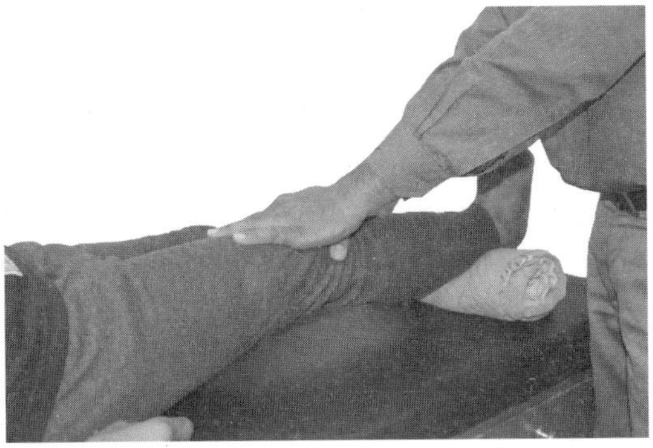

Fig. 24.14: Knee joint posterior capsule stretching

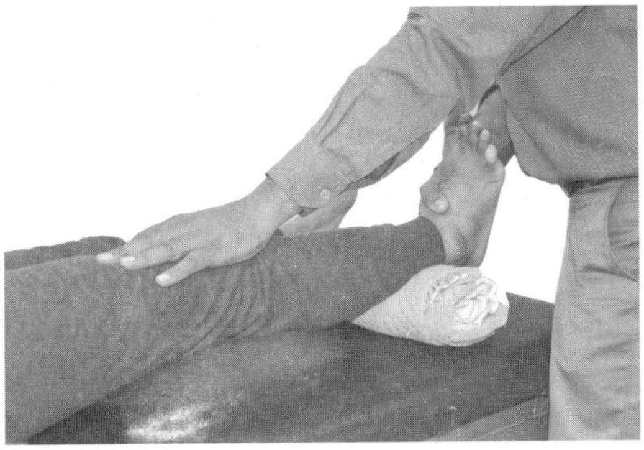

Fig. 24.15: Posterior knee joint capsule stretching with distraction of the joint

b. Quadriceps Strengthening: The towel roll is placed under the knee, and patient is instructed to extend the knee joint as much as possible. At the end range the therapist can assist the active movement. This recruits the quadriceps muscles fibers responsible for terminal extension.

c. Surge Faradic Current: Surge faradic current may also be beneficial in improving the extension lag by stimulating and recruiting the quadriceps muscles fibers. The patient is instructed to contract the muscle simultaneously with the current as much as possible.

ii. **Exercises to Improve Flexion:** The patient lies prone and therapist stands at the side of the patient. The knee joint is flexed upto the range where limitation starts. This position is held firmly and the patient is instructed to extend the knee joint. The therapist applies resistance against the concentric contraction of the muscles. Several repetitions are performed till a significant improvement in the flexion is achieved. Hot pack along the length of the quadriceps may prove more significant results (Fig. 24.16).

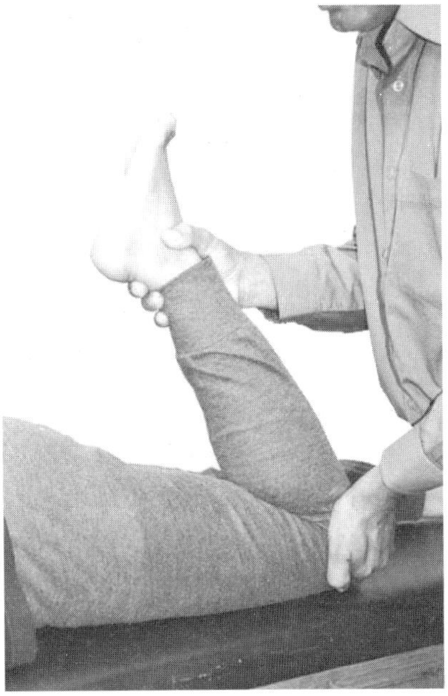

Fig. 24.16: Exercise to improve flexion

4. Weight Loss

The osteoarthrosis is a degenerative disease which is more common in weight bearing joints. The articular cartilage of the obese patients transfer more weight, hence, these patients have more chances of disruption of the proteoglycans and collagen fibers. The cartilage looses its physical properties and eventually there is loss of full thickness of the cartilage. The patients who attend the swimming pool, and do the regular walking can reduce the weight of the body. Avoiding oil content in the diet may also help in reducing the fat. Successful weight loss dramatically relieves pain and symptoms in the arthritic knee joint.

5. Activity Modification

Any activities which place more stress on the cartilage should be avoided.

i. Discontinue high impact activities, change to low impact.

ii. Avoid stair climbing, kneeling and squatting.

iii. Do not use low chair.

iv. Use western toilets.

6. Orthotic Management, Aids and Appliances

The assistive devices and orthotic aids such as knee braces, are used to improve functions of moveable parts of the body or to support, align, prevent, or correct deformities. Splints or braces help in correcting joint alignment and weight redistribution.

i. **Shoe Modification:** It has been observed that the patient with flat foot (loss of medial arch of the foot) complain pain in the medial or anterior aspect of knee joint. The flat foot changes the direction of weight distribution in the joint and also alters the quadriceps angle as it produces internal rotation of the tibia. The flat foot is possible if the intrinsic muscles of the foot are weak. The problem can be solved out by raising the medial arch of the shoe. In young population medial arch can be developed by some form of exercises and electric stimulation. These patients may do the exercise such as pulling the towel with the toes and walking on sand. But it is difficult to develop the arch in the middle aged population, therefore raising medial arch of the shoe can correct the alignment of the tibia and reduce the pain and symptoms.

ii. **Cane on Opposite Hand:** By holding the cane with opposite hand, the arthritic leg is progressed forward to the body with the cane. The weight of the body is taken on the cane and arthritic knee simultaneously, hence the load of the arthric knee is transferred to the stick or cane.

iii. **Knee Cap:** It provides passive stability to the knee joint and may be worn while walking and climbing stairs. It should not be made habit as it may decrease the strength of the muscles.

iv. **Braces:** Some custom made braces are beneficial in unloading the joint especially when unilateral compartment is affected. The unilateral joint space can be increased significantly by using a mechanical device "screw" and transferring the weight on the brace instead of joint. The disadvantage of braces is that they are very expensive, and most of the patients quit wearing quickly secondary to bulkness and inconvenience. Some patients may also be benefited from a light neoprene knee sleeve, which may improve proprioceptive feedback.

7. Hyaluronic Acid Injections

Hyaluronic acid injections are having limited value in relieving pain and symptoms. They appear to work best before there is bone-on-bone crepitus. Studies have shown that these injections are of equal benefit of non-steroidal anti-inflammatory drugs. However, other studies show that hyaluronic sodium to be no better than placebo.

8. Supplements

It is believed that the supplements such as glucosamine, and chondroitin sulphate (cartigen, free flex fort) helps in regenerating the cartilage, however no studies claim such results. The supplements are moderately expensive with no side effects. These supplements are initially advised for three months, and if found no improvement may be discontinued or if patients wish to try and derive great benefit they may use for more than three months.

SURGICAL INTERVENTION

The patients who do not get benefited with the conservative treatments and present constant pain and symptoms may be elected for surgical intervention.

Arthroscopy

The patients with normal mechanical alignment who fail to respond to a conservative management (administered at least for 3-6 months) and mild to moderate arthritis (grade 2 and 3 on radiographs) may be considered for arthroscopic debridement. The arthroscopic procedure should be considered palliative, temporary for patients with arthritic knee joint.

As the degenerative disease progresses, the degenerated articular cartilage and synovial tissue release pro-inflammatory cytokinase that induces chondrocytes to release lytic enzymes leading to degradation of type-2 collagen and proteoglycans. The arthroscopic procedure (lavaging) may "dilute" or "wash out" these inflammatory mediators, although the effect is temporary. Grade 2 and 3 osteoarthrosis with osteophytes, tibial spine pain and extension lag may be benefited from arthroscopic procedure of osteophyte removal and notch plasty.

Good prognosis can be expected if the patients present with short duration mechanical symptoms, effusion, loose bodies and relevant osteophytes but with normal alignment.

Post Arthroscopic Physiotherapy: The focus should be on the restoration of the strength and range of the joint.

a. Strengthening: Gluteus sets, quadriceps sets, VMO sets, ankle pump, straight leg raising and side leg raising exercises should be advised thrice daily. Exercises should be progressed to mini squat, cycling, jogging and running as patient shows improvement in the sign and symptoms.

b. Stretching: Iliotibial band, lateral patellar retanaculam, quadriceps, gastrocnemius, iliopsoas and posterior capsule of the knee joint should be stretched.

Osteotomy

The involvement of medial compartment of the knee joint produces varus deformity as the full thickness of the articular cartilage is lost. These patients may be advised for a valgus producing, high tibial osteotomy. Patients with greater than 10 degrees of varus may undergo supracondylar osteotomy which do not interfere with subsequent total knee replacement. However, eventually, a total knee replacement requires in the due course of time, for this reason osteotomies are performed rarely.

Total Knee Replacement (TKR)

The replacement of both the articular surfaces with the foreign material (implant) has become choice of treatments now-a-days. Patients with incapacitating pain, functional impairment, flexion deformity or contracture, valgus, varus deformities and those who failed to respond to the fair trial of conservative treatment require total knee joint replacement.

Total knee replacement consists of three main components: the femoral component, the tibial component, and the plastic spacer also known as polyethylene. All these components are known as implant or prosthesis. The selection of the implants depends on the underlying disease, progression of the disease, destruction of the joint surfaces, age and health of the patient (Fig. 24.17).

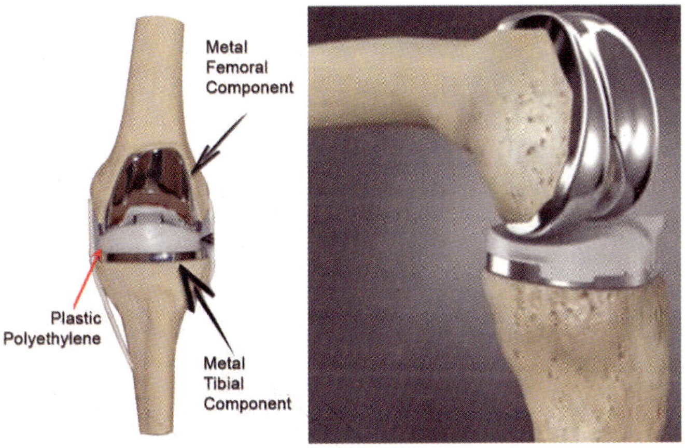

Fig. 24.17: Femoral and tibial components

Types of Implants or Prosthesis

There are three types of implants or prosthesis constrained, unconstrained and semi-constrained.

Constrained Prosthesis: Constraint is defined as the effect of the elements of knee implant design that provides the stability needed to counteract forces about the knee after arthroplasty in the presence of a deficient soft tissue envelop. Determining the amount of constraint necessary can be challenging (Fig. 24.18).

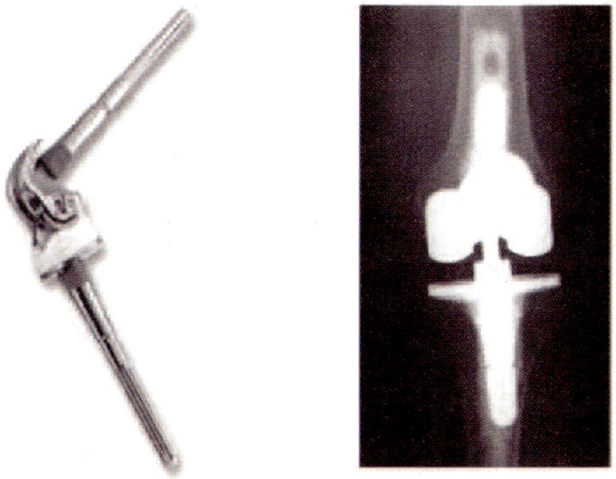

Fig. 24.18: Constrained prosthesis

Tibial and femoral components are linked together with a hinged mechanism. These are used when the knee is highly unstable and the ligaments will be unable to support other types of prostheses. This is rarely a first choice option. Constrained prostheses are reserved for severely damaged knees. Typically they are used in elderly patients undergoing revision arthroplasty. Due to the higher amount of mechanical stress put on hinged prostheses, they are not expected to last as long as other less constrained designs.

Unconstrained Prosthesis: Like an endoprosthesis for unicompartmental knee arthroplasty, an unconstrained device is used to replace only a very small portion of the articular surface or a very thin surface layer of tissue, leaving the anatomical structure of the joint intact. Designed to use the PCL, and referred to as PCL-sparing prostheses. The components are not linked and rely on the patients own ligaments and muscles for stability. A groove is present in the posterior aspect of the tibial prosthesis for the native PCL.

Semi-Constrained: A semi-constrained prosthesis is used for superficial joint replacement. There are two types of semi-constrained prosthesis. One requires excision of the posterior ligament, whereas the ligament is spared by the others. Both PCL retaining and PCL substituting knee prosthesis are successful with success rate of 95% (Fig. 24.19).

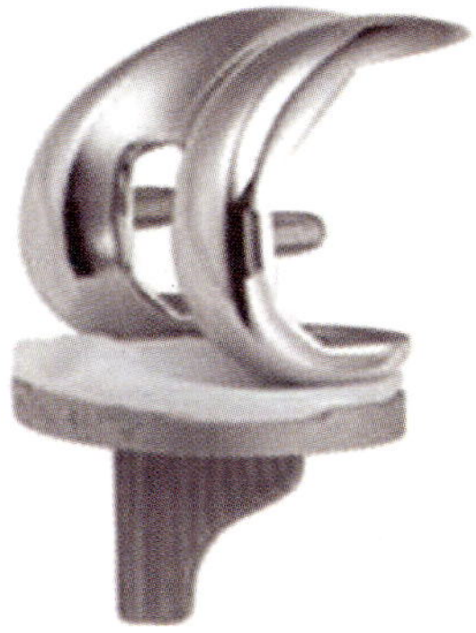

Fig. 24.19: Cruciate retaining design

In Japan, the posterior cruciate sparing type of semi-constrained prosthesis is most frequently used whereas, in the United States, stabilized prostheses that require excision of the posterior cruciate ligament have been used most commonly, possibly because of the different health care system from that in Japan. These prostheses have more inherent stability by virtue of a variety of design techniques, including placement of large central anterior tibial spine that articulates with a rectangular box like opening between the condyles of the femoral component. The posterior portion of the box is formed by a transverse metal cam that prevents posterior tibial subluxation when the knee is in extension (Fig. 24.20).

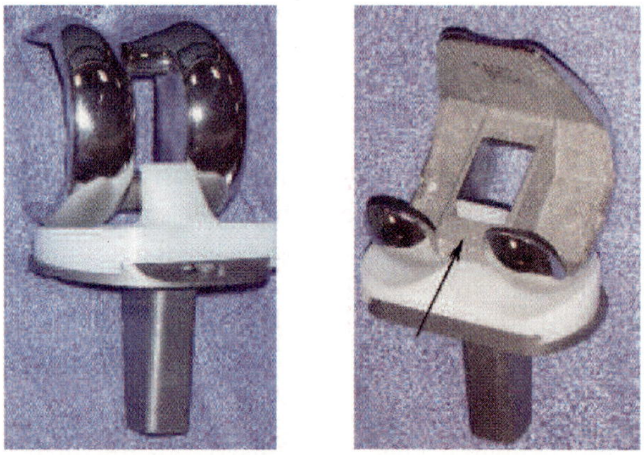

Fig. 24.20: Posterior stabilized design of semi-constrained prosthesis

Techniques of Implant Fixation

Cemented, cementless or hybrid prosthesis may be selected for the surgery. The selection of prosthesis depends upon the age, health and integrity of the bones. Semi-constrained prosthesis are used for most of the patient as these may correct flexion contracture upto 45 degrees and angular deformities upto 25 degrees. The total expected life span of the prosthesis is considered of 15-20 years, however, it may be decreased if the patient is young and dynamic. On the other hand the life span of the prosthesis is increased if the patient is sedentary (Figs. 24.21 and 24.22).

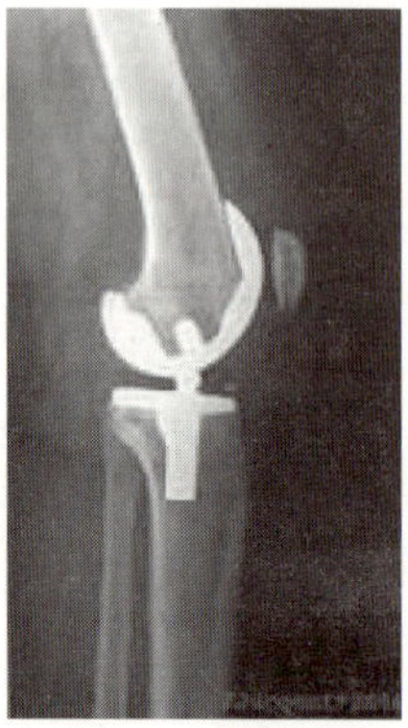

Fig. 24.21: X-ray—Total knee joint replacement

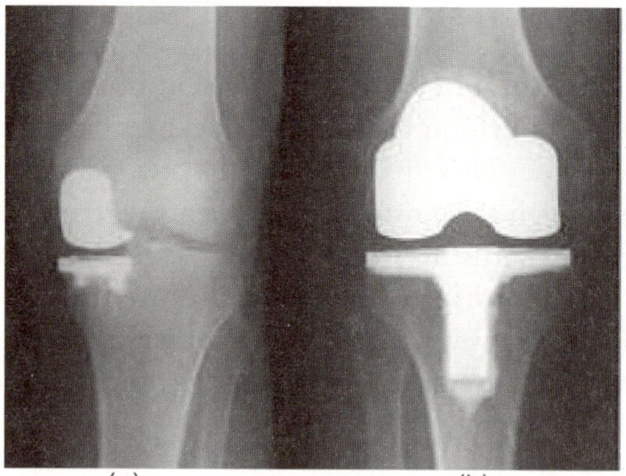

(a) (b)

Fig. 24.22: X-ray—(a) Uni-compartment replacement, (b) Total knee replacement

Pre Operative Physiotherapy

a. **Restoration of Range of Motion:** The muscle energy and PNF techniques such as hold relax, contract relax and reciprocal inhibition help in relaxing the muscle and improving range of motion. Anterior and posterior glides with distraction and stabilization (proximal part of the joint) helps in stretching of the joint capsule and regaining range of motion.
b. **Restoration of Muscle Strength:** To restore the strength the exercises such as quadriceps sets, gluteus sets, ankle pump, SLR, side SLR, and mini squat should be administered and taught to the patient to do at home.
c. **Breathing Exercises:** Deep breathing and spirometer exercises are taught well before the operation to improve cardiovascular endurance.

Post-Operative Physiotherapy

As soon as patient comes out of the operation theatre he or she is allowed to walk as per tolerance or as advised by the surgeon. The exercises such as quads sets, gluteus maximus sets, ankle pump, SLR, side SLR and hamstring sets are started from the day one, two to three times daily. The patients should achieve 90° of flexion at the end of 14th day of operation. Following should be the goals of therapist:

1. **Reduction in Pain:** Ice pack, cryotherapy on mediolateral joint or along the length of quadriceps. It should not be placed directly on the stitch line.
2. **Restoration of Strength:** Initially isometric quads sets, hamstrings sets, gluteus maximus sets, ankle pumps, SLR and side SLR should be started from the day one twice daily. The closed kinetic chain exercises such as mini squat may also be initiated following discharge of the patient. The strengthening exercises in high sitting (isotonic) with resistance may produce pain and symptoms, hence, should be initiated without the resistance and progressed to the resistance as the sign and symptoms improve.

Breathing Exercises: Deep breathing and spirometer exercises are started from day of operation to improve lungs volume and to remove secretion.

3. **Restoration of Range of Motion:** Patient should achieve at least 90° of flexion in the 14 days of operation. To improve flexion the patient is placed in supine lying position, therapist stands at the side of the leg which is being treated. Therapist holds the ankle with one hand and grasps the knee joint with other hand. The patient is encouraged to flex the knee joint as much as possible. Therapist should make efforts in increasing range of motion actively by commanding him such as yes very good, you are doing very well. In case, if patient finds difficulty in achieving flexion upto 90° at the end of second week, the therapist may go for reciprocal inhibition of the quadriceps. In high sitting position, the knee joint is flexed as much as possible, at the point where limitation starts the knee joint is stabilized and ankle joint is held firmly with the other hand. Now the patient is instructed to flex the knee joint against the resistance. The strong contraction of the hamstrings will allow quadriceps muscles to relax and helps in improving flexion range of motion. After removal of the stitches (usually after two weeks), hold relax, and contract relax of the quadriceps may be initiated to improve flexion range. The reciprocal inhibition technique is only indicated if there is severe muscle spasm and pain which does not allow the patient to contract quadriceps (contract relax, hold relax), hence, hamstrings are contracted to relax the quadriceps muscles.

   Passive movements may increase post-operative pain, spasm and symptoms; hence, these should be avoided at initial stage.

4. **Extension Lag:** Following total knee replacement pain and spasm is the common complaints of patient. Patient keeps the leg in flexed position by placing pillow under the knee joint as it relieves pain. This results in decrease in active terminal extension known as extension lag. To correct extension lag a pillow is placed under the ankle joint and a posterior directed force is applied to the knee joint with distraction. Several repetitions of posterior directed force help in regaining full extension of the knee joint. Quadriceps strengthening also helps in achieving full extension.

COMPLICATIONS AFTER TKR

Patellofemoral Joint Osteoarthritis

The degenerative process may also involve the underlying surfaces of the patellofemoral joint. Pain and stiffness in the anterior aspect of knee which aggravate with the activities such as squatting, stair climbing, descending, running and jumping are the common features of the patellofemoral arthrosis. If the tibiofemoral joint is intact and only patellofemoral joint is involved the patient will not complain pain while level walking as the patellofemoral ground reaction forces are almost negligible in level walking. On the other hand patient with tibiofemoral and patellofemoral will complain pain in both stair climbing and level walking. Extension lag may also present as the disease progresses (Figs. 24.23 and 24.24).

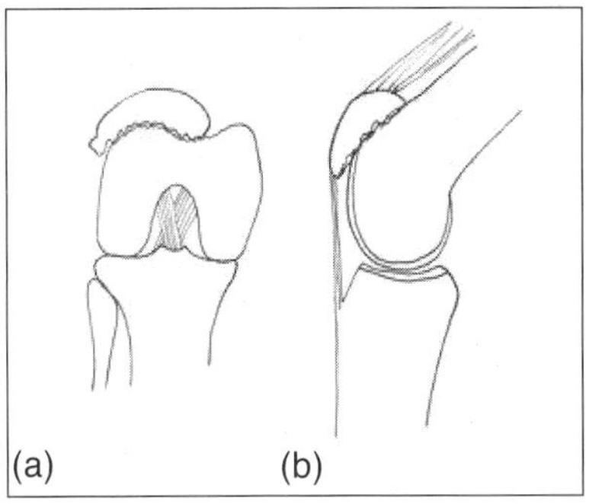

Fig. 24.23: Patellofemoral osteoarthritis a. anterior posterior view, b. lateral view

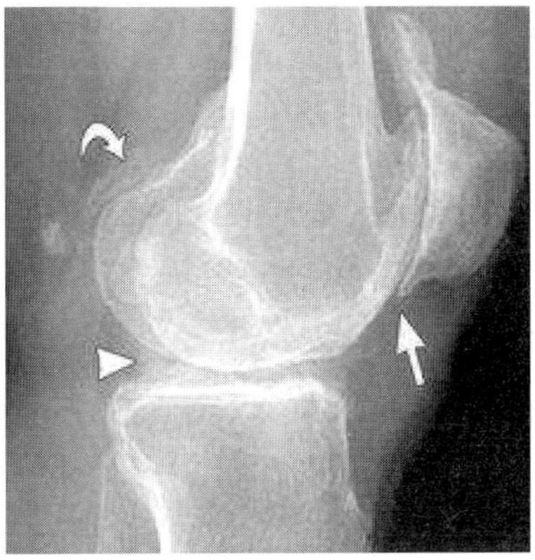

Fig. 24.24: X-ray–Lateral view, patellofemoral osteoarthritis

Patellar Mal Tracking

Normally patella moves on the trochlear groove of the femur. Lengthening or shortening of the muscles displace the patella from trochlear groove to one of the epicondyles of the femur. Therefore ground reaction forces of the patello-femoral joint shifts to either of epicondyles, which leads to disruption of cartilage of one of the epicondyles of femur. The most widely accepted theory regarding the cause of patellofemoral pain suggests that the symptoms are the result of excessive patellofemoral joint stresses owing to abnormal patellar tracking. The patellar mal tracking is thought to generate excessive stress on the medial or lateral epicondyle of femur resultant the patellofemoral joint reaction forces alter and the contact area between the patellofemoral joint surface decreases. This causes pain, irritation and degeneration in the articular cartilage. The following factors contribute to the patellar mal tracking:

i. **Weakness of Hip External Rotators:** Insufficient contraction of hip external rotators may allow internal rotators to rotate the femur internally (ante version). This will increase the Q angle and allow the patella to move on the lateral epicondyle of the femur during knee flexion.

ii. **Weakness of Gluteus Medius and Maximus:** One of the most common causes of the patellar mal tracking is weakness of the gluteus maximus and gluteus medius muscles. Weakness of these muscles causes the femur to fall inwards during the stance phase, thus increasing the Q angle, and so the lateral pull on the patella.

iii. **Weakness of the Quadriceps:** Weak quadriceps unable to keep the patella deeply into trochlear groove of the femur and resultant contact area of the patellofemoral joint is decreased, which leads to increase in stress on another area of the joint surface.

iv. **Pes Planus or Flat Foot: Foot Pronation or Flat Foot:** The tibia rotates laterally in mid stance to achieve full extension of the knee joint. This is known as screw home mechanism. Flat foot rotates the tibia medially which would actually decrease the 'Q' angle, and the lateral forces acting on the patella. Eventually the screw home mechanism is altered. To compensate for the lack of tibial external rotation caused by the failure of the foot to resupinate, the femur would have to internally rotate on the tibia such that the tibia was in a relative external rotation. Theoretically compensatory internal rotation of the femur would permit the screw home mechanism to allow for knee extension. In turn excessive internal rotation of the femur would move the patella medially with respect to the ASIS and tibial tuberosity, thereby increasing the 'Q' angle and the lateral component of the quadriceps muscle vector.

v. **Pes Cavus (High Arched Foot Supination):** It provides less cushioning during the stance phase, which can place more stress on the patellofemoral mechanism particularly in running.

vi. **Tightness of Tensor Fascia Lata (TFL):** The vastus medialis oblique works as a medial dynamic stabilizer for the patella. Weakness of a VMO allows lateral stabilizers to pull the patella on the lateral epicondyle of the femur. The patella tracks on the lateral epicondyle of femur instead of on the trochlear groove which predisposes the patellofemoral joint to osteoarthrosis. Iliotibial band is one of the lateral dynamic stabilizers of the patella. The short iliotibial band tilts and pulls the patella laterally as one of slip of the iliotibial band called the lateral retinaculum fibers attach into the lateral border of the patella.

vii. **Good Leg Arthropathy:** This is common in the patients whose one leg is short. Because of shortening of leg patient walks with the normal leg flexion. Normally during stance phase the knee remains extended which reduces ground reaction forces on the patellofemoral joint. Flexion during stance phase increases ground reaction forces on the patellofemoral joint and predisposes the joint to osteoarthrosis.

Patellar Mal Tracking Tests

The test should be done in full extension. In this position patella typically rests just lateral to the midline. As soon as the knee joint moves into flexion at around 10 to 20 degrees, the patella centers into the trochlear groove and proceeds to track in a relatively smooth and straight path with progressive knee flexion. In patients with patellar mal tracking the patella remains on the lateral epicondyle upto 30 degree of knee flexion and then suddenly jumps into the trochlear groove with a jerk and click sound.

This follows a J path and also knows as *J sign*. Patellar mal tracking may be associated with patellar tilt. Tightness of lateral structures, such as lateral retinaculum, vastus lateralis, or iliotibial band may cause lateral tilt of the patella. Normally the lateral border of the patellar can easily be elevated 0-20 degrees above the medial border. Less than 0 degree elevation of the lateral border of the patella suggests patellar tilt. In full extension the patella is observed carefully and patient is asked to contract the quadriceps. The test is considered positive for lateral tilt if the patella shifts (displacement) laterally.

Clark Sign: Patient lies supine with both the knees extended, therapist stands at the side, places one hand on the supracondylar aspect (patella) of the knee joint. The patella is pressed hard against the condyles and patient is asked to contract the quadriceps. The contraction of quadriceps causes compression of the patella on the trochlear grove against the resistance applied by the therapist. If the compression of patella produces pain, it is considered positive for patellofemoral joint osteoarthrosis. Therapist shall hold the patella firmly on the condyles and prevent the movement of patella otherwise it may aggravate symptoms.

Radiographic Evaluation of Patellar Instability

An axial image, typically a merchant (knee flexed 45 degrees and X-ray beam angled 30 degrees to axis of the femur) or skyline view may be the most significant.

Sulcus Angle: A sulcus angle less than 150 degrees is considered normal. Patients who have sulcus angle more than 150 degrees complain patellar instability. To measure the sulcus angle a line is drawn along the medial and lateral vall of the trochlea. The angle formed between them is ermed as sulcus angle (Fig. 24.25).

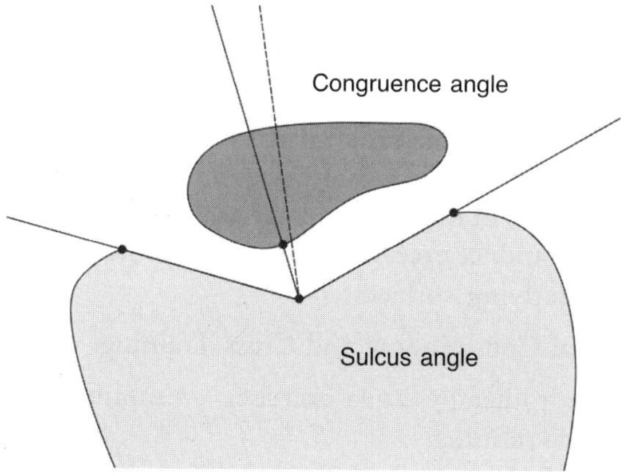

Fig. 24.25: Congruence angle and sulcus angle

Congruence Angle: One line is drawn from the apex of he trochlear groove bisecting the sulcus and second *line is rawn from the apex of the groove, the apex of the patella.* The ngle formed between these two lines is the congruence ngle which is described as – 6 degrees ± 6 degrees normal.

Patellofemoral Angle: The angle is formed by the two nes. One line is drawn along the lateral wall of the trochlear roove and the second *line is drawn along the articular surface f the lateral patella facet.* The lines should roughly be arallel. Divergence of the lines is measured as a positive ngle and is considered normal, whereas convergence of e lines is measured as negative and indicates the presence f abnormal patellar tilt (Fig. 24.26).

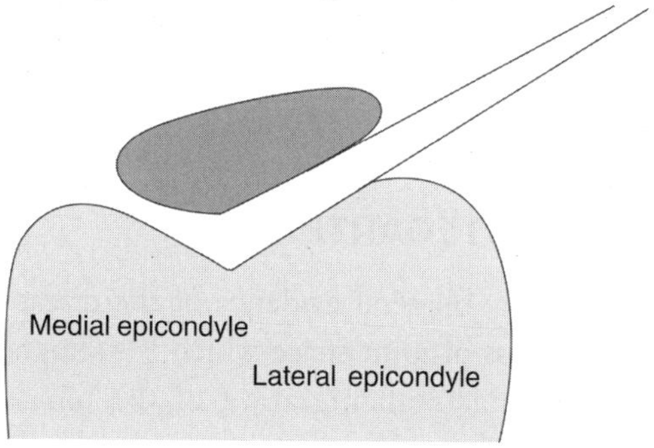

Fig. 24.26: Patellofemoral angle

reatment

he aims of treatment are of many folds:

Approximately, 70% patients with patellofemoral osteoarthrosis improve with conservative treatments.

Relief of Pain: Firstly treatment is directed to relieve pain by using physical modalities. To relieve pain ultrasound can be used on the lateral retinaculam, and patellofemoral joint line. Shortwave diathermy, cryotherapy and paraffin wax bath are also found effective in patellofermoral dysfunctions.

3. **Stretching Exercises:** The second part of treatment is to improve the patellar tracking which involves stretching of the short muscles. The second part of the treatment is sometimes overlooked but is extremely helpful and important in patients with flexibility deficit. Iliotibial band, quadriceps and hamstrings flexibility deficit are common in these patients, especially in patients with chronic patellofemoral osteoarthrosis. Static structures such as lateral retinaculam and patellar ligaments are also become tight. Restoration of flexibility can play important role in patients with patellofemoral osteoarthrosis (Figs. 24.27 and 24.28).

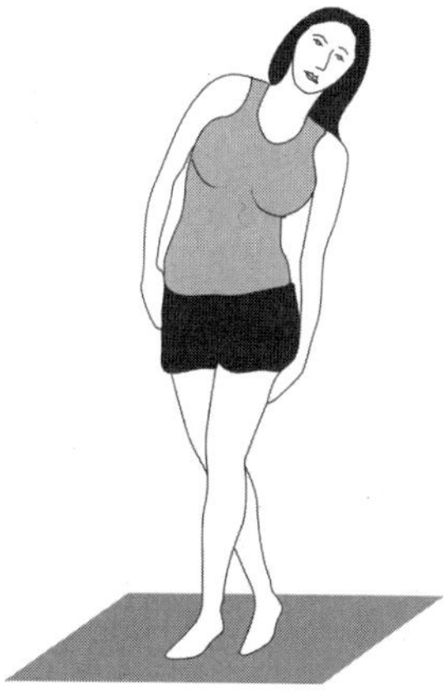

Fig. 24.27: Iliotibial band stretching

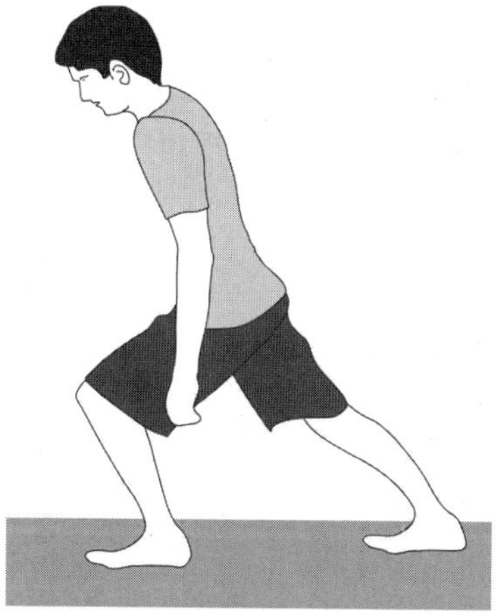

Fig. 24.28: Gastrosoleus stretching

4. Strengthening Exercises
   a. *Quadriceps Sets:* In sitting with the knee straight a towel roll is placed under the knee joint. While pressing the towel down the knee is extended fully. The position is held for at least 6 seconds. After 6 seconds of contraction muscles is relaxed. 30-40 repetitions may be performed thrice daily.
   b. *Gluteus Maximus Set:* In sitting with the knee straight a towel roll is placed under the knee joint.

The patient is instructed to press the towel down and hold it for at least 6 seconds. 30-40 repetitions may be performed thrice or twice daily.

c. *Ankle Pump Exercise:* While keeping towel roll under the knee the ankle joint is moved up and down.

d. *Straight Leg Raising:* While keeping the leg straight the patient is asked to raise it above around 60-70 degrees at the hip joint.

e. *Side Leg Raising:* The extended leg is taken out of the bed at around 20 degrees of the hip joint (side lying). In the next step the patient is placed on unaffected side lying and the affected leg is raised upto 70 degrees. Several repetitions are performed.

f. *Vastus Medialis Obliques (VMO):* Vastus medialis obliques inserts on the medial aspect of the patella at 55 degree angles. This orientation of VMO, makes it dynamic stabilizer of the patella. Weakness of the vastus medialis may allow lateral stabilizers to pull the patella laterally. This is one of the causes of the lateral maltracking of the patella. In high sitting position a towel roll is placed between the thighs. Patient is asked to press the towel between the thighs (hip adduction) and then extend the knee joint upto the full range. Some studies show that if dorsiflexion is added to the extension more VMO muscle fibers can be recruited. The hip joint is adducted during the extension as the VMO muscle fibers are the extension of the adductor muscle. Adduction of hip joint can strengthen the adductors and helps in improving the strength of the VMO (Fig. 24.29).

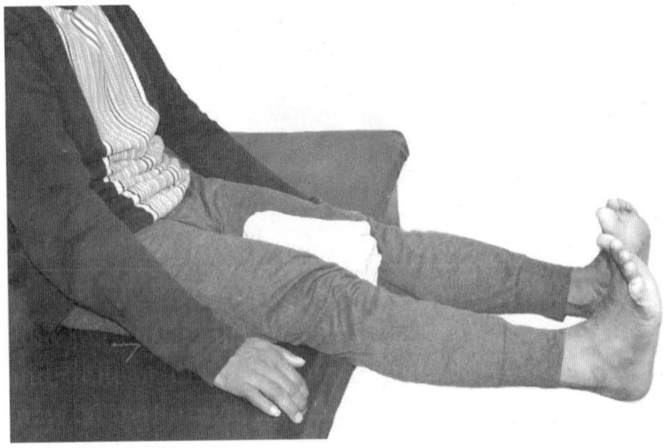

Fig. 24.29: VMO strengthening

g. *Gluteus Maximus Strengthening:* Patient lies prone with both the knees extended. While maintaining the knee extension, hip joint is extended upto full range. The extension is maintained at end range for at least six seconds. 15-20 repetition, twice daily can be performed.

h. *Hip Lateral Rotators Strengthening:* Patient lies prone with knee flexion to 90 degree. Therapist stands at the side, holds the leg at the ankle join and resists, external rotation of the hip joint.

i. *Mini Squatting:* This is the close kinetic chai exercise which helps in improving the stimulatio of the proprioceptors. Therapist must emphasise o the mini squat only upto 15-30 degrees as it doe not increase the ground reaction forces significantly Increase in the angle of knee joint beyond 30 degree can produce excessive load on the patellofemoral join underlying surfaces.

5. **General Conditioning and Cross Training:**
   i. Hydrotherapy, aqua exercises, swimming and dee pool running.
   ii. *Cycling:* Initially without resistance or as per toleranc of the patient.

6. **Activity Modification:** The ground reaction forces o the patellofemoral increase during the knee flexion.
   i. *Level Walking:* Negligible body weight.
   ii. *Stair Climbing:* 4 times of body weight.
   iii. *Squatting:* 7-8 times of body weight.
   iv. *Mini Squatting:* 2-3 times of body weight.

Hence, any activities which place more stress on th cartilage should be avoided.

a. Discontinue high impact activities, change to lo impact.
b. Avoid stair climbing, kneeling and squatting.
c. Do not use low chair.
d. Use western toilets.

HIP JOINT OSTEOARTHRITIS

78% patients show bilateral evidence of the disease. The is non-uniform loss of joint space which is radiographical identified as supralateral migration of the femoral he within the acetabulum. Early osteoarthritic changes affe the superior compartment of the femoral acetabulum. vacuum phenomenon is produced within the joint, loss cartilage is seen on the supralateral space of the joint, wi maintenance of normal cartilage axially and medially. the disease progresses (in advanced stage) there may extensive, non-uniform loss of joint space. Occasionally lar subchondral cysts may also be observed which is originat in the acetabulum and they are frequently referred as Egge cyst. As the result of cartilage loss and migration of t head within the acetabulum the head becomes incongru with the acetabulum. Osteophytes develop medially the femoral head to fill the incongruity. A ghost line of t original femoral head is often identified. The weight bearing axis is shifted from its normal position to the medial neck of femur and new bone is added along the medial cortex. The osteoarthritis begin in the roof of the acceptable rather than in the femoral head itself because cysts only appear after denudation of the overlying articular cartilage.

Radiographical Grades of Hip Osteoarthrosis

0 – Normal.

1 – Possible narrowing of joint space medially and possible osteophytes around the femoral head.

2 – Definite narrowing of joint space inferiorly, definite osteophytes and slight sclerosis.

3 – Marked narrowing of joint space, osteophytes, some sclerosis and cyst formation, and deformity of femoral head and acetabulum.

4 – Gross loss of joint space with sclerosis and cysts, marked deformity of femoral head and acetabulum and large osteophytes.

(Adopted from the Council for International Organization of Medical Sciences, 1963)

Cyst formation which may be intrusion or contusion type or both is common in hip osteoarthritis. The intrusion cyst is seen immediately subchorally and may have a wide, narrow or radiographically absent communication with the joint space. The contusion cyst is totally enclosed within the bone and may be farther from the joint space unlike intrusion cyst. A cyst may also be present before there is actual cartilage loss. A cyst may collapse, producing a bizarre configuration of the femoral head.

Secondary Hip Osteoarthritis

The persons with congenital or developmental abnormalities are more prone to the secondary osteoarthritis and the presentation of secondary osteoarthritis is usually 10 years earlier than the usual presentation of the primary osteoarthritis.

Common Conditions are: Hip dysphasias, slipped capital femoral epiphysis, Legg-Calve-Perthes disease, femoral neck abnormalities and primary protrusion acetabulii.

Clinical Features

Patient complaints pain during the activities and stiffness after activities or prolonged rest, which may last for 30 minutes. As the disease progresses the joint range of motion is decreased and there is feeling of instability of the joint. Crepitus and trendelenburg sign, firm swelling and tender points around the joint margin may be present.

Overuse Syndromes of the Knee (OSKs): These involve the extensor mechanism and are grouped together under the term Jumpers Knee. Patellar tendinitis is the most common among these patients, typically presenting with pain near the insertion of the tendon at the pole of the patella (Fig. 24.30).

Iliotibial Band Friction Syndrome: The iliotibial band inserts at the Gerdy tubercle on the anterolateral aspect of the proximal tibia. It has small attachments to the lateral patellar retinaculam and to the biceps femoris. During full extension to flexion, the iliotibial band shifts from a position anterior to the lateral femoral condyle to a position posterior to the epicondyle. The transition occurs at about 30 degrees of the knee flexion. In running, the repetitive flexion and extension causes iliotibial band to pass back and forth over the lateral femoral epicondyle. This may cause irritation in the band at the insertion and develop bursitis. The patients with iliotibial band friction syndrome typically presents with pain on anterior to the lateral femoral epicondyle associated with running and jogging (Fig. 24.31).

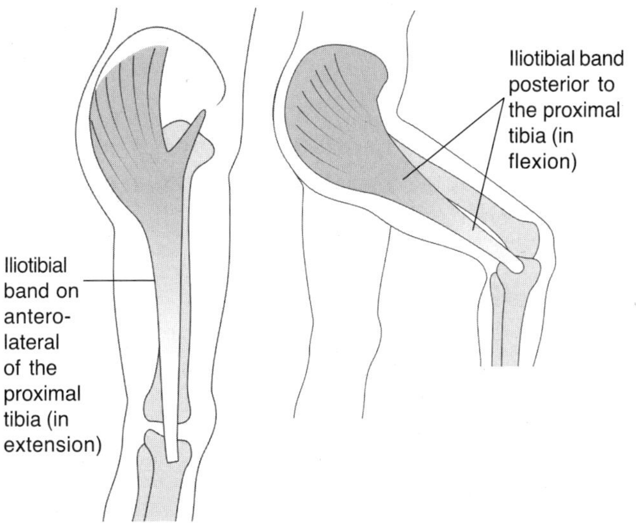

Fig. 24.30 **Fig. 24.31**

Diagnosis

The classical clinical test for hip joint osteoarthritis is internal rotation of the hip joint with flexion which may be limited and painful.

Patrick Test: Also known as figure four test is performed in supine lying. Ankle joint of the leg which is being tested is placed on the thigh of the contralateral leg, the knee joint of the tested side is pushed gently downward. This maneuver may place large stress on the hip joint and patient may experience pain. Test should be avoided on patients with severe osteoporotic changes (elderly).

Management

Reduction of Body Weight: Obese patients should be advised to reduce the weight so that load on the cartilage can be relieved.

Use of Cane: Cane in the opposite hand can significantly reduce the weight on the hip joint. In normal walk without the cane, the ground reaction forces (resultant force) across the hip joint is three times of the body weight because the force of the hip abductors acts on the greater trochanter to offset body weight and levels the pelvis in single stance.

Use of Supplements: Glucosamine and chondrotin sulphate (cartigen, free flex fort) may be advised, however their efficacy is not proved scientifically.

Modalities: Moist heat therapy, interferential therapy by using the analgesic effect (80 – 100 Hz) and short wave diathermy may be advised for relief of pain and muscle relaxation.

Exercises: Stretching: Abductors and capsule (IR and ER). Strengthening: Gluteus maximus, mediums. Quadriceps and abdominals: Straight leg raising, side leg raising, prone leg raising, knee to chest active, mini squat (30 degrees knee flexion).

Walking: Walk is the safe exercise which strengthens all the muscles of the extremity and also helps in reducing the body weight. One hour walk five times a week is advisable.

Exercises in Water: Exercises in water are beneficial for the patient those have severe symptoms or become non-ambulatory. Initially exercises are started for a short period of time. Non-ambulatory patients are instructed to stand up for a period which is comfortable for them, then rest is given. The ambulation period is increased gradually as per tolerance of the patient. Once the patient gains confidence and feels less pain then partial weight bearing started outside of the pool.

Bicycle Ergometer: Initially it should be without resistance for 15 minutes three to four times a week. The resistance is increased as per tolerance of the patient. It helps in improving strength of the lower extremity muscles and cardiovascular stamina.

I.P. JOINTS OSTEOARTHRITIS

Osteoarthritis affects primarily distal and proximal interphalangeal joints with relatively sparing of the metacarpophalangeal joints. There is non-uniform loss of joint space and formation of osteophytes. Osteophytes produces stretching on the periarticular structures. The soft tissue swelling associated with osteophytes in the PIP joints and DIP joint is known as Bouchard node and Heberden's node respectively. Osteophytes project laterally or medially and proximally. Cyst formation is rare.

Management: Patients with PIP and DIP joint osteoarthrosis are managed with superficial heating modalities such as PWB and contrast bath. To restore the strength and ROM, PNF techniques such as hold relax, contract relax and stretching exercises are recommended. Hand gripper and hand exercises may be advised for hand muscles strengthening.

RHEUMATOID ARTHRITIS

Rheumatoid arthritis is a chronic inflammatory disease of the synovium which is characterized by exacerbation and remission. It is a systemic disease which involves heart, lungs, blood vessels and eyes.

Etiology

The cause of rheumatoid arthritis remains unknown but it is believed that an immunological response takes place in the synovial tissues. An unknown, presumably exogenous, antigen enters (encounters) into the defender cell. The lymphocyte, which is transformed into a large plasma cell, secretes (manufactures) antibodies. These antibodies, antigen and complement combine to form a complex, which is also known as immune complex. Scavenger phagocytic cells, contain small enzyme-producing sacs (lysosomes) that destroy the immune complex, however some of the lysosomes escape from phagocytic cells and their proteases attack the cartilage and synovium. The immune complex is responsible for the inflammation in the synovium. The destruction of the tissues (synovium and cartilage) produces some debris which invites further phagocytic activities to remove the debris. Hence, more phagocytic activities leave more enzymes which produce more destruction and further, inflammation, and the arthritic process becomes self-perpetuating.

Pathogenesis and Pathology

Under the examination of electronic microscope of the synovium, the lining of synovium consists of three types of synovial cells, e.g., type A, type B and type C. Type A cells mainly the phagocytic cells are engaged in destroying of complex, in the synovial fluid. Type B, which resembles fibroblast and are believed to synthesize protein and hyaluronic acid. Type C, are also known as undifferentiated cells, have the properties of both A and B.

The early stage of inflammation causes dilatation of the venules and capillaries. The leucocytes pass into the tissue spaces and then into the synovial fluid. This consequence leads to inflammation in the synovium (synovitis). Early hyperemia, edema, and swelling occur in the synovium and lining cells proliferate until they are three or more layers (multiply) thick. The underlying tissue is infiltrated with lymphocytes and plasma cells. All these lead to a thickened synovial membrane.

The inflamed synovium forms a pannus a granulomatous mass, that grows over and destroys cartilage, tendon and ligaments. The pannus is formed at the peripheral part of synovium. The pannus of granulation grows progressively and extends over the cartilage surface. In the process of inflammation the cartilage is absorbed (by the pannus) and replaced with the fibrous connective tissue. Vascular granulations are also formed in the marrow which extend into the articular cartilage surface. There is destruction of the cartilage and it becomes thin and deficient. The articular part is mainly covered with the fibrous pannus. The granulation tissue also extend toward the opposite articular cartilage surface bridging the joint with other granulation tissue resulting a fibrous ankylosis (Figs. 24.32 to 24.34).

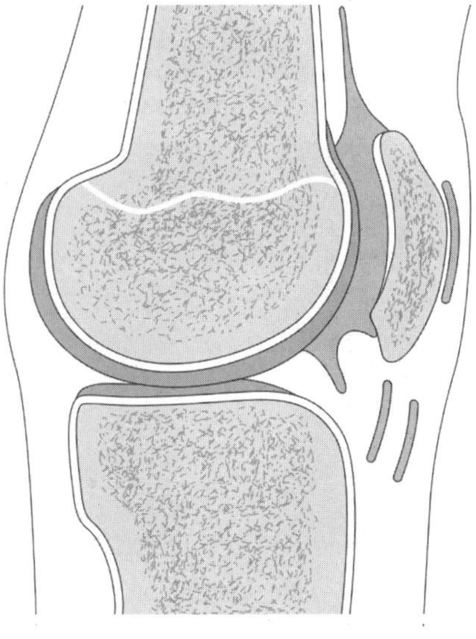

Fig. 24.32: Normal synovium and cartilage

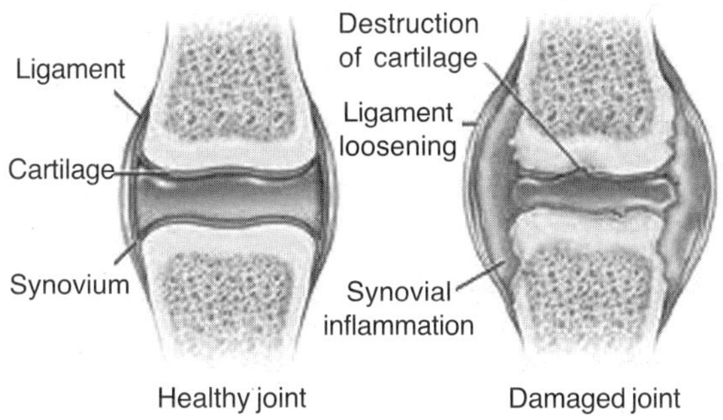

Fig. 24.33: Normal and damaged synovium and cartilage

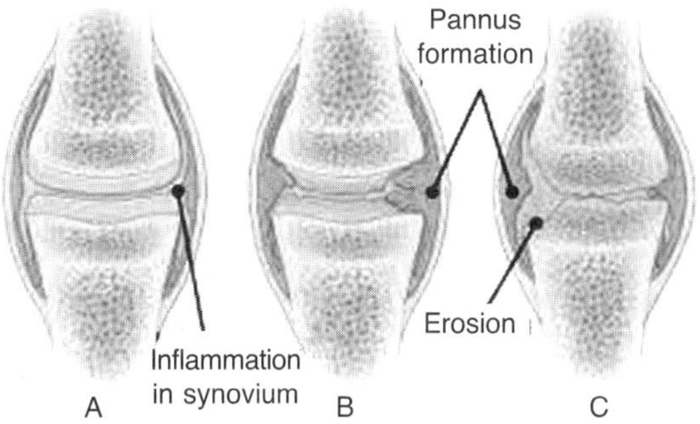

Fig. 24.34: Pannus

The synovium also extend into the peripheral part of the joint, putting pressure on the capsule, ligaments and tendons. The ligaments and tendons may sublux or rupture/tear causing muscular imbalance and joint deformity.

Subcutaneous Nodules: Subcutaneous nodules are composed of a typical basic rheumatoid unit consisting of a central necrotic zone, a surrounding layer of large mononuclear cell radially arranged (pallisade formation), and an outer zone of dense connective tissue with marked round-cell infiltration. Subcutaneous nodules are formed over the extensor surface such as forearm and tibia. They may be present in 20% of patients. Vasculitis is commonly found in rheumatoid arthritis and it is responsible for various skin lesions and may be a feature of early rheumatoid nodule formation (Fig. 24.35).

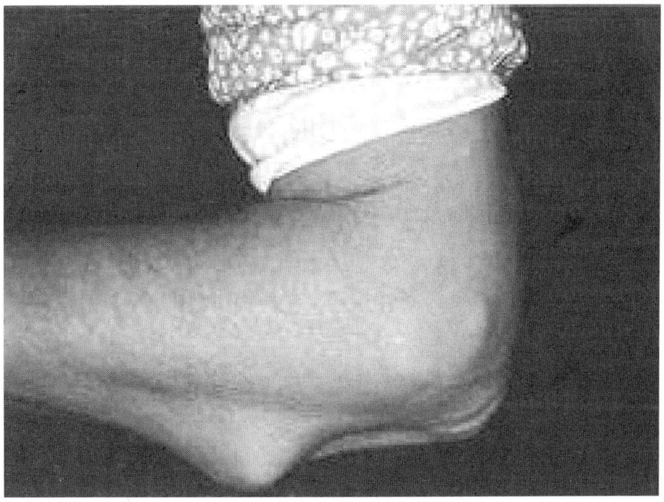

Fig. 24.35: Subcutaneous nodules

Clinical Features

1. Morning stiffness.
2. Pain on movements.
3. Symmetrical joint swelling.
4. Subcutaneous nodules.
5. Increased E.S.R.
6. Positive R.A. factor.

7. Muscle tightness and contracture.
8. Joint deformities.
9. Osteoporosis.

Diagnostic Criteria for Rheumatoid Arthritis

These are given by American Rheumatoid Association.

The diagnostic criteria are mentioned as under:

1. Morning stiffness.
2. Pain on movement or tenderness in atleast one joint.
3. Swelling: It may either be soft tissue thickening or synovial fluid in atleast one joint.
4. Swelling in atleast one other joint.
5. Symmetrical joint swelling with simultaneous involvement of both the sides of the joint. For an example if there is swelling in the left wrist joint the patient should also have swelling in the right wrist joint.
6. Subcutaneous nodules over bony prominences (on the extensor surfaces).
7. X-ray typical of rheumatoid arthritic.
8. Positive RA factor or latex fixation test.
9. Poor mucin clot.
10. Characteristic histologic changes in synovial membrane.
11. Characteristic histologic changes in nodule.

Based on the aforesaid eleven criteria the diagnosis may be classified as classical, definite, probable and possible.

Classical RA: The classical diagnosis cannot be made in the early stages as it requires aforementioned any seven criteria present for six weeks.

Definite: This needs five diagnostic criteria for atleast six weeks.

Probable: This needs three criteria out of eleven and these must be present for four weeks.

Possible RA: This diagnosis needs two of the following criteria which must be present at least for three weeks.

1. Morning stiffness.
2. Tenderness or pain on motion with history of recurrence persistence for three weeks.
3. History of swelling of joint.
4. Subcutaneous nodules.
5. Elevated erythrocyte sedimentation rate.

Laboratory Findings

An ESR is elevated particularly during an active period of inflammation, the rate continue to rise but to a lesser degree.

- Hypochromatic normocytic anemia is frequently associated. The white cell count remains normal.
- Serum from patients with rheumatoid arthritis contain a substance of unknown composition, the rheumatoid factor, in the presence of y globulin, is capable of agglutinating certain strains of streptococci, sensitized sheep cells and latex particles (Figs. 24.36 and 24.37).

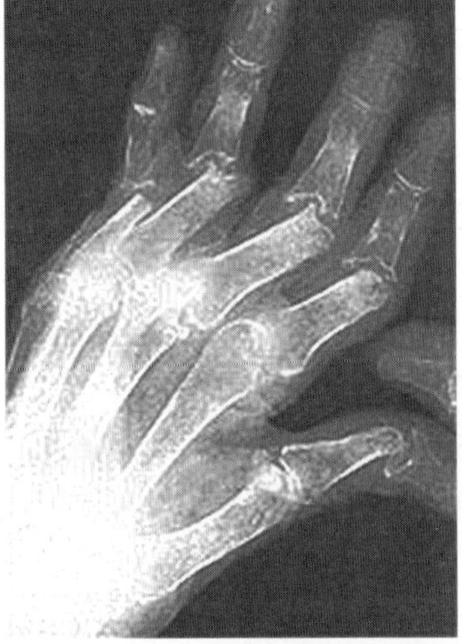

Fig. 24.36: X-ray–Rheumatoid arthritis with destruction of bones

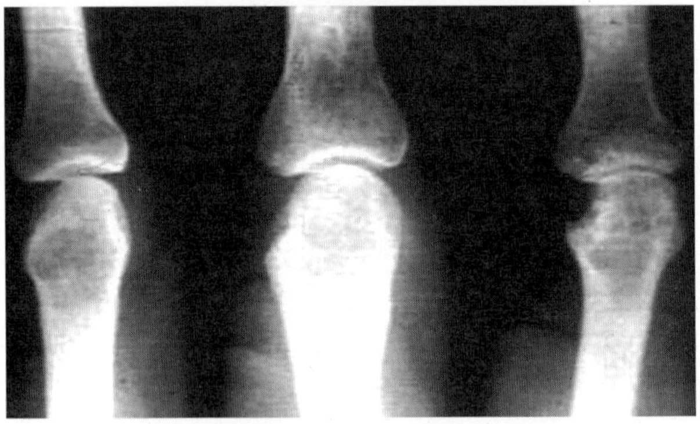

Fig. 24.37: X-rays–RA with destruction of peripheral cartilage and bone

Extra-Articular Manifestations: Apart from intra-articular structures, rheumatic arthritis also involves the other structure, known as extra-articular manifestations. These are not seen in the early stages of disease but as the disease progresses it may cause manifestations in the heart lungs, blood vessels, eyes, nerves and muscles. These manifestations are as following:

1. **Pulmonary:** Nodules, pleural effusion, bronchitis.
2. **Vascular:** Digital arthritis, ulcer, visceral arthritis.
3. **Systemic:** Fever, weight loss, fatigue, susceptibility to infection.

4. **Musculoskeletal:** Muscle wasting, bursitis, tenosynovitis, osteoporosis, synovitis.
5. **Hematological:** Anaemia, thrombocytosis, eosinophilia.
6. **Cardiac:** Pericarditis, myocarditis, endocarditis.
7. **Nodular:** Sinuses, scleritis.
8. **Neurological:** Cervical cord compression, compression neuropathies, mononeuritis-multiplex.
9. **Ocular:** Episcleritis, sclerotic.
10. **Lymphatic:** Lymphadenopathy, splenomegaly, fatty's syndrome, amyloidosis.

Deformities in Rheumatoid Arthritis

The inflammatory process involves the synovium that becomes edematous and thickened. The synovium forms the pannus which extends over the cartilage and absorbs and replaces it with fibrous connective tissues.

The edematous and thickened synovium extends into peripheral structures such as capsule, ligaments, fibrous sheath and tendons. This process damages and weakens the capsule and supporting structures. There is migration of the fat, pad, capsule and tendons. The joint becomes unstable and predisposes to deformities. The inflammatory process also causes rupture or tear of the tendon which leads to muscular imbalance and deformities. Weakening and lengthening of the static structures (ligaments and joint capsule) and rupture of the muscles in the inflammatory process, produces deformities.

Deformities of Hand and Fingers

The rheumatoid arthritis involves the proximal interphalangeal, distal interphalangeal and metacarpophalangeal joints.

Ulnar Drift: It is the ulnar deviation of the metacarpophalangeal joints. The main cause of ulnar drift is sinovitis. The flexor tendons enter fibrous sheath at angle, exerting ulnar and palmar pull that is resisted in the normal hand. Weakened and elongated joint capsule and ligaments loose the restraining power against the ulnar and palmer pull. Joint capsule and ligaments resistance to displacing force is lost. Extensor tendons are displaced in an ulnar and palmer directions, resulting base of proximal phalanx moves into ulnar and palmar direction (Figs. 24.38 to 24.40).

The disease affects the joint in two ways:

1. The inflammatory process (inflammatory infiltration) weakens and damages the capsule and supporting structures.

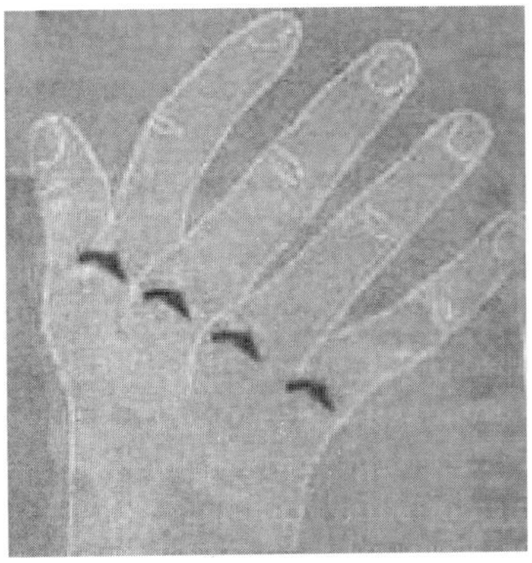

Fig. 24.38: Ulnar drift deformity

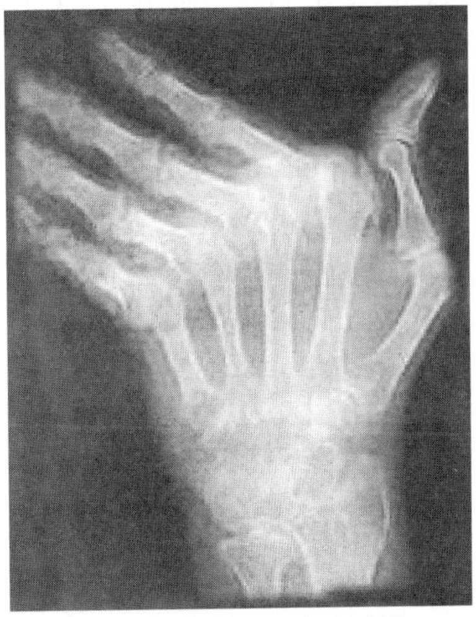

Fig. 24.39: X-ray ulnar drift

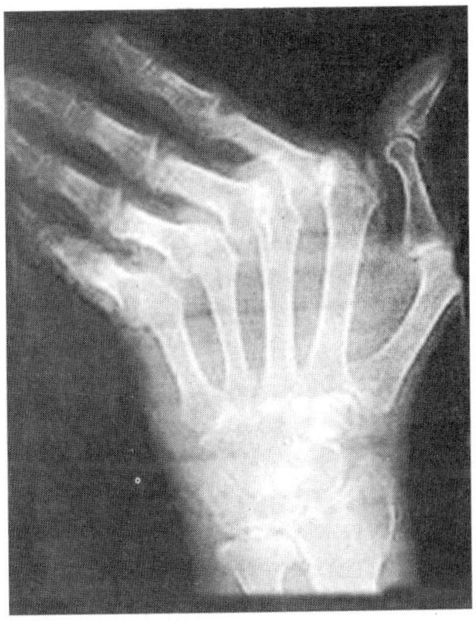

Fig. 24.40: X-ray ulnar drift

2. Edematous and thickened synovium extends into the periarticular structures and puts excessive load on them. The extensor tendon hoods are loosely fixed and vulnerable to disruption. The ligaments and capsule looses their restraining power against the ulnar forces– allowing tendons to pull across the joint in a way that enhances ulnar deviation and volar subluxation. As

resistance to displacing force is lost extensor tendons are displaced into ulnar and palmar directions.

Swan-Neck Deformity (SND)

An SND is a deformity in which the PIP joint goes into hyperextension and DIP joint into flexion. The severity of deformity depends upon the loss of PIP flexion and DIP range of motion. Though SND is very common in rheumatoid arthritis, it may also occur following injury and trauma. The inflammatory process affects the joint in two ways:

i. Synovitis of the PIP may lead to rupture of the flexor digitorum superficial tendon which allows PIP joint into hyperextension because of muscular imbalance. The hyperextension causes tension in the flexor digitorum profundus which pulls the DIP joint into flexion and predisposes the joint into SND.
ii. The inflammatory process involves the proximal interphalangeal (PIP) joints. Chronic intra-articular swelling due to synovial hypertrophy and fluid places an excessive pressure on the volar and dorsal capsule. There is dorsal migration of the volar band, which produces hyperextension at the PIP joint. Hyperextension at PIP joint causes tension in the profundus tendon that pulls the distal interphalangeal joint into flexion (Fig. 24.41).

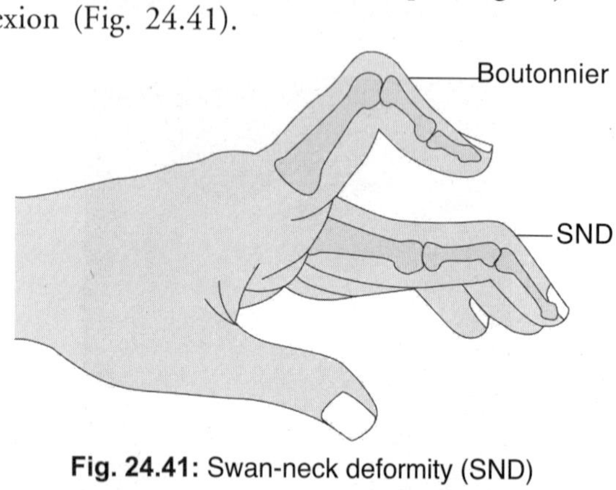

Fig. 24.41: Swan-neck deformity (SND)

Boutonniere or Button-Hole Deformity

Boutonniere deformity is very common after SND in rheumatoid arthritis, it may also occur following injury and trauma. The PIP joint goes into flexion and DIP joint into hyperextension.

The main cause of the Boutonniere deformity is the synovitis which usually affects the PIP joint. The inflammatory process damages and weakens the capsule and supporting structures. The edematous (hypertrophied) synovium distends to the dorsal capsule and also displaces the *anterior surface*. There is rupture of the central slip of the extensor digitorum communis that limits the effectiveness of it as an extensor of middle finger. The PIP joint goes into flexion which in turn *increase tension* distal extensor slip, which pulls DIP into hyperextension (Fig. 24.42).

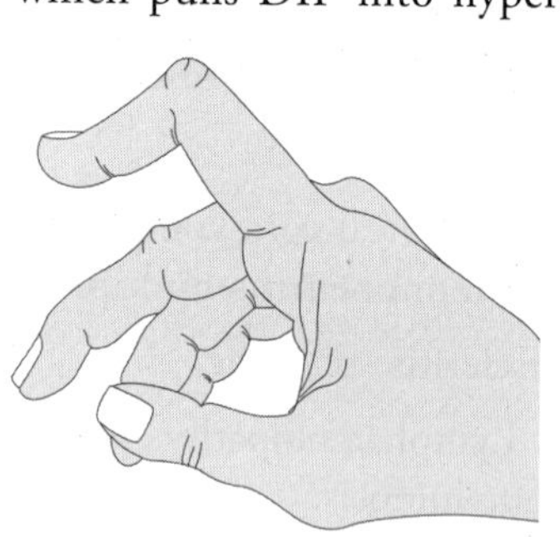

Fig. 24.42: Boutonniere or button-hole deformity

Mallet Finger

Mallet finger is the flexion deformity of distal interphalangeal joint mostly of little finger but other fingers may also be affected. The deformity usually occurs in rheumatoid arthritis, but trauma and injury to the DIP joint may also cause similar deformity.

Chronic intra-articular swelling due to synovial hypertrophy and fluid in the DIP joint extends into the dorsum of the little finger which damages and weaken the capsule and supporting structures. There is pressure on the distal attachment of the extensor tendon due to which may lengthen or rupture the extensor tendon and removes the extension force. Due to loss of extension force the flexor digitorum profundus pulls the DIP into flexion (Fig. 24.43).

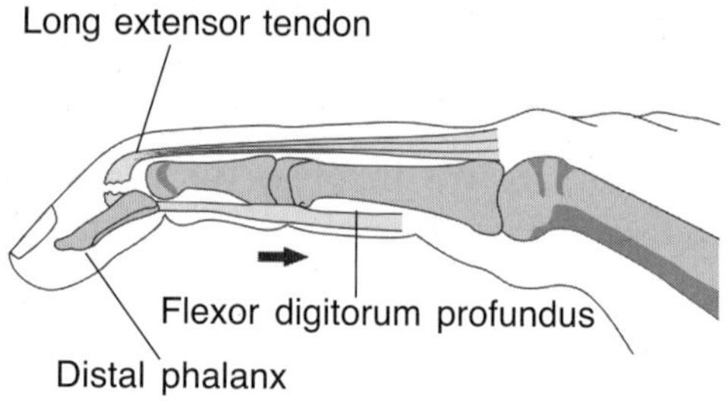

Fig. 24.43: Mallet finger

The deformity is graded as mild, moderate and severe depending on the active loss of flexion range.

Mild: Partial active extension of DIP (Partial rupture of extensor tendon).

Moderate: No active extension of DIP, passive extension possible (Complete rupture of tendon).

Severe: No active and passive extension, fixed DIP flexion (Contractor of profundus).

Wrist

The wrist joint is also involved frequently in rheumatoid arthritis. Initially swelling in the wrist joint is present due to synovitis (synovial fluid) but as the disease progresses periarticular synovial thickening swelling may also be seen. Erosions may develop in all the carpal bones.

In the inflammatory process the synovium becomes edematous and thickened and forms the pannus which absorbs and replaces the bones with the fibrous connective tissues. Eventually there is destruction or collapse of the carpal bones at the radial side which will produce radial deviation of the metacarpals. The carpal bones may sublux towards the volar surface, and step like deformity will appear at the wrist joint (Fig. 24.44).

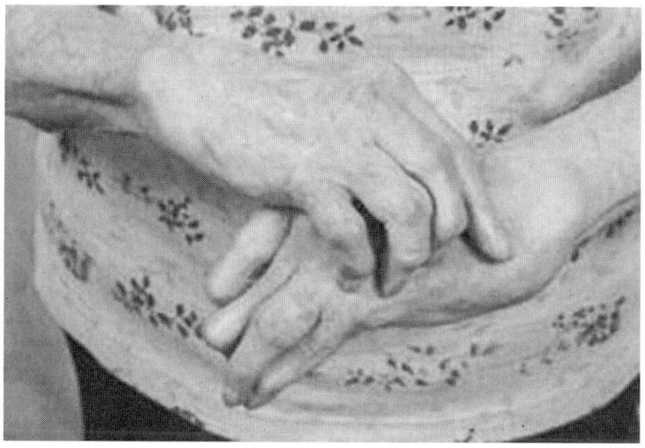

Fig. 24.44: Step deformity

The inflammatory changes also involve the synovium of the flexor tendons which enter into the carpal tunnel with the median nerve. The ischemia and swelling in the synovium of the tendons will increase the pressure within the tunnel and produce carpal tunnel syndrome with pain, numbness and tingling in finger supplied by the median nerve.

Elbow Joint

The inflamed and thickened synovium may bulge into the medial and lateral epicondyles of humerus and olecranon fossa. The olecranon fossa becomes obliterated and limits the extension of the elbow joint. The inflammatory process will destroy the anterior margin of the articular surface of the proximal ulna, allowing the olecranon to migrate in a cephaled direction.

Deformities of Lower Extremity Joint

Fore-Foot-Hallux Valgus, Hammer and Claw Toes: Chronic intra-articular swelling due to synovium hypertrophy and fluid causes broadening of the fore foot and separation of the toes, with capsular and ligamentous laxity. The weight bearing on the inflamed joint can cause dislocation of the metatarsophalangeal joints. The flexor tendons migrate and becomes functional extensors. Proximal phalanges and plantar fat pad are drawn laterally. This progressive muscular imbalance leads to hammer and claw toe deformities of the four lesser toes (Figs. 24.45 and 24.46). The lateral stability of the great toe is decreased. The great toe migrates laterally and develops hallux valgus deformity.

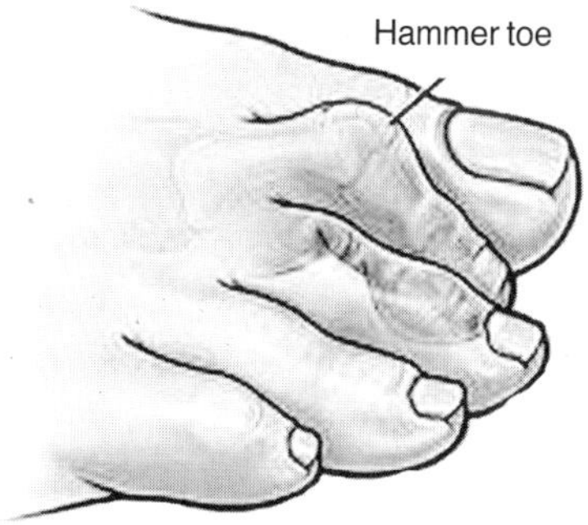

Fig. 24.45: Hammer toes

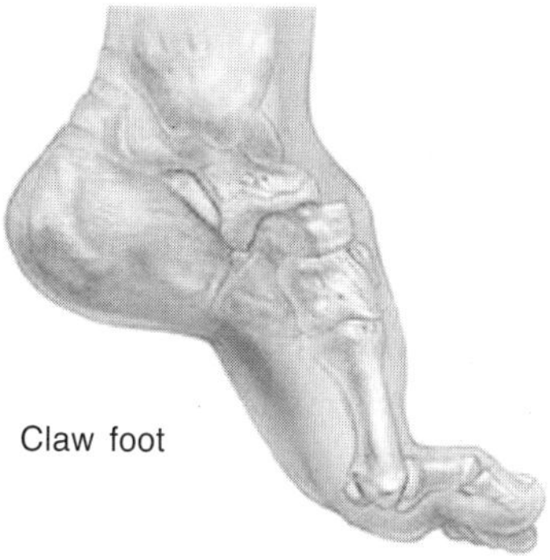

Fig. 24.46: Claw toes

Hind Foot: The hind foot does not develop marked deformities, but the inflammatory process may cause plantar fasciitis, bursitis and spur. The weight bearing on the inflamed and swollen joint may aggravate the symptoms, and may cause excessive pronation.

Ankle: In the early stage of the disease synovitis of the tibialis anterior, peroneii and tibialis posterior is common, however, no clinical evidence is seen but surgical is there. A sausage shaped swelling is seen along the length of the tendon. As the disease progresses it may destruct the cartilage and replace with fibrous connective tissues. The ligamentous laxity produces joint instability. Erosion of the ligamentous insertion can also be seen between tibia and fibula and the talus.

Knee Joint Deformities: The knee joint is frequently involved in rheumatoid arthritis which produces combination of deformities. Potter's knee describes the typical rheumatoid arthritic knee that includes flexion contracture, popliteal cysts, posterior subluxation and dislocation of tibia, valgus and external rotation of the tibia (Figs. 24.47 and 24.48).

- In the early stage of rheumatoid arthritis synovitis alters the centre of motion of the tibiofemoral joint. Intra-

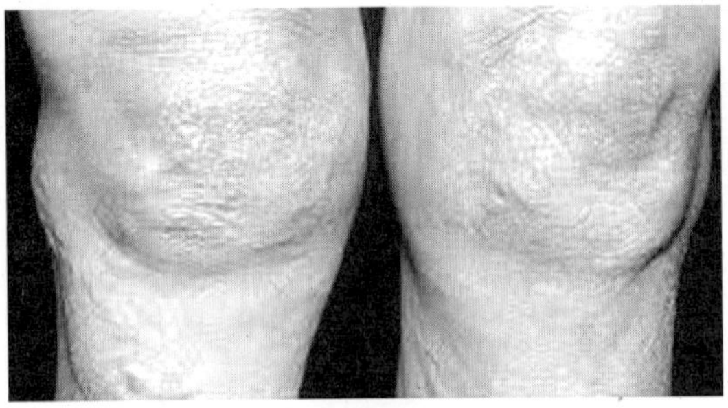

Fig. 24.47: Knee joint swelling

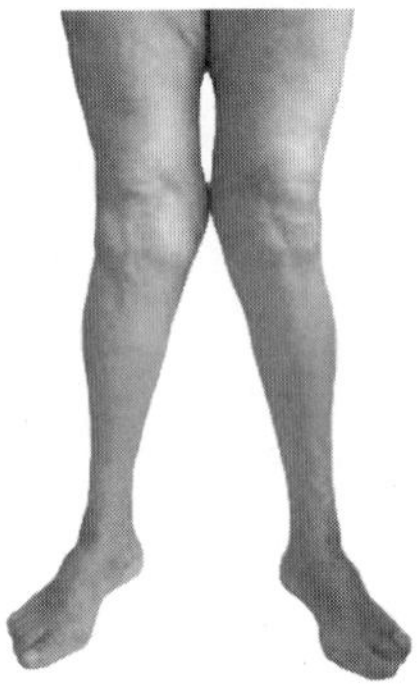

Fig. 24.48: Potter knee deformity

articular swelling due to synovitis increases in volume. The weight bearing on the swollen and inflamed knee joint can allow the synovial fluid to pass into popliteal fossa, where it forms a popliteal cyst. Sometimes the popliteal cyst which contains synovial fluid may burst and passes the fluid into the semi-membranosus and semi-tendinosus bursa. This produces intense pain in the posterior knee joint which sometime *mistaken with thrombophlebitis.*

After establishing the cause of the popliteal cyst the treatment should be directed to the cause as well as to the prevention of rupture of the cyst. Patients with rheumatoid arthritis should be advised not to put the weight on the leg. Cryotherapy and interferential therapy may help in relieving pain, swelling and symptoms. Strengthening exercises such as quadriceps sets, gluteus maximus sets, hamstrings and ankle pumps are advised to avoid disuse atrophy of the muscles. Injection of steroids into the cyst may also be recommended.

Patients with meniscal tears who do not respond to the conservative treatment, are advised for arthroscopic intervention or open excision. The recurrence rate of open popliteal cyst excision varies widely, with studies reporting frequent recurrences.

- As the disease progresses the synovium becomes thickened and edematous, and forms pannus that extends into the cartilage (peripheral part) and covers the peripheral part of it. The pannus absorbs and replaces the cartilage with fibrous connective tissue. The destruction of the cartilage can cause collapse of femoral or tibial condyles. As the cartilage wears crepetus is the evident throughout the movement.
- All components of the knee complex are involved such as medial, lateral and patellofemoral joint. Pain and spasm in the hamstrings limit the terminal extension resultant knee joint is maintained slightly in flexion. In non ambulatory patients hamstrings develop contracture which pull the tibia posterior on the femur; this produces subluxation or dislocation of the tibia. Quadriceps becomes weak due to prolong elongation.
- The destruction of the cartilage produces mediolateral instability and knee valgus. The spasm in tensor fascia lata (TFL) pulls the tibia towards lateral rotation and produces tibial external rotation in 50% cases. This causes a shortening of the lateral structure and permanent elongation of medial structures. Therefore, the rheumatoid arthritis affects the knee joint markedly and develops flexion contracture, posterior subluxation and dislocation, valgus and external rotation of the tibia.

Hip Joint: Initially joint destructions are not seen but patients may have complain of pain, stiffness, and limitation in the range of abduction and rotations. Tenderness can be palpated on the posterior and superior aspect of the joint due to trochantric and gluteus maximus bursitis. As the disease progresses patients may develop antaligic gait and Trendelenburg's sign. Swelling may be visible in the groin and femoral triangle.

In advanced cases osteoporosis occurs and the femoral head pieces the acetabulum. Avascular necrosis of the femoral head can cause collapse of the area. Eventually a true leg length discrepancy will occur.

Shoulder Joint: Initially synovial effusion may be seen due to synovitis, which may limit shoulder abduction. The inflammatory changes involve the subacromial and subdeltoid bursa, which will further produce pain and limitation in the range of motion.

The destructive changes and swelling also put an excessive pressure on the tendons of rotator cuff muscles. The rupture of the rotator cuff muscles tendon will allow the head of humerus to migrate superiorly to the acromial arch. The suprahumeral space will decrease, and the supraspinatus and sub-acromial bursa will be impinged (impingement syndrome) between the head of humerus and acromian arch. The range of motion will be limited in all three planes.

Spine: The lumbar and thoracic spine does not involve significantly in rheumatoid arthritis. The most of destructive changes take place at the atlantoaxial joint. The inflammatory changes rupture the transverse ligament which holds the odontoid to the atlas. This will produce vertical subluxation or upward translation of the dens. The subluxation of C_1 and C_2 is one of the complications an may lead to compression on spinal cord, the patient may experience numbness and tingling in the arms and legs. The therapist should not advice mechanical traction to the rheumatoid arthritic patients, if X-ray shows subluxation between atlas and axis, patient could be given soft collar or hard collar and be referred to the orthopaedician for surgical intervention such as fusion of C_1 and C_2.

MANAGEMENT OF RHEUMATOID ARTHRITIS

Physical Therapy Assessment

Cardiopulmonary Assessment: Rheumatoid arthritis is a systemic disease which involves not only joints but also other organs such as heart, lungs, blood vessels and eyes, therefore, therapist should assess the functions of vital organs before administering treatment.

Musculoskeletal Assessment: Each joint is to be examined for erythema, warmth, pain, tenderness, temperature, swelling, range of motion, crepetus, contracture, tightness and deformities.

Gait and Posture Assessment: The involvement of hip, knee and ankle joint lead to tightness, contracture and deformities in the lower extremities. In turn, there is reduced range of motion, reduced velocity and increased energy expenditure. The muscles are required to work more for acceleration of swing phase to bring the leg forward. The cadence drops to 72.5 steps per minute or more. The stride length is also reduced. Due to pain patient walks with the stiff knee (antalgic gait) and bending to the same side (Trendelenburg sign).

The Therapist Should Focus on the Following Goals

1. **Education:** The therapist should tell the patient that this is a progressive disease which cannot be cured but it can be prevented to the further progression by taking some measures.

   Energy conservation principles, work simplification techniques, exercise programs, and joint protection techniques should be taught to the patients. They must learn these management techniques and then continue to practice them through out their life.

   Fatigue is one of the features of rheumatoid arthritis. In order to avoid fatigue patient should be encouraged to organize time, task and rest periods. The position such as sitting which saves upto 25% energy should be preferred over standing. The patient should use large joint and body weight to achieve tasks. Long handled equipments increase the range of hand function and decrease the amount of bending and energy required. Electronic light weight equipments also decrease the amount of time and energy required.

2. **Relief in Pain and Spasm:** The pain and stiffness is mainly of protective in nature. There is overuse (sustained contraction) of the muscles to prevent movement at the joint. The therapist should focus on reduction of muscle guarding by using the cryotherapy and superficial heating modalities such as infra red rays, moist hot packs and paraffin wax bath. PNF techniques of slow reversal, reciprocal inhibition, hold relax and contract relax may be found of valve in reduction of pain and spasm. Exercises in water not only help in relieving of pain but also play important role in improvement of range of motion and muscle strength. In patients with acute pain where ESR is extremely high and patients find difficultly in doing hold relax and contract relax they may be taught reciprocal inhibition; as it consists isometric contraction of antagonistic muscles that is useful in relaxing the agonists group of muscles. The electrotherapy modalities such as short wave diathermy should not be advised as it may increase inflammation especially during the exacerbatory phase. Instead of SWD, pulsed diathermy or curapulse is advised. Interferential therapy of analgesic mode 80-100 Hz helps in relieving pain and muscle spasm.

   The physiotherapeutic management in relief of pain should be considered as temporary but it is the crucial step that helps in preventing tightness; contracture and deformities. Patients should learn and receive the treatment such as cold pack, hot pack, PWB and muscle relaxation exercises at home in order to prevent muscles guarding, tightness and contractures.

3. **Protection of Joints:** Activities of daily living may put excessive pressure on the painful and swollen joints. These joints become more vulnerable to damage and instability. Hence, activity that produces pain lasting more than 1-2 hours indicates joints are being overstressed and needed to be protected. To provide the dynamic stability to the inflamed joints, these joints should be supported well with work splint particularly when muscle strength is inadequate. For activities of daily living the patient should be advised to use the body weight and large joints to push the large objects instead of hands. Patient should also be advised to maximize the effect of gravity (e.g., use a laundry chute to eliminate carrying and stairs) for daily activities and office work. The following points should be taught to the patient to protect the joint:

   a. Respect the pain: Pain occurs during an activity is an important indication of joint protection.

b. Maintain adequate muscle strength and range of motion.

c. Avoid holding one position for any undue length of time.

d. Use correct patterns of movements.

e. Avoid the position in which deformity occurs.

4. **Prevention of Deformities:** Development of deformities in patients with rheumatoid arthritis is very common, as pain, swelling and muscle spasm encourage the patient to adopt the posture which relieves symptoms. Later there will be change in the length of muscle fibers, periarticular structures and decrease strength of muscle. The muscle strength is essential to support damaged joint. Pain, however, should not be ignored as doing so can lead to further damage and discomfort. Rheumatoid arthritis affects interphalangeal joints of hands, wrist and foot swelling in 90 percent of patients. Deformities are mainly caused by swelling and proliferation of the synovium into the particular structures. This, in turn, causes destruction of cartilage, erosion of bones, ligamentous laxity and rupture or tear of the muscle tendons. This lead to muscular imbalance and deformity. To prevent muscular imbalance and deformities the joint should be held in such a position that not only reduces load on the muscle tendon but also helps in relieving pain and symptoms; especially during an acute phase. The splints, proper positioning, and passive stretching, play crucial role in preventing deformities and relieving in pain and symptoms.

Splints

These are very useful in acutely inflammable joints. Improved biomechanical designs and the introduction of light weight, strong, low temperature material that are resistant to wear have provided the client with a wide array of splints. There are two types of splints–resting and dynamic.

Resting Splints: These are very effective in reducing the protective muscle guarding that is responsible for deformity. The resting splints should be worn at night and predetermined periods during the day. Splint use should continue full time for duration of flare and removed at least once a day for skin hygiene and gentle active movements. The splint should be well fitted, padded over the bony prominences to avoid pressure. These are usually made of plaster of Paris which are easy to apply. The therapist should explain the application procedure to the patients and in case of redness, pressure sores they should use soft materials between the splint and treatment part. The weight of splint also puts an additional stress on the extremity and may cause pain and fatigue, hence, the splint should be as light weight as possible.

Generally, for the upper extremity, splint is applied in 10-30° wrist extension, slight lunar deviation, interphalangeal joint in 5° flexion, metacarpophalangeal joint should be just off full flexion. Thumb should be abducted and opposed. However the position of hand and wrist may vary somewhat by practitioners (Fig. 24.49).

Wrist splint–Neutral or slight extension, Unlar deviation–5°, Ulnar drift–Should be corrected, Meta carpophalangeal joints–Should be just off full flexion, Thumb–Abducted and opposed.

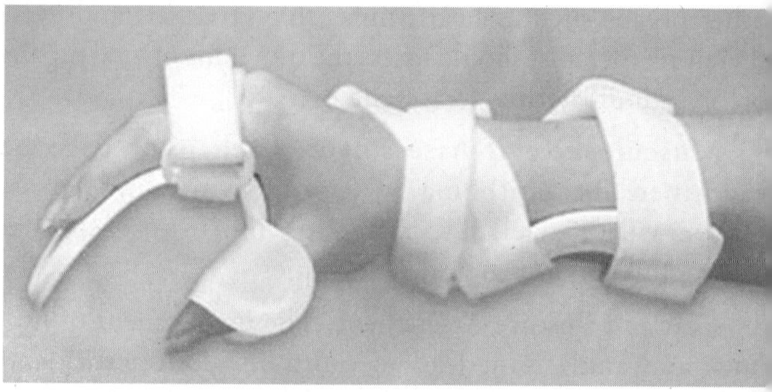

Fig. 24.49: Wrist (resting) splint

Swan Neck Splint: To restrict unwanted PIP hyperextension and to prevent swan neck deformity a proximal interphalangeal hyperextension block splint is used. The patients with swan neck deformity usually finds difficulty in performing activities with the hand. The swan neck splint not only blocks the PIP joint in slight flexion but also allows patient to flex the PIP joint more efficiently which helps in performing activities with the hand. For short term or trial purposes a custom fabricated thermoplastic material can be used but for long-term use an adjacent finger, commercial products made from metal or polypropylene are often recommended as they are more durable, less bulky, more easily cleaned, and more cosmetically appealing (Figs. 24.50a and b).

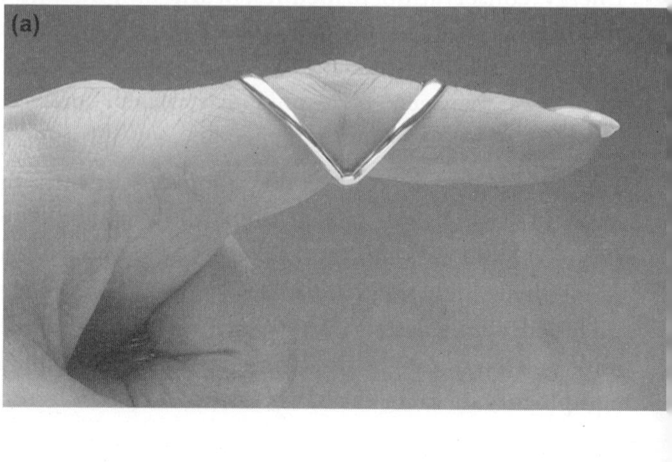

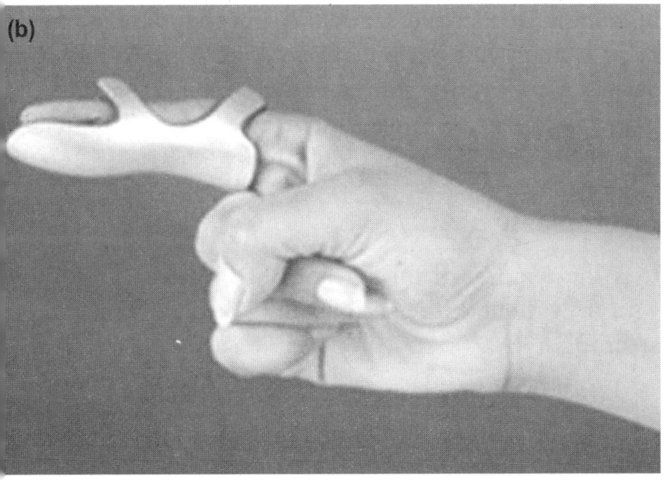

Figs. 24.50a and b: Splints for swan neck deformity

Boutonniere Splint: To prevent the boutonniere deformity the proximal interphalangeal joint is blocked in the extension and distal interphalangeal joint is left free to flex. The splint is very useful in prevention of deformity if the deformity is flexible (Fig. 24.51).

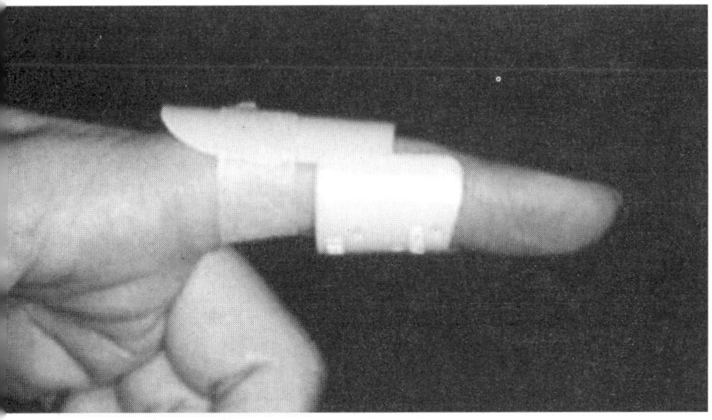

Fig. 24.51: Boutonniere splint

Knees: The knee is kept straight in 5° of flexion and then a back slab is applied from distal ischial tuberosity to the proximal heal.

Ankle and Foot: To prevent the deformities at ankle joint, a back slab is applied which extends from the neck of fibula to the tip of toe. The ankle joint should be at neutral with no valgus or varus.

5. **Correction of Deformities:** Rheumatoid arthritis is a progressive disease which develops deformities in the later stages; however, efforts are made in prevention of deformities. Once the deformity is established there is shortening (concave side) and lengthening (convex aspect) of the soft tissues. To correct the deformity the lengthened muscles are required strengthening and shortened muscles require stretching. Serial plaster, serial splinting, orthoses and dynamic splints are used to correct the deformities.

Serial Plaster: To correct the flexion contracture of the knee joint, a POP cast is applied over the deformed joint. The cast is split after 2-3 days on the concave (popliteal) side and separated as far as possible using the uncut POP on the convex side as a hinge. After cutting on the concave side the knee joint is extended as much as possible (as per tolerance of the patient) and wedges are inserted on the split POP to maintain the achieved position. The whole part is secured by a POP bandage. It is repeated once before the entire plaster has to be replaced.

Orthosis: Swelling due to synovitis and synovium hypertrophy places stretch on the periarticular structures such as ligaments, tendons and capsule that may rupture or lengthen. This whole phenomenon produces ligamentous laxity and joint instability. The orthosis provides not only passive stability to the joint but also holds the joint in functional position (Fig. 24.52).

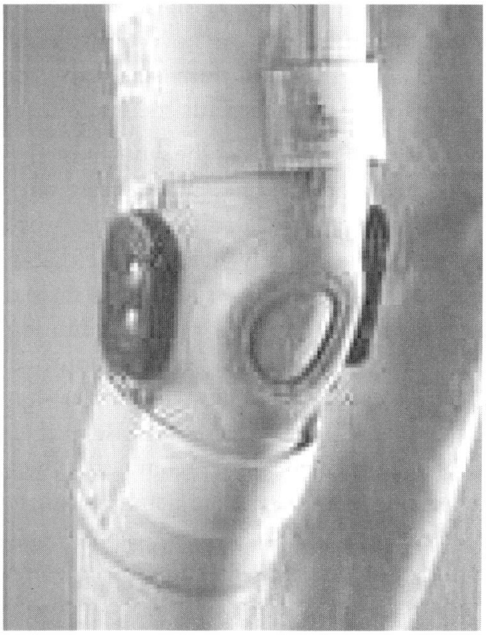

Fig. 24.52: Knee orthosis

6. **Maintenance and Restoration of Joint Range of Motion:** During exacerbatory period active assisted, hold relax, and contract relax exercises are advised to maintain the range of motion. Passive movements may increase the pain and symptoms therefore these should be avoided. Hold relax, contract relax and slow reversal exercises are found effective in increasing range of motion of the joint. For an example to improve the flexion contracture, the therapist extends the knee joint as much as possible and holds it firmly. The patient is asked to contract the hamstrings against the resistance of at least six seconds, followed by rest of same period. This exercise helps in lengthening of the hamstrings and increasing in

extension of the knee joint. Several repetitions of hold relax or contract relax may be performed until a significant improvement in the range is achieved. The exercise in water (hydrotherapy) also helps in improving range of motion.

7. **Maintenance and Improvement of Posture:** Core strengthening, upper back extensors and peripheral muscle strengthening, should be taught to the patient to improve posture. Exercises in water also help in improving posture.

Surgical Management

If pain and symptoms are not relieved with a fair trial of conservative treatment including drugs then patient may be elected for surgical intervention. Relief in incapacitating pain, restoration of joint stability and improvement in activities of daily living are the main objectives of the surgery. The progression of the stages of the rheumatoid arthritis decides the choice of surgery. Synovectomy, arthroplasty and arthrodesis are the common surgical procedures recommended to the patients with rheumatoid arthritis.

Synovectomy: The removal of the synovium relieves pain in almost all rheumatoid joints and at least temporarily halts progression of the local disease. The procedure is usually recommended in early stages of the disease where other structures of the joint remain intact except of synovium. In synovectomy the site of immunoglobulin synthesis is removed to prevent the formation of immune complexes that cause tissue destruction by activating lysosomal hydrolases. This will also decrease in the synovial rheumatoid factor, IgG/Igm ($7^s/19^s$ complex). The removed synovium usually regenerates completely within 60 days. The regenerated synovium once again capable of secreting synovial fluid, but the synovial function is considerably reduced. The regenerated synovium is again susceptible to inflammation (synovitis).

Post Operative Synovectomy: Breathing exercises, intensive coughing, hold relax, general strengthening exercises are initiated to improve posture and gait. The synovectomy is usually recommended to the knee, MCP wrist and elbow joint. To achieve the range of motion, an ice towel can be placed on the spasmodic muscles, and contract relax exercises are performed. For an example, to improve flexion of knee joint an ice pack is placed along the length of quadriceps and knee is flexed as much as possible. The therapist holds the leg firmly and asks the patient to extend the leg. The contraction is held at least for six seconds followed by relaxation. After relaxation new flexion range is achieved and same procedure is repeated. Several repetitions are performed to improve the range of motion. In case of severe muscle spasm reciprocal inhibition helps in improving flexion range of knee joint. As the spasm decreases in severity contract relax exercises may also be performed. Passive movements often increases protective muscle spasm, therefore, should be avoided.

Arthroplasty

It is the removal of one or both of the articular surfaces with or without a foreign implant. There are four types of arthroplasty:

- Excision arthroplasty.
- Interposition arthroplasty.
- Partial joint replacement (arthroplasty).
- Total joint replacement (arthroplasty).

Excision Arthroplasty: The aim of excision arthroplasty is to reduce pain in the joint. The surgery is rarely done at the hip and knee joint except salvaging procedure. If the procedure is advised for knee joint, it is usually associated with arthrodesis.

The excision arthroplasty involves the rejection of periarticular bone and the space thus formed becomes (created by surgical procedure) filled with scar tissues during the healing process. The procedure creates unstable joint due to reduction of the ligaments and joint capsule.

The excision arthroplasty has a great benefit in the rheumatoid foot as it completely relieves persisting pain, disability, metatarsalgia and subluxation of the metatarsophalangeal joint. For excision of the metatarsal head and proximal part of proximal phalanx a fowler's compression excision arthroplasty is performed. For hallux valgus keller's excision arthroplasty is the choice of surgical procedure.

Post Operative Excision Arthroplasty: The emphasis is given on the footwear. The therapist should assess the foot accurately and review footwear. The weight bearing should be as per tolerance and as advised by the surgeon. Strengthening exercise of intrinsic muscles may be initialled after first week of operation. The faradic foot bath should be started after one month of the surgery. It helps in strengthening of the intrinsic muscles as well as in reducing the swelling of the foot. In cases of swelling in the ankle and foot faradism under pressure may also be used.

Interposition Arthroplasty: Interposition arthroplasty involves debridement of joint. In this procedure the space created with debridement is filled with fat pad, fascia or foreign material, which cover only one joint surface. The procedure is usually done at shoulder joint as replacement of shoulder is unlike hip and knee joints. Pendular exercises are initiated in the first week of the surgery upto 3 weeks. After three weeks isometric exercises may be initiated if advised by the concerned surgeon.

TOTAL HIP REPLACEMENT

It is the replacement of both the articular surfaces of the joint with the foreign implants. The pain is eliminated completely by replacing both the articulating surfaces. The restoration of hip motion improves gait and reduces stress on the back and knee joint (Fig. 24.53).

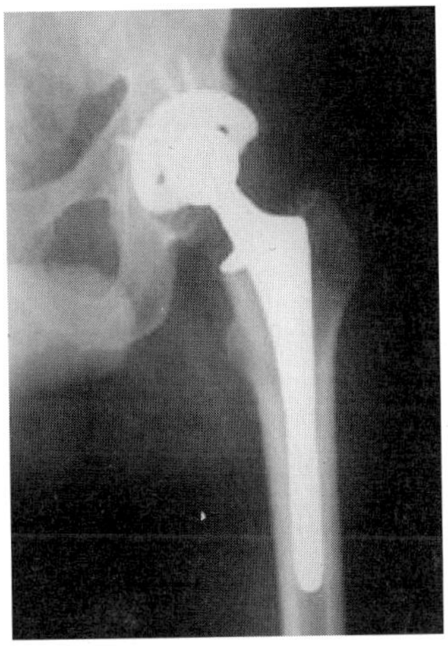

Fig. 24.53: Total hip replacement

Indications of THR

1. Persistent and debilitating pain with destruction of joint surfaces and with gross deterioration in activities of daily living and a fair trial of conservative treatment fails to improve the symptoms.
2. Failure of prior surgery.
3. Avascular necrosis.
4. Neck of femur fracture.
5. Hip arthrodesis in a poor functional position associated with increase in back or knee pain.
6. Osteoarthrosis-grade-4.

Contraindications of THR

1. Acute infection in the joint.
2. Systemic infection.
3. Malignant tumors that do not allow adequate fixation of the components.
4. In adequate bone mass.

Relative Contraindications of THR: Absent or relative insufficiency of the abductor mechanism and progressive neurologic deficit.

Approaches: The hip joint can be approached from anterior, lateral and posterior view. All three approaches have advantages and disadvantages; but lateral approach is preferred over other.

> **Osteotomy:** The patients who have leg length discrepancy may require osteotomy of the femur. It may be done for alignment correction, either angular or rotational shortening, such as a calcar episiotomy or sub-trochanteric shortening; or *exposure, such as trochanteric osteotomy or slide.* These patients should not be allowed to do SLR and side SLR unless and until the concerned surgeon advises.

Who Can Be Elected for THR? The implant used in the surgery has a projected life span of less than 20 years, hence the patients of more than 60 years are usually elected for the THR. Younger patients may also be elected for the THR if their functional status is severely compromised and persistent pain becomes intolerable. As the young patients demand more physical activities, therefore the life span of the implant is reduced further (less than 20 years). These patients require a revision surgery later in their life (after 20 years of THR).

Types of Implants

There are three types of prosthesis–Cemented, non-cemented and hybrid.

Cemented: Cement is placed between the bone and the prosthesis, therefore, stability is provided by the cement. The cemented prosthesis is as strong as it will ever be 15 minutes after insertion. The cemented components can support weight immediately after surgery. The implant achieves an adequate stability to allow an immediate full weight bearing with a cane or walker. However, some surgeons believe that weight bearing restriction should be there at least upto 6 weeks, as the bone is damaged by mechanical and thermal trauma during the surgery.

Non-Cemented Prosthesis: The implant tends to be more expansive and technically demanding to implant; however, they are easier to revise when they fail. The implant is inserted into the bone by press fit method. The stability is usually achieved by tissue on growth or in growth into the implant. The maximum stability is achieved in the 6 months of the surgery.

Weight Bearing Restrictions: The patients with non-cemented are allowed to toe touch weight bearing with the walker for at least 6 weeks. The walker is removed after 6 weeks and stick is advised further unless and until patient achieves good hip abductor mechanism and also confidence.

It usually takes 4-6 weeks. These patients may do stairs by the end of 3 months, however, stair climbing may be allowed before 3 months, if the concerned surgeon permits.

The patients with cemented implant may be allowed full weight bearing with the walker as soon as they come out of the operation theater. The walker may be removed after 4-6 weeks and a stick is given. Patients can do the stairs after 6 weeks of the surgery, however, it should be advised by the concerned surgeon.

Precautions

- No cross leg sitting.
- No internal rotation.
- No hip adduction.
- No hip flexion beyond 100°.
- No low chair (>22 inches) (Figs. 24.54a to g).

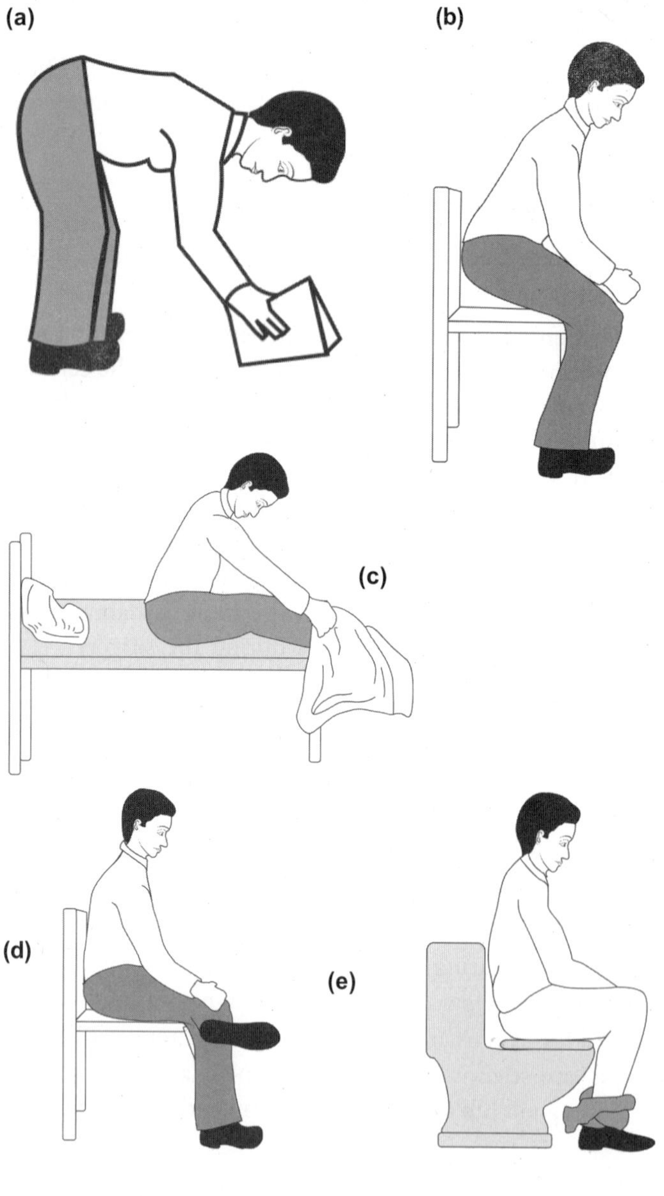

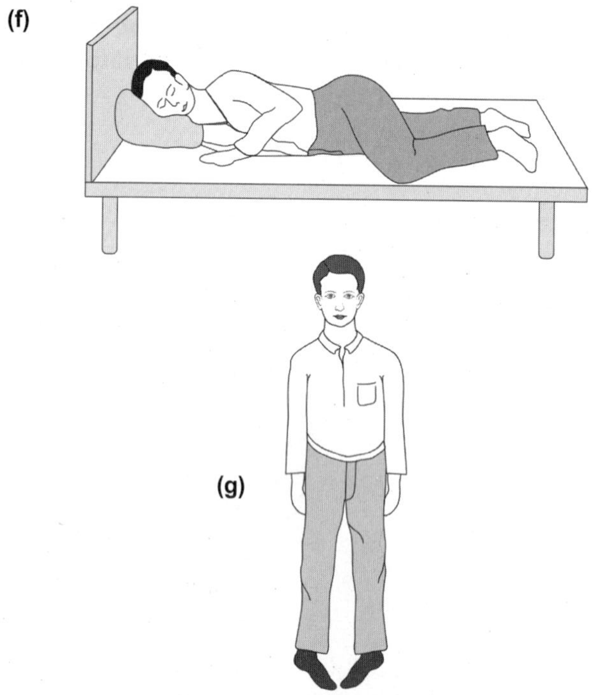

Figs. 24.54a to g: Prevention following THR

Post Operative Total Hip Replacement Management

Brace: The hip joint is guarded in the orthosis or wedge to prevent adduction of the hip as the joint is more vulnerable to dislocation in adduction. The brace may be removed during the exercise; however, it should be worn at night and predetermined period of day.

Exercises: The following exercises are initiated from day one:

i. *Quadriceps Sets:* For 6 weeks.

ii. *Gluteus Maximus Sets:* For 6 weeks.

iii. *Ankle Pump Exercises:* For 6 weeks.

iv. *Straight Leg Raising:* This exercise can produce very large *out-of-plane* loads on the hip, hence, it should be avoided, however, if it is advised, it should be performed with assistance in the first four weeks.

v. *Side SLR:* The exercise has an important role in improving abductor mechanism; initially it should be done in the supine position by bringing the leg out of the edge of the couch with assistance by the therapist. As the strength improves therapist may resist the movement. Exercise may be progressed to the side lying. In case of trochanteric osteotomies, the exercises should be avoided unless and until the concerned surgeon advises.

vi. *Stairs:* Stair climbing and descending also depends upon the type of implant. The patients with cemented implant may be allowed to climb the stairs after 6-8 weeks. Whereas patients with non-cemented implant should do stairs after 3 months only.

vii. *Sitting on Chair:* Both cemented and non-cemented patients are advised to use a chair of at least 22 inches height (for an average height person). Low chairs allow the hip to flex beyond 100 degrees, that may cause dislocation of the joint.

viii. *Weight Bearing:* Full weight bearing with the walker is allowed to the patients with cemented implant, whereas patients with cement less implant are advised to touch weight bearing with the walker for at least 6 weeks. Weight bearing on the operated side may also be limited if the greater trochanter is removed. The walker is removed and stick is advised till the patient gains confidence and abductor mechanism. It is usually given after 4-6 weeks (four weeks for the cemented and six to eight weeks for the cementless patients).

ix. *Stretching:* The hip flexors are of tonic muscles, and have tendency of getting shortened. *Thomas Stretch:* To stretch the iliopsoas muscles, the patient is placed in supine position and the unaffected leg is flexed at hip and knee joint as fully as possible. This will stretch the opposite iliopsoas muscles (extended leg). To stretch the iliopsoas muscles, the therapist should not extend the operated hip joint as it may cause implant to dislocate.

x. ***Exercises to Improve Hip and Knee Flexion:*** After hip joint arthroplasty there is severe reflexive spasm in the quadriceps muscles which limit the hip and knee flexion. In supine ICE towel or ICE pack is placed along the length of the quadriceps muscles and reciprocal inhibition is started. The technique is very much effective particularly in severe muscle spasm conditions where contract relax or hold relax are not possible. In this technique, to break the spasm in the quadriceps, the knee and hip is flexed as much as possible. The position is held and simultaneous strong isometric contraction of hip extensor and hamstrings are also performed. These isometric contractions will help in relieving quadriceps and iliopsoas muscle spasm, which improves hip and knee flexion. After 3-5 days of significant improvement in quadriceps muscle spasm, the reciprocal inhibition is progressed to hold relax and contract relax exercises. Passive stretching sometimes increases the muscle spasm hence, should be administered with caution.

25

SHOULDER INJURIES

STABILITY OF THE SHOULDER

Shoulder comprises 20 muscles, 3 bony articulations, 3 soft tissue moving surfaces (functional joints) that permit the greatest mobility of any joint area found in the body. The large humeral head articulates with the glenoid fossa. The support and stabilization of the shoulder joint primarily depends upon the static and dynamic stabilizers. The static stabilizers are the non-contractile structures such as—coracohumeral ligament, glenohumeral ligament, joint capsule and labrum itself. Osseous stability of the glenohumeral joint is enhanced by the fibrocartilaginous labrum, which functions to enlarge and deepen the glenoid socket while increasing the conformity of the articulating surfaces. The dynamic stabilizers are the contractile structures basically rotator cuff muscles. These stabilizers (static and dynamic) keep the head of humerus in the glenoid fossa and prevent excessive translation of head of humerus to the anterior, posterior and superior directions. The mobility is however at the expense of structural stability (Figs. 25.1a to c).

Masten *et al.* Describe Following Concepts of the Stability of the Shoulder

Balance, concavity and compression, superior stability, adhesion-cohesion, glenohumeral suction cup, limited joint volume and capsuloligamentous constraints.

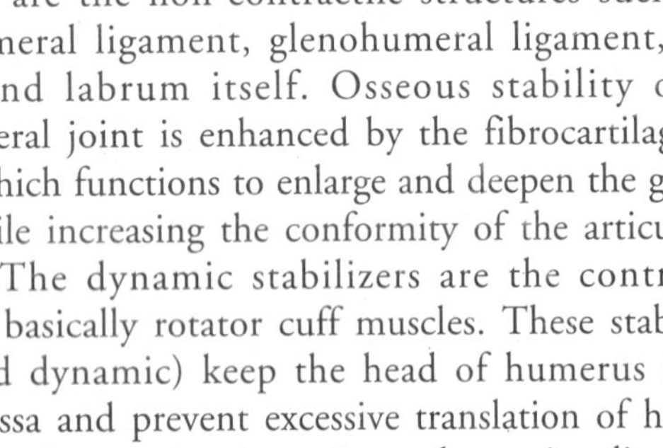

Fig. 25.1a: Static stabilizers of shoulder

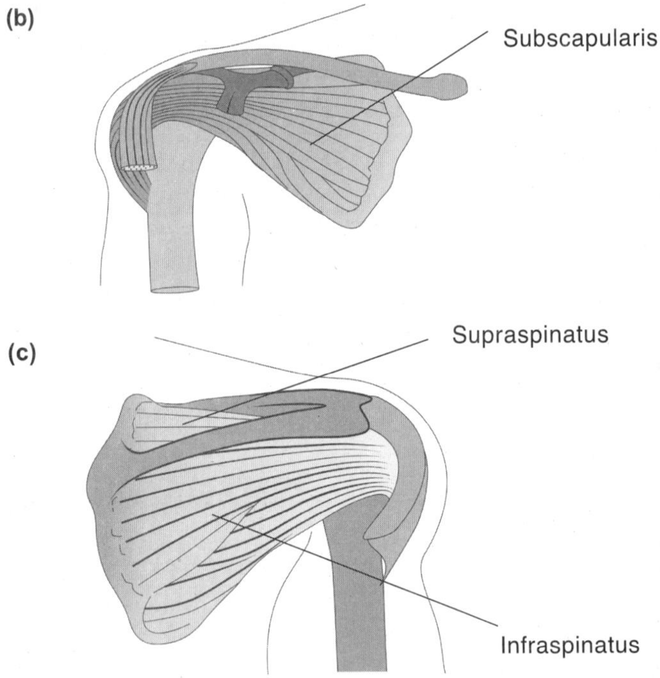

Fig. 25.1b and c: Dynamic stabilizers

Balance

Balance refers to the passage of the net joint-reaction force on the humeral head through the center of the glenoid fossa. The key components of balance include alignment of the humerus with the glenoid center line, facilitated by the surface arcs and areas of the glenoid and humeral head and by the muscles that position the glenoid and humerus relative to each other—namely, the rotator cuff and scapular stabilizers. The balance can be affected by the area of the glenoid, malalignment of the scapula and muscular imbalance.

Concavity and Compression

This refers to the stabilizing effect of the depth of the concave glenoid fossa on translation of the convex humeral head. The concavity and compression concept is strengthened by the three factors:

a. Increased thickness of the glenoid articular surface at the periphery of the glenoid relative to its center.
b. Glenoid labrum; and
c. Compressive forces produced by the rotator cuff muscles on the joint.

Superior Stability

It refers to the superior stability of the glenoid cavity, that plays major role in resisting proximal migration of the humeral head. During elevation of the arm the deltoid pulls the head of humerus up and superiorly which is resisted by the rotator cuff muscles and the superior stability of the shoulder. Therefore, even with a torn rotator cuff muscles (supraspinatus) this component can resist the upward migration of the head of the humerus. The superior stability of the shoulder can be affected by the deficient superior glenoid and the biceps labral anchorage.

Adhesion-Cohesion

Adhesion-cohesion is a mechanism by which fluid on coated articular surfaces provides an intrinsic adherence between the articular surfaces. The adhesion-coherent mechanism may be affected by changes in the fluid chemistry due to inflammatory disease, loss of thickness of the articular surfaces due to degenerative disease, and alterations in the contact areas.

Glenohumeral Suction Cup

The glenohumeral suction cup effect depends upon the tendency for matched concave and convex surfaces with a flexible periphery to center and stabilize after expressing any intervening air and fluid, thereby forming a seal. Deficiencies of the glenoid labrum or of the margin of the glenoid can adversely affect this stabilizing mechanism.

Limited Joint Volume

The normal glenohumeral joint is a potential space which has minimal synovial fluid and has an inherent negative pressure. A sealed joint ensures an increase in this negative pressure with attempted distraction, thus increasing the joint reactive force independent of other muscular forces. The stability of the shoulder is decreased if the synovial fluid is increased due to trauma, inflammation, and laxity of the capsule.

Capsuloligamentous Restraints

The joint capsule and ligaments surrounding of it provides static stability not only during the elevation but also during the rest when the arm is at side. The other concepts of Masten and *et al.* (balance, concavity and compression, superior stability, adhesion-cohesion, glenohumeral suction cup, and limited joint volume) contribute to the stability particularly during the midrange but the capsuloligamentous restraints contribute to the stability throughout the range of motion. The glenohumeral ligaments are ideally positioned thickenings within the capsule that serve to check large forces encountered within the capsule during specific arm positions and activities. The laxity of the capsuloligamentous restraints produces instability.

Movements

Shoulder is one of the complex joints in the body which requires smooth and coordinated movement of the sternoclavicular, acromioclavicular and scapulothoracic joints. The elevation of shoulder requires 30° to 40° elevation of clavicle and 60° external rotation of scapula. The scapula forms a stable base from which all shoulder movements occur, therefore, correct positioning of scapula on the thoracic wall is an essential for efficient and powerful glenohumeral joint movements. Abnormal scapula alignment and movement (dyskinesis) may result in pain in the shoulder joint with difficulty in overhead movements of the arm.

The shoulder permits greatest mobility in almost all directions. The mobility is, however, at the expense of structural stability. The following important movements take place in the shoulder during overhead activities mentioned in Table 25.1.

Table 25.1

Movement	*Plane*	*ROM*	*Muscles*
Flexion	Sagittal	0°-180°	Prime movers - Deltoid (anterior) secondary movers - Biceps brachii, Pectoralis major
Extension	Sagittal	0°-45°	Prime movers - Deltoid (posterior) Secondary movers - Latissimus dorsi
Abduction	Frontal	0°-180°	Prime movers - Deltoid middle secondary movers - Supraspinatus
Adduction	Frontal	180°-0°	Prime movers - Latissimus dorsi
External rotation	Transverse	0°-90°	Prime movers - Supraspinatus, infraspinatus
Internal rotation	Transverse	0°-80°	Prime movers - Subscapularis
Horizontal adduction		90°-45°	Prime movers - Pectoralis major

Rarely does a single muscle act in isolation at the shoulder complex. Muscles work in "Teams" to produce a highly coordinated action that is expressed over multiple joints. Because of the nature of the functional relationship among muscles, paralysis or weakness of any muscle often disrupts the natural kinematics sequencing of the shoulder.

Scapulohumeral Rhythm

In 1934, the term scapulohumeral rhythm was introduced by Codman to describe the smooth, integrated movement of the humerus, scapula and clavicle.

During elevation of the arm smooth coordinated 120 degrees movement occurs at the humerus and 60 degrees at the scapula to the total movement of 180 degrees of elevation of the arm (Fig. 25.2).

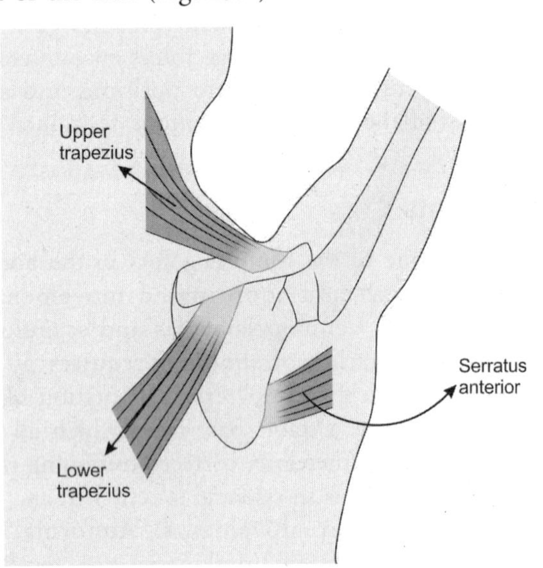

Fig. 25.2: Scapulohumeral rhythm

Scapulohumeral rhythm is divided into three phases as initial phase (0 and 60 degrees), middle phase or critical phase (60 to 140 degrees) and final phase (140 to 180 degrees).

Initial Phase of Elevation: The initial phase of elevation is referred as setting phase of the elevation. The instantaneous centre of rotation (ICR) is located near the root of the scapula. The relative contribution from scapula rotation during this phase is considerably less than from glenohumeral (3.29:1). The pull of deltoid produces an upward shear force on the humeral head, which is counteracted by the transverse compressive forces of the rotator cuff muscles. The sternoclavicular joint permits movement at the scapula by rotating 4 degrees for each of 10 degree rotation of the shoulder abduction. Movement in the acromioclavicular joint occurs in the thirty degrees of the initial phase, thereafter; it ceases and reoccurs at 135 degree of elevation.

Middle Phase of Elevation: This phase is also known as critical phase as shear and transverse forces are generated at the peak level in this phase. The deltoid continues to produce upward shear and noted maximum at 110 degrees. Supraspinatus activity peaks at 100 degrees of elevation and rapidly diminishes thereafter whereas subscapularis activity decreases substantially after 130 degrees. In addition to that the movement at the scapula takes place more than the humeral rotation at this phase.

The resultant acting force at 90 degrees of elevation with shear and compressive forces equals. The greatest relative motion at scapula occurs between 80 and 140 degrees of arm abduction and the rotation of glenohumeral to scapulohumeral has been calculated to be 7.1 to 1 in the critical phase of elevation. This important external rotation of the scapula during critical phase is mainly provided by the force couple generated by trapezius upper fibers and levator scapulae (upper portion) and serratus anterior and lower fibres of trapezius (lower portion). During the middle phase of elevation, ICR of scapula begins to migrate towards the acromioclavicular joint. Movement in the acromioclavicular joint reoccurs after 135 degrees.

Final Phase (140-180 degrees): The movement at the scapula decreases considerably during this phase and mostly movement occur at the glenohumeral joint at the ratio of 1:3.49. The rotator force arm of the upper trapezius muscles are just supportive at this stage, however lower trapezius muscles and serratus anterior continues to increase in activity during the final phase of elevation acting as upward rotator and opposing the force of the upper and middle trapezius.

ANTERIOR INSTABILITY

The term "shoulder instability" constitutes a spectrum of disorders that includes dislocation, subluxation and laxity. Anterior instability is the most common form of glenohumeral instability and may be associated with nerve injury. The head of humerus may excessively translate into anteriorly, posteriorly or inferiorly. Multidirectional instability is the combination of two or more than one instability.

Laxity: Laxity is defined as an unwanted translation of the head of humerus with symptoms. However, laxity may be considered as a normal translation of the head of humerus in the glenoid fossa if it is asymptomatic.

Subluxation: Subluxation is a partial loss of the articulation to the degree that symptoms are produced. It is caused by repetitive trauma, or direct blow to the shoulder.

Dislocation: Dislocation is defined as complete loss of the humeral articulation with the glenoid fossa as a result of acute trauma or seizures. The shoulder may dislocate anteriorly, posteriorly or inferiorly.

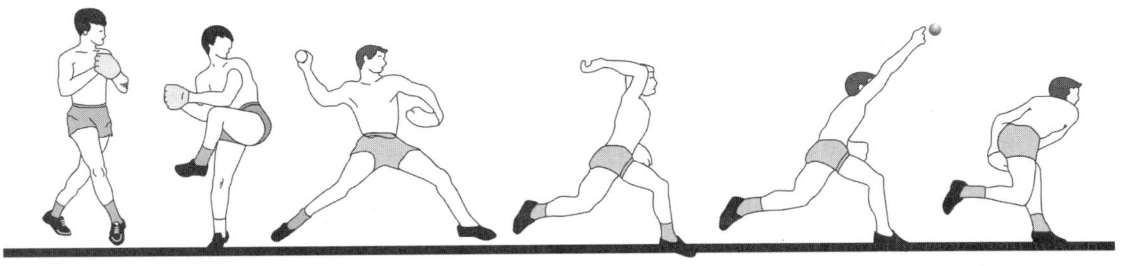

Fig. 25.3: Throwing phases

Anterior Instability in Overhead Athletes

During elevation of the arm the head of humerus is maintained in the glenoid fossa by the static and dynamic stabilizers. The shoulder sacrifices stability for the mobility and, as a result is the most common unstable joint in the body. Anterior instability is an unwanted translation of the head of the humerus anteriorly with respect to the glenoid fossa.

Over 90% instability of shoulder occur anteriorly, usually with the arm in abduction and external rotation. This position abduction and external rotation represents the "weakest position" of the glenohumeral biomechanically and is the "classic position" for anterior instability.

Overhead athletic activities require repetitive motions with the arm in at least 90º of flexion or abduction with an external rotation of the shoulder (Fig. 25.3).

The throwing motion and its related biomechanics is divided into its six stages—wind up, early cocking, late cocking, acceleration, deceleration and follow through. In late cocking when the body rapidly moves forward, the dominant shoulder achieves maximal abduction and external rotation. Significant torque and forces are placed on the anterior stabilizers of the shoulder. At the extreme elevation (flexion/abduction) with external rotation head of humerus pushes anterior stabilizers (anterior joint capsule, anterior glenohumeral and coracohumeral ligaments) into anteriorly. Prolonged repetitive stresses on the anterior stabilizers can cause hyperlaxity of the capsule and glenohumeral ligament (anterior stabilizers) and eventually there is an excessive anterior translation of the head of humerus. The posterior capsule becomes tight which limits the internal rotation.

Due to anterior instability the rotator cuff muscles develop secondary inflammatory response (rotator cuff tendinitis). Rotator cuff tendinitis produces pain in the shoulder. The stabilizing ability of the rotator cuff muscles decreases. At the end, the shoulder joint loses its static and dynamic stability; there is excessive translation of the head of humerus, further contributing to the instability.

Clinical Features

Athletes usually complain pain in the anterior aspect of the shoulder joint. In the late cocking phase they experience apprehension and sometimes hold the shoulder with the non-dominant hand in the adduction position. Pain may referred down the lateral arm. The internal rotation is decreased due to posterior joint capsule tightness. In neglected cases the range of motion may decrease in all three planes.

Assessment

The shoulder girdle is observed from anterior, posterior and lateral views.

Anterior View: The shoulder girdle is viewed from anterior for:

(i) Swelling, subluxation and dislocation of glenohumeral, sternoclavicular, and acromioclavicular joints; and

(ii) Wasting of pectoralis major, deltoid and biceps brachii.

Lateral View: The examiner should observe excessive protraction of the scapula and sulcus sign. A depression between humeral head and acromian arch indicates inferior subluxation of the head of humerous. The position of the head on the cervical spine is also viewed from lateral view.

Posterior View: The shoulder girdle is viewed from back for:

(i) Scapulothoracic joint: The medial border of the scapula extends from spinous process of second thoracic vertebra to spinous process of seventh vertebra. The inferior angle and medial border of the scapulae should be equidistance from the spine. The scapula rests on the thoracic wall. Weakness of serratus anterior allows medial border of scapula to move away from the thoracic wall which is known as winging of the scapula. Sometimes the parascapular muscles are not developed fully or they are replaced by fibrous band; allows scapula to displace superiorly (high), the condition is termed as Sprengel's scapula (high) or descended scapula. Usually affected scapula is smaller and medially rotated than normal.

(ii) Scapular postural changes such as downward rotation, and anterior tilting should also be observed as these are consistent with the shoulder pain and instability. The long term changes in muscle length correspond to long term changes is scapular posture. The patients with downward rotation of scapula present with the medial border of scapula closer to the thoracic midline than the corresponding superior medial border. These patients have insufficient scapula upward rotation, essential for the overhead activities.

(iii) Wasting or weakness of scapular muscles supraspinatus, infraspinatus and parascapular muscles serratus anterior muscle, rhomboid, trapezius middle and lower fibres is also viewed from posterior view.

Active Movements: Active range of motion of the glenohumeral and scapulothoracic joints should be observed carefully.

Resisted Isometric Movements: To reproduce the symptoms, the muscles are contracted isometrically against the resistance. Isometric movements elicit pain if there is tendinitis or impingement.

Passive Movements: Passive movements are performed to reproduce the symptoms if active movements fails to do so. The passive movements are performed to examine the end feel, muscle tightness and contracture. The movements are performed in relaxed position with proper stabilization of the scapula as lot of trick movements are possible in the shoulder joint.

Palpation: The glenohumeral, sternoclavicular and acromioclavicular joints are examined for tenderness. Therapist can use thumb or pisiform aspect of the wrist to apply pressure on the joint, if patient complains pain the site is suspected for possible area of pain and symptoms.

Test for Anterior Instability

Stability of the shoulder is provided by static and dynamic stabilizers. Static stabilizers are the non-contractile structures such as coracohumeral ligament, glenohumeral ligament, acromioclavicular ligament, joint capsule and labrum itself. The dynamic stabilizers are basically rotator cuff muscles such as supraspinatus, infraspinatus, teres minor and subscapularis. Weakness or laxity of these stabilizers may cause shoulder instability and may produce symptoms such as pain, instability and apprehension. The following maneuvers are performed to test the stability of the shoulder:

Apprehension Test (Crank Test)

This test is performed to evaluate the anterior stability of the shoulder. Test may be performed in supine, standing or sitting position but supine lying is preferred over standing and sitting as patient feels more comfortable and relaxed (Fig. 25.4).

Position of Patient: Supine, shoulder at the edge of table.

Position of Examiner: Stands at the side of the shoulder which is being examined. The examiner holds the elbow of the patient at 90° of flexion and abducts the shoulder to 90° with slight horizontal abduction.

Procedure: While maintaining the above position the examiner brings the shoulder into external rotation, and further, abduction and horizontal abduction is added. This position simulates the most common position of subluxation or dislocation in the patient with symptomatic anterior instability. In case of anterior instability the patient reacts by expressing concern or anxiety or apprehension, and sometimes, prevents the external rotation with other hand. This test produces pain in patients with subtle cases of anterior instability, but it does not produce true anxiety or apprehension. Pain is a suggestive but not diagnostic of anterior instability. For diagnosis of anterior instability patient must complain apprehension; therefore the test has modified into relocation and release test.

Relocation Test: It is the extension of the anterior apprehension test. To perform this, the examiner places the shoulder joint in the apprehension position (abduction, horizontal abduction and external rotation), until the patient feels apprehension or pain. While maintaining this position the examiner places the free hand on the anterior aspect of the shoulder joint and then the head of humerus is pushed posteriorly into the glenoid fossa. This relocates the head of humerus from subluxed position to glenoid fossa. If patient reports reduction or resolution in apprehension, then it confirms the anterior instability. After pushing the head of humerus into the glenoid fossa the apprehension disappears and now the shoulder can be abducted, externally rotated and extended further (Fig. 25.5).

Release Test: It is the sequence of the relocation test. When the posterior directed force is released gradually the symptoms of apprehension returns which further confirms the anterior instability of the shoulder joint (Fig. 25.6).

Anterior Drawer Test

Anterior drawer test is performed to draw the head of humerus anteriorly against the anterior stabilizers. Normally, it is resisted by the anterior stabilizers.

Position of Patient: Sitting with the arm hanging loosely.

Position of Examiner: Standing at the side of shoulder joint. To test the right shoulder joint the examiner stabilizes the scapula with left hand and holds the head of humerus with right hand. While maintaining the position the head of humerus is pushed anteriorly. In normal subject the head of humerus may be translated anteriorly upto 25% of the width of the glenoid. If the head of humerus can be translated more than 25% of the width of the glenoid then test is considered positive for anterior instability. Patient

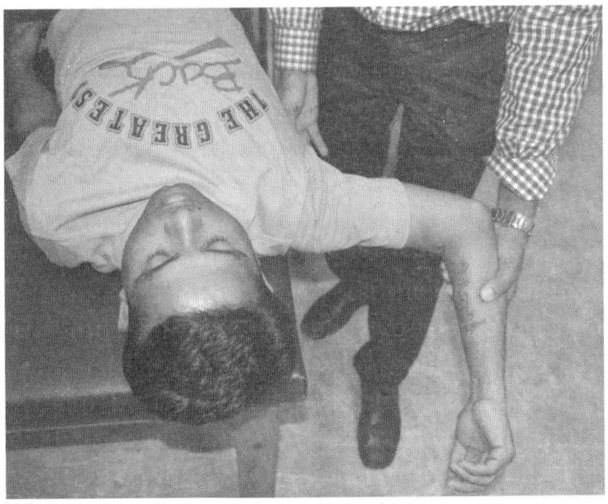

Fig. 25.4: Anterior apprehension test (crank test for anterior instability of the shoulder joint)

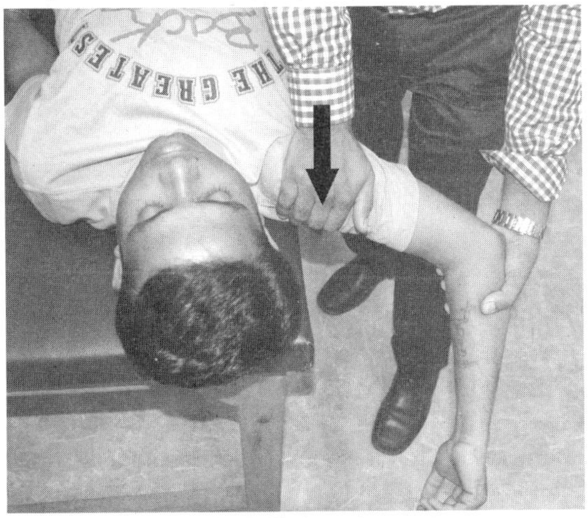

Fig. 25.5: Relocation test

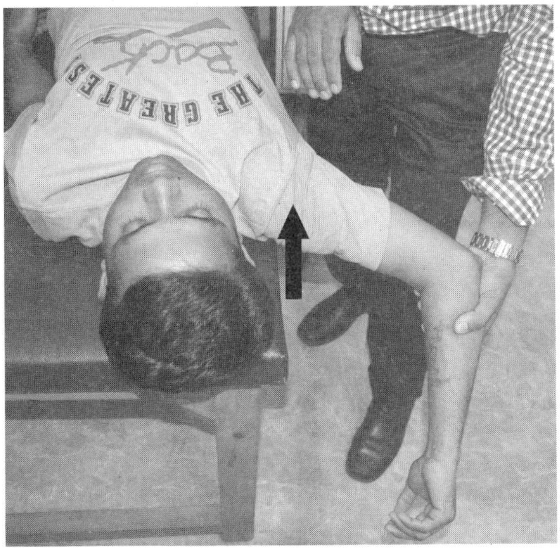

Fig. 25.6: Release test

may complain apprehension. To test the posterior instability a posterior directed force is applied to translate the head of humerus posteriorly. In normal subjects the head of humerus can be translated posteriorly upto 50% of the width of the scapula. In case of more than 50% translation of the width of the glenoid a posterior instability may be considered (Fig. 25.7).

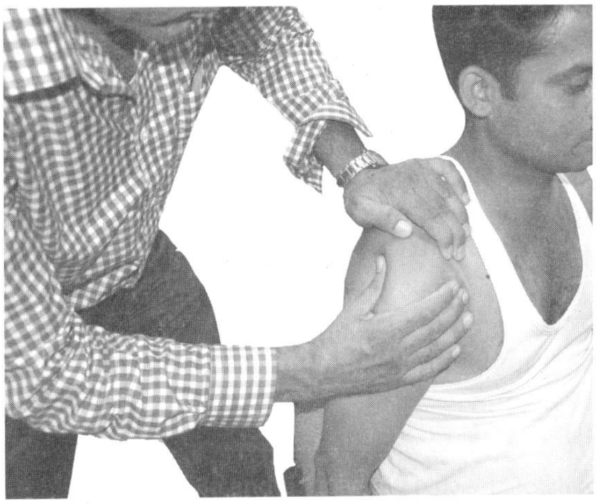

Fig. 25.7: Anterior drawer test

Load and Shift Test

This test is similar to the anterior drawer test but it is performed in supine position with slight abduction range.

Position of Patient: Supine, shoulder is slightly out of the plinth with slight abduction and extension.

Position of Therapist: Standing at the side which is being examined, facing the shoulder joint (anteriorly). To examine the patient's right shoulder, the examiner holds the forearm with right hand and grasps the head of humerus with left hand (Figs. 25.8a and b).

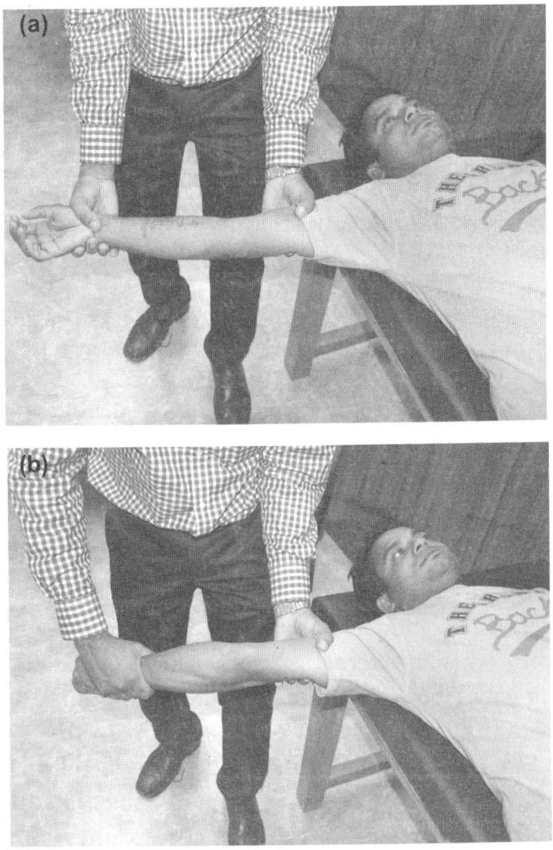

Figs. 25.8a and b: Load and shift test

Procedure: While maintaining above position (slight abduction and extension) an anterior head of humerus directed force is applied with the right hand to translate anteriorly. The amount of translation is assessed as in the anterior drawer test. The position of shoulder may be changed until the position of greatest laxity is found. For posterior instability the head of humerus is pushed posteriorly and an amount of translation is assessed as in the posterior drawer test. The test may be performed in various positions until the position of greatest laxity is found.

Management

The goals of the therapist are of restoring shoulder stability (static and dynamic), and reducing pain, apprehension and improving strength of rotator cuff and parascapular muscles.

Immobilization: The patients with anterior instability rarely require shoulder immobilization. It may be advised if the patient complaints pain and apprehension in the painful arc with rotator cuff tendinopathy. The shoulder is immobilized in the sling just to avoid the overhead activities. However, passive range of motion may be performed throughout the range of motions.

Precaution: The athlete must take precautions to avoid stress on the anterior stabilizers of the shoulder such as anterior joint capsule, anterior glenohumeral ligament and coracohumeral ligament. Patient must avoid extreme ranges of elevation with external rotation until shoulder achieves pain free stability. Shoulder hyperextension is contraindicated as it stretches the anterior stabilizers.

Relief of Pain: To decrease pain, cold packs or hot packs can be used for 15-20 minutes per treatment session, thrice or twice daily. Interferential therapy with the frequency of 80-100 Hz over the shoulder girdle muscles may be beneficial in relieving pain and symptoms.

Strengthening Exercises

Sub maximal isometric exercises of biceps, deltoid, rotator cuff muscles, and parascapular muscles are started in pain free range. These muscles may also be strengthened with the surge faradic currents.

Rotator Cuff Strengthening: Rotator cuff strengthening should be started in the pain free range of motion. Isometric exercises in arm adducted position should be preferred over the overhead. For external rotators patient stands close to the wall with elbow flexion to 90 degrees. The dorsal aspect of the hand and forearm rests on the wall. While maintaining the position in the shoulder adduction patient rotates the shoulder externally against the wall for six seconds. Several repetitions of isometric contraction may be performed to strengthen the supraspinatus and infraspinatus muscles. To strengthen the subscapularis muscle (internal rotator) the patient places the palmar aspect of hand and forearm on the wall. While maintaining the shoulder in adduction, the patient rotates the shoulder internally against wall. Several repetitions of isometric contractions may be performed (Figs. 25.9a to h).

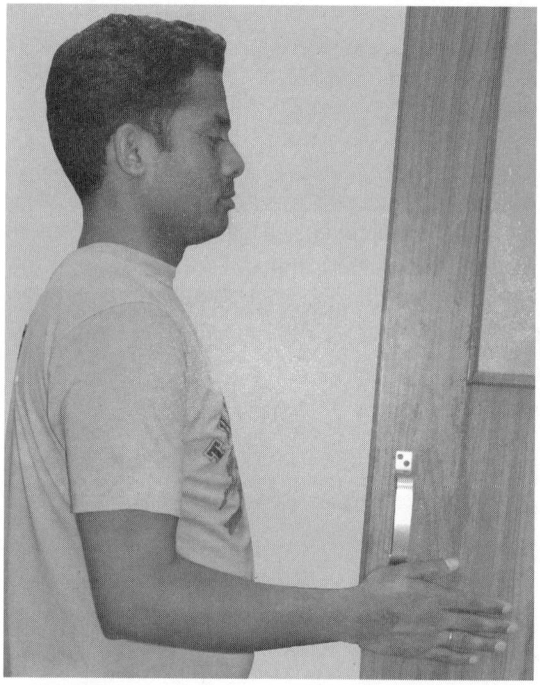

Fig. 25.9a: External rotators isometric strengthening against the wall in standing

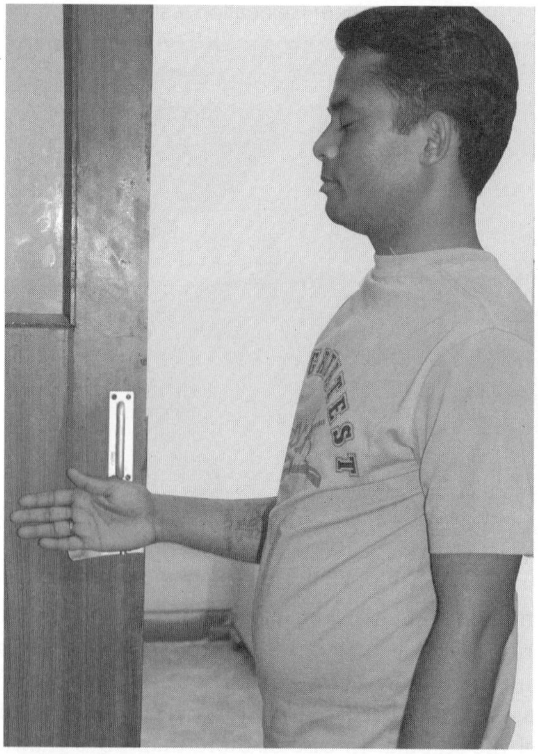

Fig. 25.9b: Internal rotators isometric strengthening against the wall in standing

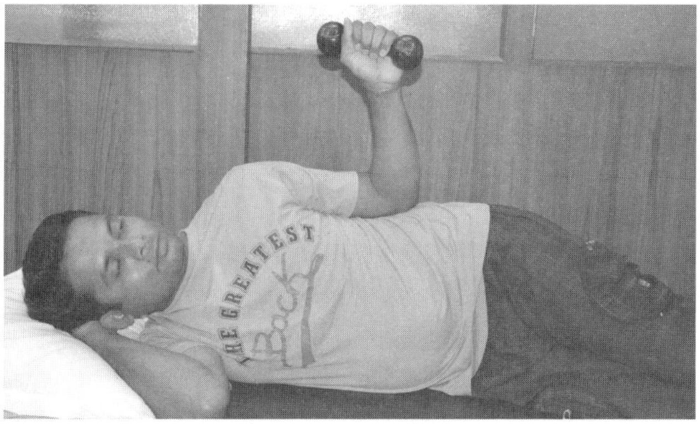

ig. 25.9c: External rotators strengthening in side lying with umbbell

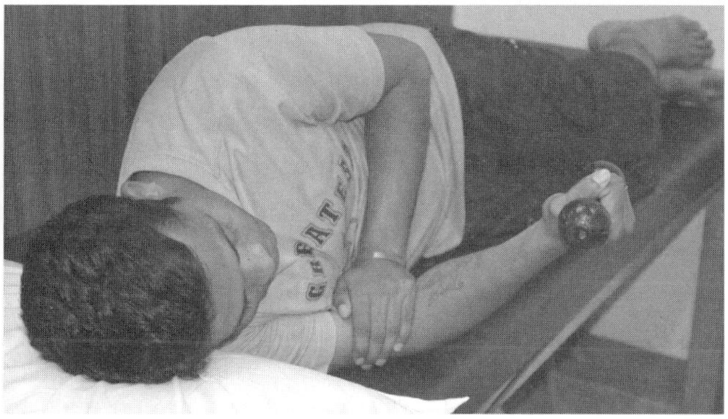

ig. 25.9d: Internal rotators isometric strengthening in side lying

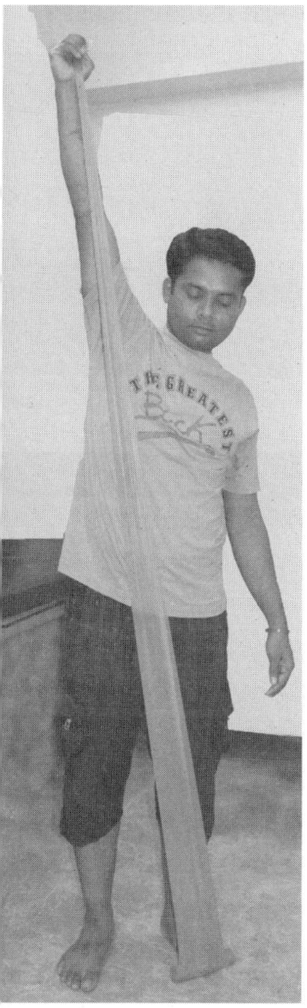

ig. 25.9e: Di flexion pattern ith theraband

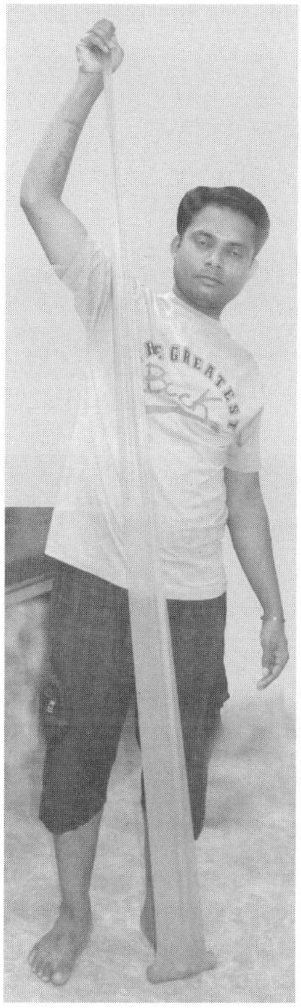

Fig. 25.9f: Diextension pattern with theraband

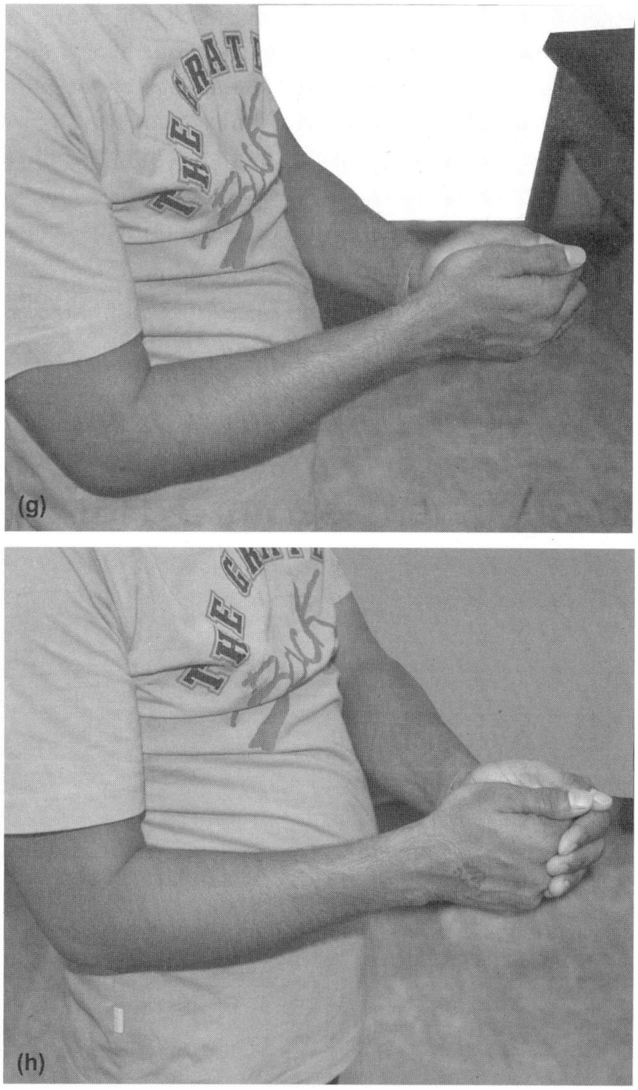

Figs. 25.9g and h: Self strengthening with resistance in sitting with elbow flexion. Other hand grasps the distal forearm

The strengthening of shoulder rotator culf muscles should begin in close kinetic chain. The close kinetic chain–exercises are preferred over the open kinetic as the joint is more stabilized in the position.

With the improvement in the sign and symptoms the exercise is progressed to the open kinetic chain exercise with the tubing, dumbbells or theraband. In standing position the patient places one end of the theraband under the opposite foot and holds the other end of the theraband. While maintaining the position the shoulder is flexed, abducted and rotated externally in the diagonal 2 pattern. Several repetitions may be performed.

Scapula Stabilizers Strengthening: To strengthen the levator scapulae, trapezius and rhomboids the patient lies in a sitting position with both the arms at the side of body. Patient holds the elbows with the hands. Forearms rests on the tummy. While maintaining the position the patient retracts both the shoulders. This exercise should be advised if there is pain in the overhead activities. As the symptoms improve the exercise is progressed to the prone lying. Patient lies prone with the shoulder out of the edge of the plinth and arm hanging downward. While maintaining the position patient elevates the arm in sagittal plane upto full range. The end range is held for at least six seconds followed by relaxation. In the next step the exercise is performed in the scaption plane, and then in the horizontal. Several repetitions are performed until the muscles go in a fatigue state. Exercises of both the scapula stabilizers may be performed in the same position with little modification. In prone position the head is taken out of the plinth. While maintaining the position of the head in line with the spine, both the shoulders are elevated in the scaption plane. With improvement of the strength the exercise may be performed with the light dumbbell (Figs. 25.10a to h).

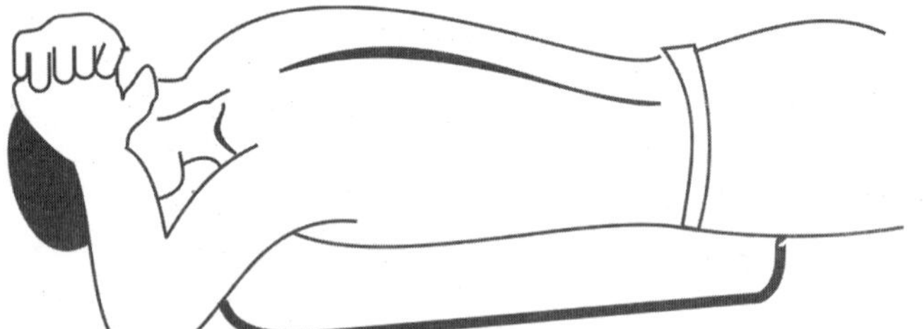

Fig. 25.10a: Trapezius and rhomboids strengthening, prone, head slightly out of the couch and hands on the occiput. Patient raises the elbows above the shoulder level and holds for the count of six. Thirty repetitions with brief rests between each ten repetitions. This exercise helps in strengthening of the rhomboid and middle trapezius

(b)

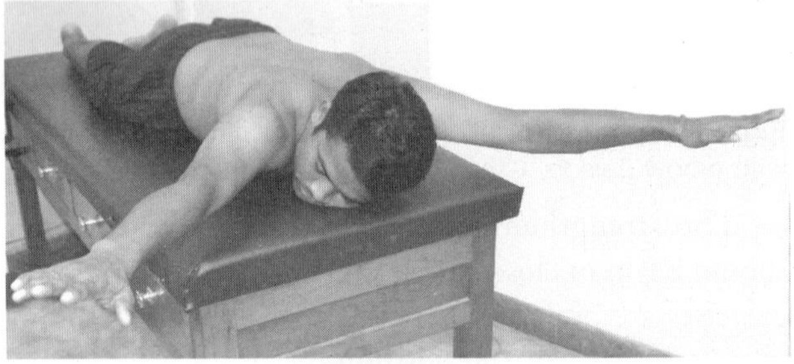

(c)

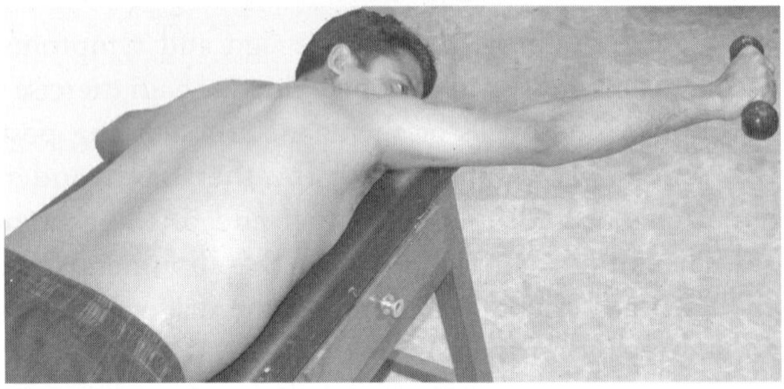

Figs. 25.10b and c: Prone, head is slightly out of the edge of the couch, shoulders are raised in a scaption plane with elbow extension. With the improvement over the time in the strength of the muscles the patient can lift the shoulders in scaption plane with the dumbbell. Thirty repetitions with brief rests between each ten repetitions. This exercise strengthens the trapezius lower fibers

(d)

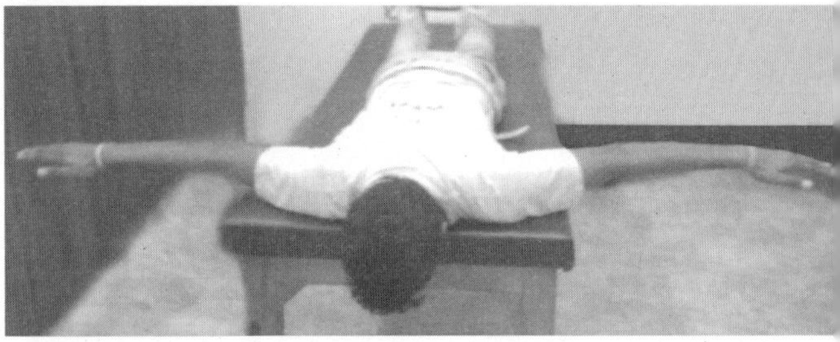

(e)

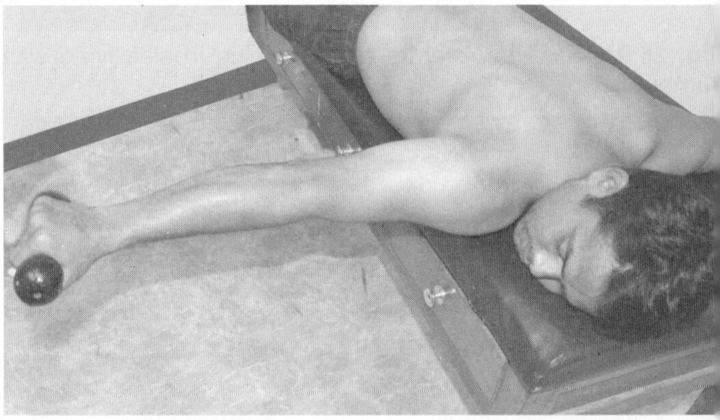

Figs. 25.10d and e: Prone, head is slightly out of the edge of th couch. Shoulders are raised horizontally to the level of shoulde blades. Thirty repetitions with brief rests between each te repetitions. This exercise helps in strengthening of the middl trapezius. With the improvement over the time in the strength c the muscle the exercise can be done with the dumbbells

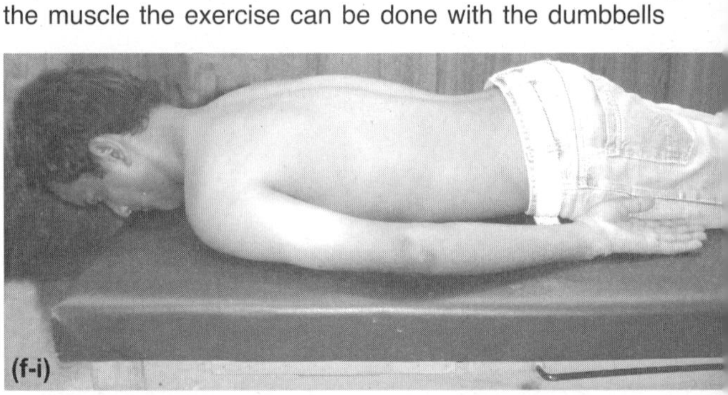

(f-i)

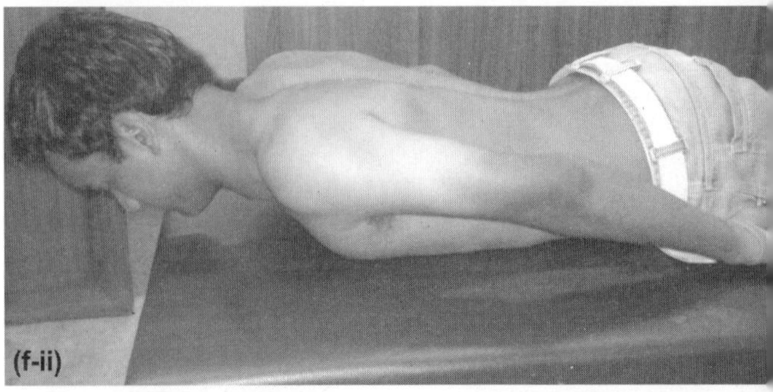

(f-ii)

Figs. 25.10f(i-ii): Prone with both the hands at the side of th body. Patient retracts the shoulders as much as possible withou changing the position of the hands. With the improvements i the strength, the therapist can apply resistance against th retraction. Thirty repetitions with brief rests between each te repetitions

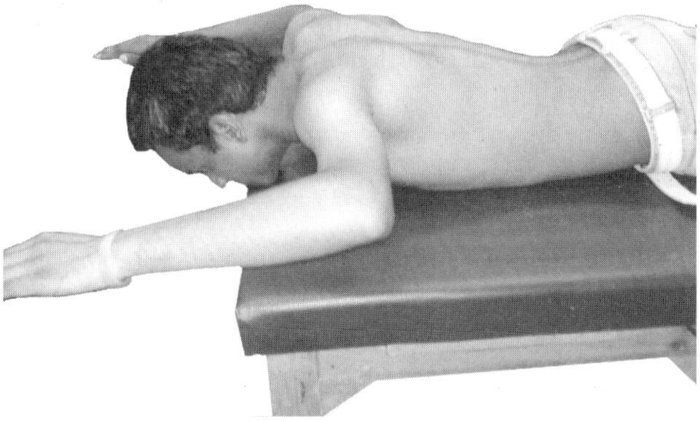

Fig. 25.10g: Prone with head slightly out of the edge of the couch. Elbows flexed to 90 degrees. Patient raises the shoulder horizontally above the shoulder blade level

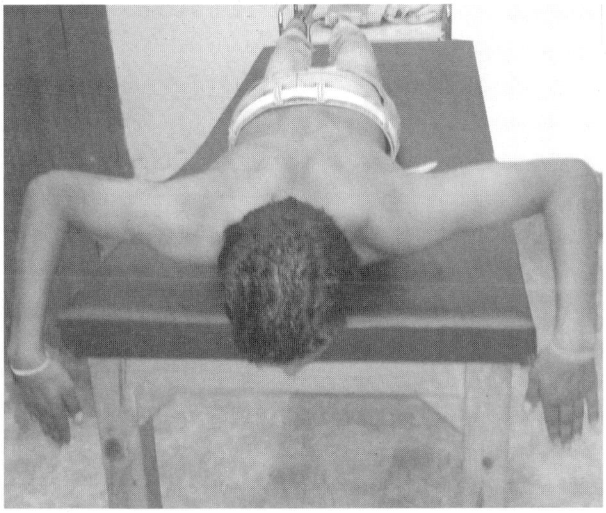

Fig. 25.10h: Rowing, rhomboid strengthening

Strengthening of the serratus anterior muscle is one of the major goals of the rehabilitation as its function is not only the stabilizing scapula on the thoracic wall but also plays important role in external rotation of the scapula. To strengthen the serratus anterior muscle the exercise should progress from minimal load. The patient lies in a quadruped with the hips and shoulders directly on the knees and hands respectively. Then the patient lifts the opposite hand off the plinth bringing to the level of the shoulder. The supported shoulder should not alter any position. While maintaining the quadruped position patient moves hips and shoulders forward on the knees and hands and then the opposite hand is lifted off the ground upto the level of the shoulder. In further progression patient is positioned in a quadruped position and hips are brought to the neutral by bending the knees while the shoulders remain on the hands. In the last step of exercise the patient assumes the quadruped position and then brings the hips and knees to the neutral position, now patient stationed on the hands and toes. The chest is brought to the floor by bending the elbows. Several repetitions are performed till the muscles fatigue (Figs. 25.11a to i).

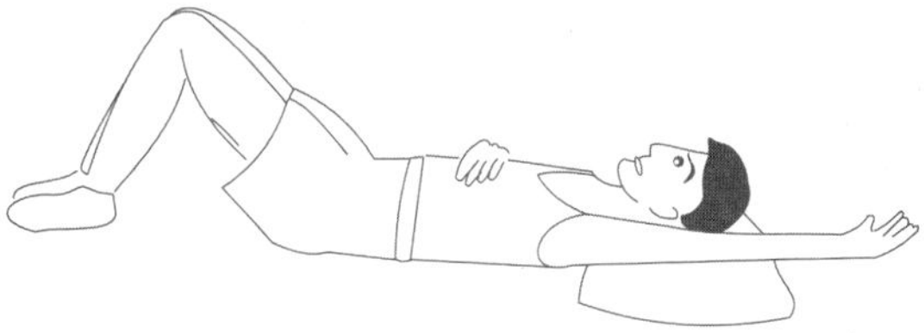

Fig. 25.11a: Serratus anterior strengthening, supine with knees flexion. Patient flexes and extends the shoulders alternately throughout the range of motion in a controlled manner

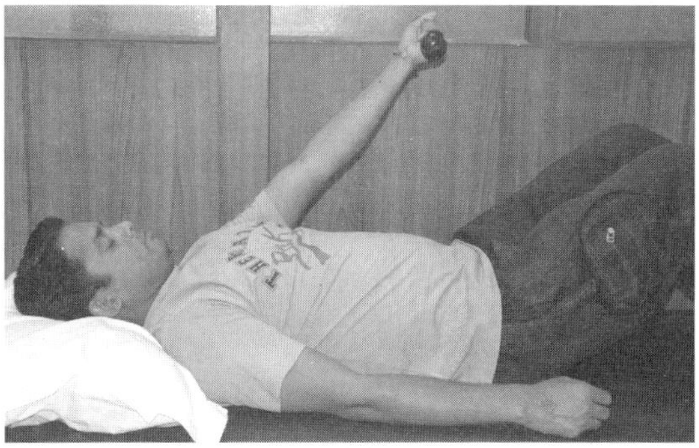

Fig. 25.11b: Supine with knees flexion. Patient flexes and extends the shoulder joint throughout the range of motion in a controlled manner with the dumbbell

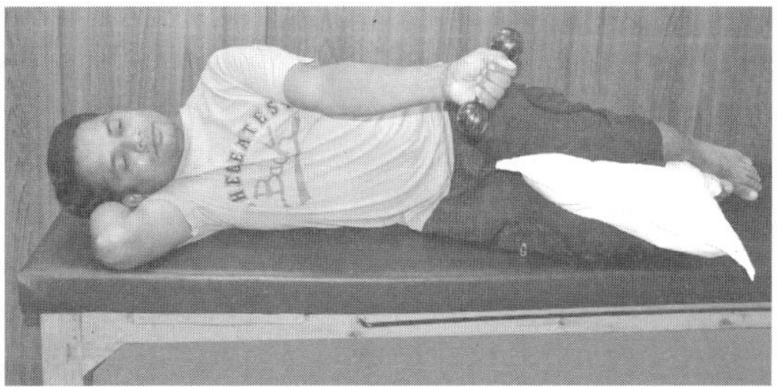

Fig. 25.11c: Side lying with pillows under the uppermost leg flexed. Patient flexes and extends the shoulder joint throughout the range of motion in a controlled manner in a scaption plane

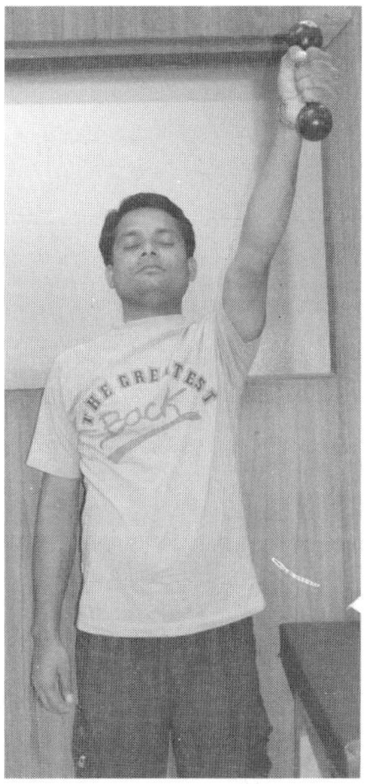

Fig. 25.11d: Sitting or standing with back supported on the wall. Patient flexes and extends the shoulder joint throughout the range of motion in a controlled manner with the dumbbell

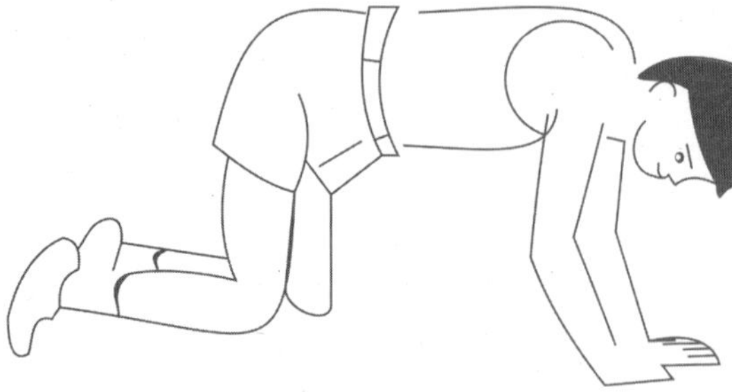

Fig. 25.11e: Quadruped position with hips directly over knees and shoulders directly over the hands

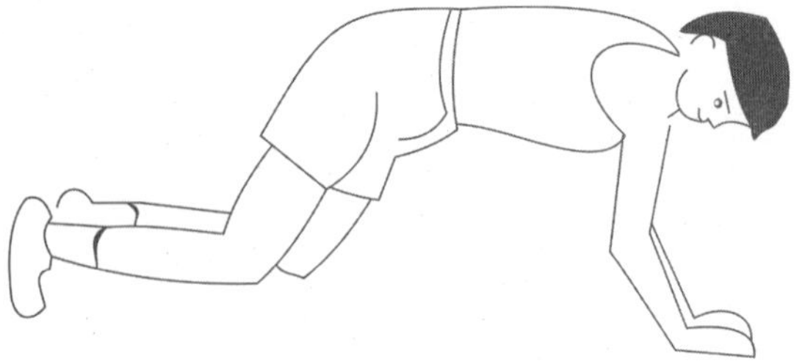

Fig. 25.11f: Quadruped position with hips slightly in front of the knees and shoulders directly over the hands

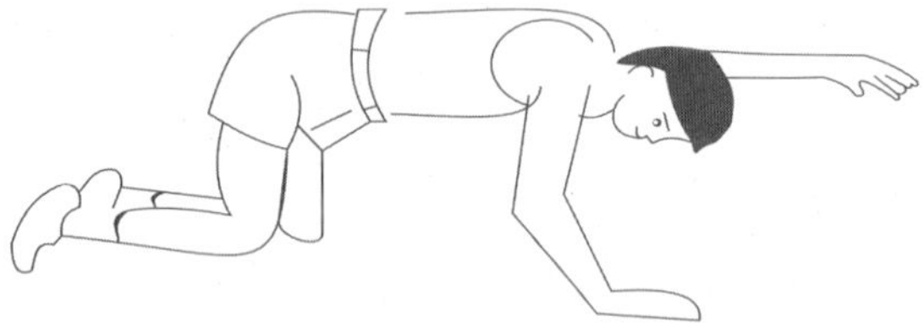

Fig. 25.11g: Quadruped position with hips slightly in front of the knees and shoulders directly over the hands and patient raises the arms alternately to the level of the shoulder

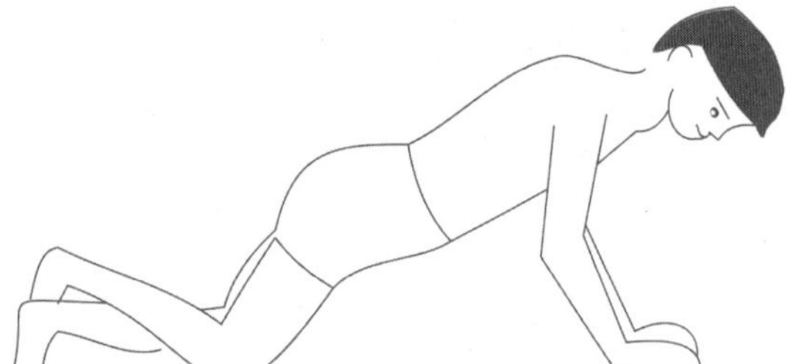

Fig. 25.11h: The weight of the body remains on the knees and hands

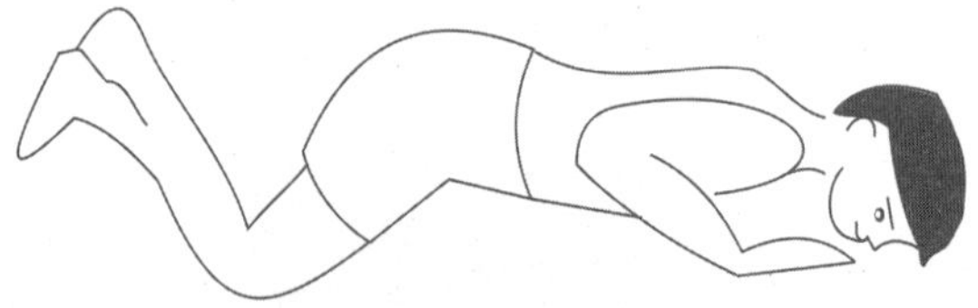

Fig. 25.11i: Push ups, while maintaining the position of the spine and hips at neutral, the patient slowly lowers the body towards the floor by flexing the elbow joints

Deltoid Strengthening: In standing position the patient abducts the shoulder with or without the dumbbell (Figs. 25.12a to e).

(a)

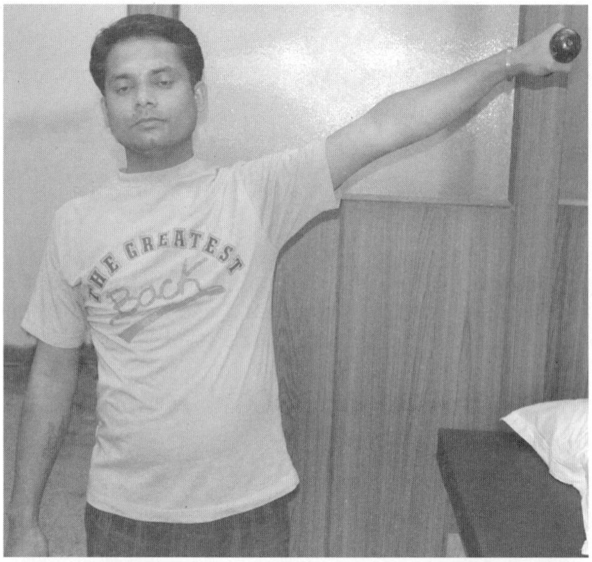

(b)

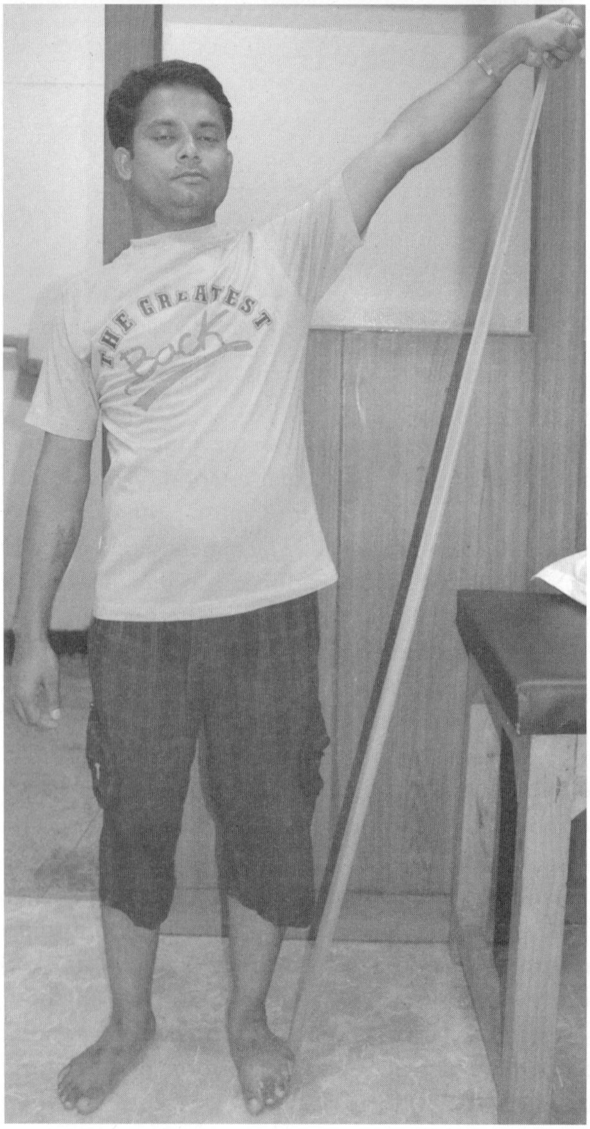

(c)

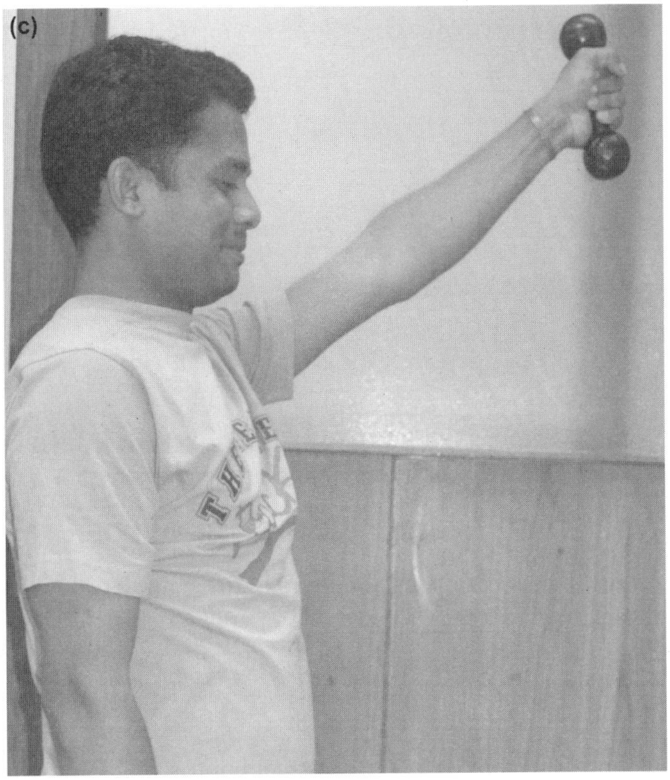

(e)

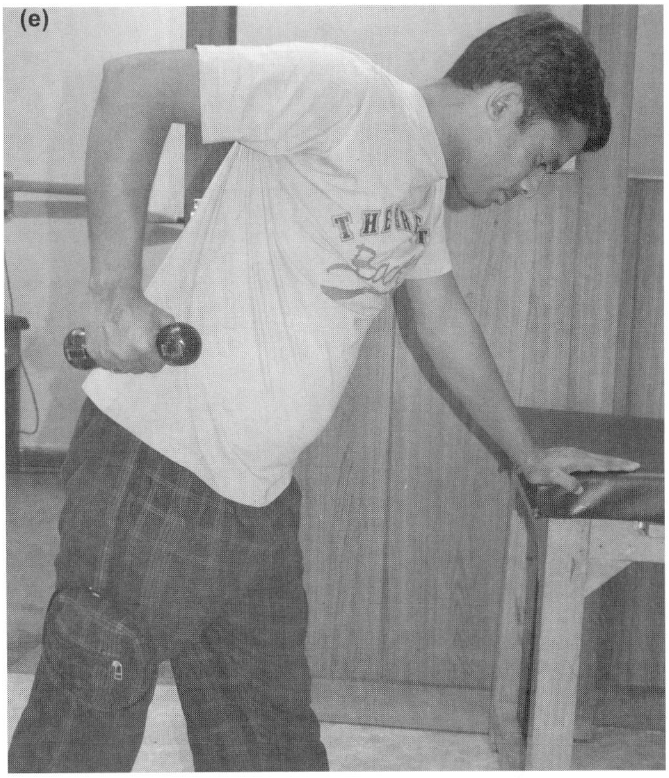

(d)

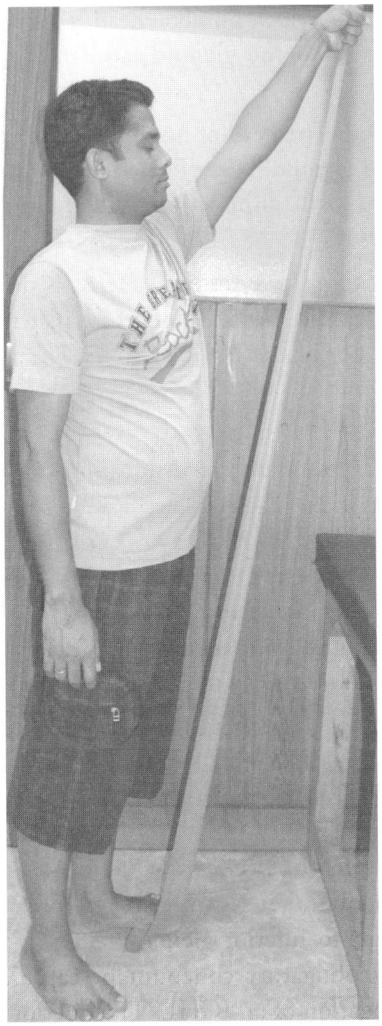

Figs. 25.12a to e: Deltoid strengthening

Biceps Strengthening: In standing or sitting position with the arm adducted the elbow joint is flexed with the appropriate weight of dumbbell (Figs. 25.13a and b).

(a)

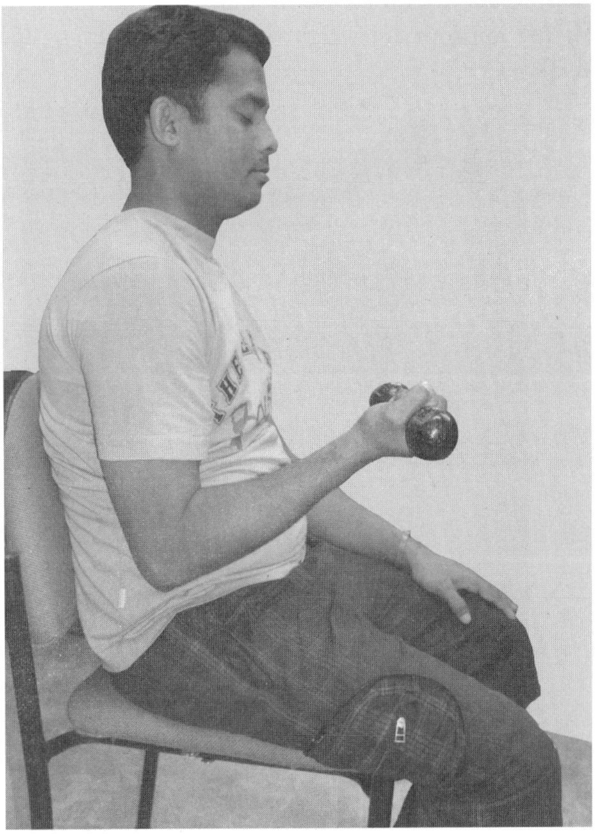

(b)

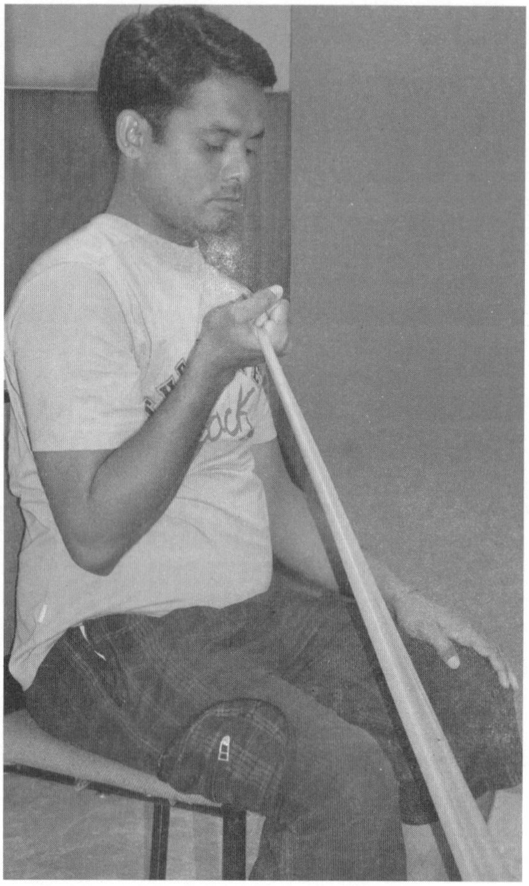

Figs. 25.13a and b: Biceps strengthening

Triceps Strengthening: In standing or sitting position with shoulder flexion the elbow joint is extended and flexed with the appropriate weight of dumbbell (Figs. 25.13c and d).

(c)

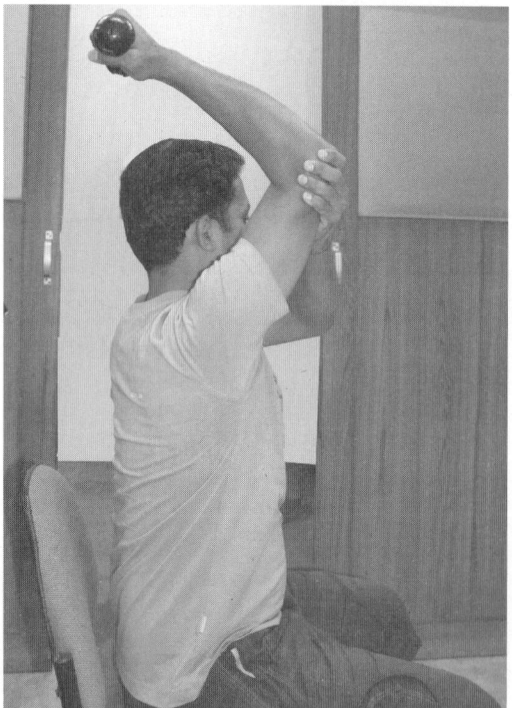

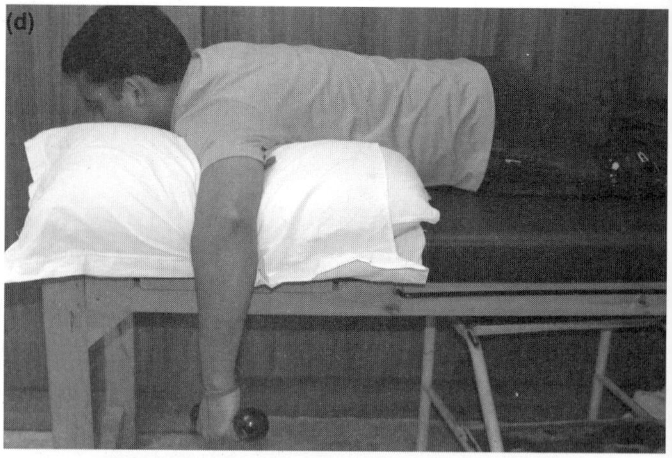

Figs. 25.13c and d: Triceps strengthening

ANTERIOR DISLOCATION OF SHOULDER

Anterior dislocation of shoulder is the complete loss of articulation between the head of humerus and glenoid fossa. The head of humerus is displaced anteriorly as the anterior stabilizers of glenohumeral joint disrupts. Anterior dislocation is of three types as described below:

a. **Sub-Coracoid:** It is the most common type of anterior dislocation in which humeral head is displaced anteriorly with respect to the glenoid, and inferior to coracoid process.

b. **Subglenoid:** The head of humerus is displaced anteriorly below the glenoid fossa. These types of dislocations are associated with either a glenoid fracture or anterior glenoid rim.

c. **Subclavicular:**The head of humerus is displaced medial to the coracoid process and rests just inferior to the lower border of the clavicle.

Pathophysiology

The patients with shoulder dislocation may present with many findings, such as Bankart lesion, Hill Sachs lesion, anterior glenoid rim damage, capsular redundancy, subscapularis deficiency, and glenoid fossa deficiency. These findings can occur alone or in combination with other lesions. Sometimes few patients may present with a history of anterior dislocation with absence of any pathological findings.

a. **Bankart Lesion:** In 1923, Bankart had described the "essential lesion" in patients with post traumatic anterior glenohumeral instability as the "detachment of the capsule from the fibrocartilaginous glenoid ligament". Avulsion of the anteroinferior glenoid labrum at its attachment to inferior glenohumeral ligament (IGHL) causes an obligatory concomitant capsular disruption, with elongation of an IGHL. The inferior glenohumeral ligament heals in redundant position in upto thirty percent patients; but no healing takes place in the disrupted avulsed anteroinferior glenoid labrum, which is the primary cause of recurrent dislocation of the shoulder. However, no single lesion is responsible for the recurrent dislocations of the traumatized shoulders. Baker *et al.* advised a system of classification for the Perthes-Bankart lesion as follows:

- Type I-Pure capsular lesion.
- Type II-Partial labral detachment.
- Type III-Complete detachment of the inferior glenohumeral labral complex.

b. **Hill Sachs Lesion:** This type of lesion occurs upto 40% in patients with anterior dislocation and upto 80% of recurrent anterior dislocations. The indentation fracture of the posterolateral humeral head occurs during this type of anterior dislocation of the shoulder. The head of humerus impacts against relatively hard anterior glenoid. Sometimes this lesion is confused with the normal bare area of the posteroinferior aspect of humeral head (Fig. 25.14).

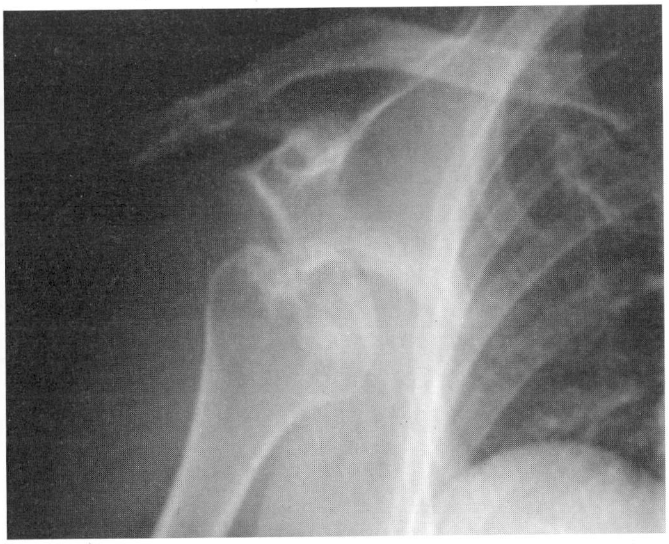

Fig. 25.14: Hill Sachs lesion

Epidemiology

First time shoulder dislocation can occur at any age although they tend to occur most frequently in the second and sixth decades. However, an average age of initial shoulder dislocation is in early thirties. Twenty-five percent patients with shoulder dislocation present with the family history of the similar problem (Fig. 25.15).

Mechanism

The shoulder joint may dislocate when a strong force such as a traumatic injury puts an excessive load on the labrum, capsule and ligaments. Ninety-five percent shoulder dislocations are resulted from a sudden wrenching movement during sport, by falling on to an outstretched arm, and from motor vehicle accidents. An individual falls on an outstretched hand, forcing the arm into abduction and external rotation, levering the humeral head out of the glenoid fossa. This is the most vulnerable position of the shoulder for dislocation.

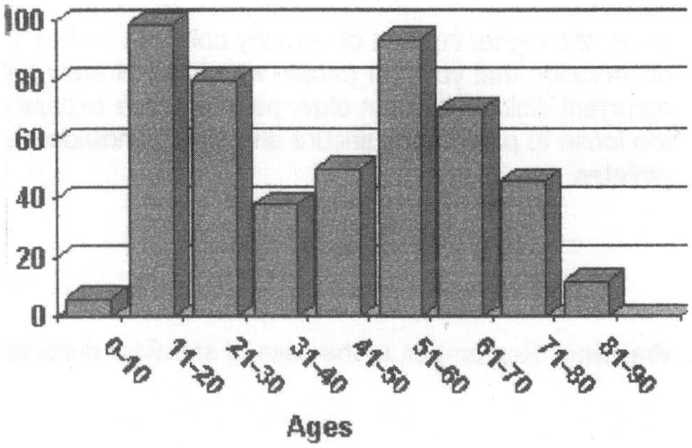

Fig. 25.15: Rate of shoulder dislocation according to the age

Clinical Features

Patient usually complaints apprehension or instability and often feel that he or she is at the risk of shoulder dislocation. They learn the positions that reproduce and ease the symptoms and tend to lean towards the affected side. The arm is held in the adduction and internal rotation positions by the contralateral extremity.

Patient experiences pain in the anterior aspect of the shoulder joint. It aggravates in abduction with external rotation and slight extension. These positions put excessive load on the joint capsule and ligament (IGHL). In long standing cases weakness and atrophy of the scapular and parascalar muscles with loss of motion in all three planes may also be seen.

Physical Examination

The shoulder joint is examined for pain, swelling, erythema, temperature, crepitus and range of motion. To test the anterior instability, anterior apprehension (crank test), relocation, release, and anterior drawer tests should be performed as these tests are having good sensitivity. The cross chest adduction test is also helpful in diagnosing anterior dislocation. In patients with anterior shoulder dislocation cross chest adduction will be limited and painful.

Imaging Studies

X-rays are taken in three views such as true AP view also known as Grashey view, scapula view and axillary view to confirm the anterior dislocation. Internal and external rotation views may also be taken as these provide oblique visualization of the shoulder joint, with the humeral head overlapping the glenoid rim. Stryker-Notch view is taken to confirm the Hill Sachs lesions. It is obtained with the patient supine. This view provides good details of the posterolateral margin of the humeral head. MRI is the choice of the imaging modality for soft tissue injury. It has 91% sensitive in detecting capsule-labral injury in the early post-dislocation phase (Fig. 25.16).

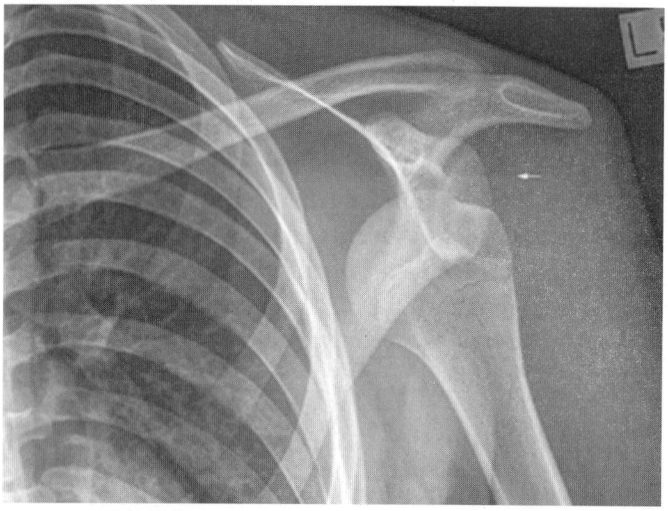

Fig. 25.16: X-ray anterior shoulder dislocation

Management

1. **Shoulder Reduction:** The dislocated shoulder is reduced as soon as possible. There are several techniques of reducing the shoulder. Early treatment of the shoulder dislocation should be directed to eliminate the static structure stretch, compression on the nerves, and muscle spasm. Some patient's shoulder reduced without the medication while others require muscle relaxants or anaesthesia. Many techniques have described by the physicians since hippocrates to reduce the shoulder dislocation few techniques are described as under:
   a. *Hippocrates Technique*: Hippocrates described the technique where physician placed his foot on the chest wall and used it as a counter traction. The arm is rotated internally and externally to disengage the head of the humerus.
   b. *Stimson's Technique*: The patient is positioned prone with the dislocated arm hanging freely out of the edge of the table. Approximately 5-6 pound weight is tied on the wrist. The shoulder is reduced after 15-20 minutes.
   c. *Milch's Technique*: The patient is positioned on the back. The dislocated arm is flexed and externally rotated. The therapist places his thumb on the head of humerus and gently pushes the head of humerus into the glenoid fossa (Fig. 25.17).

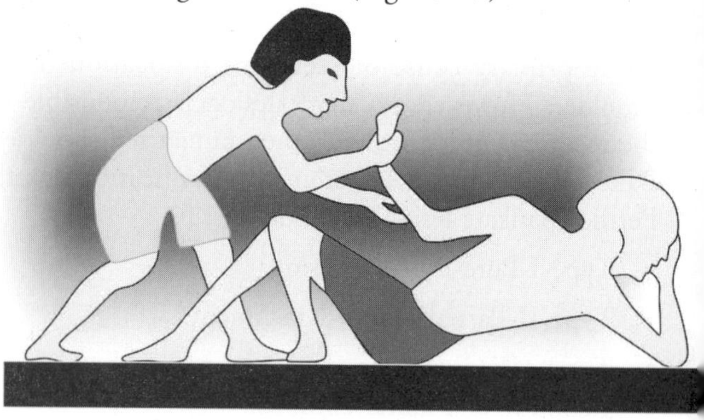

Fig. 25.17: Milch's technique of shoulder reduction

   d. *Matsen's Preferred Method*: The patient lies on the back. An assistant stands at the normal shoulder. A belt is wrapped around the chest of the patient and waist of the assistant. The practitioner stands at the dislocated shoulder near the waist of the patient. The practitioner holds the patient's elbow with flexion at 90°. A second belt is wrapped around the practitioner's waist and looped over the patient's forearm. While maintaining the position the practitioner leans backward against the belt. A steady traction along the axis of the forearm usually causes shoulder reduction (Fig. 25.18).

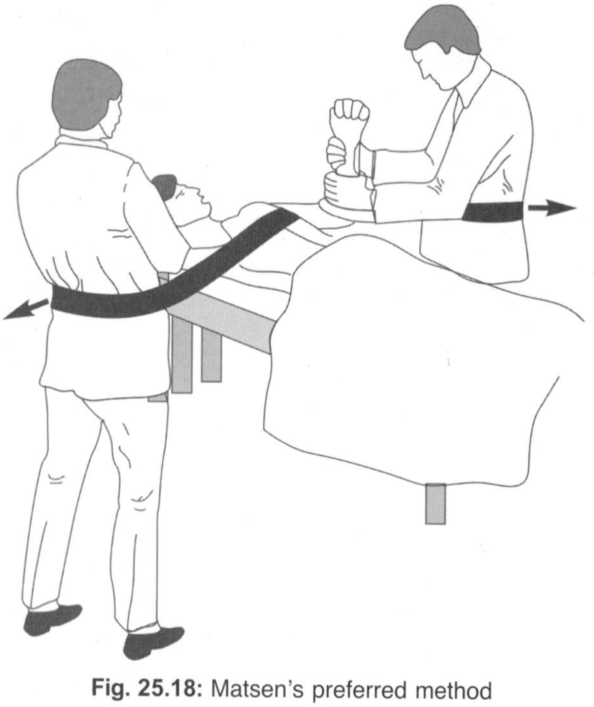

Fig. 25.18: Matsen's preferred method

2. **Immobilization:** After reduction, the shoulder is immobilized in a sling, which may be removed during the exercises. The immobilization depends upon the age of the patient (Fig. 25.19).

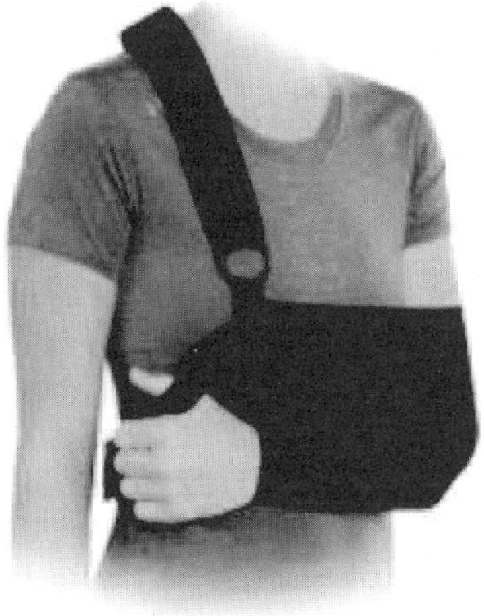

Fig. 25.19: Shoulder immobilization in sling

i. Below 20 years : Shoulder is immobilized for 3-4 weeks.
ii. Between 20 and 30 years : Shoulder is immobilized for 2-3 weeks.
iii. Between 30 and 40 years : Shoulder is immobilized for 10 days to 2 weeks.
iv. Above 40 years : Shoulder is immobilized for 3-5 days.

Recurrent Dislocations

One of the complications of primary dislocation is recurrence dislocations of the shoulder. Row found significantly higher recurrence rate in young patients. The recurrence rate of shoulder dislocation is decreased as the age is increased.

i. Those younger than 10 years had a recurrence rate of 100%.
ii. The recurrence rate is decreased to 94% in patients aged between 10 and 20 years.
iii. Between 20 and 30, the recurrence rate is found 79%; and
iv. Between 30 and 40, the recurrence rate is found 50%.

Some authors found that the recurrence rate is higher in athletes than the non-athletes. Most of the studies found that the recurrence rate of shoulder dislocation is higher in younger patients than the older patients. This is because of the arrangements of the collagen fibers and change in collagen that occurs as people grow older. In newborn, type III collagen is produced and the fibers formed from this type of collagen are supple and elastic. As the age progresses the collagen producing cells make less type III collage fibers and convert to synthesizing another form of collagen type I fibers. The type I collagen fibers contain sulfur groups that have a high tendency to cross link and form bridges between the collagen filaments, causing the fibers they comprise to be relatively tough and non-elastic. This changing ratio of collagen type I and III throughout the body is so reliable that the chronological age of an individual can be determined by analyzing the collagen type III content of a skin sample (Fig. 25.20).

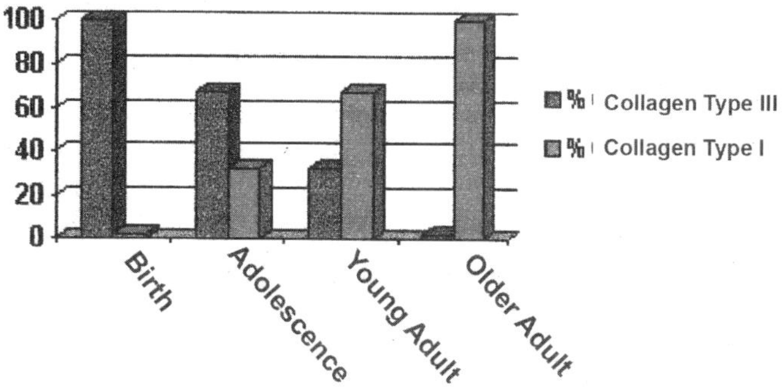

Fig. 25.20: Distribution of collagen fibers I and type II according to the age

3. **Exercises:** The exercises are divided into four phases:
   i. *Phase I: 01 week to 03 weeks*: This phase is crucial for maintaining the strength and range of motion in pain free range. Hold relax or isometric exercise of deltoid muscles, rotator cuff muscles, and para-scapular muscles (scapular stabilizers) such as serratus anterior, rhomboids, and trapezius muscles are initiated. Elevation with external rotation and hyperextension must be avoided as these movements place greater stress on the anterior stabilizers of the shoulder.
   ii. *Phase II: 3 weeks to 4 weeks*: The exercises may be progressed to the contract relax or isotonic and closed kinetic chain exercise of the deltoid, rotator cuff muscles and scapular stabilizers.
   iii. *Phase III: 4 weeks to 8 weeks*: The closed kinetic chin exercises are progressed to the open kinetic chain exercises and light isotonic dumbbell exercises of the deltoid, rotator cuff muscles and scapular stabilizers.
   iv. *Phase IV: 8 weeks to 12 weeks:* The aim of physiotherapist here is to improve the strength, power, endurance, range of motion and proprioceptive neuromuscular control of the shoulder and shoulder girdle musculature. The open kinetic and isotonic dumbbell exercises remain same as phase III. Upper body ergometer, proprioceptive training of the joints and proprioceptive neuromuscular facilitation patterns are initiated to achieve the aims.
   v. *Phase V*: The aim of the treatment at this phase is to prepare for gradual return to functional and sport activities. The therapist explains exercises such as plyometric exercises to the patient to perform at

home. When patient returns to the sport or office he should take brief period of rest during the sport activities. The maximum improvement is expected by 6 months.

4. **Operative Options:** The patients who experiences three or more episodes of recurrence of the shoulder dislocation after primary dislocation are the right candidates for the surgical intervention. A relative indication for the surgical intervention is young population; especially professional athlete who is participating sports activities actively.The early surgical intervention will reduce the risks of the recurrent instability and allow the athletes to return to sport at the earliest. There are several surgical interventions for the anterior dislocation of the shoulder. The traditional open Bankart repair is the standard of core of open stabilizing procedure with a recurrence rate of less than 5%. The recurrence rate of arthroscopic stabilization is highly variable from 0 to 45%. Few operative options are mentioned as under:
   a. *Bristow Procedure*: A small fragment of the coracoid process is removed and is attached with the anterior scapular neck. Active and passive range of motion may be initiated after 4 days of the procedure.
   b. *Putti Platt Procedure*: The procedure basically tightens the anterior capsule and subscapularis muscle with subsequent loss of the external rotation. It has been described as a "vest over pants" fashion along with a "double-breasted" technique. The lateral part of the subscapularis muscle is cut vertically and removed from its insertion part. The remaining medial stump of the subscapularis is attached to the lesser tuberosity of the humerus with thick absorbable mattresses sutures across the stumps so that they overlap on tightening the medial stump lying over the lateral one. The arm is immobilized in full internal rotation for three weeks. Full external rotation is never regained. In 1976, Morrey and Janes reported an 11% recurrence of dislocation following surgical repair. A 10-year follow-up was completed by Salomonsson *et al.* and identified that of the thirty patients who returned the questionnaire, 15 had an episode of instability defined either as a redislocation or a subluxation. The studies have reported that Putti Platt procedure alters the forces on the glenohumeral joint. This increases the load on the posterior aspect of the joint with potential to create an abnormal posteroinferior humeral head subluxation. This also contributes to the secondary osteoarthritis of the glenohumeral joint.
   c. *Eden-Hybinede Procedure*: This procedure is similar to Bristow. About 2 cm × 3 cm bone graft is removed from the coracoids process and attached to the anterior surface of the scapula. The arm is immobilized in the adduction and internal rotation. No external rotation for at least 3 weeks is allowed.
   d. *Bankart Arthroscopic Procedure*: The torn edges of the labrum are removed to reveal fresh labrum. A small hole is drilled into the bone to receive the anchor. The anchor is pushed into the drilled hole. Four sutures are attached to the anchor which is used to reattach the labrum to the glenoid. A guidewire is passed under the labrum. A suture and guidewire is retrieved through the cannula to be knotted together. The suture is then safely pulled under the labrum by the guidewire. The sutures are knotted to close the Bankart lesion and the ends of the suture are then cut. The procedure is repeated until the labrum is completely reattached to the glenoid. In the due course of time the sutures are dissolved and the static stability of the shoulder is restored by the Bankart arthroscopic procedure.

Post Operative Management After Anterior Stabilization Procedure

Phase-1 : 0-4 Weeks

a. *Sling*: Shoulder is immobilized in a sling, in adduction and internal rotation, especially at night. Sling can be removed for exercises.
b. *Range of Motion*: Flexion is increased gradually and achieved upto 140 at the end of 4th week. No passive external rotation and active internal rotation is performed.
c. *Control of Pain*: To control pain ice pack can be used around the shoulder for 20 minutes per session for 5-6 times daily.
d. *Strengthening*: Grip strengthening, external rotator cuff strengthening (within the prescribed range of motion) no internal rotators strengthening.

Phase-2 : 5-8 Weeks

Criteria to Progress to Phase 2: Patient should have minimal pain and discomfort with the exercises. No sensation or finding of instability.

a. Shoulder sling is discontinued.
b. Ice packs continue to control pain and symptoms.
c. Patient can progress to forward flexion upto 160, external rotation 50 and abduction 70.
d. Rotator cuff and scapular stabilizer strengthening

Exercises are progressed to the open kinetic chain exercises with theraband. No internal rotator strengthening.

Phase-3 : 8-12 Weeks

Criteria for Progression: The patient should have minimal pain and discomfort with exercises. Significant improvement in the strength of the rotator cuff and scapular stabilizers.

a. Pain is relieved by ice packs.

b. *Range of Motion*: At this phase patient achieves full active and passive range of motion equal to the contralateral shoulder. Capsular stretching may be beneficial in case if range of motion is not regained.

c. *Strengthening*: Similar to the phase II rotator and scapular stabilizers. Upper body ergometer for upper extremity endurance and PNF patterns for proprioceptive training may be added. Plyometric exercises with the ball to improve the functional activities are beneficial in this stage.

- **Maximum improvement after anterior stabilization is expected by 12 months but patients can return to sports by 6 months.**

POSTERIOR DISLOCATION OF THE SHOULDER

'osterior instability may be described as a symptomatic xcessive posteriorly and laterally translation of the head iumerus with respect to the glenoid fossa. On the axial K-ray the head of humerus is displaced toward the acromian or away from the ribs. The posterior instability may be anged from abnormal translation to the subluxation and lislocation. The posterior instability is far less common han the anterior instability because of significant stability rom muscular and static stabilization (glenoid fossa).

Posterior instability can either be a traumatic or traumatic. Traumatic instability typically follows a distinct iistory of true dislocation, or subluxation, sustained during significant injury. Traumatic posterior instability (posterior dislocation) of the shoulder is very rare, it typically tems from episodes of generalized muscle contraction, such s seizure or severe electric shock. Following posterior lislocation there is strong sustained contraction of the dductors and internal rotators, which keep the shoulder t lateral chest wall with internal rotation. Patients with a raumatic posterior instability do not reveal any history of raumatic injury but these patients fall into younger age ide and associated with sports activities such as throwing, ennis, cricket bowling, rugby and swimming. These ctivities place significant stress on the static stabilizer that eventully cause laxity of the joint capsule, ligaments and labrum. Subsequent posterior instability produces pain in the shoulder that limits range of motion and decreases strength of the rotator cuff muscles. The weakness of the rotator and parascapular muscles contributes further to the posterior instability of the shoulder.

Clinical Features: The posterior shoulder dislocation patient usually presents with shoulder adduction and internal rotation along with prominence of the humeral head on the posterior shoulder. Athletes with posterior instability complaint pain in the posterior aspect with exercising. Posterior translation of the head of humerus with respect to the glenoid and jerk can be noted. Sometimes posterior instability may be confused with subacromial bursities as pain occurs in the flexion with internal rotation.

Evaluation: The traumatic posterior dislocation is less commoner than the anterior dislocation, however, episodes of seizure, electric shock and strong contraction of the muscles especially adductors, and internal rotators can cause posterior dislocation of the shoulder. Standard shoulder radiographs do not demonstrate posterior displacement of the humeral head. Therefore, this diagnosis is missed acutely about 50 percent of the time. The loss of external rotation is the main clinical feature of the dislocation. The athlete involved in repeated overhead sports activities may complaint weakness of the posterior rotator cuff muscles which is in turn causes posterior instability. Offensive linemen are particularly vulnerable to this injury because of the forward-flexed and internally rotated shoulder position needed for blocking (Figs. 25.21a and b).

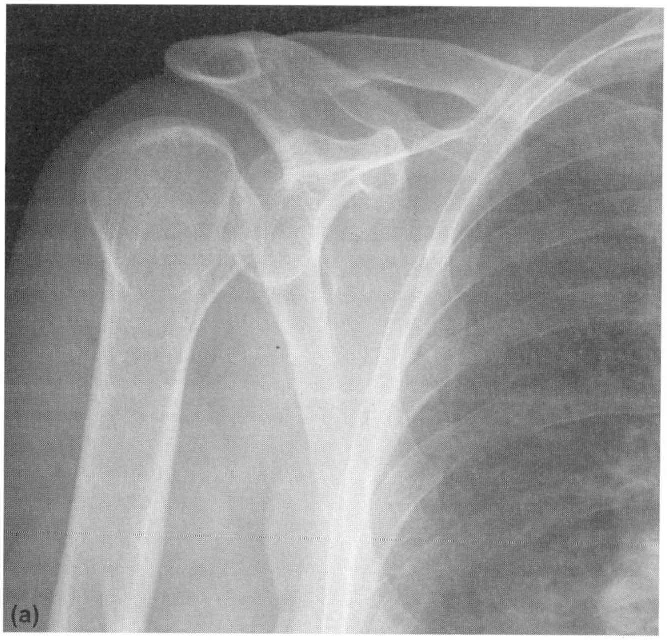

(b)

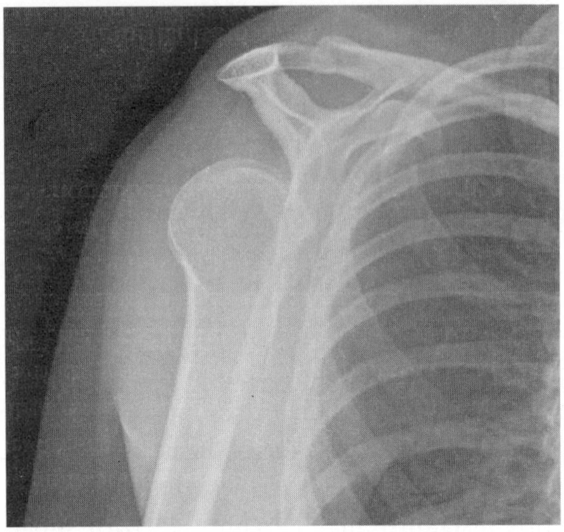

Figs. 25.21a and b: X-ray posterior dislocation of the shoulder

Tests for Posterior Instability

There are two provocative tests to reproduce the symptoms of the patient if posterior instability is present.

Jerk Test: *Position of Patient:* Sitting with shoulder and elbow flexion to 90°, and full medial rotation.

Position of Examiner: Standing, facing the patients shoulder (anterior aspect). The examiner holds elbow with one hand and places other hand on the same side of scapula of the patient. A posterior directed force is applied through the elbow, and then the arm is moved horizontally across the body. If therapist feels sudden jerk, then the test is considered positive for posterior instability. A second jerk is felt as soon as the arm returns to the starting position (Fig. 25.22).

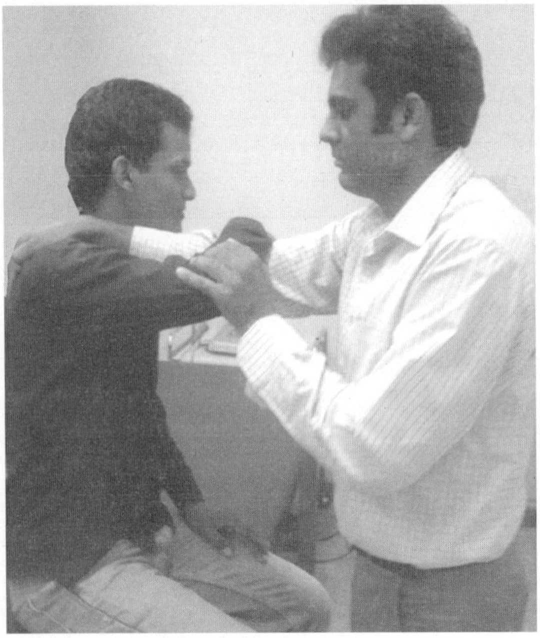

Fig. 25.22: Jerk test

Circumduction Test: *Position of Patient:* Standing.

Position of Examiner: Stands behind the patient, places one hand on the top of the shoulder and grasps the arm of the patient with other hand. The examiner initiates circumduction by bringing the patient's shoulder into extension and slightly abducted position. The examiner brings the patient's arm on the top and then the front of the patient into flexion and adduction position. This is the position of risk for posterior dislocation and in patient's with posterior instability the head of humerus is subluxed posteriorly or produces the symptoms of pain and apprehension (Fig. 25.23).

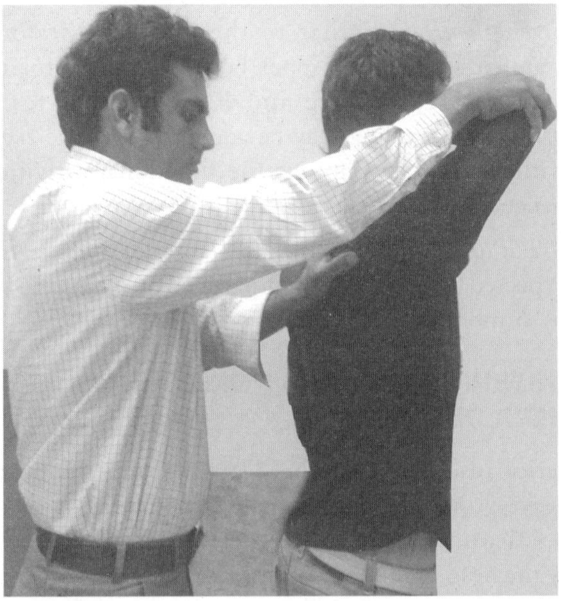

Fig. 25.23: Circumduction test for posterior dislocation of the shoulder

Posterior Apprehension Test: The test is similar to the jerk test. The patient lies supine and shoulder and elbow i flexed to 90°. The examiner holds the elbow joint with one hand and stabilizes the scapula with other hand. While maintaining the above position a posterior directed force i applied through the elbow. The patients with posterior instability complaints pain or apprehension in the posterior directed force (Fig. 25.24).

Management

Reduction: In sitting positions, the hand is placed on the lumbar spine with elbow flexion. Therapist places one hand on the posterior aspect of the head of humerus and other hand grasps the flexed elbow joint. While maintaining the position of elbow, an anterior directed force is applied on the humeral head to bring it to the glenoid fossa.

After reduction the shoulder is immobilized in a sling or brace in an externally rotated position. Internal rotation

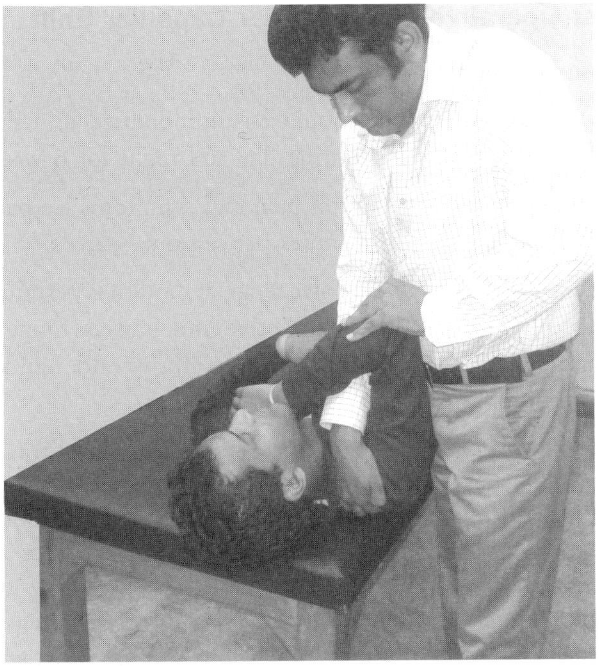

Fig. 25.24: Posterior apprehension test for posterior dislocation of the shoulder

and horizontal cross chest adduction places stress on the posterior joint capsule, therefore, these should be avoided. Pendulum exercises should be initiated in a painfree range of motion. Submaximal isometric of deltoid (anterior, middle and posterior) external and internal rotators in the adduction are beneficial in improving the strength.

- With significant improvement in the range of motion and pain, the submaximal isometric exercises should be replaced with isotonic with therabands and tubing. Rowing in prone and wall press in standing help in strengthening parascapular muscles.
- As soon as patient gains full painfree range of motion in all three planes the aforesaid exercises are added with plyometric training and D2 flexion and extension patterns.

The athletes with posterior instability due to repeated trauma to the posterior capsule demanded by the sports activities usually respond to the conservative treatment. These patients rarely require sling, but elevation with internal rotation, cross chest adduction and extreme extension should be avoided to accelerate the posterior capsule healing. The exercises for athletes with posterior instability are mainly of strengthening of deltoid, rotator cuff muscle, parascapular (serratus anterior, rhomboids, trapezius (all fibers), which are explained at anterior instability.

Failure to respond to the conservative treatment, may require, surgical intervention; capsular suture plication, and posterior capsule shift.

INFERIOR INSTABILITY

It is the symptomatic excessive, inferior translation of the head of humerus with respect to the glenoid fossa. Inferior instability can either be subluxation or dislocation of the shoulder. Inferior humeral dislocation also known as luxatio, is extremely uncommon, accounting for less than 1% of all shoulder dislocations. Forceful hyper abduction of the shoulder causes impingement between head of humerus and acromian and places extreme stress on the inferior joint capsule. The inferior joint capsule disrupts and allows head of humerus to dislocate inferiorly. The shoulder may also dislocate posteriorly if there is an axial force on the abducted shoulder.

The patients with inferior shoulder dislocation presents with severe pain and pain is aggravated with movements. The affected arm "locked" in varying degrees of abduction. Classically the shoulder is hyperabducted with the elbow flexion and resting on top of or behind the head. The head of humerus can be palpated over the lateral chest wall. Standard closed reduction is not done as it may cause humeral shaft or neck fracture and injury to the vessels. Surgical open reduction is the choice of reduction of inferior shoulder dislocation.

Complications

1. 50-60% patients will have brachial injury.
2. Axillary artery injury, thrombosis.
3. Rotator cuff tears.
4. Glenohumeral and inferior capsule disruption.
5. Fracture of humeral shaft or head.

Test for Inferior Laxity or Instability: *Position of Patient:* Sitting with the arm hanging loosely.

Position of Examiner: Stands or sits behind the patient, places one hand on the superior aspect of the shoulder. The other hand groups the distal arm of the patient.

Procedure: The examiner pulls the patients arm downwards. In normal subjects when the arm is distracted downward no sulcus or gap is formed between the acromian arch and head of humerus. The presence of sulcus indicates inferior laxity or instability (Fig. 25.25).

MULTIDIRECTIONAL INSTABILITY

It is the symptomatic instability in more than one directions: anterior, posterior or inferior. However, there may be a predominance of one direction, typically anteroinferior or posteroinferior. Patients with generalized laxity of the ligaments associated with weakness of the rotator cuff usually demonstrate multidirectional instability.

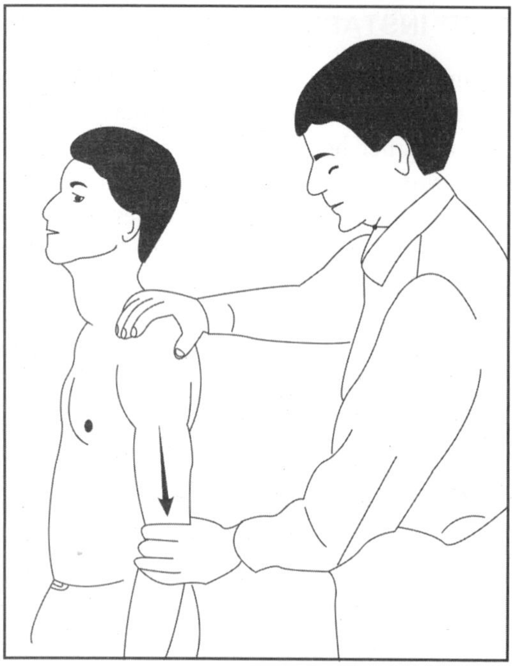

Fig. 25.25: Sulcus sign for inferior instability

Patients with multidirectional instability complaints pain, weakness and instability in overhead activities. These patients often report history of laxity in other joints demonstrated by frequent ankle sprain or recurrent patellar dislocation. Labral grind, SLAP (superior labrum from anterior to posterior), and anterior apprehension tests are helpful in diagnosing the multidirectional instability.

Management

Conservative: The conservative treatment is focused on the strengthening of the rotator and scapular stabilizers.

Surgical Intervention: The surgical intervention is considered if an extensive trial of exercises for at least 6 months fails to relieve the sign and symptoms. The patients with multidirectional instability are recommended for open inferior capsular shift.

Open Inferior Capsular Shift: The purpose of this approach is to balance tension on all sides of the glenohumeral joint and surgically reduce capsular volume. The procedure is effective particularly in patients with multidirectional instability as it reduces the laxity of the capsule in all the directions. The capsule is retracted from the subscapularis in a medial to lateral direction. It is then incised from the glenoid margin forming a T shaped incision. The inferior capsule leaf is shifted to the superiorly and superior capsule is shifted to inferiorly and attached to the respective margins by various types of the fixation devices.

Post Operative Open Inferior Capsular Shift

Phase-I : 0-6 Weeks

a. *Immobilization*: The shoulder is immobilised in a sling or gunsling orthosis during day and night for 6 weeks.
b. *Relief of Pain*: To control pain and symptoms ice packs can be used for 20 minutes per session.
c. *Range of Motion*: No passive range of motion is permitted throughout the Phase I. Active and passive range of motion of other joints such as elbow and hand is initiated.
d. *Strengthening*: The isometric exercises in sling of rotator cuff and scapular stabilizers may be initiated in a closed kinetic chain positions.

Phase-II : Weeks 07-12

a. *Range of Motion*: Patient achieves upto 140 degree flexion, 40 degree external rotation and 70 degree abduction.
b. *Strengthening*: Rotator cuff, scapular stabilizers and deltoid strengthening are progressed to the open kinetic chain with the theraband or tubing.

Phase-III : 3-6 Months

a. *Range of Motion*: Patient achieves full range of motion. Glides to stretch the capsule may be initiated with precaution if range is limited.
b. *Strengthening*: Upper body ergometer for upper extremity endurance and PNF patterns for proprioceptive training may be added. Plyometric exercises with the ball to improve the functional activities are beneficial in this stage.

SHOULDER IMPINGEMENT SYNDROME

The term shoulder impingement syndrome (SIS) was introduced by Neer in 1972, which described as "impingement of long head of biceps and supraspinatus tendon" between the head of humerus and acromial arch.

Subacromial Space: Subacromial space or suprahumeral space is formed between the superior surface of the humeral head and inferior arch of the acromian process. The tendons of supraspinatus and long head of biceps and subacromial bursae lie in the subacromial space. In healthy shoulders the normal subacromial space is considered as 10 mm. A distance (between head of humerus and acromian arch, subacromial space) of less than 6 mm is considered pathologic for impingement (Figs. 25.26a and b).

(a)

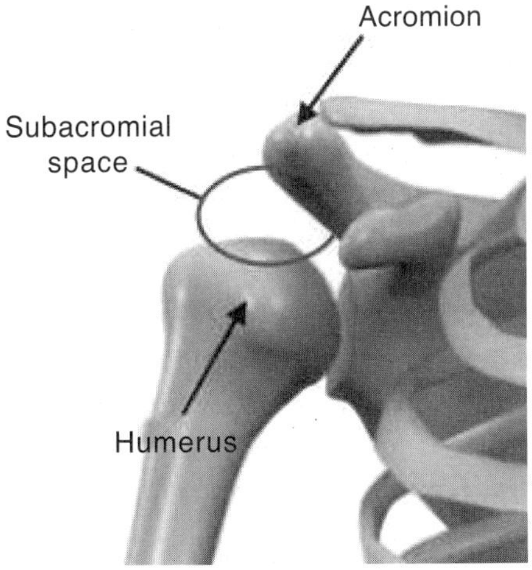

(b)

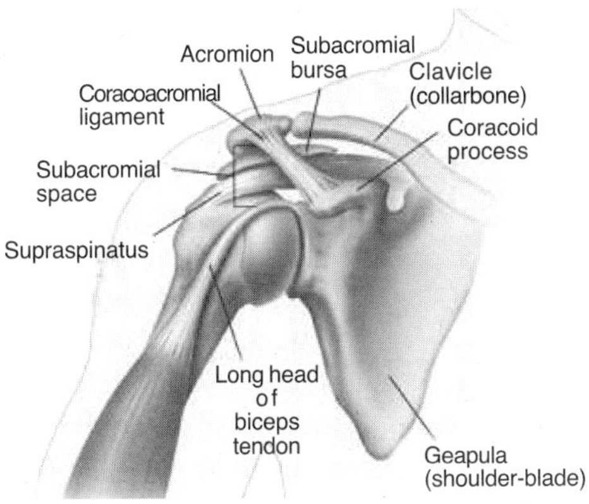

Figs. 25.26a and b: (a) Subacromial space, (b) Static and dynamic stabilizers of shoulder

Coracohumeral Compartment: This space is identified by Patte. This is the space between greater tuberosity and lesser tubercle in which subscapularis bursa, subscapularis tendon and subcoracoid bursa are situated. In resting position with arm rotating medially, the distance between tip of the coracoid and the most prominent part of the lesser tubercle has been measured to be approximately 8.7 mm in healthy shoulders. Decreased in coracohumeral space to 6.8 mm is considered to be potential for the coracohumeral impingement, the space may be decreased due to trauma or fracture of the tip of the coracoid process.

Mechanism

In overhead activities the rotator cuff muscles spin, rotate, and depress the head of humerus, thus maintaining the suprahumeral space. Overuse of these muscles in overhead activities may cause weakness. The weak rotator cuff muscles fail to spin, rotate, and depress the head of humerus adequately. Therefore, the head of humerus migrates superiorly to the acromion arch, decreasing the subacromial space and causing compression of the soft tissues such as: tendon of supraspinatus and long head of biceps and subacromial bursa between superior surface of the humeral head and inferior arch of the acromion process.

The parascapular muscles retract and rotate the scapula during overhead activities which provides room for the rotating humerus, thus maintaining the subacromial space. The excessive use of the shoulder girdle muscles may cause weakness of the parascapular muscles, resulting in inadequate external rotation of the scapula. Therefore, during overhead activities there is elevation of the arm but no external rotation of the scapula which leads to decrease in subacromial space. Eventually compression of the soft tissues such as: tendon of supraspinatus and long head of biceps and subacromial bursa between superior surface of the humeral head and inferior arch of the acromion process.

Factors Contribute to the Impingement

Several factors can contribute equally to the impingement, which are divided into extrinsic and intrinsic:

A. Extrinsic

These factors affect the suprahumeral space from outside. The extrinsic factors may include anteroinferior one third of the acromion, muscular imbalance, postural changes and precipitating factors including training errors and occupational or environmental hazards.

i. **Acromion Anomaly:** The anteroinferior one third of the acromion is thought to be the causative factor in mechanical wear of the rotator cuff through a process called impingement. Neer believed that the tendon of supraspinatus and long head of biceps are repeatedly compressed when the arm is elevated in the forward flexion (functional arc of elevation of the arm). There are three types of acromion, namely flat, curved and hooked. Neer has found no impingement with the flat acromion; most of impingement patients (70%) were present with hooked acromion.

ii. **Muscle Imbalance:** The movements of the scapula and humerus in elevation are primarily controlled by the scapular and parascapular muscles. There are two force couples formed in the upper corset to control the movements are termed as scapula force couple and glenohumeral force couple.

Force couple: A force couple is defined as two forces of equal magnitude but in opposite direction that produces rotation on a body.

Scapula force couple: The scapula force couple is formed by the two portions of parascapular muscles. The upper portion is formed by the upper fibers of the trapezius, and the levator scapulae. The lower portion of the scapula force couple is formed by the lower fibers of the trapezius and lower fibers of the serratus anterior. Simultaneous contraction of these two groups of muscles produces a smooth rhythmic motion to rotate the scapula along the posterior thorax during elevation of the arm. This external rotation (upward rotation) of the scapula provides not only a room for the rotating humerus but also provides a stable base of support for the rotating humerus to allow the humeral head to maintain its normal pathway or rotation along the glenoid. Weakness of these parascapular muscles may lead to inadequate elevation of the scapula (external rotation of the scapula) which in turn does not provide room for the rotating humerus. The greater tuberosity will stuck to the acromion and the suprahumeral space is compromised which in turn compresses the tendons of supraspinatus and long head of biceps (Figs. 25.27a and b).

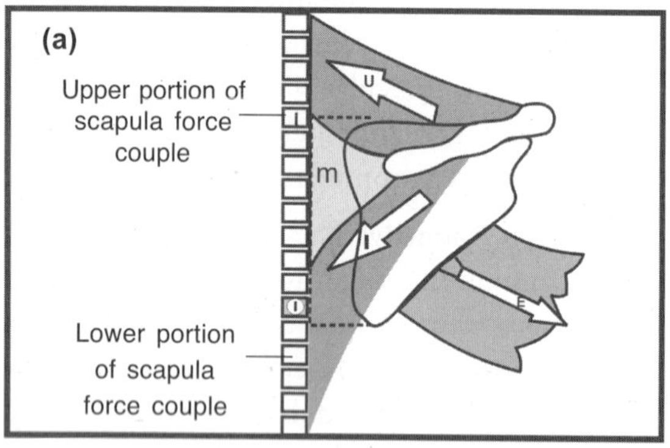

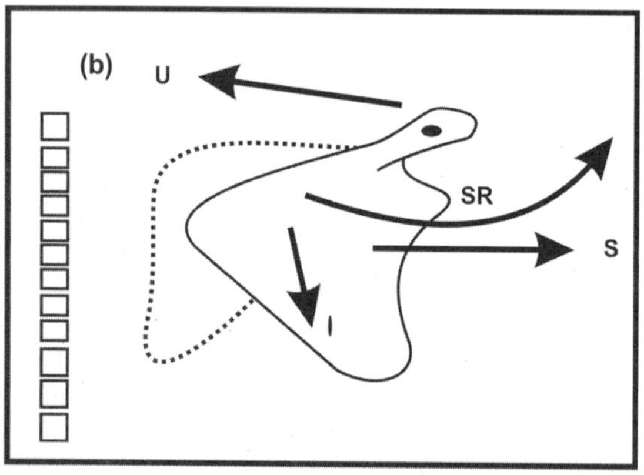

Figs. 25.27a and b: (a) Scapula force couple muscles, (b) Scapula external rotation following contraction of the scapula force couple muscles

Glenohumeral force couple: The glenohumeral force couple is formed by the scapular muscles. One portion of the force couple is formed by the lateral fibers of the deltoid and other portion is formed by the rotator cuff muscles. Simultaneous contraction of these two groups of muscles causes elevation of the humerus with an intact suprahumeral space. The result is that the rotator cuff muscles in effect "steer" the head of humerus along the glenoid during the elevation of the arm. The force generated by the middle fibers of the deltoid pulls the head of humerus upward which in turn is resisted by the strong contraction of the rotator cuff muscles thereby the suprahumeral space is maintained throughout the range of motion. Weakness of the rotator cuff muscles fails to counteract the force of the middle fibers of the deltoid, therefore, the center of rotation of the humeral head migrates 6 mm or greater to the superior direction. The suprahumeral space is compromised and the tendons of supraspinatus and long head of biceps and subacromial bursa are impinged (Fig. 25.28).

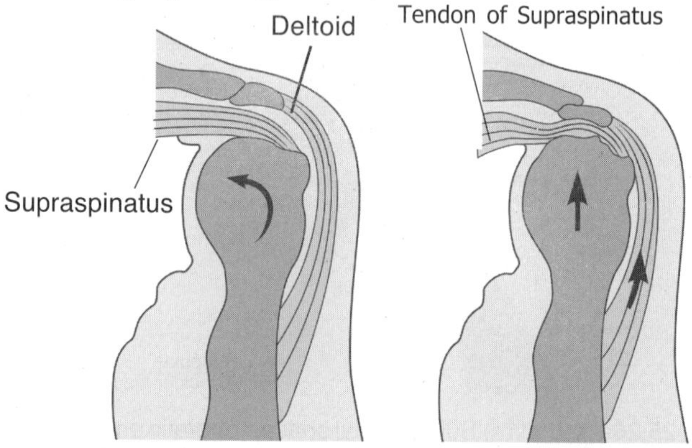

Fig. 25.28: Glenohumeral force couple muscles

iii. **Postural Changes:** The postural changes seen in the upper corset can adversely affect the force couple mechanism about the shoulder with potential pathomechanical changes. The common postural changes associated with shoulder are protracted and rounded shoulders with internal rotation and forward head posture typically seen in upper crossed syndrome.

iv. **Precipitating Factors:** The individuals involved in overhead activities such as baseball pitching, painting, cricket bowling, and tennis (overhead shots) are in the risk of the impingement syndrome. These activities may weaken the rotator cuff muscles as of overuse and thereby the rotator cuff muscles fail to depress the head of humerus downward during the elevation.

B. Intrinsic Factors

These are the changes which take place within the joint and contribute to the reduction of the joint space. Glenohumeral joint is a synovial joint which is involved in the degenerative process. There is loss of the thickness of the articular surfaces, in turn osteophytes are formed. The subacromial bursa and tendons get impinged as the subacromial space is compromised by the formation of the osteophytes. Degenerative changes in the acromioclavicular joint cause osteophyte formation, which may project to the glenohumeral joint and reduce subacromial space. Furthermore, the vascularity of the rotator cuff muscles may also contribute to the impingement. Approximately 1 centimeter medially to the insertion of the supraspinatus tendon is believed to be relatively avascular. Codman has referred this as a *"critical zone"*. The studies have suggested that the most of degenerative changes of the supraspinatus tendon take place in this zone and this is intensified by aging.

Types of SIS

Primary Impingement Syndrome: This type of impingement is common in older than 40 years and less commonly found in the athlete population. These patients complain pain in the shoulder and arm particularly in the anterior aspect of the shoulder and lateral aspect of the arm with inability to sleep on the affected side. As the condition progresses they also complain pain and weakness in the overhead activities. The common causes include:

a. Degenerative changes (osteophyte formation) in the glenohumeral and acromioclavicular joints (Fig. 25.29).

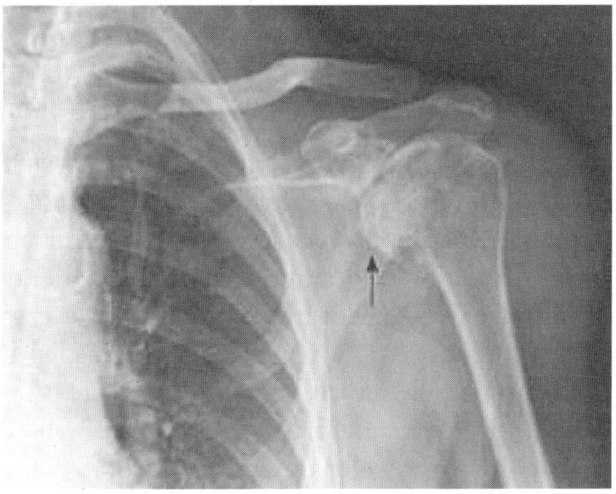

Fig. 25.29: Degenerative changes (osteophyte formation)

b. Congenital hooked acromion process (Fig. 25.30).

c. Congenital prominent tuberosity.

d. Rotator cuff tendon thickening from calcific deposit or after trauma/surgery.

Secondary Impingement Syndrome: This type of SIS is more usual in younger population between 20 and 40 years. These patients are involved in the overhead sports activities such as cricket bowling, baseball, swimming, volleyball and tennis. The symptoms remain same as primary SIS but weakness of the shoulder girdle muscles is most dominant. Patients experience a feeling of the arm going dead. The common causes include: weakness of the rotator cuff muscles and scapular stabilizer. These muscles provide dynamic stability to the glenohumeral and scapulothoracic joint.

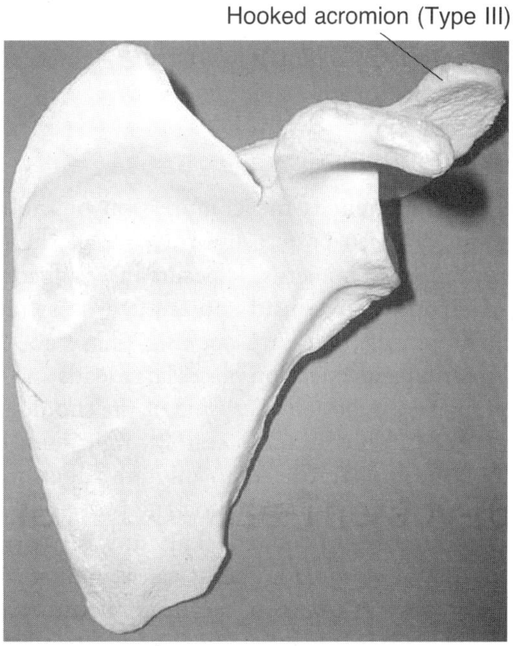

Fig. 25.30: Congenital hooked acromion process

Progressive Stages of SIS

Stage-I: Edema and Inflammation

Typical Age:
- Younger than 25 years but may occur at any age.

Physical Signs:
- Tenderness over the greater tuberosity and along the anterior-ridge/acromion.
- Painful arc of abduction between 60° and 120°.
- Positive impingement sign.
- Decrease ROM with significant subacromial inflammation.

Stage-II: Fibrosis and Tendinitis

Typical Age:
- Between 25 and 40 years.

Physical Signs:
- Crepitus of soft tissues.
- Catching sensation with lowering of the arm at approximately 100°.
- Limitation of active and passive range of motion.
- Inability to participate in overhead activities.
- Symptoms of Stage I.

Clinical Course: Not reversible by modification of activity.

Stage-III: Bone Spurs and Tendon Ruptures

Typical Age:
- Greater than 40 years.

Physical Sign:
- Atrophy and weakness of shoulder girdle muscles.
- Limitation of active range of motion is more pronounced.
- Significant restriction in use of affected upper extremity.

- Biceps tendon involvement.
- AC joint tenderness.

Clinical Course: Not reversible.

Internal Impingement

Internal impingement is the compression of the rotator cuff tendons between posterosuperior edge of the glenoid labrum and head of humerus. It occurs in younger athletes who participate in overhead sports such as swimming, baseball, or tennis. The late cocking phase abduction, external rotation and extension places large loads and casuses microtrauma to the posterior capsule of the shoulder joint. The posterior capsule becomes scarred, tight, and painful and causes the humeral head to migrate superiorly in a higher position than usual in the cocking phase of throwing or when abducted and rotated. This unwanted superior translation of the head of humerus cause impingement of rotator cuff muscle between the head of humerus and posterior glenoid. In the later stages of the condition the posterior capsule become tight which reduces the internal rotation of the shoulder, causing stiffness, pain and increasing the risk of developing injuries to the under surface of the rotator cuff or superior shoulder labrum (SLAP lesions) by a "peel back" mechanism. Athletes with internal impingement are considered at risk to develop a superior labrum from anterior to posterior (SLAP) lesion.

Clinical Features

The diagnosis of internal impingement is based on the subjective assessment including careful observation of the shoulder and history, and objective assessment.

Posterior Shoulder Pain: Chronic-diffuse posterior shoulder girdle pain is the chief complaint of the throwing athletes with internal impingement, but pain may also be localized to the joint line. The patient may describe onset of posterior shoulder pain, particularly during the late cocking phase of throwing.

Decrease in Throwing Velocity: A progressive decrease in throwing velocity or loss of control and performance in the overhead athlete.

"Dead Arm": Some signs of the pathologic process include a so-called "dead arm", the feeling of shoulder and arm weakness after throwing, and a subjective sense of slipping of the shoulder.

Muscular Asymmetry: Overhead athletes and throwers in particular often have muscular asymmetry between the dominant and the non-dominant shoulder.

Muscular/Neuromuscular Imbalance: A common finding is muscle imbalances in the shoulder complex as well as improper neuromuscular control of the scapula.

Increased Laxity: A patient with isolated internal impingement may have an increase in global laxity or an increase in anterior laxity alone of the dominant shoulder.

Anterior Instability: Patients may have instability symptoms, such as apprehension or the sensation of subluxation with the arm in a position of abduction and external rotation.

Scapular Dyskinesis

Kibler, 1991, observed consistent and abnormal scapular postural changes and altered scapular kinematics in overhead athletes with shoulder impingement and coined the term Scapular Dyskinesis. Burkhart, Morgan, and Kibler, 2003, observed consistent asymmetrical malposition of the scapula in throwing athletes with shoulder impingement and these investigators coined the term SICK Scapular Syndrome. (Scapular malposition, inferior medial border prominence, coracoid pain and malposition and dyskinesis scapular movement) (Fig. 25.31).

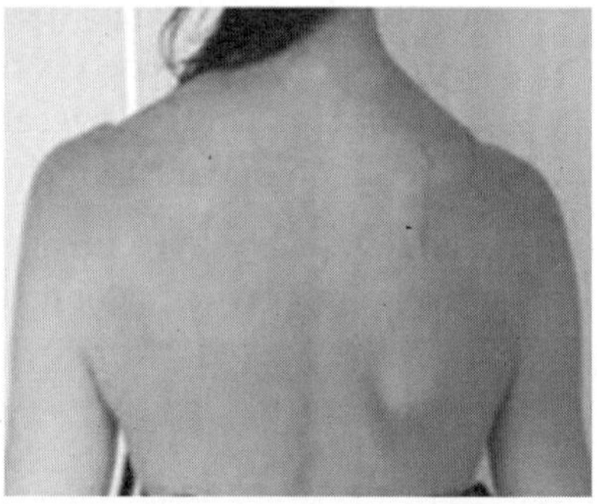

Fig. 25.31: Right Inferior angle of Scapula Prominent. Asymmetrical malposition of the Scapula

Sahrmann, 2002, observed scapular postural changes of downward rotation and anterior tilting in patients with primary impingement. According to her downward scapular rotation syndrome occurs when the inferior medial border of the scapula is closer to thoracis midline than the corresponding superior medial border. She observed that patients with a chronically downwardly rotated scapular position had insufficient scapula upward rotation during overhead elevation of the arm, with resulting subacromial pain and impingement. Sahrmann theorize that long term changes in muscle length correspond to long term changes in scapular posture. The result is a change in muscle balance and force couple capabilities of the scapular muscles to produce outward scapular rotation.

Test for Impingement Syndrome

Impingement Sign

The examiner flexes the shoulder passively, at the end of flexion range, if patient complaints pain, the possible cause of pain is considered as impingement.

In the next step of test leidocaine is injected to subacromial space and then the passive shoulder flexion is performed. If pain is relieved by injecting leidocaine, the test is considered positive.

Impingement Test

The examiner flexes the shoulder passively upto the full range of motion. If patient complaints pain at the end range of motion the test is considered positive for impingement syndrome (Fig. 25.32).

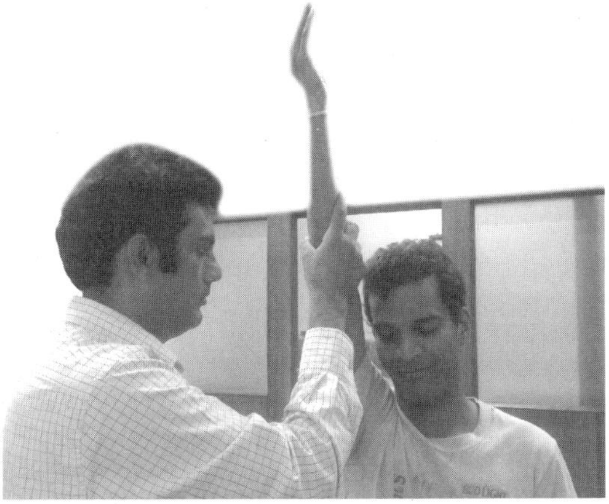

Fig. 25.32: Neer impingement test

Modified Impingement Test

Neer has modified its previous test and added the internal rotation to the flexion. The internal rotation brings greater tuberosity of humerus under the acromion arch. If the internal rotation provokes the symptoms, the test is considered positive for impingement syndrome (Fig. 25.33).

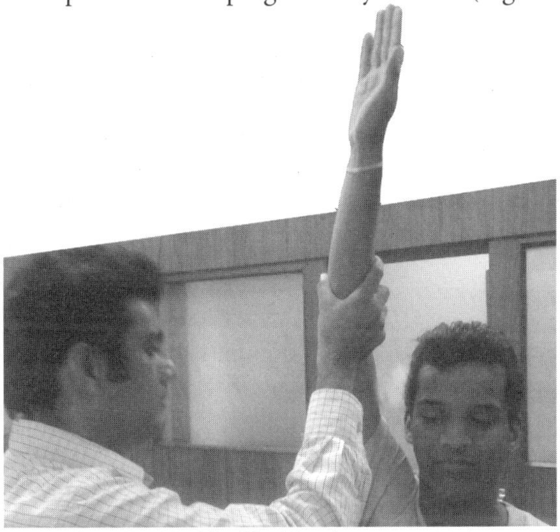

Fig. 25.33: Modified impingement test

Howkins Kennedy

In sitting or standing patient is asked to flex the elbow and shoulder to 90°. Examiner stands at the side which is being examined, stabilizes the shoulder with one hand and holds the flexed arm at the elbow joint. The shoulder is rotated medially. Reproduction of pain and symptoms indicates impingement syndrome. The medial rotation brings the greater tuberosity under the acromion arch and reproduces symptoms in case of inflamed bursa or tendon. This test has a good sensitivity; hence, it is preferred over impingement test (Figs. 25.34a and b).

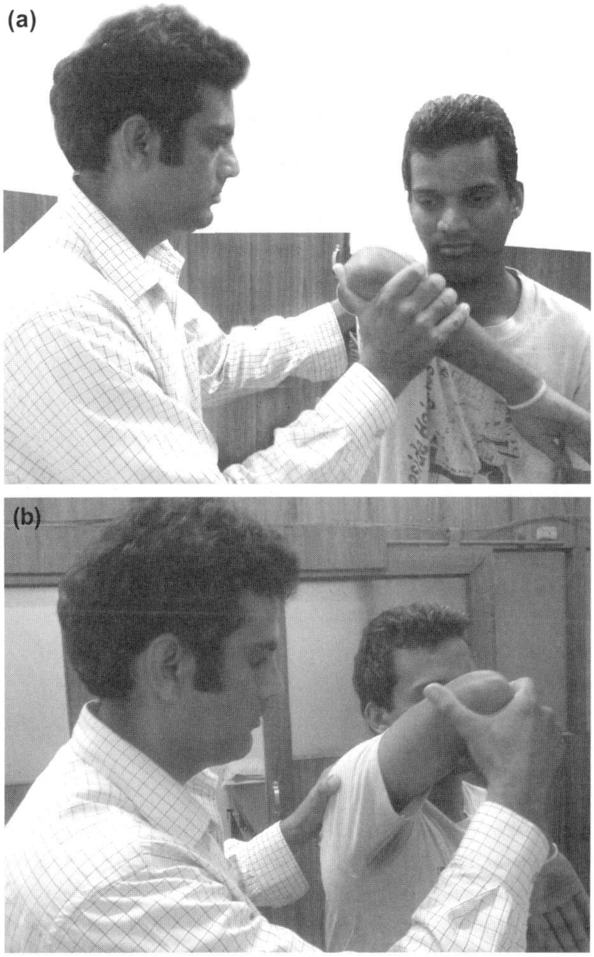

Fig. 25.34a and b: Howkins Kennedy test

Drop Arm Test

In standing the patient's arm is abducted passively to 180° by the therapist, then patient is asked to lower the arm actively in a controlled manner. After 100° patient fails to control the arm and drops it suddenly. This indicates supraspinatus tear. Sometimes patient tries to hold the arm with other hand to control it.

Empty Cane

The patient stands comfortably with both the shoulders elevated to 90° in scaption plane (between flexion and abduction) and full internal rotation (thumb pointing downwards). The therapist stands in front of the patient and holds both the hands of the patient. The patient is asked to elevate the shoulder in the scaption plane against the resistance applied by the therapist. The test is positive if the maneuver aggravates pain in the shoulder (Fig. 25.35).

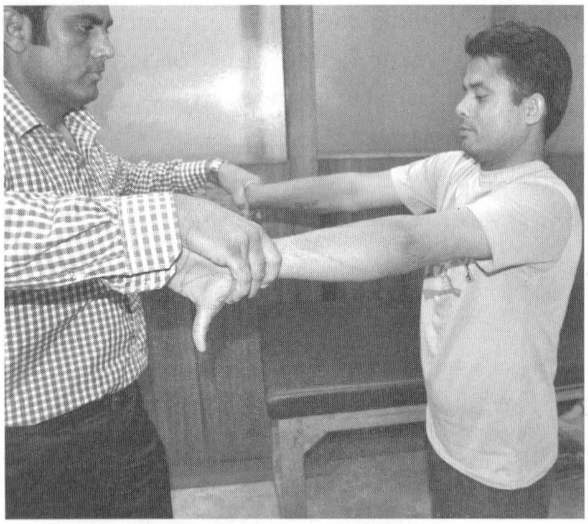

Fig. 25.35: Empty cane test

Management

Conservative Non-operative: The conservative management for both primary and secondary impingement syndromes are same. The aim of treatment is to relieve pain, improve range of motion, improve posture, correct the abnormal kinematics and strengthen the shoulder girdle muscles.

Immobilization: Usually not required.

Precautions: Loss of dynamic stability of the shoulder allows head of humerus to migrate superiorly to the acromion process that impinges the soft tissues between the head of humerus and acromion arch. Hence, overhead activities may require absolute restriction, however, to maintain the range of motion passive exercises are performed throughout the range.

Relief of Pain: To relieve pain, patients can use hot water bag or cold pack for at least 15 minutes twice daily for 2-3 weeks or till the symptoms improve. Hot pack can be followed by cold pack (10 min. each).

Shoulder Girdle Conditioning Program: Prolong pain in the shoulder may cause disuse atrophy of the shoulder girdle muscles. The muscles unable to produce adequate force to perform movements of the body. The functional performance such as activities of daily living, instrumental activities of daily living, recreation, leisure activities, and sport are compromised grossly. The conditioning program of all the major group of muscles helps in improving in the strength of the shoulder girdle muscles.

Strengthening Exercises

Pain and stiffness decrease the contraction of the muscles which in turn can reduce the strength. Initially strengthening (sub maximal isometric) exercises are started in pain free range of motion. The closed kinetic exercises are preferred over the open kinetic chain exercises. As the patient reports improvement in the sign and symptoms the open kinetic chain exercises can be started but these should be with the minimal resistance in pain free range. The progressive resistive exercises are started with the dumbbells (10 repetitions X 03 sets daily for 5 days a week). The resistance is increased every week, till the muscles gain good strength or equal to contralateral extremity. The shoulder girdle muscles such as rotator cuff, serratus anterior, rhomboids, trapezius all fibers and levator scapulae are required to be strengthen.

Following strengthening regime can be used:

1. Diagonal pattern (D2) Flexion and Extension.
2. Dumbbell exercises for deltoid and supraspinatus. The initial abduction is provided by the supraspinatus upto 30°. Abduction beyond 30° is provided by the deltoid middle fibers. All fibers of deltoid may be strengthen with the dumbbell.
3. Prone shoulder abduction for rhomboids diagonal pattern (D2 flexion).
4. Prone shoulder extension for latissimus dorsi.
5. Internal and external rotation at 90° abduction.
6. Biceps strengthening with dumbbell.
7. Dumbbell exercises for triceps and wrist extensors.
8. Serratus anterior strengthening.
9. Press ups.
10. Rowing.

Stretching Exercises

Pain in the shoulder joint limits the range of motion. The joint capsule, ligaments and muscles become tight. With the time the range of motion will be limited in all three planes. Patients find difficulty in combing, fastening bras and reaching overhead activities. To improve range of motion the therapist should work on flexibility of the joint capsule, ligaments and muscles. These structures are required to stretch either by the patients themselves or by the therapist. Following self-stretching exercises may be performed.

Mobilization

To place significant force on the capsule, ligaments and muscles the joint is mobilized with the glides.

Internal Rotation: Internal rotation is commonly decreased in patients with impingement and anterior instability as posterior capsule becomes tight. To improve right side internal rotation the patient lies supine position with the shoulder abduction and elbow flexion to 90°. The therapist stands at the side of the patient. Superior aspect of the shoulder rests on the therapist thigh. Therapist holds the elbow with the right hand and places his left hand on the anterior aspect of the shoulder. The shoulder is abducted to 90° and rotated internally as much as possible with the elbow flexion to 90°. At the range where further movement is not possible because of pain, and tightness of the posterior capsule it is maintained at this position. While maintaining the position the therapist glides the head of humerus posteriorly with the left hand. Several glides are performed to place significant stretch on the posterior capsule (Figs. 25.36a and b).

(a)

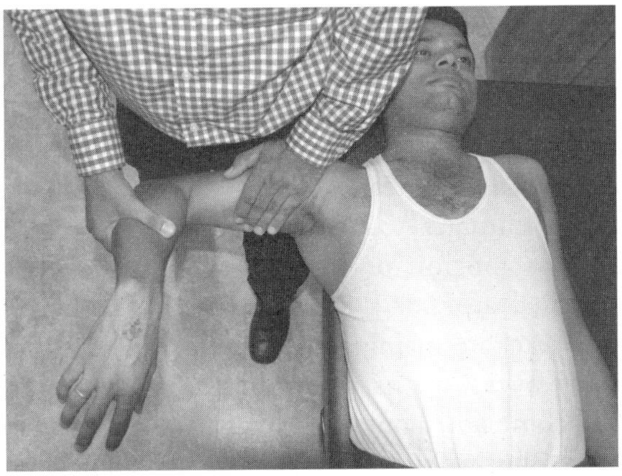

(b)

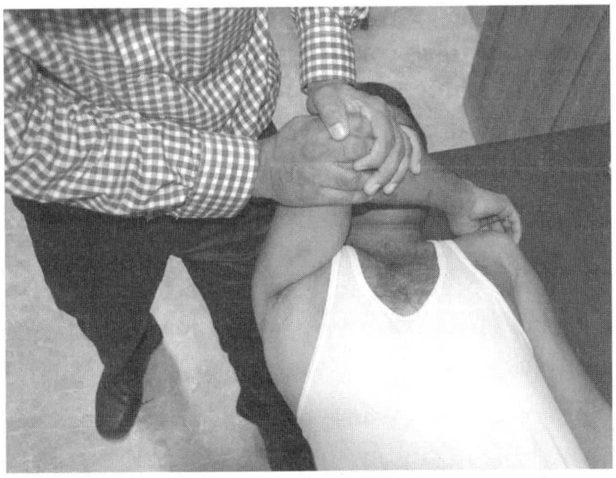

Figs. 25.36a and b: Posterior capsule stretching to improve internal rotation of the shoulder

External Rotation: External rotation is not affected severely in patients with impingement syndrome, but in Stage III it is also limited. To improve external rotation the patient lies supine with the shoulder out of the edge of the couch. The therapist stands at the side of the patient. For right shoulder the therapist stands at the right side and places right hand on the anterior and posterior aspect of the shoulder. Patient's elbow is held with the left hand. The shoulder is abducted to 90°. While maintaining the position the shoulder is rotated externally as much as possible and at the point where limitation starts the head of humerus glided anteriorly. The shoulder should be stabilized with the right hand to prevent protraction. Practically anterior glide is not effective hence, it is rarely applied (Fig. 25.37).

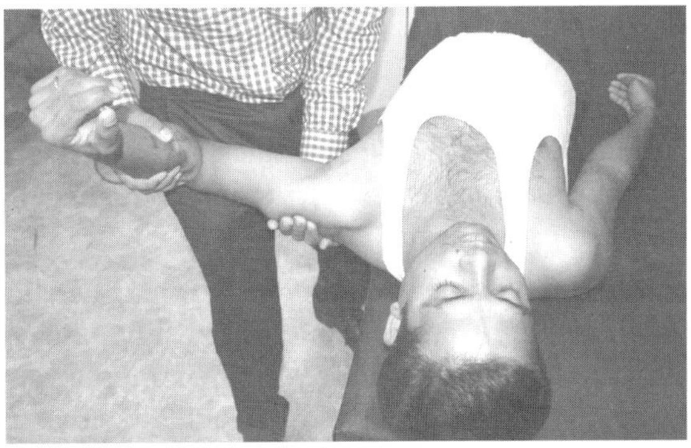

Fig. 25.37: Anterior and inferior capsule stretching to improve external rotation of the shoulder

Abduction: To improve abduction range the patient lies supine. For right side abduction the therapist stands at the right side and places left hand on the shoulder. The left hand grasps the arm firmly. The shoulder of the patient rests on the thigh of the therapist. The shoulder is abducted as much as possible and then the head of humerus is glided inferiorly. Several repetitions are performed to place significant stretch on the inferior capsule.

Flexion: The patient lies in a supine with the shoulder out of the edge. Therapist stands at the side of the patient. Shoulder is flexed with the one hand as much as possible. The other hand glides the capsule anteriorly and inferiorly (Fig. 25.38).

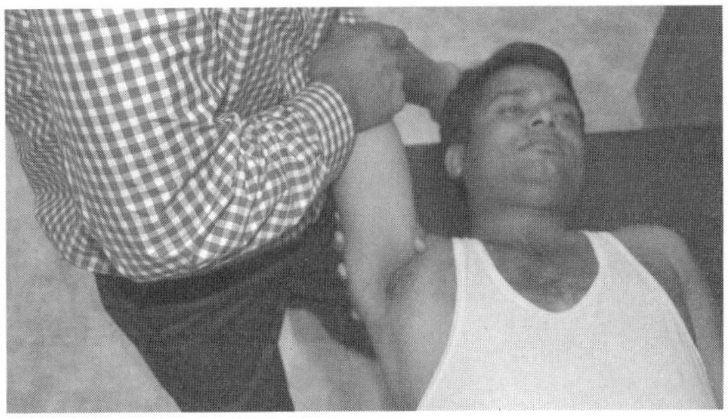

Fig. 25.38: Anterior and Inferior capsule stretching to improve flexion of the shoulder

Surgical Intervention

Patients with impingement syndrome usually respond to the conservative treatment. Surgical intervention is required if a fair trial of conservative treatment at least for one year fails to improve the symptoms. Main aim of the surgery is to increase the subacromial space. Surgical procedure involves removal of the subacromial spurs and anterolateral acromion.

ROTATOR CUFF INJURIES

The rotator cuff muscles are a group of muscles including supraspinatus, infraspinatus, subscapularis and teres minor. This group of muscles help in depressing, rotating and gliding the head of humerus in the glenoid fossa during elevation of the arm. The tendons of these muscles are situated in the subacromial space between head of humerus and inferior surface of the acromion process. The tendons injured due to decrease in the subacromial space, weakness of the parascapular muscles, overuse of the scapular and parascapular muscle and in the process of degeneration. Rotator cuff injuries are mainly tendinopathies and tear that can either be partial or full thickness. A rotator cuff injury can include any type of irritation or damage to the rotator cuff muscles or tendons.

Rotator Cuff Tears: A rotator cuff tear may be of one or more of the tendons of the four rotator cuff muscles. The tendon of the rotator cuff muscles are commonly torn and of the four the supraspinatus most frequently affected as it passess between the acromian arch and head of humerus. Supraspinatus and infraspinatus tendons fuse 1.5 cm proximal to their insertion. Tears in supraspinatus is more commoner and they are more frequently found near to the tendons bony insertion. As the tear in the supraspinatus increase in size it involves the infraspinatus tendon also due to their common insertion. Tear usually occurs at its insertion at the greater tuberosity. Many patients with rotator cuff tear remain asymptomatic. The frequency of rotator cuff tear is increased with age. There is a progressive mechanical failure of the tendon to meet the physical demands placed upon it (Figs. 25.39a and b).

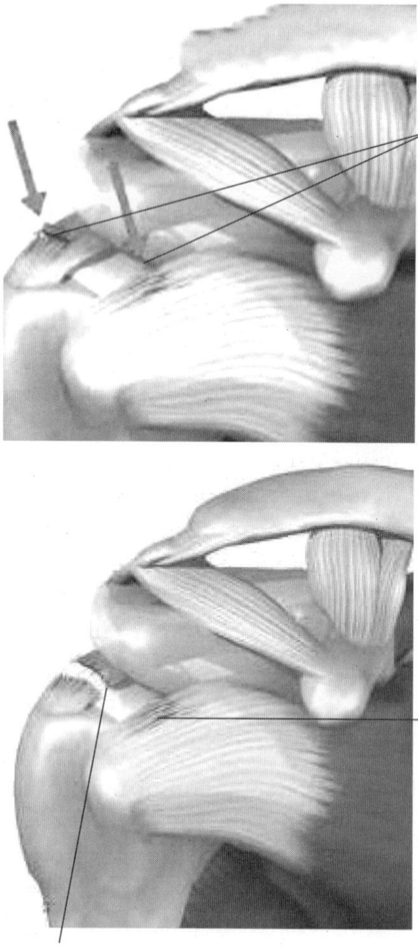

Figs. 25.39a and b

The rotator cuff tears are may be partial or full thickness. Partial tears are often appears as fraying of an intact tendon. Full thickness tears are "through-and-through". These tears can either be pin point, or large button hole with involvement of majority of tendons, where the tendons still remains substantially attached to the humeral head and thus maintain functions. If full thickness tears detach from the humeral head that may cause loss of motion and function of the shoulder.

Mechanism: The tear of rotator cuff tendons may either be acute or chronic. Acute tears occur as a result of sudden, high stress motion or impact, such as a fall on the outstretched arm, or a heavy lift with a jerky motion. Chronic tears are mainly as the result of wear that occurs gradually over time as a natural part of degenetration. Initially dominant shoulders show partial tears without the symotoms but as the age progresses the non-dominant shoulders may also involve in the process of degeneration and show tears which increase in size over the time. Number of factors contribute to the rotor cuff tear but degenerative changes and gradual repetitive microtrauma or stresses are the most common causes of the tear. Overhead activities such as throwing, rowing, weightlifting, painting etc produce microtrauma to the joint capsule, and subacromial bursa which predispose rotator cuff muscles to the degenerative changes and tear. The tear may progress to the full thickness over the time.

The second major cause of the rotator cuff tendon tear is impaired blood supply to the tendon of the rotator cuff especially supraspinatus tendon. In old age the blood supply to the rotator cuff tendons considerably decreases which impairs the natural ability of repairing of the tendons especially in the individual involved in the overhead activities. Eventually this leads to microtear or partial tear of the supraspinatus tendon.

The third cause of the tear is the impingement of the tendons that may cause micro tear, partial tear or full thickness tear. The tendon of the rotator cuff muscles especially supraspinatus may get impinged between the head of humerus and the acromion arch. The nature of mechanical activities such as bowling in cricket, swimming, tennis, baseball, and throwing are the most common activities contribute to the impingement. Rotator cuff tears following secondary impingement usually begins in the fourth decade of the life. This cause of tear is considered as an extrinsic factor whereas other factors such as degeneration, impair blood supply are considered as intrinsic factors.

Pathophysiology: The pathogenesis of rotator cuff tear is multifactorial and likely results from a combination of intrinsic, extrinsic and environmental factors. The small tears of the rotator cuff show features consistent with an attempt to heal such as increase fibroblast cellularity, blood vessel proliferation and the presence of a significant inflammatory component. However, these features of attempting healing (reparative and inflammatory changes) diminishes as the size of tear and amount of tendon degeneration increases over time. As the degenerative changes progress the tendons show thinning of the collagen fibers, a loss of collagen structure, myxoid degeneration chondroid metaplasia, and fatty infiltration. Marked edema and degeneration was seen in large and massive tears, wich more often showed chondroid metaplasia and amyloid deposition. Tissue from large and massive tears is of such a degenerative nature that it may be a significant cause of re-rutpture after surgical repair and could make healing improbable in this group.

The normal supraspinatus tendon has the proteoglycans or glycosaminoglycans of tendon fibrocartilage which suggests that it has capacity of adaptation to mechanical force (tension, compression and shear), act on the rotator cuff tendons in the shoulder. This functional adaptation may have an important consequences for the structural strength of the supraspinatus tendon and to influence the ability of the tendon to repair after injury. Unfortunately in old age it has been noticed that there is decreased in concentration of glycosaminoglycans, chondroitin sulphate and dermatan.

As the tear increases in size, the total collagen contents decrease, while there is a significant increase in the proportion of type II and type III collagen relative to type I collagen. This changes in collagen composition continues with a transformation of matrix from large organized fibrils to smaller disorganized fibrils with decreasing mechanical and physical properties of the collagen fibers. Eventully disintegration begins in the collagen fibers and proteoglycans and they fail to resist the repetitive microtrauma.

Clinical Features

The patients with acute rotator cuff tears usually reveal the history of mechanism of injury. Pain in the shoulder with or without radiation to the lateral arm, difficulty in lifting arm above the shoulder level, and weakness of scapular and parascapular muscles are the common features of rotator cuff tear. External rotation with resistance increases pain and symptoms. Passive movements may be full and pain free but in long standing cases these would be limited in all three planes with disuse atrophy of the shoulder girdle muscles.

Patients with chronic rotator cuff tear often present with gradual onset of pain in the shoulder with difficulty in moving the arm above the shoulder level. Passive motion is full initially in three planes but it may be associated with subacromial crepitus. Patient finds difficulty in lowering the arm actively from overhead position. Weakness of scapular and parascapular muscle with atrophy in the supraspinatus and infraspinatus fossa may also be seen. Patients complaint of pain in the empty can test. Howkins Kennedy and Neer impingement may also be beneficial to perform as these tests detect the impingement syndrome with or without tear of the rotator cuff.

Ultrasonography (US) has been shown to be an effective imaging modality in the evaluation of both rotator cuff and non-rotator cuff disorders, usually serving in a complementary role to magnetic resonance imaging of the shoulder.

An MRI examination of the shoulder may help to demonstrate a rotator cuff tear, its size and degree of retraction.

Plane radiographs may show degenerative changes in the articular cartilage, calcification of the tendon and collapse of the bone associated with rotator cuff tear.

Special Tests

These tests are performed on the patient to put the load on the structure so that the concern structure can reproduce the symptoms.

i. **Biceps Tendinitis Evaluation: Yargason Test:** It is performed to test the bicipital tendinitis. Patient sits comfortably on stool with the elbow flexion to 90° and forearm fully pronated. The therapist holds the hand and elbow and simultaneously resists the forearm supination and elbow flexion. If the maneuver reproduces pain in the shoulder joint, it suggest bicipital tendinitis (Fig. 25.40).

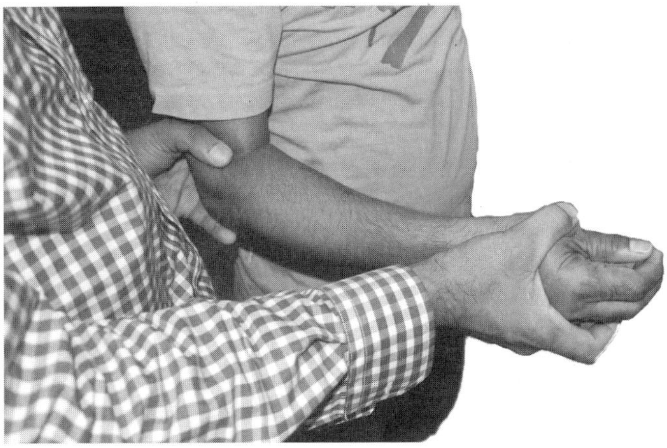

Fig. 25.40: Yergason's test for bicipital tendinitis

ii. **Speed Test:** The patient stands comfortably with both the shoulders flexed to 90° in scaption plane and forearm fully supinated. Therapist holds both the hands and resists the shoulder elevation with forearm supination (Fig. 25.41).

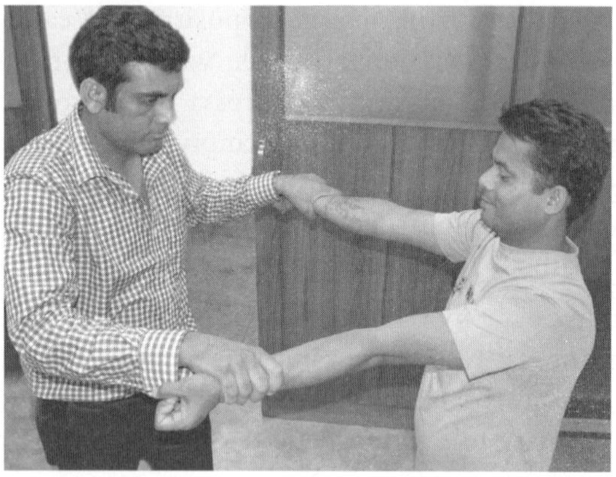

Fig. 25.41: Speed test for bicipital tendinitis

iii. **Biceps Load Test for SLAP:** The patient lies supine with the shoulder abduction to 90°. The examiner stands at the side of the shoulder which is being examined; and grasps the arm at the elbow and hand. The shoulder is rotated externally till the patient feels apprehension. When the patient becomes apprehension during external rotation, the examiner stops the external rotation, and asks the patient to flex the elbow against the resistance. If apprehension is exchanged and becomes more painful, the test is considered positive for SLAP lesion (Figs. 25.42a and b).

(a)

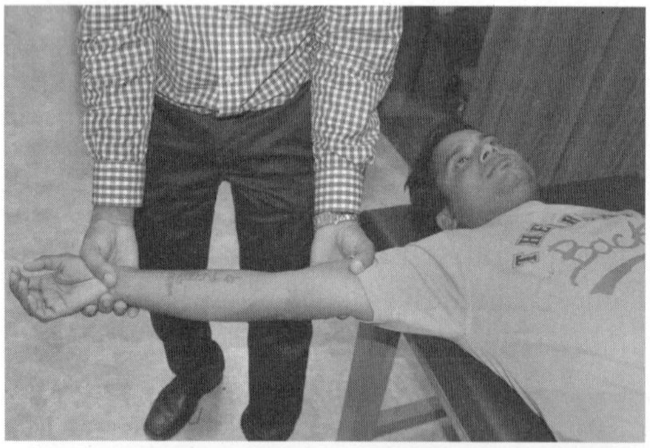

(b)

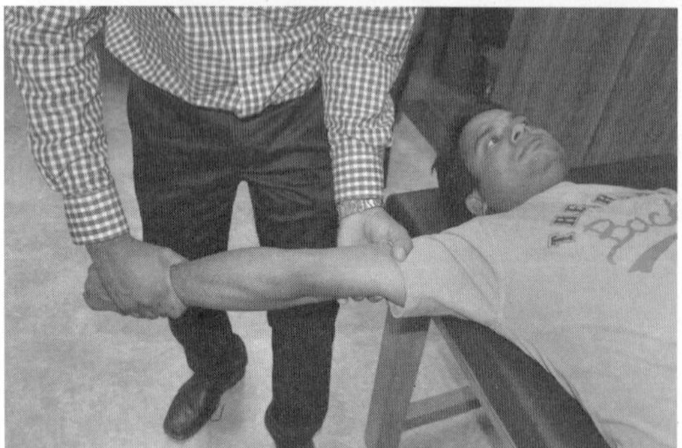

Figs. 25.42a and b: Biceps load test for superior labrum from anterior to posterior

iv. **Painful Arc Syndrome:** In an active flexion and extension, patient feels pain between 120 and 100 degrees. This particular arc is painful because in this range load on the rotator cuff muscles during active flexion and extension increases. The shoulder is abducted passively upto 120°, and the patient is asked to lower the arm actively in a controlled manner. If patient complaints pain between 100° and 80° test is considered positive for rotator cuff tendinitis (Fig. 25.43).

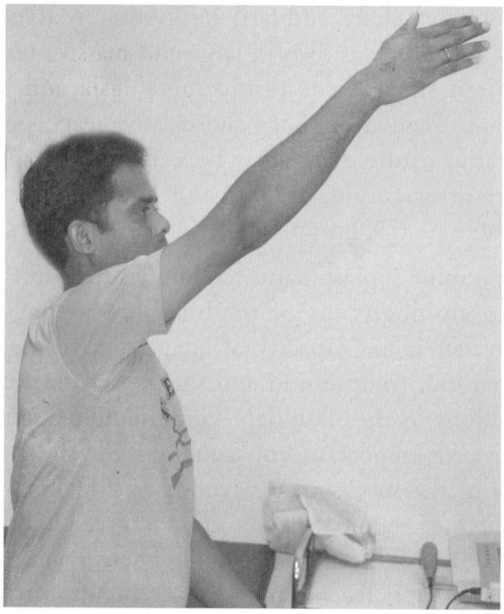

Fig. 25.43: Painful arc syndrome in flexion

v. **Apley's Scratch Test:** The test is performed to assess the shoulder external and internal rotations. The patient stands comfortably, places one hand on the opposite shoulder and tries to touch the superior aspect of the opposite scapula. In the next step the hand is placed on the back and slides up to touch the inferior angle of the scapula. If patient can reach to the scapula the external and internal rotations are considered normal (Figs. 25.44a and b).

vi. **Test for Infraspinatus and Teres Minor Tendinitis:** Patient stands comfortably with the arm at the side (adducted) and elbow flexion to 90°. Examiner stands at the side and resists the external rotation of the shoulder. If the patient complaints pain against the resistance of external rotation of the shoulder, it indicates tendinitis of infraspinatus or teres minor (Fig. 25.45).

vii. **Test for Subscapularis Tendinitis (Lift Off Test):** Patient sits comfortably on the stool with the hand (dorsum aspect) on the lower back region (lumbar spine). Patient is asked to lift the hand off the back. Inability to lift the hand off the back suggests injury to the subscapularis muscles. The test cannot be performed on the patients

(a)

(b)

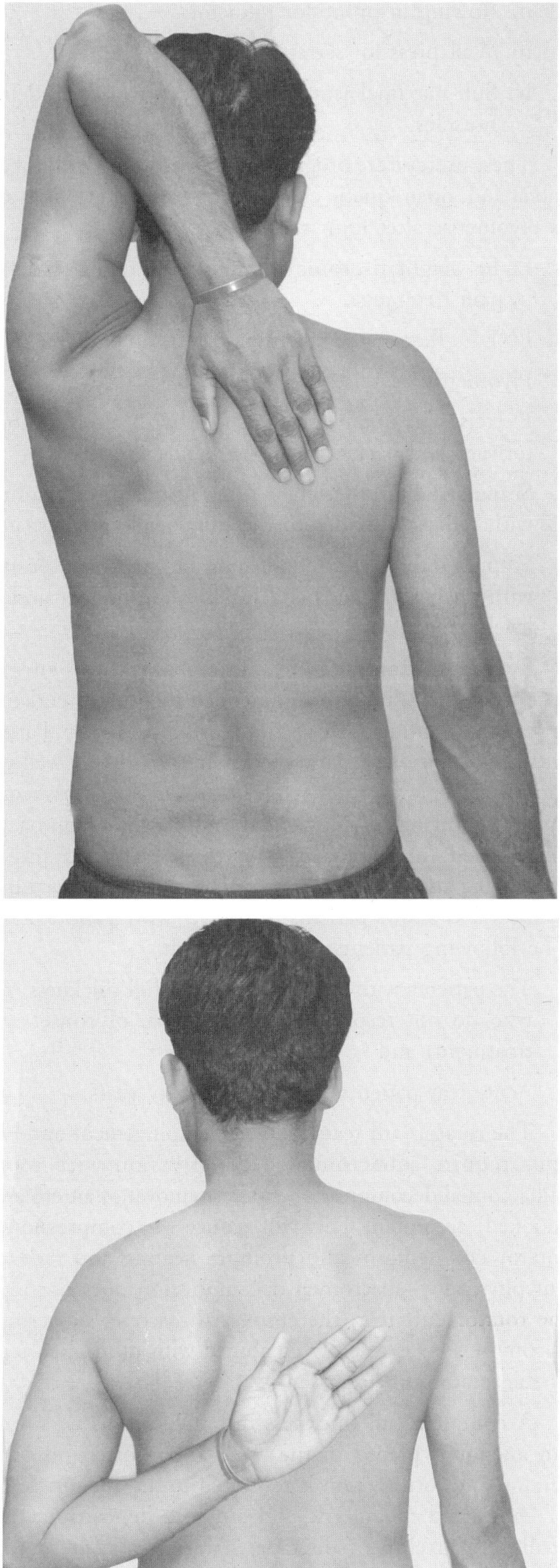

Figs. 25.44a and b: Apley's scratch test

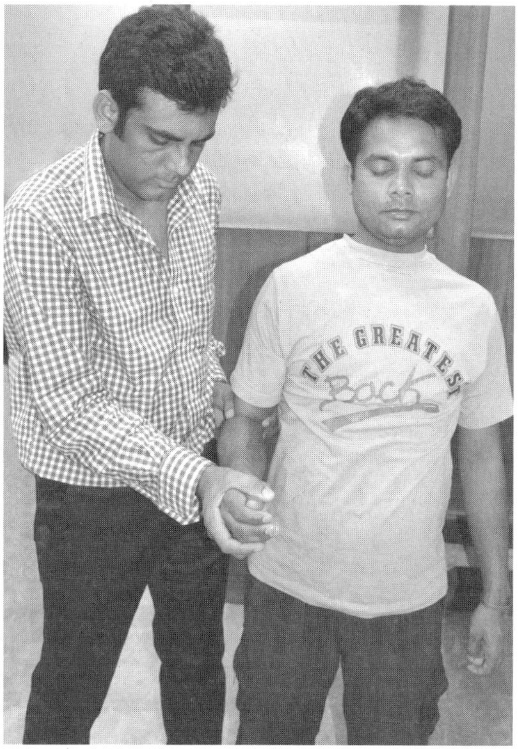

Fig. 25.45: Infraspinatus and teres minor tendinitis test

who have limitation in the internal rotation. For these patients modified lift off test is performed. In this version patient places the hand (palmar aspect) on the abdomen and rotates internally against the resistance. If patient complaints pain, it suggest subscapularis tendinitis (Figs. 25.46a and b).

(a)

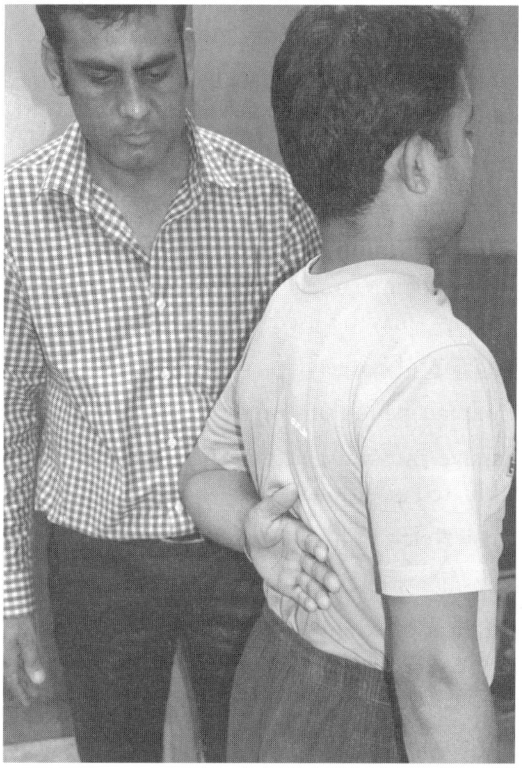

(b)

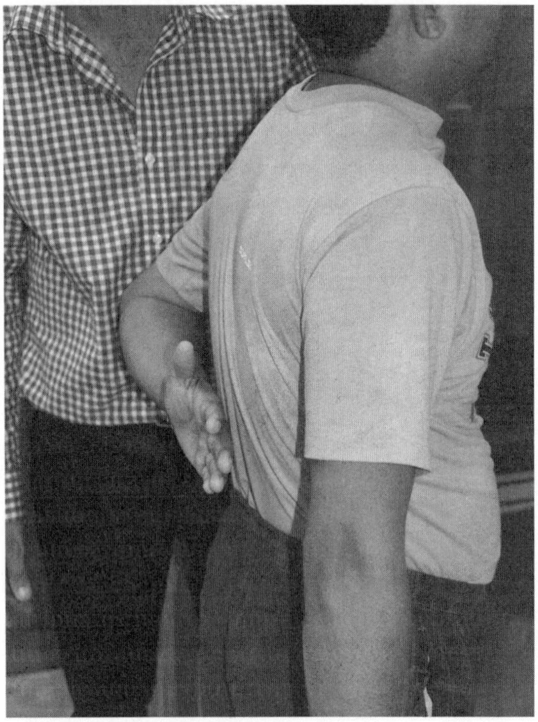

Figs. 25.46a and b: Lift off test

Management

Conservative: The patients with chronic rotator cuff tear follow a fair trial of conservative treatment for at least six months. These patients do not require surgical repair until and unless there is an acute tear of a chronic injury.

1. **Precautions:** Following precautions should be taken to avoid excessive stress on the rotator cuff muscles.
   i. No exercises in scapular (empty can) plane.
   ii. No overhead elevation with internal rotation.
   iii. No hyperextension.
2. **Immobilization:** The chronic rotator cuff tears patients do not require sling or braces to immobilize the shoulder however, this may be advised for comfort for short period.
3. **Control of pain:** To relieve pain moist heat therapy and cryotherapy may be used alternately.
4. **Restoration of range:**
   i. Codman pendulum exercises.
   ii. Passive internal and external rotation in the arm adducted position.
   iii. Passive elevation with external rotation.
   iv. Capsular stretching.
5. **Restoration of strength:**
   i. Sub-maximal isometric strengthening of rotator cuff muscles in arm adducted position to avoid strain in the tendons.
   ii. Rowing in prone for retractors.
   iii. Wall press for serratus anterior.
   iv. Sub-maximal isometric contraction of the deltoid muscles.

These exercise are progressed to the isotonic with tubing theraband, open kinetic chain and functional exercises such as plyometric after four weeks.

a. Light weight (isotonic) dumbbell exercises of deltoid in pain free range.
b. PNF Di flexion and extension pattern in pain free range.
c. Plyometric exercises.
d. Exercises in quadruped position with alternate body forward and backward on the hands and knees.
e. Scapula stabilizers strengthening in quadruped position with raising of hands to the shoulder level alternately.
f. Scapula stabilizers strengthening in quadruped position with raising of hands and legs to the shoulder and hip level respectively.

Surgical Management: There are three surgical approaches commonly recommended for rotator cuff tear—arthroscopic, mini open and open surgical repair. Patients with small tear or partial tears can be treated very well with the arthroscopic approach while large or massive tears require open surgical repair. Now-a-days arthroscopic approach is being used for repair of even the large tears and for mobilizing many of the retracted tears. The procedure is painless and allows patients to recover with a short period. The following patients may be elected:

i. The patients with chronic (partial or full thickness) tear who do not respond to the fair trial of conservative treatment; and
ii. Acute tear patients below age of sixty years.

The rotator cuff tears following impingement and bone spur require subacromial decompression with repair. Subacromial decompression consist removal of anterolateral (hooked) acromian. This will reduce the compression on rotator cuff tendons and promote healing and recovery but physically subacromial decompression does not repair the rotator cuff tear, therefore, arthroscopic subacromial decompression is recently combined with mini open repair of the rotator cuff tears.

A complete full thickness tear involves tissue sutures. An anchor is placed in the bone at the insertion of the tendon and torn tendon is resutured to the anchor. In case of chondroid metaplasic and amyloid deposition, mesh (collagen, artelon or degrade material) may be used to reinforce the repair. The mini open technique is preferred over open surgical approach as it requires tear through a deltoid splitting approach, which causes minimal injury to the deltoid muscles and produce better results. The open surgical repair procedure requires detachment of a portion of the deltoid.

Post Arthroscopic and Mini open Repair Management: The rehabilitation of rotator cuff tears repair consist immobilization, relief in pain, restoration of range of motion, restoration of strength and functional strengthening.

Phase I 0 to three weeks

i. **Immobilization:** Sling is recommended to immobilize the shoulder during the day for one week and at night at least for 6 weeks. The sling is removed for the exercises.
ii. **Mobilization:** Pendulum exercises started within 48 hours of the operation in the pain free range of motion. Passive internal and external rotation in painfree range with the arm adducted and elbow flexed to 90 degrees.
iii. **Restoration of strength:** Sub-maximal isometric contraction in pain free range of deltoid (anterior, posterior and lateral), rotator cuff muscles and parascapular muscles.

Phase II Four weeks to six weeks

i. Sling continue at night.
ii. Progress to open kinetic chain exercises with theraband or tubing or dumbbell as per weight tolerance within the pain free range of motion.
iii. Rowing in prone for retractor muscles strengthening.
iv. Wall press for serratus anterior strengthening.

Phase III Seven weeks to three months (early intermediate phase)

i. Continue strengthening exercises of rotator cuff with tubing, rowing in prone for retractors with dumbbells and wall press.
ii. Anterior, posterior and inferior glides to stretch the capsule and increase range of motion.
iii. Progress to light functional activities.

Phase IV Three months to six months (Advanced strengthening)

i. Functional activities.
ii. Plyometric exercises.
iii. Swimming.
iv. Return to play with warm up and conditioning exercises.

Prognosis

Rotator cuff tears is the degenerative process which affects people often in the fifth decade of life. Many studies have shown the people with rotator cuff tear remain asymptomatic, however, micro tears are progressed to the partial and large rotator cuff tears over the time, and 20% patients of whose tears enlarges remain asymptomatic and 80% patients eventually develop symptoms gradually. The high rate of tear prevalence in asymptomatic individuals suggests that rotator cuff tears could be considered a "normal process of degeneration" rather than of an apparent pathological process.

ADHESIVE CAPSULITIS

Adhesive capsulitis is a condition of glenohumeral joint in which the non-contractile structure joint capsule becomes inflamed and tight. In 1946, Naviaser had surgically explored 10 cases of stiff shoulders, and found absence of glenohumeral synovial fluid and redundant axillary fold of the capsule, as well as thickened and contracted joint capsule which had become adherent to the humeral head, thus he used the term adhesive capsulitis. On microscopic examination he found reparative inflammatory changes in the capsule.

Etiology

The etiology of adhesive capsulitis or frozen shoulder remains unknown, however, evaluation of anatomic, histologic, and surgical specimens from patients with idiopathic frozen shoulders demonstrate that the disease often involves inflammation in the glenohumeral joint capsule. Although, most of authors describe that limitation in the range of motion of glenohumeral joint in chronic phase is not due to capsular adhesions. Instead, pathologic data confirm an active process of hyperplastic fibroplasia and excessive secretion of type III collagen fibers, that cause tightness in the coracohumeral ligament, soft tissues in the rotator interval, the subscapularis muscle, and the subacromial bursae.

The contractures in patients with frozen shoulder are identical to those seen in a Dupuytren contracture of the hand. These contractures have a classical feature of progressive loss of range of motion of the joint. Despite these histopathologic similarities, the favourable and regressive outcome of adhesive capsulitis differ from the unfavourable and progressive outcome of Dupuytren disease. The studies have also found presence of autonomic sympathetic dysfunction in the upper extremities in patients with isolated idiopathic frozen shoulder. The studies have found similar histologic findings in joints affected by complex regional pain syndrome and frozen shoulder. Both the conditions have similar risk factors such as trauma, diabetes, thyroid disease and dyslipidemia.

Epidemiology

The prevalence of adhesive capsulitis in the general population is reported to be 2%, however, the unselected individuals with diabetes may have prevalence rate of upto 11%. The most significant association with insulin dependent diabetic patient is the risk of developing of adhesive capsulitis in their life is approximately 40%. The disease may affect bilateral shoulders in as many as 16% of patients. Both the shoulders may be affected, either simultaneously or sequentially. The contralateral shoulder is usually affected within 5 years of disease.

Adhesive capsulitis is also associated with medical conditions such as, hyperthyroidism, ischemic heart disease, inflammatory arthritis and cervical spondylosis.

Adhesive capsulitis affects females more than males with the female to male ratio of about 1.4:1. The females are affected somewhat earlier than the males; with the mean age of onset are 52 years for females and 55 years for males. There is no racial variation seen in the patients with adhesive capsulitis.

Clinical Features

Stiffness and pain with progressive loss of both active and passive movements are the dominant features of adhesive capsulitis. Initially patients with adhesive capsulitis complaint pain at night with sleep disturbance but in the advance phase pain decreases in intensity and also patients feel less discomfort in sleeping, however active and passive range of motions are decreased in all three planes. The loss of range of motion occurs in a typical capsular pattern–external roation, abduction, flexion and internal rotation. Reverse scapulohumeral rhythm is the classical feature of the adhesive capsulitis in late phases. Pain may radiate down the lateral aspect of arm. The symptoms of adhesive capsulitis usually progress gradually over a number of months or years. The symptoms may also vary greatly from person to person. Adhesive capsulitis is classically characterized by three phases which can sometimes be difficult to distinguish.

Freezing Phase: Patients typically experience stiffness and dull ache, deep situated pain that may increase to a sharper with certain movements or activities. The pain is usually more severe at rest and at night and often aggravates when the patients turn side on the affected shoulder. This keeps the patient awaken for hours. To relieve pain, patient uses hot water bag. The range of motion is not limited in this phase. This phase lasts upto 2-9 months.

Frozen Phase (3-18 months): This phase is also known as progressive stiffness phase in which range of motion decreases gradually over the time. Progressive limitation in range of motion occurs in a capsular pattern, such as external rotation, abduction, flexion and internal rotation. The intensity of pain is decreased gradually but pain at night remains a common complaint especially when the patient turns on the affected side. The intensity of referred pain from shoulder to lateral arm also decreases. The activities of daily living are grossly compromised, patient finds difficulty in combing hair, reaching into the back pocket, washing the opposite shoulder, taking off the inner wears and fastening the bra.

Thawing Phase: It is the last stage of adhesive capsulitis characterized by minimum pain, gross limitation in range of motion and slow recovery in range. Patients may demonstrate reverse scapulohumeral rhythm.

Differential Diagnosis

It is not easy to differentiate the adhesive capsulitis from other conditions as pain stiffness, and loss of range of motion are present in all the shoulder conditions. However, based on some clinical and radiological findings adhesive capsulitis can be differentiated from other shoulder conditions. Rest pain, night pain, sleep disturbance with loss of external rotation are the distinguished features of adhesive capsulitis, moreover, all the resisted movements of shoulder remain pain free.

Impingement Syndrome: External rotation is not limited in the initial phase. End range flexion with internal rotation elicits pain. Painful arc, empty cane and Hawkins Kennedy tests are positive in patients with impingement syndrome. These tests are negative in adhesive capsulitis.

Rotator Cuff Tendinitis: Resisted movements are painful. Painful arc syndrome will also be positive. Patients complaint pain in the mid range. The passive flexion may be full and pain free.

Anterior Instability: Patient feels instability rather than pain. Pain is present in the posterior deltoid because of overuse and eccentric contraction to prevent anterior translation of the head of humerus. There is no limitation in external rotation, instead of that internal rotation is decreased as posterior capsule becomes tight.

Therapist asks the chief complaint to the patient and establishes a pleasant relationship so that he or she can take history. Therapist asks questions related to the complaint, which helps in making a provisional diagnosis.

Management

The degree of pain and disability caused by idiopathic frozen shoulder is highly variable and depends on the stages of the disease. Sometimes the physical modalities and exercises fail to improve the symptoms. Therefore, the treatment to adhesive capsulitis should be multifactorial. It should consist physical modalities, therapeutic exercises, medications, intra-articular injections and surgical intervention if it is needed. Following should be the goal of treatment:

1. Relief of pain.
2. Maintenance of range of motion.
3. Maintenance of muscle strength.
4. Restoration of range of motion.
5. Restoration of muscle strength.
6. Correction of posture.

Relief of Pain: Adhesive capsulitis is a painful condition that often causes great frustration for both patients and clinicians. Pain progresses over time, hence, the physical modalities being used for relieving pain may not be effective at one time. Hot packs, ice packs and interferential therapy may be beneficial in relieving pain and symptoms. Ultrasound of 1MHz may also help in relieving pain, and increasing extensibility of the joint capsule. Hold relax and contract relax exercises should be initiated to reduce the spasm of shoulder girdle muscles. Soft tissue manipulation and pendulum exercises also help in relieving pain and muscle spasm. If patient do not respond to the modalities and soft tissue manipulation he or she should be referred to orthopedic surgeon for non-steroidal anti-inflammatory drugs and corticosteroids. Unfortunately the progression of the disease cannot be halted with the aforesaid treatments, therefore, patient should be educated about the progression of the disease so that he or she should be continued with the treatment. Although some patients recover in 2 months without entering into phase; however, other may enter into frozen phase and have symptoms upto 24 months.

Maintenance of Range of Motion: In the freezing phase pain is the main complaint of the patient. The limitation in the range of motion is not the usual feature of freezing phase. But because of pain, patient starts avoiding end range movements, that can limit the range of motion of joint in the frozen phase. Hold relax, contract relax and passive range of motion, gentle glides and pendular exercises should be started to maintain the range of motion. Exercises to maintain the range of motion should be continued unless and until there is significant improvement in pain and sumptoms.

Maintenance of Muscle Strength: Isometric exercises of rotator cuff muscles and scapular stabilizers are initiated to maintain the strength of muscles.

Restoration of Range of Motion: Range of motion is limited because of tightness of the muscles, ligaments and joint capsule. To improve range of motion muscle relaxation technique and glides are administered to increase the flexibility of muscles, ligaments and joint capsule.

PNF Techniques: Hold Relax and Contract Relax: These techniques are beneficial in relaxing the muscles. To improve the external rotation, patient is placed in a comfortable position, and shoulder is rotated externally as much as possible. With an appropriate stabilization the internal rotators (subscapularis muscle) are allowed to contract isotonically (contract relax) against the resistance. Several repetitions of contract relax are performed to improve external rotation.

To improve flexion, patient lies in a comfortable position, and shoulder is flexed as much as possible. With an appropriate stabilization, the extensors are contracted against the resistance (contract relax). Several repetitions of contract relax are performed to improve flexion range.

To improve abduction, the patient lies in a comfortable position and shoulder is abducted as much as possible. With an appropriate stabilization the shoulder is adducted isotonically against the resistance (contract relax). Several repetitions are performed to improve abduction range.

To improve internal rotation, the patient lies in a comfortable position, and shoulder is rotated internally as much as possible. With an appropriate stabilization the shoulder is rotated externally against the resistance. Several repetitions of contract relax may be performed to improve internal rotation.

The muscle relaxation techniques are followed by muscle stretching and capsule glides to achieve maximum results.

Hold relax and reciprocal inhibition techniques may also be performed to relax the muscles in case of severe muscle spasm.

Mobilization

The patients with adhesive capsulitis usually present with capsular pattern. Initially the anterior capsule adheres to the humerus followed by inferior and posterior. To improve range of motion, the capsule must be stretched. To stretch the capsule the joint is distracted and glided with significant force.

Capsule Stretching: The loss of range of motion in patients with adhesive capsulitis is mainly due to tightness in the capsule. Initially anterior joint capsule becomes tight which limits the external rotation of the shoulder but as the disease progresses inferior and posterior part of capsule also becomes tight. The joint capsule can be stretched with the glides after placing the joint in an extreme limitation range. Shoulder joint capsule stretching techniques are explained in Chapter 7.

26

CERVICAL SPINE

CONCISE ANATOMY

The cervical spine is comprised seven vertebrae. C_1vertebra also known as atlas does not have body and spinous process and it serves as a ring or washer that the skull rests upon and articulates in a pivot joint with the dens or odontoid process of C_2. The atlas is composed of two arches anterior (thick) and posterior arch (thin), and two prominent lateral masses. Each lateral mass has a superior and inferior articular facet joint. Superior articular facets are kidney shaped, concave, and face upward and inward, these articulate with the occipital condyles. The inferior lateral articular facet joints are relatively flat face downward and inward and articulate with the superior facets of the axis. According to Steele's rule of thirds, at the level of the atlas, the odontoid process, the subarachnoid space, and spinal cord each occupy one third of the area of the spinal canal (Figs. 26.1a, b, 26.2 and 26.3).

C_2 vertebra also known as axis has a large body which contains the odontoid process (dens). The odontoid process to the atlas is held in place by the transverse ligament. The apical, alar, and transverse ligaments, by allowing spinal column rotation, provide further stabilization and prevent posterior displacement of the dens in relation to the atlas. Fifty percent rotation (45 degrees) of the cervical spine occurs at the atlanoaxial joint.

(a)

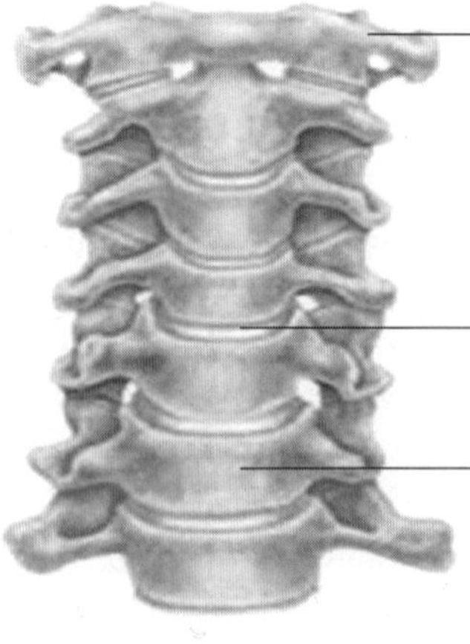

(b)

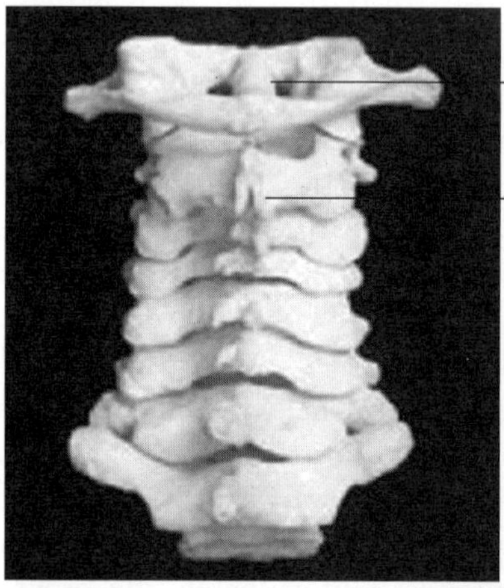

Figs. 26.1a and b: Cervical spine a. Anterior view, b. Posterior view

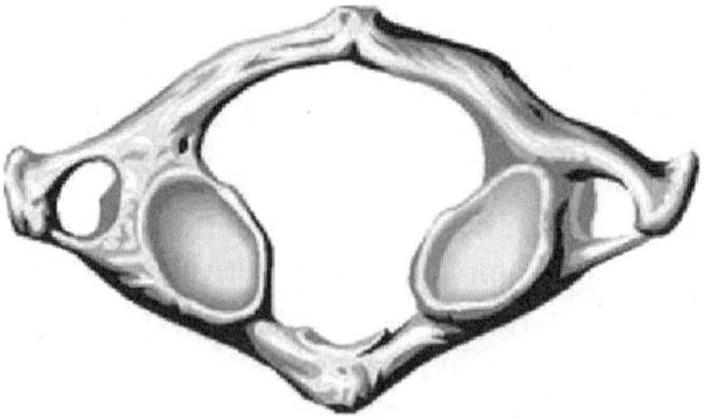

Fig. 26.2: Atlas

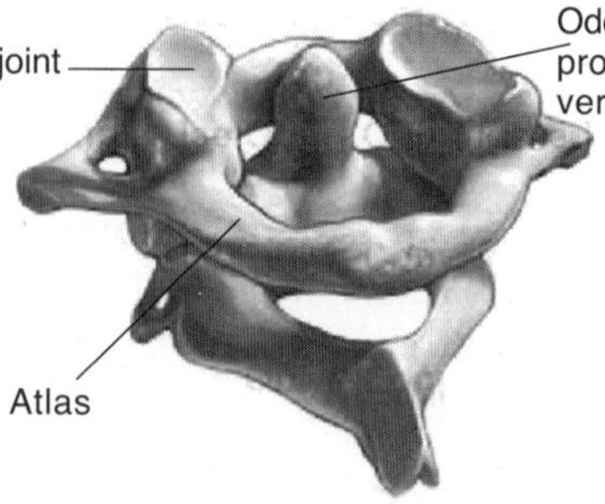

Fig. 26.3: Atlas articulation with axial vertebra superior view

Stability

The static stability of the upper cervical spine is mainly provided by the external and internal ligaments. The external ligaments consist of the atlanto-occipital, anterior atlanto-occipital, and anterior longitudinal ligaments. The internal ligaments have 5 components:

i. The transverse ligament holds the odontoid process in place against the posterior atlas, and prevents anterior subluxation of C_1 on C_2.

ii. The accessory ligaments arise posterior to and in conjunction with the transverse ligament and insert into the lateral aspect of the atlantoaxial joint; the apical ligament lies anterior to the lip of the foramen magnum and inserts into the apex of the odontoid process.

iii. The paired alar ligaments secure the apex of the odontoid to the anterior foramen magnum.

iv. The tectorial membrane is a continuation of the posterior longitudinal ligament to the anterior margin of the foramen magnum.

v. The 3 cm × 5 mm accessory atlantoaxial ligament not only connects the atlas to the axis but also continues cephalad to the occipital bone; functionally, it becomes maximally taut with 5-8° of head rotation, lax with cervical extension, and maximally taut with 5-10° of cervical flexion.

The lower cervical spine is made up of five vertebrae from C_2 to C_7. Each vertebra from C_2 to C_7 has a body which is concave on its superior surface and convex on its inferior surface. The spinous processes of C_3 to C_6 are usually of bifid, whereas the spinous process of C_7 is nonbifid and somewhat bulbous at its end.

Facet Joints

The facet joints in the lower cervical spine are most noticeable near the pedicles. These are diarthrodial synovial joints with fibrous capsules surrounded by a capsule of connective tissue and produces synovial fluid to nourish and lubricate the articular cartilage. The C_0-C_1 and C_1-C_2 joints are innervated by anterior rami of the first and second cervical spinal nerves, whereas, C_2-C_3 facet joint is innervated by two branches of the posterior ramus of the third cervical spinal nerve. Each C_3-C_4 to C_7-T_1 is innervated by the medial branches above and below (Figs. 26.4a and b).

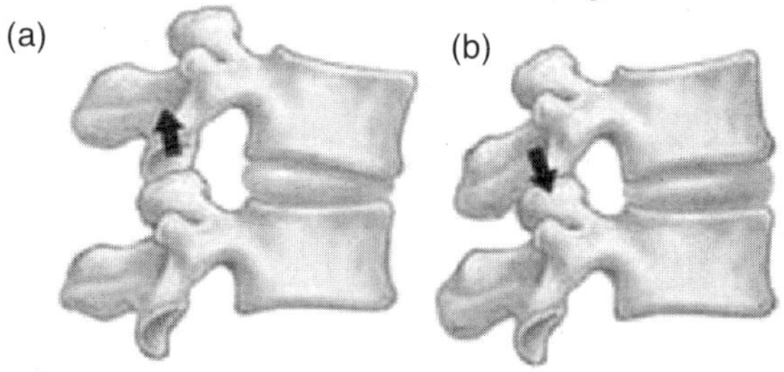

Figs. 26.4a and b: Intervertebral disc a. upslide, b. down slide of the facet joints

Movements: Movement in the cervical spine occurs in all three planes as flexion, extension and rotation, these are mentioned in the Tables 26.1 to 26.4.

Table 26.1: Movements of the facet joints of cervical spine

Movement	*Plane of movement*
Flexion	The upper facet slides up and forward on the lower facet
Extension	The upper facet slides down and back on the lower facet
Side flexion	The upper facet slides down and back on the same side and up and forward on the opposite side
Rotation	The upper facet slides down and posterior on the same side and up and anterior on the opposite side

Table 26.2: Approximate range of motion of cervical spine (Craniocervical region) in degrees

Joints	*Flexion*	*Extension*	*Axial rotation*	*Side flexion*
Atlanto-occipital	5	10	Negligible	5
Atlantoaxial	5	10	40-45	Negligible
Intracervical region (C_2-C_7)	35	60-70	45	35
Total range of motion at craniocervical region	45	80-90	90	40

Table 26.3: Muscles of the craniovertebral region

Muscles	*Action(s)*
Rectus capitis posterior minor	Atlanto-occipital extension
Rectus capitis posterior major	Craniovertebral complex extension
Superior oblique	C_0-C_1 ipsilateral side flexion and extension
Inferior oblique	C_1-C_2 ipsilateral rotation
Rectus capitis lateralis	C_0-C_1 joint ipsilateral side flexion
Rectus capitis anterior	C_0-C_1 joint flexion

Table 26.4: Muscles and their action/movements of lower cervical

Muscles	*Action(s)/Movement(s)*
Longus coli	Flexion, ipsilateral rotation, ipsilateral side flexion
Longus capitis	Flexion, ipsilateral rotation
Scalenes anterior	Flexion, contralateral rotation, ipsilateral side flexion
Scalene medius	Ipsilateral side flexion, contralateral rotation
Scalene posterior	Ipsilateral side flexion, contralateral rotation
Sternocleidomastoid	Flexion, contralateral rotation, ipsilateral side flexion and extension
Trapezius upper fibers	Ipsilateral side flexion, contralateral rotation and extension
Levator scapula	Ipsilateral side flexion and ipsilateral rotation
Splenius, capitis and cervicis	Extension, ipsilateral rotation and ipsilateral side flexion
Spinalis, capitis and cervicis (inconsistent—blends with semispinalis)	Extension
Semispinalis, capitis and cervicis	Contralateral rotation and extension
Longissimus, capitis and cervicis	Extension, ipsilateral rotation and ipsilateral side flexion
Iliocostalis cervicis	Extension and ipsilateral side flexion
Interspinalis	Extension
Multifidus	Extension, contralateral rotation
Rotators	Extension and ipsilateral rotation
Intertransversarii	Contralateral rotation

PROLAPSED INTERVERTEBRAL DISC

Intervertebral Disc

The intervertebral disc is the largest avascular structure in the body which is situated between two vertebral bodies. It is composed of annulus fibrosus (AF), and a nuclease pulposus (NP). It is reinforced peripherally by an end plate. As it is the largest avascular structure in the body its nutrition depends on diffusion. It receives its blood supply from the two closest vessel sources, which are those beneath the vertebral end plate and those at the periphery of the annulus fibrosus. Certain movements possible those in and out of the flexion, may facilitate nutrition of the disc (one of the benefit of exercise may be to facilitate the nutrition of the intervertebral disc). The intervertebral disc has a blood supply upto 8 years, thereafter, they are dependent for their own diffusion of tissue fluids. As the intervertebral disc is an avascular and its nutrition depends upon the diffusion and movements its healing transpires, but complete healing takes months to years (Fig. 26.5).

Pathomechanics

Disc herniation is the protrusion of the nucleus pulposus of the disc through the annulus fibrosus. The nucleus pulposus is a non compressible gelatinous material of the disc which absorbs and transfers the weight to the adjacent vertebra. As the load of the body comes on the nucleus pulposus it may protrude anteriorly, posteriorly, or laterally but fortunately it is prevented by the annulus fibrosus. The annulus fibrosus is strengthened and reinforced by the end plate. Therefore, in spite of protrusion to the anteriorly or posterolaterally that the nucleus pulposus transfers the weight to the adjacent vertebra. Unfortunately, forward bending of the cervical spine places excessive load on the posterior annulus fibrosus and on the end plate. If the movement is combined with jerk, twist or injury it may rupture the annulus fibrosus and end plate and the nucleus pulposus may protrude through the ruptured annulus fibrosus to the posterolaterally, where it can put significant pressure on the nerve roots.

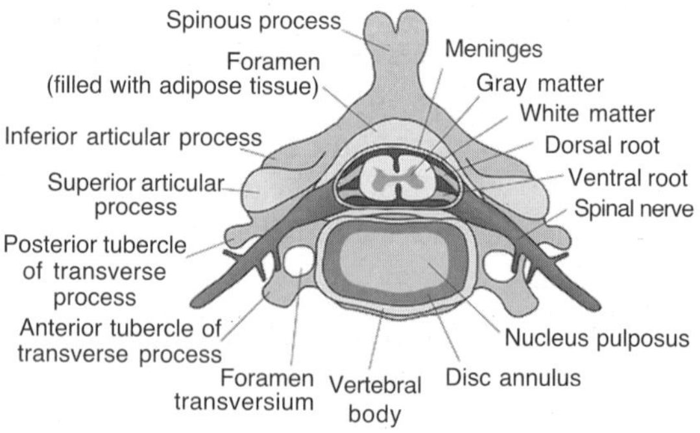

Fig. 26.5: Normal disc image

Disc herniation in the cervical spine occurs most commonly at the C_5-C_6 and C_6-C_7 vertebral levels, and radicular symptoms are experienced in the course of C_6 and C_7 nerve roots. There are two mechanisms which may cause disc herniation. First, the disc herniation may result from general wear and tear, such as when performing jobs that require constant sitting or involves forward bending movements. Such types of activities elongate and weaken the annular fibrous and end plate, which may in turn later stages allow the nucleus pulposus to herniate through the annulus fibrosus. This is a slow process of the disc herniation. The second mechanism, involves the jerk or sudden injury to the disc which causes nucleus pulposus herniation through the annulus fibrosus posterolaterally that may put pressure on the nerve roots to produce radicular symptoms. Since there is not a lot discs material (size of the disc) between the vertebral bodies in the cervical spine, the discs are not usually very large. The size of the vertebral foramen from where the nerve roots pass are also not that great, which means that even a small cervical disc herniation may impinge the nerve and cause significant radicular symptoms (Fig. 26.6).

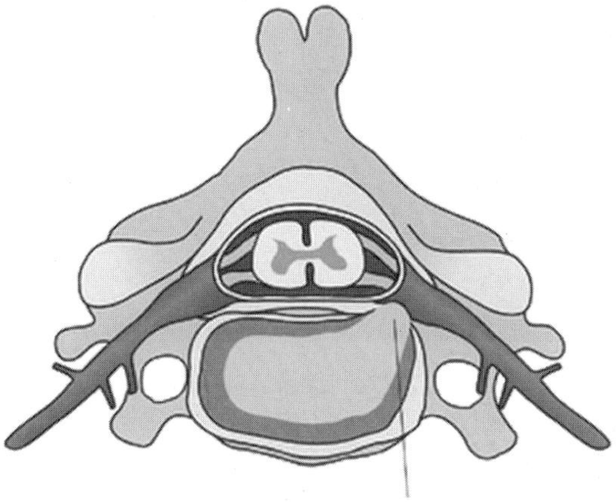

Fig. 26.6: Intervertebral disc herniation causing nerve compression

Clinical Features

A cervical herniated disc may produce pain either in the cervical region or in the arm or both that depends upon the severity of the disc herniation and pressure on the nerve roots. In case of posterolateral herniation with significant nerve root compression the area of symptoms will be as below:

1. C_4-C_5 **Intervertebral Segment:** Pain and weakness will be in the course of the C_5 nerve root (deltoid region) it usually does not cause numbness and tingling sensation.
2. C_5-C_6 **Intervertebral Segment:** It is one of the most common sites, involves C_6 nerve root. Pain numbness, tingling sensation may be experienced in the course of the C_6, i.e., thumb of the hand. Adequate pressure on the C_6 nerve root can cause weakness in the biceps and wrist extensor muscles. The biceps jerk may diminish.
3. C_6-C_7 **Intervertebral Segment:** Pain, numbness and tingling sensation is experienced in the course of the C_7 nerve root, i.e., posterior aspect of the arm and middle finger. It may cause significant weakness in the triceps and finger extensors. This is also one of the most common levels for a disc herniation. Triceps jerk may diminish.
4. C_7-C_8 **Intervertebral Segment:** This may produce weakness in the finger flexors and numbness and tingling sensation in the forearm (ulnar side) to the little finger of the hand.

Symptoms: Patients experience more pain and symptoms in the arm and shoulder. To avoid pain and stretching in the nerve the patient keeps the shoulder elevated, which further contributes to the spasm in the upper fibers of trapezius muscle of the same side but relieves tension in the nerve. Diffused type of tenderness may be present on the neck. The patient bends the cervical spine to the opposite side to avoid pressure on the nerve roots which in turn produces cervical scoliosis or list. In patients with acute radiculopathy the symptoms such as pain, parasthesia, numbness and tingling sensation are the common symptoms. Weakness and loss of jerks may also be present in long standing cases. Patients report that their symptoms decrease when they place their hand on the top of the head, as this position decrease the tension in the nerve roots. The symptoms are aggravated by the neck movements particularly by flexion which opens the posterior intervertebral space that allows disc to protrude posteriorly. Sneezing and coughing also aggravate the symptoms.

Assessment

Observation: Normally the chin should be in line with the sternum (manubrium), the ears should be in line with the shoulders and the forehead vertical in the cervical spine. Deviation such as side flexion and rotation due to torticolis or muscle spasm should carefully be observed from anterior view. Other postural deviations such as Klippel Feil syndrome (fusion of the some cervical vertebra usually C_3-C_5), forward head posture (poking chin), torticolis should also be observed.

Shoulder Elevation: Usually the dominant shoulder will slightly be lower than the non-dominant side, spasm or injury can cause elevation of the shoulder to provide protection and relief in the symptoms.

Shoulder Protraction: Shoulders may be protracted due to weakness of the depressors and retractors (rhomboids).

Scapula Winging: The medial border of the scapula may also be raised on thoracic wall due to weakness of the serratus anterior.

Rounded Shoulders: The rounded shoulders may be associated with forward head posture. It is common in long standing and chronic cases.

Muscle Wasting: Muscle wasting usually does not seen but in long standing cases it may be observed on the scapular, parascapular and muscles supplied by the corresponding nerve root. The motion may be limited and painful in all three planes in later stages.

List: It is the most common feature of the prolapsed intervertebral disc which can be observed in acute and chronic cases. The patient bends the neck to the opposite side to relieve the pressure on the nerve roots. In long standing cases the muscles of the concave side becomes tight and produces scoliosis in the cervical spine (Figs. 26.7a to e).

Palpation: *Tenderness:* Tenderness may be present on the para-vertebral regions and on the spinous processes.

Passive Movements: Passive ranges may be limited with the abnormal end feels. The therapist palpates each structure to reproduce the symptoms so that the site where from pain is originated may be determined. Passive

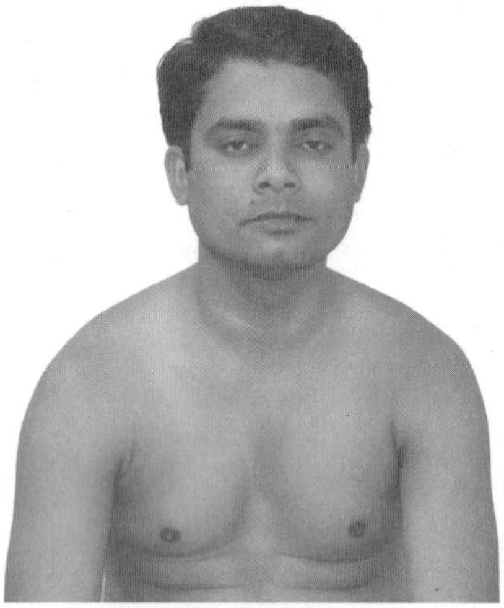

Fig. 26.7a: Anterior view

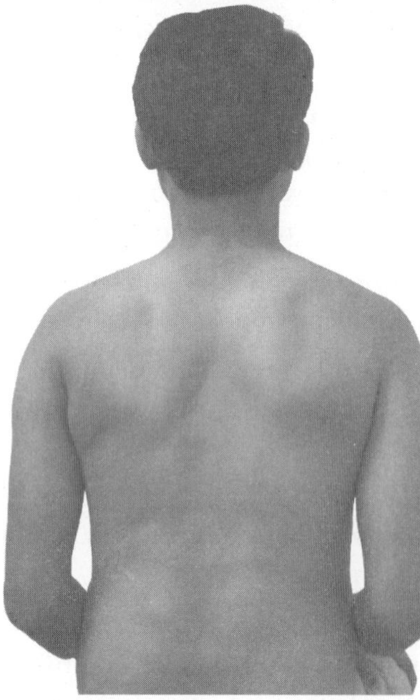

Fig. 26.7b: Posterior view

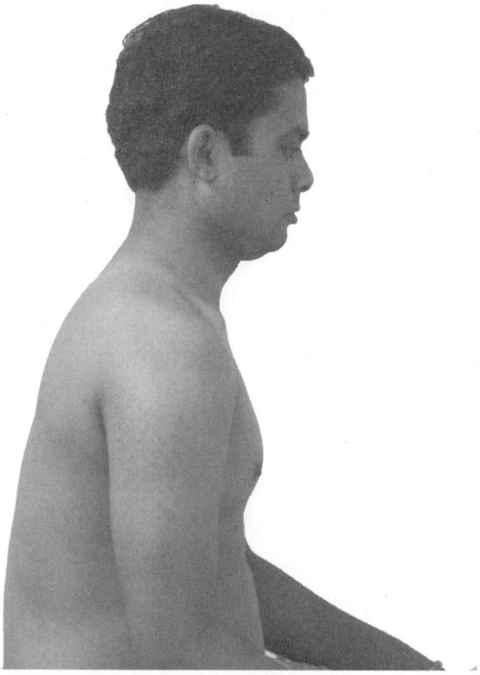

Fig. 26.7c: Lateral view

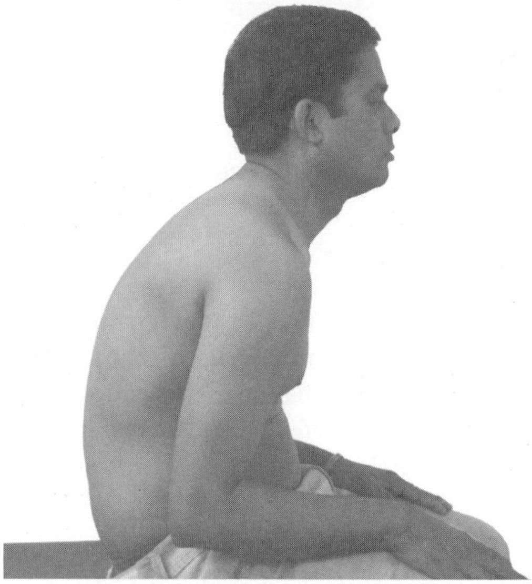

Fig. 26.7d: Forward head posture

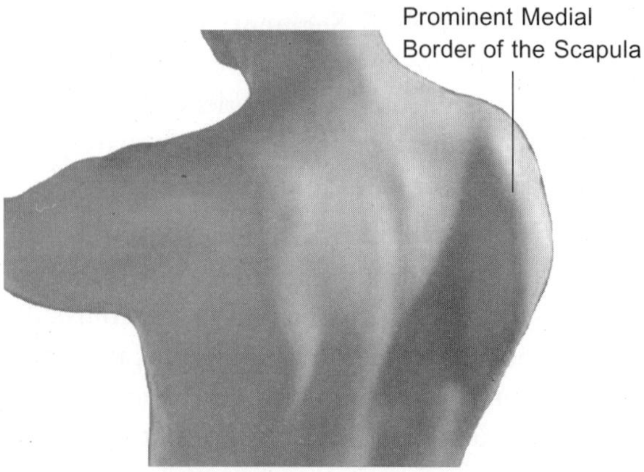

Fig. 26.7e: Winging of the scapula

ıovements are performed to determine the end feel. Patients ıay play tricks on the therapist by performing ompensatory movements at other joints, therefore, to etermine the motion at the cervical spine the distal egments should be stabilized. To test the flexion at the ervical spine the examiner should first flex the upper cervical pine and then (while maintaining it), the lower cervical pine is flexed. Limitation in the range of motion determines ss of upper cervical spine flexion. The other movements ıould also be tested passively.

Capsular Pattern: The examiner should also note hether a capsular pattern is present or not. The capsular attern is the limitation of side flexion with rotation. The ıovements at each segment during side flexion and rotation ay be felt by palpating the adjacent transverse process on ıch side.

Identification of the Transverse Process of the C_1: The xaminer places the thumb and index finger on each side f the mastoid process and then moves the finger and ıumb inferiorly and anteriorly until a hard bump is alpated on each side (usually below the ear lobe and just ehind the jaw) (Figs. 26.8a and b).

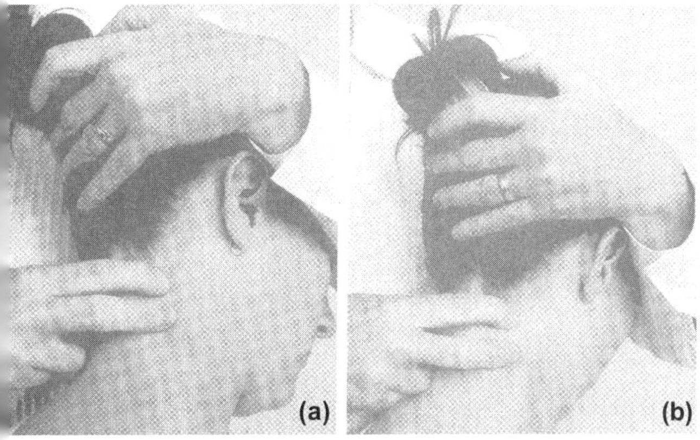

igs. 26.8a and b: Identification of the transverse process of e C_1

Identification of the C_7 Vertebra: The spinous process f the C_7 vertebra is prominent and it can easily be lentified by placing the thumb on the spinous process.

If the passive movements with over pressure fail to produce the symptoms, the examiner may with great care, rogress to the combination of movements.

Special Tests: Special tests are performed to reproduce ıe symptoms.

Foraminal Compression and Distraction: Patient sits n the stool with both arms hanging at the side of the ody. Therapist stands behind the patient and places both ıe hands on the top of the head of the patient. While aintaining the neck in neutral position the therapist pplies downward pressure through the body to the head. The test is considered positive if patient experiences radicular symptoms with the pressure. It suggests radiculopathy due to soft disc herniation or due to degenerative changes putting pressure on the nerve roots. If symptoms such as pain aggravates in the cervical spine without radiation it may be due to arthritic changes without radiculopathy (Figs. 26.9 and 26.10). In the next process the therapist changes the position of hands and places on occiput and under the chin and distracts the cervical spine by applying upward force. If it relieves symptoms, then confirms the radiculopathy.

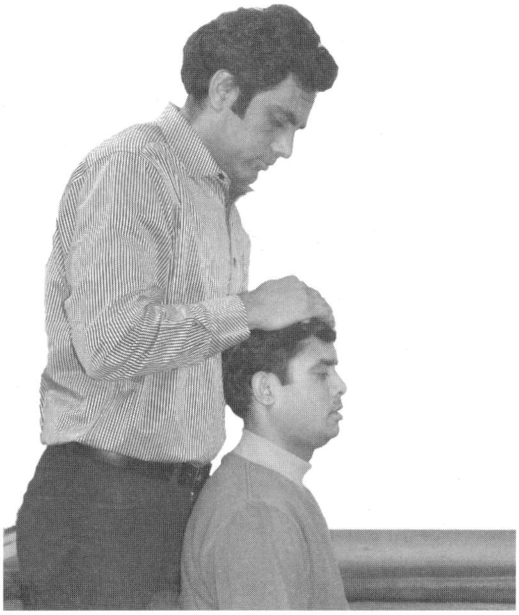

Fig. 26.9: Foraminal compression test

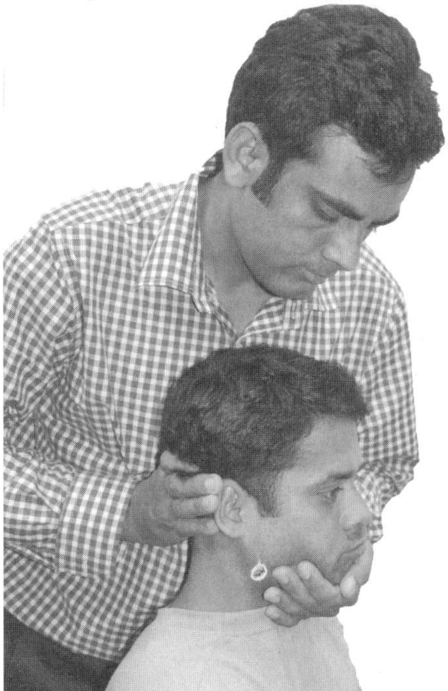

Fig. 26.10: Foraminal distraction test

Spurling Test

Also known as quadrant test is very useful in reproducing the symptoms in the cervical spine. Patient remains in sitting position as foraminal distraction and compression test. Therapist stands behind the patient and places both the hands on either side of the head of the patient. The head is extended, flexed to the affected side, and rotated (same side) and a downward pressure is applied through the body and arms and is maintained for 30 seconds for delayed onset of symptoms. The test is considered positive if it reproduces radicular symptoms to the same side. This suggests radiculopathy due to soft disc herniation or degenerative changes causing compression on the nerve roots. If the test aggravates pain on the same side of the side flexion and rotation without radicular symtoms, it suggests changes in the facet joints and outer part of the disc (Figs. 26.11a to c).

Upper Limb Tension Tests

Upper limb tension tests are known as brachial plexus tension tests, were first described by Elvey. The tests were designed to put the pressure on the neural structure of the upper extremity similar to straight leg raising test for lower extremity. These are divided into three tests according to the course and distribution of the upper extremity spinal nerves (brachial plexus).

(a)

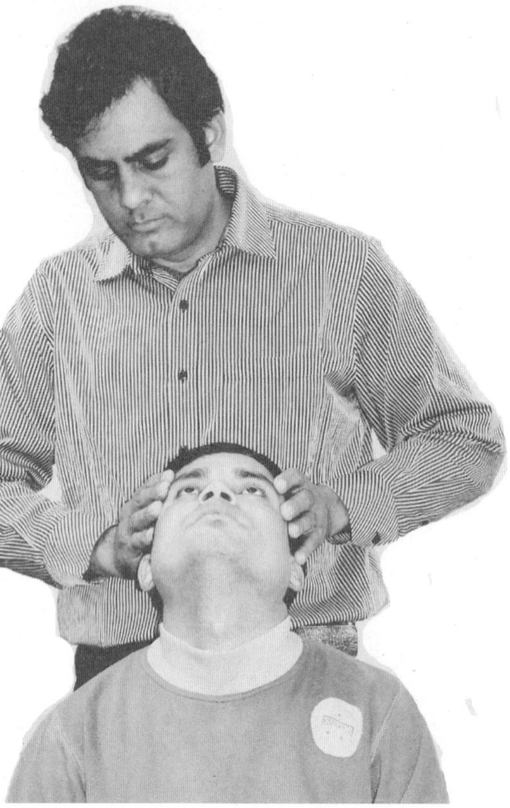

(b)

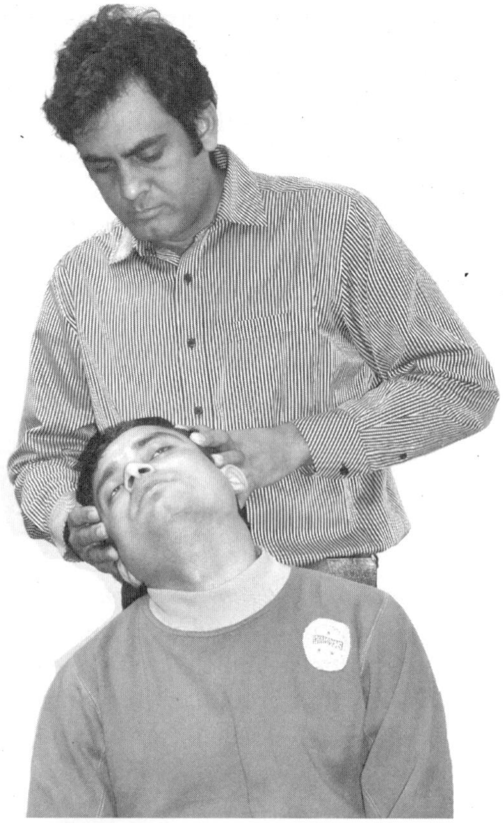

(c)

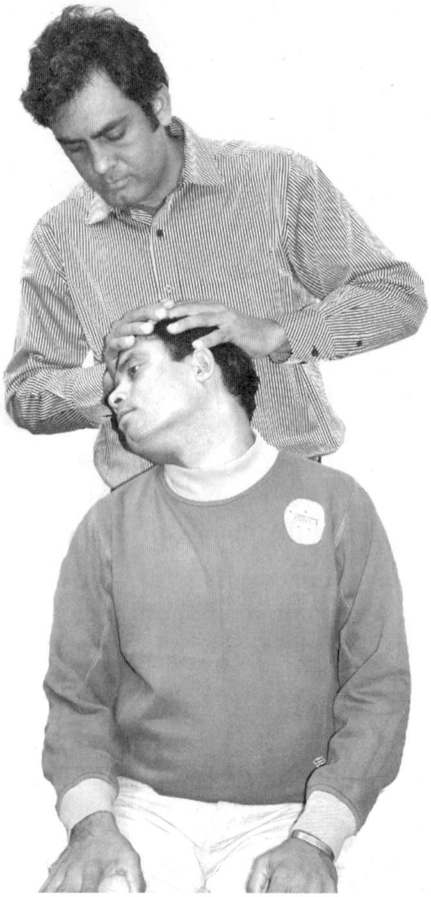

Figs. 26.11a to c: Spurling test

Upper Limb Tension Test$_1$: This test is also known as median nerve dominant test. It is designed to test the median nerve roots of C_5, C_6 and C_7. Patient is positioned in a supine lying and therapist stands at the side of the patient which is being tested. To test the right side, the therapist holds the right hand of the patient with his right hand and grasps elbow joint with the left hand. Therapist depresses the shoulder with the thigh. The shoulder is brought into the 110 degree abduction. While maintaining the shoulder depression with the right hand, the fingers, wrist and elbow are extended, followed by supination of the forearm. The neck is bent first to the affected side and then to the opposite side. The test is considered positive if the neck bending toward the affected side relieves the symptoms, and neck flexion to the opposite side aggravates the symptoms.

The true radicular involvement would radiate the symptoms to the lateral arm deltoid and mid arm (C_5), down the dorsal radial aspect of the forearm to involve the index finger and the thumb (C_6), and centrally down the forearm to involve the dorsum of the hand and the long finger (C_7) (Fig. 26.12).

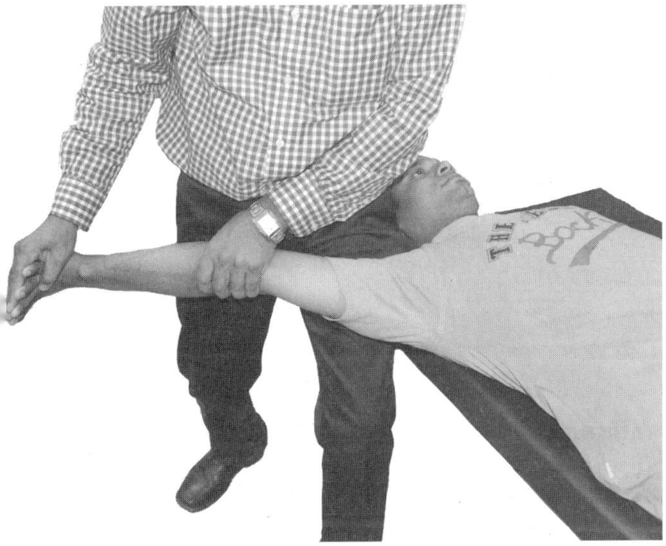

Fig. 26.12: Upper limb tension test$_1$, median nerve dominant

Upper Limb Tension Test$_2$: This test is designed to place significant tension on the nerve roots of C_6 or C_7 to provoke the radicular symptoms. There are two variants of this test, one is median nerve dominant and other is radial nerve dominant.

Median Nerve Dominant Test: The patient is positioned in supine with the scapula out of the edge of the table. The therapist stands close to the shoulder joint which is being tested. The shoulder is depressed with the help of the thigh inferiorly. For an example, to test the right median nerve the therapist holds the arm of the patient with the left hand and the hand with the right hand. The shoulder joint is depressed, abducted and rotated externally to 90 degrees. While maintaining the above position the therapist extends the wrist joint. The test is considered positive if the maneuver produces radicular symptoms to the course of C_6 and C_7 nerve roots (Fig. 26.13).

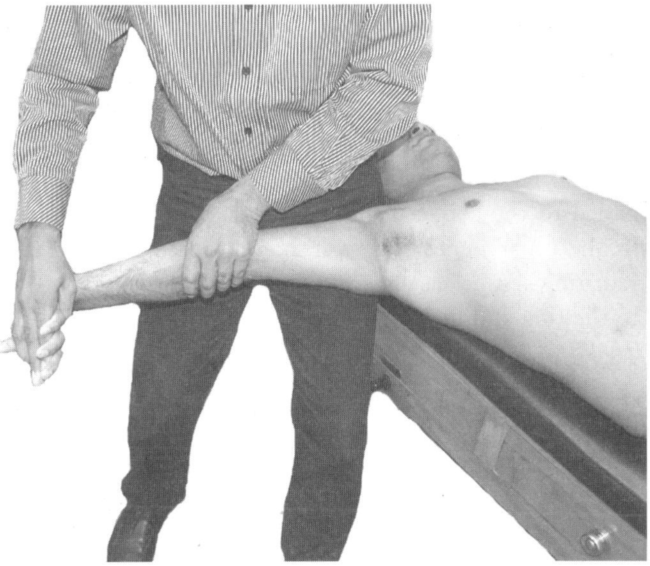

Fig. 26.13: Upper limb tension test$_2$, medial nerve dominant

Radial Nerve Root Dominant Test: The position of patient, therapist and arm remains same as median nerve dominant test. Shoulder is abducted to 10-20 degrees and rotated medially instead of externally as was in median nerve dominant test with wrist flexion. The test is considered positive if the radicular symptoms are produced particularly to the radial nerve distribution (Fig. 26.14).

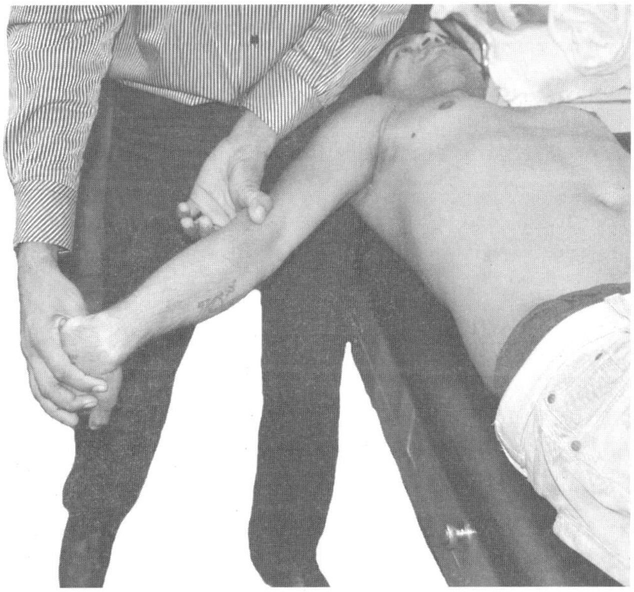

Fig. 26.14: Upper limb tension test$_2$, radial nerve dominant

Upper Limb Tension Test$_3$: The upper limb tension test 3 is designed to place the tension on the nerve roots of the ulnar nerve C_8 and T_1. It is also known as ulnar nerve dominant test. The patient is positioned in supine and therapist stands at the side of the patient, facing the shoulder. To test the right ulnar nerve the therapist stands toward the same side and places right hand on the top of the patient's shoulder and grasped the left hand of the patient with his or her left hand. The patient's flexed elbow rests on the anterior thigh of the therapist. While maintaining the shoulder depression and elbow flexion the therapist abducts the shoulder joint upto 90 degree with external rotation. At the last an extension of the elbow is added to the above maneuver to place significant tension in the ulnar nerve. The test is considered positive if the radiating symptoms aggravate down the arm past the elbow to the ring and little finger (C_8) or into the axilla (T_1) (Fig. 26.15).

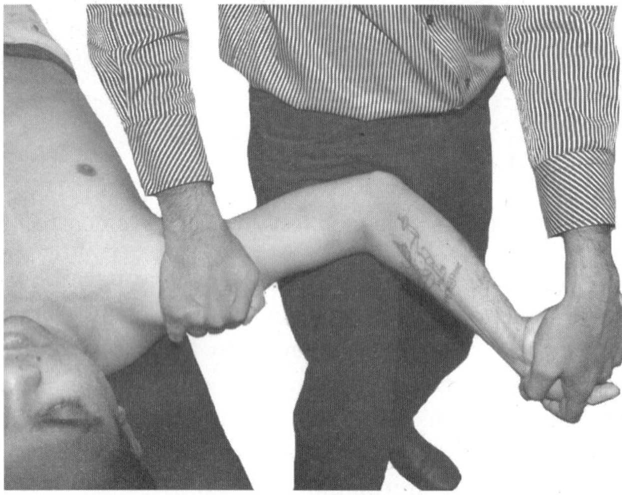

Fig. 26.15: Upper limb tension test$_3$, ulnar nerve dominant

Box 26.1: Vertebrobasillary insufficiency

Disc and facet joint degenerative changes may project the osteophytes laterally and posterolaterally or anteriorly, which can compress and distort the vertebral artery. Compression on one side vertebral artery rarely produces the symptoms because blood supply to the brain is compensated by the other vertebral artery. Osteophytes which project to both the vertebral arteries and cause significant compression and distortion can produce symptoms such as vertigo or giddiness dysarthria, visual symptoms (diplopia) and ataxia with episodes of syncope. The symptoms are aggravated by the neck movements particularly by extension with rotation.

Due to its close proximity to cervical vertebra, the artery is at risk of kinking with neck motions, especially in the presence of degenerative changes.

Course: The vertebral artery enters at the C_6 vertebral foramen and runs through it to C_2.

Examination: Patients present with the symptoms of vascular such as drop-attack, diplopia, dizziness etc. Headache is not the dominant feature, however, pain may be felt in the cervical spine due to degenerative changes. The movements of the cervical spine will aggravate an VBI symptoms.

Test: The test must be performed prior to any manipulative technique specially if there are the symptoms of VBI. The patient is placed in supine position with the head off of the edge of the couch. Therapist stands at the top of the head of the patient and places both hands on either side of the patient's head. The head is rotated to the right side followed by side flexion and extension. The patient is instructed to keep the eyes open and hold the position for atleast 10-15 seconds. During this period the therapist may busy the patient in simple conversation rather than asking the symptoms of the VBI. In case of positive VBI, patients will complain dilatation of pupil, nystagmus, distress, dizziness, slurred speech, visual disturbances or any other untoward occurrence.

Note:

- Test must be performed with cautious, sometimes it may be fatal and can cause death by blocking/ kinking the artery.
- Positive VBI is the absolute contraindication of any kind of joint manipulation, such as thrust at the end etc.
- Therapist may administer aspirin or raise the legs in case of positive test to avoid unwanted danger.

Muscle Strength Testing/Myotomes (Figs. 26.16a to i)

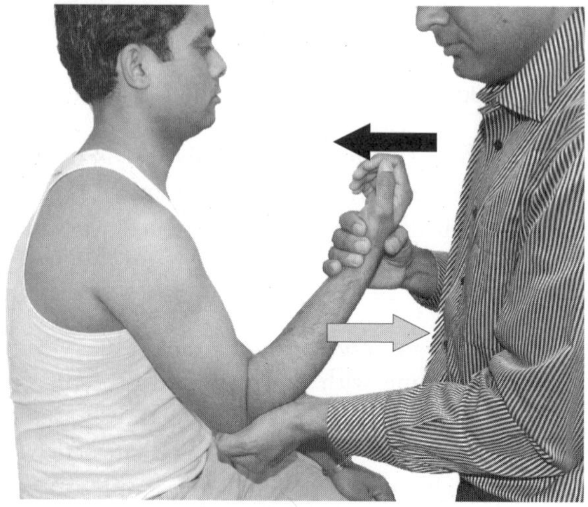

Fig. 26.16a: Biceps

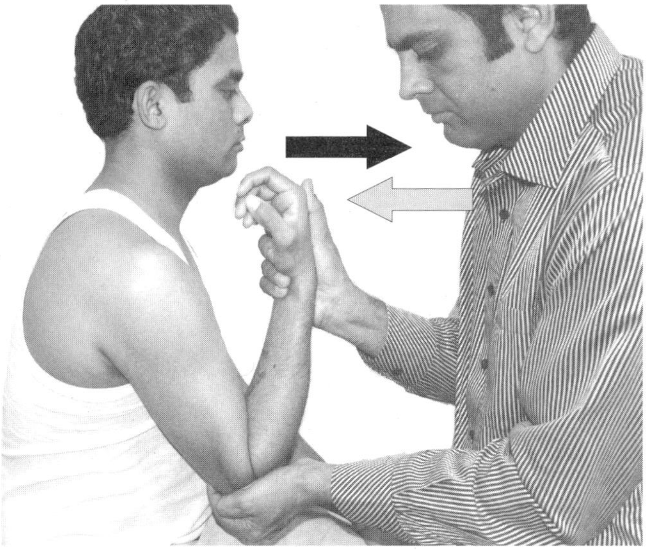

Fig. 26.16b: Triceps

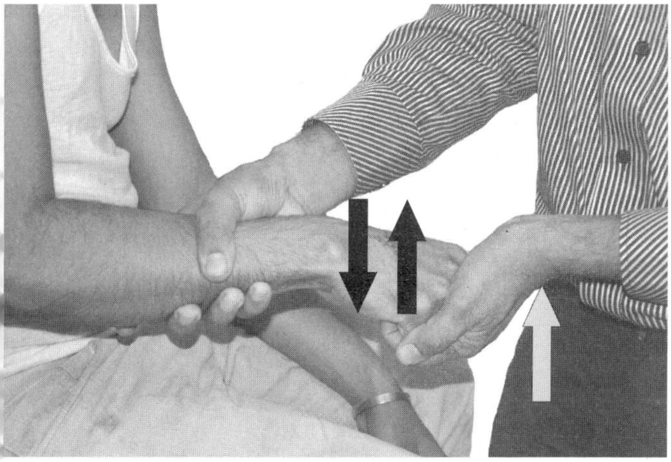

Fig. 26.16c: Wrist flexors

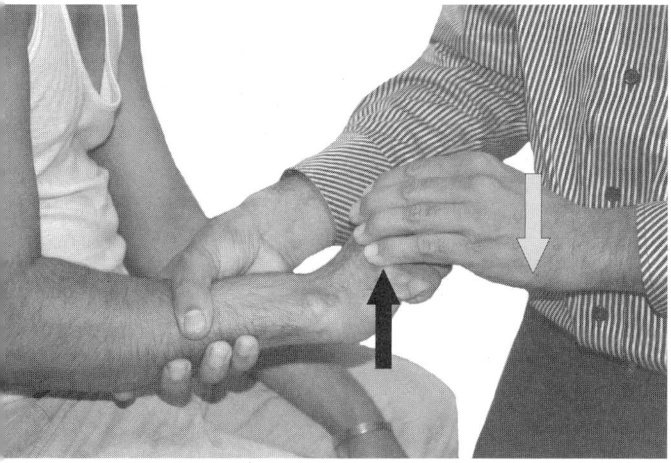

Fig. 26.16d: Wrist extensors

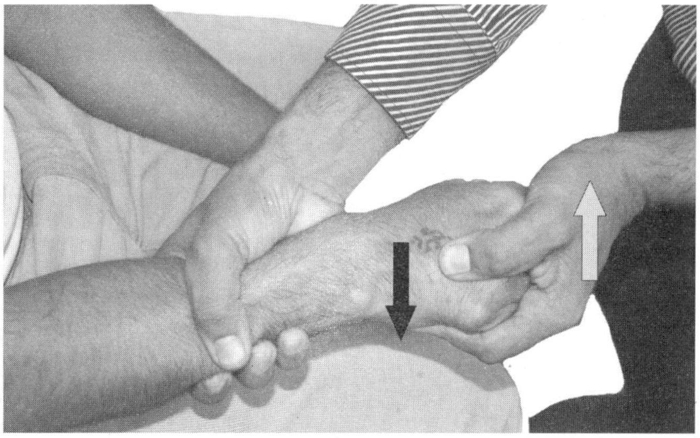

Fig. 26.16e: Wrist ulnar deviators

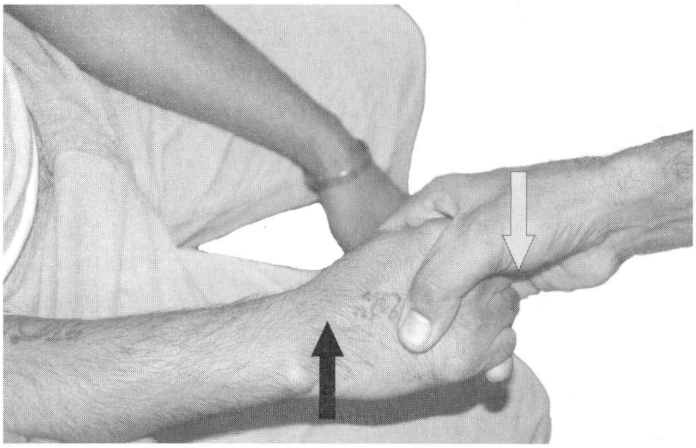

Fig. 26.16f: Wrist radial deviators

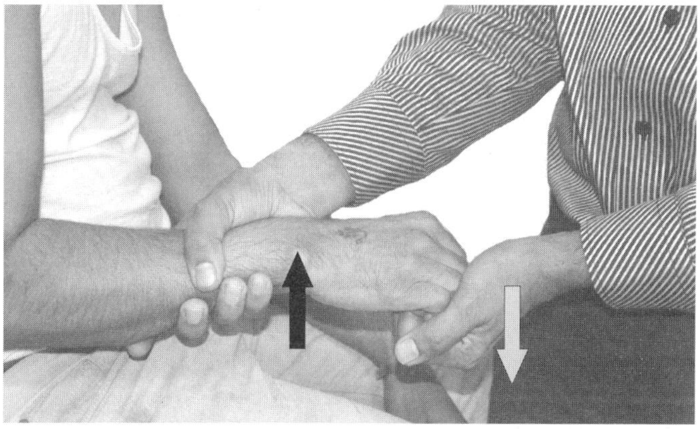

Fig. 26.16g: Finger flexors

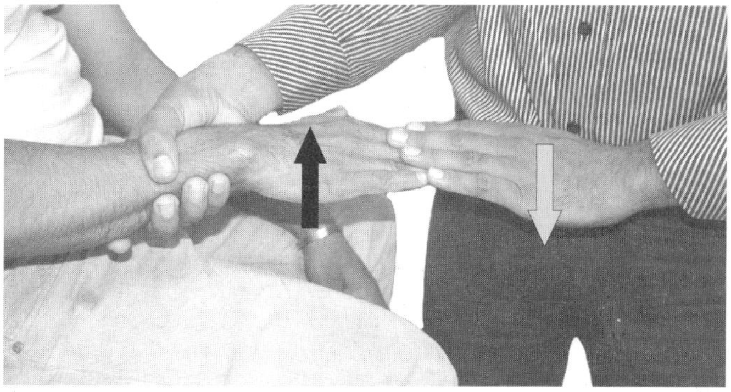

Fig. 26.16h: Finger extensors

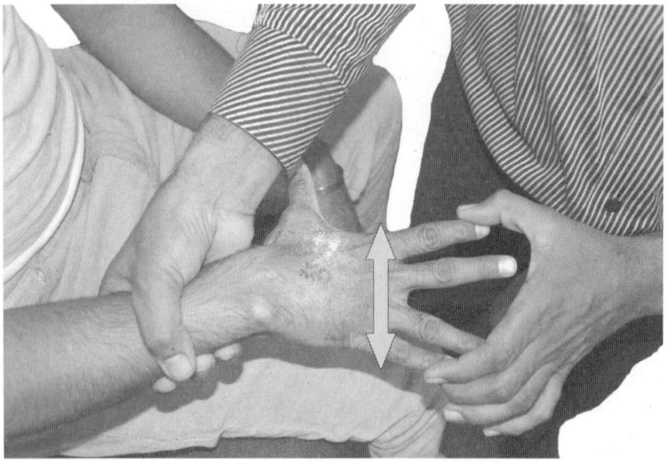

Fig. 26.16i: Finger abductors

Deep Tendon Reflexes: Biceps, triceps or supinator jerk may be diminished or lost (Figs. 26.17 to 26.19).

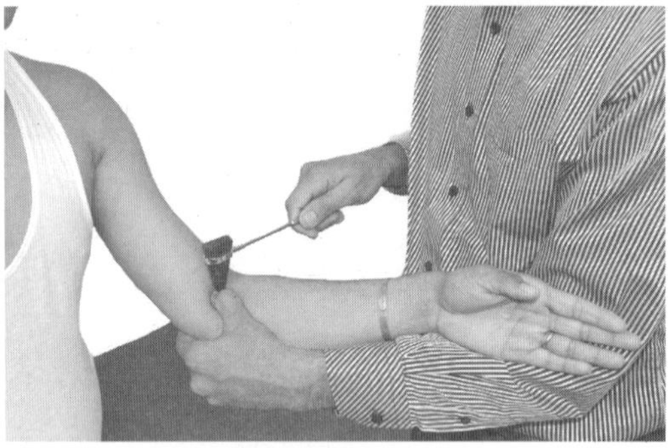

Fig. 26.17: Biceps jerk

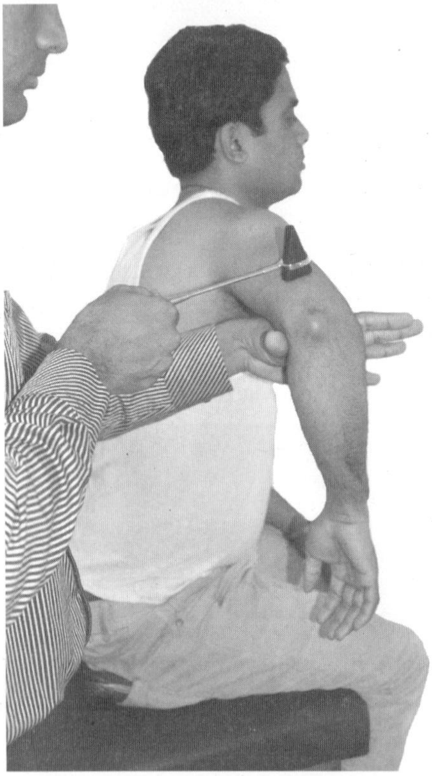

Fig. 26.18: Triceps jerk

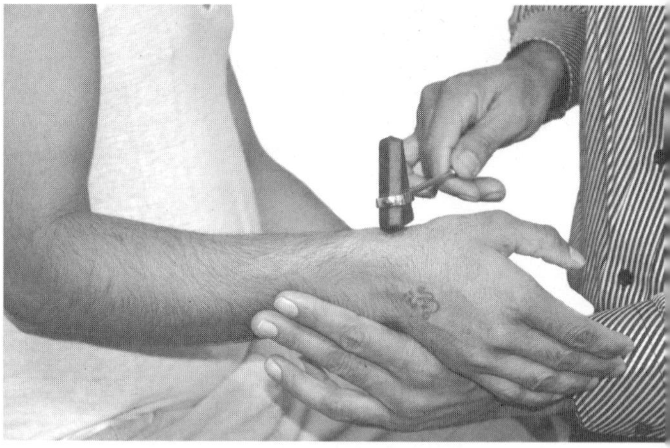

Fig. 26.19: Supinator jerk

Dermatomes: Sensation may be decreased or lost of a particular dermatome in longstanding cases (Fig. 26.20).

Management

1. **Spontaneous Resorption of Sequestrated Intervertebral Disc:** Acute radiculopathy improves rapidly with conservative treatment. This is because the soft disc herniation, with time and treatment can shrink (resorption) and disappear. Orief T, Orz Y, Almusrea KA conducted the study on radicular pain due to sequestrated disc herniation of cervical and lumbar disc.

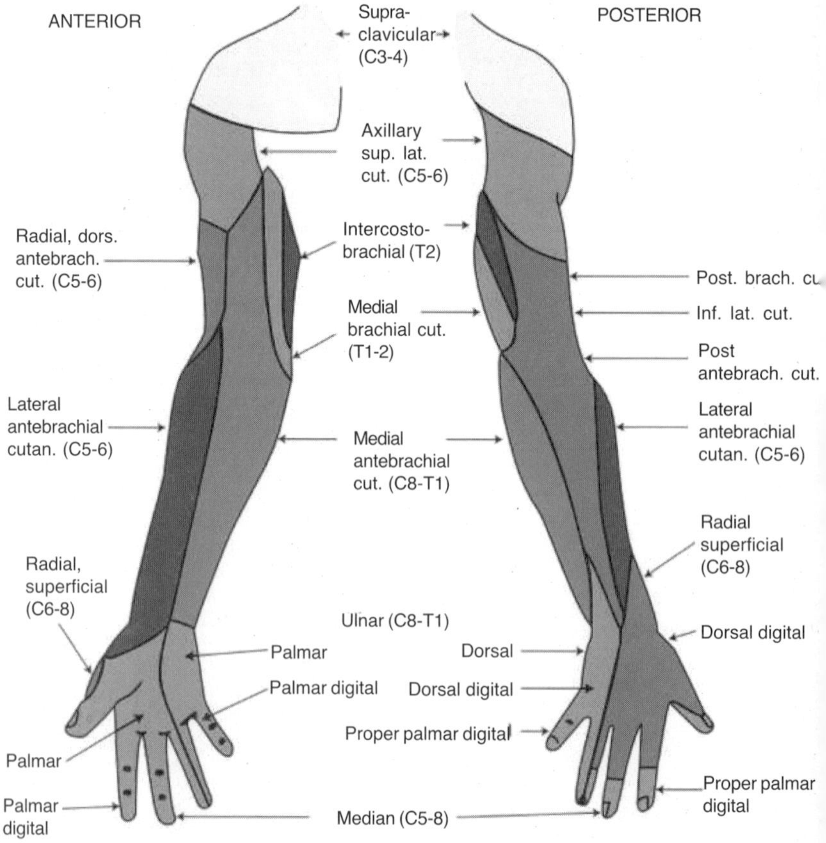

Fig. 26.20: Dermatomes upper extremity

The patients were managed conservatively. All patients recovered from their radicular pain within three to four weeks and it was correlated with resorption of their sequestrated intervertebral disc herniation as documented in their follow-up magnetic resonance imaging (MRI) at 4-6 months. They found that sequestered disc herniation has potential for regression which can clearly be demonstrated by magnetic resonance imaging because of having higher water content, and therefore, may regress through both dehydration and inflammation-mediated resorption. They suggested conservative treatment in the initial course of the sequestrated of disc herniation for at least two months before recommending the surgical intervention unless severe neurological deterioration take place.

2. **Control of Pain and Spasm:** Moist heat therapy which helps in relieving muscle spasm should be recommended and it can be used by the patient twice or thrice daily for atleast 15-20 minutes per session at workstation or house. Transcutenous Electrical Nerve Stimulation (TENS) (pocket type) which stimulates A large diameter and blocks the A delta fibers at gelatinous is also beneficial. However, it is less recommended now-a-days.
3. **Immobilization of Cervical Spine:** The patients with acute radiculopathy are advised cervical collar (soft or hard). The cervical collar which distracts the intervertebral joints helps in reducing the intradiscal pressure and protrusion of the nucleus pulposus on the nerve roots. In case of moderate disc prolapse soft collar is advised to prevent the movements at the cervical spine, thus preventing the intervertebral disc to further prolapse. But in case of severe disc prolapse and involvement of more than one segment (constant symptoms not relieved by placing the hand on the head or by other measures), hard collar is advised which immobilizes and keeps the cervical spine in distracted position thus helps in reducing the pressure on the nerve roots (Figs. 26.21 and 26.22). The use of cervical collar for prolong period of time can cause adverse effects such as disuse atrophy of the muscles hence, it should be advised only for short period of time.

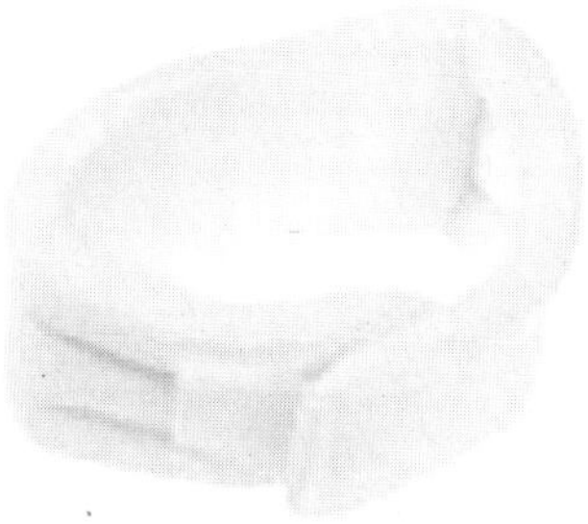

Fig. 26.21: Soft cervical collar

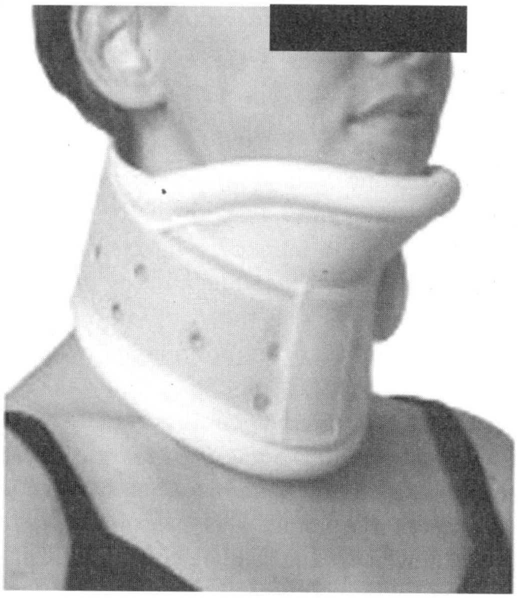

Fig. 26.22: Hard cervical collar

4. **Stress Reduction:** Emotional and physical stresses can increase tension in the neck muscles and interfere with or delay the recovery process. Patient should be advised to eliminate stress as much as possible by placing the non-urgent jobs on hold, obtaining counseling for major life stresses and seeking support from family, friends and health providers.
5. **Cervical Pillow:** In case of straightening of the cervical spine due to spasm, an H-shaped pillow is placed under the nip of the neck to maintain the cervical lordosis (Figs. 26.23a and b).

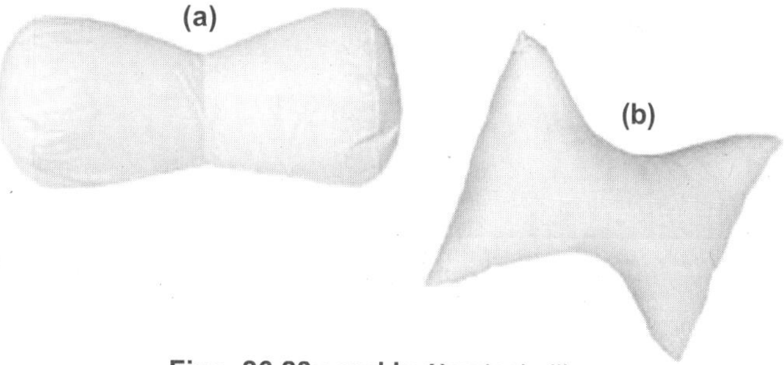

Figs. 26.23a and b: Cervical pillows

6. **Activity Limitation and Posture Modification:**
   a. Avoid sitting posture in the same position for prolong period of time.
   b. Maintain good posture by holding head up and keeping shoulders back.
   c. Use the chair arm rests to keep the shoulder slightly shrugged.
   d. Sleep with neck in a neutral position.

e. Place small pillow under the nape of the neck to maintain the cervical lordotic curve.

f. Place enough pillows to keep the neck straight in line with body (side lying).

7. **Traction:** It is one of the most important treatments for an acute radiculopathy. Traction is the most effective means to stretch the supporting ligaments of the neck. Distraction of the intervertebral joint by the mechanical device helps in relieving the symptoms. It should be recommended in the flexed position approximately 15-20°, for lower cervical spine as flexion will open the intervertebral foramen that will allow disc to shrink back to its normal position. Some patients find difficulty in attending the clinics therefore; they may be advised cervical traction at home. They can purchase a cervical traction kit available in the market. The kit is placed on the wall and patient should use it in slightly neck flexed position. Intermittent traction may help in reducing circulatory congestion and relieve pressure on the dura, blood vessels and nerve roots in the intervertebral foramen. Removing pressure on the blood vessels will improve the blood circulation, remove noxious chemical irritants and decrease pain and other symptoms (Fig. 26.24).

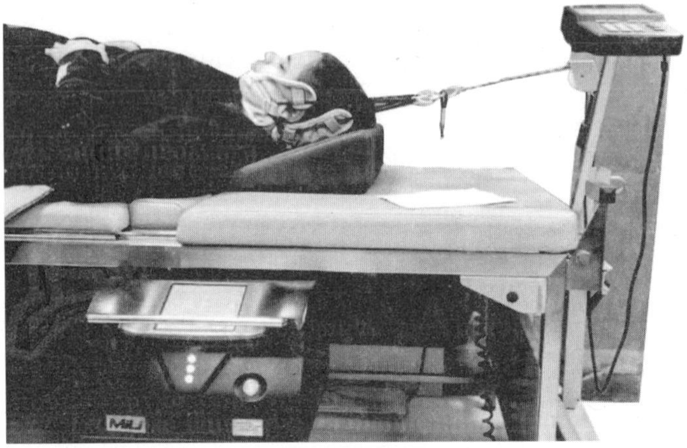

Figs. 26.24: Traction

8. **Exercises:** Exercises should begin as the acute pain starts subsiding. The collar is removed and exercise which relieves the symptoms should be repeated several times. The therapist must note that any movement particularly flexion which aggravates the symptoms must be avoided. Repeating exercises in pain free range helps in centralizing the symptoms. Patients with severe degree of disc prolapse will also have malalignment of the facet joints. These patients will improve with the conservative treatment but pain will persist at the end ranges of motion especially in extension and side flexion. Sustained natural apophyseal glides may help in improving the pain and range of motion but it should be advised a the stage where radicular symptoms subside.

a. *Strengthening:* The weak muscles such as deep necl flexors, rhomboids, serratus anterior and trapeziu middle and lower fibers are strengthened (Figs 26.25 to 26.28).

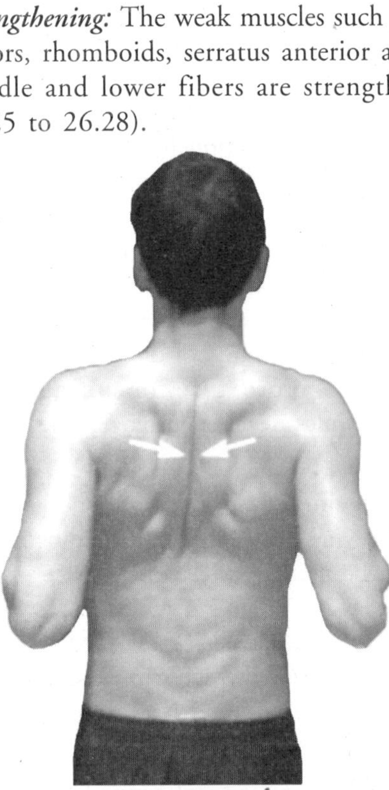

Fig. 26.25: Rhomboids and trapezius middle in standing

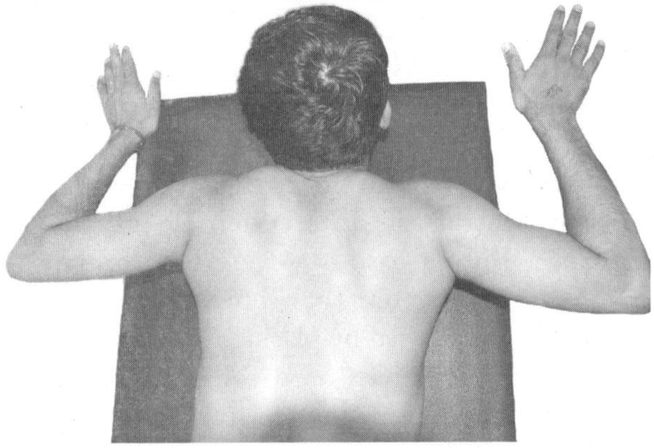

Fig. 26.26: Rhomboid in prone

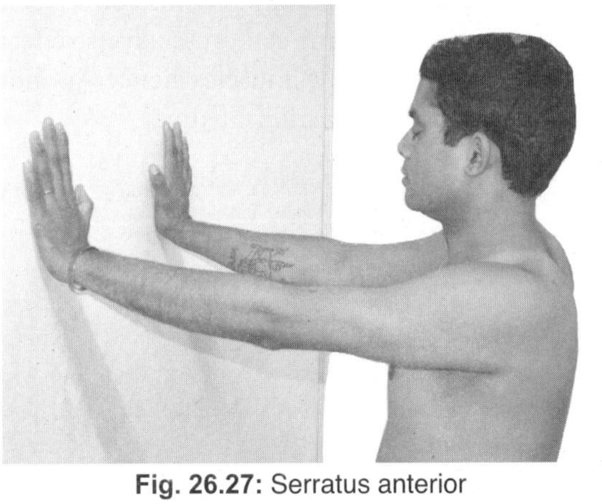

Fig. 26.27: Serratus anterior

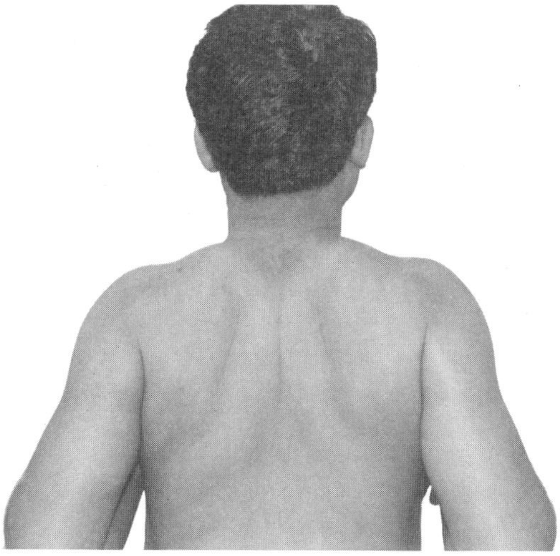

Fig. 26.28: Trapezius middle in sitting

b. Stretching: The tight muscles such as levator scapulae, trapezius upper fibers, erector spinae, and pectoralis major should be stretched to improve the flexibility (Figs. 26.29 and 26.30).

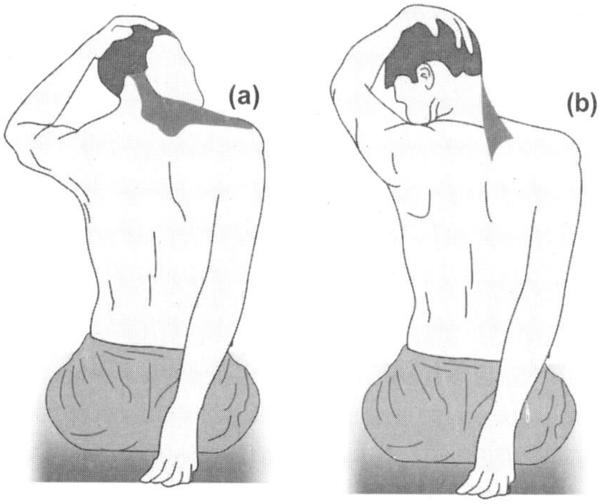

Figs. 26.29: Stretching a. Levator scapulae, b. Trapezius upper

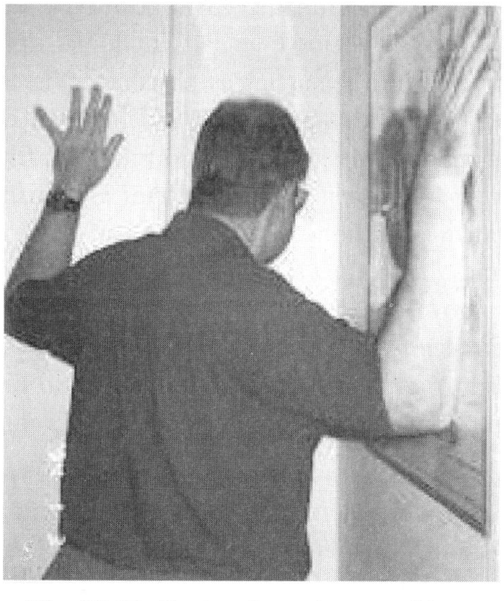

Fig. 26.30: Pectoralis major stretching

c. Non-Weight Bearing Bias: The patients with soft disc herniation are often more comfortable with the traction, soft or hard collar and lying down. Perhaps this relieves the load on the facet joints and also reduces pressure on the nerve roots by reducing the intradiscal pressure. For such patients traction and rest may be the choice of treatment until the patient feels comfortable in weight bearing. The patient is progressed to weight bearing as healing improves and he or she begins to tolerate weight bearing.

d. Adverse Effects of Rest: Rest in collar increases intradiscal pressure with the time; the nucleus potentially can absorb more water contents to equalize pressure (imbibition). On the other hand, lying with flexed spine allows the imbibed fluid to accumulate posteriorly in the intervertebral disc where there is greater space. When patient stands, pain and symptoms from a disc protrusion are accentuated, because, accumulated fluid in the disc spaces will increase the intradiscal pressure. Therefore, to avoid exacerbating symptoms absolute rest during acute phase should not be advised. Rest for 1-2 days may be advised, but it should be interrupted with short intervals of exercises.

e. Extension Exercise Bias: Patients with cervical disc protrusion are often comfortable and may have partial or full relief with extension of the neck. The patients with extension bias often assume a flexed posture with or without neck side flexion. The impairment may be due to a contained intervertebral disc lesion, fluid stasis, injury to the facet joints, or a muscle imbalance from a faulty flexed posture.

f. McKenzie: New Zealand based physical therapist Robin Anthony McKenzie had developed and launched the concept in 1981 which he called Mechanical Diagnosis and Therapy (MDT). An MDT is a system encompassing evaluation, diagnosis, and treatment for the spine and extremities. It primarily uses self treatment strategies and minimizes manual therapy procedures. He states that self treatment is the best way to achieve a lasting improvement in the sign and symptoms. The long term goal of McKenzie concept is to teach the patients how to treat themselves and manage their own pain for life by using exercises.

In the process of diagnosis he performs repeated movements on the cervical spine or lumbar spine and finds the movement which relieves the symptoms from distal to proximal part of the area. As an example, for soft disc herniation (acute radiculopathy) there are the movements which relieve and aggravate the symptoms. The movements which relieve the symptoms become the diagnostic tool. In the process of therapy the movement which relieves the symptoms from distal to proximal is performed repeatedly, while the movement which aggravates the symptoms is discarded. The goal of the therapy part is to centralize the patient's pain and symptoms in the neck rather than treat pain that is localized in a specific area. As an example, for a patient with acute cervical radiculopathy, whose chief complaint is pain in the arm and forearm, the extension movement of the neck is performed repeatedly to decrease the radicular symptoms from forearm, arm, to the neck rather than directing the treatment to the arm and forearm.

The mechanical diagnosis and therapy concept categorizes the clinical presentations of the patients into subgroups which are not based on anatomy. Based on the categorization the patient is instructed on specific exercises to gradually decrease the pain and symptoms.

There are mainly three types of syndromes—Postural, Dysfunction and Derangement.

i. **Postural Syndrome:** It is the result of positions or postures those place significant stress on the intervertebral discs, ligaments, capsule and muscles. The pain is localized and not reproduced with the movements, but if the movements at end ranges are maintained for sustained periods of time may reproduce the pain and symptoms. The postural syndrome is very much common in the population whose job requires prolong sitting. Posture is worst while working on the computers, reading and even driving. People who work on computer in slouch posture and read or drive with a forward head posture create enormous stresses on the muscles, ligaments, tendon, discs and facet joints of the cervical spine. 8-10 lbs weight creates no stress on the neck if the head is on the midline of the neck (normally the ears position directly over the tip of the acromion process). If the head moves one inch forward to the midline it can create an extra 10 lbs stress on the neck. Hence, the patients with forward head posture carry an extra weight between 10 lbs and 30 lbs or more. The forward head posture leads to long term muscle strain, disc herniations and nerve root compression. McKenzie consists a set of exercises for this syndrome which include chin tuck or neck retraction, neck extension and expansion in sitting, and neck extension and expansion in standing.

a. *Chin Tuck or Neck Retraction:* This exercise is also known as double chin exercise. The head is drawn backwards without the chin lifting up. The patient keeps the chin tucked in and down and draws it back as far as it can be done comfortably. The position is held for six seconds at the end range. Exercise is repeated ten times. This exercise helps in strengthening and will align the neck itself with the rest of the spine, and releases the pressure on the muscles, ligaments and discs (Fig. 26.31).

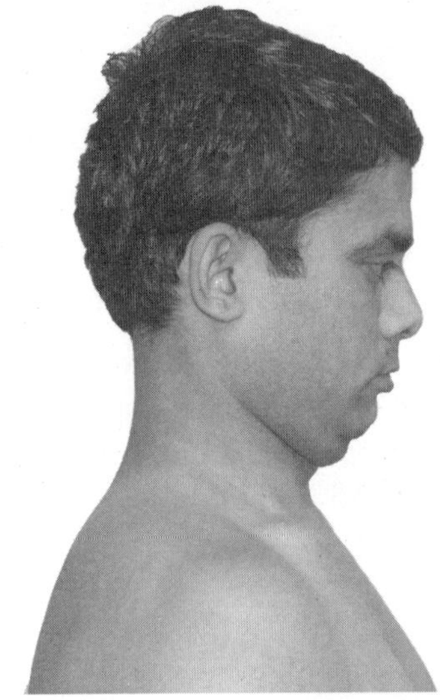

Fig. 26.31: Chin tuck or neck retraction

b. *Neck Retraction and Expansion in Sitting:* The exercises not only releases the pressure occurs in slouched posture but also releases the strain on the muscles. This exercise produces the movement at the discs which helps in lubrication of the fluid and nutrition to the discs. The neck retraction and expansion in sitting is the extension of the chin tuck exercise. The patient sits on the stool comfortably and draws the head backwards without lifting the chin up. The chin tucked in position is drawn back as far as it is possible. Patient looks up gradually toward the roof as far as possible. It is essential to keep the chin stays down and in, even during the head tilts. After holding this position for five seconds, the patient relaxes the muscles and brings to the starting position. The exercise can be repeated ten times. In the next step of the exercise as the symptoms improve, the head is turn side to side with the neck retraction and expansion. Ten repetitions can be performed. Patient should be taught to breathe and relax during the exercise (Figs. 26.32 and 26.33).

c. *Neck Retraction and Expansion in Supine:* This exercise is recommended to the patients who find difficulty in performing the chin tuck exercise in sitting positions. The patient lies supine, head is taken out of the edge of the table. Head is drawn

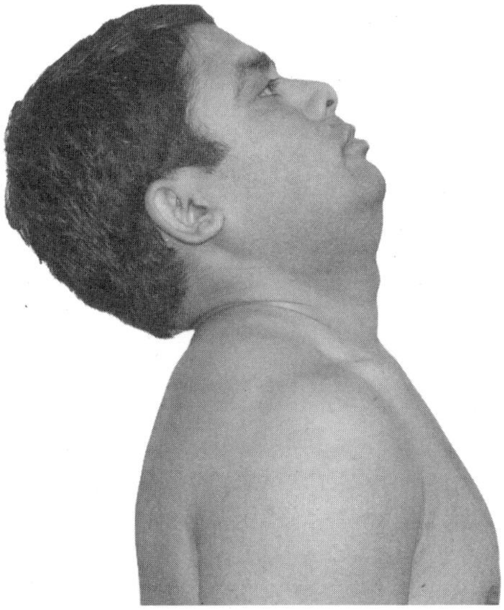

Fig. 26.32: Neck retraction and expansion in sitting up

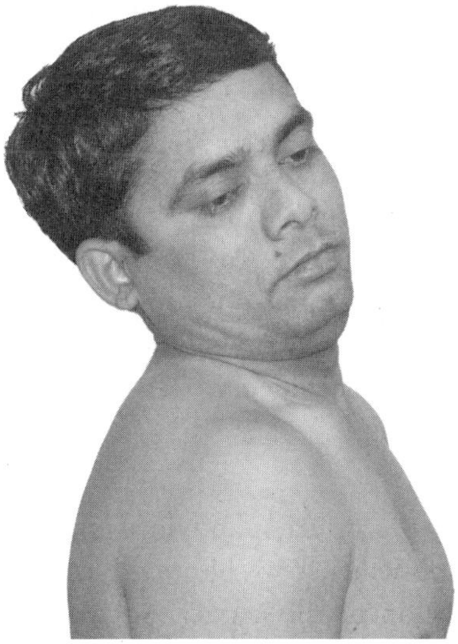

Fig. 26.33: Neck retraction and expansion with side flexion in sitting

back on the neck as far as possible and the position is held at least for five seconds. It can be repeated ten times 2-3 times daily (Fig. 26.34).

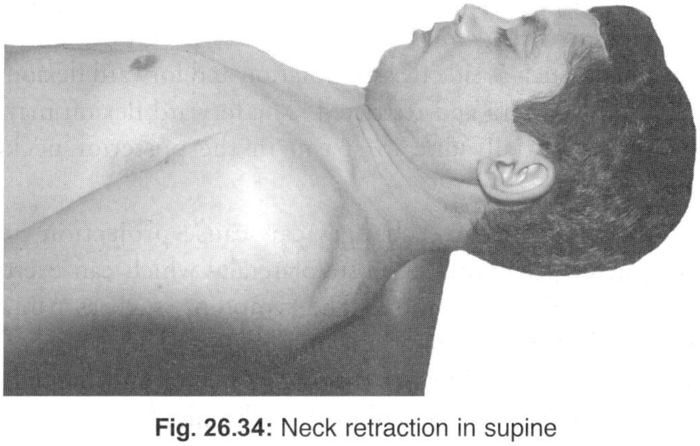

Fig. 26.34: Neck retraction in supine

ii. **Dysfunction Syndrome:** In this syndrome patients present with pain and limitation in the motion at the end ranges. Due to poor posture there is shortening or scarring or adherence of the connective tissues which limit the motion at the end ranges. A dysfunction may be intermittent or chronic, but its hallmark is a consistent movement loss and pain at the end range of motion. The movements hardly produce pain and symptoms in the initial and mid range. Exercises which can stretch the muscles or break the adhesions are usually effective. Treatment is focused on tissue remodeling which require regular exercises. The improvement in the sign and symptoms is slow because the process of tissue remodeling progresses slowly. In addition to the stretching exercises the postural correction exercises are the cornerstone of the dysfunction syndrome.

iii. **Derangement Syndrome:** This category is the most common syndrome that presents clinically. Hallmark of derangement syndrome is its sensitivity to certain movements and its preference for particular movement pattern. When these movements such as flexion and or extension are performed, the symptoms either aggravate or relieve. The derangement syndrome is very common after the prolapsed intervertebral disc. The radicular symptoms which are originated from the neck are experienced in the arm and forearm. It is not uncommon for the patient to experience rapid reduction in the radicular symptoms immediately during the assessment. Treatment for the patients with derangement syndrome, as with the postural and dysfunction syndromes, is directly guided by the patients response to these provocative assessment movements.

iv. **Manual Therapy:** Manual mobilization such as maitland and mulligan can also be started as patient shows improvement in the radiculopathy symptoms. The techniques are explained in cervical spondylosis/disc degeneration.

CERVICAL DISC DEGENERATION

The disc is relatively a non-compressible gel, comprises proteoglycans, collagen fibers and water. The physical ability to absorb the weight of the body depends on its proteoglycan water complex. The disc degeneration is a gradual process which begins usually after fourth decade of the life but in some cases such as traumatic or pathological, it may commence even in fourth decade of the life. The degenerative changes in the disc increases as the life progress, but it is not essential that these changes will produce symptoms. Some people remain asymptomatic throughout their life though degenerative changes can be seen on X-rays. On the other hand people with minimal degenerative changes may have symptoms and seek intervention. This depends upon the adaptability of the body. As the disc degeneration is a slow process, the body adapts the changes hence, no symptoms are produced in the due course of time, but a trauma or injury to the cervical spine can cause stress on the changes and the symptoms are produced.

In the process of degeneration the nucleus pulposus loses its water binding capacity and becomes compressible and less able to absorb and transfer the weight or load to the annulus. In turn the annular collagen fibers break down and cease to function as weight absorber, the result is desiccation of the nucleus with fragmentation and tear or fissuring of the annulus (Figs. 26.35 to 26.37).

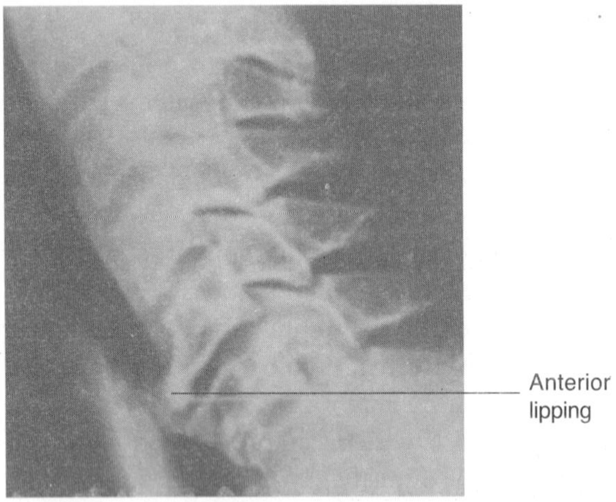

Fig. 26.35: Spondylosis with anterior lipping

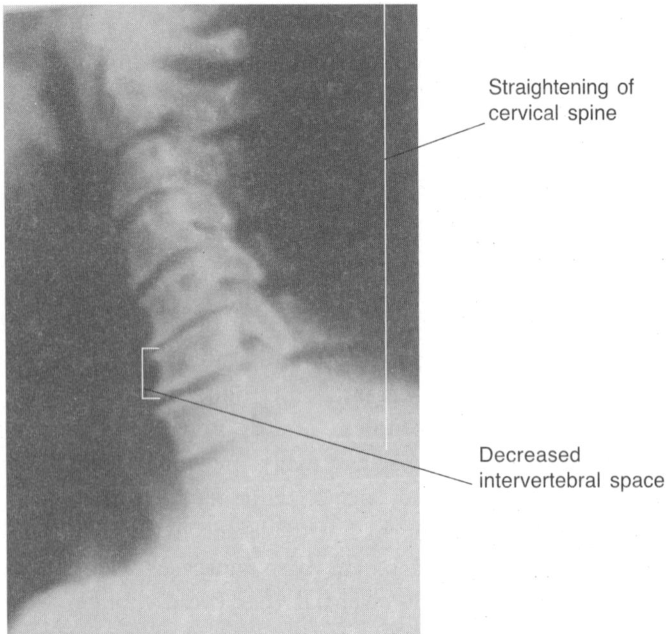

Fig. 26.36: Disc degeneration with reduced intervertebral space between C_5-C_6 and C_6-C_7 and anterior lipping

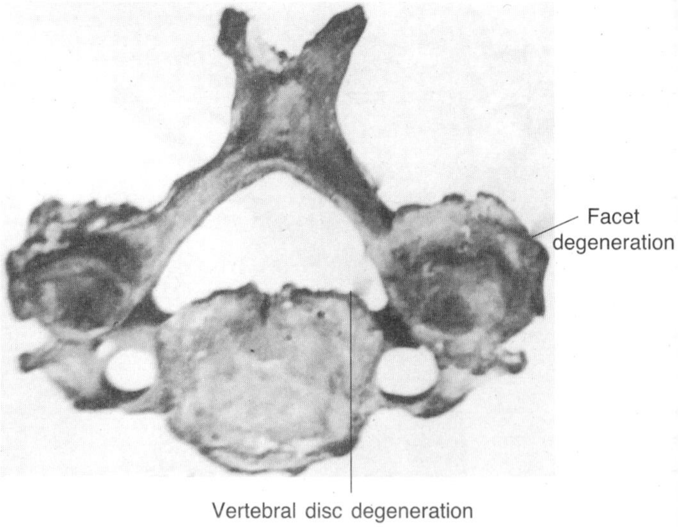

Fig. 26.37: Disc degeneration with facet joint degeneration

Due to fragmentation, desiccation and fissuring, the height of the disc is decreased. The annular fibers may bulge into the nerve roots and cord territory and abnormal movement occurs in the mobile segment due to instability. In an attempt at repair and stabilization, fibrotic changes occur in the nucleus. Stabilizing osteophytes occur at the margin of the disc spaces. In the next process of disc degeneration, the desiccated nuclear material may or may not rupture through a tear in the annulus to cause nerve root or cord pressure (Table 26.6 and Flowchart 26.1).

Clinical Features

The patients with cervical spondylosis experience pain in the cervical spine which may be in the central part or on paravertebral region of the cervical spine. Initially pain is localized but may radiate down the arm or forearm and hand if there is nerve root compression. Activities which hold the neck in extension such as shaving, painting, putting on shoes and shocks, knitting, reading with bifocals or half moon glasses, using telephone or even excitedly watching cricket match on television may precipitate, aggravate and perpetuate the symptoms. These activities put excessive stress on the posterior pillars (facet joints). Initially extension is restricted with pain but as the disease progresses other movements such as side flexion, rotation and forward flexion will also be painful and restricted. The forward flexion may be limited initially due to spasm in the posterior neck muscles.

Gross degenerative changes can cause projection of osteophytes posteriorly or posterolaterally which can exert pressure on the nerve roots. The symptoms such as pain, parasthesia, tingling sensation, numbness and weakness of the muscles may be felt at the arm, forearm and hand(s) which are termed as radiculopathy (chronic).

Table 26.6: Stages of intervertebral disc degeneration

Stages	*Nucleus pulposus*	*Annulus fibrosus*	*Facet joint*	*Result*
Normal	Proteoglycan/water	Collage fibers structure with high tensile strength	Smooth gliding	Nucleus absorbs forces and transfers to annulus. Smooth pain free movement
Stage I	Loss of water, breakdown of proteoglycans	Fissuring and tearing of fibers	Synovitis, hypomobility	Intermittent axial pain
Stage II	Nuclear protrusion	Fissuring, disc resorption	Capsular laxity and subluxation	Axial and radicular pain
State III	Desiccation and narrowing	Osteophyte formation	Osteophyte formation	Minor axial pain and neurological compromise

Flowchart 26.1: The normal disc

The normal disc is composed of collagen – Proteoglycan complex and fluid which maintain its physical properties such as height, shape and structure

↓

As the age progresses, disc loses its water binding capacity and becomes compressible

↓

The disc loses its physical properties (height, shape and structure), and the intervertebral space is decreased (instability). Load is transferred to the posterior pillars (facet joints). Dysfunction and subluxation of the facet joints, facet joint synovitis/capsulitis occurs

↓

Patients experience localized pain and limitation in the movements. Muscle guarding (muscle spasm) further contribute to the limitation in the range of motion

↓

Formation of osteophytes which may project anteriorly, posteriorly and posterolaterally. The osteophytes project to the nerve roots may cause significant pressure on the neural tissues

↓

Neural tissue compression, numbness, tingling sensation, radicular pain, down the arm. Decrease biceps or triceps jerks(s), decrease muscle power

Assessment

Pain and stiffness in the cervical spine with restriction of extension and other range of motion are the common complaints of the patients with cervical disc degeneration or spondylosis. Middle aged group people are generally involved. Disease progresses with gradual onset.

Observation: The chin should be in line with the sternum (manubrium); the ears should be in line with the shoulders and the forehead vertical on the cervical spine. Deviation such as side flexion and rotation due to muscle spasm should carefully be observed from anterior view. Other postural deviations such as Klippel Feil syndrome (fusion of the some cervical vertebra usually C_3-C_5), forward head posture (poking chin), should also be observed.

Usually the dominant side shoulder will slightly be lower than the non-dominant side, spasm or injury can cause elevation of the shoulder to provide protection and relief in the symptoms. The rounded shoulders may be associated with forward head posture.

Muscle Wasting: Muscle wasting may be seen in long standing cases it may be observed on the scapular and para-scapular region. Shoulders may be drooped and protracted due to weakness of the depressors and retractors (rhomboids), the medial border of the scapula may also be raised on thoracic wall due to weakness of the serratus anterior. Extension is limited initially but other movements may also be limited and painful in all three planes in later stages.

Special Tests

A. **Foraminal Compression and Distraction:** Patient sits on the stool with both arms hanging at the side of the body. Therapist stands behind the patient and places both the hands on the top of the head of the patient. While maintaining the neck in neutral position the therapist applies downward pressure through the body to the top of the head. If patient experiences radicular symptoms with the pressure it suggests radiculopathy and the test is considered positive. If symptoms such as pain aggravates in the cervical spine without radiation it may be due to osteoarthritic changes in the cervical spine.

B. **Spurling Test:** Also known as quadrant test is very useful in producing the symptoms in the cervical spine with or without radiculopathy. Position of patient remains sitting as foramen compression and distraction test. Therapist stands behind the patient, places both the hands on the top of the head of the patient. The head is extended, bent and rotated to the affected side (same side) and a downward pressure is applied through the body and arms. If it aggravates pain on the same side of the side flexion and rotation, it suggests degenerative changes in the facet joints and outer part of the disc to the same side. If the test reproduces radicular symptoms, it suggests chronic radiculopathy due to degenerative changes causing compression on the nerve roots. The spurling test has good sensitivity to the radiculopathy.

C. **Alar-Odontoid Integrity:** Patient is positioned in a comfortable sitting with arms hanging freely on the sides. Therapist stands on the same side of alar-odontoid ligament and places the thumb of one hand lateral to the spinous process of C_2 vertebra and other hand on the top of the head.

Procedure: To test the left ligament the therapist bends the patient's head to the left side (same side). The side flexion of the head should produce immediate and simultaneous rotation of C_2 to the same side as of side bending, which is palpated as movement of spinous process of C_2 in the direction opposite of the side bending (Fig. 26.38). A test is considered positive if the motion of C_2 spinous process is absent. It is the indication of rupture or lax of alar ligament or fracture of the odontoid process.

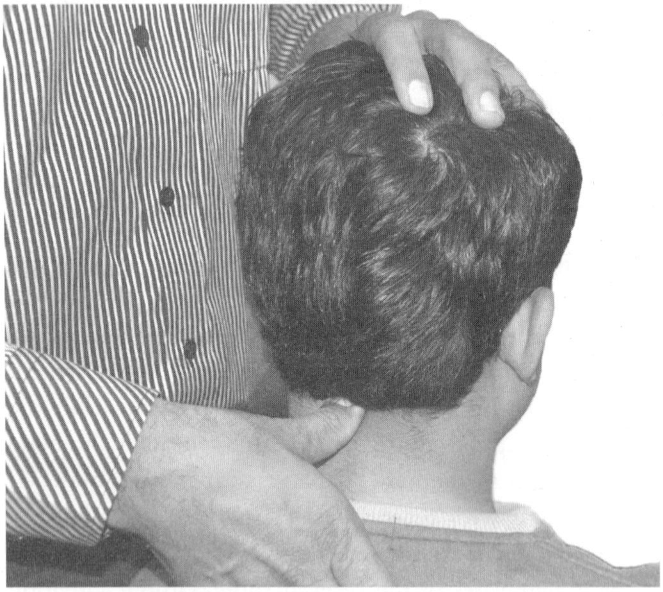

Fig. 26.38: Alar odontoid integrity test

D. **Transverse Ligament Test:** In case of lax or ruptured transverse ligament, it is recommended to have the patient perform the self test, as it is a very serious condition and can be a fatal. For self testing, patient sits comfortably on the stool with both the hands hanging freely at the sides. Patient is asked to gently nod the head. Therapist looks for any signs or symptoms of cord compression such as nausea, bilateral arm symptoms etc.

E. **Sharp Purser Test:** The patient sits comfortably, and therapist stands at the side of the patient. Therapist places stabilizing hand on the occiput and forearm around the temporal region. The thumb of the mobilizing hand is placed on the spinous process of axis.

Procedure: The patient actively performs forward bending to his or her comfort. Therapist applies a posterior to anterior force on the axis. A positive test is the feeling of occiput and atlas sliding back on axis, often with a click sound, indicating reduction of subluxation of occiput and atlas (Fig. 26.39).

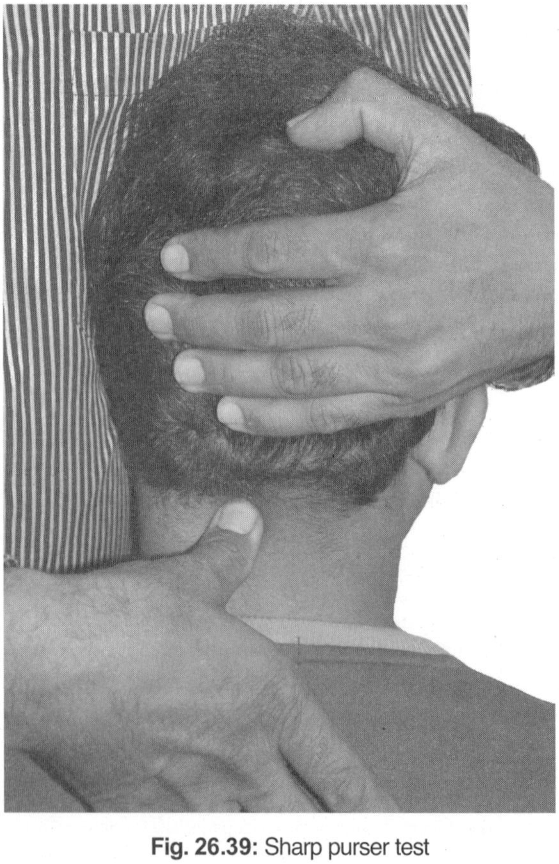

Fig. 26.39: Sharp purser test

Differential Diagnosis

Acute Radiculopathy: Patients with acute radiculopathy (soft disc herniation, a sudden process) experience more symptoms in the arm, forearm and hand, while patients with chronic radiculopathy (degenerated disc herniation a gradual process of disc degeneration) experience more pain and symptoms in the neck rather than in the arm and forearm. Moreover, acute radiculopathy is commoner in young age group with onset of unilateral symptoms. On

Box 26.2: Thoracic Outlet Syndrome

Introduction: Thoracic outlet syndrome is a compression of the brachial plexus or subclavian artery or subclavian veins in the outlet formed by the scalene muscles on three sides and cervical rib on the fourth side at the upper thorax. The subclavian veins are rarely involved in the syndrome as they pass beneath the thoracic outlet.

Causes: The neurovascular bundle which passes through the thoracic outlet gets compressed if the outlet is narrowed due to spasm in the anterior and middle scalene muscles, or if the shoulder girdle is depressed. The common causes of thoracic outlet syndrome include physical trauma from a car accident, repetitive injuries from a job such as frequent non-ergonomic use of a keyboard, sports-related activities, anatomical defects such as having an extra rib and pregnancy. The athletes who frequently raise their arms above the head such as swimmers, volleyball players, shuttlecock players, baseball pitchers, and weightlifters may be at the risk of thoracic outlet syndrome.

Types: There are three types of thoracic outlet syndromes classified according to the involvement of the structures. The compression occurs of three anatomical structures (arteries, veins and nerves), can be isolated, or–more commonly–two or three of the structures are compressed to greater or lesser degrees.

a. **Neurogenic Thoracic Outlet Syndrome:** It accounts 95% of all cases of thoracic outlet syndrome. This type of syndrome includes the compression of brachial plexus. The symptoms are of pain, parasthesia, tingling sensation and weakness of the thenar and hypothenar muscles.
b. **Arterial Thoracic Outlet Syndrome:** It is due to compression of the subclavian artery.
c. **Venous Thoracic Outlet Syndrome:** This type of syndrome occurs due to subclavian vein compression.

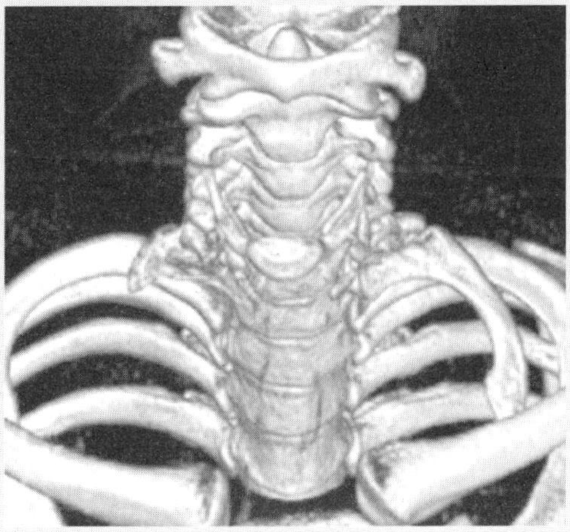

Sometimes the thoracic outlet syndrome is classified by the name of the structure which produces compression on the neurovascular bundle.

Scalenus Anticus Syndrome: The spasm in the scalene muscles particularly anterior and middle scalene can reduce the outlet and can put significant compression on the brachial plexus or/and on the subclavian artery.

Cervical Rib Syndrome: Some people are born with an extra incomplete and very small cartilaginous rib. It is known as cervical rib because it is originated from the cervical (seventh) vertebra. This rudimentary rib causes fibrous changes around the brachial plexus nerves, inducing compression and causing the symptoms and signs of thoracic outlet syndrome.

Costoclavicular Syndrome: The thoracic outlet is narrowed between the clavicle and the first rib and the symptoms of neurovascular bundle compression are produced.

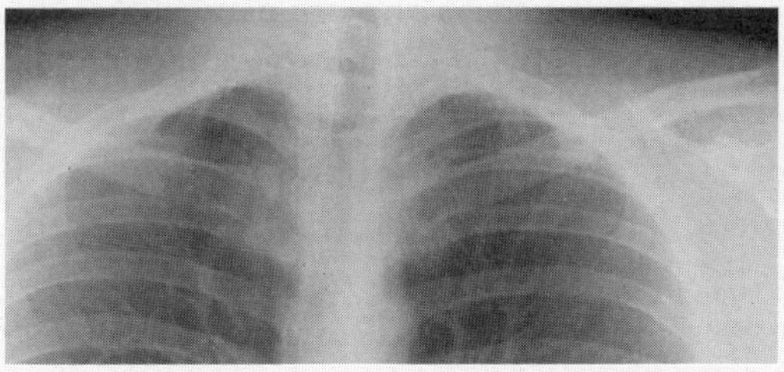

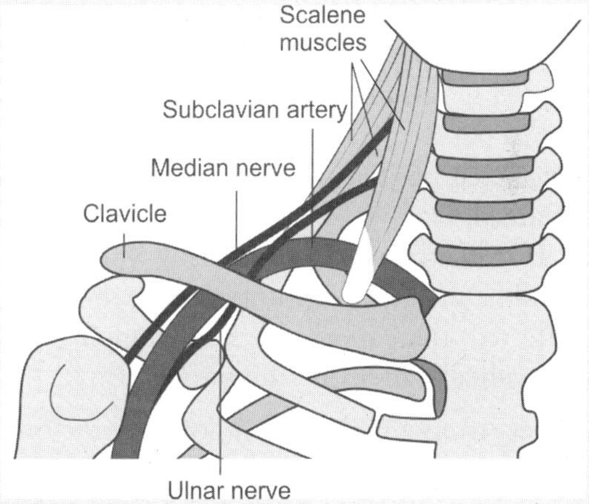

Symptoms: The symptoms either neurogenic or vascular or both types be present. Thoracic outlet syndrome mainly affects the upper extremity. The neurogenic symptoms such as pain, parasthesia, numbness are almost always present, and can be sharp, burning, or aching. It can involve only part of the hand (as in the 4th and 5th finger only), all of the hand, or the inner aspect of the forearm and upper arm. Pain can also be felt in the side of the neck, the pectoral area below the clavicle, the axillary area, and the upper back

Contd.

Contd.

(i.e., the trapezius and rhomboid area). Tenderness on the anterior scalene muscle (pectoral area) may also be present. The vascular symptoms such as discoloration of the hands (one hand colder than the other hand), swelling, and weakness of the hand and arm muscle are commonly present. A painful, swollen and blue arm, particularly when occurring after strenuous physical activity, could be a sign of a venous compression or subclavian vein thrombosis called Paget-Schroetter Syndrome.

Examination: The patients with thoracic outlet syndrome usually complaint pain, weakness, heaviness and swelling in the hand. The symptoms are aggravated after the activities. Patients commonly find difficulty in performing overhead activities. A cervical rib may be seen on the X-rays.

a. **Adson's Test:** The patient sits on the stool with both the hands hanging freely on either side. The neck is rotated and flexed to the opposite side. Therapist stands behind the patient and palpates the radial pulse with one hand. While keeping the pulse palpated the extremity is abducted and extended to the 30 degrees. The patient is instructed to take the deep breath. The test may be considered positive, if the therapist finds diminished or feeble radial pulse.
b. **Roos Test:** In a comfortable sitting position, the patient is asked to abduct the shoulders to 90 degrees with elbows flexion to 90 degrees. Patient is instructed to open and make the fist of both the sides as fast as possible at least for three minutes. The test is considered positive if patient complaints heaviness and finds difficulty in keeping the arms at 90 degrees. The affected arm will drop gradually while the normal side will be maintained. In case, where, both the sides are affected, the patient will start dropping both the arms gradually after one minute.
c. **Doppler Arteriography:** With probes at the fingertips and arms, tests the force and "smoothness" of the arterial flow through the radial arteries, with and without having the patient perform various arm maneuvers (which causes compression of the subclavian artery at the thoracic outlet). The movements can elicit symptoms of pain and numbness and produce graphs with diminished arterial blood flow to the fingertips, providing strong evidence of impingement of the subclavian artery at the thoracic outlet.

Management: The patients with thoracic outlet syndromes are managed with the conservative treatment. This includes mostly exercises but for symptomatic relief in pain and symptoms the heat modalities may also be advised. If the patients do not respond to the fair trial of conservative treatment, surgical intervention is the last choice, which may include resection of cervical rib.

Conservative Treatment: This includes stretching, strengthening exercises and heat therapy. The muscles which keep the shoulder girdle elevated and retracted such as trapezius (upper, middle and lower) fibers, rhomboids, serratus anterior are need to be strengthened in order to avoid pressure on the neurovascular bundle. The core muscle strengthening also plays important role in the management of thoracic outlet syndrome as it helps in correcting kyphotic anomaly of the upper back. The pectoralis major, scalene (anterior, middle and posterior) and extensors of cervical should be stretched. Continuous mode of ultrasound therapy of 1Mhz over the scalene muscles with the intensity of 1watt per centimeter square may be useful in increasing the extensibility of the scalene muscles. Hot pack may also help in decreasing the muscle spasm.

Neural Tissue Mobilization: The patients with thoracic outlet syndrome often involve compression of a large cluster of nerves, typically resulting in motor and/or sensory impairment throughout the arm, forearm and hand. Neural tissue mobilization given by David Buttler, Australian based physical therapist also known as neural gliding or buttler neural tissue mobilization is considered to be very effective in terms of stretching and mobilizing affected nerve fibers. It is performed in a similar manner of D2 flexion pattern of proprioceptive neuromuscular facilitation (PNF). The patient lies supine with the shoulder out of edge of the couch. The therapist stands at the side and grasps the hand of the patient and elbow joint. The shoulder joint is depressed appropriately and arm is rotated externally with the elbow extension. While maintaining the aforesaid position the therapist abducts and flexes the extremity over the shoulder.

Surgical Management: It may be advised to the thoracic outlet syndrome patients who presents with cervical rib. It involves removal of the cervical rib, scalene muscles and any compressive fibrous tissue which causing pressure on the neurovascular bundles. However, no surgical option should be considered until all non-invasive approaches have been exhausted.

ie other hand the chronic radiculopathy occurs in the iiddle aged group of patients which may be unilateral or ilateral.

Anzina Pectoris: Similar symptoms of radiculopathy are roduced but patients with anzina pectoris experience pain n the left anterior chest. The symptoms are relieved by king isosorbite trinitrate drugs orally.

Thoracic Outlet Syndrome: Patients with thoracic outlet yndrome present with mixed type of symptoms ieurovascular). In addition to neurological symptoms atients also experience heaviness and swelling. These atients present with drooped shoulders and tenderness n the anterior chest (over the anterior scalene muscle) -ray findings may reveal cervical rib.

Ianual Therapy

. **Distraction of Occipito-Atlanto and Atlantoaxial Joints:**

Position of Patient: Sitting on the treatment table or stool.

Position of Therapist: The therapist stands at the side of the patient opposite to the joint being mobilized. To mobilize the right side facet joint of OA and AA the therapist stands at the left side of the patient and places right hand (stabilizing) on the transverse process of the atlas for OA or articular rim of axis for AA facet joint. The mobilizing hand is around the base of the occipital. The therapist stands with 30-40° knee flexion.

Procedure: The therapist cradles the head between the mobilizing hand and stabilizing hand on his chest and extends the knees to produce cranial force or distraction of facet joints of OA and AA (Figs. 26.40 and 26.41).

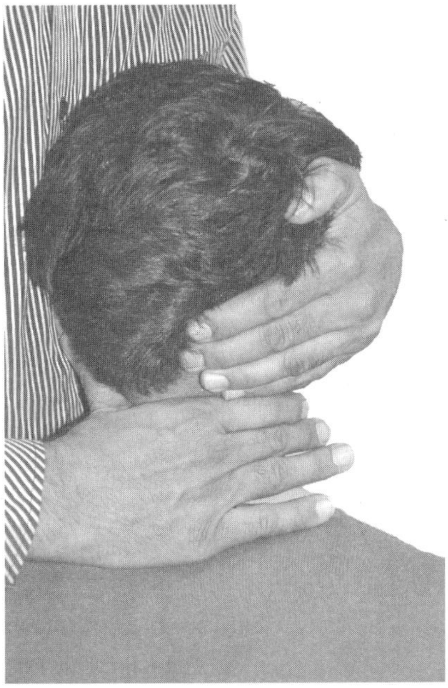

Fig. 26.40: Position of hands

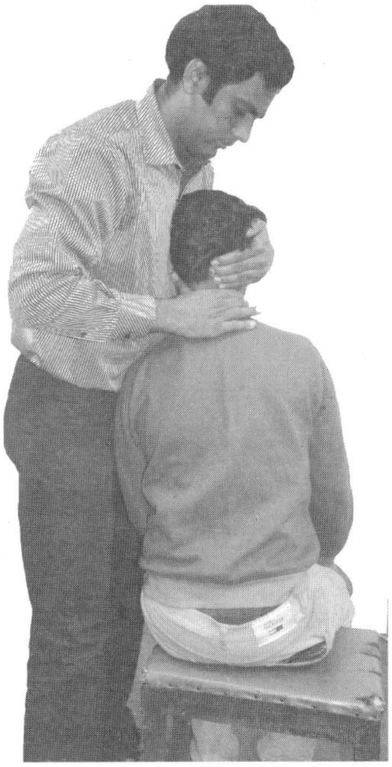

Fig. 26.41: Occipito-atlanto and atlantoaxial distraction

B. **Mobilization (Maitland):** Maitland mobilization is one of the conventional mobilization techniques which is always performed in a relaxed position.

Position of Patient: Supine, head remains off of the couch, arms at the side of the body.

Position of Therapist: Therapist stands at the top of the head. Left hand grasps the occiput and right hand holds the chin. The patients head rests on the belly of therapist. A paper or napkin may be placed between the head and belly for cosmetic purposes. Therapist stands with slight knees bent. This intermittent cervical manual traction helps in improving the range of motion of intervertebral and facet joints.

a. ***Distraction:*** While maintaining the above position the therapist distracts the head with the help of body. End range may be held for at least 6-10 seconds. 10-15 repetitions may be performed (Fig. 26.42).

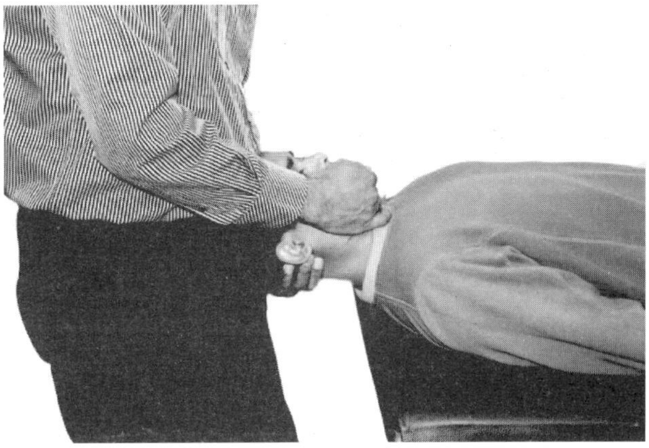

Fig. 26.42: Distraction

b. *Side Flexion:* While maintaining the traction the head is taken to the left side up to the full range or till the restriction starts and then to the neutral position, the pressure may be released. Then the head is taken to the right side with the traction. The traction is maintained throughout the range of motion till the head comes to the neutral position. When the head is taken to the left and to the right the therapist should have wide stance and should move the body with the head without changing the stance (Fig. 26.43).

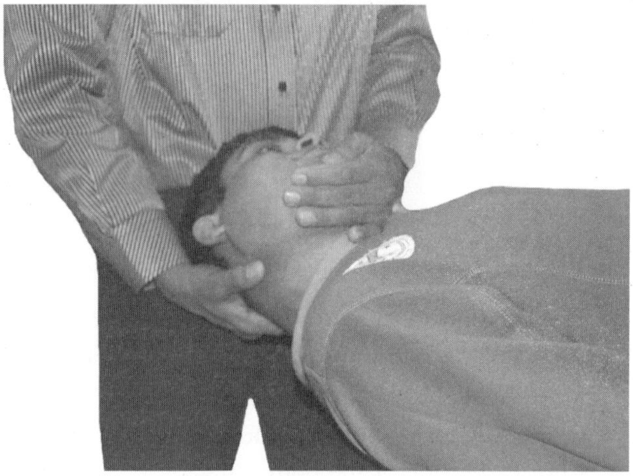

Fig. 26.43: Side flexion

c. *Rotations:* While maintaining the traction in the neutral position the head is rotated to the left and then to the neutral and to the right. The traction is maintained throughout the range until the head is brought to the neutral position (Fig. 26.44).

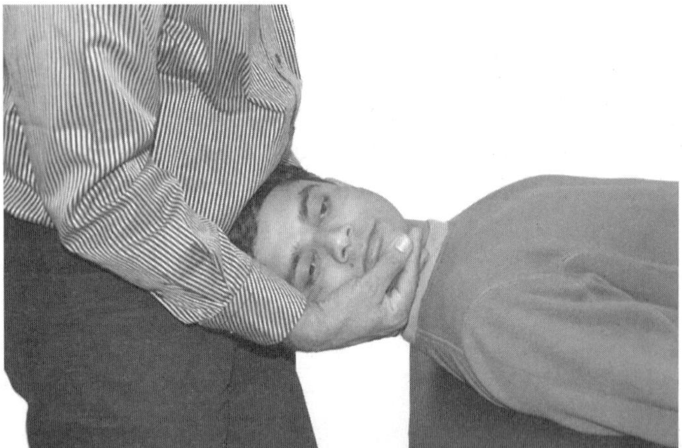

Fig. 26.44: Rotation

d. *Forward Flexion:* In neutral position traction is applied with both the hands and the head is taken to the forward flexion in full range of motion or upto the restriction starts. The traction is maintaine throughout the range of motion until the head come to the neutral position (Fig. 26.45).

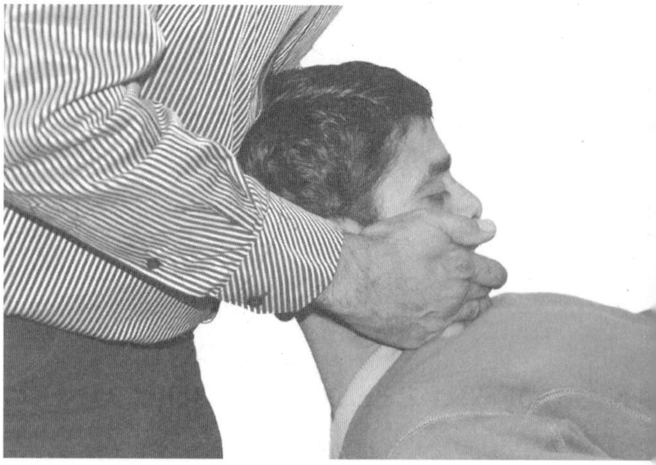

Fig. 26.45: Forward flexion

e. *Extension:* While maintaining the traction the hea is taken to the extension in the full range of motio or till the restriction starts. The traction i maintained throughout the range of motion (Fig 26.46).

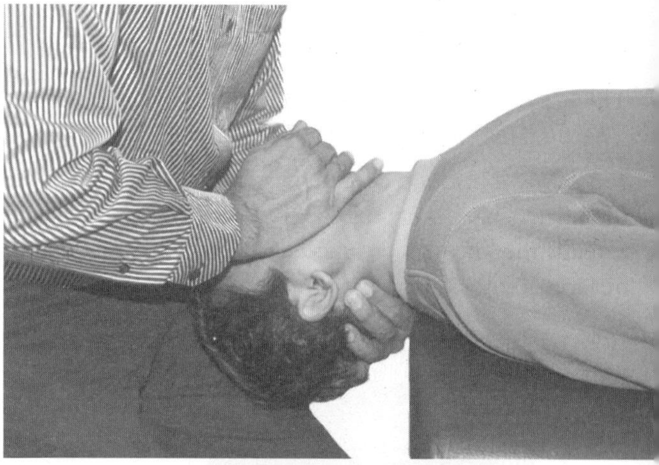

Fig. 26.46: Extension

C. **Posterior Anterior Central Vertebral Pressure:** T mobilize the vertebral column, pressure is applied o the spinous process with the thumbs.

Position of Patient: Prone, forehead rests on the palm c the hand of the patient. Chin is tucked fully i particularly for C_1, C_2 and C_3 vertebra.

Position of Therapist: Therapist stands at the head of th patient. Thumbs are held in opposition and back t back (to reinforce). The tip of the thumb pad is place on the spinous process of the vertebra which is bein mobilized. The fingers are placed on either side of th neck.

Procedure: While maintaining the position of neck and the hands, the therapist applies gentle pressure through the arms and body to the spinous process which will produce oscillatory movements in the mobile vertebral segment. The mid-cervical area requires less pressure to mobilize than the upper and lower cervical area. The procedure can also be performed with lateral flexion and rotation of the cervical spine. It is termed as combined technique (Figs. 26.47a to c).

D. **Posteroanterior Unilateral Vertebral Pressure:** To mobilize the vertebral column pressure can also be applied on the transverse process with the thumb through the body.

Position of Patient: Prone, forehead rests on the hands of the patient with chin tucked well in.

Position of Therapist: The therapist stands at the side of the neck of the patient, places one thumb on the posterior surface of the articular process (transverse process) to be mobilized. The fingers may rest on the neck of the patient.

(a)

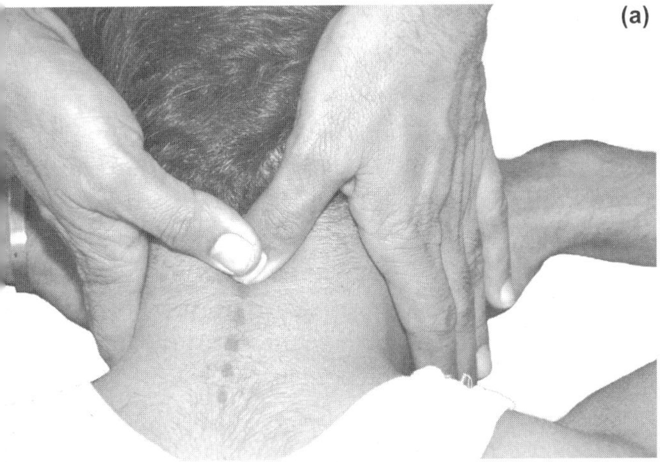

(b)

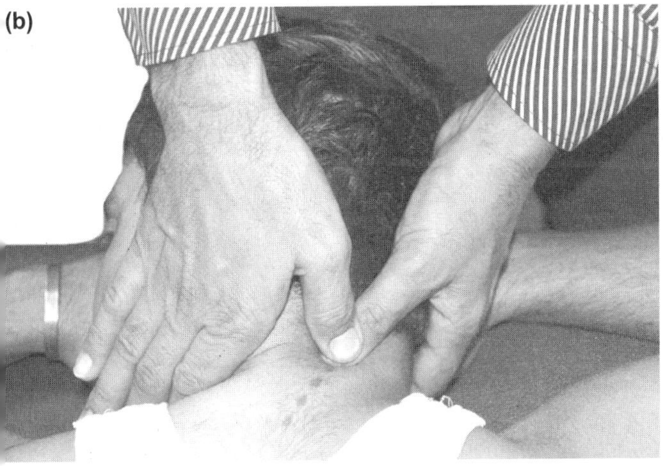

(c)

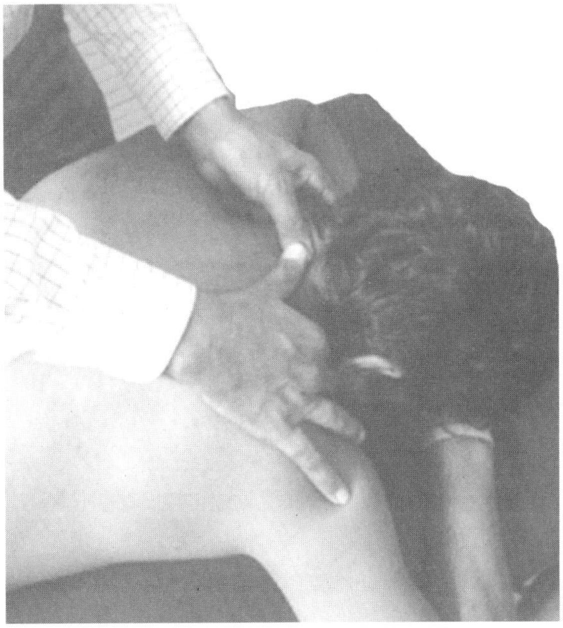

Figs. 26.47a to c: PA central pressure technique, a. in neutral, b. in rotation, c. side flexion

Method: While maintaining the above position of the neck and thumb a gentle pressure is applied through the arms and body to the posterior surface of the articular process; which produces oscillatory movements at the mobile vertebral segment. The technique is useful in unilateral pain with limitation in the range of motion (Fig. 26.48a). *The posteroanterior unilateral vertebral pressure technique can also be applied with rotation of the cervical spine. As an example for a patient who complains pain in the cervical spine and the origin of that is from the C_2 and C_3 segment. The patient's neck is turned to the left at 30 degree rotation; therapist places the thumb on the left posterior surface of the articular (transverse) process of the C_2 vertebra. The pressure is directed through arms and trunk to the articular surface which produces oscillatory movements at the C_2 and C_3 segment. This helps in increasing the range particularly symptoms arising from the $C_2/_3$ mobile segment. It is usually performed on the side of the pain or restriction* (Fig. 26.48b).

E. **Transverse Vertebral Pressure:** To mobilize the vertebral column; pressure is applied on the lateral aspect of spinous process with the thumb.

Position of Patient: Prone with forehead rests on the hands of the patient. The chin is tucked in (moderate degree) to reduce the cervical lordosis.

Position of Therapist: The therapist stands at the side of the patient. The thumb of one hand is placed on the lateral side of the spinous process of the vertebra, while thumb of other hand is placed on the thumb of first hand to reinforce it. The fingers rest on the neck and head.

(a)

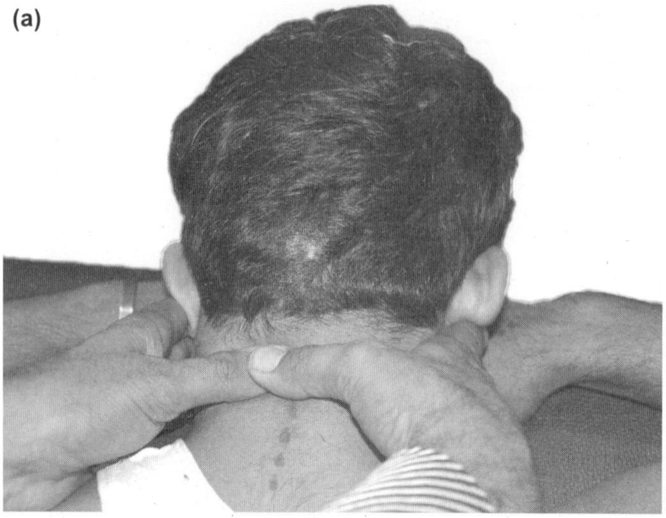

(b)

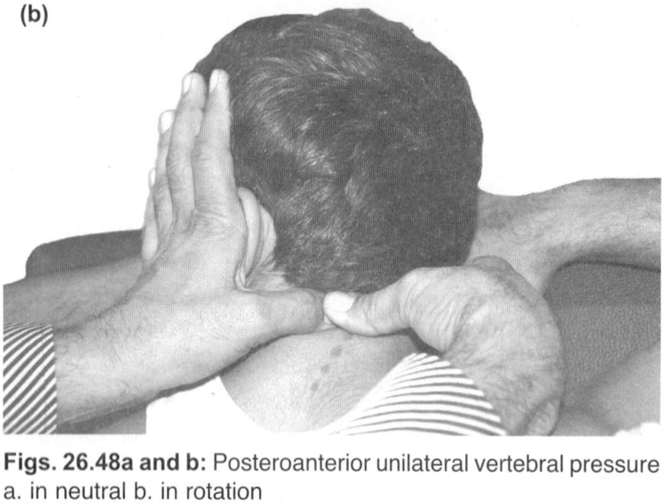

Figs. 26.48a and b: Posteroanterior unilateral vertebral pressure a. in neutral b. in rotation

Procedure: A gentle pressure is applied through the trunk and arms to the lateral side of the spinous process which produces oscillatory movements at the mobile segment. The technique is useful in unilateral painful conditions particularly originated due to degenerative changes in the vertebral column. The pressure is directed from the non-painful side to the painful side. For an example if patient has pain and symptoms on the right side, then the therapist stand at the left side and place thumb on the left lateral side of the spinous process (Fig. 26.49).

F. **Sustained Natural Apophyseal Glides (SNAGs):**

Position of Patient: Sitting on a height adjustable stool.

Position of Therapist: The therapist stands at the side of the patient for a C_2/C_3 vertebral segment; the therapist stands on the right side of the shoulder of the patient. The right index and middle finger is placed on the base of the occiput; the middle phalanx of right little finger is placed over the spinous process of axial vertebra. The thenar eminence of the left hand is placed on the left little finger.

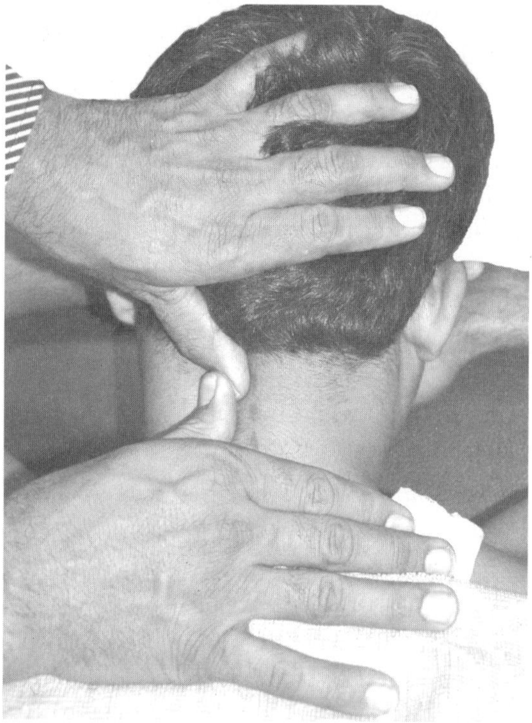

Fig. 26.49: Transverse vertebral pressure–left thumb on left sid of spinous pressure

Procedure: While stabilizing (cradling) the head betwee the therapist right arm and the chest a gentle pressur through the left hand is applied to the (left little finger spinous process of the axial vertebra for at least 5-1 seconds. Similar glides of 8-10 repetitions may b performed. The pressure created from left arm an thenar eminence to the little finger thrusts the secon vertebra (axial) anteriorly on the first (atlas) and i pressure is sufficient it may also thrust the first vertebr (atlas) forward on the occiput (Fig. 26.50).

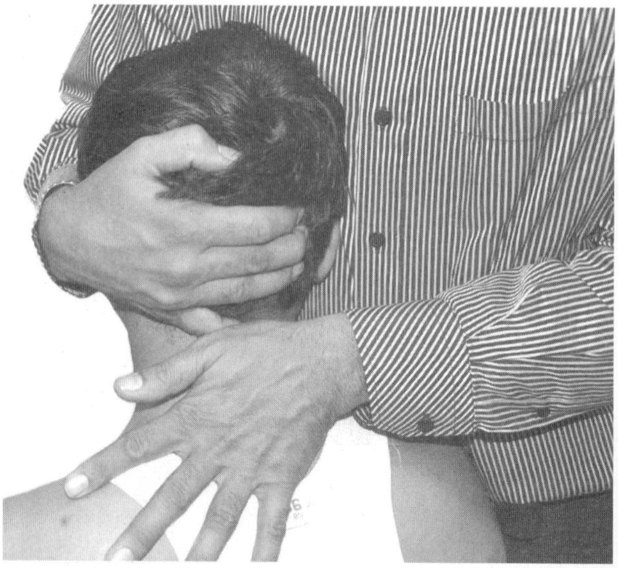

Fig. 26.50: SNAG to improve pain and range of motion at C_1 an C_2 mobile segment

Strengthening Exercises

1. **Deep Neck Flexors (Nodding or Chin Tuck Exercise):** This exercise is the cornerstone for the cervicogenic headache patients with forward head posture.

   Position of Patient: Sitting on a stool.

   Position of Therapist: Therapist sits on the stool and faces the patient. He demonstrates the exercise to the patient. Therapist can place one hand on the chin and other hand on the head to facilitate the movement.

   Procedure: The patient is instructed to tuck the chin in. Some patients find it difficult to perform in the desired direction, therefore, the therapist stabilizes the head with the right hand and pushes the chin back as much as possible with the left hand. The chin tuck exercises produce flexion at the upper cervical spine. At the end range of motion (full flexion) the patient is asked to hold the position for atleast six seconds. Three sets each of ten repetitions may be performed twice or thrice daily till the hyperextension of the upper cervical spine is corrected. The exercise should be an active in order to strengthen the deep neck flexors (Fig. 26.51).

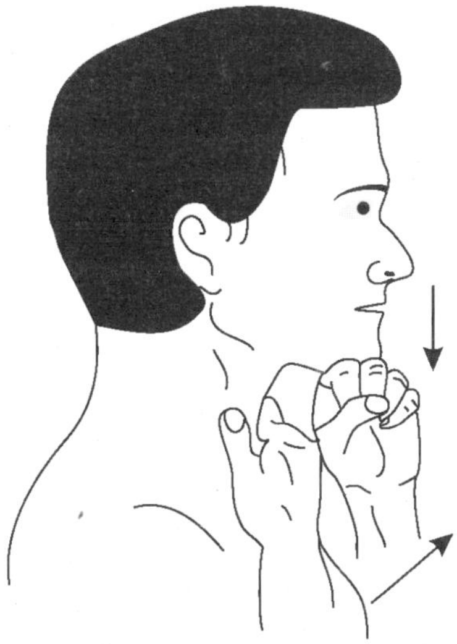

Fig. 26.51: Deep neck flexors exercises

2. **Trapezius (Middle and Lower Fibers) and Rhomboid (Retractors):** These muscles are the stabilizers of the scapula and play important role in keeping the scapula on the thoracic wall. The trapezius muscles (middle and lower) contribute to the force couple during the elevation of the arm. In sitting position with arms at side and hands resting on the thighs, the patient is asked to take the shoulder girdle back as much as possible without changing the position of hands. Therapist may stand behind the patient and place the hands on the patient's shoulder blades (scapula). The patient is asked to take the shoulders back against the resistance applied by the therapist (Fig. 26.52).

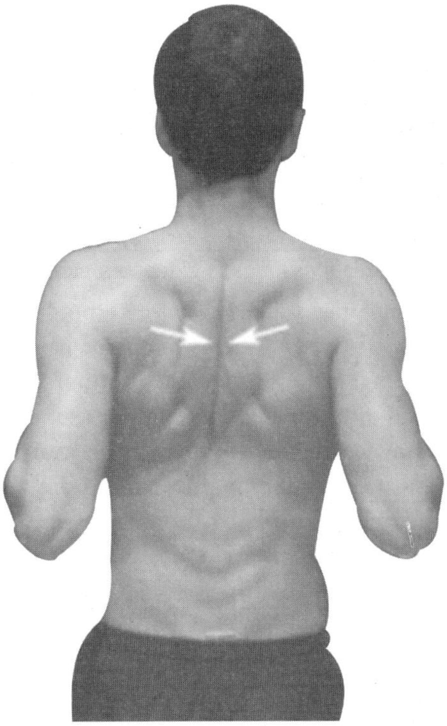

Fig. 26.52: Trapezius and rhomboids strengthening

3. **Serratus Anterior:** The patient stands against the wall flexes both the shoulders to 90° and places both the hands on the wall. Wall is pushed without changing the position of the hands. This may be repeated several times twice or thrice daily until the scapula is stabilized on the thoracic wall properly. Weakness of serratus anterior muscle can cause winging of the scapula (Fig. 26.53).

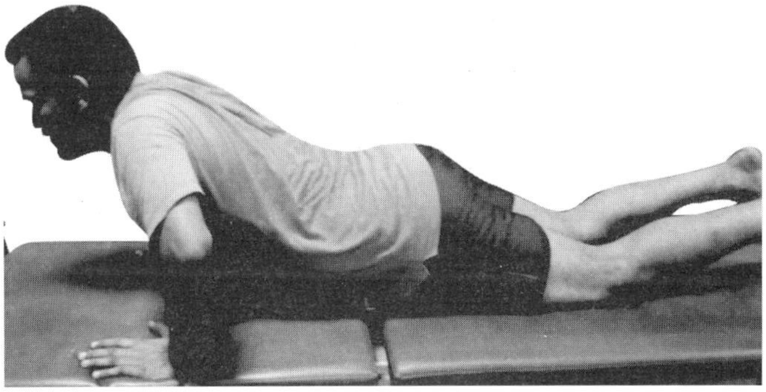

Fig. 26.53: Serratus anterior strengthening

4. **Upper Thoracic Extensors or Erector Spinae Muscles:** The upper thoracic erector spinae muscles are the phasic type of muscles which are having tendency of weakness and lengthening.

   Position of Patient: Prone lying with both hands at the side of the body. Patient is instructed to raise the head and upper thoracic spine and hold at least for six seconds (Fig. 26.54).

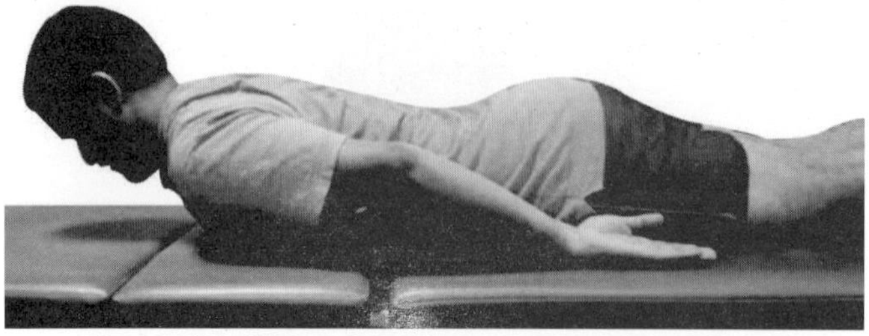

Fig. 26.54: Upper thoracic extensors strengthening

5. **Trapezius Upper Fibers:**Trapezius upper fibers are the tonic type of muscle fibers which are having tendency of shortening; however, in some postural problems such as drooped or protracted shoulders or rounded shoulders the muscles go in the lengthening position. To correct the posture the trapezius upper fibers are also need to be strengthened. In sitting position patient places both hands on the thigh and elevates the shoulders as much as possible which is held at end range at least for six seconds. Therapist can place both hands on the top of shoulders and can resist the shoulder elevation (Fig. 26.55).

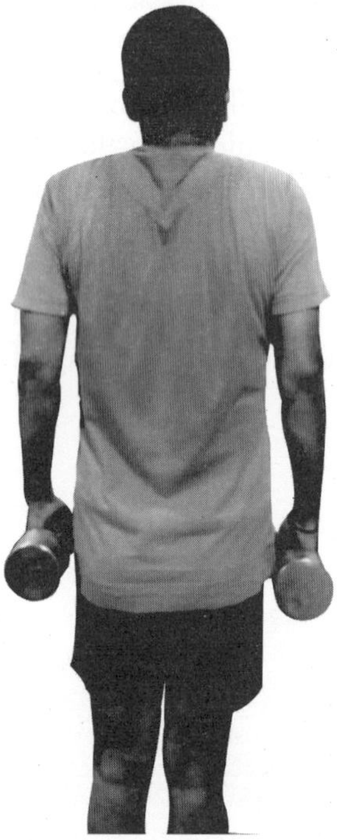

Fig. 26.55: Trapezius upper fibers strengthening

6. **Multifidus, Gluteus Maximus and Transverse Abdominis Strengthening:** See core strengthening program in Chapter 27.

Stretching Exercises

1. **Posterior Neck Muscle Stretching:** These are the tonic muscles which become shortened and cause hyperextension at the cervical spine (upper) following degenerative changes and pain.

Position of the Patient: Supine lying.

Position of Therapist: Stands at the end of the plinth (at head of the patient). The patient's head rests on the therapist thigh. The therapist grasps the occiput with the left hand and the chin with the right hand. Therapist bends the knees slightly to allow the COG to pass behind the trunk and to avoid the stress on the back.

Procedure: The therapist pushes the chin backward with the right hand. While maintaining the chin tuck in position the neck is flexed and is held at least for 6-10 seconds for significant stretching (Figs. 26.56a and b).

(a)

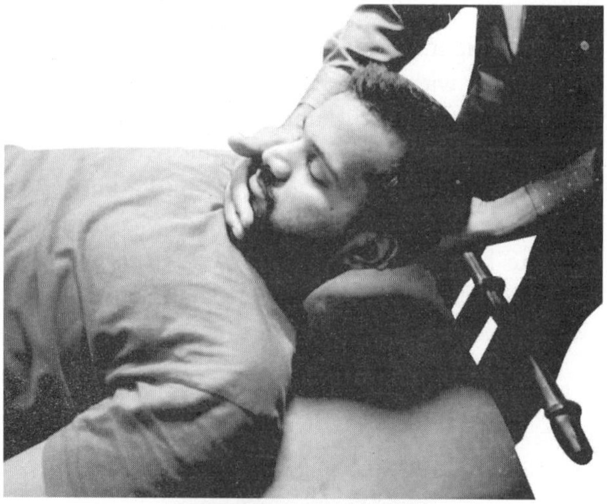

(b)

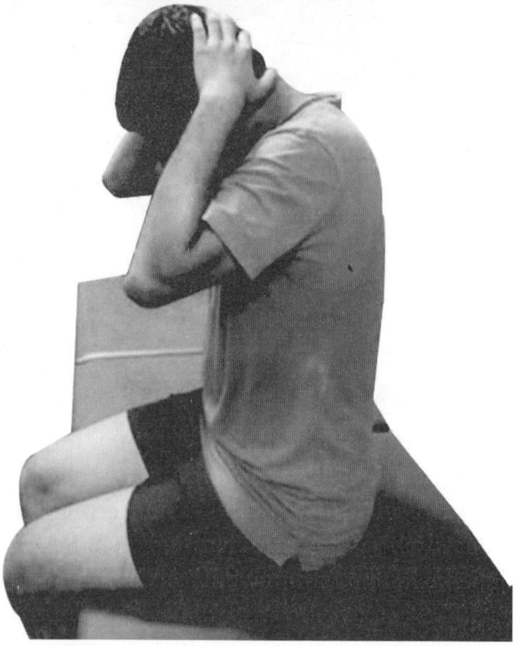

Figs. 26.56a and b: a. Posterior neck muscles stretching in supine, b. Posterior neck muscle stretching in sitting

2. **Pectoralis Major:** In a standing or sitting position patient abducts the shoulders at 90° and then takes them back horizontally. Therapist can assist the patient and apply

overpressure at the end range of motion. The exercise should be performed cautiously by patients with anterior instability. The patients may also perform the exercise by taking the shoulders backward at the 90 degree (Fig. 26.57).

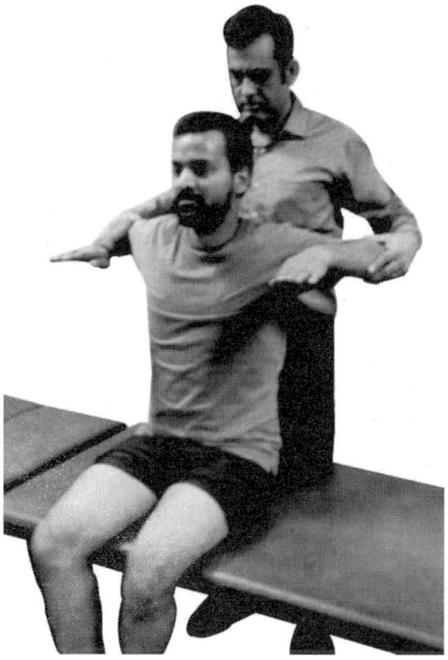

Fig. 26.57: Pectoralis major stretching

3. **Levator Scapulae and Trapezius Upper Fibers:** *Position of Patient:* Sitting with comfortable back rest. The head is rotated to the opposite side.

   Position of Therapist: Therapist stands behind the patient. To stretch the right levator scapulae muscle the therapist stands behind the patient and places right hand on the patient's right shoulder and the left hand grasps the occiput (slightly to the right side).

   Procedure: While stabilizing the right shoulder with the right hand, the neck is flexed to the left shoulder with left rotation (Figs. 26.58 and 26.59).

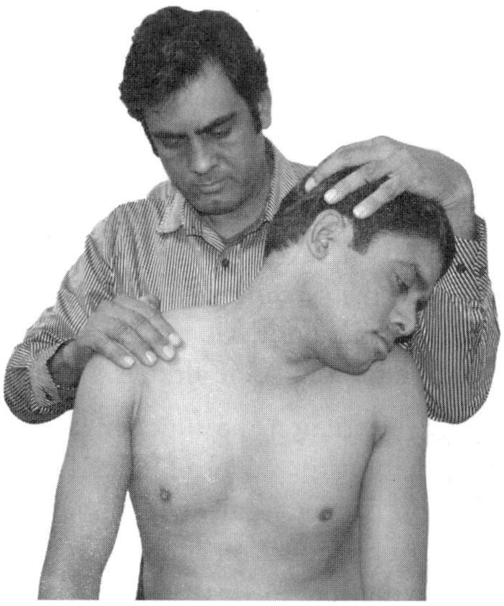

Fig. 26.58: Levator scapulae stretching in sitting

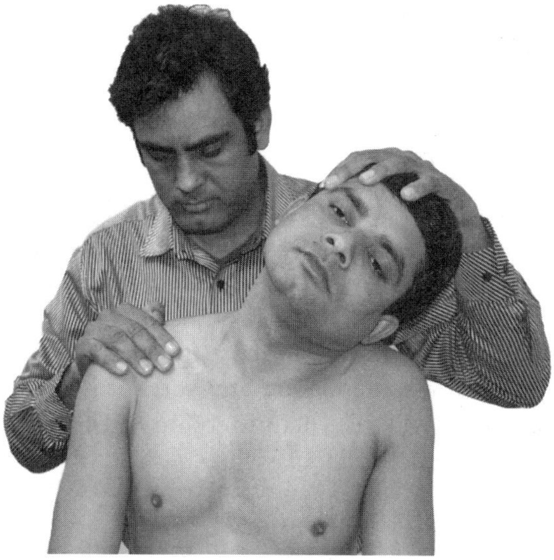

Fig. 26.59: Trapezius upper fibers stretching

4. **Soft Tissue Manipulation:** The flexibility of the extensors can also be increased with soft tissue manipulation such as wringing, squeezing and kneading.

Modalities

Moist Heat Therapy: This is one of the beneficial modalities helps in relieving pain and spasm and improving in flexibility of the muscles. The hot water bags easily available in the market may be used by the patient for at least 15-20 minutes twice daily. Patient should find the comfortable position such as sitting, prone or supine.

Short Wave Diathermy: Short wave diathermy is one of the effective modalities to produce the heat to the deep structures such as ligaments, tendons and capsule. It helps in improving extensibility of the tissues.

Ultrasound Therapy: Therapeutic ultrasound of 1 MHz, intensity between $1W/cm^2$ and $1.5W/cm^2$ with continuous mode shown good results in patients with cervicogenic headache. The continuous mode causes some heating effect which helps in improving the flexibility of the extensor muscles.

Mechanical Traction

Position of Patient: Supine with hip and knees flexion at 90°. A towel roll is placed under the upper cervical spine. Cervical spine is flexed forward at least to 20° to place significant traction at the lower cervical spine, while maintaining this position a cervical halter is put on. An intermittent traction is more effective than the sustained traction as it produces stretching and relaxation of the static stabilizers of the spine. This may be recommended for at least 15 minutes of duration per treatment session. However, static traction is preferred over the intermittent to the patients with soft disc herniation as it helps in relieving sustained pressure on the nerve roots. To place significant traction in the upper cervical region, the neck should be at neutral position.

Surgical Management

The patients with soft disc herniation usually recovers with conservative treatment, but involvement of multiple level of disc herniation may cause severe motor and sensory nerve deficit. Such small percentages of patients require surgical intervention. The common surgical procedures for intervertebral disc herniation are: anterior decompression and fusion (ADCF), Laminectomy, Laminactomy-facetectomy and Laminoplasty.

Post Surgical Management

The post surgical treatment is divided into three phases:

Phase I: During the phase I the patient is advised to put on cervical collar, however, the collar may be removed for the exercises and modalities. The collar may be soft or hard that depends upon the surgical procedure. To decrease pain and spasm, cryotherapy is advised initially for 15 minutes thrice daily. Soft tissue manipulation such as wringing and squeezing is performed on the trapezius upper fibers and posterior neck muscles. Gentle stretching of erector spinae trapezius and levator scapulae if the surgeon permits may be initiated in pain free range. Strengthening exercises of deep neck flexors, serratus anterior and rhomboids in the form of isometric should also be started. Exercises which aggravate the symptoms should be discontinued immediately.

Phase II: To progress to the phase II, the patient should have minimal pain and spasm; and improved neuro-muscular control, range of motion or may be limited with pain in the end range. Grade 2 and 3 mobilization to improve the range of motion and intensive isometric may also be initiated at this stage to regain normal posture. Resistance may be applied manually.

Phase III: To progress to the phase III, the patient should restore full range of motion and neuromuscular control without pain and symptoms. The patient is withstand the demands of activity, work and practice. The exercises such as PNF techniques, dynamic strengthening, and conditioning programme in conjunction with activity, work, or practice are initiated during this phase.

FACET JOINT HYPOMOBILITY

The movements in the mobile segment greatly depends upon the orientation of the facet joints, hence, these are determined largely by the direction in which the articular joints face. The zygapophyseal joints (facet joints) face or slant upward and posteriorly at an angle of 45 degree, lying halfway between the horizontal and the frontal plane. Such a slant would seem to favour rotation and lateral flexion and to be unfavorable to flexion and hyperextension. However, flexion and hyperextension occur as freely as lateral flexion while rotation from the second cervical vertebra down occur only as moderate in terms of range of motion (Table 26.7).

Table 26.7: Facet joint movements in the cervical spine

Movement	*Plane of movement*
Flexion	The upper facet slides up and forward on the lower facet
Extension	The upper facet slides down and back on the lower facet
Side flexion	The upper facet slides down and back on the same side and up and forward on the opposite side
Rotation	The upper facet slides down and posterior on the same side and up and anterior on the opposite side

The facet joints in the cervical spine are diarthrodial synovial joints with fibrous capsules, surrounded by a capsule of connective tissue and produces synovial fluid to nourish and lubricate the articular cartilage.

Clinical Features

The patients with facet restriction usually present with the complaint of pain and limitation in the flexion or extension combined with side flexion and rotation. The patients reveal the history of sudden jerk or quick movement followed by pain and limitation in the range of motion in a typical pattern. For an example, following sudden jerk or movement injury; the neck may stuck in the forward flexion with right rotation and right side flexion. The quadrant test (spurling) will be positive. Tender points may also be present on corresponding facet. The facet hypomobility produces two types of restrictions–opening and closing.

Opening and Closing Facet Joint Restriction

Following jerk, twist or sudden movement there is excessive slide of one of the facet joints. The excessive sliding of the facet stretches the facet capsule and stucks in a new position which may limit the range of motion either in flexion or in extension. The flexion opens the facet joint; hence restriction in flexion is termed as opening facet restriction. On the other hand the extension closes the facet joint hence, restriction in the extension is termed as closing facet restriction. These restrictions flexion or extensions are often combined with rotation and side flexion.

In an opening restriction the superior facet joint does not glide up and forward on the inferior facet, thereby limiting the flexion of that segment. In a close restriction the superior facet stucks in flexion and unable to glide down and backward on the inferior facet, thereby, limiting the extension of that segment.

Management

The treatment is aimed at smooth gliding of the facet joint in the treatment plane. Many techniques have been developed to bring the smooth gliding of the facet joint back to the normal. Before exploring the techniques the practitioners should be aware of the orientation of the facet joints plane and should also practice on the normal subjects before administering to the patients.

1. **Mobilization:** This has translatory and oscillatory glides performed on the patients in a most comfortable position.

   a. *For Opening Restriction:* The patient is positioned prone with the forehead resting on a towel with the cervical spine in pain free position. The therapist stands at the side of the facet which is being mobilized. For a patient who has a C_6 and C_7 level facet opening restriction on the right side, the therapist stands on the right side and places the thumb on the superior aspect of the C_6 and C_7 facet and applies pressure in the direction of the treatment plane. The oscillating glides are applied at end range which may last upto 30-60 seconds three to five times per treatment session (Fig. 26.60).

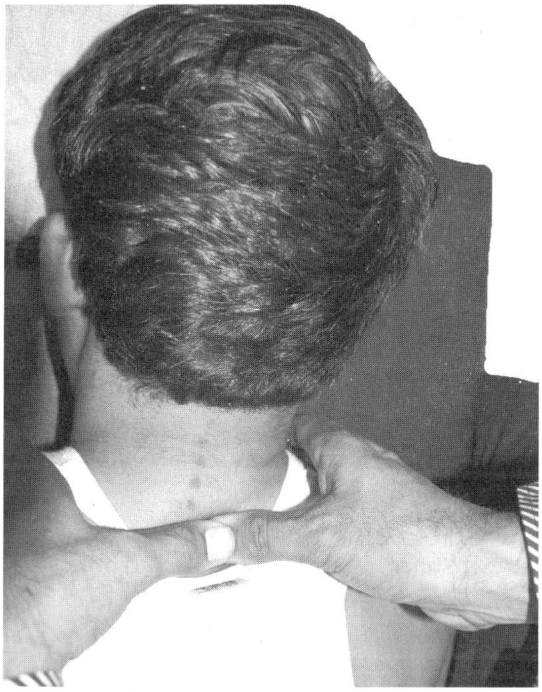

Fig. 26.60: Mobilization for opening restriction of C_6-C_7 facet joint

   b. *For Closing Restriction:* The position of patient remains same as for opening restriction. Therapist stands at the level of head, and places the thumb on the superior facet of the segment. For a patient who has closing restriction at right C_6 and C_7 segment, the therapist stands at the right side of the segment which is being mobilized and places the thumb on a superior facet of the C_6 and C_7 segment. The therapist applies a force down and backward in the treatment plane (Fig. 26.61). Several repetitions (60 oscillations per minute) may be performed to improve range of the facet joint.

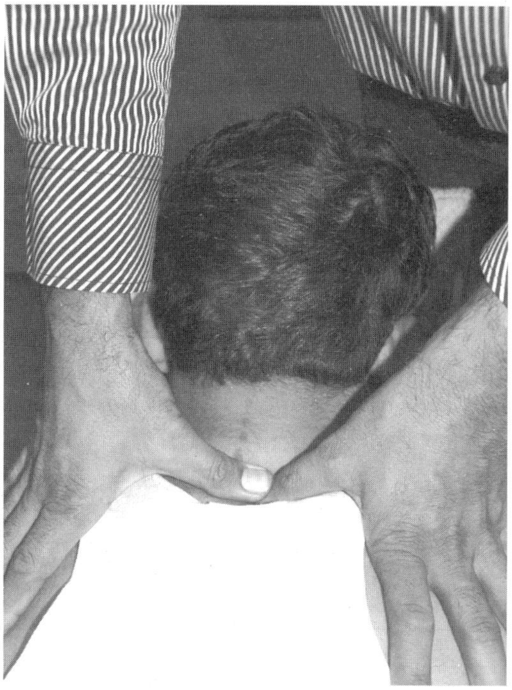

Fig. 26.61: Mobilization for closing restriction of C_6-C_7 facet joint

2. **Muscle Energy Techniques:** The muscle energy techniques involve isometric contraction of muscle or group of muscles which are responsible for loss of range of motion. If right side flexion and rotation is limited, the left side flexors and rotators are allowed to contract isometrically, as they are holding the neck to the left side flexion rotation. This strong isometric contraction causes same degree of relaxation that improves pain and range of motion.

   a. *For Opening Restriction:* The patient has limitation in the range of flexion with rotation and side flexion. For a patient with right C_6 and C_7 opening restriction the patient may have restriction in the flexion, left side flexion and left rotation.

   Position of Patient: Supine; head out of the edge of the table. The therapist stands at the head. Head of the patient rests on the waist or thigh of the therapist. Therapist places right hand on the chin and left hand under the occiput, and then brings the neck in the extreme restricted positions (flexion, left side flexion and left rotation).

   Procedure: While maintaining the above position the therapist instructs the patient to move the head into extension, right side flexion and right rotation against the resistance for 3-6 seconds applied by the therapist. The patient is allowed to relax the muscles. In the next step, the neck is again brought into the further improved positions (flexion, left side flexion and left rotation). Therapist maintains the position and again instructs the patient to bring the neck into extension, right side flexion and right rotation against the resistance (isometric) applied by the therapist for 3-6 seconds. Several isometric contractions may be performed to reduce the muscle spasm and increase the range of motion (Figs. 26.62 and 26.63).

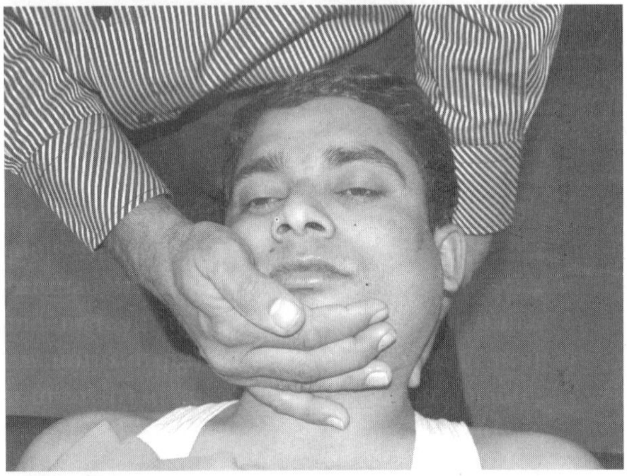

Fig. 26.62: Muscle energy technique for opening restriction at the level of right C_6-C_7

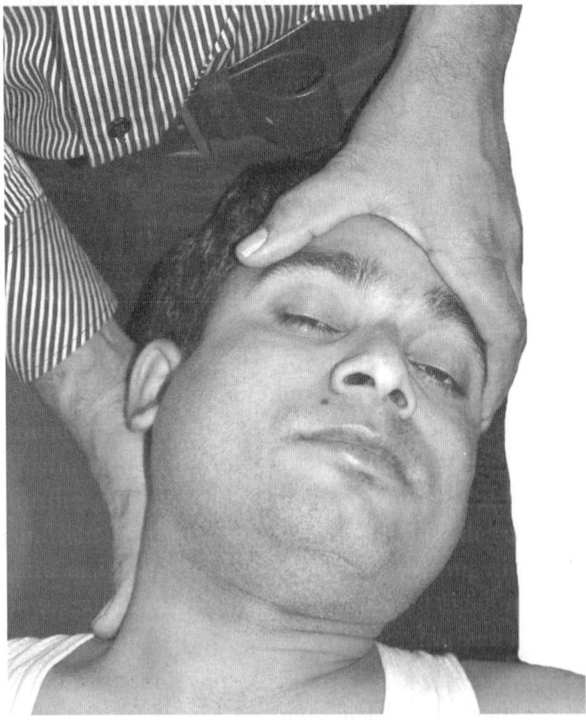

Fig. 26.63: Muscle energy technique for closing restriction at right side C_6-C_7

b. ***For Closing Restriction:*** For a patient with right side C_6-C_7 closing facet restriction, the extension, right side flexion and right rotation may be limited. In this case the neck will be stiff in flexion, left side flexion and left rotation. To perform the technique the patient is positioned in supine with the head out of the edge of the table. Therapist stands at the head, and places right hand under the occiput and left hand on the forehead (fingers on the forehead and hypothenar on the left side of head). The head of the patient rests on the therapist's thigh or waist. Therapist instructs the patient to bring the neck in the extreme limited positions (extension, right side flexion and right rotation).

Procedure: While maintaining the above position the therapist instruct the patient to move the head into flexion, left side flexion and left rotation against the resistance (isometric) applied by the therapist for 3-6 seconds. Patient is instructed to relax the muscles and neck is brought into the further improved positions (extension, right side flexion and right rotation). The therapist maintains the positions and instructs the patient to bring the neck into flexion, left side flexion and left rotation against the resistance applied by the therapist for 3-6 seconds. Several repetitions of isometric contractions may be performed to improve pain and range of motion.

Box 26.3

Muscle Energy Techniques: Strong isometric contraction of spasmodic group muscles is followed by same degree of relaxation of the same group of muscles.

3. **Side Glide Mobilization for Opening Restriction:** The patient lies supine with the head out of the edge of the table. Therapist stands at the top of the head of the patient and makes a *web space* of both the mobilizing and stabilizing hands. The stabilizing hand is placed on the distal and the mobilizing hand on the proximal part of the restricted mobile segment. For a C_6-C_7 segment opening restriction, the stabilizing hand is placed on the C_7 vertebra (distal part of mobile segment) and the mobilizing hand is placed on the C_6 vertebra (proximal part of the mobile segment). The patient's head rests on the therapist thigh or waist.

   Procedure: The therapist flexes the cervical spine with distraction to allow the mobile segment to open as much as possible. A gliding force is applied with the mobilizing hand towards the same side of the facet joint at the proximal mobile segment. This allows opening of the facet joint of the C_6-C_7 mobile segment opposite of the mobilizing hand, and closing of same side of the facet joint of the C_6-C_7 mobile segment (Fig. 26.64).

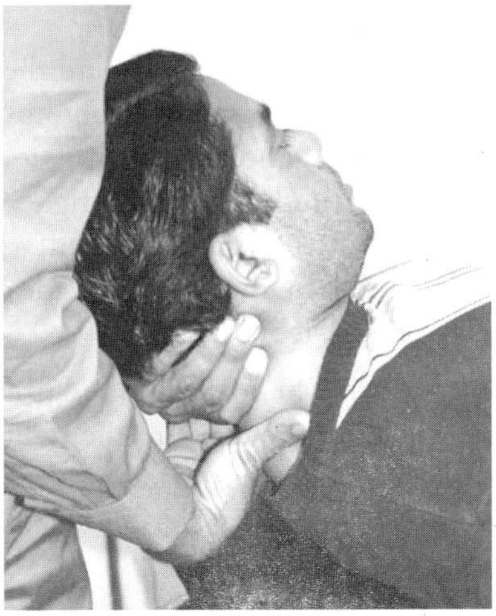

Fig. 26.64: Side glide mobilization for opening restriction

4. **Sustained Natural Apophyseal Glides (SNAGs):** The much talked about technique SNAG has been given by Brain Mulligan, a Neazeland based physical therapy practitioner. These techniques are performed in weight bearing positions. These are very effective if the therapist can identify the exact site of facet dysfunction. The thumb is placed under the spinous process or direct on the facet and then it is glided in the treatment plane. Patient may have relief in sign and symptoms instantly. Unlike Maitland and other conventional techniques which are performed in most relaxed position (lying), the SNAGs are performed in the weight bearing position either in sitting or standing because when improvement in the sign and symptoms are achieved in a functional position they are likely to be retained. These mobilization techniques may also be performed with the movements (active or passive). At the end of active range of motion the therapist applies gentle overpressure. The important part of the technique is that the therapist should identify the location where from pain is originated, then the spinous process of the superior vertebra is palpated and thumb is placed under that. The therapist applies pressure through the thumb up in the direction with the movement along the treatment plane.

   a. ***SNAGs to Improve Rotation and Decrease Pain Associated With It:*** For an example C_5 and C_6 is the intervertebral joint where from pain is originating and that is also limiting the rotation. The therapist places the medial border of one of the thumbs under the spinous process of C_5 and it is reinforced by other thumb. The spinous process of C_5 is pushed up in the direction of treatment plane through the reinforced thumb and then the patient is instructed to rotate the neck to the restricted painful direction. At the end of limitation a gentle overpressure is applied and is held atleast for 6-10 seconds. The head is returned to the neutral position with the gentle pressure. Improvement in the pain and range is assessed and several repetitions are performed. In case where pain aggravates, the therapist should stop and perform the technique on other level or discontinue (Fig. 26.65).

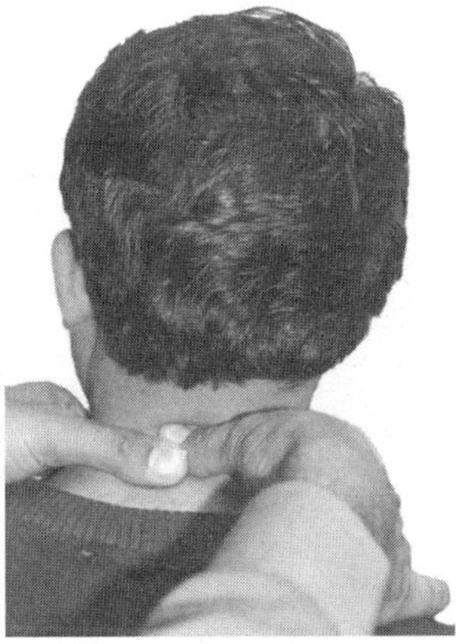

Fig. 26.65: SNAGs to improve rotation

   b. ***SNAGs to Improve Flexion and Decrease the Pain Associated With It:***

   Position of Patient: Sitting on a stool.

   Position of Therapist: Therapist stands behind the patient, faces the cervical spine. Similar to previous technique therapist identifies the site where from pain is originating, for an example C_6 and C_7 is the site. The medial border of the thumb is placed under the spinons process of C_6. The spinous process of C_6 is pushed up and anteriorly along the treatment plane with the thumb and patient is asked to flex the neck forward. At the end of restriction overpressure is applied and is held for few seconds. The neck is then returned to the neutral position with the pressure (Fig. 26.66).

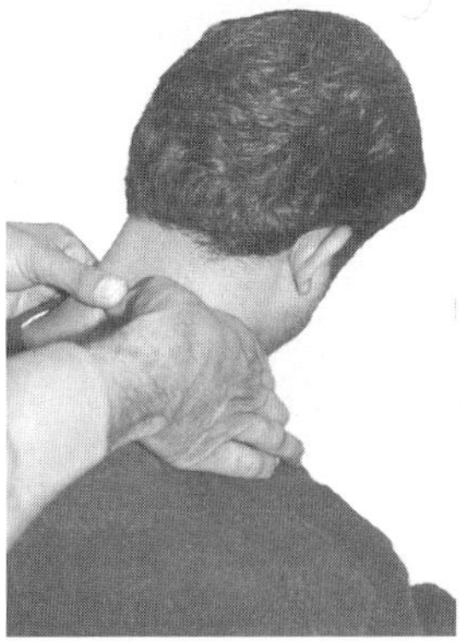

Fig. 26.66: SNAGs to improve flexion

c. ***SNAGs to Improve Extension and Decrease Pain Associated With It:*** Similar to the previous technique (flexion), medial border of thumb is placed under the spinous process of the mobile segment, and the spinous process of the superior vertebra is pushed up along the treatment plane and patient is instructed to extend the cervical spine. At the end of motion where restriction starts, the therapist applies overpressure and sustains for few seconds. The cervical spine is then taken into the neutral position (Fig. 26.67).

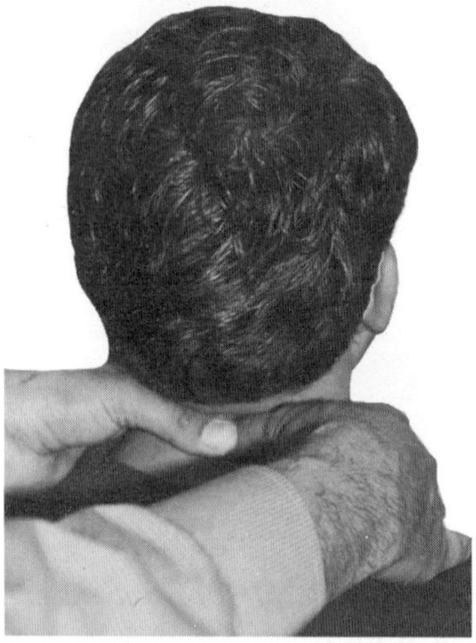

Fig. 26.67: SNAGs to improve extension

d. ***SNAGs to Improve Side Flexion and Reduce Pain and Symptoms Associated With It:*** The position of patient and therapist remains same as above. The therapist places thumb under the spinous process of the superior vertebra and pushes it up along the treatment plane. Patient is instructed to bend the neck to the restricted and painful side. At end of restriction the therapist applies overpressure and sustains for few seconds. The neck is then returned to the neutral position with the pressure (Fig. 26.68).

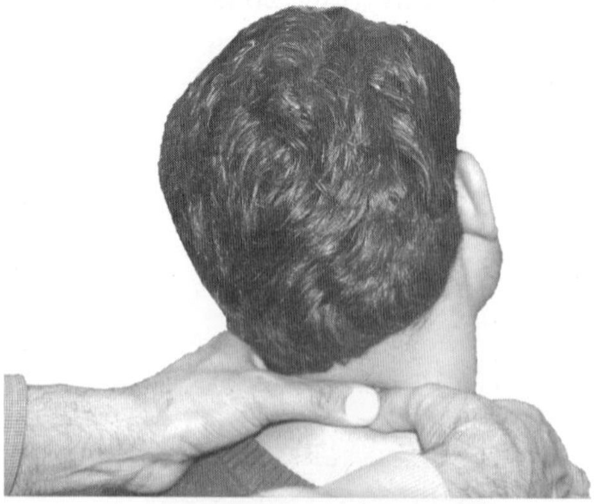

Fig. 26.68: SNAGs to improve side flexion

e. ***Spinal Mobilization With Arm Movement:***

Position of Patient: Sitting on a stool with the shoulder abduction to 90°.

Position of Therapist: Stands behind the patient. The facet which is producing the symptoms is identified. For example C_4 and C_5 is the site where from symptoms are produced to the right shoulder and aggravated with the arm movement. The therapist places the thumb on the left lateral side of the spinous process of C_4 vertebra.

Procedure: The therapist applies pressure on the spinous process to rotate it to the right and sustains it and allows the patient to adduct the shoulder joint horizontally with elbow flexion (Fig. 26.69).

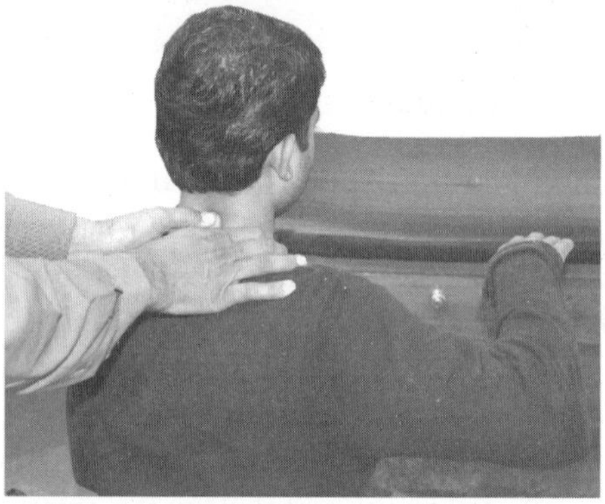

Fig. 26.69: Spinal mobilization with arm movement

f. ***Facet Down Slide:*** Patient lies supine with the head out of the edge of the table. The therapist places mobilizing hand under the neck with second metacarpophalangeal joint directly on the posterior pillar (apophyseal joints or transverse process) which is being mobilized.

Procedure: While maintaining the above position; the neck is bent to the same side of the facet which is being mobilized. As soon as the movement reaches its limitation and patient starts complaining pain, the therapist glides the facet joint in the plane of facet through second MCP joint. The technique is effective in closing facet restriction and improving pain and range of motion. Therapist should be more cautious when it is used in acute inflammation and muscle guarding. It should be discontinued in case pain is aggravated (Fig. 26.70).

g. ***Facet Up Slide:*** The position of patient and therapist remains same as facet down slide.

Procedure: The neck is flexed to the opposite side of the facet which is to be mobilized upto the pain and limitation starts. To glide the facet joint, the therapist creates a force to the superior and anterior

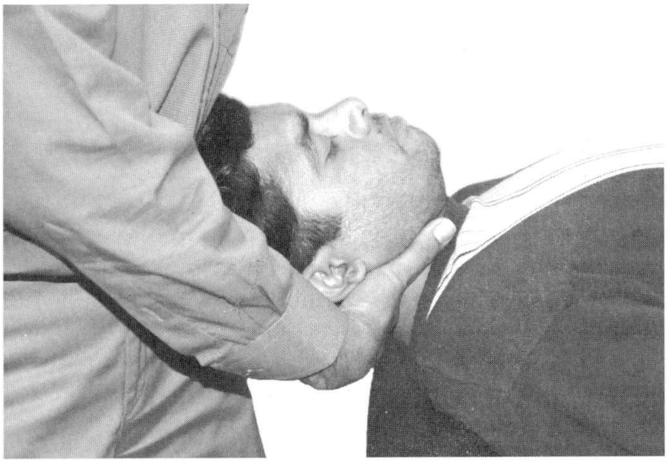

Fig. 26.70: Facet down slide mobilization

direction (towards the opposite eye) in its treatment plane. Facet up slide helps in opening facet restriction (Fig. 26.71).

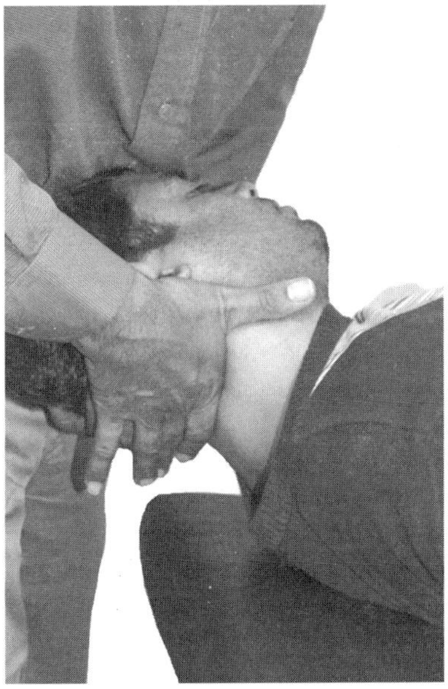

Fig. 26.71: Facet up slide mobilization

CERVICOGENIC HEADACHE (CH)

Introduction: Cervicogenic headache is described as a syndrome that is "a final common pathway" not an entity. Thus CH is a syndrome that can have many contributing factors. The World Cervicogenic Headache Society has defined CH as referred pain perceived in any part of the head and caused by a primary nociceptive sources in the musculoskeletal tissues that are innervated by the C_1, C_2 and C_3 spinal nerves. Pain associated with CH has been attributed to physical impairments of the joint, muscle and neural structures in the cervical region, and in particularly the upper cervical region.

The studies have demonstrated that the patients with CH had significantly less strength and endurance of the deep neck flexors compared to age-matched controls. They have also identified a decrease in strength of the deep neck flexors in patients with CH; when compared to able bodied individuals. In a recent clinical study involving patients with CH, Jull *et al.* (JOSPT, 2005) compared the effect of specific active exercises directed at improving the strength and endurance of the deep neck flexors to manual therapy, or a combination of active exercise and manual therapy, displayed better outcomes than a control group who received no treatment. In particular, the group who received active exercise improved in both pain behavior and strength of deep neck flexors.

Pathomechanics: A forward head position with increased extension of the upper cervical region is commonly observed. This extended alignment is of particular importance because some investigators have described how cervical extension may contribute to increased stress on the cervical facet joints as a result of approximation of the facet joint surfaces. It has also observed that patients with CH frequently extend their neck when they perform unilateral or bilateral shoulder flexion (Jan, 2005, JOSPT) (Figs. 26.72a and b).

(a)

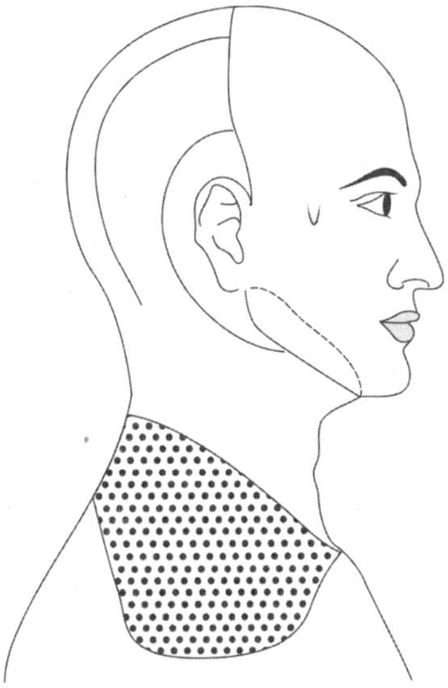

(b)

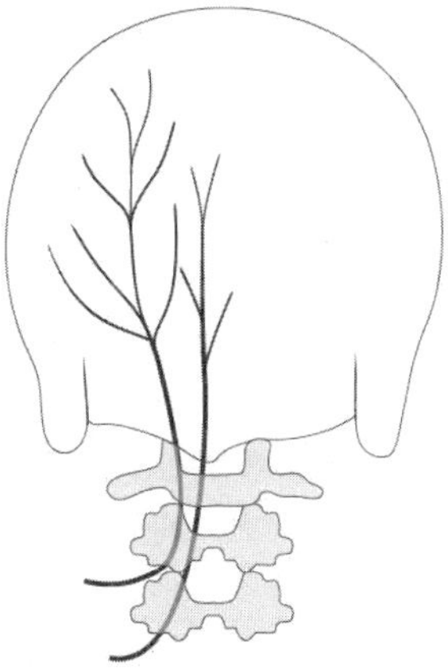

Figs. 26.72a and b: C_2 and C_3 nerve supply

In the scapulothoracic region it has been noted that patients with CH often display an alignment of scapular abduction and depression indicating lengthened levator scapulae and trapezius muscles. This scapular alignment is often associated with concomitant weakness of some or all portions of the trapezius as well as the rhomboids and levator scapulae (Mary Kate Mc Donnell *et al.* 2005, Jan JOSPT). This suggests that impairments not only lies in the cervical region, but also in the scapulothoracic and lumbar region, may be important to consider when treating a patient with cervicogenic headache. The compensatory head position associated with a slumped, round upper back results in extension of the cervical spine (hyperextension of the upper cervical spine). The tight muscles (erector spinae) will produce hyperextension at the C_0-C_1, C_1-C_2 and C_2-C_3, which cause approximation of the posterior pillars (facet joints). This will irritate the pain sensitive structures, territories of the anterior and posterior rami of C_1, C_2 and C_3 which distribute the pain in the suboccipital, temporal and supraorbital region.

Common Characteristics of Cervical Headache

- The cervicogenic headaches are most often unilateral but as the disease progresses these can become bilateral.
- Tenderness can be palpated over the facet joint ipsilateral to the headache which may be present bilaterally with the time.
- The extensor muscles show tightness and limit the cervicocranial flexion and produce some sort of stretching feeling in the neck.
- Soft tissue manipulation and hot water fomentation improves the symptoms.
- Pain is perceived in the occipital, temporal or supraorbital regions.
- Pain does not change the location as it is common in migranous headache.
- Extension will aggravate the symptoms as it causes further approximation to the facet joints and irritation to pain sensitive structures.
- *Cervicogenic headache* is similar to migraine headache due to the ipsilateral pain and the typical migraine like symptoms such as nausea, vomiting and ocular. It differs from migraine in two ways:

1. It never alternates sides.
2. Initiates from neck.

Box 26.4

Migraine

A typical migraine headache is unilateral and pulsating lasting from 4 hours to 72 hours.

Symptoms: Nausea, vomiting, photophobia–increased sensitivity to light, phonophobia–increase sensitivity to sound. Approximately 1/3rd of people who suffer from migraine headache perceive an auro-unusal visual, olfactory, or other experience that are the signs that the migraine will soon occur.

Pathophysiology: Cause is idiopathic. An accepted theory is that is a disorder of the serotonergic control system, a PET scan demonstrated the aura coincides with diffusion of cortical depression consequent to increased blood flow (upto 300% greater than baseline).

There are some migraine headache variants, some originate from the brainstem (featuring inter cellular transport dysfunction of calcium and potassium), and some are genetically disposed.

Types of Cervicogenic Headache

A. **Occipital – Headache:** The greater occipital nerve which is a both sensory and motor, supplies the semispinalis and splenius capitis muscles. Pain is experienced in the occipital and can radiate to vertex. It corresponds to the territories of the posterior rami of C_2 and C_3 facet joints. *It represents 20% of cervicogenic headaches.*

Friction Sign of Scalp: It consists of pressing firmly with the pad of the fingers against the scalp and mobilizing it with small to and fro motions. Maneuver is painless in normal scalp, but it is very disagreeable and even painful in the cases of an occipital headache of cervical origin (Fig. 26.73).

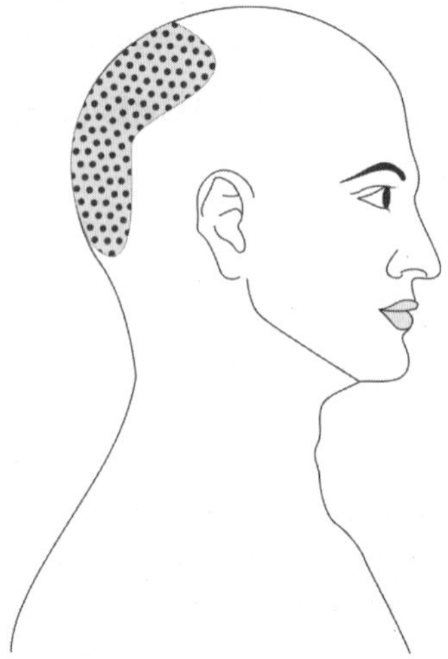

Fig. 26.73: Occipital cervicogenic headache

Clinical Features

- Tenderness present on the ipsilateral to C_2-C_3 facet joint.
- The territory that is painful to friction can correspond to the posterior ramus of C_3 and C_2.
- C_3 – innervates – paramedian zone.
- C_2 – innervates – lateral part of the occiput, it can be more diffused but it does not go beyond the bi-auricular line. The periauricular region also receives innervations from anterior rami of C_2-C_3.
- The extension of the neck can reproduce the symptoms.
- Upper cervical goes into hyperextension and lower into flexion.
- Shoulder becomes rounded and protracted.
- The thoracic spine assumes in a kyphotic posture.

B. **Occipito Temporomaxillary Headache (5%):** It is felt on the retroauricular mastoid and parietal region and radiates towards the inferior maxilla. Tenderness and pain presents on ipsilateral to the C_2 and C_3. The painful scalp in the retroauricular territory is innervated by the superficial cervical plexus (anterior ramus of C_2, sometimes of C_3). The angle of jaw is innervated by the anterior ramus of C_2 and C_3, not by the trigeminal nerve. Friction sign on the scalp (retroauricular) and pinch rolling at the angle of Jaw is positive (Fig. 26.74).

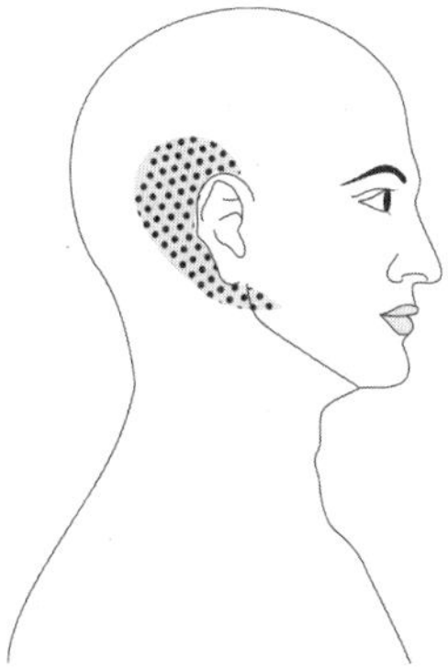

Fig. 26.74: Occipito temporomaxillary cervicogenic headache

C. **Supraorbital Headache (67%):** The topography of the pain is usually supraorbital, sometimes occipito-supraorbital, and in a few cases retro-orbital.

Eyebrow Sign: The eyebrow is pinched between the thumb and index finger and kneaded and rolled like a cigarette. It is explored from one end to the other, going over the forehead skin. In patients with *supraorbital headaches* the roll is painful and thickened throughout all or part of the brow on the side of the usual headache, generally the side of C_2-C_3 articular pain (Fig. 26.75).

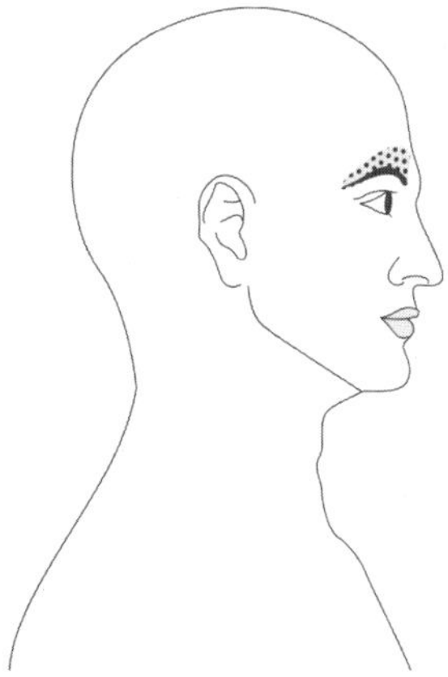

Fig. 26.75: Supraorbital cervicogenic headache

Chick Sign: Sometimes pain may also be experienced in chick. When the skin of the neck is rolled and pinched they complaint tenderness below the maxilla. Facial pain syndrome is also has origin from the cervical spine. The syndrome is relieved by mobilizing and manipulating the cervical spine and muscles.

UPPER CROSSED SYNDROME

Janda named this syndrome "Upper crossed" because when the weakened and shortened muscles are connected in the upper body, they form a cross. The upper crossed syndrome involves the tightness of the trapezius (upper fiber), upper cervical extensors, pectoralis major and levator scapulae and weakness of the rhomboids, serratus anterior, middle and lower trapezius and deep neck flexors (Fig. 26.76).

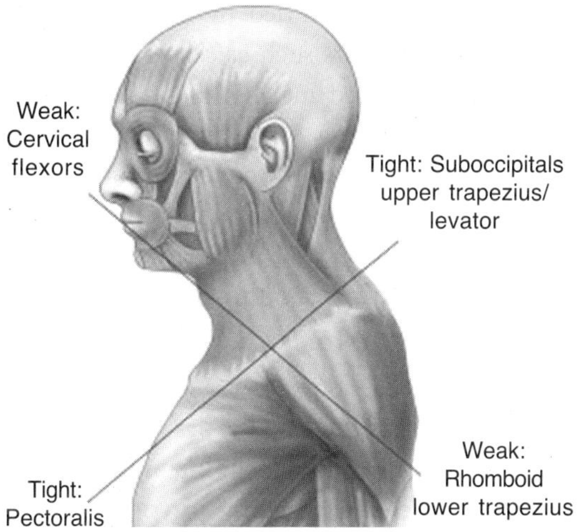

Fig. 26.76: Upper crossed syndrome

This muscular imbalance produces elevation and protraction of the shoulders, winging of the scapula and protraction of the head (forward head). Upper crossed syndrome places stress on cervical cranial junction, the C_4-C_5 and T_4 segments and the shoulder due to altered motion of the glenohumeral joint (Table 26.8).

Table 26.8: Upper crossed syndrome

Weak muscles	*Shortened muscles*
- Serratus anterior	- Pectoralis major
- Lower and middle trapezius	- Upper trapezius and levator scapulae
- Deep neck flexors	- Sup occipitalis
	- Sternocleidomastoid

Clinical Features

The patients with upper cross syndrome exhibit forward head posture, rounded and protracted shoulders with kyphosis of the upper dorsal spine. There is significant decrease in active flexion of upper cervical spine, extension of upper dorsal spine, and retraction of the shoulders. The strength of the deep neck flexors, serratus anterior, trapezius upper and lower, upper dorsal extensors, and rhomboid is found decreased when compared with the normal subjects. There is shortening of the pectoralis major and minor, and extensors of upper cervical extensors. Scapula may show anterior lipping with elevation of the inferior angle on the thoracic wall. The external rotation of the scapula may decrease during elevation and may hamper the scapulohumeral rhythm. Patient may complaint pain in the terminal flexion and abduction due to impingement as the scapula does not provide room to the rotating humerus.

Kim Christiansen (chiropracticener) states that "postural patterns are maintained by a complex arrangement of proprioceptive input modified by habits, somatotype and even psychogenic factors such as self esteem". Christiansen proposed that sustained malalignment results in muscular imbalance (shortening and lengthening of group of muscles). The end result of muscular imbalance is development of common postural patterns, such as forward head posture, elevation and protraction of the shoulders, protraction of head, increase thoracic kyphosis and cervical lordosis.

Ideally, when the posture is viewed from the side in standing, the plumb line should pass through the earlobe, midway through the shoulder joint, midway through the trunk, greater trochanter, slightly anterior to the mid point of the knee joint and slightly anterior to the ankle joint. In patient with upper crossed syndrome and cervicogenic headache the plumb line passes anterior to the shoulder joints and if the distance of the plumb line is high from the shoulder to the anterior, the condition may be graded as severe. If the distance of the plumb line from the shoulder to the anterior is very low the syndrome may be graded as mild and the patients may remain asymptomatic.

Management

The treatment of the upper cross syndrome should include postural correction exercises mainly strengthening of the weak muscles and stretching of the short muscles. The forward head is realigned by strengthening of the deep neck flexors, upper dorsal extensors, retractors of scapula, and serratus anterior. The pectoralis major, minor and upper cervical extensors should also be stretched to improve the flexibility.

1. Strengthening
   a. Deep neck flexors.
   b. Rhomboid.
   c. Trapezius upper, middle and lower.
   d. Serratus anterior.
   e. Levator scapulae.
2. Stretching
   a. Pectoralis major and minor.
   b. Upper cervical extensors.

CERVICAL SPONDYLOLITIC MYELOPATHY

The gross osteoarthritic changes in the cervical spine due to disc and intervertebral joint osteoarthritis may project the osteophytes into the spinal canal and can contribute to narrowing of the canal. It is not at all uncommon for a patient with myelopathy to have associated radicular symptoms and produce the mixed type of symptoms such as lower motor neuron and upper motor neuron lesion symptoms. A pure myelopathic syndrome is rarely produced by the chronic disc degeneration with posterior osteophytes alone. A pure myelopathic syndrome within the cervical spinal cord is produced if the degenerated changes are combined with a congenital small bony spinal canal, degeneration in the cervical motion segment with annular bulging and osteophytes, facet joints hypertrophy ligamentum flavum infolding, abnormal cervical segment motion (i.e., forward or backward subluxation, and vascular impairment of the substance of the spinal cord.

The congenital small bony spinal canal, degeneration in the cervical motion segment with annular bulging and osteophytes and facet joint hypertrophy cause compression while vascular impairment causes ischaemia in patients with cervical spondylolitic myelopathy.

Clinical Features

The patients with cervical spondylolitic myelopathy present with mixed type of symptoms in the upper and lower extremities.

Upper Extremities: In upper extremity two types of adicular and myelopathic symptoms are produced. The ower motor neuron lesion (radicular) symptoms are xperienced in the course of nerve root whose nerve root is ompressed in process of osteophytes or spurs. The upper notor neuron (myelopathic) symptoms are produced below he lesion.

In the process of degeneration the osteophytes will roject posteriorly to the nerve roots and then to the spinal ord, therefore, below the lesion (at spinal cord) the ymptoms will be myelopathic but at same level of lesion vhere nerve root is compressed there will be lower motor euron (radicular) type of symptoms such as pain, aresthesia, weakness, and diminished reflexes. The nyelopathic symptoms will be same as upper motor neuron uch as exaggerated reflexes, increased muscle tone, spastic gait and spastic weakness in the hand often described as lumsiness (Figs. 26.77a to c).

(a)

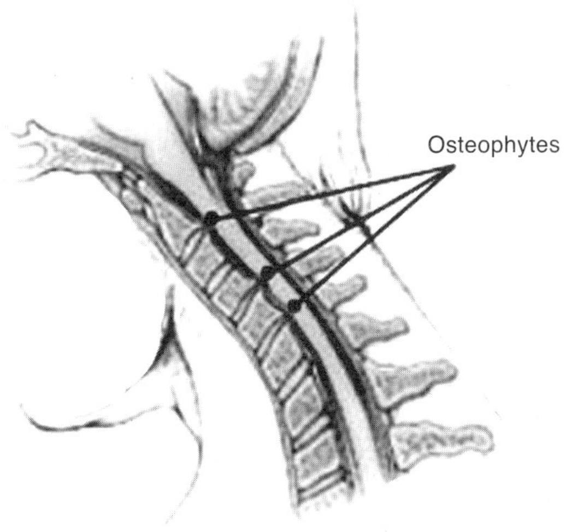

(b)

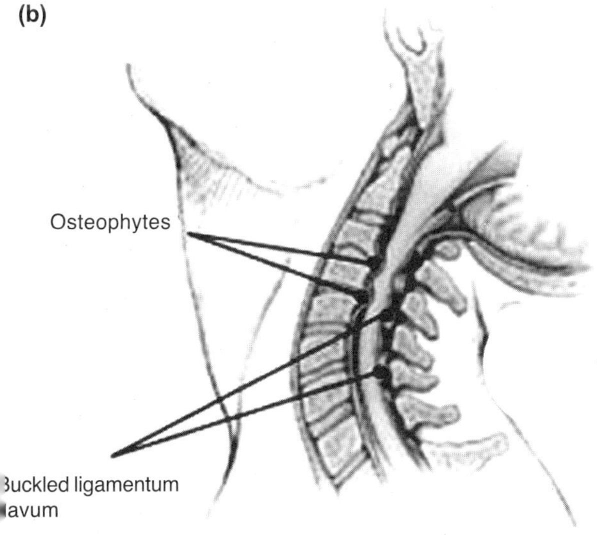

(c)

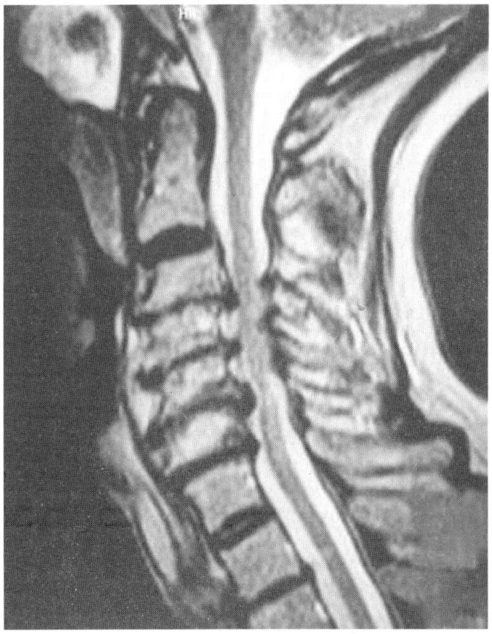

Figs. 26.77a to c: Cervical spondylolitic myelopathy

As an example osteophytes at C_5-C_6 may compress the C_6 nerve root and can cause pain, weakness and diminished biceps reflexes, and paresthesia in the thumb and index finger. This is because of lower motor neuron lesion in C_6 nerve root. The lesion in the C_6 nerve root remains below the anterior horn cell, therefore, the lower motor neuron lesion symptoms are produced, whereas, compression on spinal cord will produce upper motor neuron symptoms because, corresponding nerves are compressed above their anterior horn cells.

Lower Extremities: In the lower extremities symptoms will be upper motor lesion type. The patients find difficulty in walking, stair climbing and scuffing of shoes. As the disease progresses the gait becomes broadbased and jerky. Patients often flex the cervical spine to open the intervertebral foramen in order to relieve the symptoms.

Conservative Management

The patients with CSM do not respond significantly to the conservative treatments. Symptoms such as pain and spasticity can be reduced temporarily by advising hot water fermentation and passive movements respectively. Core strengthening should be taught to maintain the posture. Gait should also be improved.

Cervical Traction: Manual and mechanical traction will not improve the myelopathic symptoms but it may help in stretching of the ligaments and other soft tissues and in maintaining the range of motion. Traction may help in relieving the pressure on the nerve roots and in improving the symptoms of radiculopathy. It rarely helps in improving the symptoms of myelopathy.

Strengthening Exercises: Strengthening of weak muscles such as deep neck flexors, rhomboids, trapezius and serratus anterior should be taught to prevent disuse atrophy of the muscles.

Surgical Management

Surgical intervention should only be advised when the symptoms are deteriorating and patients are having difficulty in performing activities of daily living. It is not there that surgical intervention will reverse the myelopathic deficit completely, but it is advised to improve the functions of patient and to stop further progression of the disease. The surgical procedures demand removal of the posterior vertebral bodies, removal of the lamina, removal of the ligamentum flavum and decompression of the nerve roots.

TORTICOLIS (WRY NECK)

Torticolis is a side flexion with rotation of the neck due to tightness or contracture of the sternocleidomastoid muscle. It is almost always a condition in children and is a symptom and/or sign not a disease. Torticolis may also occur as a result of intracranial lesion or intraspinal pathology. The torticolis may be of several types but the most common torticolis are congenital muscular, spasmodic and paralytic (Fig. 26.78 and Flowchart 26.2).

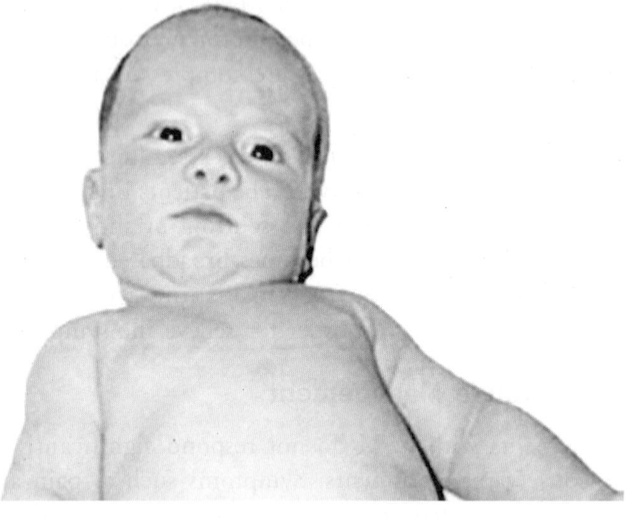

Fig. 26.78: Torticolis

Paralytic Torticolis

Unilateral cervical muscle movement in poliomyelitis is rather unusual. When it does occur the head is rotated towards the side of paralysis.

Spasmodic Torticolis

Severe spasm and pain in SCM, trapezius and splenius muscle may produce torticolis in adult patients. These patients often associated with severe psychiatric disturbances.

Flowchart 26.2: Pathoanatomy

Breech or difficult forceps deliveries
↓
Trauma to the muscle(s) (SCM)
↓
Ischaemia of the muscle
↓
Venous occlusion
↓
Fibrosus and contracture
↓
Neck turns and bends

Congenital Muscular Torticolis

The shortening or tightness of the sternocleidomastoid muscle will flex the neck to the same side and rotate it to the opposite side. The exact cause is unknown but it is believed that following factors may contribute to the torticolis.

a. Intrauterine malposition.
b. Heredity.
c. Breech delivery or difficult forceps delivery.
d. Acquired muscular ischaemia/some maldevelopmental deficits in the muscle.
e. Malposition in the uterus.

Examination

Children do not complain pain and other symptoms however, mother or family members notice after two weeks of the birth that the head of the child is not on the neck it is flexed and rotated. A soft non-tender mass is frequently palpated within the substance of the involved sternocleidomastoid muscle. The overlying skin and subcutaneous tissues are freely movable and separated from the mass, which generally attains its greatest dimension during the first six weeks of the life. Then mass gradually disappears and leaves the sternocleidomastoid muscle injured and contracted, which is frequently overlooked.

Clinical Features

The face becomes flattened and underdeveloped on the ipsilateral side. The face is smaller on the side of contracture

The parieto-occipital region on the contralateral side of the skull also flattens. If the torticolis is left without treating, the facial and skull deformities increase due to inability of the soft tissues to keep pace with the bony growth of the skull and cervical spine. The corners of the eye and mouth are drawn down, eye itself appearing smaller than that on the sound side, and of a different shape. The nose deviates slightly towards the affected side. Shortening of bilateral sternocleidomastoid muscles is very rare but if present, the head is then bent forward, and kyphosis is a complication.

Management

Soft Tissue Manipulation: Stroking and finger kneading is performed on the sternocleidomastoid muscle where swelling is noticed.

Passive Stretching: It is one of the best treatments in terms of improvement in flexibility of the muscle. The child is placed supine on the plinth with the head out of the edge. The therapist holds the head well with both the hands. For a left torticolis child the head is rotated to the same side (left side) and then flexed to the opposite side (right side), as much as child allows or tolerates. The stretched position is held for at least six seconds to allow maximum effects of stretching. Several repetitions may be performed in a session. Sometimes child will cry or struggle with the maneuver, hence, the stretching should be quick. The therapist can also teach the same to the patient care givers to perform the exercise at home. Precautions should be taken not to hurt the child.

Manual Traction: As the child grows older, traction may also be indicated. In a supine position with head out of the edge the therapist holds the chin and occiput of the child and distracts the cervical spine, which must be held for at least six seconds to allow the maximum effect of stretching.

Surgical Intervention

Torticolis in older children is very rare or if it is present it may be due to neglected congenital torticolis or may be an acquired. These children do not respond to the soft tissue manipulation and stretching, they must be treated by surgical intervention. The sternal and clavicular head of the sternocleidomastoid muscles are divided close to their origins, and any contracted bands of fascia are also severed. After releasing the contracted muscle and fascia, the head is positioned in the overcorrected position with the help of splint, orthosis or plaster of paris until the stitches are removed (at least for 10-14 days).

Postoperative stretching exercises should be started after removal of the stitches or after consultation with the surgeon. Initially exercises should be mild in intensity. In sitting or supine position the head is bent to the opposite side with rotation to the same side of the operated muscle. The intensity of exercise may be increased as the healing improves.

MANUAL THERAPY FOR THE THORACIC SPINE

Similar to cervical and lumbar spine degenerative changes take place in the thoracic spine also. Symptoms such as pain and limitation in the range of motion particularly in rotation are the dominant clinical features of the degenerative changes of the thoracic spine. Following pain and symptoms the patients adapt a posture which relieves the symptoms. This is the first step of malalignment or faulty posture. As the disease progresses the patient develops "upper crossed syndrome". This involves hyperextension at the upper cervical, protraction at the shoulders and flexion at the lower cervical and upper thoracic spine kyphosis. These are two points where patients feel more stresses. Sometimes a hump can also be seen on the upper thoracic spine. T_2 and T_3 segment bears more unwanted stresses.

It is thought that manual therapy at thoracic spine can improve the mobility and pain at cervical, thoracic and sometimes at the shoulders. The improvement in the mobility of the thoracic spine, significantly takes stress off adjacent, hyper mobile cervical spine or shoulder joints.

SNAGs to Improve Rotation at Upper Thoracic Spine: Patient sits on a stool with the hands clasped behind the neck. For a patient with pain and limitation in the right rotation due to D_{10} and D_{11} mobile segment, the therapist stands behind the patient, wraps left arm around the chest. The ulnar border of the right hand is placed under the spinous process of D_{10} vertebra. The patient is instructed to rotate the neck to the right side as much as possible. During the movement (right rotation) the spinous process of D_{10} vertebra is pushed up and superiorly. The right hand around the chest encourages the movement and also helps in applying overpressure if indicated (Fig. 26.79).

SNAGs to Improve Flexion: Patient sits on the stool with the hands resting on the thighs. For a patient with pain and limitation in the flexion range, resulting from lesion in the D_{10} and D_{11} mobile segment, the therapist stands behind the patient (slightly to the right side) and wraps the left arm around the trunk at the level of D_{10} and D_{11} level. The ulnar border of the right wrist is placed under the spinous process of D_{10}, which applies gliding force along the facet plane. The patient is asked to flex the thoracic spine as much as possible within the painfree range.

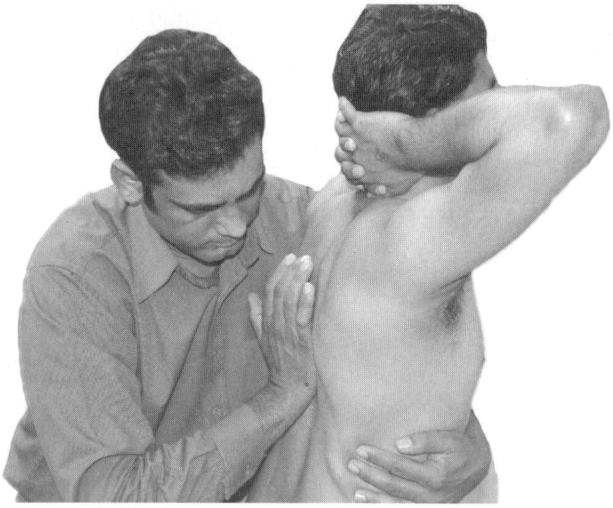

Fig. 26.79: SNAGs to improve rotation at upper thoracic spine

The gliding force is applied through the wrist while the left arm acts as a fulcrum for flexion. The gliding force is maintained throughout the range of motion till the movement returns to the neutral (Fig. 26.80).

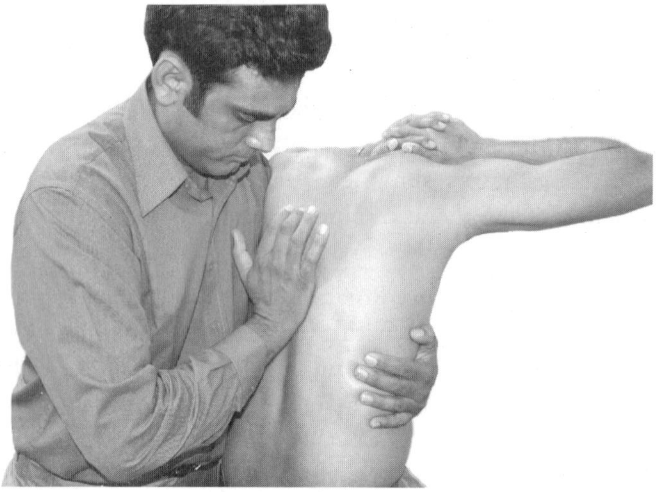

Fig. 26.80: SNAGs to improve flexion at upper thoracic spine

To improve an extension the position of the patient, therapist, and hands remain same as for flexion. The patient is asked to extend the spine as much as possible within the painfree range. The gliding force is applied through the ulnar border of the wrist throughout the movement till the movement returns to the neutral position (Fig. 26.81).

Upper Thoracic Thrust Manipulation: The patient sits on a stool comfortably with the hands clasped behind the neck. The therapist stands behind the patient with slight flexion of the knees, and loops the hands through the patients arms and places over the patient's hands. A towel

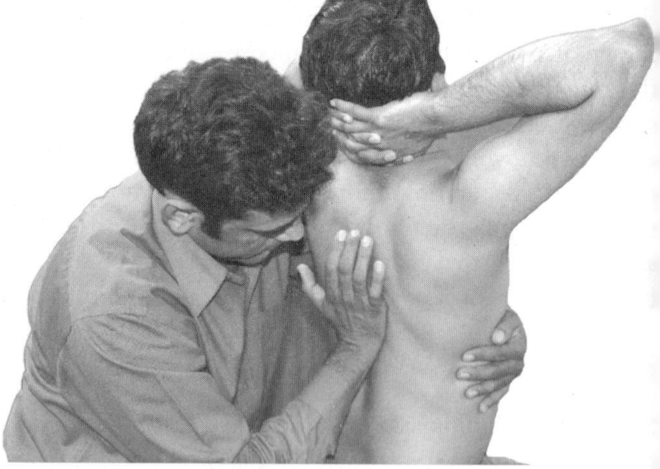

Fig. 26.81: SNAGs to improve extension at upper thoracic spine

or sheet can be placed between the therapist chest and patient's back for cosmetic purposes. The therapist chest should rest on the patients back. A thrust is delivered to the upper thoracic spine by leaning backward and extending the knees. The technique is discarded if patient complains discomfort and pain in the shoulders. This technique not only improves pain and range at upper thoracic but also helps in relieving pain in the cervical spine.

Mid Thoracic Thrust Manipulation: The patient sits comfortably on a stool with both the hands grasping opposite scapula (posterior shoulder), so that the elbows are parallel and rests on the lower sternum. The therapist stands behind the patient and grasps the patients lower elbow. A small towel may be placed on the desired segment between patients back and therapists chest. The therapist takes up slack by adducting the arms, retracting the shoulders and pushing the chest to the desired segment (thoracic spine). A high velocity thrust is delivered by the therapist through the patients arms from anterior to posterior direction.

Thoracic Thrust Manipulation in Standing: The patient stands with both the hands clasped behind the shoulders on scapula. The therapist stands behind the patient places a small towel piece between his chest and the patient's thoracic spine, grasps the patient's lower elbow. Similar to the mid thoracic thrust manipulation, therapist takes up slack by adducting the arms, retracting the shoulder girdles and pushing the chest to the patients thoracic spine. While maintaining, position the therapist produces high velocity thrust by lifting the patient with extension of knees and leaning backward.

27

LOW BACK PAIN

INTRODUCTION

Back pain is a complex phenomenon and it is not always possible to determine its source reliably as it may originate from several structures of the mobile segment. However, it is possible to recognize basic patterns and presentations of pain and this certainly helps to facilitate provisional diagnosis. Pain experienced in the spine with radiation such as sciatica, may have one or more of four origins: Spinal, vascular, visceral and psychogenic.

The hectic life-style (daily busy schedules) long and indefinite working hours are eventually the predisposing factors to various health and stress related ailments among metropolitan youth. People do not find time to walk even for a mile, this life-style causes loss of flexibility of the muscle fibers.

The most common cause of back pain is a minor strain to muscle and/or ligament, but people suffering from this type of back pain usually do not seek medical treatment as most of these soft tissue injuries resolve naturally. Sometimes injury or strain to the muscle and ligament can cause further damage to the mobile segment that leads to dysfunction of the apophyseal joint and intervertebral joint, the exact balance being uncertain.

Almost 80% of the population experience low back pain sometimes in their life, that each year 2% to 5% of adults seek treatment or lose time from work because of low back pain. Some of these individuals become disabled and need long term treatment, therefore, we can realize how significant an issue of low back pain is in our society. At least 70% patients recover completely within one month but some are prone to the recurrence of low back pain.

To manage the low back pain we have specialists: such as spine surgeons, physicians, physical therapists and occupational therapists. With all this high energy and intellect dedicated to the low back pain care, the society can expect improved results. The reasons of our failure to cope with the low back pain may be following:

(a) It is fact that we are dealing with the symptoms.

(b) Subjective low back pain is not always associated with objective physical findings.

It is, therefore, necessary to have a very clear concept of possible source of pain when presented with the problem of a patient seeking relief from the irksome burden of constant low back pain. In order to differentiate these lesions and to facilitate a provisional diagnosis, the clinician must diligently elicit an accurate and lucid history, and conduct a routine subjective and objective physical examinations.

Classification of Low Back Pain

Pain experienced in the low back region with or without peripheral radiation is a symptom not a disease, which may have origin within or outside of the spine. The causes of low back pain are many but it may broadly be classified into four major groups:

1. Spondylogenic.
2. Viscerogenic.
3. Vasculogenic.
4. Psychogenic.

Spondylogenic Referred Pain: The spondylogenic type of pain is originated from the spine itself due to trauma, pathology or degeneration. It is a non-radicular pain which originates from any of the components of mobile segment including facet joints, intervertebral joint, the intervertebral disc, muscles, ligaments, and the dura mater. Similar type of pain may also be referred from viscera to the low back region, proximal thigh and groin; therefore, it is important to distinguish the spondylogenic referred pain from visceral referred pain. The spondylogenic pain is deep dull aching which is relieved by rest and aggravated by the movements of the lumbar spine. The local tender points may not be elicited.

Radicular Pain: The radicular pain is a type of mechanical low back pain which has origin in the intervertebral foramen (nerve roots) and experienced in the course of the nerve root/s. It is characterized by pain, parasthesia, numbness (anaesthesia), loss of reflexes and muscle power. Sometimes the symptoms are more severe in the legs then in the spine.

Viscerogenic Low Back Pain: Viscerogenic back pain may originate from viscera such as kidneys, the pelvic viscera, lesions of the lesser sac, and retroperitoneal tumors. The pain perceived in the low back region is referred from the viscera, neither is aggravated by activities or movements of lumbar spine, nor is relieved by rest. Indeed, with severe pain, the patient whose symptoms are visceral in origin, will walk around to get relief.

Vascular Low Back Pain: Pathological changes in the vessels and arteries (vascular bundles) may produce similar symptoms as of sciatica or spinal pain. The symptoms may be boring type of deep-situated lumbar pain unrelated to activities (abdominal aortic aneurysms). Superior gluteal artery insufficiency may produce buttock pain of claudication nature. The important feature of abdominal aortic aneurysm and superior gluteal artery insufficiency is that symptoms aggravate by walking and relieved by rest. While walking pain may radiate from the buttocks to the leg. However, pain is not aggravated by the activities such as bending, stooping, lifting etc. In patients with intermittent vascular claudication pain is experienced in the calf, which is aggravated while walking and relieved by standing still. In patients with neurogenic claudication or spinal canal stenosis pain is similar to peripheral claudication and is frequently initiated and aggravated by the act of walking a short distance, however, not relieved by standing still.

Psychogenic Low Back Pain: Although pure psychogenic back pain is rarely seen in clinical practice but failure to consider it in the assessment of low back pain might lead to serious errors in diagnosis and management. The patients with psychogenic back pain are very anxious, tend to overexpose their problem. They are usually demonstrative, the hands being used to point out various painful areas almost without prompting. The pain distribution is often atypical and not specific to the particular dermatome. The reflexes are almost always hyperactive and hypersensitive to the touch. Diffuse tenderness even to slightest touch will be presented. In such patients, although the task may be difficult, the therapist must be prepared to accept the possibility of an underlying pathological process and investigate its probability thoroughly.

ANATOMICAL AND PATHOLOGICAL ASPECTS

The spine is a flexible, multisegmental column bridging the interval between the base of the skull and the pelvis. It maintains not only the posture but also protects the neural structures. In addition to this it allows movements in the vertebral column.

The Mobile Segment

The mobile segment of the lumbar spine is of static stabilizers which are divided into two parts anterior and posterior segments. The anterior mobile segment contains anterior longitudinal ligaments, intervertebral joints, intervertebral discs, and intervertebral bodies. The posterior mobile segment contains posterior longitudinal ligaments, apophyseal joints, interspinous and supraspinous ligaments. The mobile segment works as a single functional unit during movements and rest. If any one structure of mobile segment is damaged due to trauma or in the degenerative process, it can decrease the stability of the lumbar spine and can contribute to the low back pain and symptoms (Figs. 27.1a and b).

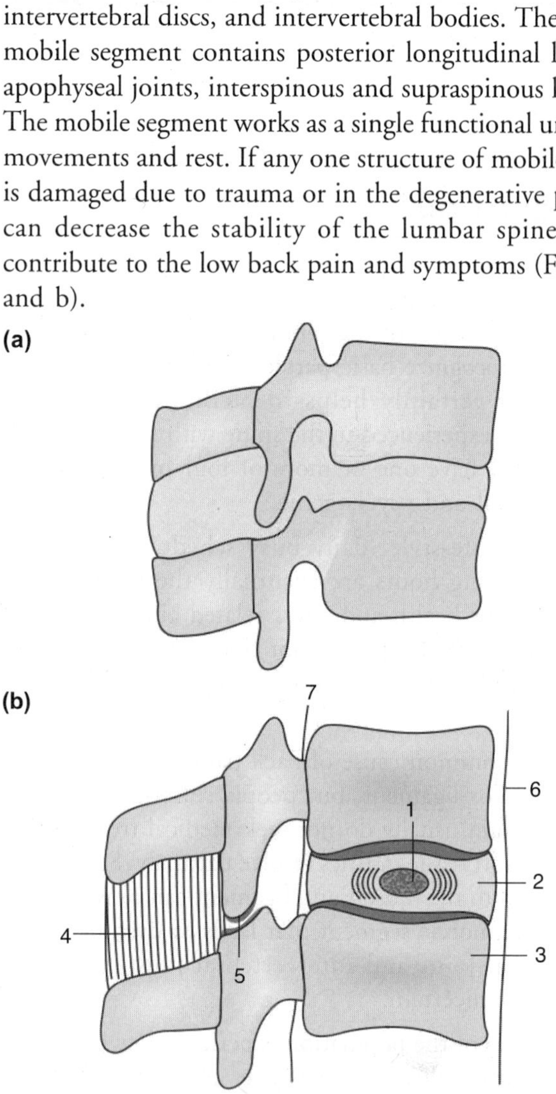

Figs. 27.1a and b: Mobile segment (1) Nucleus pulposus, (2) Annulus fibrosus, (3) Vertebral body, (4) Interspinous ligament, (5) Facet joint, (6) Anterior longitudinal ligament, (7) Posterior longitudinal ligament

Box 27.1: Minor Intervertebral Derangement (MID)

Theory of Maigne: Maigne pointed out that the functional ability of the mobile segment depends intimately upon integrity of the I.V.D. Thus if the disc is injured, other elements of the segment will also be affected. For an example, disc herniation reduces the intervertebral joint space, which in turn causes approximation of facet joints and laxity in the ligaments.

/ertebrae

Γhe lumbar spine has got five vertebrae with posterior :oncavity joined with the sacrum vertebra. The vertebral oodies are connected to the intervertebral discs, and the ıeural arches are joined by the facet joints. The size of the ertebral bodies increases from first lumbar vertebra to the ifth lumbar vertebra as the load increases from L_1 to L_5. The lumbar vertebrae have massive bodies, suitable for upporting the entire superimposed weight of the head, runk and arms. The total mass of five lumbar vertebrae is ıpproximately twice that of the seven cervical vertebrae Fig. 27.2).

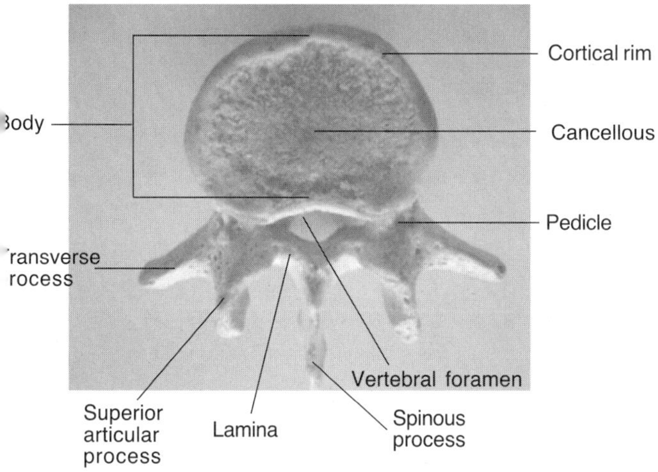

Fig. 27.2: Lumbar vertebra

Facet Joints

There are two facet joints at each mobile segment. The rticular surface of the facets of the lumbar vertebrae is riented nearly vertical. The superior facets are moderately oncave, facing medial to posteromedial. The facet surfaces f the upper lumbar region tend to be oriented close to the agittal plane. The superior facet surface in the mid to lower umbar region tends to be oriented midway between the agittal and frontal planes.

The inferior articular facets are slightly convex, facing enerally lateral to anterolateral. These are reciprocally natched to the shape and orientation of the superior rticular facets. The inferior facets of L_5 articulate with the uperior facets of the sacrum and the joints are typically riented much closer to the frontal plane than the other umbar facet joints articulations. The anteroposterior umbosacral stability to the lumbosacral junction is rovided well by the L_5 – S_1 apophyseal joints.

The facet joints typically demonstrate changes with ging. The change may result from forces related to the evelopment of bipedal gait in early childhood. Side-to-side joint asymmetry is common in adults and *lead articular troops, i.e.,* developmental alteration in the joints shape in a certain percentage of the population. Some investigators feel that tropism may alter the biomechanics and increase the forces in some portions of the intervertebral discs, thereby predisposing them to injury (Fig. 27.3).

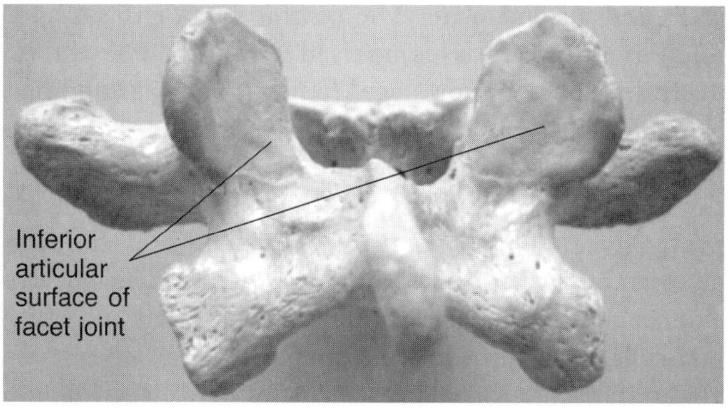

Fig. 27.3: Lumbar vertebra showing the facet surfaces

The facet joints are richly innervated from the medial branch of the posterior primary rami. The capsule of the facet joint receives a number of tiny branches from two segmental nerves. The malalignment of the facet joints causes stretching of the capsule, and produces dull to severe pain depending upon the severity of malalignment. The facet joints can produce pain in the low back region and that may be referred to any part of the lower limb as far as the calf and ankle but most commonly pain is referred to the gluteal region, proximal thigh and groin. The entrapment of the medial branch of posterior ramus can occur and could refer pain to the structures that it innervates.

Apophyseal Glides During Spinal Movements

The facet joints glide to facilitate the lumbar movements. In case of facet joints malalignment these can block the movements of lumbar spine.

During Flexion: The upper facet slides up and forward on the lower facet that opens the facet joint.

During Extension: The upper facet slides down and back on the lower facet that closes the facet joint.

During Side Flexion: The upper facet slides down and back on the same side to the movement "closing the joint" and up and forward on the side opposite of the movement (opening the joint).

During Rotation: The upper facet moves up and anterior on the opposite of the movement (opening the facet) and moves down and posterior of the same side of the movement (closing the joint).

Intervertebral Disc

The intervertebral space of the lumbar spine involves portions of two vertebral bodies and an intervertebral disc. The intervertebral disc is the largest avascular structure of the body which is situated between two vertebral bodies. It comprises annulus fibrosus (AF), a nuclease pulposus (NP) and an end plate. The central part of the disc, a nucleus pulposus is comprised 70% to 90% water, depending on a person's age. It functions as a modified hydraulic shock absorber that dissipates and transfers loads between consecutive vertebra. The nucleus pulposus is thickened by relatively large branching proteoglycans. Each proteoglycan is an aggregate of many water binding glycosaminoglycans linked to core proteins. The nucleus also contains type II collagen fibers, elastic fibers and other non-collagenous protein. The annulus fibrosus consists of 10 to 20% concentric layers or rings of collagen fibers. The end plate is associated more strongly with the IVD then with the vertebral body. It is situated on the superior and inferior part of the intervertebral disc. It is the weakest part of the intervertebral disc in compression (Fig. 27.4).

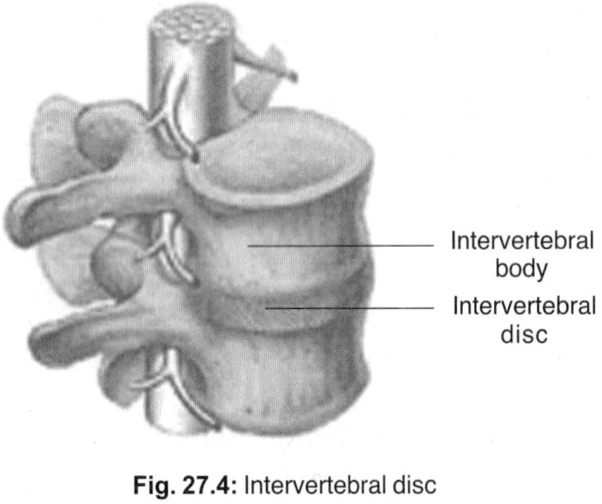

Fig. 27.4: Intervertebral disc

The intervertebral disc is the largest avascular structure of the body and its nutrition depends on diffusion. It receives its blood supply from the two *closest vessel sources,* which are those beneath the vertebral end plate and those at the periphery of the annulus fibrosus. Certain movements possible those in and out of the flexion, may facilitate nutrition of the disc (one of the benefits of exercise may be to facilitate the nutrition of the intervertebral disc). The intervertebral discs have a blood supply upto 8 years, but, thereafter, they are dependent on diffusion of tissue fluids. As the intervertebral disc is avascular and its nutrition depends on the diffusion and movements its healing transpires, but complete healing takes months to years.

The disc was generally believed to be non pain sensitive and consequently inert structure. Recently it has been found that the superficial layer of the annulus fibrosus in the lumbar region has significant innervations from the sinuvertebral nerves and stimulation of those nerve endings can result in pain.

As the load is transmitted to the nucleus through the hyline cartilage plate the load of axial compression is distributed not only in vertical direction but also radially throughout the nucleus as well. The intervertebral discs add considerable stability to the vertebral column as well as being shock absorber (Flowchart 27.1).

Flowchart 27.1: Mechanism of load transmission

Body weight and muscle contraction increases load on the disc

↓

The end plate moves inward and toward the nucleus pulposus

↓

The nucleus pulposus deforms radially and against the annulus fibrosus

↓

The annulus fibrosus becomes tensed and stretched within the walls of rings of collagen and elastic fibers

↓

The annulus fibrosus creates a pressure back to the nucleus pulposus and end plates

↓

The load passes to the next vertebral segment

Flowchart 27.1

The stability to the vertebral column is primarily provided by the structural configuration of the collagen fibers within the annulus fibrosus. The annulus fibrosus is the part of intervertebral disc primarily composed of collagen fibers. The collagen fibers are organized in such a way that they inhibit radial expansion of the nucleus pulposus. They are arranged in multiple concentric layers, with fibers in every other layer running in identical directions. The orientation of each collagen fiber is about 30° + 90° = 120 degrees from the vertical.

The compressive forces on the intervertebral disc are generated by the body weight and the contraction of the muscles, they push the end plate inward and toward the nucleus pulposus. The nucleus pulposus deforms radially and against the annulus fibrosus. The annulus fibrosus becomes tensed and stretched within the walls of the rings of collagen and elastic fibers. The internal resistance reinforces the walls of the annulus fibrosus. The entire mechanism creates pressure back to the nucleus pulposus and end plates, reinforces the entire disc and passes the load to the next vertebra.

Movements

Osteokinematics and Arthrokinematics: The range of motion of the lumbar spine differs at various levels as it depends on orientation of the facets of intervertebral joints. The movement does not occur independently at one motion segment but it involves the combined action of several motion segments.

Spinal coupling: Movement of the vertebral column in one plane is usually associated with an automatic and at times nearly interceptible movement in another plane as well. (During axial rotation and lateral flexion the spinal coupling takes place) (Figs. 27.5, 27.6 and Table 27.1).

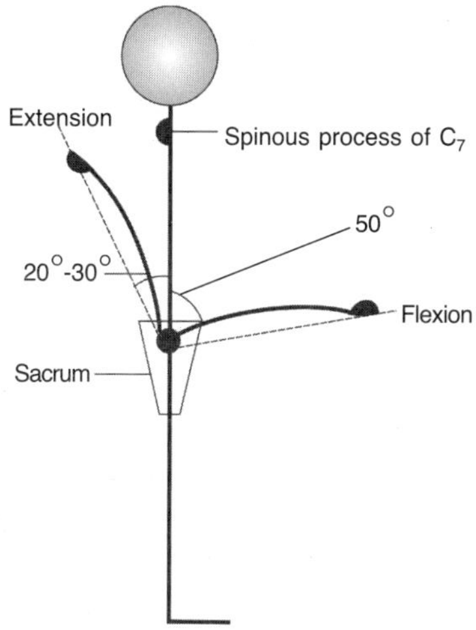

Fig. 27.5: Lumbar spine flexion and extension

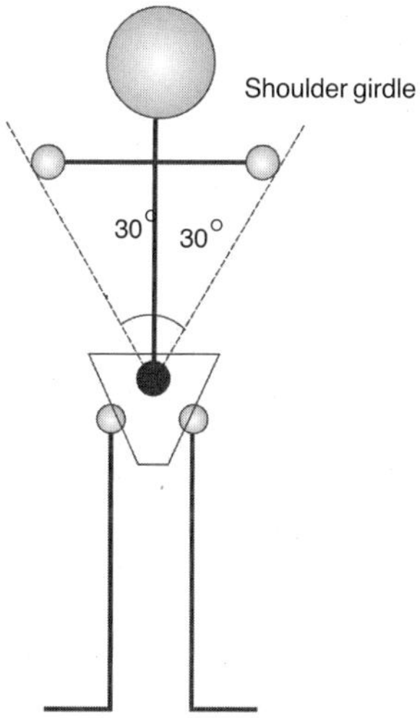

Fig. 27.6: Lumbar spine range of motion (side flexion)

Table 27.1: Movements of the lumbar spine

Movement	*In degrees*	*Plane*
Flexion	50	Sagittal
Extension	20-30	Sagittal
Rotation	05	Horizontal
Lateral flexion	30 (Each)	Frontal plane

Ligaments

The various ligaments of the lumbar vertebral column form a continuous, dense, connective tissue stocking surrounding the vertebrae, and extending to the sacral area. In humans the ligament can best be described as a fan. It extends between borders of the spinous process of adjacent vertebrae. These are divided as under:

1. Neural arch ligaments
   - Ligamentum flavum.
   - Interspinous ligament.
   - Supraspinous ligament.
2. Articular capsular ligament.
3. Ligaments ventral to the facet joints
   - Anterior longitudinal ligament.
   - Posterior longitudinal ligament.
4. Intertransverse ligament.
5. Ileolumbar ligament (Fig. 27.7).

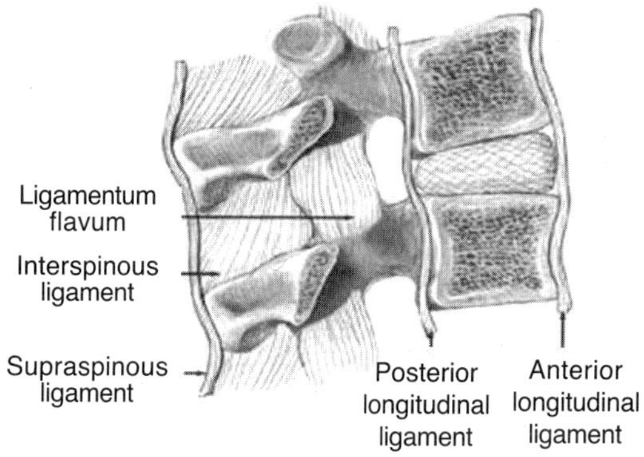

Fig. 27.7: Ligaments of the lumbar spine

Ligamentum Flavum

This ligament is composed of elastic fibers (80%) and collagenous fibers 20%. The elastic fibers imparting the ligament its yellow color and flexible nature forms a significant portion of roof of the spinal canal. The ligamentum flavum bridges the interlaminar interval attaching to the interspinous ligament medially and the facet capsule laterally. Superiorly it attaches to the anterior surface of the lamina above and inferiorly it establishes a cup-like grasp on the superior margin of the lamina below.

Normally, the ligament maintains a taut configuration, stretching for flexion and contracting its elastic fibers at neutral, therefore it provides a roof for the vertebral canal that does not buckle during extension-flexion movements of the vertebral column (in this way it covers but never infringes on the epidural space).

With aging the elastic fibers of the ligamentum flavum decrease in number and concomitant increase in the density of collagen fibers. These events favor the deposition of calcium in the ligamentum flavum which leads to hypertrophy. There is buckling of the ligamentum flavum and encroachment on the spinal canal potentially contributing to spinal stenosis. Ossification of the ligament is associated with increasing age, and the presence of cauda equina syndrome. *Chondrogenesis in the ligament appears more associated with the presence of spondylolisthesis.* Eventually the ligament loses its elastic properties which contributes to the development of adolescent idiopathic scoliosis.

Supraspinous and Infraspinous Ligaments

The anterior border of the ligament is the continuation of ligamentum flavum and posterior border thickens to form the supraspinous ligament which is further anchored to the thoracolumbar fascia. The fan shaped arrangement of the ligament not only allows the ligament to expand without rupture but also prevents the separation of vertebral column during flexion. The supraspinous ligament is tightly adhering to the posterior border of the lumbar spines and interspinous ligament.

Anterior Longitudinal Ligament

It runs the whole length of the anterior aspect of the spine and attaches to anterior annular fibers of each disc.

Posterior Longitudinal Ligament

It extends from the base of occiput (as the membrane tectorial) cervical to the sacrum caudally. The ligament is much thinner both in width and thickness than the anterior longitudinal ligament in the lower lumbar region, therefore, the main opposition to flexion of the lumbar spine comes from ligament flavum. This contributes to the lumbar disc problem at lower region.

Intertransverse Ligaments: Intertransverse ligaments are centrally membranes that extend between an adjacent transverse processes. These ligaments constitute a part of fascia system which separates the ventral compartment muscles from posterior muscles.

Iliolumbar Ligament: The iliolumbar ligament is a substantial ligament that binds the transverse process of the L_5 vertebra to the sacrum and resists forward sliding, lateral flexion and axial rotation of the L_5 vertebra on sacrum. Initially the ligament is muscular and represents the L_5 components of iliocostalis lumborum and as age progresses it undergoes fibrous metaphasis.

Muscles

The structural unit of the skeletal muscle is the muscle fiber, a cylindrical cell with hundreds of nuclei. Each muscle is composed of many hundreds of muscle fibers, which provide stability and mobility to the mobile segment. Weakness or tightness of the muscles can alter the stability and mobility of the mobile segment.

The Lumbar Multifidus: The lumbar multifidus is the largest and most medial muscle of the lumbar muscles and consists of repeating series (five separate bonds) of fascicles that stem from the laminae and spinous processes of the lumbar vertebrae and exhibit a constant pattern of attachments caudally.

The deepest fibers of the muscle in the lumbar arise from the posterior inferior aspect of the each vertebral lamina and articular capsule of the facet joint. The deep fibers insert into the maxillary process two levels below the deep fiber of the L_5 lamina inserts on an area on the sacrum just above the first dorsal sacral foramen as the L_5 lamina has no maxillary process (Figs. 27.8a to f).

Dick N and *et al.* department of rehabilitation sciences and P.T. Ghent University, Campus Hymens, state by using MRI study that the deep multifidus has a higher percentage of slow twitch fibers compared to the superficial multifidus. *No differential reenlistment has been found following trunk extension with and without pain induction.*

The superficial fibers have combined effect on the spine, they exert compression loading of the spine to enhance its stiffness and produce an effective moment arm for extension of the lumbar spine and control the lumbar lordosis. The laminar deep fibers can be considered to stabilize the two overlying functional segments. They control intervertebral shear and torsion via intervertebral compression. The attachment of the deep fibers of multifidus to the facet joints have an advantage in allowing multifidus in keeping the capsule from being impinged during movements caused by the multifidus.

Decrease in the size of the multifidus has been constantly documented in people with low back pain. Wallwork TL and *et al.* conducted study aimed at to compare both the size (cross-sectional area) and the ability to voluntary perform an isometric contraction of the multifidus muscle at four vertebral levels in 34 subjects with and without chronic low back pain by using the ultrasound imagings. The study shown a significantly smaller cross-sectional area of the multifidus muscle for the subjects in the chronic low back pain group compared with normal healthy subjects at the L_5 vertebral level and a significant smaller percent

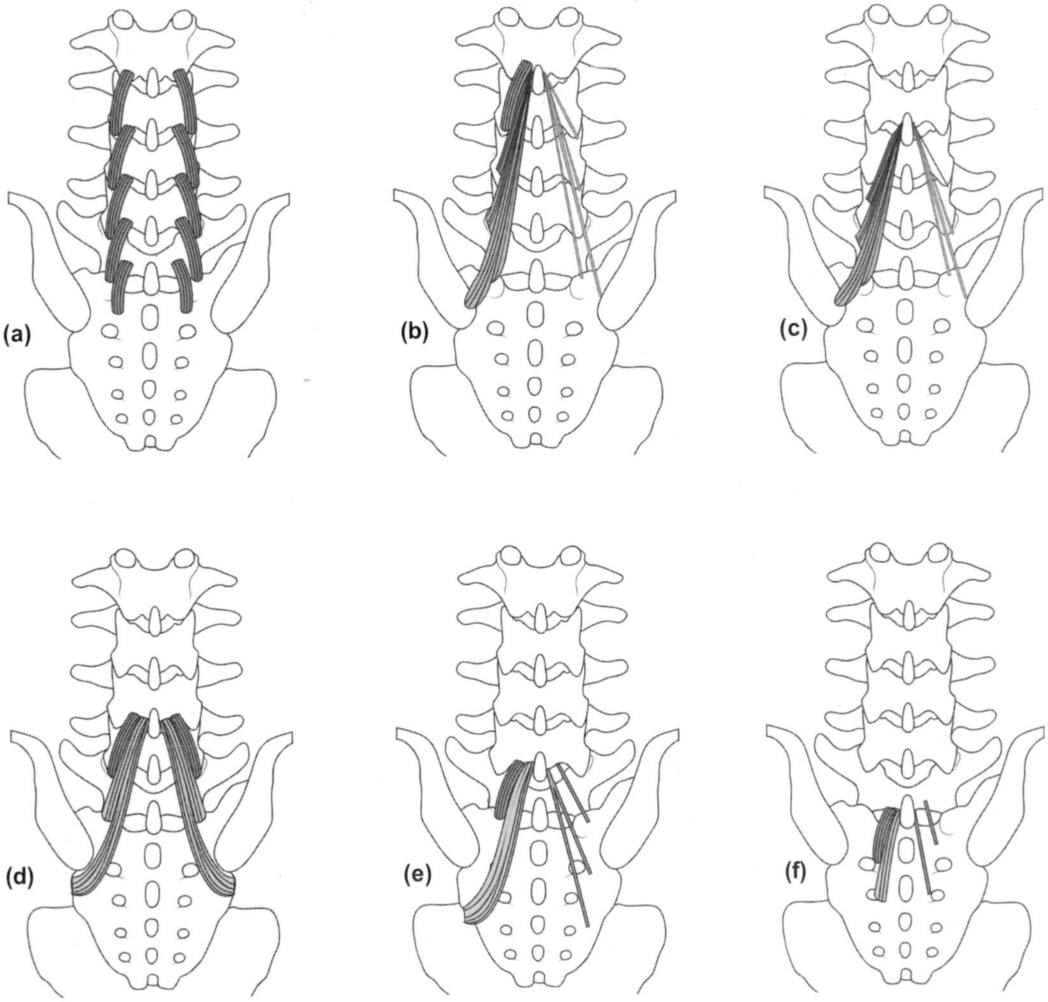

Figs. 27.8a to f: The component fasciculus of multifidus a. The laminar fibers of multifidus, b to f. The fascicles from L_1 to L_5 spinous process, respectively

thickness contraction for subjects with the chronic low back pain group of the same vertebral level.

Hides J, Gilmore C, *et al.* have also conducted the similar type of study by recruiting 40 asymptomatic and 50 chronic low back pain subjects. Their results showed that the greatest asymmetry between sides was seen at the L_5 vertebral level in patients with unilateral pain presentation. The smaller multifidus cross-sectional area was ipsilateral to reported side of pain in all cases.

Recent advances in the understanding of the biomechanics of low back pain have highlighted the importance of muscular stabilization of the "neutral zone" range of motion in the low back area. The lumbar multifidus muscles (LMN) are important stabilizers of this neutral zone and dysfunction in these muscles strongly associated with low back pain. The dysfunction is as a result of pain inhibition from the spine, and it tends to continue even after the pain has resolved, likely contributing to the high recurrence rate of low back pain.

The oblique abdominals are the primary rotators of the spine. The horizontal rotation occurs after *impaction* of the contralateral facet joint only if an appropriate shear force is applied to the intervertebral disc. The horizontal vector of the multifidus, however, is so small that it is unlikely that the multifidus would be capable of exerting such shear force on the disc by acting on the spinous process. Muscle training directed at teaching patients to activate their multifidus is an important feature of any clinical approach to the low back pain patients.

Transverse Abdominis: Studies have shown that strengthening of transverse abdominis helps in decreasing the pain and symptoms of low back pain as it is a key stabilizer of the lumbar spine. A coordinated contraction of the transverse abdominis, diaphragm, and pelvic floor muscles contributes to both unloading and stabilization of the lumbar spine. The transverse abdominis is optimally aligned for a posterior pull on the abdominal fascial complex.

This posteriorly directed pull, especially around the slightly pressurized abdominal cylinder, compliments the more angled pulls of the external and internal abdominal oblique muscles. Thus the pull of the abdominal muscles cinches the abdomen with a corset-like effect and brings the abdominal contents posterior against the spine, which serves as another check to anterior shear of the lumbar vertebrae.

The fascicles of transverse abdominis originate from the inner surface of the lower six costal cartilages, the lumbar spine via the thoracolumbar fascia, the anterior two third of the inner lip of the iliac crest, and the lateral third of the inguinal ligament. The fascicles insert into the linea alba (Fig. 27.9).

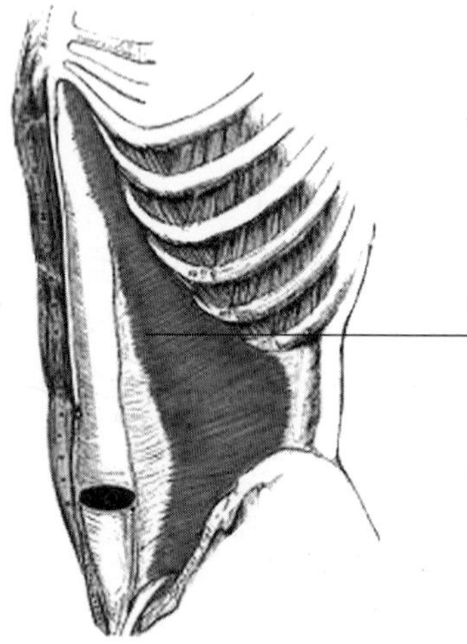

Fig. 27.9: Transverse abdominis

Thoracolumbar Fascia System

The muscles of the lumbar spine are enveloped by three layers of the fascia known as thoracolumbar fascia. The fascia consists of collagen fibers oriented in a variety of directions, with no particular orientation predominating. It is a dense network consisting of three layers of connective tissues–posterior, middle and anterior, which enclose the erector spinae, multifidus and quadratus lumborum muscles. Thoracolumbar fascia extends from the sacrum to the upper back and neck and is prominent in the low back region (Fig. 27.10).

Posterior Layer of the Thoracolumbar Fascia: The posterior layer of the thoracolumbar fascia is formed by the apponeurosis of the latissimus dorsi. It is thickest and strongest of the three layers which is attached to the spinous processes. It is a bilinear layer consisting of superficial and deep portions. The superficial portion is formed by the tendons of the ipsilateral latissimus dorsi, passing caudally and medially.

The deep portion is formed by the tendons of the contralateral latissimus dorsi, passing downwards and laterally. The posterior layer extends into the thoracic region

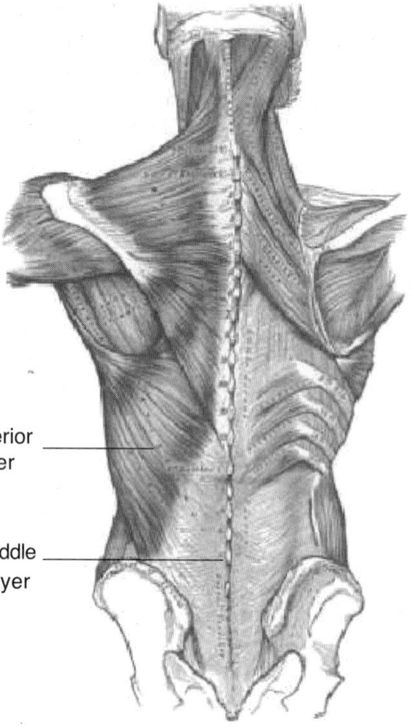

Fig. 27.10: Thoracolumbar fascia consisting three layers

and lies posterior to the erector spine and multifidus muscles. The posterior layer of the thoracolumbar fascia is designed to transmit forces between the shoulder girdle, lumbar spine, pelvic girdle and lower extremity.

The Middle Layer of the Thoracolumbar Fascia: It is attached to the lumbar transverse processes and separates the deeper lumbar portion of the erector spinae muscle from quadratus lumborum muscles. It consists of tendinous fibers of the transverse abdominis. Between the transverse processes these tendons interlace to form the middle layer of thoracolumbar fascia.

The Anterior Layer of the Thoracolumbar Fascia: It is the thinnest layer of the thoracolumbar fascia which covers the anterior surface of the quadratus lumborum muscle and is formed by the deep fascia of this muscle.

The tension in fascia is created as a result of contraction of the muscles, which is within the fascial envelop. The increase in fascial tension results in stiffening of the spinal column which contributes to the stability of the spinal column. The coordinated contraction of the diaphragm, the transverse abdominis and pelvic floor muscle increases the stiffness (stability) of the spine by increasing intra-abdominal pressure.

There is a functional relationship between the shoulder girdle, abdominal musculature and the lateral raphe of the thoracolumbar fascia. There is continuation of the abdominal fascia with the thoracolumbar fascia. It is therefore, easy to visualize that abdominal or the oblique ventral muscle tendon sling has an impact on the function or tension of the thoracolumbar fascia and vice versa. The pectoral apponeurosis of the abdominal muscles often cross the midline to blend with the abdominal fascia on the opposite side and the superficial aspect of the rectus sheath.

ASSESSMENT

For an effective management of low back pain, assessment remains cornerstone of the clinical practice. It includes subjective and objective examination, provisional diagnosis and intervention.

General Information

The purpose of the medical practice is to relieve suffering. The first responsibility of the clinician is to understand the patient's problem irrespective of his or her religion. During the general information the clinician obtains the following information from the patient:

1. Age.
2. Sex.
3. Occupation.
4. Height : Weight ratio.
5. Reaction to stress and pain.

Consideration of Age

The prevalence of the certain conditions are at the certain ages. The disc degeneration starts at around age of 40 years, while onset of ankylosing spondylitis is before the age of 40 years. The patient over the age of 50 years presents with low back pain may be considered for the malignant disease, while, the patient below the age of 25-30 years with low back pain is considered for the mechanical, infective or traumatic such as dysfunction at the intervertebral disc, apophyseal joints, ligaments, postural problems and malalignment and ruled out for the degenerative disease.

Sex

While obtaining general information, clinician must consider the sex of the patient. The prevalence of ankylosing spondylitis is higher in the males than females. If a female presents with a low back pain she may be considered for dysmenorrhoea, urinary and pelvic infection etc.

Occupation

People involved in the activities such as lifting and carrying objects may have dysfunction of the intervertebral disc, facet (apophyseal) joints etc., the prolong shortening of muscles and ligament to the concavity side and lengthening of the muscles and ligaments to the convexity side.

Subjective Examination

During subjective examination the examiner gathers information from the patient by asking questions such as: What is the problem? When it started? How it started? etc. The information collected during the subjective examinations depends on a greater extent by the quality of communication between the examiner and patient. Therefore, the examiner should establish a pleasant relationship with the patient to get an accurate information from the patient. Attempts are made to gather accurate information from the patient so that these may give clues in making the diagnosis and in designing scheme of management. The examiner should ask the relevant questions. Every question need'nt be asked otherwise the patient will get irritated and may distort the information. The subjective examination involves following:

A.

a. Chief complaint.
b. Onset of signs and symptoms.
c. Mechanism of injury.
d. Duration of symptoms (complaint).
e. Area of symptoms.
f. Nature and quality of pain and symptoms.
g. Severity or intensity of the pain and symptoms.
h. Depth of pain and symptoms.
i. Irritability.
j. Behavior of pain and symptoms.
k. History
   - Previous history of treatment for pain and symptoms.
   - Past medical history including history of surgery, if any.

B. Observation of:

i. Posture from all three planes.
ii. Movement (active).
iii. Swelling, redness, erythema and muscle atrophy.
iv. Deformity.
v. Gait.

Chief Complaint

Why has the patient referred for the treatment?

a. Pain.
b. Stiffness.
c. Giving way.
d. Instability.
e. Weakness.
f. Loss of function.
g. After:
   i. Trauma.
   ii. Surgery.
   iii. Manipulation under anesthesia (MUA).
h. Differential diagnosis.

Onset of Symptoms

The pain and other symptoms may start with gradual or sudden onset. Symptoms start with gradual onset indicates an active pathology such as infection or inflammation if they do not subside with the rest. The mechanical back pain such as disc degeneration and faulty posture has the gradual onset but they respond to the rest and heat modalities. The symptoms start with sudden onset speaks about traumatic lesion, and there is probability of the injury to the ligaments, intervertebral disc, apophyseal joints or muscle tear/rupture etc.

Mechanism of Injury

The patient explains how the injury took place. If patient is able to reveal the exact mechanism of injury, the clinician/examiner can reach to the exact site/structure level. Following mechanisms of injury are mentioned as under:

Forward Bending and Lifting the Heavy Weight: During forward flexion the line of gravity falls anterior to the midline which increases the extension moment arm, and requires more muscle work to stabilize the spine and lift the object. Initially the individual tries but fails to generate that much force in the midway, resulting tear of the muscles and posterior static stabilizers, that enables the intervertebral disc to prolapse posterior, and causes dysfunction at the facet joints.

Area of Symptoms: It is useful to record the area of the pain by using a body chart, because this helps in a quick visual reference. The patient may complain of more than one symptoms.

Severity or Intensity of Pain: The patient is asked to indicate according to the description as charted or number which best describes the intensity of their pain, from its least and at its worst.

- Mild.
- Moderate.
- Distressing.
- Horrible.
- Excruciating.

Depth of Pain: The depth of pain may give some indication as to the structure at fault but, like quality of pain, this can be misleading.

Irritability: This is the length of time for which the person has to perform the activity to increase the pain, and conversely how long it takes before the pain settles to its former intensity. It can be measured as high, moderate or low.

High Irritability: The aggravating factor causes the pain to increase very quickly or instantly and then the pain takes a long time to settle down.

Moderate Irritability: The aggravating factors take longer to increase the symptoms.

Low Irritability: The aggravating factor can be performed for a long time before exacerbating the patient's symptoms and then as the activity stops, the symptoms subside rapidly.

Behavior of Symptoms

Aggravating and Relieving: The movement or posture that produces or increases the symptoms.

Positional Factors: Most musculoskeletal pain is mechanical in origin and is therefore, made better or worse by adopting particular positions or postures that either stretch or compress the structure that causes pain.

Time Factors: Certain pathologies tend to be more painful at characteristic times of the day, for example, chronic changes are characteristically painful and stiff initially and arising from sleep.

Duration of the Symptoms

Constant: The symptoms persist all the time and there is no relief while rest and during activities.

Example: In inflammatory/infective conditions the patient complaints pain in the day and night. Sometimes the symptoms are less severe in the day probably due to engagement in the activities.

Intermittent: Any relief in the symptoms even for a few minutes or low.

Example: Mechanical pain. The patient complains less severe to no pain while resting in a particular position which releases the stress/load on the damaged structure.

History

Previous Treatments: Has the patient received any treatment for this condition in the past, if yes what treatment has been taken? Was it effective? or Was the improvement partial or total?

Past Medical History: Has the patient suffered any major illness? This might affect the tissues and be a contraindication to particular treatments.

Examples:

i. Respiratory.

ii. Cardiac disease.

iii. Diabetes.

iv. Rheumatoid arthritis.

Is the patient receiving or *received oral* steroid medication? The patients having chronic respiratory diseases, inflammatory bowel diseases or RA, may receive oral steroid therapy. This treatment affects bone and produces tendency towards bruising. Medication used in the past or using for the present condition should also be noted.

Physical Observation: After taking the history next element of lower back pain assessment is careful physical observation of the patient posture. Here the examiner notes down the abnormalities of the posture and restriction in the active range of mention, if any, and the patterns of movements (such as compensatory movement and muscle substitutes to show the maximum results. The best way to find the abnormalities in the posture and movements is to have the normal picture of the posture and movements in the mind (practice to observe the posture and movements on normal subjects) or compare it with the normal. This is known as system review. For an instance the examiner finds the pulse rate of the patient 99 per minute and when it is compared with normal it is termed as tachycardia but if the examiner does not have the normal value in the mind it cannot be said that it is high. The posture is reviewed (observed) from anterior, lateral and posterior view. During an observation the patient should be undressed.

Observation of the Posture from Anterior View: (Fig. 27.11)

The curve of the thoracic and cervical may also be viewed as it may change in order to compensate the lumbar spine curve.

Posterior View: Lateral tilling of *pelvis, unequal length of the legs, pelvic up slip and down slip, lumbar lordosis and side flexion (both sides) are observed from this view* (Fig. 27.12).

Observation of the Active Range of Motion: All active movements are observed from anterior, posterior and lateral view.

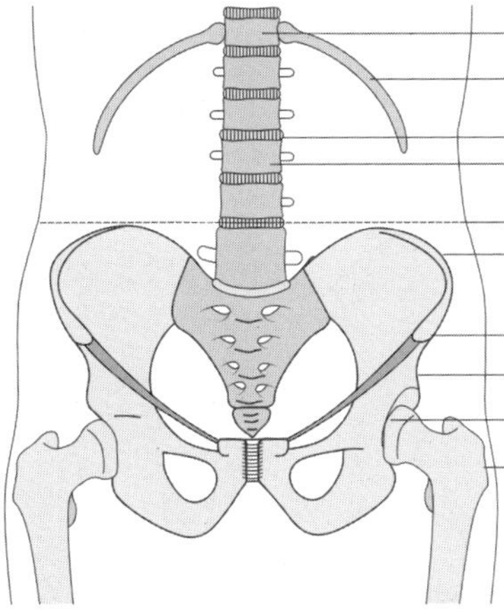

Fig. 27.11: Physical observation from anterior view

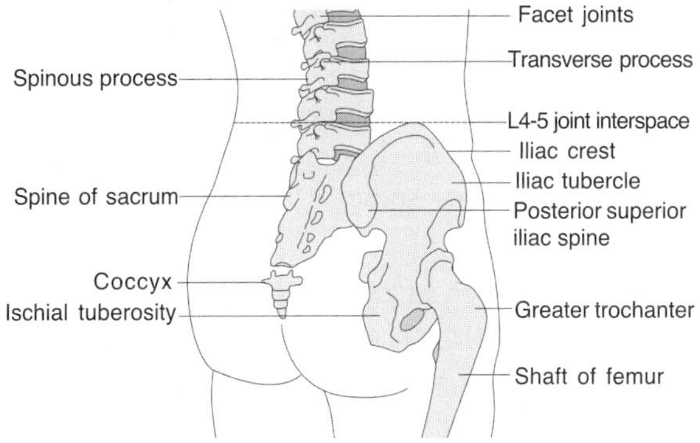

Fig. 27.12: Observation from lateral view

The lumbopelvic rhythm is the coordinated movement of the lumbar spine and hip during trunk flexion and extension. Ideal lumbopelvic rhythm is such that motion at the lumbar spine should be accompanied by motion of pelvis rotating over the hip. An appropriate rhythm is a lumbar flexion of 30° and anterior pelvic tilt (hip flexion) of 60°. In forward bending lumbar spine flexes first and when it reaches to its limit (30° flexion) pelvis starts rotating anteriorly on the hip joints. The total lumbopelvic rhythm is approximately 90° flexion of lumbar spine and pelvis on the hip joints (Fig. 27.13a). When the person returns to

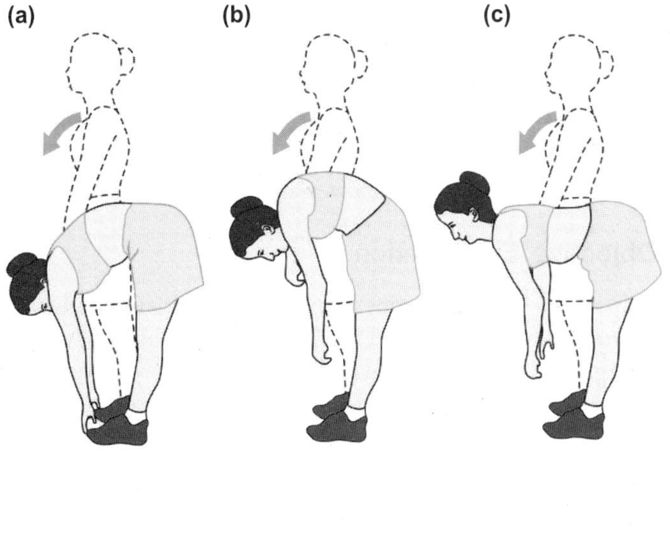

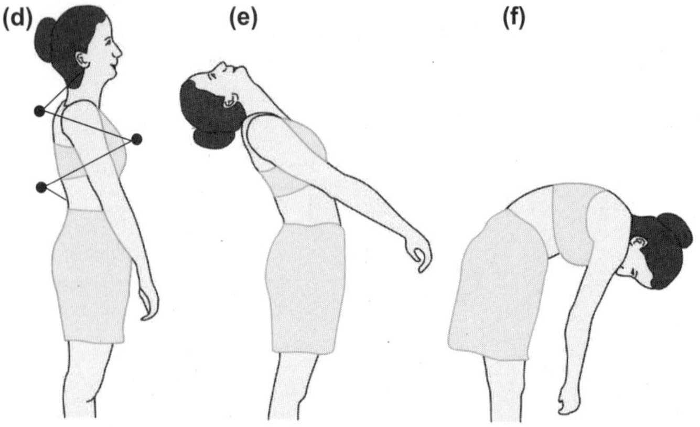

Figs. 27.13a to f: (a) Normal lumbopelvic rhythm (Flexion and Extension), (b) Short hamstrings limiting anterior pelvic rotation on the hip joint, compensating by hyperlordosis, (d) Short lumbar extensors, limiting lumbar flexion, compensating by excessive anterior pelvic tilting on the hip. (d to f) Returning to the neutral and then to the extension

its erect standing from lumbopelvic flexion, the pelvis starts rotating posteriorly on the hip joints which is followed by extension of the lumbar spine to its neutral position (Fig. 27.13b).

Several factors such as tight hamstrings, erector spinae and excessive kyphosis can alter the lumbopelvic rhythm.

Observation of the Gait: The gait is observed from anterior, posterior and lateral views. The abnormality in the gait may be due to pain or weakness. The following conditions may alter the gait:

(i) *Prolapsed intervertebral disc with radiculopathy:* The patients will bend the trunk to the opposite side to relieve the pressure on nerve roots. He or she walks with slight hip and knee flexed position with more weight on the toes of the affected side this relieves the tension in the sciatic nerves.

(ii) *Facet block or malaligned:* The patient walks with flexed lumbar spine with slight bending to the opposite side. The spine will be fixed in one position, no significant movement is taken place beyond that position. Overall the patient walks with stiff back to the flexion.

(iii) *Chronic low back pain with lower crossed syndrome:* The hip joints remain slightly in flexed position with anterior tilling of the pelvis and exaggerated lumbar lordosis. Sometimes knees bucking inwards may also be noticed after a short walk.

Objective Examination

Palpation: The examiner should have the knowledge of anatomical structure and surface anatomy area which is being palpated. The lower back region is palpated to determine the level of the lesion and to detect the abnormalities in the bone structure (such as spina bifida and spondylolisthesis) and to establish the nature of the problems. There are two methods of palpation (i) Use of the tips of the thumbs and (ii) Use of the pisiform pad of hand. Which method and when it should be used depends on the area which is being examined. For small and delicate structures, tips of thumb or finger can be used but for larger areas such as glutei and lumbar both methods can be used. If the pressure is not sufficient with the thumb or pisiform pad than the other hand can be used as reinforcement.

The examiner should palpate the structures slowly and carefully starting with light pressure initially and working into high pressure to palpate deep structures. The palpation should start from distal part of the lesions and then progress to the central part so that the examiner has some idea of what to expect. Any difference or abnormality should be noted.

The examiner should be able to:

i. Determine differences in tissue tension, e.g., effusion, spasm.
ii. Distinguish differences in tissue texture.
iii. Identify shapes, structures and tissue type and thus detects abnormalities.
iv. Feel variations in temperatures and pulse.
v. Feel tremors and fasciculation.
vi. Feel dryness or excessive moisture of the skin.

The examiner must ensure that the area to be palpated is as develop a clear picture of what released as possible exactly (the structure) being palpated.

The lumbar spine is also palpated to determine the:

(i) **L_4 and L_5 Level:** The patient must be relaxed in prone lying with an adequate exposure of the lumbosacral spine. Therapist stands behind the patient and places the fingers on the top of the iliac crests and thumbs at the same level of the midline of the back which crosses the level of fourth and fifth lumbar disc interspace. After palpating the top of the iliac crests an imaginary line is drawn from top of the left iliac crest to the top of the right iliac crest. The imaginary line where it crosses the lumbar spine is the intervertebral disc space between fourth and fifth vertebrae and the spinous process of fourth lumbar vertebra. After palpating the spinous process of fourth lumbar vertebra the spinous process of L_3, L_2 and L_1 can be palpated by moving upward (Figs. 27.14 and 27.15).

(ii) **Posterior Superior Iliac Spine and S_2 Level:** Moving down from the top of the iliac crest, two depressions can be observed, these are the posterior superior iliac spines. When these are connected with an imaginary line, the line where it crosses the spine is considered as the second sacral verterbra. The other sacral vertebra

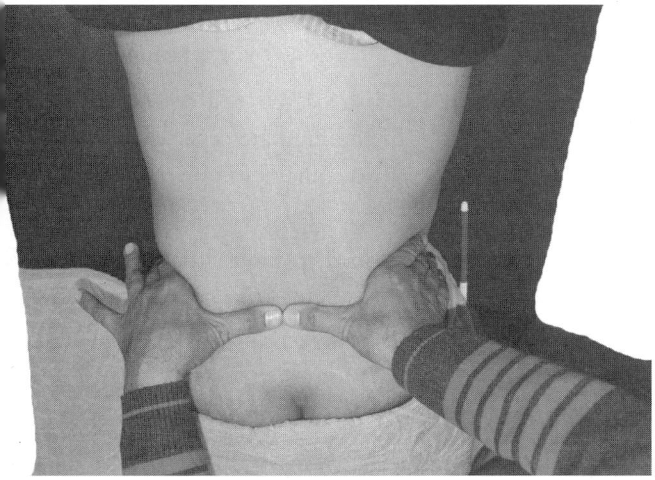

Fig. 27.14: Determination of the L_4/L_5 intervertebral space

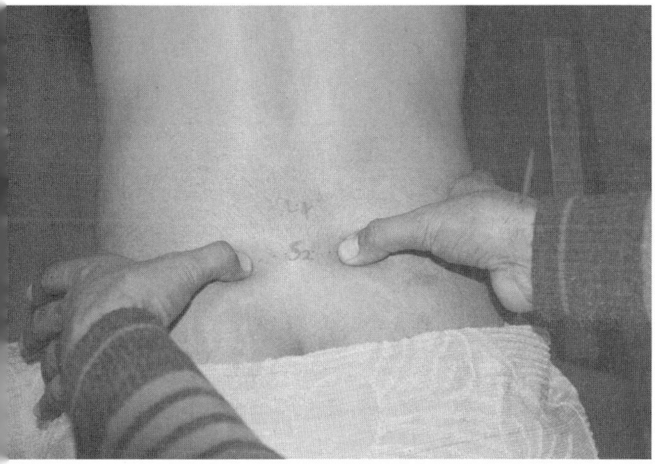

ig. 27.15: Determining posterior superior iliac spine and S_2 evel

can also be palpated by moving up and down of the second sacral vertebra.

Special Tests

The therapist must interpret the data collected during the history and subjective examination. Based on the interpretation of the data it should be decided by the therapist which test and when it should be performed. The tests are performed to reproduce the symptoms. Tests those are not related to the symptoms should not be performed as it may discomfort the patient unnecessarily. A proper history taking and effective subjective assessment will allow the therapist to move forward to the exact special tests needed to perform to reproduce the symptoms and to confirm the diagnosis.

Quadrant Test: It is a useful compressive provocation test designed to determine if the origin of the pain is truly in the lumbar spine. The test should be performed when patient has no radicular symptoms but localized in the lumbar spine and active and passive movements fail to reproduce the symptoms. The quadrant test places greater stress on the articular pillars of the apophyseal joints, the posterior and lateral wall of the disc and posterior longitudinal ligament.

The patient stands comfortably and therapist stands behind the patient and places both hands on the shoulders of the patient. The therapist must ensure that the patient should not bend the knees throughout the procedure.

Procedure: The test is performed in three steps: (Figs. 27.16a to c)

1. While keeping the hands on the patient's shoulders, the therapist instructs the patient to extend the lumbar spine to its limit and applies over pressure by the hands.

(a) (b) (c)

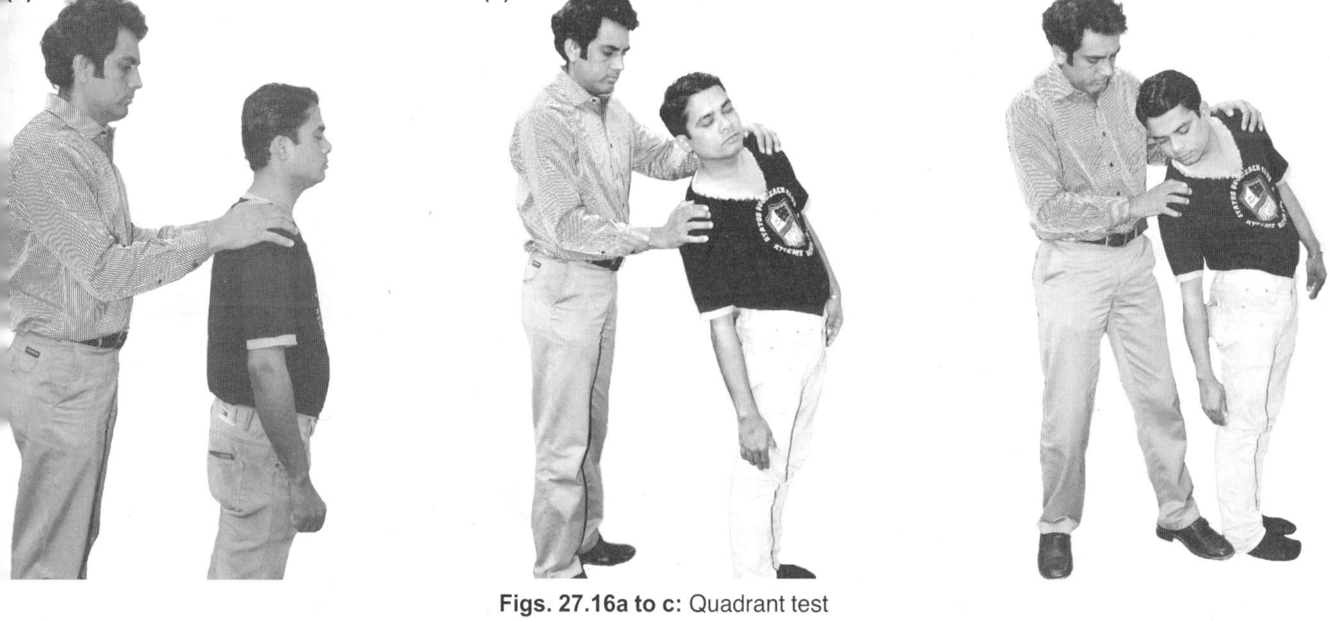

Figs. 27.16a to c: Quadrant test

2. The lumbar spine is bent (side flexed) to the affected side (painful side).

3. The last step is to rotate the lumbar spine to the painful side.

These three movements–extension, side flexion and rotation which place greater stress on the posterolateral part of the facet joint, intervertebral disc, and posterior longitudinal ligament are held at least for 20 seconds to allow for a delayed response. If patient complaints pain then the test is considered to be positive and indicates involvement of the forementioned three structures.

Slump Test: It is a provocative test performed on the patient who has pain in the lumbar spine with or without leg pain, especially if leg pain includes posterior thigh pain. The test is designed to put the tension on sciatic nerve.

The patient is positioned in high sitting and therapist stands at the side of the patient which is being examined. The test is performed in five steps (Figs. 27.17a to e).

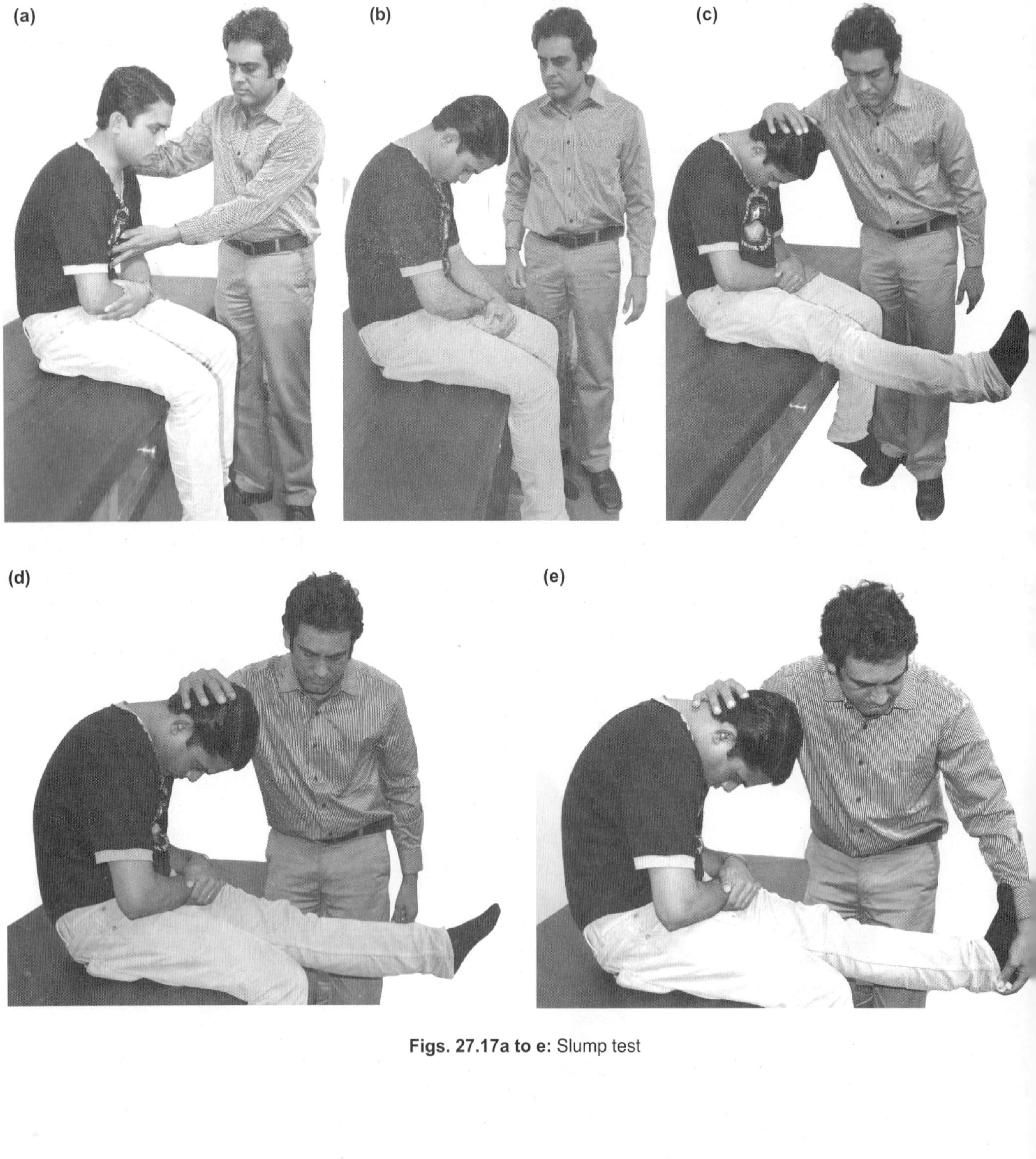

Figs. 27.17a to e: Slump test

. The patient slumps forward without excessively flexing the trunk. The test is negated by excessive flexion of the back from the lumbar area.

i. The patient now places the chin on the sternum.

ii. While maintaining the slump position and neck forward flexion, the patient is asked to extend the unaffected knee joint first and then the affected knee joint. In both the cases (sciatica and hamstrings tightness) terminal extension will be limited and painful. The position is held for 20 seconds to allow delayed response.

v. Further tension in sciatic nerve can be added by dorsiflexion of the ankle joint of the affected side, if it reproduces pain and symptoms in the back and posterior thigh, it may be due to sciatic nerve stretching or due to hamstrings tightness.

v. Passive dorsiflexion is also added to the last step. If it aggravates the symptoms in the posterior thigh and back, this further confirms, sciatic nerve root compression (sciatica).

To rule out the hamstrings pain from sciatic origin, knee extension is maintained and the patient is asked to extend the neck to its neutral position.

a. If the pain disappears and patient is able to extend the knee joint, it is probably of spinal origin as the neck extension reduces the tension in the dura and indicates disc pathology or dura tethering (sciatica).
b. If pain persist (even after neck extension) it is due to hamstrings tightness.

Significance: It is the useful screening test for differentiating hamstrings stretch from sciatic nerve stretch (Fig. 27.18).

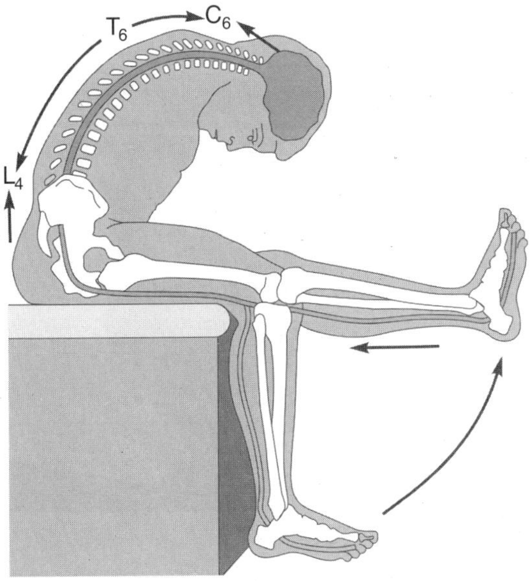

Fig. 27.18

The Straight Leg Raising (SLR) Test

The straight leg raising test is designed specially to put the tension in the sciatic nerve and dura to reproduce the symptoms. Initially it was performed only by raising the legs but now it is modified and dorsiflexion and neck flexion are added to it (similar to slumps test).

SLR is a sciatic nerve stretching test performed by the therapist passively by raising the leg with knee extension. During the procedure the patient is asked to relax the quadriceps and not to raise the leg actively. As the test is designed to increase the tension in the sciatic nerve it is considered negative or normal if the patient complaints pain before 35 degrees and after 75 degrees of hip flexion. This is because upto 35 degrees hip flexion, no tension increases in the sciatic nerve and the nerve remains relaxed. The tension in the sciatic nerve starts increasing after 35 degrees of hip flexion upto 75 degrees of hip flexion and again after 75 degrees tension in the sciatic nerve cannot be increased further therefore SLR is considered positive only if the patient's symptoms are reproduced between 35 and 75 degrees.

Procedure: The patient lies in supine and therapist stands at side of the leg which is being examined. The therapist holds the leg at ankle with one hand and stabilizes the pelvic with other hand (Fig. 27.19).

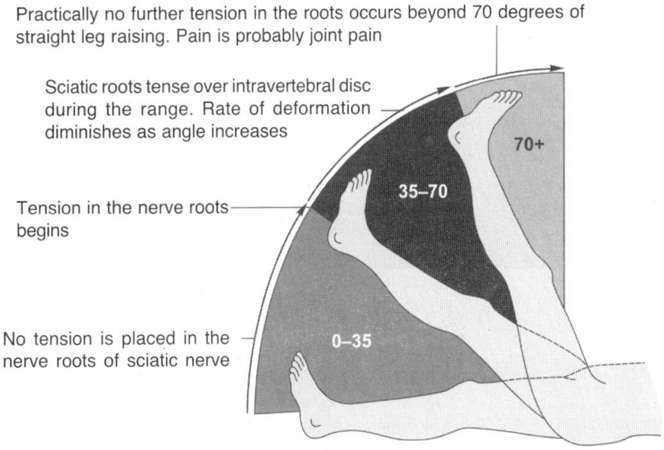

Fig. 27.19: The straight leg raising (SLR) test

The patient is instructed to relax the quadriceps and allow the therapist to raise the leg. The patellar movements can be checked by the stabilizing hand, if patella moves free then it is considered that the quadriceps muscles are relaxed. The therapist raises the leg gradually and notices the range where patient's symptoms aggravate. For example the pain and symptoms are aggravated at 60 degrees then the test is considered to be positive at 60 degrees.

For further confirmation the hip joint range is maintained at 60 degrees and sudden passive dorsiflexion is added to the SLR. If the dorsiflexion aggravates the symptoms, it further confirms the sciatic nerve pain. This is also known as Lasegue's test (adding dorsiflexion to SLR). If the passive dorsiflexion does not increase the posterior thigh pain symptoms then the pain is likely due to hamstrings tightness. Further tension in the sciatic nerve and dura can also be increased with neck flexion (Figs. 27.20a to d).

Significance: The test is an excellent sign of dural and irritation by lumbar disc protrusion. The test places a varying degree of tension on each of the lumbar spinal nerve roots in the dural sleaves from L_4 to S_2 but specially on S_1 nerve root.

Crossover Sign or Cross SLR: The normal leg is raised passively with the knee extension. If the patient complaints of radicular pain and symptoms on the contralateral leg it is known as crossover sign. This is present in patients with large soft disc protrusion. If the crossover sign is positive, it indicates surgical intervention as a choice of treatment.

Quick Tests: The tests are performed to examine the L_4 and S_1 nerve roots. The patient is asked to walk quickly and efficiently for 2-3 minutes.

a. ***Walking on Heels:*** The patient is asked to walk quickly and efficiently for 2-5 minutes on the heels. If patient cannot walk and drops the fore foot then the involvement of L_5 nerve root may be considered.

b. ***Walking on Toes:*** The patient is asked to walk on the toes as much quick as possible for 2-3 minutes. Inability of walking on toes indicates weakness of the gastrosoleus and compression on the S_1 nerve root.

Deep Tendon Reflexes

The deep tendon reflexes are performed to test the integrity of the nerve roots.

a. **Patellar Tendon Jerk:** The patellar tendon jerk is elicited to test the integrity of the L_3 nerve root. The L_3 and L_4 nerve roots supply the quadriceps muscles. The lower

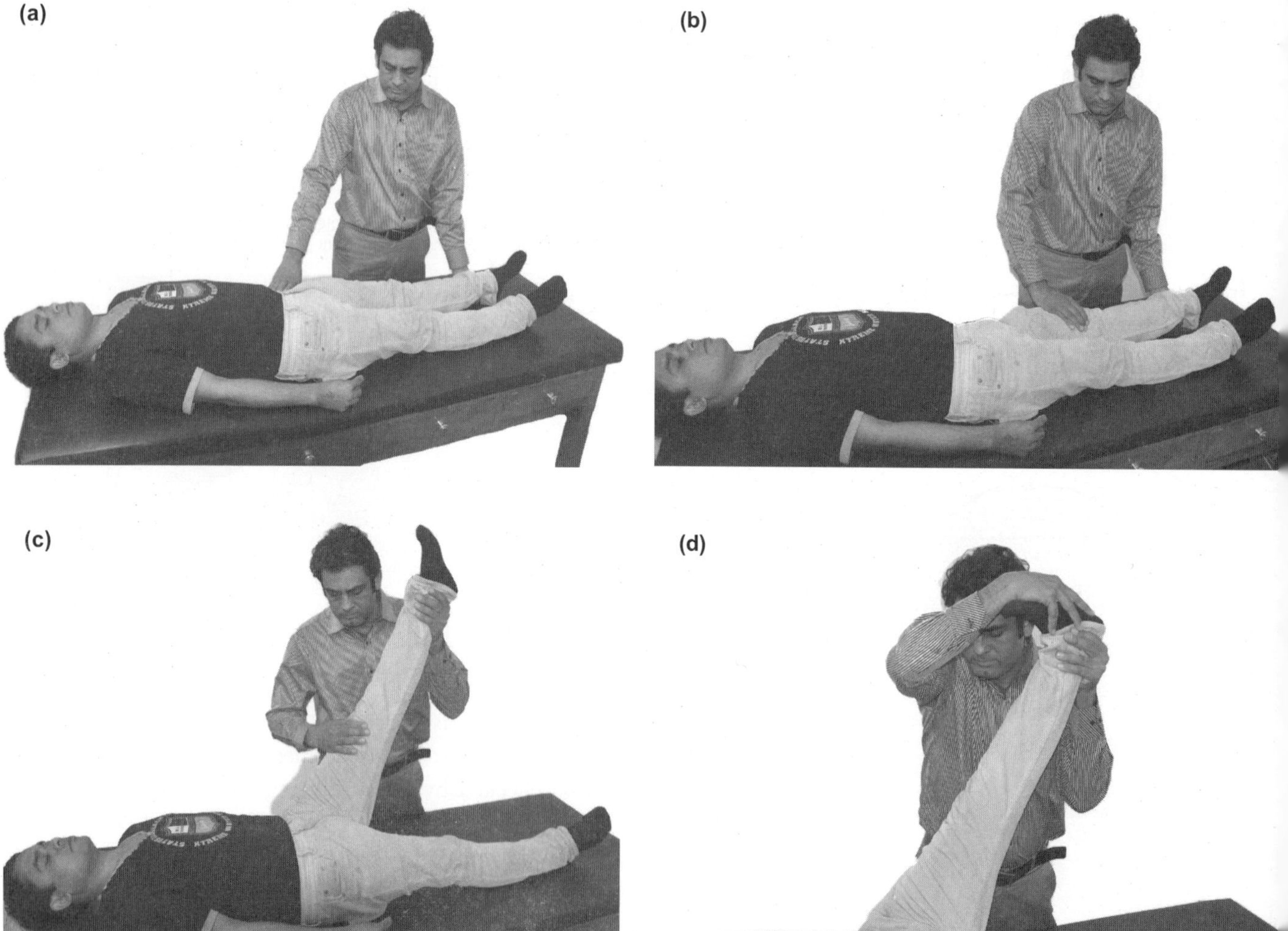

Figs. 27.20a to d: SLR, Lasegue's test

part including patellar tendon is supplied by L_3 nerve root. Compression on the L_3 nerve root can diminish the patellar tendon. The patellar tendon jerk/reflex will be absent if the motor nerve severely compressed. To test the patellar tendon reflexes the patient lies in high sitting position. The patient should look straight and not at the knee joint. The therapist stands at the side of the knee joint. The patellar tendon (between patella and tibial tuberosity) is felt. Therapist holds the percussion hummer with the right hand in loose grasp and strikes the patellar tendon. The movement should take place in the wrist joint only. Both sides of the patellar jerks can be tested without changing the position (therapist). Some patients do not relax the quadriceps muscles and the results vary. These patients should be kept busy in talking or asked to clench their teeth or grasp the hands to divert the attention to allow the muscle to relax. The therapist should deceive the patient and strike the tendon to get exact results. This is known as Jendrasik maneuvre (Fig. 27.21).

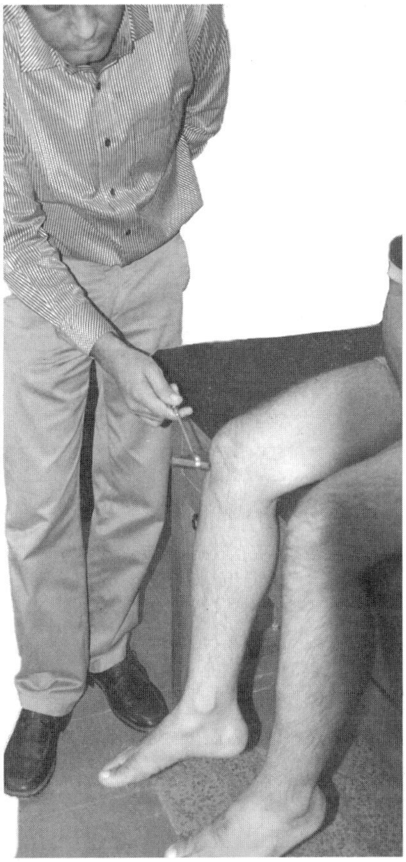

Fig. 27.21: Patellar tendon reflexes

b. **Ankle Jerk:** To test the integrity of the S_1 nerve root, the ankle jerk is tested.

Position of Patient: High sitting or prone with knee flexion upto 30°–40°.

Position of Therapist: Stands at the side of the patient, places left hand under the leg. Achilles tendon is palpated and then strike with the hammer with right hand. The therapist can test both side of Achilles tendons without changing the position and compare with the normal (Fig. 27.22).

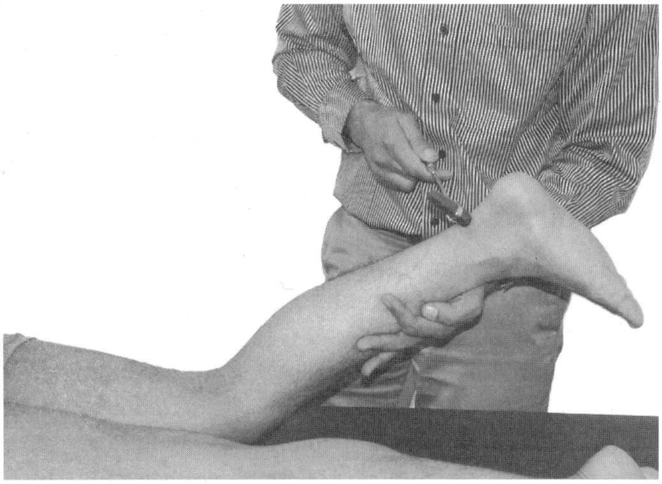

Fig. 27.22: Ankle jerk

POSTURAL PAIN

Pathology, poor work station and injury can produce pain in the lower back region. The patient finds the compensatory movements or positions that reduce the pain. The compensation or adaptations lead to systemic and predictable patterns of muscular imbalance. The primary muscles responsible for specific joint movement may become weak or inhibited causing synergistic muscles to become hyperactive. The antagonistic group of muscles loses their flexibility and become tight.

The central nervous system regulates tonic and phasic muscle groups which oppose each other in action. The tonic muscle group functions as a facilitator while the phasic muscle groups work as inhibitor. The tonic muscles are also known as postural, have primary function to maintain upright (trunk) posture and the phasic muscles are responsible for rapid motions. Due to segmental dysfunction, pain and malalignment, the postural muscles become tight whereas, the phasic muscles have tendency to go into lengthened state, resulting in muscular imbalance, which eventually causes chronic pain and disability.

This situation alters the cooperative harmonious relationship between muscles and fascia leading to imbalance and articular compensation which further contributes to the change in movement patterns. The altered movement pattern is a movement pattern in which a change occurs in the coordination of the muscle firing sequences for a specific group of muscles facilitating a specific joint movement. *As a result of abnormal physiologic movements, motion patterns involving the fascial planes is altered, i.e., the paravertebral fascia of the cervical spine continues with the thoracolumbar fascia and is affected by its abnormal function. It means that cervical spine aberrant coupling patterns may be a function of abnormal thoracolumbar fascia loading.*

If the posture is not corrected in the initial stage the patient will continue to adapt the most suitable posture which will ease the symptoms and gradually develop a typical abnormal posture known as lower crossed syndrome.

Lower Crossed Syndrome

Lower crossed syndrome is a postural distortion syndrome affecting the lower kinetic chain (lumbopelvic, hip complex, knee and ankle). The patient usually presents with anterior pelvic tilt, increased lumbar lordosis (sway back) and flexed hip joints. There is stress on the L_5-S_1 vertebral segment which produces pain and discomfort in the lumbar spine. This progresses to instability of the sacroiliac joints with increased lumbosacral angle, knee pain (anterior) and piriformis tightness (Figs. 27.23a and b) and (Table 27.2).

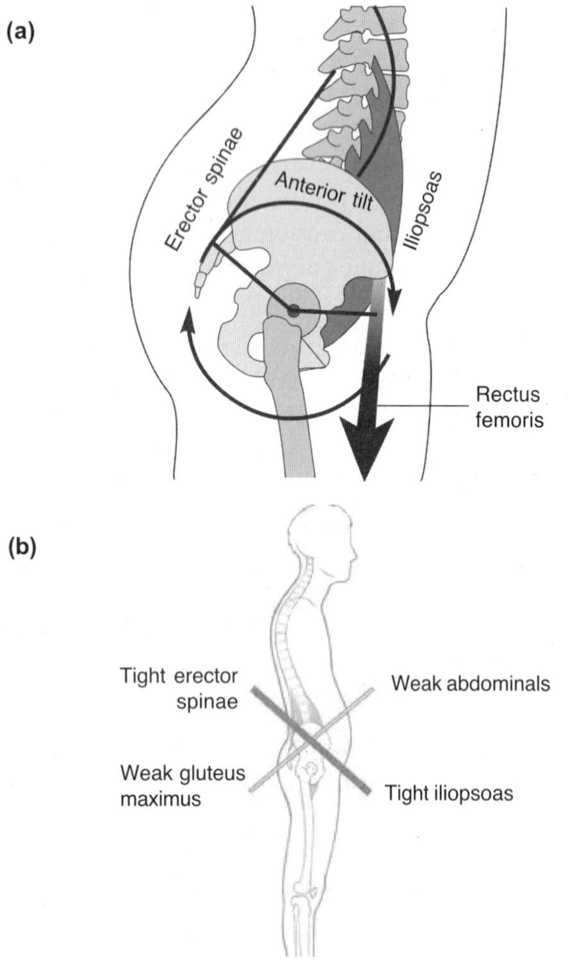

Figs. 27.23a and b: Lower crossed syndrome

Table 27.2: Lower crossed syndrome

Tight or facilitated muscles	*Weak or inhibited muscles*
Iliopsoas	Rectus abdominis oblique
Rectus femoris	Gluteus maximus
Tensor fascia lata	Gluteus medius
Adductor group	Hamstrings
Erector spinae	
Gastrocnemius	

Tonic Muscles: These types of muscles contain slow twitch type I fibers, a_2 motor neuron, high capillary density and high number of spindles. These fibers show slow fatigability and have tendency to become shorten due to dysfunction. These are involved in oxidative metabolism.

Phasic Muscles: These are fast-twitch type II fibers, contain a_1 motor neuron, low capillary density and less number of spindles. These fibers show fast fatigability and have tendency to become weak due to dysfunction. These muscles involved in glycolytic metabolism (Table 27.3).

Table 27.3: Tonic and phasic muscles

Tonic muscles	*Phasic muscles*
Lower extremity/pelvic area	Lower extremity/pelvic area
Biceps femoris	Vastus medialis
Semitendinosus	
Semimembranosus	
Iliopsoas	Vastus lateralis
Rectus femoris	Gluteus medius
Tensor fascia lata	Gluteus maximus
Adductor brevis	Tibialis anterior
Adductor magnus	Peroneal group
Gracilis	
Quadriceps femoris	
Adductor longus	
Gastrocnemius	
Soleus	
Trunk and shoulder girdle	Trunk and shoulder girdle
Cervical and lumbar erectors	Rhomboid muscles
Quadratus lumborum	Trapezius (ascending portion)
Scalene muscles	
Pectoralis major	Trapezius (horizontal portion)
Levator scapulae	
Trapezius (descending portion)	Pectoralis major (sternal portion)
Biceps brachii (short and long head)	Triceps brachii
	Thoracic erectors

Clinical Features

Patients with lower cross syndrome exhibit anterior tilting of the pelvis, hyperlordotic lumbar spine and bulging abdomen. These manifestations are mainly due to the muscular imbalance. There is weakness of abdominals and gluteus maximus, and shortening of the quadriceps, iliopsoas and erector spinae (extensors of the lumbar spine). The hyperlordosis of the lumbar spine causes approximation of the facet joints which results in pain the paravertebral region. Pain from the facet joint may also be referred to the paravertebral region, gluteal area, groin, posterior, and lateral thigh. Patients also feel pain in the anterior knee joint as the patella shifts superiorly due to shortening of the quadriceps muscles. There is a compensatory curve in the upper dorsal spine (kyphosis), rounded and protracted shoulders and forward head. Therefore, many of the patients with lower cross syndrome develop upper cross syndrome and vice versa if not treated at the right time.

Physical Tests

Upper crossed syndorme is diagnosed primarily on the basis of clinical findings. The provocative tests help in exaggerate the symptoms and provide clues to locate the sources of pain.

Quadrant Test: The test is perfomed in the standing. Examiner stands behind the patient and places hands on both the shoulders of the patient. While maintaining the position the therapist extends side flexes and rotates the trunk to the painful side. All the combined movements are held at the end range for fifteen seconds for delayed onset of symptoms. This position places stress on the lateral part of the disc and same side of the facet joint. Test is considered positive if patient complaints pain.

Thomas Test: There is a hyperlordotic curve in the lumbar spine which results in anterior tilting of the pelvis. The iliopsoas of both the sides show tightness. Thomas test in the supine, with contralateral knee and hip flexion (knee to chest) raises or flexes the affected hip joint in case of shortening of hip joint. However, the affected hip joint remains at neutral in case of normal cases when the hip and knee joint is flexed.

Management

The treatment of the lower cross syndrome includes postural correction exercises mainly strengthening of the weak muscles and stretching of the short muscles. The aim of the treatment should be re-align the lumbar spine by strengthening of the abdominal and stretching of the erector spinae muscles so that the excessive load on the facet joint can be alleviated. Core strengthening program which is described at Page No. 583 of the lumbar spine which includes curl up, side curl up to strengthen the rectus abdominis, and obliqus, and transverse abdominis activation exercises for increasing the intra-abdominal pressure (IAP), and decreasing the intradiscal pressure is helpful in improving the posture. Posterior tilting exercises such as isometric gluteus maximus, hamstrings and isometric curl up are also beneficial. The stretching of lumbar erector spinae, iliopsoas, and quadriceps should be the priority of the therapist to improve flexibility of these muscles. The strengthening and stretching should also progress to the upper back if there is a compensatory upper cross syndrome.

1. Pelvic posterior tilting exercises in crook lying and in standing.
2. Williams flexion antilordotic exercises.
3. Erect sitting from slouched posture.
4. Curl up and reverse curl up.
5. Side curl up.
6. Abdominal hollowing and abdominal tuck in.
7. Mini squatting.
8. Hamstrings sets.
9. Thomas stretch.
10. Quadriceps stretching.
11. Erector spinae stretching (Figs. 27.24a to k).

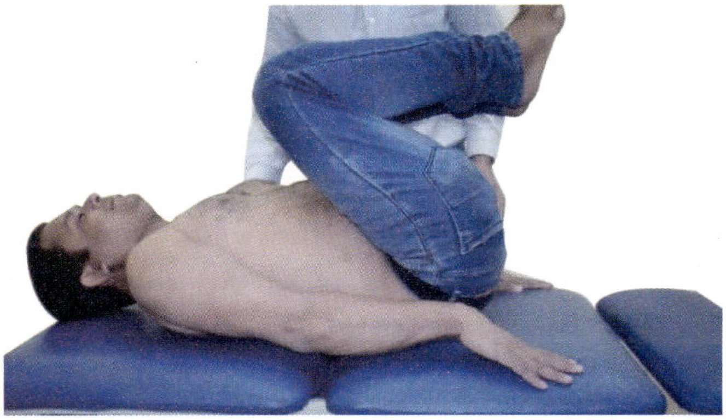

Fig. 27.24a: Posterior pelvic tilt in supine

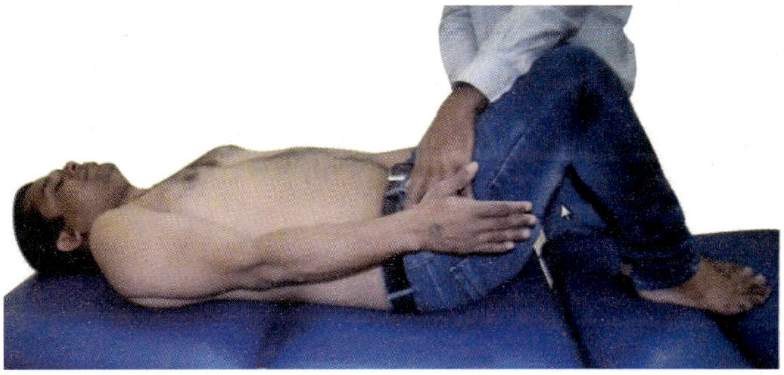

Fig. 27.24b: Anterior pelvic tilt in supine

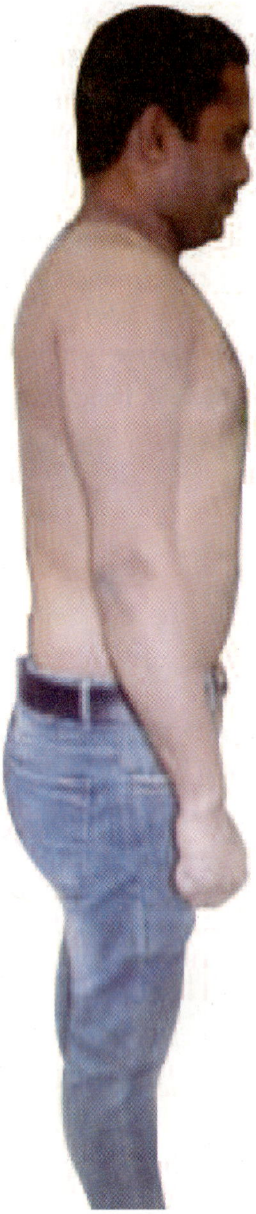

Fig. 27.24c: Glutei squeeze and posterior pelvic tilt in standing

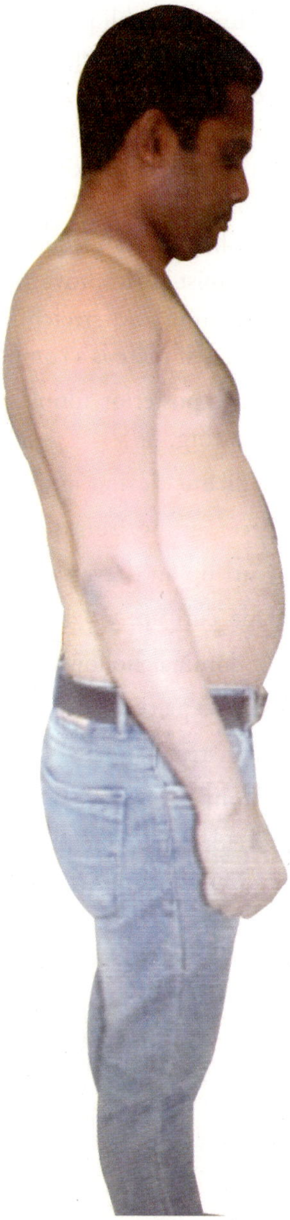

Fig. 27.24d: Anterior pelvic tilt in standing

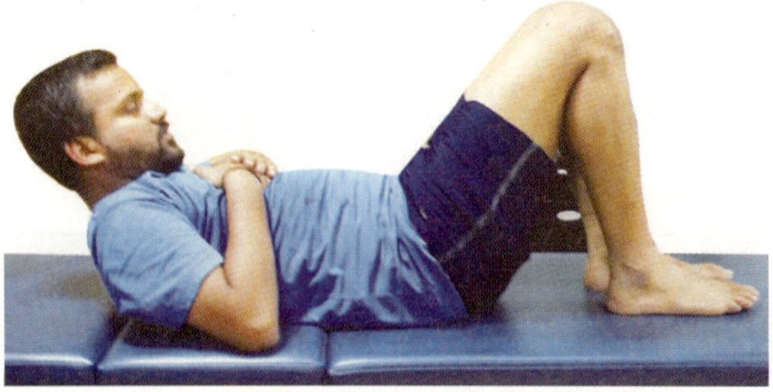

Fig. 27.24e: Curl up

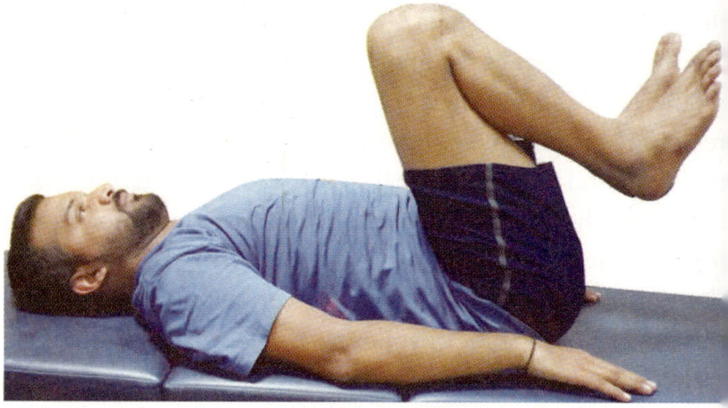

Fig. 27.24f: Reverse curl up

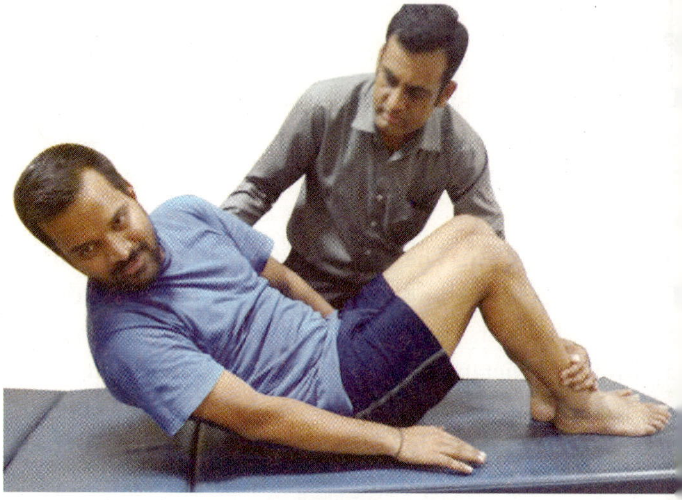

Fig. 27.24g: Side curl up

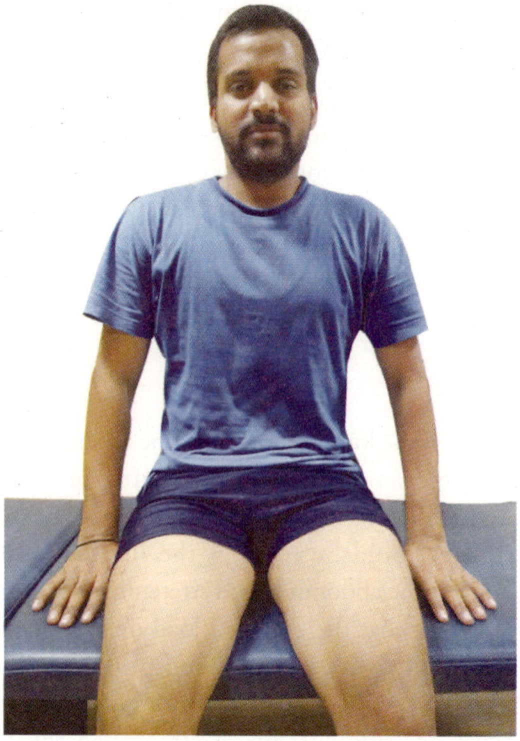

Fig. 27.24h: Abdominal hollowing

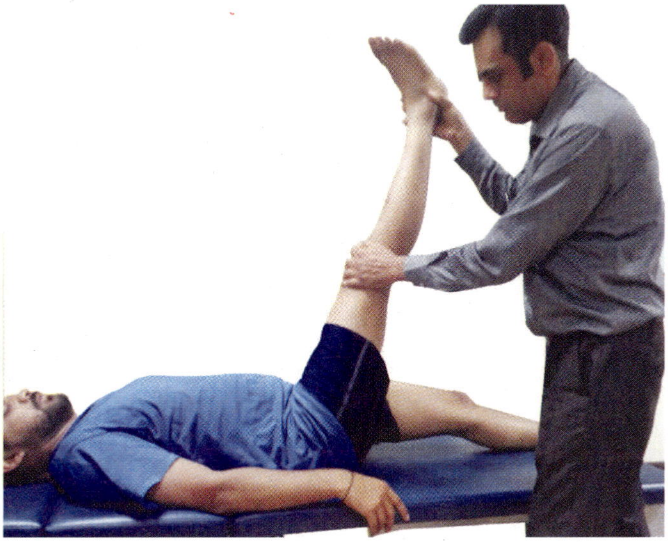

Fig. 27.24i: Hamstrings stretch

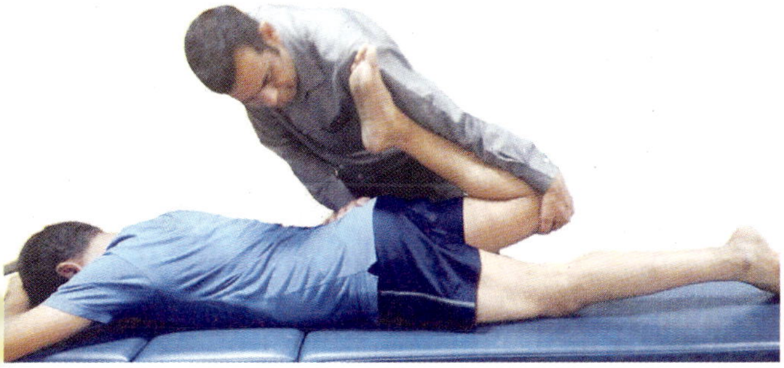

Fig. 27.24j: Quadriceps stretch curl up

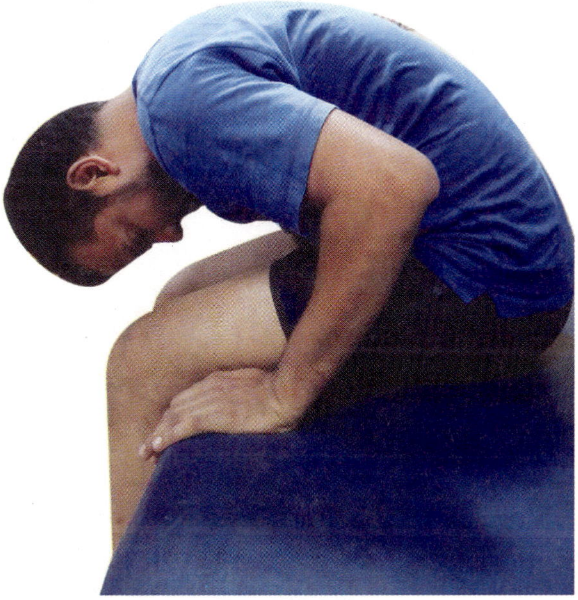

Fig. 27.24k: Erector spinae muscle stretching

SCIATICA

Sciatica is a symptom not a disease and is usually describes any painful condition along the course of the sciatic nerve. It may either be neuralgic or neuritis.

Neuralgic Sciatica is due to an external pressure on the nerve usually before it leaves the pelvis, as from a spinal cord tumor that exerts pressure within a canal, or metastatic tumors (that press the root, plexus or trunk), osteoarthritic spondylosis of the lumbar spine, prolapse intervertebral disc, and sacroiliac strain etc.

Neuritis Sciatica: It is an inflammation of the sheath or connective tissue surrounding the axons themselves. Sciatic neuritis may be due to generalized toxaemia, from alcoholism or lead or arsenic poisoning, or it may be a result of systemic diseases, such as diabetes or syphilis. It is most commonly an interstitial neuritis, but in some cases the inflammation may spread to the axons, and set up a parenchymatous neuritis.

Prolapse Intervertebral (Soft) Disc (PIVD) Sciatica

A prolapsed intervertebral disc or a disc protrusion is a herniation of the nucleus pulposus posteriorly or posterolaterally or centrally through the annulus fibrosus. This may occur at any level of the spine but most often it occurs at the lumbar spine L_4 and L_5 levels usually in young adult life.

Pathomechanics: When an individual lifts a heavy object with forward flexion, excessive pressure is generated in intervertebral space. The center of gravity falls anteriorly, requires more muscle work from the extensors. If the load which is being lifted exceeds the force generated by the muscles, the muscles get strained which in turn transfers load to the posterior longitudinal ligament. The posterior vertebral segment opens excessively which allows nucleus pulposus to prolapse through the annulus fibrosus. The anterior part is compressed and the posterior part opens out. This tends to squeeze the nucleus pulposus posteriorly or posterolaterally. With or without undue stress the herniation may enlarge and impinge on a nerve root, thus producing symptoms and signs such as tingling sensation, numbness and weakness along the nerve root known as acute radiculopathy. The compressed nerve root becomes edematous, enlarged and often adherent to the protrusion. The extruded material from a ruptured disc appears to be more prone to irritate the tissue and set up an inflammatory reaction, with edema. There is increased redness on the dural sheath as well as on the epineurium.

Stages of Disc Protrusion

The disc may prolapse from mild to severe degree which is described in five stages:

1. **Protrusion:** Initial distention of the annulus occurs with posterior displacement of the nucleus, causing protrusion of the intervertebral disc (Figs. 27.25a to d and 27.26a and b).

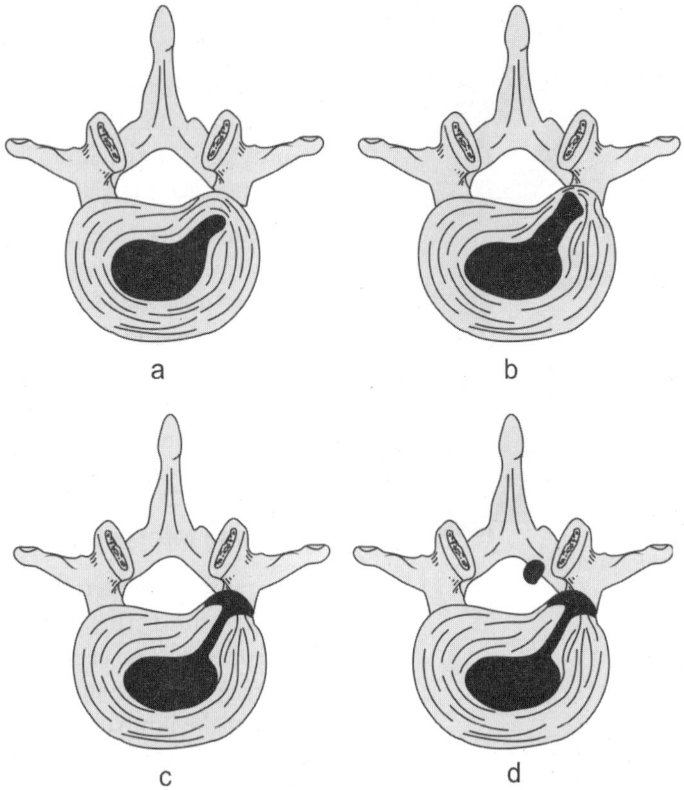

Figs. 27.25a to d: Stages of disc protrusion: a. protrusion, b. prolapse, c. extrusion, d. sequestrum

2. **Dehydration**, desiccation with early degeneration of the disc material.
3. **Herniation or Prolapse:** The radial tear of the annulus allows the nucleus to completely protrude posteriorly within the annulus and rest underneath the longitudinal ligament.
4. **Extrusion:** Subsequent protrusion through the annulus results in an extruded or uncontained disc herniation.
5. **Sequestration:** Eventually, a piece of the nucleus separates and migrates to form a sequestered herniation. The sequestrated disc material through both the annulus and posterior ligament free to move within the spine.

Symptoms

The chief complaint of the patient is pain either sudden or gradual in onset. It is gnawing or burning and may be continuously present which occur in paroxysms. Pain is

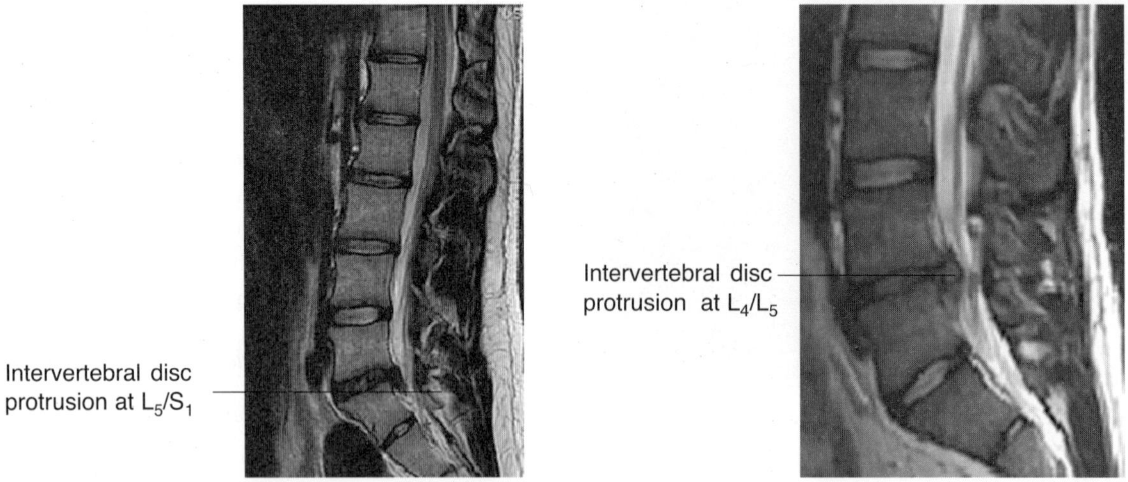

(a) L_5 and S_1 disc protrusion (b) L_4 and L_5 disc prolapse

Figs. 27.26a and b: MRI showing disc prolapse and dural compression often extremely severe especially in the leg and is worsened in any position that causes pressure on the nerve root such as sitting. Pain commences in the lumbar spine and radiates down the buttock, and posterior thigh which may never reach below the knee joint; but it may involve any or all branches of the nerve in its course. Special points of tenderness known as valley's points are found on the nerve and its branches: between the ischial tuberosity and the greater trochanter, at the center of the posterior aspect of the thigh, just lateral to the middle popliteal space, the middle of the calf and last just behind the medial malleolus. Straight leg raising and Lasegue's sign may be positive in all cases. In severe cases patient walks on the affected side toes with the knee flexion and list is often produced. Muscle atrophy, parasthesia, hyperesthesia, loss of ankle jerk may also be seen.

Clinical Features

Pain: Pain is the most dominant feature which is more in intensity in the thigh and buttock rather than in the lumbar region. It is aggravated in any position which causes pressure on nerve roots such as sitting or which stretches the nerve such as standing on heels with knees straight. Diffuse tenderness may be present.

Gait: With severe symptoms the patients walk on toes with hip and knee flexion to avoid stretching on nerve. This produces a limp, but relieves pain while walking. The pelvis is lifted upon the affected side and a compensatory scoliosis list may develop.

Parasthesia: Parasthesia, most often described as 'pins and needles' is present in one or another in majority of cases, which may be localized by the patients.

Sensation: Some patients have complaints of diminished feeling of sensation partial or complete (rare) and numbness. Loss of other sensations–cold and warmth–although often demonstrable.

Muscle Wasting: Muscles which are innervated by the compressed nerve roots may show some degree of weakness and muscle wasting. For example compression of fifth lumbar nerve root may cause weakness in the extensor hallucis longus (EHL).

Deep Tendon Reflexes (DTRs): Loss of tendon reflex depends upon the severity of nerve root compression. Occasionally, the ankle jerk may be absent but even a slight reduction in the response to the threshold stimulus may be of significance.

Posture: The most common change in the lumbar spine is flattening of the lumbar curve, quite frequently noticeable even in relatively mild cases. Very rarely there may be an increase in lumbar lordosis.

Circumduction Test: Forward flexion of spine or circumduction away from the affected side may produce pain. This suggests lateral displacement of the nerve root. Flexion towards affected side does not stretch the root and is a movement of relative ease. A root stretched over the summit of the protrusion would give pain of flexion straight forwards, the more reliably the test indicates sideways displacement of the root. Straight leg raise test (SLR), Lasegue's test, Quadrant test may also be performed.

MANAGEMENT

There is a gradual resorption of the herniated disc without surgical intervention. The larger disc herniations were found to have more resorption. This favorable natural history shows why upto 75% of patients with confirmed, painful herniated discs recover without surgery within 6 months. These patients have found to have less recurrence rate than the patients who have managed with surgical intervention.

Box 27.2
"Cause of the cause": Unfortunately the sciatic nerve pierces the piriformis muscle in 10 percent population. Spasm and pain in the piriformis muscle is the most commonly associated with lumbar spine, sacroiliac and hip joint pathology. The piriformis muscle stabilizes the pelvis with increased motion in the sacroiliac joints or other forms of pelvic instability. Due to inflammation in the muscle, edema develops in the belly of muscle and passive external rotation will produce pain particularly at the end range as it stretches the tight muscle.

Relief of Pain: Sometimes in cases of insidious-onset, the gluteus medius muscle becomes weak; this may contribute to Trendelenburg gait and exacerbates the problem. After proper muscle testing, if the muscle is found weak it should be strengthened with resisted and closed kinetic chain exercises.

Cryotherapy for duration of at least 20 minutes may allow greater penetration and helps in healing of inflammation particularly in acute symptoms. Moist heat packs, shortwave diathermy, and interferential therapy may be advised to relieve pain and symptoms.

Bed Rest: Rest used to be the choice of the treatment in the past, but recent studies have shown that rest for more than three days has no healing effect but it encourages the muscle wasting. The compressive forces in the intervertebral disc decreases in lying and with the time, the nucleus potentially can absorb more water to equalize pressure. Lying with hip and knee flexion increases the intervertebral space posteriorly which allows accumulation of imbibed fluid in posterior increased space. The accumulated imbibed fluid in the posterior space increases the intradiscal pressure and produces pain and symptoms specially when patient rises from prolong bed rest. This is the reason that absolute bed rest is not recommended.

The Royal College's General Practice Guidelines state that prolong bed rest may lead to debilitation, chronic disability and increasing disability in rehabilitation. Advice to continue ordinary activity can give equivalent or faster symptomatic recovery from the acute attack and lead to less chronic disability and less time work than 'traditional' medical treatment with analgesics as required, advice to rest, and let pain be your guide for return to normal activity. Hence, bed rest should not be recommended for simple back pain.

Box 27.3
Lateral shift: Lateral shift is the lateral displacement of the trunk and shoulders in relation to the pelvis. Displacement of the trunk and shoulders to the right side is termed as right lateral shift. The lateral shift is most commonly associated with the disc herniation with acute radiculopathy. The patient shifts or bends the trunk and shoulder to the opposite of the radiculopathy. For example the patient with left acute radiculopathy will shift the trunk to the right side to avoid pressure and irritation on the nerve root. Sometimes the muscles may also produce lateral shift.
McKenzie has described a technique to correct the lateral shift. The extension exercise alone cannot correct the lateral shift, therefore, he has described the technique which is followed by spinal extension exercise. The patient stands with the elbow flexion, and therapist stands at the side opposite to the disc herniation. In case of left lateral shift the therapist stands to the right side of the patient. Therapist places his right shoulder under the elbow and wraps both the hands around the top of the opposite pelvis. A force couple is created by pulling the pelvis with both the hands and by pushing the trunk to the midline simultaneously. The purpose of the technique is to centralize the symptoms. In case patient reports improvement in the sign and symptoms the technique should be continued followed by spinal extension exercise.
Self correction of the lateral shift: In standing, in case of right lateral shift the patient places his right hand on the right rib cage and left hand on the top of left illium. Both hands pushes the trunk and pelvis simultaneously to the midline. **In side lying:** The patient lies on the affected side, and a small pillow or towel is placed under the thorax. Patient should remain in this position till the pain centralizes. **In prone lying:** The patient lies on the prone position and therapist creates a force couple in opposite direction and glides the pelvis and thorax towards the midline.

Seventy-five percent patients with prolapse intervertebral disc resolve spontaneously within six months. Only 5-10 percent patients with persistent radiculopathy (sciatica) require surgery. These patients have 10 times higher risk of developing subsequent disc herniation compared to the general public.

Ergonomics: The initial prevention of proplapsed intervertebral disc to further progression is the major part of the treatment. The patients with prolapse intervertebral disc are taught all the positions which aggravate and relieve the intradiscal pressure. Patient should be encouraged to use the position which produces least pressure on the intervertebral disc. The below mentioned positions are described in ascending order lowest disc pressure to highest pressure:

a. ***Supine with Knees Flexion and Supported on Pillows*** (Figs. 27.27a and b)*:* This position allows the iliopsoas muscles to relax and flattens the lumbar lordosis which decreases pressure on the intervertebral disc. In acute prolapsed intervertebral disc cases this is the choice of position which should be recommended during the bed rest. In supine the load produced by the body weight is eliminated.

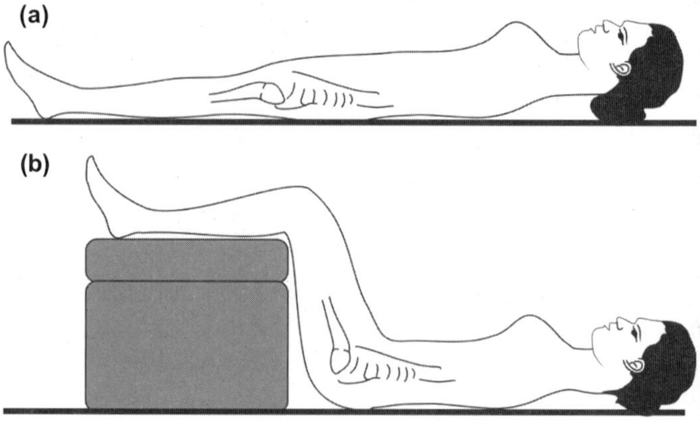

Figs. 27.27a and b: a. Supine with hip and knee at neutral b. Supine with hip and knee flexion supported on stool

b. ***Sitting with Back Rest to 90º:*** Initially when patient is moved from bed rest to sitting, it should be recommended only if the back rest support of the chair is inclined appropriately. Further placing a pillow under lumbar region reduces the intradiscal pressure. This is the ideal position for the patients with prolapse intervertebral disc who wants to attend office (Fig. 27.28). Erect sitting and sitting with forward bending increases the pressure on the nerve roots hence, it should not be advised.

c. ***Standing:*** Patients with prolapse intervertebral disc can be allowed to stand without any hesitation as this position produces 100% load on the intervertebral disc.

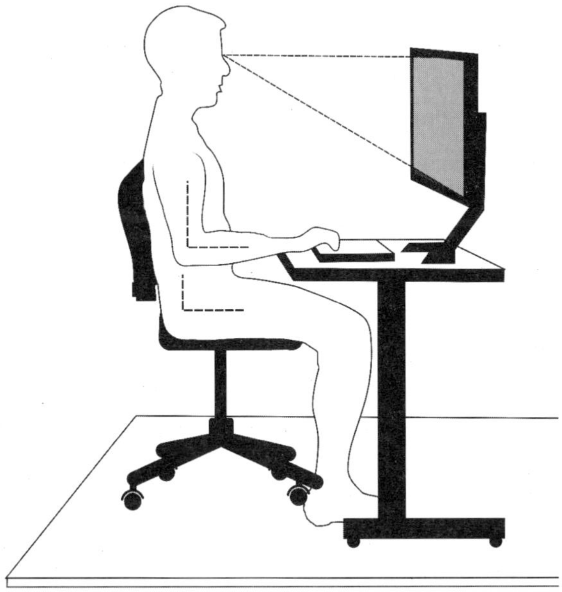

Fig. 27.28: "Ideal sitting" position

d. *Walking:* Moderate walking is safe and perhaps ideal therapeutic exercise for those with PIVD. If the speed of walking is increased from 90 steps/minute it further can increase the intradiscal pressure, therefore, walking should be advised but the speed should be limited to the normal cadence. The patient should be taught not to bend the trunk forward as it increases intradiscal pressure.

e. *Sitting:* The patients with prolapse intervertebral disc complaint pain, irritation and burning sensation in erect sitting because it increases the intervertebral disc pressure by 150%. The erect sitting should not be recommended as it may cause further disc prolapse.

f. Forward bending with weight lifting (Fig. 27.29).

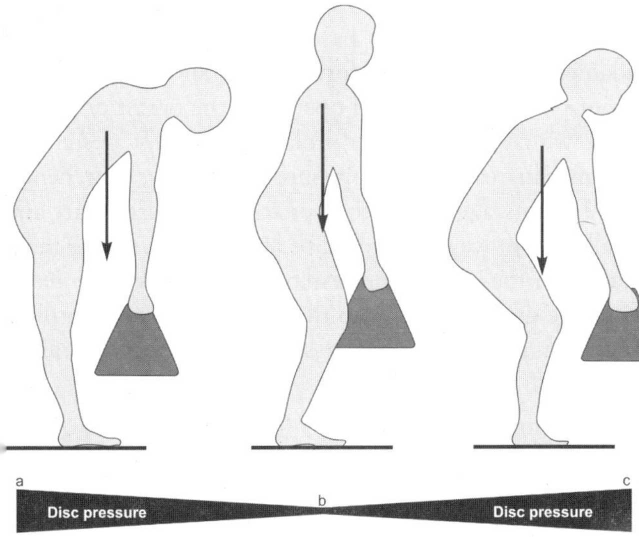

Fig. 27.29

Relative change in the pressure/load in the third lumbar disc in different positions in percentage (Figs. 27.30a and b).

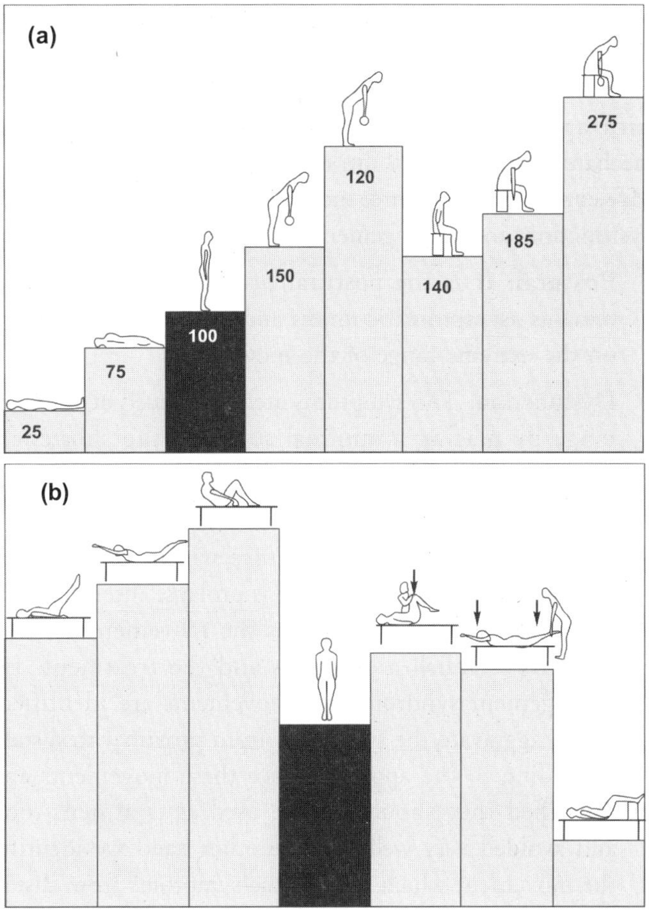

Figs. 27.30a and b

Therapeutic Exercises

As soon as patient finds improvement in the sign and symptoms exercises are started. Initially exercises which produce least pressure on the intervertebral disc should be started. These are progressed according to the improvement in pain and other symptoms of the patient. Some of the exercises can be initiated in the acute phase to decrease muscle spasm and increase range of motion.

Spinal Extension Exercises

In spinal extension the posterior part of the intervertebral space is compressed and the anterior part opens out. This tends to squeeze the nucleus pulposus anteriorly and reduces the protrusion/prolapse in the intervertebral disc posteriorly; for this reason spinal extension exercises are beneficial and safe for the patients with prolapse intervertebral disc. McKenzie has described spinal extension exercises as under:

McKenzie Method

McKenzie approach is not merely extension exercises. In its true sense, it is a comprehensive approach to the spine based on the principles and fundamentals that when understood and followed accordingly are very successful. In fact most remarkable, but least appreciated, is the McKenzie assessment process. Identification for the underlying disorders through objective findings and movements for each individual and then separating them with apparently similar presentations into definable mechanical syndromes is the key of the McKenzie approach. McKenzie has named three mechanical syndromes: Postural, dysfunction and derangement.

- **Postural:** It is the postural problem where patient remains asymptomatic unless and until a stress is given on the extreme range of the movement.
- **Dysfunction:** The symptoms are reproduced at the end range by placing a minimal stress, as the shortened structures ligaments and muscle get elongated.
- **Derangement Syndrome:** It is the anatomical disruption or displacement of the structure within the motion segment. The classical example is prolapse intervertebral disc. McKenzie approach uses the movements of the body to establish a diagnosis and the treatment. In derangement syndrome the movements are identified which aggravate the symptoms from proximal to distal. According to the approach once these movements are identified they should not be used as treatment tool and avoided very well. On the other hand we identify the movement which reduces the symptoms from distal to proximal. Such type of movements become the treatment tool and performed repeatedly. Increase in symptoms from proximal to distal is known as peripheralization, whereas, decrease in symptoms from distal to proximal is known as centralization. Movements which centralize the symptoms are performed repeatedly.

Derangement Classification

Derangement One

Central or symmetrical pain across L4/5.

Rarely buttock or thigh pain.

No deformity.

Derangement Two

Central or symmetrical pain across L4/5.

With or without buttock and/or thigh pain.

With deformity of lumbar kyphosis.

Derangement Three

Unilateral or asymmetrical pain across L4/5.

With or without buttock and/or thigh pain.

No deformity.

Derangement Four

Unilateral or asymmetrical pain across L4/5, with or without buttock and/or thigh pain and with deformity of lumbar scoliosis.

Treatment: The lateral shift is corrected first, once centralization has occur proceed as in derangement one.

Derangement Five

Unilateral or asymmetrical pain across L4/5, with or without buttock and/or thigh pain. Leg pain extending below the knee. No deformity.

Treatment: Extension principles applied. If response is slow, unilateral mobilisation/manipulation procedures are indicated.

Derangement Six

Unilateral or asymmetrical pain across L4/5, with or without buttock and/or thigh pain. Leg pain extending below the knee.

Treatment: If movements indicate the reduction is possible, treatment is commenced following the same methodology as for Derangement 4/5. After the acute episode has subsided, evaluate for nerve root adherence and treat flexion principle for nerve root adherence.

Derangement Seven

Symmetrical or asymmetrical pain across L4/5, with or without buttock and/or thigh pain, with deformity of accentuated lumbar lordosis.

Treatment: Correct deviation if present (flex in step standing). Progress to flexion in lying. Progress to flexion in standing.

McKenzie approach is based on sound principles and fundamental, for example forward flexion compresses the anterior part of the disc and opens out the posterior part of the disc which allows further prolapse of the disc posteriorly which may increase further pressure on the nerve root, hence, the symptoms aggravate from proximal to distal part and logically this movement should be avoided as it may damage further. On the other hand, extension compresses posterior part of the disc and opens up the anterior part, which plays important role in relieving symptoms from distal to proximal.

(a) ***Prone on Elbows:*** The intradiscal pressure in a prone position with upper body supported on the elbows can be decreased to 50% of the body weight. The exercise may be advised even in acute stage when the patient is on bed rest (Figs. 27.31a and b).

(a)

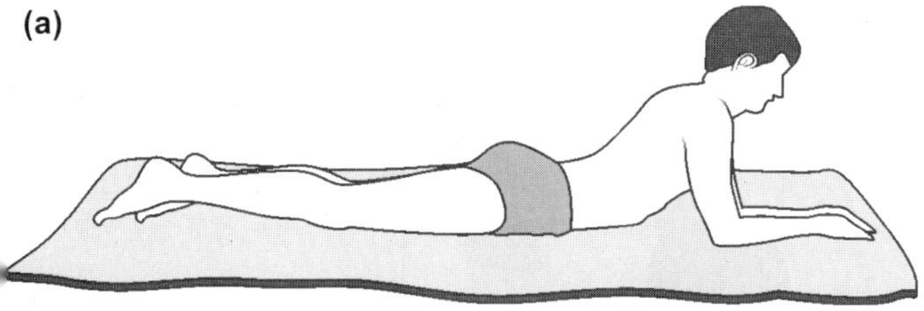

(b)

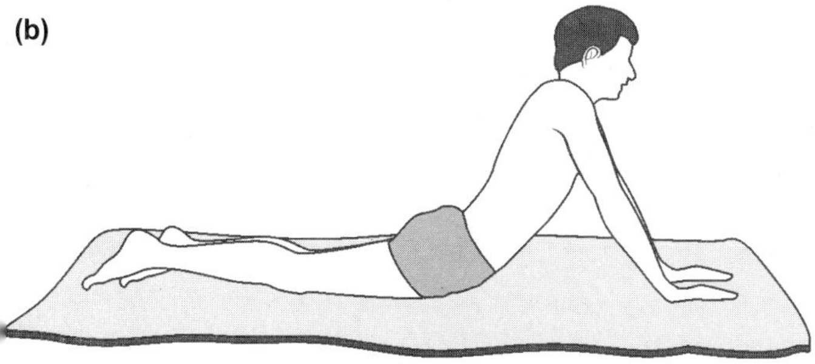

Figs. 27.31a and b

(b) Bridging: The extension of the lumbar spine in supine position with hip and knee flexed to 60°; has great benefit as it does not produce pressure on the intervertebral disc, instead of it helps in recovering from prolapse.

(c) Spinal Extension with Pillows under Abdomen: The placement of pillows under the abdomen in prone position can decrease the arch of the back and allows the disc to better resist stresses because the vertebrae are aligned with each other. Arching the back in prone position can greatly activate the erector spinae muscles but also produce such high stresses on the lumbar discs, which are loaded in an extreme position. Isometric contraction of erector spinae with pillows under the abdomen is the preferable position (Figs. 27.32a and b).

(a)

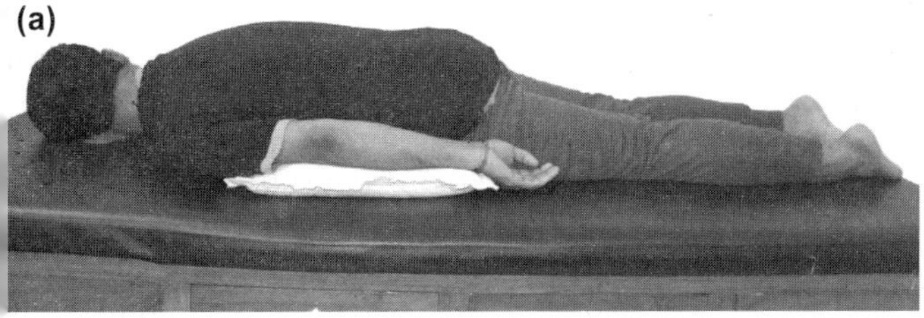

(b)

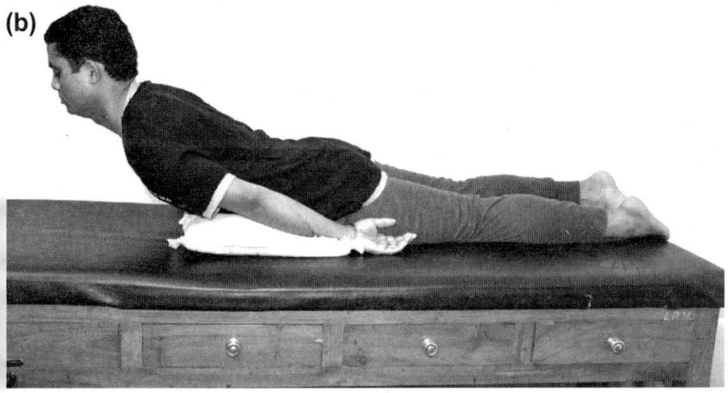

Figs. 27.32a and b: Spinal extension pillow under abdomen (a. starting, b. extension)

(d) Slump to Erect Sitting: Sitting with slight forward flexion with relaxed shoulder girdle is the slump position. When coming back to the erect sitting from slump allows strengthening of the erector spinae muscles especially upper back extensors.

Spinal Flexion Exercises: The extension exercises are progressed to flexion exercises as soon as patient achieves full range of motion in sagittal plane with minimal pain. These exercises should be progressed from the exercises which produce least intradiscal pressure to the highest intradiscal pressure. Flexion exercises are often advised to provide core stability following spinal extension exercises (Figs. 27.33 and 27.34).

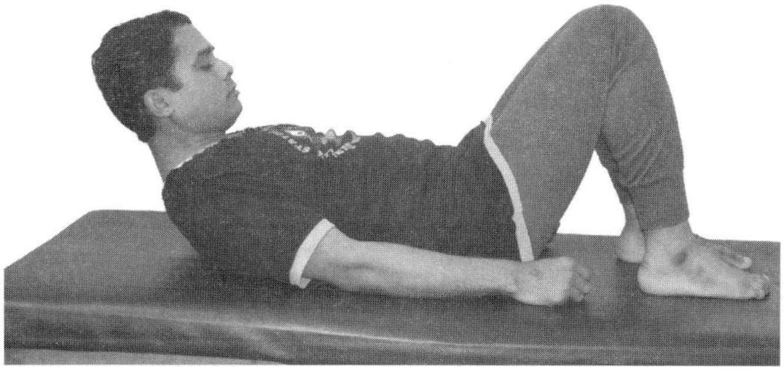

Fig. 27.33: Curl up

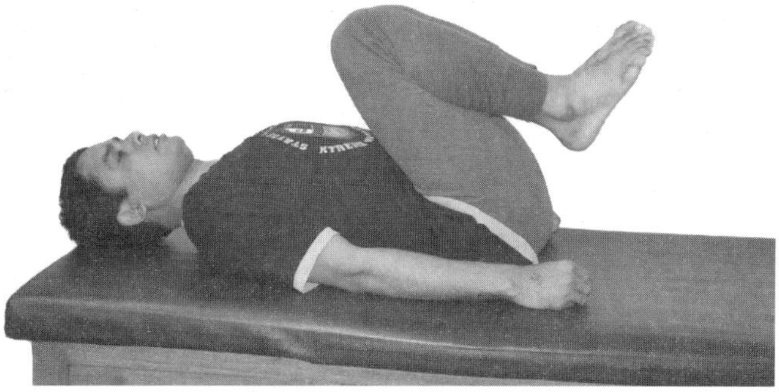

Fig. 27.34: Reverse curl up

(a) Curl up: This exercise is advised to strengthen the upper portion of rectus abdominis and external oblique muscles. In supine position with knees flexed to 90°, the head and shoulders are lifted off the plinth. The load on the lumbar spine remains minimal as the patient is allowed to clear the shoulder blades only minimizing the lumbar motion. A greater movement is produced by raising the arms or placing hands behind the head, as the center of gravity of the upper body shifts farther away.

(b) Twisting Curl up: The patient lies in supine position with one leg flexed to 90° and other leg (ankle) is placed on top of the flexed knee joint. Patient is asked to lift the head and off the shoulders from the plinth. Patient places both hands on the occiput and then turns to the opposite side of flexed knee joint.

(c) *Reverse Curl up:* Isometric reverse curl up performed, provides efficient training/strengthening of the lower abdominals, and produces moderate stresses on the lumbar discs.

Stretching Exercises: After significant reduction in pain and symptoms stretching of back extensors may be initiated. In supine position, the flexed knees are taken passively to the chest, and are repeated at least 25 times, thrice daily. This exercise is progressed to stretching in long sitting. In long sitting the patient is asked to touch the toes with the knees straight. In this position both hamstrings and back extensors are stretched. The exercise may be progressed to the standing with forward bending at knees extended (Figs. 27.35a and b, 27.36 and 27.37).

Stability of the Lumbar Spine: It can be achieved through several means: IAP, co-contraction of the trunk muscles core muscles strengthening external support and surgery.

Intra-abdominal Pressure (IAP): Intra-abdominal pressure is a mechanism that may contribute to both unloading and stabilization of the lumbar spine. IAP is the pressure created within the abdominal cavity by a coordinated contraction of the diaphragm, the abdominals and pelvic floor muscles. This creates an extension moment that lies the compression forces on the lumbar spine. The intra-abdominal pressure reduces the load on the intervertebral discs. Therefore, the patients with soft disc herniation should be encouraged to improve an IAP mechanism. The recent studies have shown that the transverse abdominis is the primary abdominal muscle responsible for intra-abdominal pressure generation.

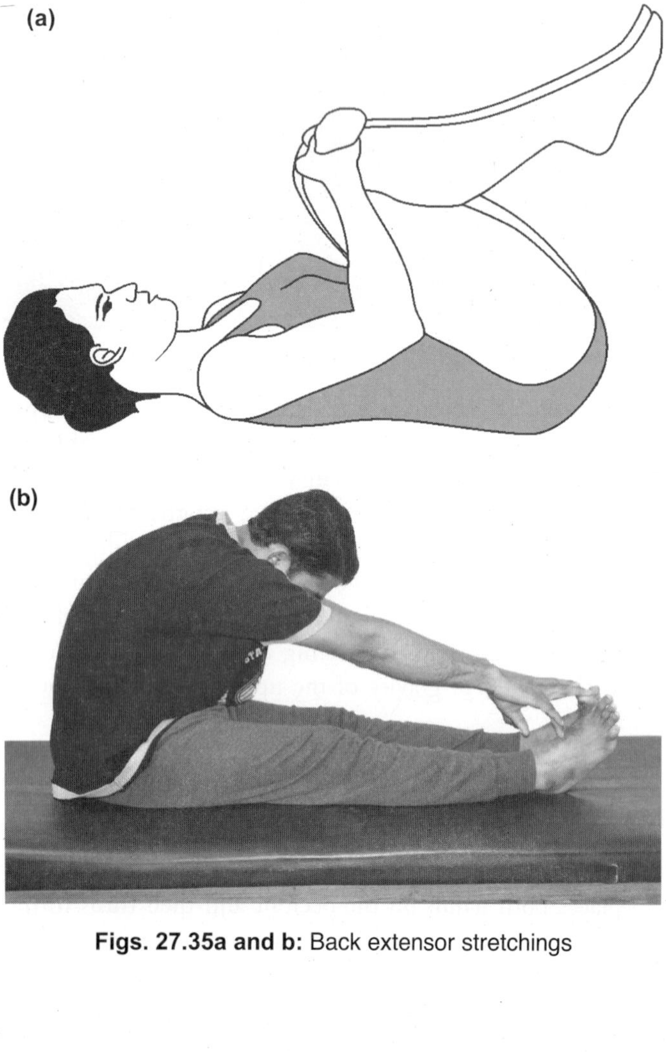

Figs. 27.35a and b: Back extensor stretchings

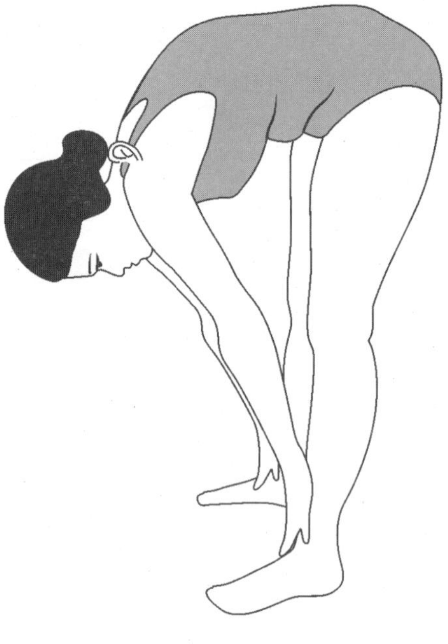

Fig. 27.36: Long sitting with toe touch

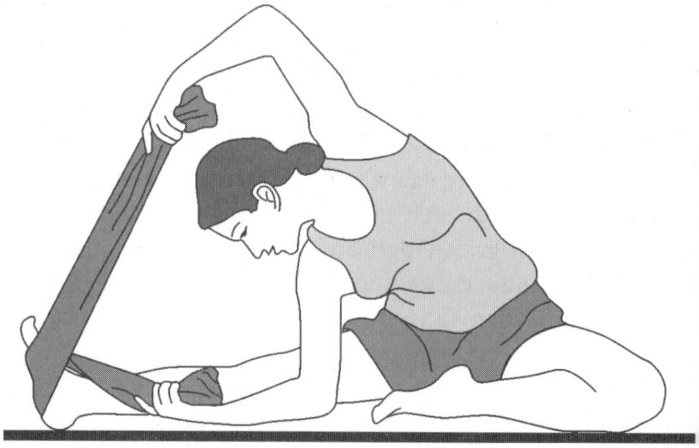

Fig. 27.37: Degenerated disc prolapsed (a) Annulus tear, (b) Circumferential tear, (c) Peripheral tear, (d) Radical tear, (e) Disc prolapsed

Stress Reduction: Emotional stresses can increase the tension in the muscle and interfere with or delay the recovery process. Try to eliminate stress as much as possible by placing non-urgent jobs on hold. Obtaining counselling for major life stresses and seeking support from family, friend or health providers.

Box 27.4: Disc Degeneration

Age: Disc degeneration can occur at any age, but it is more common in older discs, usually after forty years. As the age progressess the disc loses its water binding capacity and physical properties. There is a gross disruption of collagenous network (fibers). The disc becomes less resistant to the repeated stresses. In the process of degeneration, there is formation of tears and fissures in the annulus fibrosus and nucleus pulposus respectively.

A. **Annulus Tears:** There are three types of tears often occur in the degenerated annulus of the disc.
   (a) *Circumferential Tears:* These may represent the effect of interlaminar shear stresses, possibly arising from compressive stress concentration in older discs.
   (b) *Peripheral Rim Tears:* These are also known as 'rim lesions' consist of focal circumferential avulsions of the peripheral annulus. They are twice as common in the anterior annulus compared to the posterior, and typically affect the upper anterolateral margin of the disc. The peripheral tears may occur due to trauma.
   (c) *Radial Fissures:* These fissures commences from the nucleus and extends to the posterior or posterolateral. The radial fissures are associated with nucleus degeneration and with disc radial bulging but is not clear which comes first.

B. **Disc Prolapse:** In the process of degeneration there is formation of radial fissures of the annulus which may be associated with degeneration in the nucleus. The gross radial fissures allow the nucleus to migrate posteriorly or posterolaterally to the extent that the disc periphery is affected, then the disc is said to be prolapsed or herniated, which contains primarily the nucleus pulposus displaced down a radial fissure. The disc prolapse may be protrusion, extrusion or sequestration depending on the extent of migration of nucleus.

The degenerative process of disc has been divided into three stages with relatively destine findings:

Stage I: The first stage is dysfunction which is seen before the age of 45 and is characterized by circumferential and radial tears in the disc annulus and localized synovitis of the facet joints.

Stage II: It is the stage of instability which is common in patient between 35 and 70 years age. This stage is characterized by internal disruption of the disc, progressive disc resorption, degeneration of the facet joint with capsular laxity, subluxation and joint erosion.

Stage III: It is the stage of stabilization. The progressive development of hypertrophic bone around the disc and facet joints leads to segmental stiffening.

Adverse Effects of Bed Rest: In lying, intradiscal pressure decreases with time, the nucleus potentially can absorb more water contents to equalize pressure (imbibition). On the other hand, lying with flexed spine allows the imbibed fluid to accumulate posteriorly in the intervertebral disc where there is greater space. When patient stands, pain and symptoms from a disc protrusion are accentuated, as the accumulated fluid in the disc spaces will increase the intradiscal pressure. Therefore, to avoid exacerbating symptoms absolute bed rest during acute phase should not be advised. Bed rest for 1-2 days may be advised, but it should be interspersed with short intervals of standing.

Non-Weight Bearing Bias: The patients with soft disc herniation are often more comfortable with the traction and lying down. Because this relieves the load on the facet joints and also reduces pressure on the nerve roots by reducing the intradiscal pressure. For such patients traction and rest may be the choice of treatment until the patient feels comfortable in weight bearing. The patient is progressed to weight bearing as pain and healing improves.

Extension Exercise Bias: Patients with lumbar disc protrusion are often comfortable and may have partial or full relief with extension of the spine. The patients with extension bias often assume a flexed posture with or without side flexion. The impairment may be due to a contained intervertebral disc lesion, fluid stasis, a flexed injury or a muscle imbalance from a faulty flexed posture.

Therapeutic Modalities: SWD, MWD and moist heat therapy may also be beneficial in reduction of muscle spasm. Moist heat therapy is the most convenient and feasible modality which may be used at home also. These help in relieving pain and increasing flexibility and range of motion of the lumbar spine. Interferential Therapy at 80-100 Hz (analgesic effect) may also be advised for relieving pain and muscle spasm.

LUMBAR LATERAL SHIFT

Lumbar lateral shift is the lateral displacement of the trunk and shoulders in relation to the pelvis. According to Porter RW and Miller CG, 1986,[1] it is *undoubtedly associated with a disc protrusion* and associated with a poor prognosis for conservative management. This acute onset deformity is variously called a sciatic scoliosis or lateral shift (McKenzie RA, 1972),[2] trunk list Porter (RW, Miller CG, 1986),[1] acute lumbar/sciatic scoliosis (Weitz EM,1981)[3], *wind-sweptspine* (Grieve GP, 1981),[4] or lateral deviation (Cyriax J).[5] The lateral shift can either be to the ipsilateral (painful side) or contralateral side (away from the painful side). The majority of the discogenic patients will have contralateral lateral shift or away from the side of the pain (Fig. 27.38).

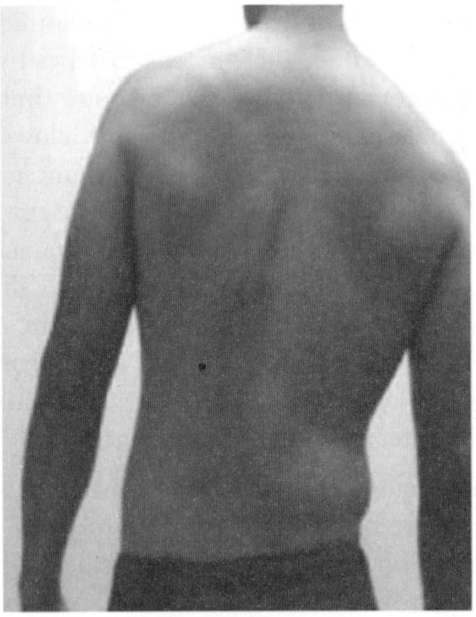

Fig. 27.38

The lateral shift may be explained either as avoidance of compression or irritation of a spinal nerve either actively or reflexively through muscle spasm (Falconer MA, McGeorge M4, Begg AC, 1948,[6] Grieve GP, 1983,[7] and White AA, III, Panjabi MM, 1990)[8] or as aberrant disk mechanics where a protrusion or herniation acts as a space-occupying phenomenon pushing the trunk away from the painful mass (McKenzie RA, May S, 2003,[9] Laslett M)[10] in a contralateral shift presentation or collapse of the upper vertebral body into a large annular fissure producing an ipsilateral shift presentation (Laslett M).

Many studies advocated that the prognosis of the lumbar lateral shift with the conservative treatment is poor. However, McKenzie has claimed that about 90% patients rapidly respond to the manual correction (McKenzie RA, 1972),[3] especially if the lateral shift is contralateral. McKenzie method of mechanical diagnosis and therapy (MDT) is one of the most common systems used in the management of spinal pain conditions.[11,12]

McKenzie has described a technique to correct the lateral shift. The patient stands with the elbow flexion, and therapist stands at the side opposite to the lateral shift. To correct the right lateral shift the therapist stands at the left side of the patient and places his shoulder under the elbow and wraps both hands around top of the opposite pelvis. A force couple is created by pulling the pelvis with both the hands and by pushing the trunk to the midline simultaneously. Both the pelvis and trunk is aligned towards midline. It is important not to exert the counterpressure at the level of the shoulder such that top-down lateral flexion movement is imparted. The impression the therapist and patient should have is that a lateral shearing motion is being imparted rather than anatomical lateral flexion. Initially, the applied pressure is gentle with rhythmic oscillations interrupted by pressure sustained for a few seconds. The therapist usually feels a solid resistance to the applied side gliding pressure at first, but over a period of time, which varies from case to case, the resistance appears to "soften" and a greater range of motion is achieved. This procedure is continued until all obstruction to the side gliding mobilization is cleared. Despite the patient's best efforts it is usual for the shift to return after leaving the clinic. Therefore, to maintain the corrected position of the lateral shift, the patient is instructed to carry out the lateral shift correction exercises at least every hour, or more often if the pain worsens, radiates away from the spinal midline, or there is an awareness of the shift returning (Mak Laslett).[1]

Once full correction of the lateral shift is achieved, the second component of the procedure follows.

Case Report

A case report published on Journal of Manual and Manipulative Therapy in 2009 conducted by Mark Laslett described examination and manual correction using the method first described by McKenzie in a patient with a large right-side contralateral shift. A 41-year-old athletic male of Chinese descent, worked as a manager of a company and was a high-level martial arts participant actively engaged in teaching. He presented with acute left-sided low back pain three days after the onset of pain during a vigorous karate training session.

The pain was confined to the left mid and lower lumbar spine without somatic or radicular pain referred into the buttock or lower extremity. The pain was aggravated by forward bending, sitting, walking, coughing and sneezing and it disturbed his sleep. Rising from chairs was especially painful and difficult. Standing still and lying down provided the best relief. Range of motion was not measured goniometrically, but movements in all directions were severely restricted by pain, except right lateral flexion and right *side gliding in standing* (MDT assessment of lateral flexion of the lower lumbar spine), which appeared normal.

According to the MDT classification system, the acute onset of a contralateral lateral shift and painful obstruction to motions attempting to correct the shift and restore extension lead to a provisional diagnosis of mechanical derangement[14-16] of lumbar discogenic pain was reasonable. The radiculopathy was ruled out as there was no sign and symptoms of numbness, muscle weakness and absent tendon reflexes.

The patient was instructed to avoid any lumbar flexion in any position, twisting or lateral flexion towards the lateral shift, and avoid asymmetrical standing with decreased weight bearing of the leg on the side of pain. Sitting was also avoided in the first few days as much as possible, however, for the activities of daily living it was not restricted.

The patient was initiated with side gliding manual technique to correct the lateral shift as mentioned above. This was followed by lumbar extension in the prone position, then standing. The patient was instructed to continue the home exercise program of two hourly side gliding and extension exercises but to add ten supine flexion (knee to chest) exercises. Before doing the flexion exercises, he was to check that no obstruction to self-correction of the lateral shift or lumbar extension had recurred. Immediately after the flexion exercises, he was to carry out lumbar extension and side gliding exercises to ensure that no recurrence of obstruction to extension or of lateral shift had developed with the flexion exercises. In the event of recurrence, he was to cease the flexion exercises and return to the shift correction and extension protocol.

In this case, correction of the lateral shift was achieved rapidly and the increase in pain experienced with the first corrective movements quickly diminished and ceased. On the third day following the initial treatment, the patient was assessed as clinically stable. Thirteen days after the initial consultation, he was reviewed again and assessed his recovery as 90% of full painless function at that time.

Mechanical Diagnosis and Treatment (MDT): A Case Study

The McKenzie Method of Mechanical Diagnosis and Therapy (MDT) is an internationally acclaimed method of assessment and treatment for spinal and extremity pain developed by New Zealand physiotherapist Robin McKenzie. It has been widely used all over the world for more than 30 years. MDT is a philosophy of active patient involvement and education that is trusted and used by clinicians and patients all over the world for back, neck and extremity problems. This approach continues to be one of the most researched physical therapy based methods available. Repeated motion testing is the hallmark of the mechanical diagnosis and treatment (MDT) system for patients with non-specific low back pain (LBP). This system has demonstrated reliability, especially when utilized by credentialled practitioners (Busanich B, Verscheure S, 2006, Hefford C, 2008, Werneke, 1999 and Kilpikoski, 2002.[17-20]

A case study conducted by Bryan Williams *et al.*[21] (2011) included a 40-year-old patient with a diagnosis of a large L5-S1 disc herniation and left S1 radiculopathy. It was worse when she bent forward, climbed stairs, or would lie prone. She noted that standing, sitting and walking would inconsistently increase her pain. Pain regularly disturbed her sleep and it was generally worse early in the morning. She reported a positive Valsalva sign; worse with coughing, sneezing, and during bowel movements. The pain was located in the left buttock and posterior thigh with paresthesia, which she scored 6/10 on the visual analog score.

The therapist used MDT examination system to evaluate the patient. Her posture was modestly slouched and featured a notable reduction of lumbar lordosis. No frontal plane was discernible. Her straight leg raise on the left was positive at 30°. This test produced concordant pain into the left lower extremity. There was no sensory deficit present. Range of motion especially extension was restricted. The lower extremity pain aggravated by extension, flexion, and side gliding to the right. The side gliding to the left abolished the buttock pain almost completely of the patient but the same aggravated after eight repetitions. Based on the findings and examination the therapist seemingly uncovered a relative lateral component in a patient with no apparent lateral shift. In the MDT system, the provisional classification for this patient is a unilateral/asymmetrical, above-knee derangement.

Intervention

Therapist chose frontal and transverse plane exercises for this patient as the movements in the sagittal plane aggravated the symptoms. The side glide movement in the standing relieved the symptoms but aggravated after eight repetitions, therefore, non weight bearing position is chosen for the exercises. The patient is placed in a left side lying (the affected side) with a pillow under the lumbar spine. Transverse plane movements towards right side performed. The combined movements of side glide towards the left and rotation towards the right side abolished the patient's pain completely and restored considerable range of motion in the sagittal plane when the patient was tested again in the standing position. The patient was sent home with instructions and a single home exercise, replicating the repeated right rotation in left side lying 6-8 times a day. The patient returned after three days only with minimal stiffness in the morning. Her range of motions improved much. Any pain she experienced was readily manageable by herself doing the repeated rotation in side lying. On the second visit she was assessed for the sagittal motion in prone on elbows and initiated sagittal loading strategy with the figure of four position. The patient was instructed to avoid flexion in the sagittal motion as this movement peripheralized the symptoms (Fig. 27.39).

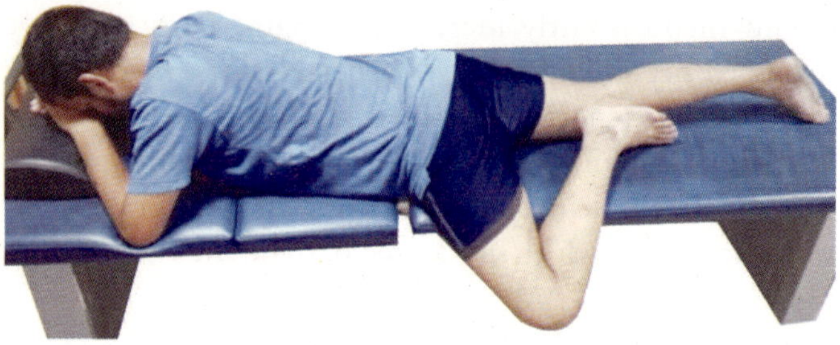

Fig. 27.39

At visit 3, 4 and 5 (1, 4 and 5 weeks after the initial visit) the patient demonstrated significant improvement in the sign and symptoms. At the sixth and final visit (six weeks since the initial evaluation), the patient was able to extend the lumbar spine in standing with no pain.

CORE STABILITY

Core stability is the combination of global and local stability system. The global stability system involves the larger and superficial muscles such as rectus abdominis, paraspinals and obliques. The local stability refers to the deep intrinsic muscles such as the transverse abdominis and multifidus. The global stability system provides mobility whereas local stability system provides segmental stability to the lumbopelvic region. Weakness of the muscles of these systems can grossly cause the loss of stability and mobility of not only the proximal (lumbopelvic) region but also the distal region (extremities). A comprehensive strengthening program of core muscles will *not only prevents injuries* but also improves the performance of the athletes who participate in sports activities.

Core muscles provide stability and mobility mainly to the lumbopelvic joints which involves the intervertebral sacroiliac and hip joints and it also *encompasses the scapulothoracic* junction. The mobility and stability of the lower extremities depend upon the core stability. For example weakness of the abdominals allows the pelvis to rotate anteriorly which causes tightness of the quadriceps and produces anterior knee pain. Anterior knees pain can cause adverse effects on the stability of the knee joint (lower extremity).

Evaluation of the Core Stability

Evaluation of muscles of lumbopelvic region before *commencing strengthening*, should be the prime objective, because it helps in determining the area where the therapist and patient needs to work more. The functional movement screen (FMS) test which *involves stepping, lunging, squatting, striding, reaching, anterior posterior core stability* are used in evaluating the core stability.

a. **Biering–Sorenson Extensor Endurance Test:** (Fig. 27.40)

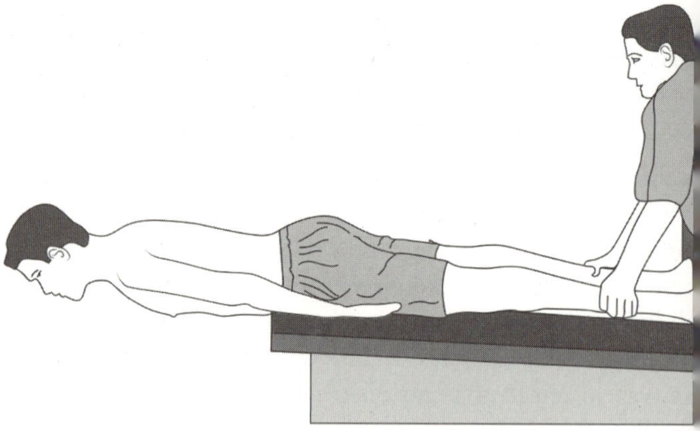

Fig. 27.40: Extensor endurance test

Position of Patient: Prone with trunk off the table.

Position of Therapist: Standing at the side of the feet of the patient, places both the hands on calves.

Procedure: The patient is asked to maintain the upper torso paralleled to the plinth (floor) time is recorded till the patient maintains the position. Once the patient falls below the level of plinth the test is completed and time is recorded.

b. **Flexor Endurance Test:** (Figs. 27.41a and b)

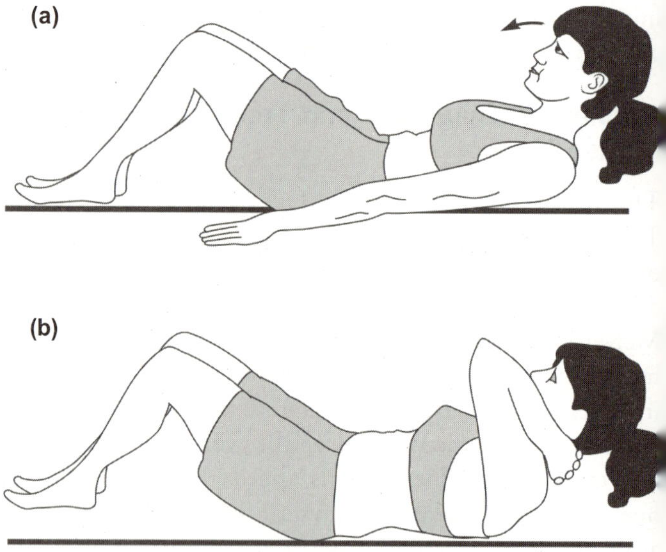

Figs. 27.41a and b: Flexor endurance test

Position of Patient: Sitting inclined with 55° angle. Hands placed on the opposite shoulders. Hips at 30° and knees flexed to 90°.

Position of Therapist: Standing, stabilizes the ankle and legs.

Procedure: The back rest removed and patient is asked to maintain the position. If patient can maintain the position without touching the back to the table (the flexors strength is considered as good). Abdominal endurance can also be tested in supine position with both the hip and knees flexion to 90 degrees. Endurance is considered fair if the subject can lift the head and shoulders ten times with both the hands at side. Endurance may be considered good if the subject clears the shoulder blades off of the ground ten times with both hands clasped behind the neck.

c. **Lateral Endurance Test:** (Fig. 27.42)

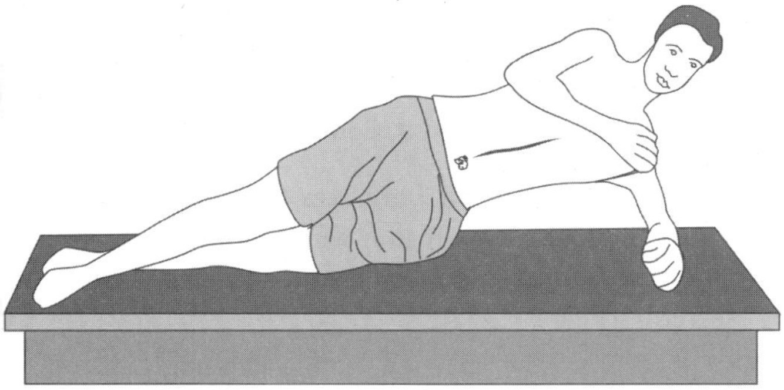

Fig. 27.42: Lateral endurance test

Position of Patient: Side lying. Top foot is placed in front of the bottom foot. The body rests on the elbow. Top hand may be placed on the opposite shoulder.

Procedure: The patient takes the hips off the plinth, so that the body comes in a straight line. The lateral stability is considered poor if the patient finds difficulty in lifting the hips.

d. **Normal Firing Pattern of the Pelvis** (Fig. 27.43)

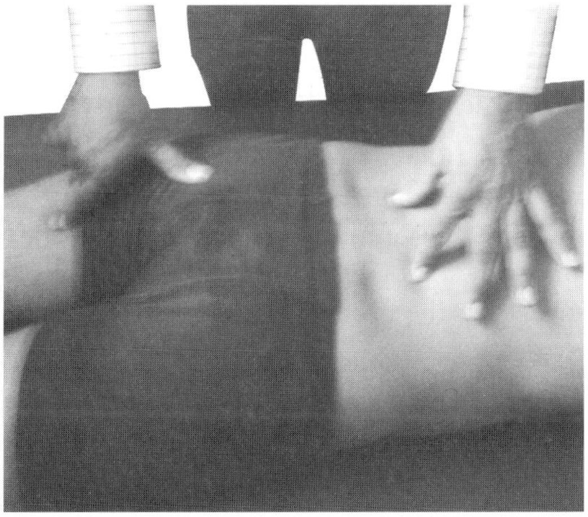

Fig. 27.43

Position of Patient: Prone lying with adequate exposure of gluteus maximus, erector spinae and hamstrings muscles.

Position of Therapist: Stands at the side, facing the lumbosacral spine. To test the left gluteus maximus therapist stands at the left side, places thumb and index finger of left hand on erector spinae of each side. The right hand thumb is placed on the gluteus maximus and little finger on the hamstrings of the same side.

Procedure: While maintaining the position of hands patient is asked to extend the left hip joint. In normal firing pattern contralateral erector spinae will fire first, followed by the ipsilateral gluteus maximus, ipsilateral erector spinae and hamstrings. If the ipsilateral erector spinae fires before the gluteus maximus this indicates an inhibited gluteus maximus.

[*Normal Firing Pattern:* Contralateral erector spinae, ipsilateral gluteus maximus, ipsilateral erector spinae and hamstrings.]

Inhibited Gluteus Maximus: Contralateral and ipsilateral erector spinae, gluteus maximus and hamstrings.

e. **Overhead Squat Test (Global Assessment Test):** It is the full body functional analysis test which tests the total kinetic chain, neuromuscular efficiency, integrated–functional strength, dynamic flexibility and involves a degree of muscular fatigue, that is why the test is known as global assessment test (Fig. 27.44).

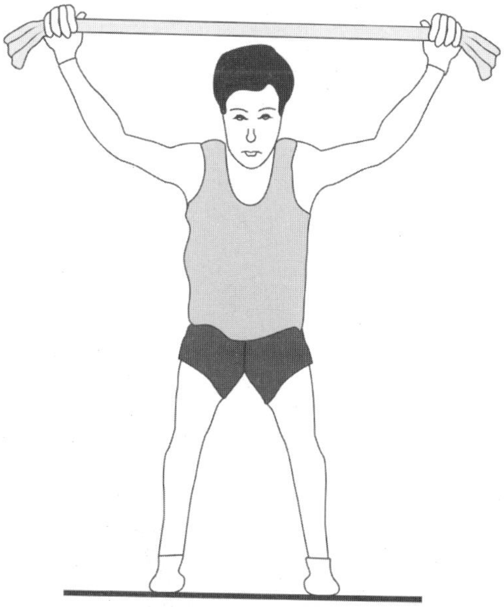

Fig. 27.44: Overhead squat test

Position of Patient: Standing with feet and shoulders (shoulders abduction 120°) apart.

Position of Therapist: Standing behind the patient, walks around during the test. Checks the feet, knees, lumbar curve, arm movement, chin elevation and stomach protrusion.

Procedure: The patient is asked to slowly squat down to a comfortable position for 6-15 repetitions.

Deviations: In case of lower crossed syndrome feet flattened, toes flaring out, knees buckling inward, and low back arching are the common deviations. These may be unilateral or bilateral.

Core Strengthening

The core stabilizers are strengthened in different positions. The exercises are progressed from minimal load to maximum load as the symptoms improve. Exercise which exacerbates the symptoms should not be performed.

Crunch or Curl up: Crunch exercises are designed to strengthen the abdominals as strong abdominals can unload the lumbar spine stress. The exercises are started with one knee flexed and other leg remains extended. The head and shoulder blades are lifted off the plinth and the hand position is changed as the crunch exercises progress. Every position is held up to 6 seconds to allow optimal contraction of the abdominals. 10 repetitions of three sets may be performed at a session (Figs. 27.45a to e).

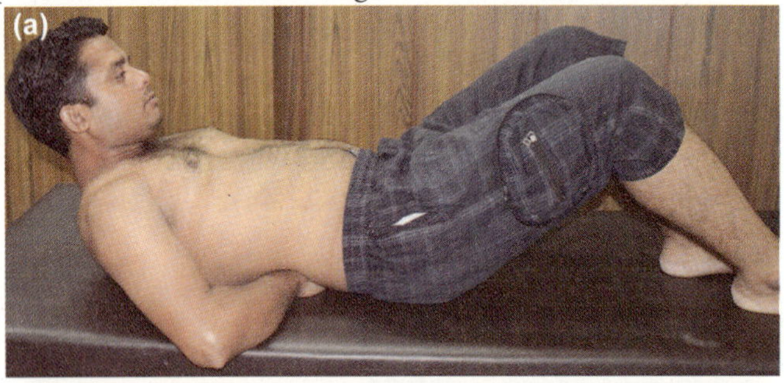

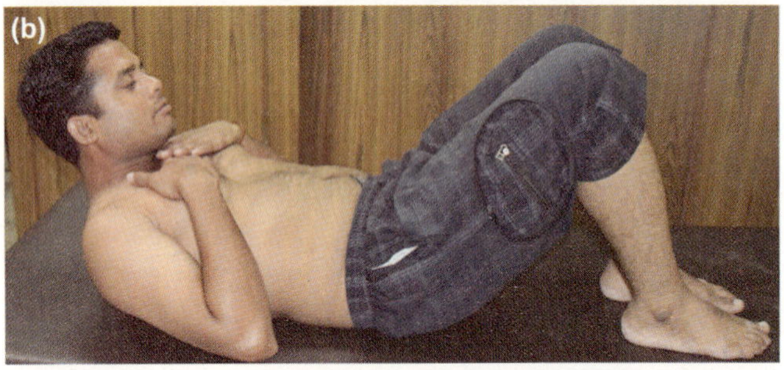

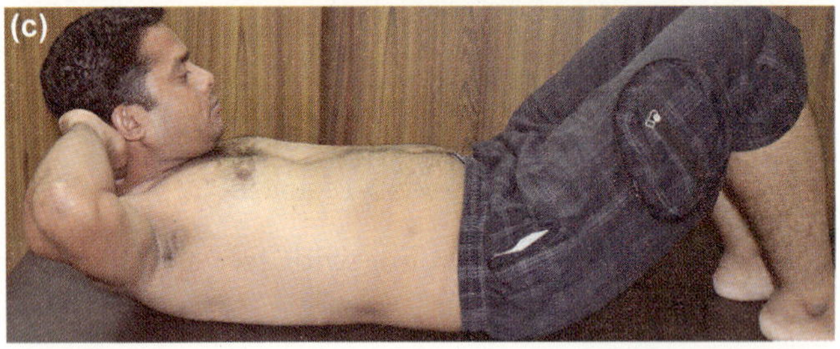

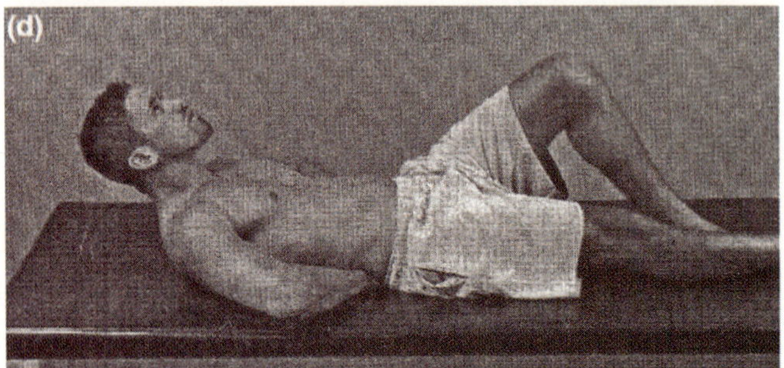

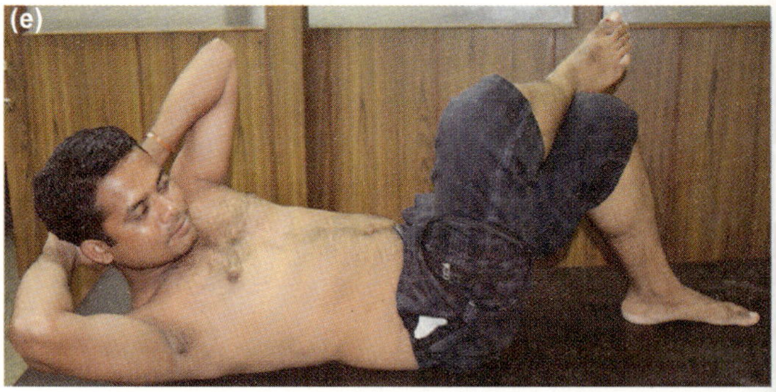

Figs. 27.45a to e: Curl up exercises

a. A supine with one or both legs flexed to 90°. Hands under the lower back region with elbows on the plinth. The head and shoulder blades lifted off the plinth for 6 seconds (Fig. 27.45a).
b. Supine with both legs flexed and hands on the chest. The head and shoulder blades lifted off the plinth for 6 seconds (Fig. 27.45b).
c. Supine with both legs flexed, head and shoulder blades lifted off the plinth, the hands are placed on the occipital region. The position is held for 6 seconds (Fig. 27.45c).
d. Supine with both legs flexed, hands placed under the lower back region with elbow lifted off the plinth. The head and shoulder blades lifted off the plinth for 6 seconds (Fig. 27.45d).
e. Supine with one leg flexed and other is raised and placed on the top of it. Both hands are placed on the head. The patient lifts head and one shoulder to opposite of the raised leg (Fig. 27.45e).

Planks: Plank exercises are designed to improve endurance and strength of the abdominal wall and the extensors including multifidus. The patient is positioned prone on elbows and then trunk, legs and arms are lifted alternatively off the ground as the planks progress (Figs. 27.46a to e).

a. Prone on elbows (90° flexed) with hips off the plinth weight is taken on the elbows, knees and toes (Fig. 27.46a).
b. Prone on elbows (90° flexion) with hip and knees off the plinth, weight is taken on the elbows and toes (Fig. 27.46b).
c. Prone on elbows, weight is on the elbows and toes. One leg is raised to the level of hip joint (Fig. 27.46c).
d. Prone on elbows, weight is on the elbows and toes. One arm is raised to the level of shoulders (Fig. 27.46d).
e. Both the legs placed on the medicinal ball and the weight of upper body is taken on the hands (Fig. 27.46e).

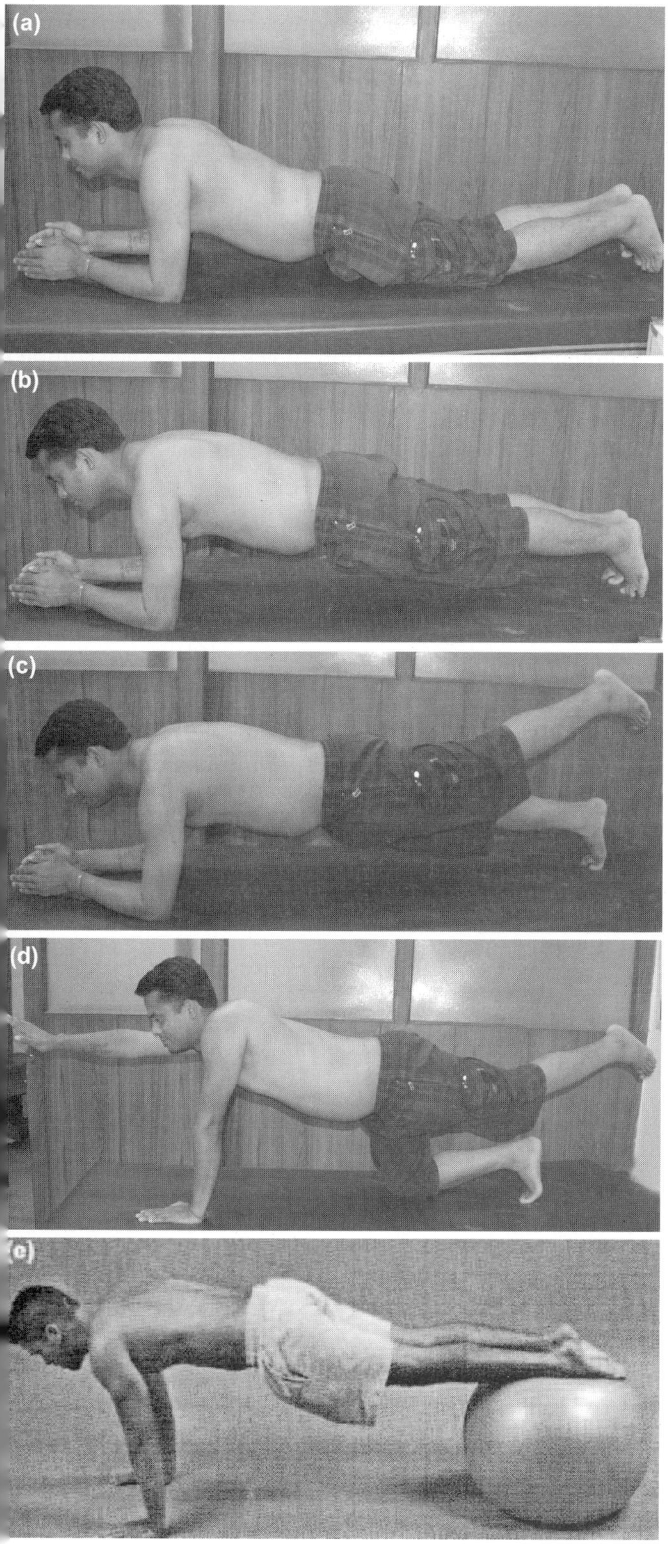

Figs. 27.46a to e: Planks

Birddog (Four-Point Kneeling) Exercises: The four-oint kneeling exercise is designed to strengthen the large umber of the core muscles such as transverse abdominis ıultifidus, internal and external obliques, gluteus maximus, rector spinae and quadratus lumborum. All exercises ommence from quadruped position and progressed to the aising of arm and leg alternatively (Figs. 27.47a to e).

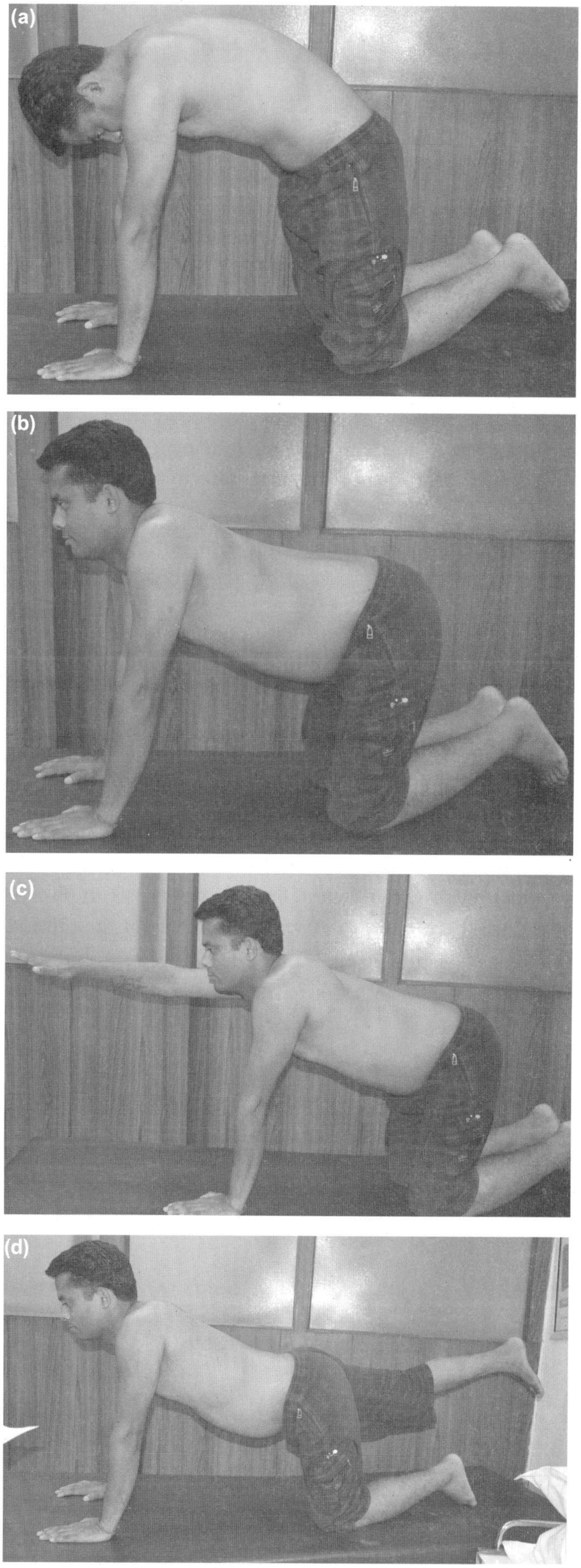

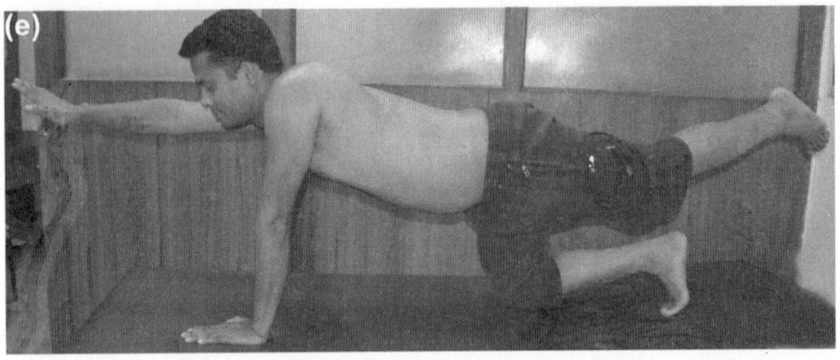

Figs. 27.47a to e: Birddog exercises

a. Quadruped position with forward flexion of the spine-camel position (Fig. 27.47a).
b. Quadruped position with extension of the trunk-cat position (Fig. 27.47b).
c. Quadruped position with trunk at neutral, one arm is raised to the level of shoulder joint for 6 seconds (Fig. 27.47c).
d. Quadruped position with trunk in neutral position, one leg is raised to the level of hip joint for 6 seconds (Fig. 27.47d).
e. Quadruped position with trunk in neutral position, left arm and right leg is raised upto the level of trunk. This is followed by right arm and left leg raising (Fig. 27.47e).

Dead Bug: Dead bug exercises are also designed to recruit the muscle fiber of rectus abdominis, external oblique, internal oblique, upper and lower extremities. The exercises are performed on mat in supine (hook) lying. The legs and arms are moved alternatively to allow the contraction of the muscles. The weight cuffs can also be added (to the patient) to increase the activity of the muscles (Figs. 27.48a and b).

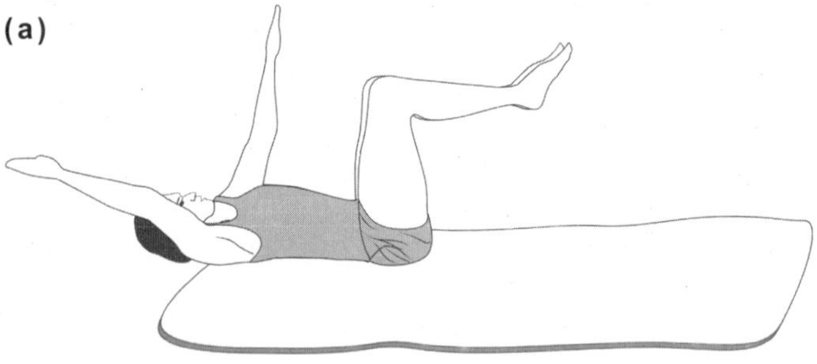

Figs. 27.48a and b: Dead bug exercises

a. Hook lying with alternate movement of the arms and legs (Fig. 27.48a).
b. Hook lying with cuff tied on the ankle joint and hands. Alternate movement of legs and arms (Fig. 27.48b).

Overhead Squat: The exercise is recommended to the athletes as it challenges and integrates all aspects of the core such as hip, trunk and shoulders. The exercise should not be recommended to the older patient with patellofemoral osteoarthritis as it increases the patellofemoral ground reaction forces on the knee complex (Figs. 27.49a to d).

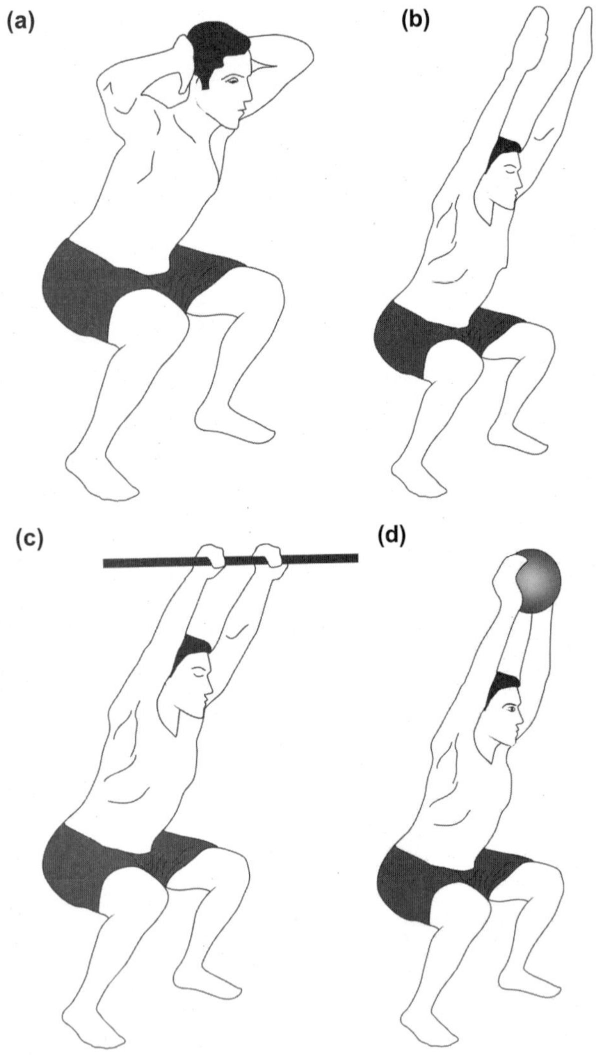

Figs. 27.49 a to d: Overhead squat

a. In standing both the hands are placed on the occipu[t] and the patient squats. The exercise should start wit[h] mini squat and progressed to half squatting. In case o[f] pain and other symptoms the exercise should b[e] discontinued.
b. In standing both the hands are raised over the head an[d] the same procedure is repeated.

c. In standing, a rod is held with both the hands over the head and the same procedure is repeated.

d. In standing, a football sized ball is held with both the hands over the head and the same procedure as above is repeated.

Transverse Abdominis Strengthening

The patient lies supine with the knees flexed. The therapist instructs the patient to pull the umbilicus in towards the spine. The exercise is repeated atleast 20-30 times thrice daily. The exercise is progressed in sitting position after significant improvement in the strength. Finally the exercise is progressed to the prone position. A tennis ball is placed under the umbilicus. Therapist instructs the patient to draw the umbilicus up and in towards the spine, attempting to lift the stomach off the tennis ball, without moving the pelvis.

Abdominal Hollowing versus Abdominal Bracing

Abdominal hollowing is the exercise in which tummy is taken in or the umbilicus is drawn up and in at the neutral position of the lumbar spine. This exercise coactivates the transverse abdominis and the internal oblique muscles and contributes to the lumbar spine stability, therefore, exercise is also known as core stabilizing exercise. Unfortunately this exercise activates only two muscles and does not activate the muscles to high enough levels to cause a training effect in healthy individuals.

On the other hand abdominal bracing is the contraction of all the abdominal muscles that constitute the abdominal wall. In this exercise the tummy is neither drawn in or taken out, the abdominals are contracted at the neutral position in a similar situation like a boxer tightens his muscles when other boxer is about to hit the abdomen wall. The abdominal bracing is believed to be superior to the abdominal hollowing in terms of recruiting more muscles while performing more challenging dynamic stability exercises. It also provides more stability to the spine during rapid perturbations.

There was much debate over effectiveness of these exercises. It is concluded that both the exercises are effective in spinal stability, but the abdominal hollowing exercise is more effective in the acute stage when pain is the concerned because it increases the abdominal pressure and in turn decreases intra-discal pressure. As the pain improves the abdominal hollowing exercise should be progressed to the abdominal bracing.

LUMBAR FACET SYNDROME

Facet syndrome is one of the major causes of low back pain which contributes 15% to 40% to the chronic back pain. Approximately 80% of patients with facet syndrome have association with prior disc disease. Pain comes suddenly with the history of trauma such as lifting weight with a sound of click in posterior pillars; which may radiate upto the buttocks but not below the knees. The pain aggravates in extension and rotation of the lumbar spine and may be by lumbar flexion.

Clinical Features

Pain is usually felt directly over the affected facet joints and referred to the buttocks, groin, and lateral and posterior thigh. Tenderness may be elicited over the affected facet joint. In majority of patients it is of diffused type. Patients with facet hypomobility often report increased pain in extension and prolonged periods of inactivity like sitting or standing.

Mechanism

The superior facet articular surface moves up and forward on the inferior facet articular surface during lumbar flexion. Lifting of heavy objects causes excessive opening of the superior facet articular surface. When the person returns to the neutral position from the lumbar flexion with the object, the superior facet articular surface fails to slide backward and downward on the inferior facet articular surface, and stucks in a particular position. The facet joint is said to be malaligned. The muscles guard the facet joint by preventing the movements of that motion segment.

Minor capsule tear can originate at the level of the posterior facet joints due to injury or trauma. There is a malalignment or subluxation of the affected facet joint. The synovium is stressed and leads to synovitis. The facet joints become inflammed and cause pain, soreness and stiffness.

The lumbar facet syndrome occurs often with the intervertebral disc protrusion. There is a gradual resorption of the herniated disc with the time, but the facet malalignment remains untreated. Patient recovers with the sign symptoms of radiculopathy, but left with facet syndrome symptoms. The facet joints become inflammed and cause pain, soreness and stiffness.

Minor Intervertebral Derangement (MID) Theory: Maigne has given this theory and pointed out that the functional ability of the mobile segment depends ultimately upon the condition of the intervertebral disc. Therefore, even a minimal change in the height of intervertebral disc due to trauma or degeneration can produce apophyseal joint dysfunction which is a reflex cause of protective muscle spasm and pain in the corresponding segment, with loss of function. There is increased load on the posterior pillars (facet joints). Extension of the lumbar spine produces approximation of the facet joint with resultant pain. The flexion opens the compressed facet joints, resulting to relief in pain.

Types of Facet Restrictions

The facet restrictions are named according to the position in which the facet joint is stuck. There are two types of restrictions. It may be stuck/restricted either in flexion or extension position, combined with side flexion and rotation. In case, the facet joint is stuck in the flexed position, which limits extension of the lumbar spine, in other words it limits the closing of the facet joint, hence it is termed as closing restriction. If the facet joint is stuck in extension with side flexion and rotation it means the flexion will be limited, hence it is termed as 'opening restriction' (Fig. 27.50).

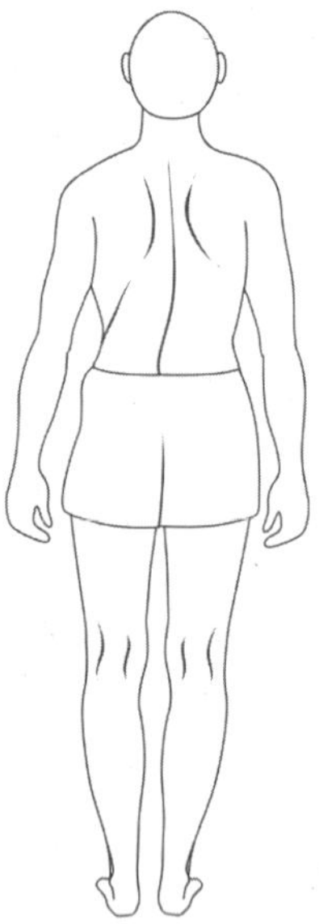

Fig. 27.50: Patient with facet joint restriction

1. **Opening Restriction:** The facet joint is stuck in extension, rotation and side flexion, so the segment has limited mobility in flexion, rotation and side bending.
2. **Closing Restriction:** If the facet joint is stuck in flexion combined with side flexion and rotation of the same side.

Management

Flexion Bias Exercises: This exercise is most commonly used in patients with facet syndrome. As per McKenzie approach the position or movement patterns that relieves the symptoms should be repeated. In these patients flexion exercise may act to reduce facet joint compression and provide stretch to lumbar musculature, ligaments and myofacial structures. The repeated flexion of lumbar spine in pain free range may centralize the symptoms in patients with facet syndrome. The cyclic range of motion exercises usually passive are the cornerstone of the McKenzie program.

Techniques for Opening Restriction

A. Left Side (L_4-L_5) Opening Restriction

Position of Patient: Left side lying.

Position of Therapist: Facing the patient.

Procedure: The therapist palpates the intervertebral space of L_4-L_5 with the right hand and flexes the hip and trunk with left hand. As soon as therapist feels the opening of L_4 and L_5 intervertebral space, he usually around 90° stops flexing the hip and spine further. The knees of the patient rest on the therapist thighs and the therapist holds the ankles of the patient with left hand. At the last step the therapist pulls the patient's feet and legs toward the patient's head, creating a side bending movement in the spine which opens the left facet joint of L_4 and L_5 and closes the right facet joint at L_4 and L_5 and improves the range of motion (Figs. 27.51a and b).

(a)

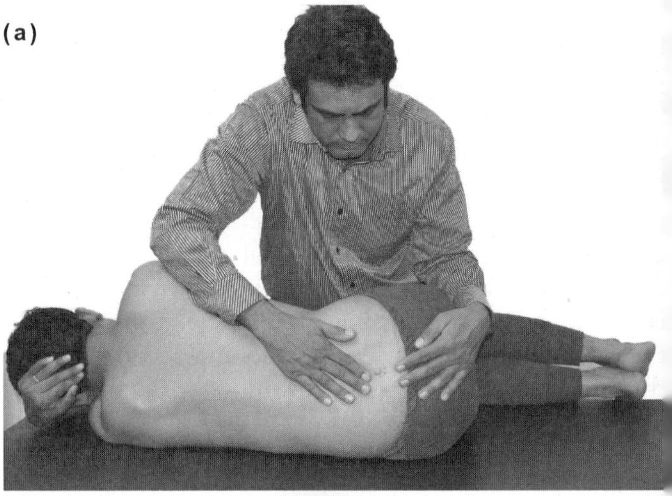

(b)

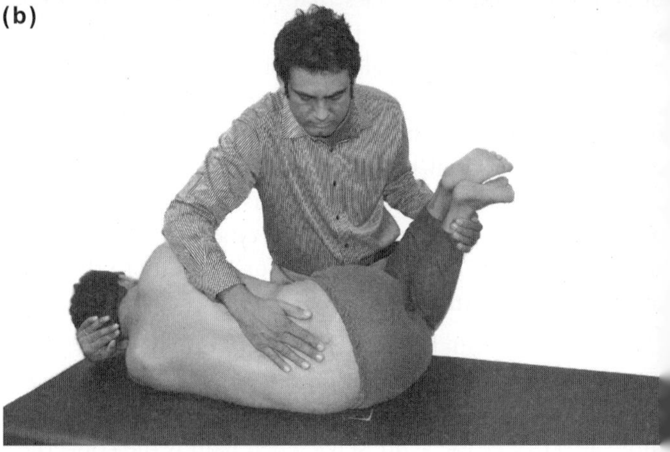

Figs. 27.51a and b: a. Left side lying with hip and knees flexion to 90°, therapist feels the opening of L_4/L_5 facet joint b. The spine is bent to the right by bringing the legs to the head to open the left L_4/L_5 facet joint

B. Both Sides (Left and Right Open Restrictions)

Position of Patient: Supine a towel roll is placed under the spine at the level of L_3. Hip and knees flexed to 100°.

Position of Therapist: Kneel standing on the plinth at the side of the patient (Fig. 27.52).

Procedure: The therapist places both the hands on the top of knees of the patient and applies downward force through the femur, creating motion at the lumbar spine. This opens both the facet joint at the level of L_3 and L_4 and increases the range of motion (Fig. 27.52).

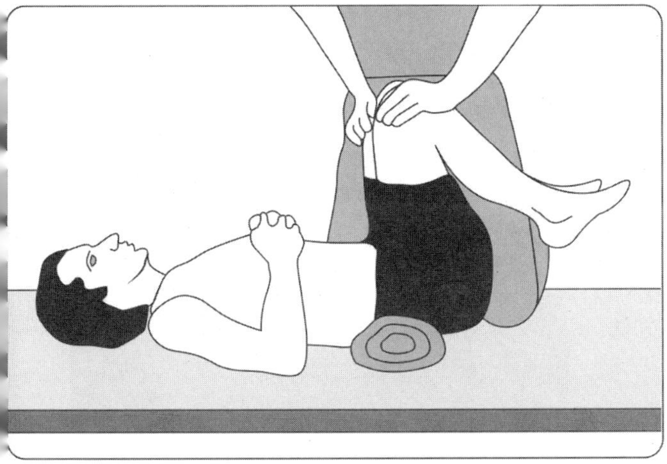

Fig. 27.52: Technique for opening restriction at left and right L_3/L_4 level

Techniques for Closing Restrictions

Common Complaints: Patient may have complaint of pain and stiffness with extension limitation.

A. **Left L_4-L_5 Level Closing Restriction**

The side flexion and rotation of the same side will be limited when patient attempts to extend the lumbar spine. Pain deviates to the opposite side of the restriction as the facet joint is stuck on that side and does not close as well as the other side.

Position of Patient: Prone with extension of the lumbar spine till the restriction starts. To maintain this position a wedge is placed under the chest of the patient. Arm rests on the wedge.

Position of Therapist: Therapist stands at the side of the patient.

Procedure: Therapist places pisiform aspect of the right hand on the spinous process of the restricted vertebra. Keeping the arms straight gentle rhythmic oscillations are applied through the arms to the vertebra (Fig. 27.53).

Note: The same procedure can be done by changing the position of wedge from chest to thighs. Rest of the procedure remains same (Fig. 27.54).

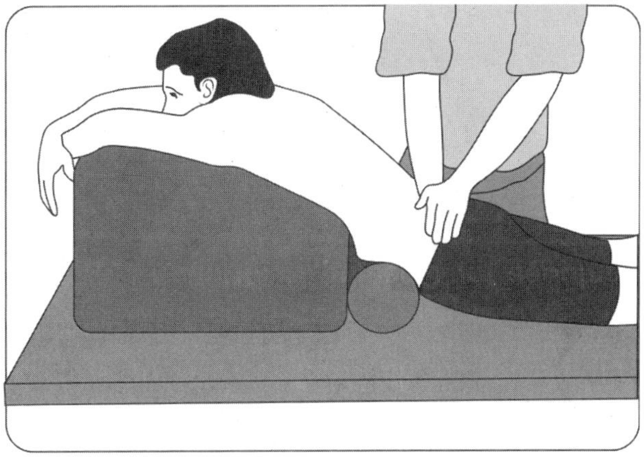

Fig. 27.53

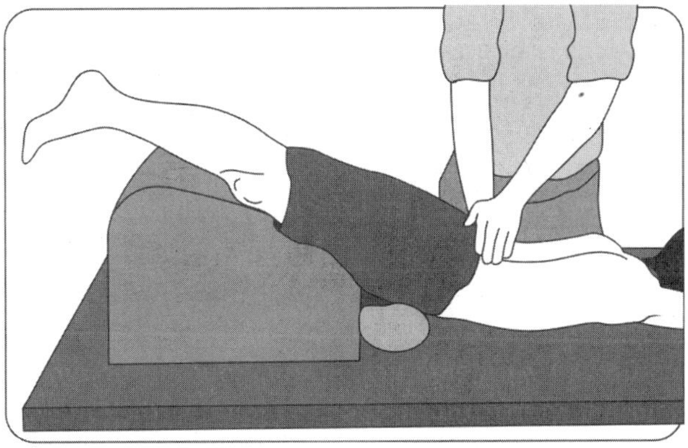

Fig. 27.54: Technique for closing restriction at L_4-L_5

B. **Physiological Mobilizations for Opening and Closing Restrictions at L_3-L_4 level**

Position of Patient: Side lying with upper most hip and knee flexed to 90-100°.

Position of Therapist: Standing facing the patient, places right arm under the axilla and right hand on the L_3-L_4 level. The therapist places left arm on the gluteal region and the fingers of left hand on the space between L_3-L_4.

Procedure: A force couple is applied through the hand creating rotation at the lumbar segment. Right hand pushes the chest backwards and left hand pulls the pelvis anteriorly. This creates a rotation on the desired segment (Figs. 27.55a and b).

(a)

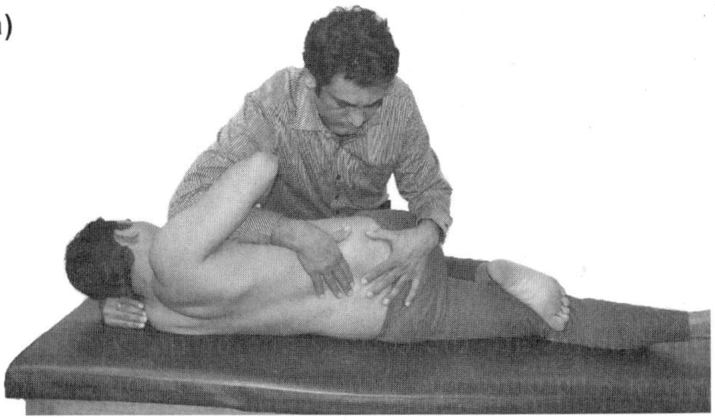

(b)

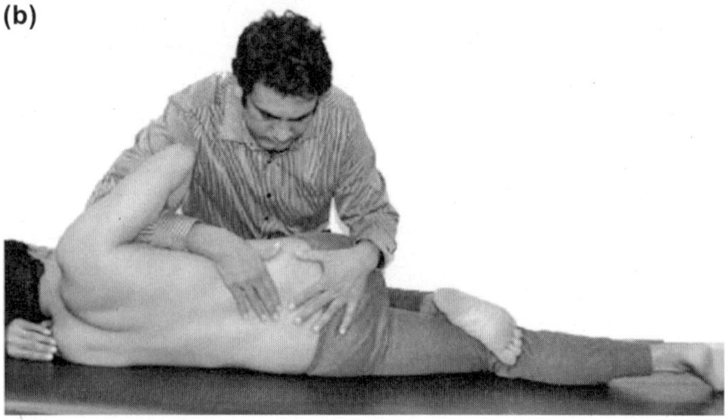

Figs. 27.55a and b: Technique for opening and closing restriction at left L_4-L_5 level

Muscle Energy Techniques for Opening and Closing Restrictions: The use of voluntary contraction of the muscles in a controlled direction against the counter force applied by the therapist can decrease the muscle spasm, and increase flexibility and range of motion.

A. **Muscle Energy Technique for Flexion Restriction (Open Restriction):** At the level of L_4-L_5 right rotation, right bending.

Position of Patient: High sitting, grasps both the hands and holds the edge of the plinth to the right side, creating forward flexion, right side flexion and right rotation.

Position of Therapist: Standing, facing the patient, places right hand on the left scapula and left hand on the right scapula.

Procedure: The patient is asked to flex, side bend and rotate the spine to the limited side as much as possible.

Therapist maintains the position at the extreme limitation range with both the hands and asks the patient to extend, rotate and bend to the left side isometrically against the resistance applied by the therapist. The whole procedure involves the sub-maximal isometric contract for 3-5 seconds followed by a relaxation. The isometric contraction and a relaxation consists of one set. After completing one set the patient should be placed further into flexion, right side bending and right rotation upto the limitation in the range begins. 3-5 repetitions should be performed (Fig. 27.56).

B. **Muscle Energy Technique for Extension Restriction of the L_4-L_5 Level Extension, Right Rotation (Right Side Flexion)** (Fig. 27.57)

Position of Patient: High sitting with right hand on the left thigh.

Position of Therapist: Standing behind the patient, places right forearm on the chest and hand on the left shoulder of the patient. Therapist places left hand on the L_4-L_5

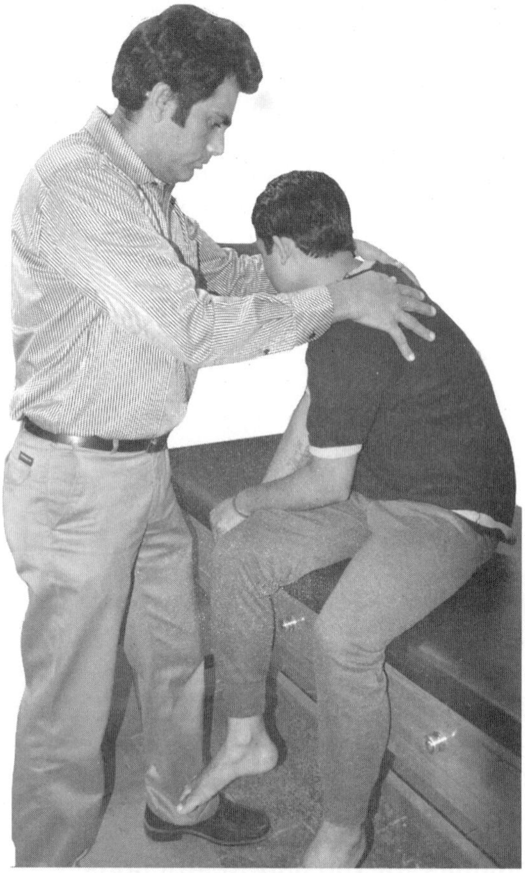

Fig. 27.56: Muscle energy technique for flexion restriction (open restriction)

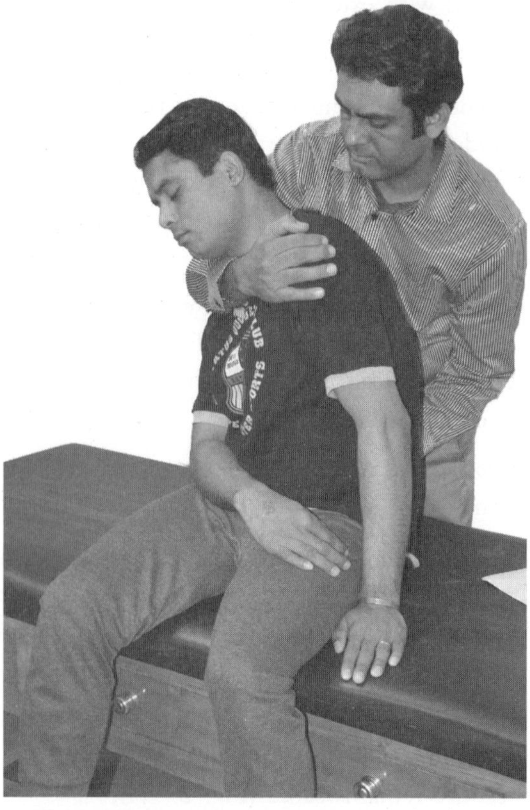

Fig. 27.57: MET for extension restriction at L_4-L_5 level

level. Spine is extended with right side flexion and rotation until the restriction is felt or symptoms start aggravating.

Procedure: Patient is asked to flex the spine with left side flexion and rotation against the resistance applied by the therapist. A submaximal isometric contraction is held for at least 3-5 seconds, followed by relaxation. The procedure is repeated 3-5 times per session.

Sustained Natural Apophyseal Glides (SNAGs)

A. SNAGs to Improve Pain and Lumbar Flexion at L_3-L_4 Segment

Position of Patient: Sitting, hands rest on the anterior thighs.

Position of Therapist: Standing behind the patient, facing the dorsal aspect of L_3-L_4 level. A belt is wrapped around the patient's waist just below the anterior superior iliac spine and over the sacrum of the therapist. The spinous process of the L_3 vertebra is palpated, and the pisiform aspect of the wrist is placed under it (Fig. 27.58).

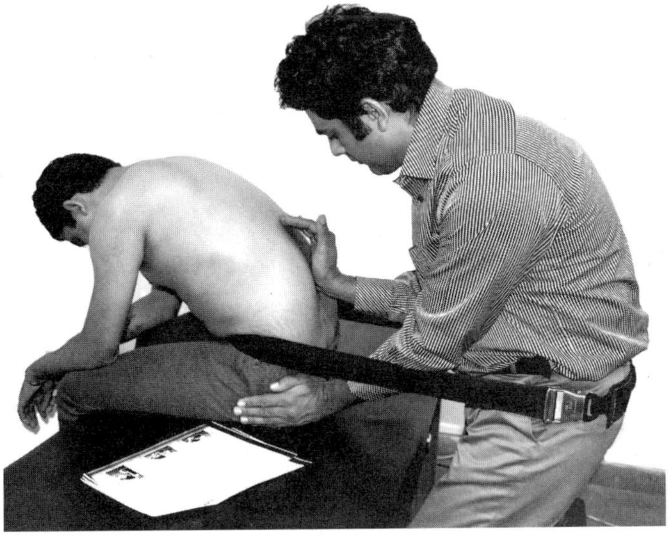

Fig. 27.58: SNAGs to improve pain and lumbar flexion at L_3-L_4 segment

Procedure: Therapist applies an accessory gliding force up along the treatment plane while the patient flexes the spine forward until the pain is felt, at this point therapist applies over pressure and is sustained for few seconds and then returns to the starting position. An accessory gliding force up along the treatment plane is maintained throughout the range of motion until the patient returns to starting position. It is unadvisable to relieve the force in the mid range, it can produce pain. As per this approach three repetitions are enough in the first visit which can significantly reduce the pain and improve the flexion range. The same can be performed on other lumbar spine segments, but for the L_4-L_5 and L_5-S_1 segments instead of pisiform aspect of wrist, medial border of thumb can be used and it is reinforced with other thumb.The same procedure may be performed in standing with slight knees extension.

B. SNAGs to Improve Extension Range and Pain at L_3-L_4 Segment

Position of Patient: Standing.

Position of Therapist: Standing, behind the patient slightly to the left side of the patient to allow the patient to extend the spine, facing the L_3-L_4 segment. The pisiform aspect of wrist is placed under the spinous process of the L_3 vertebra (superior spinous process of the segment). A belt is wrapped around the patient's and therapist's waist similar to previous technique (Fig. 27.59).

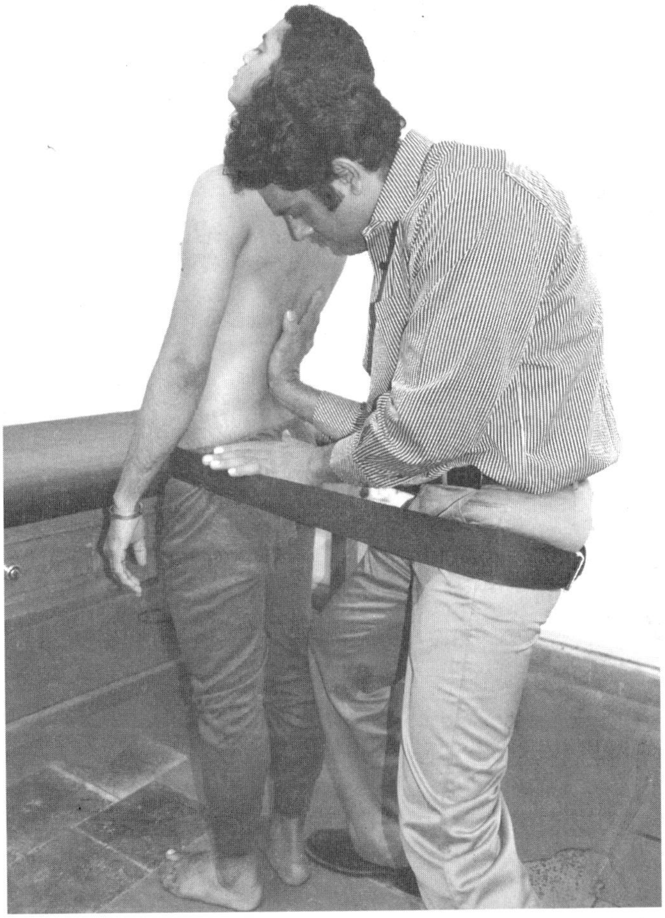

Fig. 27.59: SNAGs to improve pain and lumbar flexion at L_3-L_4 segment

Procedure: Patient extends the lumbar spine gradually and at the same time with the extension therapist pushes the L_3 spinous process up along the treatment plane; until the patient feels pain, at this point therapist applies an over pressure and is sustained for few seconds then returns to the starting position. The accessory gliding force up along the treatment is maintained throughout the range until patient returns to starting position. If the pressure/force is released in the mid range before reaching to the starting position it may produce unwanted pain and symptoms. The same procedure can be performed in sitting position for 3-5 times.

As per this approach three repetitions are enough in the first visit and patient should be called after one day. The same procedure can be performed on the other segments.

C. **SNAGs to Improve Rotation Range and Pain at L_3-L_4 Segment**

Position of Patient: Standing.

Position of Therapist: Stands behind the patient. A belt is wrapped around the patient's waist and therapist's gluteal region. The pisiform aspect of right wrist is placed over the spinous process of L_3 vertebra (Fig. 27.60).

Procedure: For restriction in rotation to the left side patient rotates the trunks to the left side. The right arm of the therapist encourages the movement. Therapist applies an accessory glide up along the treatment plane on L_3 until the pain and limitation starts. At the end range of rotation the therapist may add overpressure. An accessory gliding force up along the treatment plane must be maintained throughout the range until the patient returns to the starting position. Three repetitions in the first visit are sufficient for significant improvement.

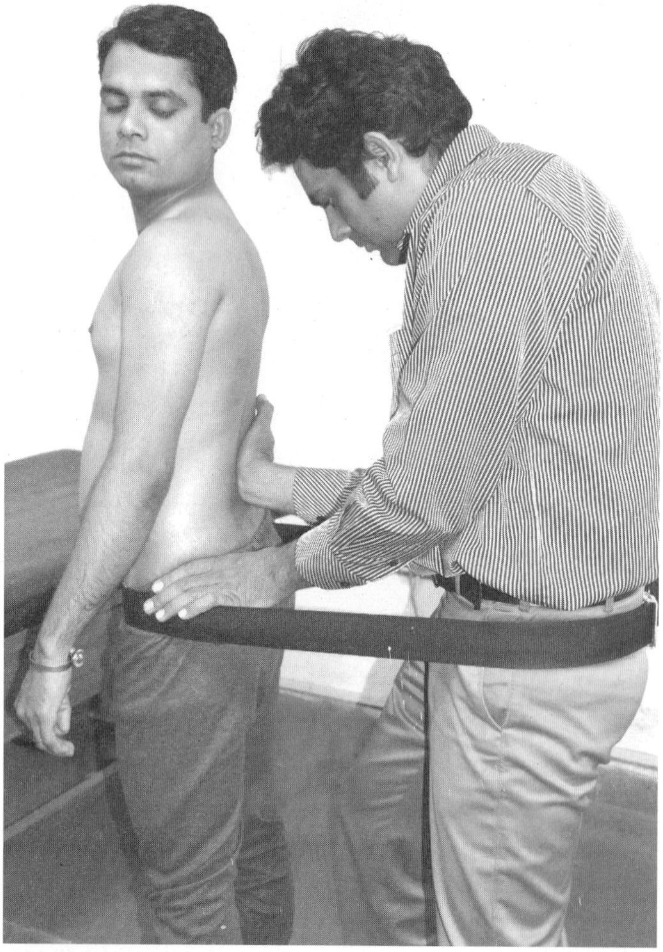

Fig. 27.60: SNAGs to improve pain and lumbar flexion at L_3-L_4 segment

D. **Self SNAGs to Improve Lumbar Flexion at L_3-L_4 Level**

In standing the patient holds the belt and wraps it around the L_3-L_4 level and stabilizes both the hands in front of the chest with the elbows flexed. Patient applies a gliding force up at the L_3-L_4 by pulling the belt with both hands. Patient maintains the gliding force and bends forward until the pain is felt, then returns to the starting position (Fig. 27.61).

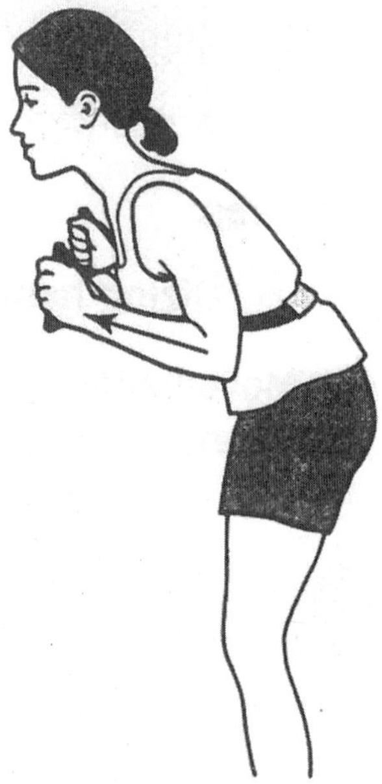

Fig. 27.61: Self SNAGs to improve flexion and pain at L_3-L_4 segment

E. **Self SNAGs to Improve Lumbar Extension at L_3-L_4 Level**

In standing position similar to previous technique, while maintaining the gliding force, the patient bends backwards until the pain is felt, then the patient returns to the starting position (Fig. 27.62).

PIRIFORMIS SYNDROME

The sciatic nerve passes underneath piriformis muscle at the level of greater trochantor. Spasm and tightness in the muscle can cause pressure on sciatic nerve. Bulky wallet in the hip pocket can also cause pressure on the piriformis muscle and in turn irritates the sciatic nerve. The

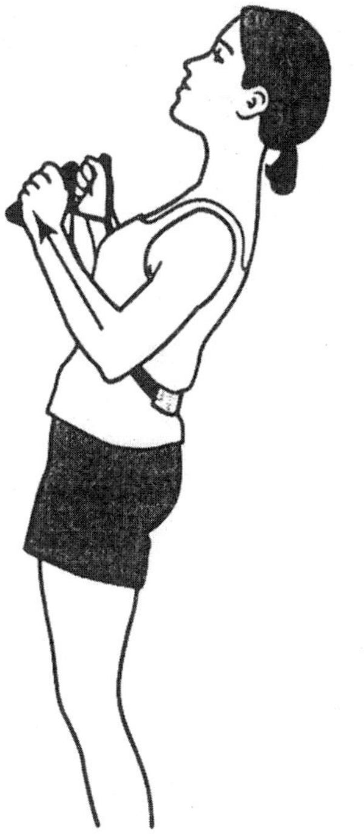

Fig. 27.62: Self SNAGs to improve extension and pain L_3-L_4 level

presentation is identical to prolapse intervertebral disc radiculopathy but pain is localized on the buttock which may radiate down the course of sciatic nerve. Symptoms aggravate in the sitting position as the wallet puts more pressure. Typical symptoms are tingling and numbness along the sciatic nerve course. Shortwave diathermy, on the gluteal region and continuous ultrasound with 1 MHZ at high intensity may help in relieving inflammation. If the root cause is tight trousers with bulky wallet the patient should be advised to wear loose trousers. Stretching of the piriformis muscle is the cornerstone of the treatment. In supine position the hip joint is internally rotated and taken to the opposite shoulder with knee flexion. If the diagnosis is correct, the patient will respond to the treatment even in one sitting of stretching (Fig. 27.63).

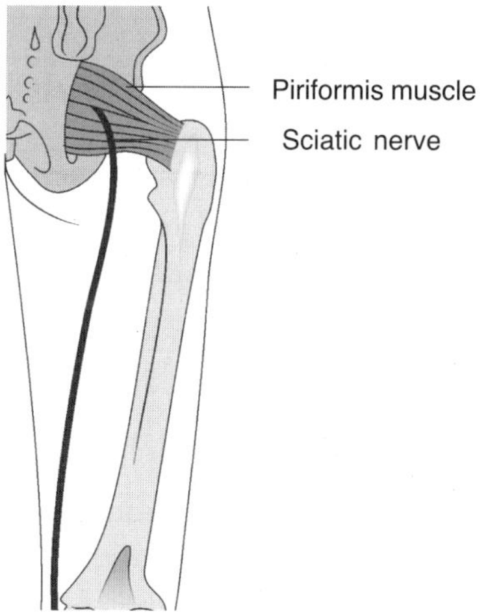

Fig. 27.63: Piriformis syndrome, piriformis muscle and sciatic nerve

SPONDYLOLYSIS

Spondylolysis is a stress fracture of the pars interarticularis. The classic theory of causation for spondylolysis has been that an individual is born with weak pars-interarticularis, and at approximately 6 years of age, a fatigue injury occurs that breaks the pars in children involved in the repetitive flexion extension activities such as back-walkovers in gymnasts causing excessive load on the pars-interarticularis (eventually fractures the pars). Later in high school with the history of weight lifting football play or the extension stresses of gymnastics or wrestling, the lateral fracture becomes irritated and symptomatic. 5% of the general population remain asymptomatic (Fig. 27.64).

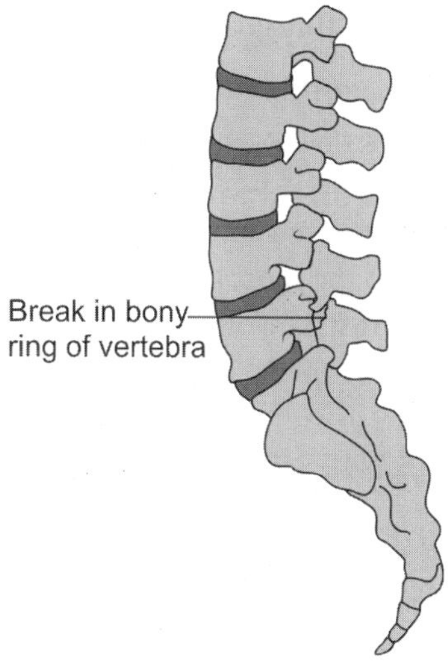

Fig. 27.64 : Spondylolysis

Clinical Features

1. Age: Usually children below *the age of eighteen years.*
2. Gradual onset, sometimes acute.
3. Hereditary predisposition.
4. Symptoms usually low back pain dominant to one side, but more often is in line with the lumbosacral junction.
   a. Occasionally posterior thigh pain with hamstrings tightness.
   b. No neurological signs and symptoms.
5. Stork test:
   (a) The patient stands on one leg with the other leg on the weight bearing knee.
   (b) While maintaining the above position the patient hyperextends the lower lumbar spine.
   (c) Reproduction of the symptoms suggest spondylolysis.
6. Single-photon emission computed tomography (SPECT) scan can show involved area.

7. Oblique radiographs may help in determining the defect.
8. The next element of investigation is C.T. scan which requires only if aforesaid techniques fail to detect the site of lesion.

Management

1. If the patient has no symptoms of low back pain (despite the results of radiographs, bone scan and C.T. scan), do not limit the activities of the patient let him play the sport.
2. If the patient's low back pain limits the sports activities then the children should be on brace.
3. In general, treatment depends upon the severity of the symptoms. Flexion exercises and generalized conditioning exercises are instituted to strengthen the core stabilizers. Once the patient becomes asymptomatic, he or she returns to the sport and to the normal activities of daily living. Most of young patients improve with the conservative treatment and surgery is not required.

SPONDYLOLISTHESIS

It is defined as slip of one vertebra on another. The forward slip of vertebra is resisted by the posterior facet joints, intact neural arch and pedicle. Normal bone plasticity prevents stretch of the pedicle and the intervertebral discs. The breakdown of this normal locking mechanism causes forward slip of the vertebra which is known as spondylolisthesis (Fig. 27.65 and Table 27.4).

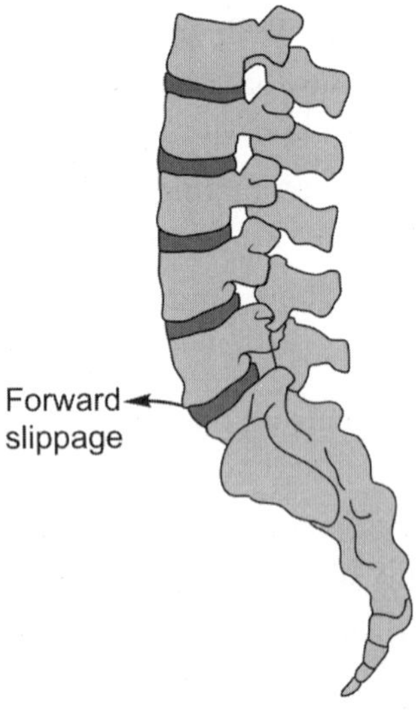

Fig. 27.65: Spondylolisthesis forward slip of L_4 vertebra or the L_5 vertebra

The amount of slip of one vertebra on another is graded in percentage as mentioned below: (Meyerding grading) (Fig. 27.66).

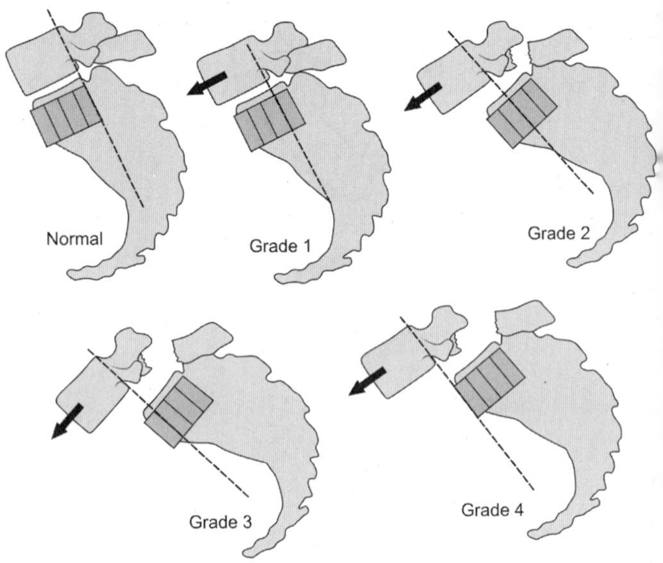

Fig. 27.66: Meyerding grading, grade 1, 2, 3 and 4

Grade I – 25%.

Grade II – 25% - 50%.

Grade III – 50% - 75%.

Grade IV – 75% - 100%.

The complete slip or dislocation of vertebra is called a spondyloptosis.

Assessment of displacement or slip of vertebra on anothe[r] is represented in percentage (%).

A/B × 100 = Slip of vertebra in percentage.

Wiltse Classification

Table 27.4: Commonly accepted clinical classification of spondylolisthesis

Type	*Classification*	*Descriptions*
I	Dysplastic	Congenital abnormalities of upper sacrum or arch at L_5
II		Lesion in pars interarticularis
III		Facet joint degeneration
IV		Fracture in areas of arch other than pars
V	Pathologic	Secondary to generalized or localized bone

Adopted from Macnab's Backache

Clinical Features

- Patients experience a sudden onset of backache with restriction in the motion of the lumbar spine, commonly associated with functional scoliosis.
- On observation buttocks look like "Heart shaped".

- Slip visualized on standing "spot" lateral.
- Often patient complaints of pain in the hamstring muscles.
- Coughing and sneezing can intensify the symptoms.
- Typical physical changes that occur in an individual with lumbar spondylolisthesis is a general stiffness of the back and tightness in the hamstrings with change in both posture and gait.
- In most advanced cases, the gait of the patient may change to give the appearance of more of a "waddle" then a walk where the individual rotates the pelvis more due to decreased flexibility of the hamstrings.

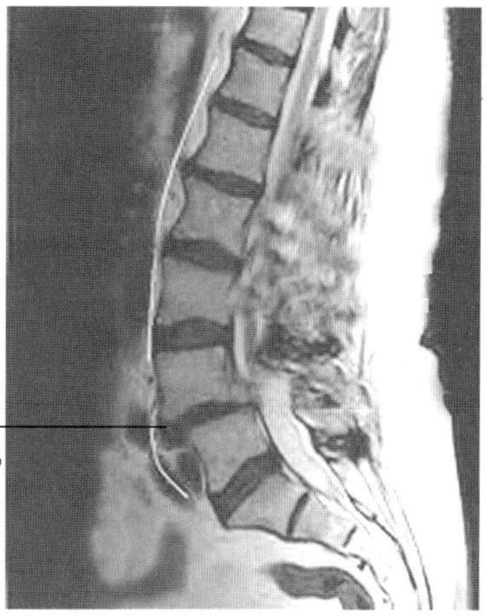

Fig. 27.67: MRI–spondylolisthesis L_4 vertebra over L_5 vertebra

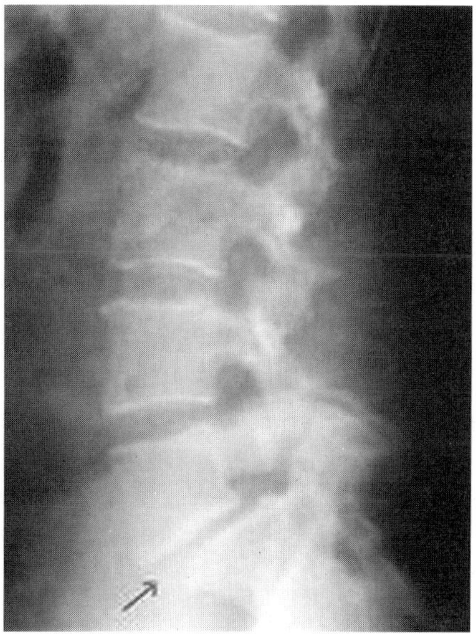

Fig. 27.68: X-ray–spondylolisthesis L_4 vertebra over L_5 vertebra

Isthmic Spondylolisthesis

Approximately 5 to 7% of population has either a fracture of the pars interarticularis or a spondylolisthesis. 80% of these patients remain asymptomatic. Isthmic spondylolisthesis occurs most commonly at L_5-S_1.

The etiology of lesion is unknown. The congenital defects in the pars interarticularis of the neural arch occurs mostly between the 5 and 7 years, and forward slipping of the vertebral body occurs between 10 and 15 years. Once this has occurred it rarely continues to many of the patients experience occasional back pain but so does the vast majority of people without isthmus spondylolisthesis.

A more contemporary theory of pain generation is excessive tension on the annulus of the inferior disc and foraminal stenosis at the level of the slip. However this theory does not explain why some patients have symptoms while others do not, since the inferior discs of all the patients are subjected to similar forces.

Degenerative Spondylolisthesis

It affects the elderly people. As the age progresses usually after fourth decade of life, degenerative changes begin in the intervertebral disc and articular cartilage of the facet joints become incompetent and allows vertebral body to slip forward on the other. Not all slips remain asymptomatic but if they are associated with spinal canal stenosis they can produce symptoms such as neurogenic claudication. But the neural arch remains intact. The degeneration causes gross segmental instability (Figs. 27.67 and 27.68).

Traumatic Spondylolisthesis

Forward slipping of a vertebral body may occur as a result of trauma to the spine. Trauma can cause dislocation of the posterior joints or a fracture of spinous process extending into the lamina of the pars interarticularis which may produce slipping of one vertebra over other. A true traumatic spondylolisthesis is very rare (fracture through pars interarticularis with forward slip of the vertebra).

Congenital or Dysplastic Spondylolisthesis

It is a true congenital spondylolisthesis that occurs because of malformation of lumbosacral junction with small, incompetent facet joints. It is associated with multiple congenital anomalies. In a true congenital or dysplastic spondylolisthesis the lesion may be either dysplasia of the upper sacrum, specifically in the facet joints, or an attenuation of pars interarticularis that gets pulled out and thinned as taught it were made of a malleable plastic. Due to lack of stability there is forward slip of the L_5 on the sacrum. As the forward slip progresses, the pars interarticularis becomes increasingly stretched, it may eventually break the pars interarticularis and produces spondylolisthesis. This break/fracture is secondary to the slip and is not the cause of spondylolisthesis.

The aforesaid concept represents a slight deviation from the Wiltse-Newman-Macnab classification. According to this theory due to lack of stability development of first sacrum of the first sacral arch, with absence or dysplasia of the superior aritcular facet of the sacrum the only lumbosacral disc prevents the forward slip of the L_5 vertebra. When the lumbosacral disc breaks there is forward slip of the L_5 vertebra with the inferior facets gliding over the rudimentary superior articular facets. In the next process slipping involves attenuation and elongation of the pars interarticularis.

Management–Conservative

Flexion Exercises: William Flexion exercises generally help in reducing the slip of the vertebra. The exercises can be performed in many positions (Figs. 27.69a to c).

(a)

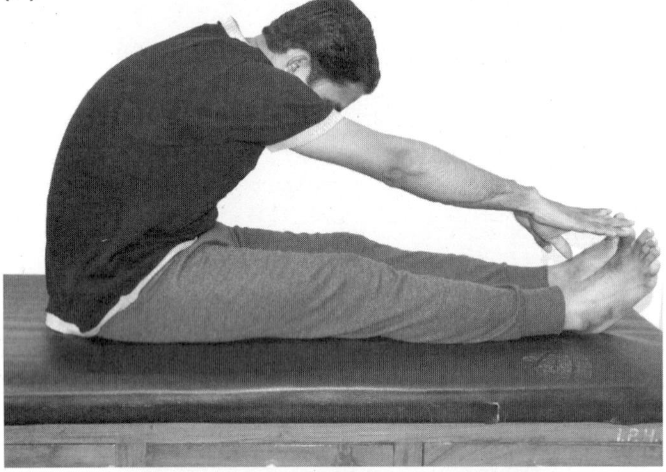

(b)

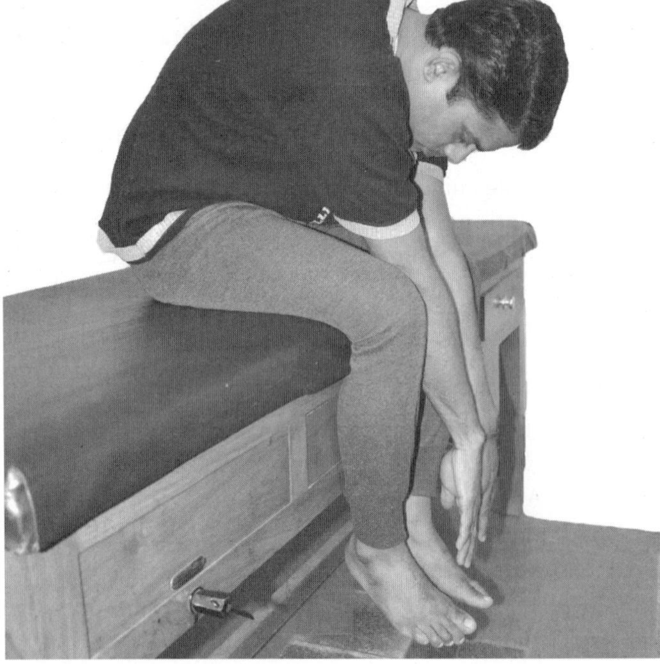

(c)

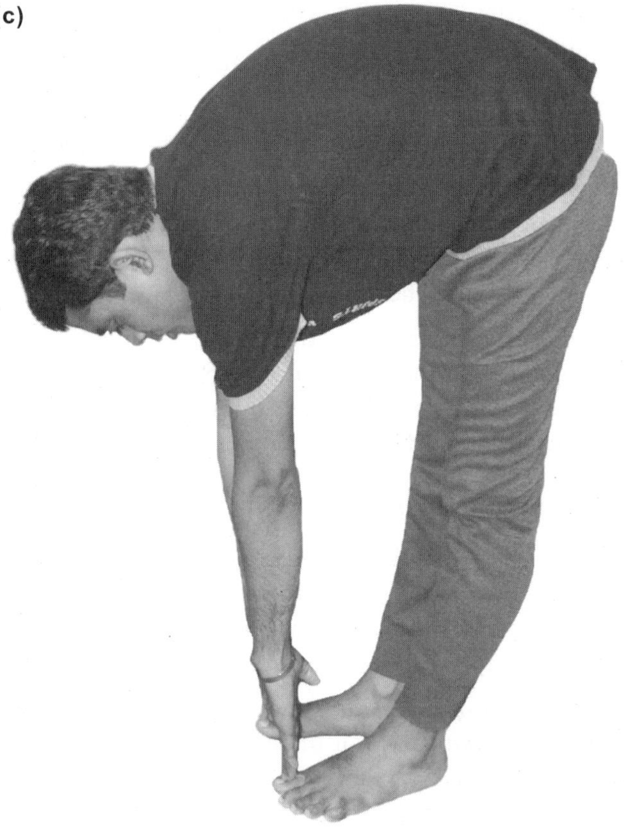

Figs. 27.69a to c: Flexion exercises, a long sitting with toe touch, high sitting with toe touch, standing with toe touch

1. *Supine lying:*
   i. The patient is asked to touch the knee to the chest alternately and then touch both the knees to the chest simultaneously.
   ii. With the flexion of both hip and knee joints the patient lifts the head and shoulders.
   iii. Bilateral straight leg raising.
2. *Long sitting:* Patient attempts to touch the toes with the fingers.
3. *Standing:* Patient attempts to touch the toes with the fingers.

Modalities: The modalities such as short wave diathermy, hot packs, electrical stimulation can ease the pain and muscle spasm.

Soft tissue manipulation of the muscles, ligaments tendon can reduce the muscle spasm and improves the range of motion. Stretching of the hamstrings and extensors increases the flexibility and improves range of motion at hip and lumbar spine.

Brace: During the stage when symptoms such as pain and instability are there the patient may be advised lumbar corset, however, it should be removed during the exercises

Once symptoms start to improve a generalized conditioning program and specific equipment based exercises are initiated to strengthen the core muscles.

Surgical Management

The young patients improve with the flexion exercises and modalities and rarely require surgical intervention.

Surgical treatment is only considered after at least 6 weeks to one year of non-operation treatment fails to improve the symptoms.

Posterior Lateral Fusion: Fusion with decompression.

SACRALIZATION

Sacralization is a *developmental anomaly* in which one or both transverse processes of the fifth lumbar vertebra generally become disproportionally large and strong. Sometimes they become so large that they extend into the base of the sacrum or ileum and form a connection with them. This union forms a foramen between the lower margin of the transverse process and the upper free edge of the sacrum instead of the normal broad and irregular cleft (Fig. 27.70).

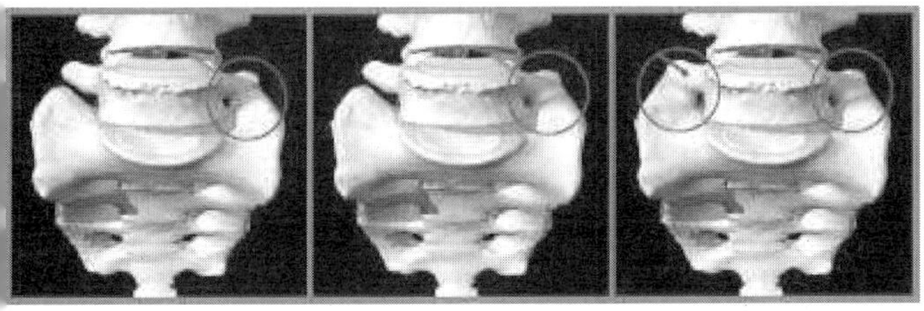

Fig. 27.70: Sacralization

INTERMITTENT CLAUDICATION

Claudication is a pain and/or cramping of the lower leg due to inadequate blood flow to the muscles. The word claudication comes from the Latin "claudicate" meaning to limp. The pain in the muscles is felt during exercises or walking, and subsides at by rest. Hence it is called as intermittent claudication as the pain comes and goes. However in severe cases the pain persists during the exercises or walk as well as at rest. Intermittent claudication may either be vascular or neurogenic.

Vascular Claudication

Vascular claudication is a condition involving insufficient blood circulation due to narrowing of the arteries in the legs.

Clinical Features

Commonly, the calf muscles are the most affected, and patients describe a cramping discomfort as characteristic of pain. In the initial stage of the disease, the patient may walk with the pain, but as the disease progresses further, this is not possible and claudicating pain causes limping which is relieved by rest. Symptoms can worsen when walking barefooted or wearing *flat slippers,* and climbing stairs or up hills. In short, symptoms aggravate whenever muscles are required to work more. Patient frequently rests in between the walk/work to relieve the symptoms. In cases where blockage is severe the pain is not relieved by rest and persists all the time.

Causes

The most common cause of vascular intermittent claudication is the atherosclerosis. There is deposition of cholesterol in the innermost layer of the artery, that decreases the diameter of the artery. Over the years the cholesterol and calcium builds up in the arteries. The narrowing or blockage of the artery will reduce the blood supply to the muscles. The muscles demand more oxygen when patient walks; the demand of oxygen is completed by the blood. In the patients with narrowing of arteries there is an inadequate blood supply to the muscles and that is why the patient starts complaining of pain during continued walk.

In some patients the blood flow is so restricted that the symptoms are not relieved even during rest. These patients also complain of night pain which disturbs the sleep. The symptoms are eased when the leg is hanged down over the edge of the bed. This is the critical stage where ischemia has developed and the leg is at risk of avascular necrosis.

Pathophysiology

The normal artery consists of three layers. The inner layer known as intima is the surface in contact with flowing. A single layer of *cells (endothelial cells) lines the whole* of the arterial (and venous) system. The initial trigger for the development of atherosclerosis is probably damage to the endothelial *cell layer lining the artery.* The damage is usually by smoking, viruses, chemicals and drugs. In the initial stage, yellow *fatty streaks* develop in the blood vessels caused by the deposition of fats in the wall. They are yellow due to deposited cholesterol. At this stage there is complaint of pain, these can progress to the development of atherosclerosis plaques. There is thickening of the innermost wall of the artery that limits the blood flow to the muscles/ tissues. The plaques are caused by the accumulation of low density lipoprotein (LDL, a type of cholesterol).The increased LDL in the blood stream will lead to transport into the artery wall where it is retained. Moreover, other cells such as monocytes are attracted towards this *attired* LDL which further accelerates the accumulation. A fibrous plaque develops as smooth muscle cells and monocyte accumulate.

Furthermore, the monocytes also transform into another cell type called macrophases which absorb the cholesterol and fats deposited in the arterial wall. The plaques can become so thick that they protrude into the artery and can interfere with normal blood flow. In more advance cases calcium is also deposited and the plaques become very hard.

Embolisation: Sometimes the plaque surface becomes ulcerated, that leads to fragmentation of the plaques. These are carried downstream to block a smaller blood vessel– this is the complication of atherosclerosis.

Collateral Arterial Supply: When the plaques become large they can block the artery completely and in that situation the blood is diverted into smaller arteries, known as collateral arteries. These small arteries, although not the major blood vessels to the leg, usually carry enough blood to prevent severe disability.

Prognosis

Overall about one third of patients with intermittent vascular claudication will improve, one third will remain stable and rest of patients will deteriorate. In majority of cases (> 65%) the symptoms will remain stable or improve.

Amputation

In the advance stage or severe cases the symptoms become constant (not relieved by rest, pain at rest and at night), and there are ischemic ulcerations (critical limb ischemia). These changes indicate that the patient has developed problems that are putting the leg at risk of amputation.

Physical Examination

The patient should be examined for high blood pressure, heart abnormalities, blockage in the arteries of neck, and abdominal aneurysms. In addition to above patient should also be examined for ulcer and colour changes of the skin.

A. **Ankle Brachial Index:** The systolic blood pressure of the arm is measured. Then the systolic blood pressure of the leg is also measured at four different sites and passes a Doppler probe over arteries in the foot. The signal emitted from the strongest artery is recorded as the cuffs are inflated and deflated. This is considered as the ankle's systolic pressure. The systolic blood pressure of the arms divided by the systolic blood pressure of the leg. The result is called the ankle-arm pressure index (API) or ankle-brachial index (ABI).

   Results: If the result is 90 or above, this result often rules out peripheral artery disease (PAD). If the result is below 90, this is usually sufficient information to diagnose the PAD. ABI between 50 and 40–highly associated with impaired leg functions. ABI below 40–highly risk of gangrene.

   Patients with ABI above 90 may further undergo *freomil test. The systolic B.P. of arm and leg* is measured following treadmil. If the ABI falls or drops, the case may be diagnosed as PAD. The lower the ABI, the greater the risk for heart attack, stroke or other serious circulatory diseases.

B. **Invasive Angiography:** It is a conventional angiography in which angiogram *uses dye, that is injected* through a catheter in the groin.

C. **Magnetic Resonance Angiography:** It is the non-invasive method which gives as accurate results as invasive angiography. Gadolinium is given through an intravenous to provide more clear images. The magnetic field and radiofrequency waves are used in this method that provides images of the arteries. MRI is the test which is used frequently in the clinical practice.

D. **Computed Tomography:** In this method X-rays are used to test the flow of blood. This is more advanced method but is used only on the patients those are contraindicated to MRA, as it causes radiation exposure.

Management

Medical: The effect of medicines on the clot is negligible, that cannot unblock the arteries. Aspirin 25 mg, clopidogrel and cilastazol are some of the drugs advised to dilute the blood or make the blood less sticky.

Symptoms and Exercises: Regular exercises can improve the symptoms and walking distance. The patients with intermittent claudication are advised to walk as much as till the pain is perceived. Once the pain becomes severe stop walking and take rest till it subsides. Again repeat the same. Measure the distance at the same pace for one week. On the next week the distance can be increased. On the third week increase the distance slightly further. This exercise program will improve the distance covered in walking. Regular exercises can help to lower the blood cholesterol levels as well as improve walk and general well-being.

Buerger Exercises: There is a good evidence that patients with intermittent claudication who take regular exercise can increase their walking distance (the distance that they can walk before they have to stop because of pain in the muscles). Buerger exercises are the postural exercises specifically recommended for patients with arterial insufficiency to enhance circulation in the lower extremity.

These exercises are also known as Buerger-Allen exercises as described by them. The exercise is started in the supine position with the legs raised to 45 degrees. Patient maintains the raised legs for three and performs ankle pump exercises for at least one minute or until blanching occurs. Once blanching occurs the leg is lowered on the treatment table at the level of the heart and again patient performs ankle pump exercises for at least one minute, and then once the feet become warm (redness appears) the leg is hanged with the knee flexion for three minutes with one minute of ankle pump exercises. If the exercise is performed for both the legs the patient has to sit and hang the legs for three minutes and do the ankle pump exercises for one minute. The patient then returns to the supine position with the lower extremities "flat" for another 3 minutes and performs an active muscle contraction for 1 minute in this position.

Cholesterol: The increased level of cholesterol low density lipoprotein (LDL) should be the patient's first priority to reduce it. The patient should cut down the fat in diet. The drugs which reduces cholesterol level in the blood should be advised.

Smoking: There are lot of evidence that tobacco is the basic cause of the trouble, moreover smoking clamps down the small collateral blood vessels and reduces the blood supply and oxygen to the tissues. The patient must make efforts to give up smoking.

Surgery

Angioplasty: Sometimes short blockages can be stretched open with a balloon in the radiology department under local anaesthesia.

Bypass Graft: In advanced stages where patients develop critical limb ischemia, the bypass graft is the choice of surgery to restore blood flow to the leg and of course to avoid amputation. The larger blockages are bypassed using a vein from the leg under general anaesthesia.

Neurogenic Claudication

It is the neurological entity which is caused by spinal stenosis or inflammation of the nerves. The neurogenic claudication is also intermittent but in severe nerve root cases, the neurogenic claudication is not intermittent but painfully persistent.

Clinical Features

Pain is felt in the unilateral or bilateral calf muscles, buttock and thigh. Pain may be associated with weakness of the thigh and calf muscles. Pain is aggravated or precipitated by walking and prolonged standing and is not relieved by resting. After few yards of walk pain starts in the back and lower extremity. To relieve the pain patient bends forward and then walks another few yards. The forward flexion opens the intervertebral foramena and reduces the pressure on the nerve roots. This is the reason that the patients with neurogenic claudication have less disability in climbing steps, pushing carts and cycling.

Spinal Stenosis

Spinal canal stenosis is the narrowing of the spinal canal with subsequent neural compression and is frequently associated with symptoms of neurogenic claudication, such as pain paraesthesia, numbness in the leg and thighs.

Pathology: Lumbar spinal stenosis usually occurs in middle aged and elderly people. It generally takes long time for the stenosis to develop and the symptoms of neurogenic claudication to appear. The symptoms of neurogenic claudication are unusual before the sixth decade of life.

The first factor which contributes to the spinal stenosis is narrowed spinal canal. However, alone (small spinal canal) rarely produces the symptoms of neurogenic claudication. The degenerative changes of intervertebral disc produce osteophytes, and also causes thickening of the ligamentum flavum. As the age progresses, usually after sixth decade of life, the thickened (hypertrophied) ligamentum flavum may bulge into the spinal canal, degenerated osteophytes also extend into the spinal canal and contribute to the significant narrowing of canal which eventually produces pressure on the spinal cord or cauda equina; resulting manifestations of neurogenic claudication.

Vertebral displacement with an intact neural arch will critically narrow an already small canal. Spondylolisthesis due to degeneration effectively reduces the canal size at the level of displacement. It is more commoner in women. Whereas, bilateral neurogenic claudication is more common in men, and approximately 50% bilateral neurogenic claudication in men is caused by degenerative spondylolisthesis.

Patients with neurogenic claudication do not have symptoms of claudication at rest as oxygen supply remains adequate, but symptoms aggravate during exercises or walking due to an inadequate oxygenation or accumulation of metabolites in the cauda eqiuna.

Many patients may have radiological evidence of spinal canal stenosis but remain asymptomatic or do not have neurogenic claudication symptoms, hence, it is not necessary for the spinal stenosis to have symptoms of neurogenic claudication, such as a large central disc protrusion can block the canal without claudication, and single level stenosis from degenerative changes at L_3-L_4, L_4-L_5 may occlude the dural sac and yet produce only back pain.

Assessment of Neurogenic Claudication and Spinal Stenosis: Not all patients with lumbar spinal stenosis have symptoms of neurogenic claudication, but usually after six decades of life, presence of leg pain in walking, classically relieves by flexion of the spine and not simply relieved by rest, are the common clinical finding of the spinal stenosis with neurogenic claudication. The studies have shown that no firm conclusion on the diagnostic performance of clinical or radiological tests can be drawn; hence expensive imaging may therefore, be unnecessary except where surgical intervention is advised. There are some physical tests useful in making the diagnosis of neurogenic claudication following lumbar spinal canal stenosis. There are the simple clinical tests of exercise tolerance either using a static bicycle or a walking test.

A. **Static Bicycle Test:** The patient is asked to lumbar extension (erect sitting, no forward flexion). After 2-3 minutes if he finds difficulty in further cycling, he or she is asked to flex the lumbar spine and do cycling. If the symptoms or leg pain relieves in forward flexion the test may be considered positive for neurogenic claudication with stenosis.

B. **Walk Test:** The patient is asked to walk with lumbar extension as much as possible. He or she is asked to flex the lumbar spine, if there is any leg pain or difficulty in erect walking. The test may be positive for intermittent claudication if the patient complains of leg pain in erect walking but feels comfortable in forward flexed walking. In the next step the patient is asked to walk on the ramp (hill) up and then down. Complaint of leg pain on walking down on the hill or ramp is the indication of intermittent claudication.

Management of Neurogenic Claudication

It is universally recommended that conservative treatments are used as the first line of treatment for patients with neurogenic claudication. A fair trial of conservative treatment relieves the pain symptomatically and increases range of motion and strength of muscles. The patient is educated about the progression of the diseases and measures to control the progression. The physiotherapist should emphasize on flexion based exercises, core stability strengthening exercises and general fitness exercises. To relieve pain superficial heat therapy, deep heating modalities such as short wave diathermy and interferential therapy are usually recommended. Surgical intervention may not always be the choice of treatment, except in cases presenting with severe and persistent pain and disability or where there are sign of progressive neurological deficit or cauda equina compression.

REFERENCES

1. Porter RW, Miller CG. Back pain and trunk list. Spine 1986;11: 596–600.
2. McKenzie RA. Manual correction of sciatic scoliosis. New Zealand Med J 1972;484:194–199.
3. Weitz EM. The lateral bending sign. Spine 1981;6:388–397.
4. Grieve GP. Common Vertebral Joint Problems. Edinburgh, UK: Churchill Livingstone; 1981.
5. Cyriax J. Textbook of Orthopaedic Medicine: Diagnosis of Soffi Tissue Lesions. 8th ed., Vol. 1., London, UK: Ballière Tindall; 1982.
6. Falconer MA, McGeorge M, Begg AC. Surgery of lumbar intervertebral disc protrusion: A study of principles and results based upon 100 consecutive cases submitted to operation. Br J Surg 1948;35: 225–249.
7. Grieve GP. Treating backache: A topical comment. Physiotherapy 1983; 69:316.
8. White AA, III, Panjabi MM. Clinical Biomechanics of the Spine. 2nd ed. Philadelphia: JB Lippincott Company; 1990.
9. McKenzie RA, May S. Mechanical Diagnosis and Therapy: The Lumbar Spine. 2nd edition Waikanae, NZ: Spinal Publications; 2003.
10. Laslett M. The McKenzie method of managing acute lumbar list, kyphosis and hyperlordosis. American Back Society Spring Symposium, 1991.
11. Battié MC, Cherkin DC, Dunn R, Clol MA, Wheeler KJ. Managing low back pain: Attitudes and treatment preferences of physical therapists. Phys Ther 1994; 74: 219–226.
12. Foster NE, Thompson KA, Baxter GD, Allen JM. Management of nonspecific low back pain by physiotherapists in Britain and Ireland: A descriptive questionnaire of current clinical practice. Spine 1999; 24:1332–1342.
13. Correction of an acute lumbar lateral shift: Maintenance of Correction and Rehabilitation: A Case Report, J Man Mani Ther 2009; 17 (2): 78-85.
14. Van Wijmen PM. The use of repeated movements in the McKenzie method of spinal examination. In: Boyling JD, Palastanga N, editors. Grieve's Modern Manual Therapy. 2nd ed. London, UK: Churchill Livingstone; 1994.
15. McKenzie RA. A physical therapy perspective on acute spinal disorders. In: Mayer T, Mooney V, Gatchel R, editors. Contemporary

Conservative Care for Painful Spinal Disorders. Malvern, PA: Lea & Fabiger; 1991.

16. McKenzie RA. The Lumbar Spine: Mechanical Diagnosis and Therapy. Waikanae. NZ: Spinal Publications; 1981.

17. Busanich B, Verscheure S. Does McKenzie therapy improve outcomes for back pain? J Athl Train 2006;41:117–119.

18. Hefford C. McKenzie classification of mechanical spinal pain: Profile of syndromes and directions of preference. Man Ther 2008;13:75–81.

19. Werneke M, Hart D, Cook D. A descriptive study of the centralization phenomenon: A prospective analysis. Spine 1999;24:676–683.

20. Kilpikoski S, Airaksinen O, Kankaanpaa M, Leminem P, Videman T, Alen M. Interexaminer reliability of low back pain assessment using the McKenzie method. Spine 2002;27:207–214.

21. A mechanical diagnosis and treatment (MDT) approach for a patient with discogenic low back pain and a relevant component: A case study.J Man Manip Ther 2011 May; 19(2):113–18.

28

SACROILIAC JOINT PAIN

A sacroiliac synovial joint comprised sacrum and ilium is a plain joint which absorbs the weight of the trunk and transfers it to the ilium and lower extremities. The joint is surrounded by number of muscles and ligaments which contribute to the stability and play an important role in shock absorption. The joint has physiologically normal ridges and depressions, which can be seen easily on X-rays. Tension in the ligaments can be increased by strong contraction of the muscles as there are fibrous connections between the ligament and muscles. For an example; there is a fibrous connection at ischial tuberosity between sacrotuberous ligament and biceps femoris muscles. Tension in the sacrotuberous ligament can be increased by contraction in biceps femoris or vice versa. The sacrotuberous ligament also has attachments to the multifidus muscle. The tension in the sacrotuberous ligament is also increased as a result of contraction (tension) in multifidus muscles. This potentially increases the ligamentous stabilizing mechanism of the sacroiliac joint.

Mobility: Many authors have different opinions on the mobility of the SI joint whether motion can occur at SI joint or not. The studies have proven that a small amount of motion range from 2 degrees to 4 degrees is possible in three planes, sagittal, frontal and transverse. The normal sacroiliac joint cartilage has intra-articular ridges and depressions; which show friction coefficient (particularly by the complimentary ridges and depressions) motion takes place within the ridges and depressions.

Under abnormal stresses the sacroiliac joint is forced into a new position, ridges and depressions are no longer complimentary. This new position can block the motion at sacroiliac joint. This blocking results to asymmetrical opposition of the SI joint surfaces and can cause unilateral SI joint hypermobility or hypomobility.

Nutation: It is also known as sacral flexion. The base of sacrum moves anteriorly and inferiorly while the apex of sacrum moves posteriorly and superiorly. The attachment of the superficial erector spinae to the sacrum provides a potential force for sacral nutation. The superficial erector spinae plays a major role in force closure of the sacroiliac joint. The rectus abdominis and biceps femoris muscles rotate the innominate or ilium posteriorly on the sacrum and produces nutation at the sacroiliac joint. The nutation provides stability to the sacroiliac joint.

Counter Nutation: Counter nutation is also known as sacral extension. The base of the sacrum moves posteriorly and inferiorly while apex moves anteriorly and superiorly. Pubococcygeus and levator ani originating from the pubic rami and inserting into the coccyx rotate the sacral base posteriorly (counter nutation). Iliacus, rectus femoris and tensor fascia lata/iliotibial band complex rotate the ilia forward or anteriorly relative to the base of the sacrum (counter nutation). The counter nutation decreases the stability of the sacroiliac joint (Figs. 28.1 and 28.2).

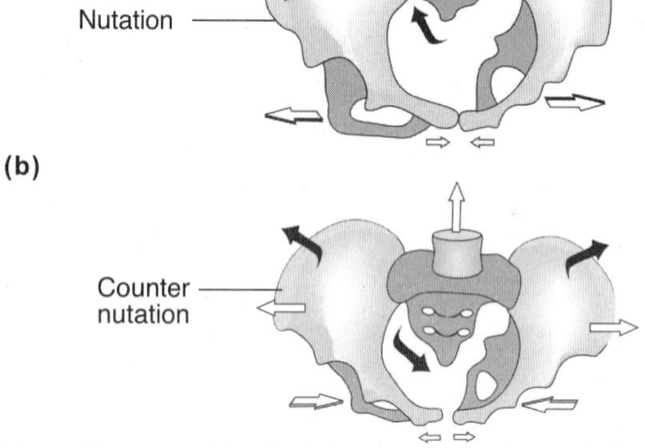

Figs. 28.1a and b: Nutation and counter nutation at sacroiliac joint, anterior view

In standing, forward flexion of lumbosacral spine causes forward rotation of the ilia and base of the sacrum (nutation). After 50-60 degrees, the ilia continues to rotate anteriorly while the base of sacrum rotates posteriorly and the apex of sacrum rotates anteriorly (counter nutation).

(a)

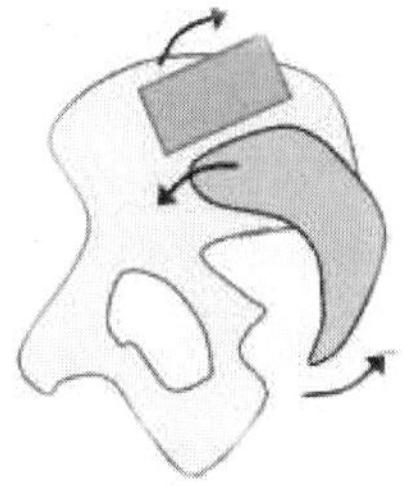

(b)

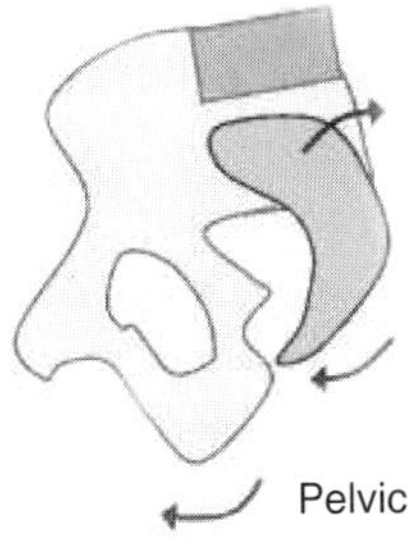

Figs. 28.2a and b: Nutation and counter nutation at sacroiliac joint, lateral view

In sitting forward flexion of the lumbar spine rotates the pelvis or ilia anteriorly with respect to the base of sacrum (counter nutation). Further, trunk flexion causes tension in the long dorsal sacroiliac ligament resulting in posterior rotation of the ilia with respect to sacrum (nutation). Hence, in sitting trunk flexion causes counter nutation initially, but it is replaced with the nutation due to tension in the ligaments.

In standing, initially, trunk extension rotates the ilia posteriorly with respect to the base of sacrum. This increases lumbar lordosis and the lumbosacral angle. In sitting, trunk extension does not rotate the ilia initially but further extension will result in anterior rotation of the ilia as tension in the sacrospinous and sacrotuberous increases.

Stability: The sacroiliac joint is stabilized by the static and dynamic structures, termed as form closure and force closure respectively. These structures help in preventing friction in the sacroiliac joint by increasing the joint friction coefficient and joint compression.

Form Closure: The shape, structure or form of the joint provides the stability.

(i) The specific anatomical structures such as interlocking ridges, grooves and roughening of the joint surfaces helps in increasing the friction.

(ii) The triangular shape of the sacrum fits between the ilia, helps in increasing compression and minimizing shear on the SI joint as its lateral arches are firmly connected to ilia, sacrotuberous and sacrospinalis ligaments, the coccygeus and piriformis muscles.

Force Closure: The force closure is a mechanism in which the stability of the sacroiliac joint is provided mainly by the dynamic stabilizers by the force generated within and outside the SI joint. The muscles such as multifidi, sacrospinalis (extensor spinae) produce anterior rotation of the base of sacrum (nutation), and the contraction of rectus abdominis and hamstrings produce posterior rotation of the pelvis (nutation) with respect to the base of sacrum. The contraction of the aforesaid muscles produce nutation which contribute to the force closure mechanism, thereby increasing the compression on the sacroiliac joint surfaces, which in turn increases the stability of the joint for load transfer. The inner unit consists of multifidi, thoracic diaphragm, transverse abdominis, and pelvic floor muscles. These specific muscles are coupled with pelvic floor muscles. The simultaneous contraction of these two groups of muscles (force couple) affects the stability of the sacroiliac joint and lumbosacral junction, and may also move the sacrum into stable or unstable position. For an example, the contraction of multifidus muscle causes nutation, whereas, contraction of iliacs and ischiococcygeus causes counter nutation.

The oblique muscles have connections with hip joint muscles via their corresponding fascia, which helps in stabilizing the SI joint. The posterior oblique muscle, latissimus dorsi connects the contralateral gluteus maximus through thoracolumbar fascia. The contraction of these two muscles produces compression on the sacroiliac joint through the thoracolumbar fascia. The internal abdominal and external abdominal oblique also known as anterior oblique, connects the contralateral adductors of the hip joint through anterior abdominal fascia. The contraction of these muscles help in the stabilizing the SI joint.

The gluteus medius and minimus and the contralateral adductors play important role in stabilizing the pelvis on the femur while standing and walking. Weakness of these muscle contribute to the instability of the pelvis and sacroiliac joints.

The erector spinae muscles are connected to the sacrotuberous ligament and biceps femoris through the deep lamina of the thoracodorsal fascia. Contraction of these muscles increases tension in the sacrotuberous ligament, which in turn compresses the sacroiliac joint and increases its stability.

PELVIC MALALIGNMENT

The stability of sacroiliac joint and positions of pelvis is greatly affected by the spine and extremities alignments. The pelvis may show rotational malalignment along with upslip. The rotational malalignment and upslip may also occur in isolation 80% and 10% respectively. The rotational malalignment may also occur in association with outflare and inflare, however, outflare and inflare may also occur in isolation.

Rotational Malalignment

The pelvis rotates anteriorly and posteriorly in sagittal plane during normal walk and activities of daily living. Excessive rotation of innominate may affect the kinetics of the lumbosacral spine. The most common presentation of rotational malalignment is that of right anterior and left posterior innominate rotation with locking of the right sacroiliac joint. The opposite sacroiliac joint (left) may show compensatory hypermobility. The studies have shown that there are two major causes of the pelvic rotation malalignment, the repeated or direct trauma and muscular imbalance. As discussed earlier, there is nutation of the sacrum during forward bending upto 50-60° in standing. Beyond 50-60° forward flexion, the base of sacrum rotates posteriorly and inferiorly (counter nutation of the sacrum), this contributes to the instability of the sacroiliac joints as relaxing of the posterior pelvic ligaments. The caudal glide of the SI joint is impaired and the joint becomes vulnerable to dysfunction. If forward bending is combined with the side bending and axial rotation, anterior rotation of the SI joint of the contralateral side is restricted due to increased tension in the sacrotuberous ligament because of strong contraction of the biceps femoris and piriformis (attached to the sacrotuberous ligament). Whereas, the anterior rotation of the SI joint, on the ipsilateral side is increased; which leads to asymmetrical loading of the spine and pelvis. There is acute pain often felt on trying to get back to the standing. This dysfunction can be prevented to some extent if the spine bends forward prior to the pelvic anterior rotation and innominate rotates posteriorly before the spine extension. This is also known as lumbopelvic rhythm (Fig. 28.3).

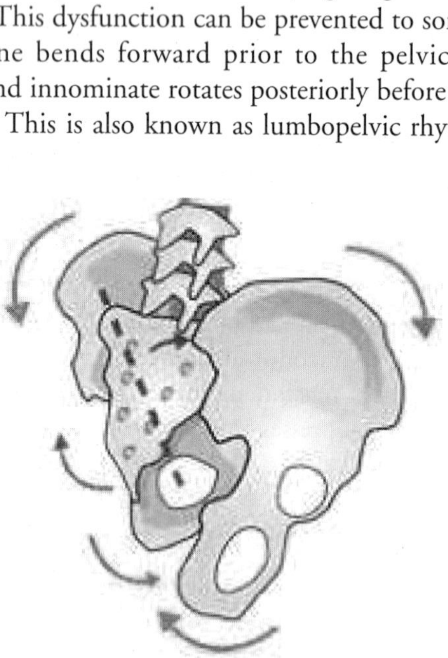

Fig. 28.3: Rotational malalignment a. Anterior, b. Posterior

The rotational malalignment either anterior or posterior also depends upon position of the innominate at the time of trauma. For example a posterior directed force at the anterior or superior aspect of the pubic bone and an anterior directed force of the level of posterior iliac crest can cause anterior malalignment of the pelvis. Similarly a posterior directed force at the anterior iliac crest and anterior directed force at the ischial tuberosity can cause posterior malalignment of the pelvis.

The forces transmitted by the extremities through the hip joints to the sacroiliac joint may also cause significant rotational malalignment of the pelvis. In this regard the position of the leg is very important at the time of trauma is to understand the exact mechanism. For an example, if the hip joint is flexed and force is transmitted from the leg to the pelvis through the hip joint, it may place significant anterior rotation of the pelvis on sacrum. These forces from the leg usually come when an athlete or individual falls on knee joint, casual jump on one leg, misses a step when going downstairs etc.

In addition to the position of extremities, the lumbar spine also contribute to the malalignment of pelvis. For example, rotation of the L_5 vertebra either left or right will put the tension on the ligaments and cause posterior rotation of the pelvis. For an instance, right rotation of the L_5 vertebra on sacrum, will rotate the right transverse process posteriorly and left transverse process anteriorly. The rotation of transverse processes put the tension on iliolumbar ligaments. Therefore the right tensed iliolumbar ligament will pull the right pelvis posteriorly, and left iliolumbar ligament pulls the left pelvis anteriorly.

Muscular Imbalance: The muscles such as gluteus maximus, medius, abdominals, psoas major and hamstrings play important role in nutation by rotating the pelvis posteriorly with respect to the sacrum. It also helps in achieving the closed packed position of sacroiliac joint. In closed packed position a joint has maximal resistance to distraction and translation or shear and demonstrates greater load bearing stability. Weakness of these muscles allows the pelvis to rotate anteriorly with respect to the sacrum and produces counter nutation. It has already been mentioned that counter nutation decreases the stability of the sacroiliac joint. This is because in counter nutation the joint goes into the loose packed position. This is a position (loose packed) of minimal congruency between the articular surfaces with greatest potential for separation of joint surfaces. The loose packed position of the sacroiliac joint is provided by the contraction of iliocostalis, tensor fascia lata and rectus femoris muscles.

Upslip and Downslip: In normal gait, the sacroiliac joint may permit pelvis to translate upward and downward approximately two degrees. Upslip and downslip are the abnormal positions of innominate in which one side of the innominate will exert excessive translation (more than two degrees) and stuck either in upward or downward direction respectively in relation to the sacrum. Upslip is more commoner than the downslip which may be 10-20% in isolation, and 5-10% in association with rotational malalignment. The upslip most commonly occurs when the traumatic force is transmitted from the extended leg through the neutral hip joint to sacroiliac joint. This mechanism produces upslip instead of rotational malalignment as the hip and knee joints remain neutral. Situation may be like falling on the foot with hip and knee neutral. Sometimes if patient falls or lands directly on the ischial tuberosity on one side, that may also cause upslip. In compare to upslip, downslip occurs rarely. The pelvis may translate excessively downward and stuck, if there is a traction force on the leg. The typical mechanism may be like one foot has sunk into a hole and the individual tries hard to extract it. This may cause excessive downward translation (downslip) of the innominate in relation to the sacrum.

Outflare and Inflare: The pelvic outflare and inflare occurs in the transverse plane around a vertical axis. The outflare and inflare of the innominate refers to the outward and inward movements respectively. Normally these movements occur in combined with rotation of the pelvis. The outward or outflare occurs with the anterior and posterior rotations of the pelvis. Inward movement or inflare also occurs with anterior and posterior rotations. For an instance, during anterior rotation of the innominate, the innominate flares out as it is allowed by the anterior widening of the sacrum. Interestingly, even in posterior rotation of the pelvis, there may be outflare of the innominate because the posterior narrowing of the sacrum glides innominate medially.

In patients with sacroiliac joint dysfunction, outflare and inflare may exist in isolation or in combination with anterior and posterior rotations. If there is an excessive outward movement of the pelvis in a transverse plane, it may stuck in an outflare position. In combined with rotation malalignment, outflare occurs with anterior rotation of the innominate and the compensatory inflare occurs with the opposite posterior rotation of the pelvis.

Sacral Torsion: It is the normal movement of the sacrum as the part of daily activities. It occurs with the movements of trunk, pelvic bones, lower extremities and by the contraction of piriformis and iliacus muscles. Excessive sacral torsion can also cause sacroiliac joint dysfunction or malalignment.

Sacral Torsion Combined with Lumbar Vertebra: The right side of the L_5 vertebra on the sacrum will rotate the right transverse process of the L_5 vertebra posteriorly and left transverse process of the L_5 anteriorly. This rotation of the transverse processes of L_5 vertebra will increase the tension on the iliolumbar ligament by virtue of their attachments to the transverse processes and ilium, which in turn bring the surfaces of L_5-S_1 facet joints increasingly closer together. If there is further rotation of the L_5 over the sacrum the L_5-S_1 facet joints compressed maximally and starts acting as a fulcrum, so that any further rotation of L_5 will now cause torsion of the sacrum around the right oblique axis. The piriformis muscle which has its diagonal orientation, inserts on the anterior aspect of the base of sacrum. This muscle rotates the sacral base posteriorly with relation to the innominate. The strong contraction or shortening of the piriformis muscle can cause torsion of the sacrum and loss of mobility between the ilium and sacrum.

Subjective Examination of Lumbosacral Spine: The important part of the assessment is the understanding of complaint of the patient as much as possible. The patient will reveal the mechanism of injury, whether the pain and symptoms started with trauma or accident. In case of trauma, was the force transmitted through extremities to trunk? If force transmitted through extremities, then what was the position of extremity? Flexed or extended? This will help in establishing the diagnosis of malalignment of sacroiliac joint.

The second part of the assessment is the careful observation of the pelvis and lumbosacral spine. This includes observation of the height of iliac crests, pubic bones, Anterior Superior Iliac Crests (ASIS), Posterior Superior Iliac Crests (PSIS), dimples of venus on the buttocks (about 1 cm above the PSIS), ischial tuberosities, inferior lateral angle of the sacrum and sacral sulci (Fig. 28.4).

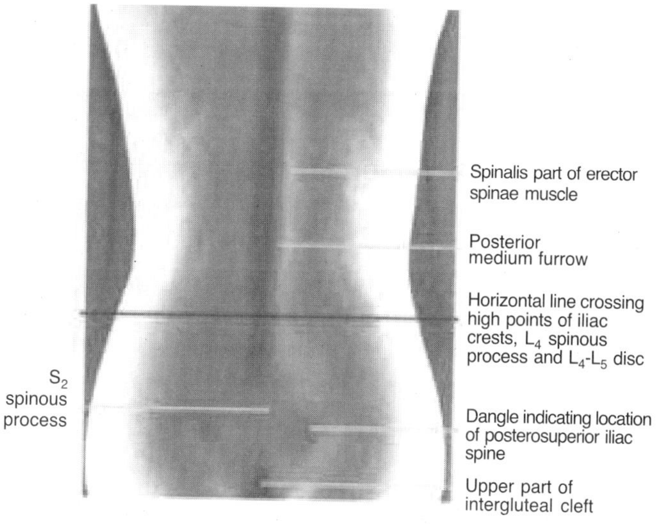

Fig. 28.4: Bony landmarks observed in sitting and lying

Pelvic Obliquity: The level of the iliac crests is observed in standing, sitting and lying. In case of leg length discrepancy, the lengthened (leg) side iliac crest will be raised in standing, but both the iliac crests will be leveled in the sitting. On the other hand, in case of malalignment the iliac crest will be raised in both standing and sitting. In more evident malalignment cases, the opposite iliac crest to that noted in standing, is raised in sitting position.

Range of Motion: The active range of motion of the lumbosacral spine is observed carefully from anterior, posterior and lateral views. In normal lumbopelvic rhythm, initially motion occurs in the end then at the pelvis. In case of tightness of extensors of spine, the innominates rotate prior to the flexion of the spine, this can produce dysfunction of the sacroiliac joint.

Observation of Outflare and Inflare: In supine position, the distance of both the anterior superior iliac spines is measured from the umbilicus. In case of presence of outflare the one side of the ASIS will have more distance from the umbilicus than the opposite ASIS (Inflare). Outflare and inflare can also be observed in prone lying. In case of outflare the corresponding posterior superior iliac spine will move inwards with respect to the midline or gluteal cleft, and for inflare the PSIS moves outward from the gluteal cleft.

The examiner should develop a hypothesis regarding the contribution of faulty lumbopelvic posture to pathomechanical cause of symptoms and the relationship of other body regions in perpetuating the faulty lumbopelvic posture. For an example a lordotic posture with anterior pelvic tilting elongates external oblique.

Objective Examination

The sacroiliac joint and innominates are palpated for tenderness, any kind of crepitus and temperature. For tenderness, the examiner can place the thumb or pisiform aspect of the wrist on the corresponding area. To deliver more force the thumb and pisiform can be reinforced with other hand thumb and pisiform respectively.

The passive movements of lumbosacral and sacroiliac joints are performed to reproduce the symptoms. In order to localize the symptoms, the examiner should test the sacroiliac joints, hip joints, lumbar spine and also supporting soft tissue structures, however, emphasis is given on sacroiliac joints and its supporting soft tissues. The tests which can compress the sacroiliac joints, are more likely to reproduce the symptoms from sacroiliac joint, and tests which distract the sacroiliac joint are more likely to reproduce the symptoms from ligaments and capsule.

Flexion and Extension Tests: The tests are designed to evaluate the movement of pelvic girdle and lumbosacral junction in standing and sitting. The therapist stands behind the patient and places tip of both thumbs on each dimples of venus (inferior aspect of the posterior superior iliac spine). In normal cases the thumbs move up in lumbosacral flexion and down in extension by an equal amount. In standing, when the lumbosacral spine is flexed, the one side of PSIS will be raised than the other. In case of upslip, the right and left PSIS still will move in unison and to an equal extent (Figs. 28.5a and b).

(a)

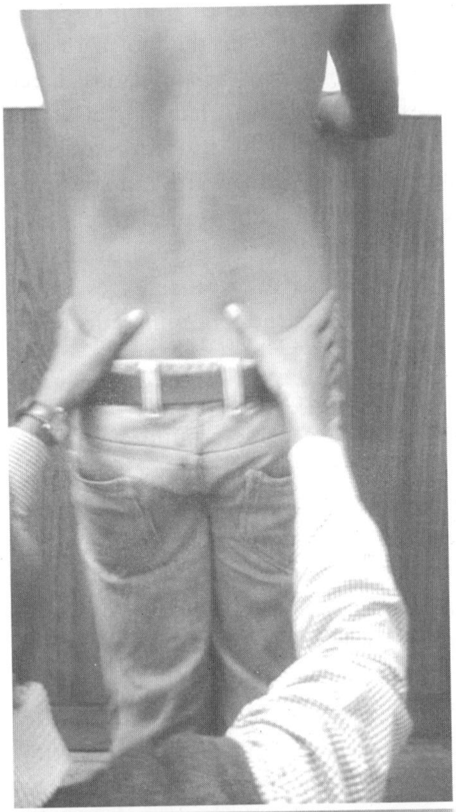

(b)

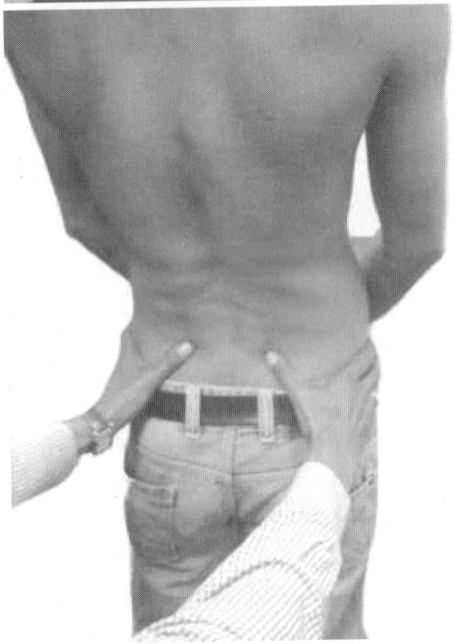

Figs. 28.5a and b: Flexion and extension test

In the presence of rotational malalignment, there is decreased movement possibly at one SI joint relative to the other or even complete loss of movement referred to as locking of the sacroiliac joint. No movement takes place at locked sacroiliac joint, instead of that ilium and the sacrum of the locked sacroiliac joint moves as one unit as on trunk flexion and extension. For an example, if right sacroiliac joint is locked, the right sacrum and ilium will move as a one unit, higher than the left on trunk flexion and lower on trunk extension. It may be concluded that the PSIS of locked or hypomobile sacroiliac joint will show more movement than the normal sacroiliac joint.

Walk Test: This test evaluates the mobility of the sacroiliac joint in non weight bearing position. The patient stands with both hands on a wall or chair to balance himself or herself. The therapist crouch down so that the eyes are at level with the sacrum and the posterior superior iliac spines. The therapist tucks each thumb up and under the PSIS on either side to firmly locate their position. To test the right sacroiliac joint, the patient is asked to stand on the left leg and flex the right hip joint upto 90 degrees, without tilting the pelvis, as if taking a marching step. The therapist notices the movements on both the sacroiliac joints. If normal, the physiotherapist would expect an PSIS on the non weight bearing right leg to rotate posteriorly and inferiorly. A test may be positive if the right posterior superior iliac spine fails to rotate posteriorly relative to the sacral base. If the hip joint (right side) is flexed further (above 90 degrees), the right PSIS moves upwards rather than downwards, this is because the locked right sacrum and right innominate (right sacroiliac joint) rotate as one unit counter clockwise in the frontal plane. If the joint is not locked completely some movements (downward rotation) can be expected, but is less on the right compared with what occurs when the test is performed on the normal left leg (Figs. 28.6 and 28.7).

Patrick or Faber Test: This is one of the provocative tests, useful in making a diagnosis of sacroiliac joint pathology. It places greater stress on the sacroiliac as well as hip joint; hence, it should not be performed on geriatric patients where osteoporotic changes are evident. The patient lies supine on the treatment couch, and affected side foot is placed on the opposite knee joint so that the hip joint (affected side) can be brought into flexion, abduction and external rotation. The therapist stands at the affected side and places one hand on the flexed knee joint and other hand on the opposite ASIS. While maintaining the position, the therapist gently presses the knee and opposite ASIS downwards simultaneously. If low back pain or buttock pain is reproduced the cause is likely to be a disorder of sacroiliac joint (Fig. 28.8).

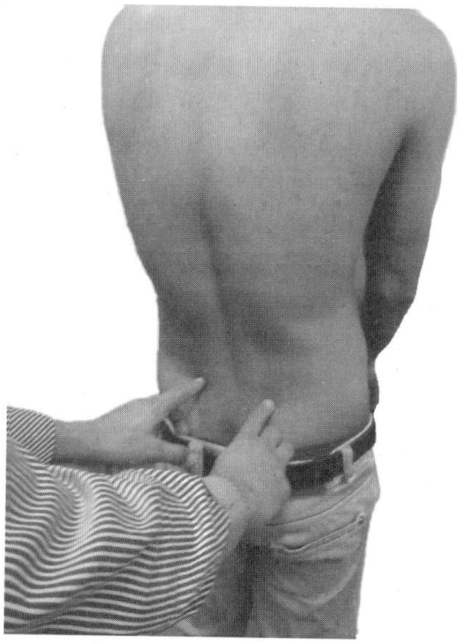

Fig. 28.6: Walk test starting, finger tips on the leveled PSIS

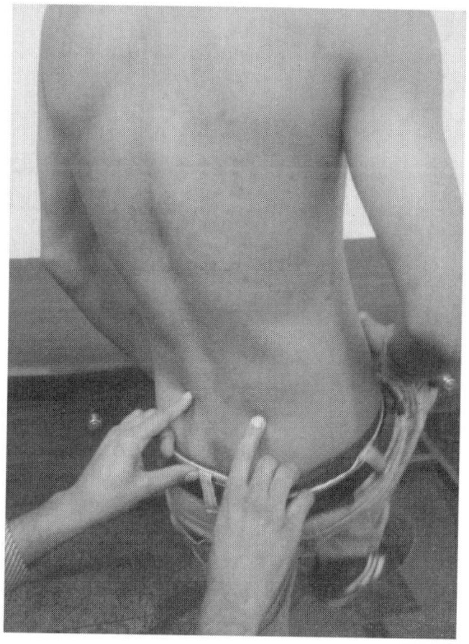

Fig. 28.7: Walk test with right hip and knee flexion, right PSIS with the finger tip moves posterior and inferior. Test is considered normal. If right PSIS moves superior and anterior instead of posterior and inferior, test is considered positive for right SI joint hypomobile

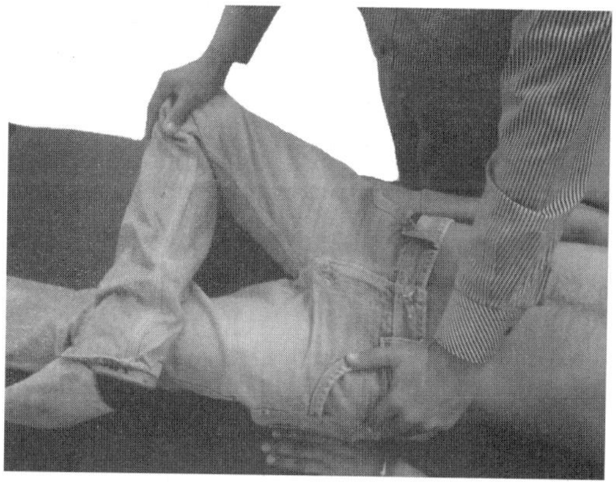

Fig. 28.8: Patrick or faber test

Winged Compression Test: The patient lies supine on the treatment couch. The therapist stands at the side and places hands on both the anterior superior iliac spine with crossed arms. The therapist separates the iliac crests with a downwards and outwards pressure. The test places compressive forces on the sacroiliac joint and provokes pain in case of sacroiliac joint pathology (Fig. 28.9).

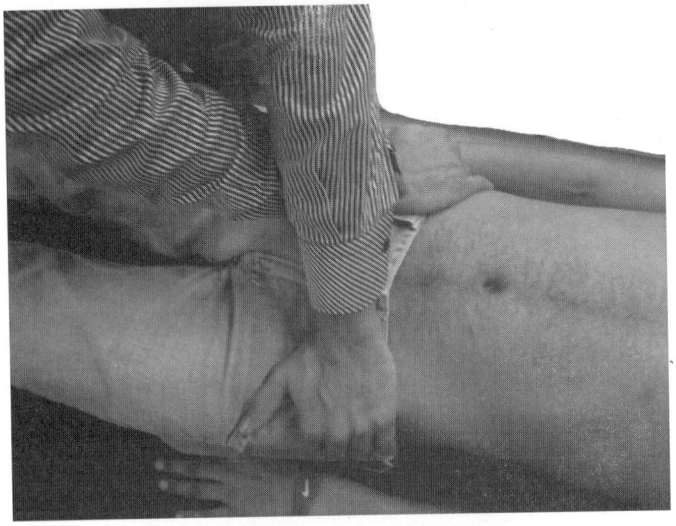

Fig. 28.9: Winged compression test

Compression and Distraction Test: The patient lies supine on the treatment couch. Therapist stands at the side and places hands on both the anterior superior iliac spine. In the first step of the test both the iliac crests are separated by pushing them downwards and outwards. In the second step of the test the iliac crests are brought towards each other by pulling them in order to relieve pressure on the sacroiliac joint. In case of sacroiliac pathology, the compression test should provoke the symptoms while distraction test relieve the symptoms.

MANAGEMENT OF SACROILIAC JOINT

Many approaches such as mobilization, manipulation and muscle energy techniques are administered to correct the alignment of the joint. The core stability strengthening programme should also be incorporated to mobilization as muscle weakness is very common following pain and malalignment of the sacroiliac joint.

Direct Oscillation (Mobilization): The patient lies supine on the treatment couch. Therapist stands at the side of the sacroiliac joint which is being mobilized; and places the heel of the right hand on the sacrum with reinforcement by the left hand. Direct oscillation is helpful in achieving nutation and counter nutation movements of sacrum with reference to the innominate. To produce nutation, the therapist places the heel (pisiform aspect) on the base of the sacrum (over the posterior proximal part of sacrum) and exerts anterior pressure through the body momentum, there should not be any movement at the wrist, elbow and shoulders. To improve counter nutation, therapist places the heel over the apex (posterior distal part) of the sacrum and exerts anterior pressure through the body.

Direct Central Pressure with Hyperextension (Mobilization): This technique is effective in correcting the posterior rotational malalignment of the innominate. The technique combines the use of anterior directed central pressure and extension of the lumbar spine through hyperextension of the hip joint with the leg. The therapist stands at the opposite side of the sacroiliac joint which is being mobilized and places heel of one hand on the posterior superior iliac spine and holds the leg with other hand at the lower thigh. The therapist hyper extends the hip joint with the one hand by using the leg as a lever and applies downward pressure with the heel of other hand. The hyperextension of the hip joint should be upto the pain free range (Fig. 28.10).

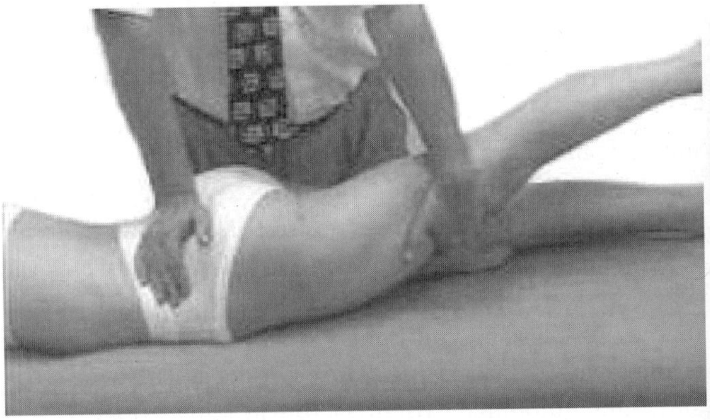

Fig. 28.10: Direct central pressure with hyperextension

Muscle Energy Techniques: The muscle energy techniques are also effective in correcting rotational malalignment of the sacroiliac joint by using the strong isometric contraction of the muscle or group of muscles.

Correction of Right Anterior Pelvic Malrotation (MET): The right anterior rotation of the innominate can be corrected by strong contraction of the right gluteus maximus muscle. The patient lies on the left side with affected side uppermost; and flexes the right hip joint in diagonal manner as much as possible. The lower leg (left) is pulled backwards to the point where sacrum just begin to move. The therapist stands at the front side of the patient and places right hand on the lumbar spine and left hand on the distal thigh to resist the hip extension. The patient is asked to grasp the table with right hand. The therapist maintains the position of the patient's trunk with the right hand and forearm and asks the patient to move the hip joint into extension. The left hand resists the movement of hip joint (Figs. 28.11 to 28.13).

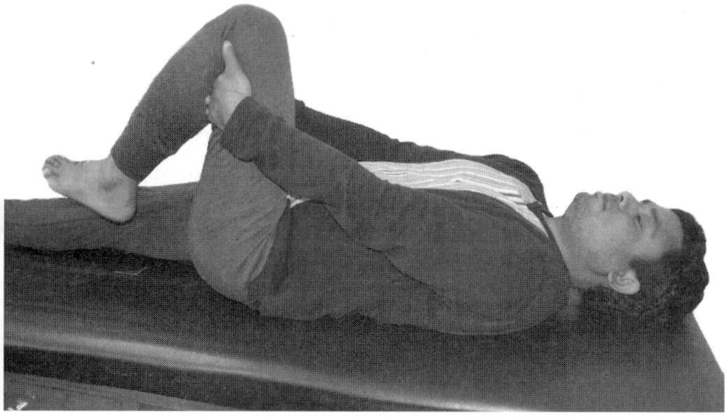

Fig. 28.11: Self-correction of left anterior malrotation by using gluteus maximus MET. The patient places the hands on the distal posterior thigh

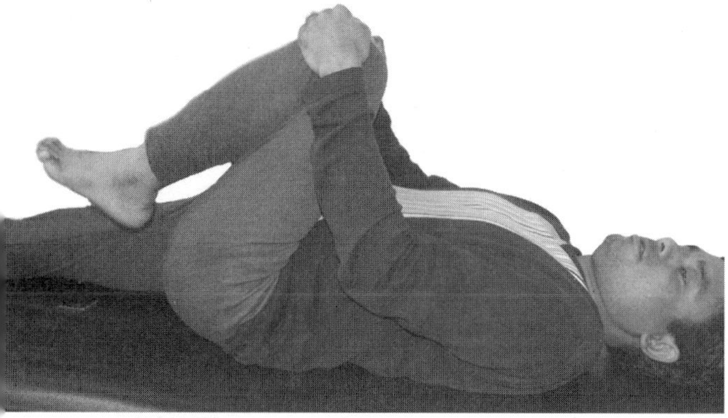

Fig. 28.12: Correction of left anterior pelvic malrotation by muscle energy technique

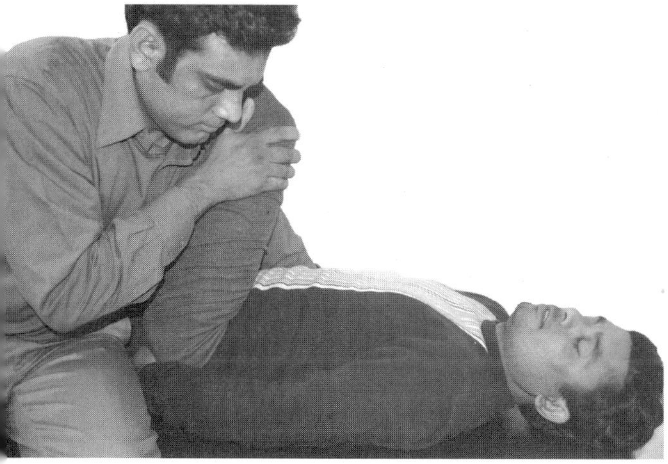

Fig. 28.13: Correction of left anterior malrotation in supine lying by gluteus maximus muscle energy technique

When thigh is free, the strong contraction of the gluteus maximus will extend the hip joint; but by resisting hip extension, the action can be reversed to the origin. Now gluteus maximus will exert a posterior rotational movement on the right innominate, as it is free to move.

The technique may also be performed in supine lying. The patient flexes the hip and knee joint as much as possible, and holds the flexed knee joint with both the hands. While maintaining the position the patient is asked to contract the gluteus maximus muscle as much as possible for at least six seconds. Several repetitions may be performed to see the desired results; and hip is taken further to the chest and opposite shoulder after every repetition. In order to produce posterior rotation on the desired innominate the distal attachment (insertion) of the gluteus maximus needs to be fixed (by holding the knees with the hands) and the proximal attachment (origin) of the gluteus maximus muscle remains free to allow the innominate rotate posteriorly during the isometric contraction.

Correction of Posterior Tilt: Muscle energy technique also helps in correcting the posterior tilt of the innominate by using the isometric contraction of the iliacus and rectus femoris muscles. For iliacus contraction patient lies supine comfortably on the treatment couch. The therapist also sits on the edge of the plinth at the affected side, approximately at the knee joint. The affected side knee and hip is flexed to 90°. Therapist places the flexed leg on his shoulder and holds the distal thigh with both the hands to block the hip flexion. The patient is asked to flex the hip joint by contracting the iliacus muscles. In order to produce anterior rotation on the innominate, the hip flexion is blocked by the therapist to rotate the innominate anteriorly. The technique may also be performed by the patient himself or herself without the assistance of the therapist by pushing the knee joint with both the hands (Figs. 28.14a to d).

(a)

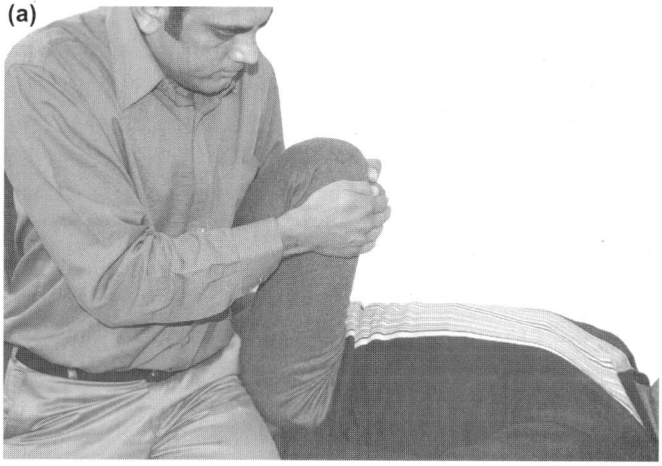

(b)

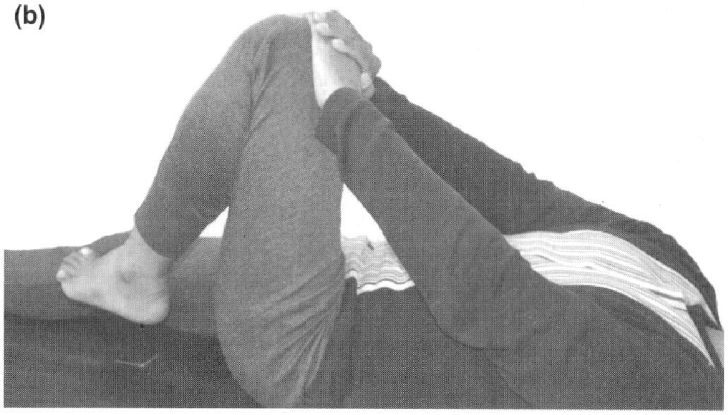

(c)

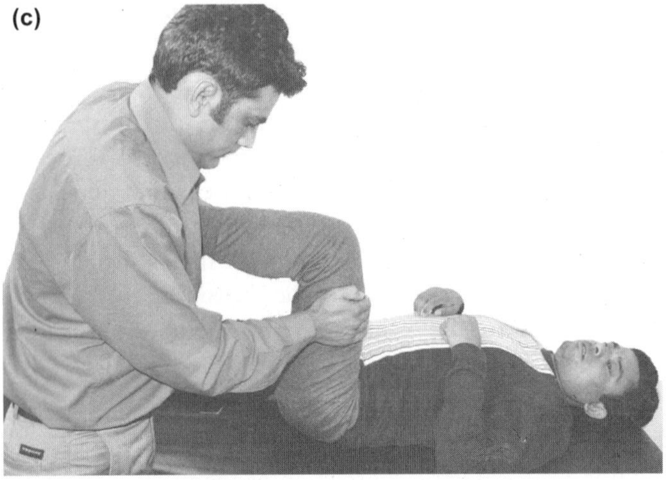

(d)

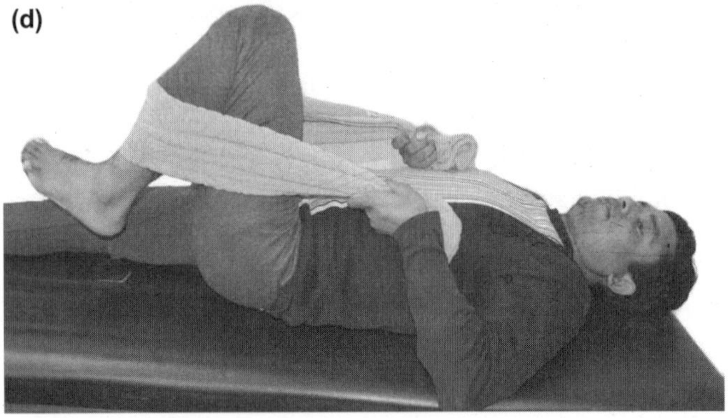

Fig. 28.14a to d: Correction of posterior malalignment by using a. iliopsoas MET, b. self-iliopsoas MET, c. rectus femoris MET, d. self-rectus femoris MET

The rectus femoris muscle originates from the anterior inferior iliac spine (AIIS) and anterior rim of the acetabulum. The muscle inserts on the superior pole of the patella and then to the tibial tubercle through patellar tendon. Rectus femoris is a principle extensor of the knee joint. It also has a secondary action on the hip joint, i.e., flexion. To correct the posterior malrotation of the innominate the distal attachments of the rectus femoris is fixed and proximal attachment is left free to produce the movement on the innominate. The patient lies supine with hip 90° flexion and knee full flexion. Therapist stands at the opposite side of the leg and holds the flexed knee and ankle joint. The patient contracts the rectus femoris as much as possible, and the therapist resists the movement and maintains the hip and knee flexion. Several repetitions may be performed to produce significant correction of the innominate on sacrum.

Sacral Thrust (Manipulation): It is the manipulative technique with a low amplitude and high velocity thrust to the base of sacrum to correct the rotational malalignment. The patient sits comfortably on the treatment couch. For left sacroiliac joint hypomobility the patient sits comfortably on the treatment couch with the left hand on the right shoulder and trunk rotation and bending to the right side. The therapist stands behind and to the right side of the patient, and places left hand on the left base of the sacrum. The therapist grasps the patient's left arm and locks the spine into side bending and right rotation including the sacrum with the right hand. This will cause the left sacral base to move forwards which can be felt with the left hand. While maintaining the position the therapist applies a low amplitude high velocity thrust with the left hand in an anterior direction. The small arc of movement must be applied at a full stretch (Fig. 28.15).

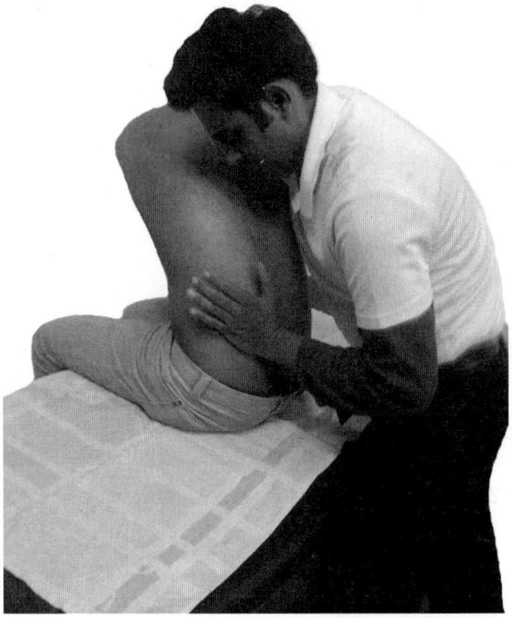

Fig. 28.15: Sacral thrust

Simultaneous Correction of Right Anterior and Left Posterior Rotation

(i) The patient lies supine with both legs out of edge of the treatment table. Patient flexes the right hip and knee as much as possible and holds at the knee joint with both the hands in order to bring it to the chest. The left leg hangs freely into the hip extension. The right hip flexion corrects the right anterior rotation as it rotates the right innominate posteriorly on the sacrum. The left leg which hangs, freely extends the left hip and rotates the left innominate anteriorly on the sacrum, corrects the posterior rotation of the left innominate (Figs. 28.16a and b).

(ii) The patient stands and places right foot up on the stool with flexion of hip and knee joint. The left foot remains on the floor with full extension of the left hip and knee joint. The patient holds the chair with the right hand. The right hip and knee flexion with slight trunk flexion rotates the right innominate posteriorly on the sacrum and helps in correcting the right anterior malrotation.

(a)

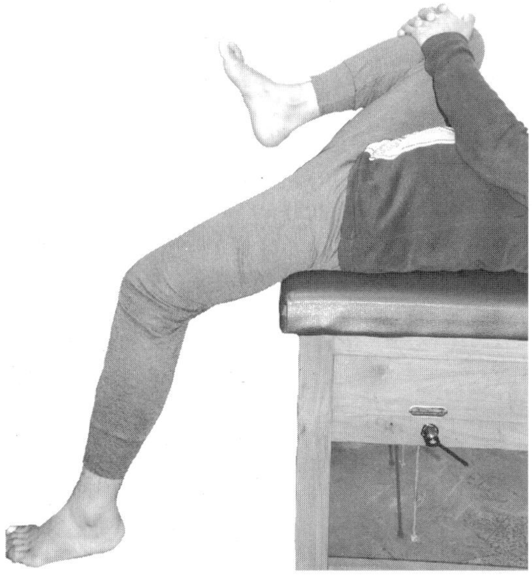

(b)

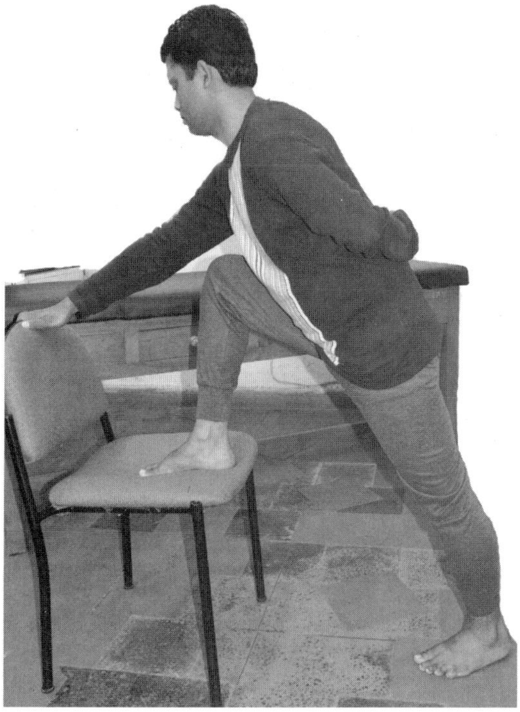

Figs. 28.16a and b: Simultaneous correction of right anterior and left posterior rotation

The left extended hip corrects the posterior rotation of the left innominate by rotating the left innominate anteriorly on the sacrum.

Correction of Upslip: The patient lies supine with the ankle joint slightly out of the table. He or she holds the table with both the hands. Therapist stands at the foot of the patient and grasps the affected side ankle firmly with both the hands, and lifts the leg slightly off the table. The therapist keeps the patient busy with conversation and then a sharp high velocity tug is applied to the leg, in the plane of the sacroiliac joint.

Note: The therapist should ensure complete relaxation of the girdle muscles. To achieve complete relaxation the therapist can flex hip and knee three to four times before the traction.

- It should not be used in case of pain in the ankle, knee or hip joint.
- The patient should be warned that there may be increased discomfort for a few days (Fig. 28.17).

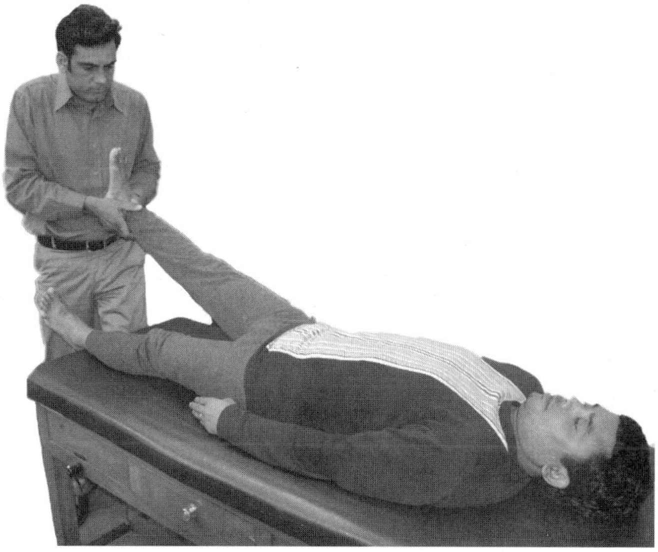

Figs. 28.17: Correction of upslip (right)

Correction of Outflare: The most common clinical presentation is existence of outflare on one side (usually with the posterior rotational malalignment) and inflare on other side (with the anterior rotational malalignment), however, outflare or inflare may exist in isolation. To correct the right outflare, the patient lies supine with both the knees and hips flexion. The right ankle is placed on the anterior aspect of the left knee joint. Now the right leg is in the position of figure of four; with abduction, external rotation and flexion of the hip joint. The therapist sits on the table at the same side, and places left hand on the lateral aspect of the right knee joint and right hand on the left knee joint. The patient pushes the therapist's left hand outwards by contracting the external rotators, abductors and extensors against the resistance applied by the therapist's left hand. Several repetitions may be performed. Each repetition should have 5-6 seconds contraction. After each contraction the therapist should flex the left leg to bring the right hip joint into more flexion, abduction and external rotation so that tension in the external rotators may be maintained (Fig. 28.18).

Correction of Inflare: The patient lies supine with both the hips and knees flexion. To correct right inflare, the right ankle joint is placed on the anterior aspect of the left

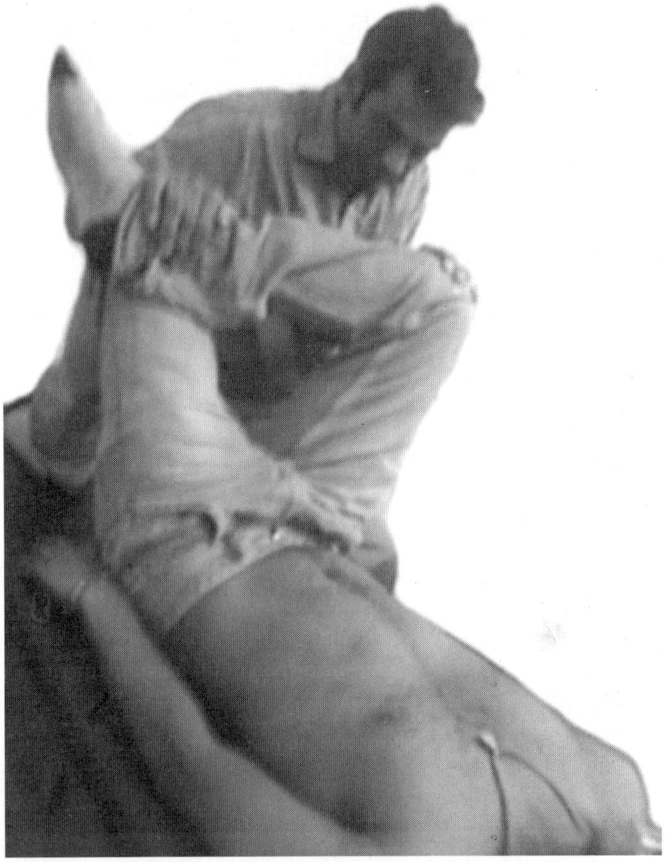

Fig. 28.18: Correction of sacroiliac outflare

knee joint. Now the right leg will be in figure of four position with hip flexion, abduction and external rotation. The therapist stands opposite of the right side, and places right hand on the medial aspect of the right knee joint and left hand on the ankle joint. The patient contracts the flexors, and internal rotators against the resistance applied by the therapist with the right hand. The contraction is followed by further progression of hip flexion and external rotation. Several repetitions may be performed (Figs. 28.19 and 28.20).

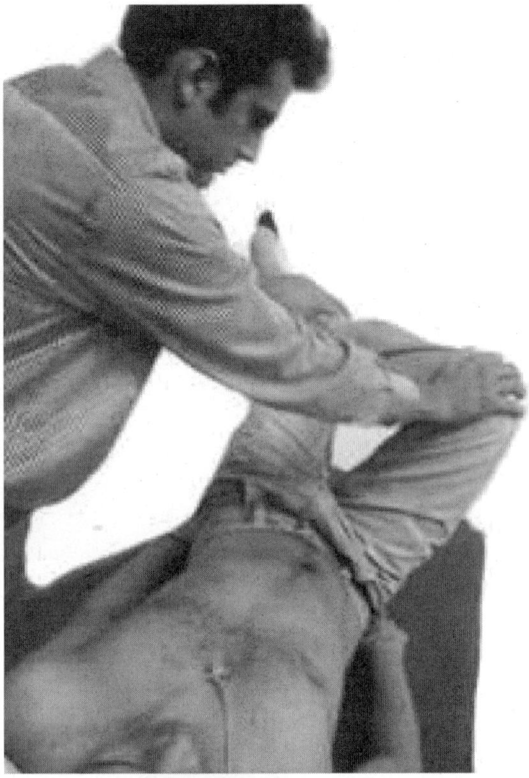

Fig. 28.19: Correction of sacroiliac inflare

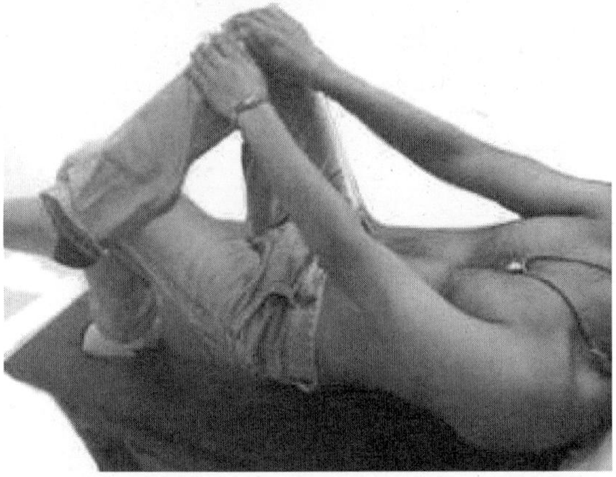

Fig. 28.20: Self-correction of sacroiliac inflare

INDEX

A

B

C